AMA MANUAL OF STYLE

A Guide for Authors and Editors 10th Edition

Cheryl Iverson, MA (*Chair*)

Stacy Christiansen, MA

Annette Flanagin, RN, MA

Phil B. Fontanarosa, MD, MBA

Richard M. Glass, MD

Brenda Gregoline, ELS

Stephen J. Lurie, MD, PhD

Harriet S. Meyer, MD

Margaret A. Winker, MD

Roxanne K. Young, ELS

AMA MANUAL OF STYLE

A Guide for Authors and Editors *10th Edition*

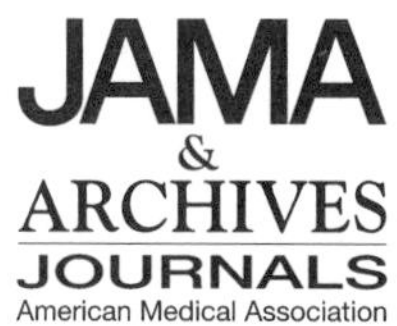

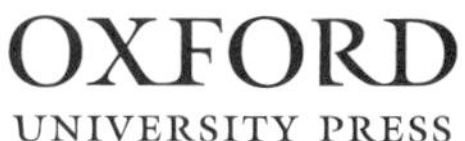

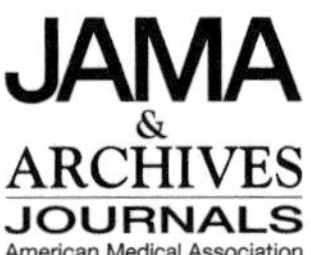

OXFORD
UNIVERSITY PRESS

Oxford University Press, Inc., publishes works that further
Oxford University's objective of excellence
in research, scholarship, and education.

Oxford New York
Auckland Cape Town Dar es Salaam Hong Kong Karachi
Kuala Lumpur Madrid Melbourne Mexico City Nairobi
New Delhi Shanghai Taipei Toronto

With offices in
Argentina Austria Brazil Chile Czech Republic France Greece
Guatemala Hungary Italy Japan Poland Portugal Singapore
South Korea Switzerland Thailand Turkey Ukraine Vietnam

Published by Oxford University Press, Inc.
198 Madison Avenue, New York, New York 10016

www.oup.com

Library of Congress Cataloging-in-Publication Data
AMA manual of style : a guide for authors and editors.—10th ed. / Cheryl
Iverson ... [et al.].
p. ; cm.
Rev. ed. of: American Medical Association manual of style. 9th ed. ©1998.
Includes bibliographical references and indexes.
ISBN 978-0-19-517633-9
1. Medical writing—Handbooks, manuals, etc. 2. Authorship—Handbooks,
manuals, etc. I. Iverson, Cheryl. II. American Medical Association. III. American
Medical Association manual of style. IV. Title: Manual of style. V. Title:
Guide for authors and editors.
[DNLM: 1. Writing. WZ 345 A511 2007]
R119.A533 2007
808'.06661—dc22 2006037192

9 8 7 6 5 4 3 2 1

Printed in the United States of America
on acid-free paper

Foreword

I never cease to be amazed by the general inability of physicians, other health professionals, and scientists to communicate through the written word. Their scholarly and creative ideas and insightful data interpretation often seem to get lost in the translation from brain to page. The sad state of this art became vividly clear to me when I was invited to become the editor of *Archives of Pediatrics & Adolescent Medicine* in 1995 and subsequently in 2000 to become the editor in chief of *JAMA*, the *Journal of the American Medical Association*. Among the reasons I was invited was that the search committees considered me to have "superior" writing skills. Good grief, I thought, we are indeed in big trouble.

My most vivid recollection of being taught formal writing was by Theresa Camorata Wozniak, my high school "English" (with those last names?) teacher. She would begin each lesson by writing something like the following on the blackboard (yes, blackboard; it was the 1950s, after all): "Do not waste time; that's the stuff of which life is made." Mrs Camorata Wozniak obviously chose to ignore—or more likely to correct—Ben Franklin's "Do not squander time, for that is the stuff life is made of." Her grammar lesson was, of course, not to end a sentence with a preposition; the moral lesson is obvious. Both remain with me to this day. However, despite this background and the hundreds of other lessons from various editors and colleagues, I still do not consider myself to have "superior" writing skills. Hence, my continuing reliance on this manual of style.

My amazement at the difficulty so many bright, accomplished health professionals have in communicating through the written word has continued to be augmented daily when I read the various manuscripts submitted to *JAMA* that reach my desk. Simply comparing the original submitted manuscript with the published version clearly illustrates the value and skills of the editors, and especially the manuscript (née copy) editors. And therein lies the value of this manual.

The issue of communicating well in writing is certainly not new, and good writing will become even more important but perhaps more challenging as the use of online written communication becomes the norm. Computer-based programs, such as spell-check, are fine for some words (unless your name is DeAngelis, which spell-check translates as "dunghill"), but grammar, punctuation, correct usage, and reference style are only a few items simply not covered reliably. But, all is not yet lost. The *AMA Manual of Style*, 10th edition, contains everything that a group of editors from the *JAMA* and *Archives* family of journals believe is essential to produce a manuscript that is well organized, clear, readable, and authoritative.

The first book on medical writing written by a *JAMA* editor was published in 1938.[1] However, the 10th edition of the manual represents the collective and updated work of editors over more than 40 years. The first edition was written in the mid-1960s when the then-editors of *JAMA* assembled and codified their collective knowledge and experience. That first volume was a trim 70 pages or so and had a green cardboard cover. Over the years, the collective knowledge and experience generated by a substantially increased number and pace of manuscript submissions plus the foundation of the previous editions' material have resulted in a much more extensive and comprehensive manual.

The 5 sections—Preparing an Article for Publication, Style, Terminology, Measurement and Quantitation, and Technical Information—are chock-full of valuable information for authors, editors, publishers, reviewers, and anyone else interested in scientific writing. If you look for information that is not found herein, please contact us so that we can add it to the next edition, which is already on the minds of those who will carry the torch to the 11th edition.

Read and understand, write and be understood, and mostly, enjoy.

Catherine D. DeAngelis, MD, MPH
Editor in Chief, *JAMA* and the *Archives* Journals

REFERENCE

1. Fishbein M. *Medical Writing: The Technic and the Art.* Chicago, IL: American Medical Association; 1938.

Preface

What's new in this edition? Below is a short response to a question that can only be answered fully through frequent use.

- A new chapter on medical indexes.
- A completely updated Nomenclature chapter, with 4 new subsections (molecular medicine, ophthalmology, psychiatry, and radiology), the latest nomenclature in many fields (eg, virology, chromosomes), molecular medicine subsections added to many fields (eg, cardiology, neurology), more material on complementary and alternative medicine, and a more international approach to drug nomenclature.
- Expanded, and now separate, chapters on manuscript preparation, visual display of data, and references. The References chapter includes almost all new examples, with about 50 examples of electronic references alone.
- A change in the policy for table footnotes from using superscript symbols to using superscript lowercase letters.
- A greatly expanded chapter on ethical and legal considerations, including just some of the following:
  - New responsibilities for authors, including identifying contributions of all authors as well as substantial contributions of nonauthors.
  - New policies on group authorship.
  - Updates on conflict of interest, including requirements for complete financial disclosure, transparency of the role of the sponsor, and independent statistical analysis for industry-supported studies.
  - New information on editorial freedom in the wake of the firings of the editors of *JAMA* and other general medical journals.
  - New policies and procedures for journal editors, including correspondence columns, corrections, and the role of editorial boards.
  - Updated definition of scientific misconduct, procedures for handling allegations of fabrication, falsification, and plagiarism and publishing retractions.
  - New information on data sharing and open access.
  - Updates on copyright and trademark, especially as they affect online publishing.
  - New privacy concerns for patients in scientific publication.
  - New case law on libel and suggestions for minimizing risk of libel.
  - Revised guidelines on advertising, including online advertising.
  - Updated information on author and editor relations with the news media and early release of information to the public.

- New subsection in the Grammar chapter, to include homonyms, idioms, colloquialisms, slang, euphemisms, and cliches.
- A decision to drop the commas previously used to set off "Jr" and "Sr."
- Inclusion of guidelines for capitalization of computer terms and intercapped compounds.
- Addition of many new terms to the Correct and Preferred Usage and to the Study Design and Statistics glossaries.
- New policy on abbreviation or expansion of state names.
- Revised policy on SI units and updated conversion table.
- New material in the statistics chapter on cost-effectiveness analysis and survey studies and requirement of clinical trial registration.
- Information on online editing and coding, with samples of a marked-up and coded page.
- Expanded typography chapter, with emphasis on improving readability.
- Updated and expanded publishing glossary and resources chapters.

As with the previous edition, nothing has been deleted and much-used chapters such as Numbers and Percentages, Punctuation, and Eponyms have been thoroughly updated.

The tradition of working with a committee of 10, begun with the eighth edition, has continued through the tenth, with committee members dividing the work at the outset, doing independent research and writing, obtaining critiques from outside peer reviewers, and providing critiques on all of each other's material. Often, several cycles of writing, reviewing, discussing, and rewriting were necessary. As with the last edition, in cases in which complete agreement among all committee members was not possible, we have agreed to disagree, with the majority opinion becoming the policy.

We have continued to attribute each chapter to a "principal author." Because we have found it impossible to otherwise assess the relative contributions of the committee members, their names appear in alphabetical order on the title page. Others who have made substantial contributions are Jeni Reiling, *JAMA,* who is the principal author of 2 updated chapters, and Bruce McGregor, who coauthored the indexing chapter. Many other people who added strength to the work are listed in the Acknowledgments section.

In the preface to the ninth edition, I expressed hope that the print book would be followed by an electronic version. That did not come to pass, but for this edition, the hope will be realized. Sign up at http://www.amamanualofstyle.com for information about a future electronic version of the *Manual.* We also welcome your comments on the manual regarding suggestions for improvement or to note corrections. Write to Cheryl Iverson at cheryl.iverson@jama-archives.org.

Cheryl Iverson, MA
Chair, *AMA Manual of Style* Committee
Chicago, Illinois
October 19, 2006

Acknowledgments

The individuals listed below reviewed part or all of the manual in draft form. Their advice and comments were invaluable in adding clarity, polish, and additional substance to the manual. Any errors are solely the responsibility of the *AMA Manual of Style* Committee.

Laura Adamczyk
Archives Journals

Karen Adams-Taylor, MS
JAMA and *Archives* Journals

Daniel M. Albert, MD, MS
Editor, *Archives of Ophthalmology*
University of Wisconsin, Madison

Lynn M. Alperin
Texas Medicine

Jessica S. Ancker, MPH
Columbia University College
of Physicians and Surgeons,
New York, New York

David Antos
JAMA and *Archives* Journals

Christine A. Arturo
American Academy of Ophthalmology,
San Francisco, California

Michael L. Callaham, MD
University of California, San Francisco

Diane L. Cannon
Archives Journals

Terri S. Carter
Archives of Surgery,
Baltimore, Maryland

Helene M. Cole, MD
JAMA

Peter Cummings
University of Washington, Seattle

Pam Diamond
Pfizer Inc, New York, New York

Judith Dickson, MS, ELS(D)
Science Editing Inc, Rockville, Maryland

John H. Dirckx, MD
Dayton, Ohio

Pierre Durieux, MD, MPH
René Descartes University and Hôpital
Européen Georges Pompidou,
Paris, France

Karl Elvin
JAMA and *Archives* Journals

Allison Frank Esposito
Dallas, Texas

Ronald G. Evens, MD
Washington University School
of Medicine, St Louis, Missouri

Lauren B. Fischer
JAMA and *Archives* Journals

Fred Furtner, MAMS
Archives Journals

Barbara Gastel, MD, MPH
Texas A&M University, College Station

Maxine A. Gere, MS
Blue Cross and Blue Shield Association,
Chicago, Illinois

Julie T. Gerke, ELS
Quintiles Medical Communications,
Parsippany, New Jersey

Erin M. Giannini
Norwich, England

Paula Glitman
Archives Journals

Robert M. Golub, MD
JAMA and *Archives* Journals

C. K. Gunsalus, JD
University of Illinois, Champaign/Urbana

Cindy W. Hamilton, PharmD, ELS
Hamilton House, Virginia Beach, Virginia

Lisa Y. Hardin
JAMA and *Archives* Journals

Wayne G. Hoppe, JD
JAMA and *Archives* Journals

Bob Johnson, ELS
WordHawk Editorial Services, Palo Alto, California

Mary Ellen Johnston
JAMA and *Archives* Journals

Sheldon Kotzin, MLS
National Library of Medicine, Bethesda, Maryland

Hope J. Lafferty, MD
Memorial Sloan-Kettering Cancer Center, New York, New York

Trevor Lane, MA, DPhil
University of Hong Kong

Diane Berneath Lang, BS
Radiological Society of North America, Oak Brook, Illinois

Connie Manno, ELS
Archives Journals

Diana J. Mason, RN, PhD, FAAN
American Journal of Nursing

Richard W. Newman
JAMA and *Archives* Journals

Kim S. Penelton-Campbell
JAMA

Margaret Perkins, MA, ELS
New England Journal of Medicine

Drummond Rennie, MD, FRCP, MACP
JAMA

Povl Riis, MD
University of Copenhagen, Copenhagen, Denmark

June K. Robinson, MD
Editor, *Archives of Dermatology*
Northwestern University, Feinberg School of Medicine, Chicago, Illinois

Roger N. Rosenberg, MD
Editor, *Archives of Neurology*
University of Texas Southwestern Medical Center at Dallas

Gale L. Saulsberry
JAMA and *Archives* Journals

Karon Schindler, MA
Emory University, Atlanta, Georgia

Philip Sefton, ELS
JAMA

Heather A. Shebel
JAMA

Valerie Siddall, PhD, ELS
AstraZeneca, Cheshire, England

Kristine B. Simmons, BA
Archives Journals

Cheryl Smart, MA, MBA
St Louis, Missouri

Joan Stephenson, PhD
JAMA

Naomi Vaisrub, PhD
JAMA

Elizabeth Wager, MA
Sideview, Princes Risborough, England

Cara M. Wallace, BS(Hons)
JAMA

Jane C. Wiggs, MLA, ELS
Mayo Clinic, Jacksonville, Florida

Flo Witte, MA, ELS
AdvancMed LLC, Lexington, Kentucky

Caroline Woods, PA-C, MS
Duluth, Minnesota

In addition, 2 others deserve to be singled out for special thanks: Catherine D. DeAngelis, MD, MPH, editor in chief of *JAMA* and editor in chief of Scientific Publications and Multimedia Applications for *JAMA* and the *Archives* Journals, for her support of the work done on this edition by members of her staff, and Nicole Netter Snoblin, Lake Forest, Illinois, who copyedited this edition as she has the 2 previous editions.

Contents

Section

1

Preparing an Article for Publication

1 Types of Articles

Effective written communication requires the author to consider the intended message and audience and use a form appropriate to both. Medical journal articles usually fit into one of the following 7 main types.

1.1 **Reports of Original Data.** Published reports of original research are the backbone of medical and scientific communications. Critical evaluation and replication of the findings of such reports are key aspects of quality control and progress in science and medicine; the clinical applications of original research are a major source of benefits for patients. Journals often categorize reports of original data as Original Articles, Original Communications, or Original Reports, section headings that emphasize the new findings such articles intend to communicate. Short articles reporting original data may be called Brief Reports. Studies that address basic issues of physiology or pathology may be called Research Reports or Clinical Investigations. In *JAMA*, articles that report preliminary findings are called Preliminary Communications.

Articles that report original research results usually follow the traditional IMRAD (Introduction, Methods, Results, and Discussion) format. Changing the acronym to AIMRAD would give appropriate emphasis to the abstract, which has become increasingly important in the era of electronic databases. Many readers scan only the title and abstract (eg, from a search of an electronic database) and often use the abstract to decide whether to obtain or read the full text of the article. This highlights the importance of the abstract in communicating a brief but accurate and informative summary of the article.[1] Structured abstracts, which provide summary information in a standard format, have enhanced value and are now required by many medical journals for all reports of original data.[2,3] (See 2.5, Manuscript Preparation, Abstract, and 2.8, Manuscript Preparation, Parts of a Manuscript, Headings, Subheadings, and Side Headings, for guidance in preparing these sections.)

1.2 **Review Articles.** Review articles collate and summarize the available information about a particular topic, in contrast to reports of original data. Review articles have great practical importance because clinicians often use them as guides for clinical decisions. This use highlights the importance of ensuring that reviews are systematic, include all relevant data, and are not overly influenced by the opinions and biases of the authors. Thus, review articles should specify the methods used to search for, select, synthesize, and summarize the information.[4] Some reviews employ meta-analysis, statistical techniques that combine quantitative results from independent studies. (See 20.4, Study Design and Statistics, Meta-analysis.) Structured abstracts for review articles give authors a helpful framework for the information that should be provided and enable readers to grasp quickly the methods, main findings, and conclusions of the review. (See 2.5.1, Manuscript Preparation, Abstract, Structured Abstracts for Systematic Reviews [Including Meta-analyses].)

1.3 **Descriptive Articles.** Descriptions, summaries, or observations that lack the systematic rigor of original research or systematic reviews may be published as Case Reports (for patient descriptions), Clinical Observations, Special Articles, or Special Communications. To merit publication, such articles should make novel observations that can stimulate research or should provide useful information about topics of particular interest to a journal's readership. Since the scientific value of single case reports is often limited, many journals prefer to consider them as Letters to the Editor and publish them only if they make a unique observation that merits more systematic investigation.[5] Some medical journals publish case reports as educational tools. Grand Rounds or Case Conference presentations published in journals typically combine descriptive case material (used to highlight clinical features of a disorder) with a review of the major issues illustrated by the case. Because of the variability of their content, there is no standard format for descriptive articles. A short abstract may be helpful and usually is written in an unstructured narrative form. Such abstracts summarize the main points of the article and are useful for inclusion in electronic databases.

1.4 **Consensus Statements and Clinical Practice Guidelines.** Governmental and private organizations often develop recommendations for the prevention, diagnosis, and treatment of various disorders. These recommendations regarding appropriate clinical decisions are usually made by a group of experts after they assess the available evidence. Recommendations may be published as consensus statements developed at a conference or as clinical practice guidelines (sometimes called *practice parameters*) developed over time. In either case, publication of the recommendations should identify the sponsor and the participating experts, explain how the participants were selected, describe the evidence that supports the recommendations, and explain the process for achieving consensus in reaching the conclusions. Structured abstracts can be helpful in summarizing this information.[6,7]

1.5 **Articles of Opinion.** Editorials are short essays that usually reflect the views of the editor or the policies of the journal. Editorials may be written by the editor, a member of the editorial staff or editorial board, or an invited author. Editorials may comment on an article in the same issue of the journal, providing additional context and opinion regarding its implications, or may deal with a separate topic of interest to the journal's readers or editors. In the past, it was common for authors of medical journal editorials not to be identified, as is still the usual practice for newspaper editorials. This has become much less common as authorship responsibility and accountability have received increasing emphasis in medical publishing. (See 5.1.3,

Ethical and Legal Considerations, Unsigned Editorials, Anonymous Articles, Pseudonymous Authors.) Journals generally do not publish unsolicited articles of opinion as editorials. Opinion pieces that represent only the views of the authors may be published in other journal sections, such as Commentary, Sounding Board, Viewpoint, or Controversies.

1.6 **Correspondence.** Letters to the Editor are an essential aspect of postpublication review. The International Committee of Medical Journal Editors has recommended that all biomedical journals provide "a mechanism for submitting comments, questions, or criticisms about published articles, as well as brief reports and commentary unrelated to previously published articles. This will likely, but not necessarily, take the form of a correspondence section or column. The authors of articles discussed in correspondence should be given an opportunity to respond, preferably in the same issue in which the original correspondence appears."[8] Published letters usually comment on an article previously published in the same journal, and replies from the authors of the article can make for lively and useful exchanges. Indeed, providing published responses to questions and criticisms is part of the responsibility of authorship.

Most journals request that such letters to the editor be sent within a specified period (often about a month) after publication of the original article. Journals rely on these reader responses as part of postpublication peer review and quality assurance. Letters should focus on the scientific, clinical, or ethical issues raised by the original article and should not include ad hominem attacks on the authors. Often 1 or 2 letters are chosen for publication as being representative of the responses to a particular article.

Letters not pertaining to a previous article may report original research data, describe a problem, or report a case. Letters reporting original research should follow the same IMRAD format as a full-length research article but in a substantially truncated length. Journals usually have strict limitations for the length and the number of references for published letters. Letters submitted for publication may be subject to review and revision, and they require statements of authorship responsibility, disclosure of conflicts of interest, and copyright transfer. Correspondents should indicate whether letters sent to the editor are to be considered for publication.

1.7 **Reviews of Books, Journals, and Other Media.** Readers of such reviews seek both an overview of the product and an assessment of its quality relative to similar works. Thus, these reviews usually include description and opinion, both of which may extend to broader issues raised by the work. There is often considerable room for individual style and expression in these critiques, but supporting evidence for the reviewer's praise or criticism is essential.

1.8 **Other Types of Articles.** Journals publish other items and articles that do not fit into any of the major categories. Examples include personal reflections and essays (eg, A Piece of My Mind in *JAMA*), news articles, poetry, obituaries, reports on conferences, and articles based on clinical photographs. Authors should examine several issues of a journal to make sure that a submission is appropriate and read the journal's instructions for authors to determine requirements regarding various types of articles.

ACKNOWLEDGMENT

Principal author: Richard M. Glass, MD

REFERENCES

1. Winker MA. The need for concrete improvement in abstract quality. *JAMA*. 1999; 281(12):1129-1130.
2. Rennie D, Glass RM. Structuring abstracts to make them more informative. *JAMA*. 1991;266(1):116-117.
3. Taddio A, Pain T, Fassos FF, Boon H, Ilersich AL, Einarson TR. Quality of non-structured and structured abstracts of original research articles in the *British Medical Journal*, the *Canadian Medical Association Journal*, and the *Journal of the American Medical Association*. *CMAJ*. 1994;150(10):1611-1615.
4. Cook DJ, Mulrow CD, Haynes RB. Systematic reviews: synthesis of best evidence for clinical decisions. *Ann Intern Med*. 1997;126(5):376-380.
5. Riesenberg DE. Case reports in the medical literature. *JAMA*. 1986;255(15):2067.
6. Hayward RS, Wilson MC, Tunis SR, Bass EB, Rubin HR, Haynes RB. More informative abstracts of articles describing clinical practice guidelines. *Ann Intern Med*. 1993; 118(9):731-737.
7. Olson C. Consensus statements: applying structure. *JAMA*. 1995;273(1):72-73.
8. International Committee of Medical Journal Editors. Correspondence. Uniform Requirements for Manuscripts Submitted to Biomedical Journals: Writing and Editing for Biomedical Publication. http://www.icmje.org. Updated February 2006. Accessed September 1, 2006.

2 Manuscript Preparation

Preparation of a scholarly manuscript requires thoughtful consideration of the topic and anticipation of the reader's needs and questions. Certain elements either are standard parts of all manuscripts or are used so often as to merit special instruction. These elements are discussed in this section in the order in which they appear in the manuscript. References are discussed separately in chapter 3 and tables and figures in chapter 4.

The preparation of any manuscript for publication should take the requirements of the intended journal into account; this may enhance the chances of acceptance and expedite publication. For the author, manuscript preparation requires familiarity with the journal to which the article is submitted. Most journals publish instructions for authors, which serve as useful guides; some journals' instructions for authors contain a manuscript checklist (see that from *JAMA*[1] [reproduced in this chapter as the Table] as an example). Some publishers also publish style manuals, which provide in-depth instruction (see 25.0, Resources). For journals that subscribe to the Uniform Requirements for Manuscripts Submitted to Biomedical Journals,[2] as *JAMA* and the *Archives* Journals do, adherence to these guidelines will be acceptable, although the individual journal may require more than the Uniform Requirements or make changes to suit its house style.

Many journals request submission of material through a Web-based manuscript submission and peer review system; many journals require such submission. Others may request materials on disk or as e-mail attachments; some may still accept printed paper copies ("hard copy") (see 6.2, Editorial Assessment and Processing, Editorial Processing).

2.1 Titles and Subtitles. Titles should be concise, specific, and informative and should contain the key points of the work. For scientific manuscripts, overly general titles are not desirable (but see also 2.1.7, Names of Cities, Counties, States, Provinces, and Countries).

Avoid: Cocaine Use and Homicide

Better: Cocaine Use and Homicide Among Men in New York City

(*Note:* The shorter, more general title might be appropriate for an editorial or an opinion piece.)

Similarly, although the subtitle is frequently useful in expanding on the title, it should not contain key elements of the study as a supplement to an overly general title.

Avoid: Psychiatric Disorders: A Rural-Urban Comparison

Better: Rural-Urban Differences in the Prevalence of Psychiatric Disorders

Avoid: Multiple Sclerosis: Sexual Dysfunction and Response to Medications

Better: Sexual Dysfunction and Response to Medications in Multiple Sclerosis

Avoid: Hospitalization for Congestive Heart Failure: Explaining Racial Differences

Better: Racial Differences in Hospitalization Rates for Congestive Heart Failure

Avoid: Cardiovascular Evaluation of Competitive Athletes: Medical and Legal Issues

Better: Medical and Legal Issues in the Cardiovascular Evaluation of Competitive Athletes

However, too much detail also should be avoided. Subtitles should complement the title by providing supplementary information that will supply more detail about the content and aid in information retrieval. Several examples of informative title and subtitle combinations appear below:

BRCA1 Testing in Families With Hereditary Breast-Ovarian Cancer: A Prospective Study of Patient Decision Making and Outcomes

Prevention of Systemic Infections, Especially Meningitis, Caused by *Haemophilus influenzae* Type b: Impact on Public Health and Implications for Other Polysaccharide-Based Vaccines

Long-term Outcome of Patients With Essential Thrombocythemia: Prognostic Factors for Thrombosis, Bleeding, Myelofibrosis, and Leukemia

Prevalence of Cutaneous Adverse Effects of Hairdressing: A Systematic Review

Subtitles of scientific manuscripts may be used to amplify the title; however, the main title should be able to stand alone (ie, the subtitle should not be a continuation of the title or a substitute for a succinct title):

Avoid: An Unusual Type of Pemphigus: Combining Features of Lupus Erythematosus

Better: Pemphigus With Features of Lupus Erythematosus

Avoid: Von Hippel–Lindau Disease: Affecting 43 Members of a Single Kindred

Better: Von Hippel–Lindau Disease in 43 Members of a Single Kindred

Phrases such as "Role of," "Effects of," "Treatment of," "Use of," and "Report of a Case of" can often be omitted from both titles and subtitles.

Avoid: Effect of Smoking on Lung Cancer Risk

Better: Smoking and Lung Cancer Risk

Avoid: Use of Gastric Acid–Suppressive Agents and Risk of Community-Acquired *Clostridium difficile*–Associated Disease

Better: Gastric Acid–Suppressive Agents and the Risk of Community-Acquired *Clostridium difficile*–Associated Disease

Sometimes, especially in randomized controlled trials, in which causality can be demonstrated, the use of such phrases as "effects of" is appropriate.

Effects of Protein, Monounsaturated Fat, and Carbohydrate Intake on Blood Pressure and Serum Lipids: Results of the OmniHeart Randomized Trial

Declarative sentences are used frequently as titles of news stories and opinion pieces (eg, "Experts Set 2005 Influenza Vaccine Policy and Plan for Unpredictable Pandemic," "Spate of Lawsuits May Finally Find Chink in Tobacco Industry's 'Impenetrable Armor'"). However, sentences in scientific article titles tend to overemphasize a conclusion and are best avoided.

Avoid: Fibromyalgia Is Common in a Postpoliomyelitis Clinic

Better: Prevalence of Fibromyalgia in Patients With Postpoliomyelitis Syndrome

Similarly, questions should not be used for titles of scientific manuscripts.

Avoid: Is Television Viewing Associated With Social Isolation? Roles of Exposure Time, Viewing Context, and Violent Content

Better: Television Viewing and Social Isolation: Roles of Exposure Time, Viewing Context, and Violent Content

Questions are generally more appropriate for titles of editorials, commentaries, and opinion pieces:

Levothyroxine and Osteoporosis: An End to the Controversy?

Toward Improved Glycemic Control in Diabetes: What's on the Horizon?

Postradiotherapy Pelvic Fractures: Cause for Concern or Opportunity for Further Research?

Randomized controlled trials should be identified in the title or subtitle because this alerts readers to the level of evidence and the study design and is helpful to researchers performing a meta-analysis:

Physical Rehabilitation for Frail Nursing Home Residents: A Randomized Controlled Trial

Other aspects of study design or methods may be included in the title or subtitle.

Sex Differences of Endogenous Sex Hormones and Risk of Type 2 Diabetes: A Systematic Review and Meta-analysis

Oxycodone for Cancer-Related Pain: Meta-analysis of Randomized Controlled Trials

Depression, Apolipoprotein E Genotype, and the Incidence of Mild Cognitive Impairment: A Prospective Cohort Study

Incidence of Multiple Primary Melanoma: Two-Year Results From a Population-Based Study

An Observational Study of Cognitive Impairment in Amyotrophic Lateral Sclerosis

Sometimes a subtitle will contain the name of the group responsible for the study, especially if the study is large and is best known by its group name or acronym or if it is a part of a series of reports from the same group (see also 14.9, Abbreviations, Collaborative Groups):

Lowering Dietary Intake of Fat and Cholesterol in Children With Elevated Low-Density Lipoprotein Cholesterol Levels: The Dietary Intervention Study in Children (DISC)

Prevention of Stroke by Antihypertensive Drug Treatment in Older Patients With Isolated Systolic Hypertension: Final Results of the Systolic Hypertension in the Elderly Program (SHEP)

Administrative Data Feedback for Effective Cardiac Treatment: AFFECT, a Cluster Randomized Trial

Some journals, such as *JAMA,* have moved away from including the study name in the title or subtitle for any but the original report of outcomes or secondary analyses that provide unique information.

Low-Fat Dietary Pattern and Risk of Invasive Breast Cancer: The Women's Health Initiative Randomized Controlled Dietary Modification Trial

For the majority of secondary analyses, having the study name in the abstract is sufficient for information retrieval. In the following example, the study participants were members of the Framingham Offspring Study, an inception cohort of the Framingham Heart Study.

Sibling Cardiovascular Disease as a Risk Factor for Cardiovascular Disease in Middle-aged Adults

2.1.1 **Quotation Marks.** If quotation marks are required in the title or subtitle, they should be double, not single (see 8.6.3, Punctuation, Quotation Marks, Titles).

Above All "Do No Harm": How Can Errors Be Avoided in Medicine?

2.1.2 **Numbers.** Follow the style for numbers included in titles as described in 19.0, Numbers and Percentages.

Educational Programs in US Medical Schools, 2004-2005

Comparison of 2 Methods to Detect Publication Bias in Meta-analyses

Skin Reactions in a Subset of Patients With Stage IV Melanoma Treated With T-Lymphocyte Antigen 4 Monoclonal Antibody as a Single Agent

If numbers appear at the beginning of a title or subtitle, they—and any unit of measure associated with them—should be spelled out. Exceptions may be made for years (see also 19.2.1, Numbers and Percentages, Spelling Out Numbers, Beginning a Sentence, Title, Subtitle, or Heading).

Primary and Secondary Prevention Services in Clinical Practice: Twenty Years' Experience in Development, Implementation, and Evaluation

Three-Day Antimicrobial Regimen for Treatment of Acute Cystitis in Women: A Randomized Trial

Seventy-five Years of the *Archives of Surgery*: 1920 to 1995

Six-Month Trial of Bupropion With Contingency Management for Cocaine Dependence in a Methadone-Maintained Population

2.1.3 **Drugs.** If drug names appear in the title or subtitle, (1) use the approved generic or nonproprietary name, (2) omit the nonbase moiety unless it is required (see 15.4, Nomenclature, Drugs), and (3) avoid the use of proprietary names unless (*a*) several products are being compared, (*b*) the article is specific to a particular formulation of a drug (eg, the vehicle, not the active substance, caused adverse reactions), or (*c*) the number of ingredients is so large that the resulting title would be clumsy and a generic term, such as "multivitamin tablet," would not do.

2.1.4 **Genus and Species.** Genus and species should be expanded and italicized in the title or subtitle and an initial capital letter should be used for the genus but not the species name, just as in the text. (See also 15.14.1, Nomenclature, Organisms and Pathogens, Biological Nomenclature.)

Elimination of a Community-Acquired Methicillin-Resistant *Staphylococcus aureus* Infection in a Nurse With Atopic Dermatitis

2.1.5 Abbreviations. Avoid the use of abbreviations in the title and subtitle, unless space considerations require an exception (see the first example below) or unless the title or subtitle includes the name of a group that is best known by its acronym (see the second example below). In both cases, the abbreviation should be expanded in the abstract and at first appearance in the text. (See also 10.6, Capitalization, Acronyms and Initialisms, and 14.0, Abbreviations.)

Prevalence of HIV-1 in Blood Donations Following Implementation of a Structured Blood Safety Policy in South Africa

Reporting of Noninferiority and Equivalence Randomized Trials: An Extension of the CONSORT Statement

2.1.6 Capitalization. Capitalize the first letter of each major word in titles and subtitles. Do not capitalize articles (eg, *a, an, the*), prepositions of 3 or fewer letters, coordinating conjunctions (and, or, for, nor, but), or the *to* in infinitives. Do capitalize a 2-letter verb, such as *Is* or *Be*. Exceptions are made for some expressions, such as compound terms from languages other than English and phrasal verbs:

Ethical Questions Surrounding In Vitro Fertilization

Permanent Duplex Surveillance of In Situ Saphenous Vein Bypasses

Choice of Stents and End Points for Treatment of De Novo Coronary Artery Lesions

Weighing In on Bariatric Surgery

Researchers Size Up Nanotechnology Risks

Universal Screening for Tuberculosis Infection: School's Out!

See 10.0, Capitalization, for overall guidelines. For capitalization of hyphenated compounds, see 10.2, Capitalization, Titles and Headings.

2.1.7 Names of Cities, Counties, States, Provinces, and Countries. Include cities, states, counties, provinces, or countries in titles only when essential, especially for results that may not be generalizable to other locations (eg, unique to that site).

Epidemic of Gang-Related Homicides in Los Angeles County From 1999 Through 2004

Equity of Use of Home-Based or Facility-Based Skilled Obstetric Care in Rural Bangladesh

Identification of a New *Neisseria meningitidis* Serogroup Clone From Anhui Province, China

Comparison of Stage at Diagnosis of Melanoma Among Hispanic, Black, and White Patients in Miami–Dade County, Florida

Gender Disadvantage and Reproductive Health Risk Factors for Common Mental Disorders in Women: A Community Survey in India

In other cases, include this geographic information in the abstract and the text only. (See also 14.5, Abbreviations, Cities, States, Counties, Territories, Possessions; Provinces; Countries.)

Avoid: Pertussis Infection in Adults With Persistent Cough in Nashville, Tennessee

Better: Pertussis Infection in Adults With Persistent Cough

Avoid: Hospitalization Charges, Costs, and Income for Trauma-Related Injuries at the University of California, Davis, Medical Center in Sacramento

Better: Hospitalization Charges, Costs, and Income for Trauma-Related Injuries at a University Trauma Center

Avoid: Prevalence of Erectile Dysfunction in Men Seen by Primary Care Physicians in Canada

Better: Prevalence of Erectile Dysfunction Seen by Primary Care Physicians

2.2 **Bylines and End-of-Text Signatures.** In major articles, authors are listed in a byline, which appears immediately below the title or subtitle. In letters, editorials, book reviews, essays, poems, and news stories, the authors' names may appear as signatures at the end of the text, rather than as a byline under the title. The authors' names and academic degrees are used, as in the byline. Further information given in the signature varies with the journal. The author should consult a recent issue for style and format.

2.2.1 **Authors' Names.** The byline or signature block should contain each author's full name (unless initials are preferred to full names), including, for example, Jr, Sr, II, III, and middle initials, and highest academic degree(s). Authors should be consistent in the presentation of their names in all published works for ease of use by indexers, cataloguers, readers, and data searchers.

If the byline includes names of Chinese, Japanese, or Vietnamese origin, or other names in which the family name is traditionally given first, some journals—and some authors—may westernize the order and give the surname last. For example, an author whose name is conventionally given as Zhou Jing, where Zhou is the surname, might list his name as Jing Zhou for publication in a Western journal, or the journal might elect to publish it that way regardless of the author's preference. For journals that choose to follow the author's preference in presentation of the order of first name (given name, familiar name) and surname, and that therefore might retain the conventional (ie, non-Western) presentation of such names in the byline, the surname may be distinguished from the first name by capital letters (eg, ZHOU Jing)[3] or some other typographic distinction (eg, **Zhou** Jing or Zhou Jing).

Alternatively, a preferred citation might be published, as suggested by Black[4] in a discussion of treatment of names of authors from Spanish- and Portuguese-speaking countries. Although this would address only the authors shown in the citation, it is a viable alternative and one that might be used for all citations or only those that might otherwise be incorrectly cited (see also 2.2.4, Multiple Authors, Group Authors).

JAMA and the *Archives* Journals favor following the authors' preferences on presentation of their names and recommend querying the author at the editing stage to ensure that the surname is properly identified in the online tagging. Online tagging is critical for accurate indexing since searching by author's surname depends on appropriate tagging by the journal and identification of surname by the searcher. (See 2.10.15, Preferred Citation Format.) See the *Chicago Manual of Style* for more details on conventional presentations of names from various cultures.[5]

2.2.2 **Authorship.** All persons listed as authors should qualify for authorship (see 5.1, Ethical and Legal Considerations, Authorship Responsibility, and 5.1.2, Ethical and Legal Considerations, Authorship Responsibility, Guest and Ghost Authors). Order of authorship should be determined by the authors (see 5.1.5, Ethical and Legal Considerations, Authorship Responsibility, Order of Authorship). According to the International Committee of Medical Journal Editors,[2]

> Authorship credit should be based on 1) substantial contributions to conception and design, or acquisition of data, or analysis and interpretation of data; 2) drafting the article or revising it critically for important intellectual content; and 3) final approval of the version to be published. Authors should meet conditions 1, 2, and 3.

Some journals (including *JAMA,* several of the *Archives* Journals, *BMJ,* and *Lancet*) may publish authors' specific contributions. See 2.10.5, Acknowledgment Section, Author Contributions.

Persons who made other contributions but who do not qualify for authorship may be listed in the Acknowledgment section (see 2.10.14, Acknowledgment Section, Additional Contributions), with their permission (see 5.2, Ethical and Legal Considerations, Acknowledgments).

If an author requests that his or her name be withheld from publication, this should be allowed only in rare cases with compelling justification. In those rare cases, the author must meet the authorship criteria, but the byline may reflect the author's desire for anonymity (see 5.1.3, Ethical and Legal Considerations, Authorship Responsibility, Unsigned Editorials, Anonymous Authors, Pseudonymous Authors).

See also 2.2.4, Multiple Authors, Group Authors.

2.2.3 **Degrees.** Journals should establish their own policies on the inclusion of authors' degrees. The policy of *JAMA* and the *Archives* Journals is as follows: The highest level of degree or professional certification will be published with each author's name. If an author holds 2 doctoral degrees (eg, MD and PhD, or MD and JD), either or both may be used, in the order preferred by the author. If the author has a doctorate, degrees at the master's level are not usually included, although exceptions may be made when the master's degree represents a specialized field or a field different from that represented by the doctorate (eg, MD, MPH).

Academic degrees below the master's level are usually omitted unless these are the highest degree held. Exceptions are made for specialized professional certifications, degrees, and licensure (eg, RN, RD, COT, PA) and for specialized bachelor's degrees (eg, BSN, BPharm) and combination degrees (eg, BS, M[ASCP]).

Generally, US fellowship designations (eg, FACP or FACS) and honorary degrees (eg, PhD[Hon]) are omitted. However, non-US designations such as the British FRCP or FRCS and the Canadian FRCPC are included. (See 14.1, Abbreviations, Academic Degrees, Certifications, and Honors, for the rationale for this policy.)

JAMA and the *Archives* Journals prefer that authors in the military, or retired from the military, use their academic degrees rather than their military titles.

2.2.4 Multiple Authors, Group Authors. When the byline contains more than 1 name, use semicolons to separate the authors' names. See also 5.1.7, Ethical and Legal Considerations, Authorship Responsibility, Group and Collaborative Authorship.

Multiple Authors. The following examples show bylines with multiple authors.

> Melvin H. Freedman, MD, FRCPC; E. Fred Saunders, MD, FRCP; Louise Jones, MD, PhD; Kurt Grant, RN
>
> John E. Ware Jr, PhD; Martha S. Bayliss, MSc; William H. Rogers, PhD; Mark Kosinski, MA; Alvin R. Tarlov, MD
>
> Thomas G. Delap, FRCS; Antonios Kaberos, MD; William E. Grant, FRCSI; Michael P. Stearns, FRCS

Individual Authors* for *a Group. When a byline or signature contains 1 or more individuals' names and the name of a group (not all members of which meet the qualifications for authorship), use *for* followed by the name of the group if the specific individuals named qualify for authorship and are writing *for* the group.

> William A. Tasman, MD; for the Laser ROP Study Group

Individual Authors* and *a Group. When a byline or signature contains 1 or more individuals' names, and the name of a group (all members of which meet the qualifications for authorship), use *and* followed by the name of the group if the individuals *as well as all the members of the group* qualify for authorship. In this case, every member of the group must qualify for authorship, and for journals with specific authorship criteria, like *JAMA* and the *Archives* Journals, every member of the group must sign a statement that he or she has met the criteria for authorship. (See 5.1.7, Ethical and Legal Considerations, Authorship Responsibility, Group and Collaborative Authorship, and 14.9, Abbreviations, Collaborative Groups.)

> Debra L. Hanson, MS; Susan Y. Chu, PhD; Karen M. Farizo, MD; John W. Ward, MD; and the Adult and Adolescent Spectrum of HIV Disease Project Group

Subgroup as Author. Occasionally a specific subgroup of a larger group will be listed as the author:

> Executive Committee for the Symptomatic Carotid Atherosclerotic Study
>
> The Writing Group for the DISC Collaborative Research Group

In this case, the names of the members of the subgroup should be clearly listed as authors and each member of the subgroup must sign a statement indicating that he or she met the authorship criteria.

Group Name and Asterisk (Linking to Named Authors). If only a group is given in the byline but not all members of the group qualify as authors, an asterisk must follow the group name in the byline and refer to an asterisk footnote at the bottom of the first page of the article. The footnote must list the actual authors or refer to the list elsewhere in the article if the list is too long to provide on the first page. Each member of this group must sign a statement indicating that he or she has met the authorship criteria.

> *Byline:* Collaborative Ocular Melanoma Study Group*
>
> *This report was prepared on behalf of the COMS Group by Marie Diener-West, PhD; Sandra M. Reynolds, MA; Donna J. Agugliaro, RN, BSN; Robert Caldwell, PA; Kristi Cumming, RN, MSN; John D. Earle, MD; Barbara S. Hawkins, PhD; James A. Hayman, MD; Ismael Jaiyesimi, MD; Lee M. Jampol, MD; John M. Kirkwood, MD; Wui-Jin Koh, MD; Dennis M. Robertson, MD; John M. Shaw, MD; Bradley R. Straatsma, MD, JD; and Jonni Thoma, RN, BSN.
>
> **Group Information:** A list of the COMS Group members as of September 30, 2000, was published in *Archives of Ophthalmology* (2001;119[7]:961-965).
>
> *Byline:* Cryotherapy for Retinopathy of Prematurity Cooperative Group*
>
> *This article was prepared on behalf of the Cryotherapy for Retinopathy of Prematurity Cooperative Group by Velma Dobson, PhD (chair); Graham E. Quinn, MD, MSCE; C. Gail Summer, MD; Robert J. Hardy, PhD; and Betty Tung, MS.
>
> **Group Information:** A complete list of the members of the Cryotherapy for Retinopathy of Prematurity Cooperative Group at the 10-year examination was published in *Archives of Ophthalmology* (2001;119[8]:1110-1118).

Note that, in conjunction with the mention of a group in the byline, reference to the names of the members of the group may be given as shown immediately above or may be given in a box in the article or at the end of the article, in the Acknowledgments. (See also 2.3.3, Footnotes to Title Page, Author Affiliations.)

Group Name in Byline, With All Group Members Qualifying as Authors. If each member of the group qualifies for authorship, the group name may be listed in the byline or signature block without an asterisk (see 2.3.3, Footnotes to Title Page, Author Affiliations, and 2.10.6, Acknowledgment Section, List of Participants in a Group Study). The group members would be listed at the end of the article or in a box within the article and would be identified as authors. (See also 5.1.7, Ethical and Legal Considerations, Authorship Responsibility, Group and Collaborative Authorship.)

2.3 Footnotes to Title Page.

Footnotes should be avoided within the text. Such explanatory material can usually be incorporated into the text parenthetically. The footnotes discussed below are those that may appear at the bottom of the first page of major articles.

2.3.1 Order of Footnotes.

The preferred order of the footnotes at the bottom of the first page of an article in *JAMA* and the *Archives* Journals is as follows (see also 22.0, Typography). *Note:* Not all articles will include all of these.

JAMA

- Author affiliations
- Death of an author (death dagger [†]) (see 2.3.2, Footnotes to Title Page, Death)

- Information about members of a group (see 2.10.6, Acknowledgment Section, List of Participants in a Group Study)
- Corresponding author contact information

> *Byline:* John A. Doe, MD; Myrtle S. Coe, MD†; Simon T. Foe, RN; for the XYZ Group
>
> *Footnotes:*
>
> **Author Affiliations**: Department of Pediatrics, Baylor College of Medicine, Houston, Texas.
>
> †Died November 3, 2005.
>
> **A List of the XYZ Group** members appears at the end of this article.
>
> **Corresponding Author**: John A. Doe, MD, Department of Pediatrics, Baylor College of Medicine, 1 Baylor Plaza, Houston, TX 77030 (jdoe@baylor.edu).

Archives *Journals*

- Author affiliations
- Death of an author (death dagger [†]) (see 2.3.2, Footnotes to Title Page, Death)
- Information about members of a group

> **Group Information**: The members of the XYZ Group are listed at the end of this article.

or

> **Group Information**: The members of the XYZ Group are listed in a box on page 100.

(In the *Archives* Journals, the contact information for the corresponding author, which is published on the first page of an article in *JAMA,* is given in the Acknowledgment section [see 2.10, Acknowledgment Section] immediately after the acceptance date.) See also 22.0, Typography.

2.3.2 Death. If an author of an article has died before the article goes to press or is posted online, a death dagger (†) should follow the author's name in the byline, and one of the following footnotes should be inserted after the affiliation footnote.

> †Died November 17, 2005.
>
> †Deceased.

2.3.3 Author Affiliations. The institutions with which an author is professionally affiliated, including locations, are given in a footnote. The authors' last names are given parenthetically in the footnote following their respective institutions. If 2 or more authors share the same last name, their initials should be used in addition to the last name to distinguish them. Title and academic rank are not included in this footnote. If all authors in the byline are affiliated with the same department and institution, there is no need to include their names in the footnote.

List the affiliations in the order of the authors' names as given in the byline, but, for ease of grouping, combine the listings of authors affiliated with the same institution (eg, if the byline includes authors A, B, and C and if authors A and C are at the same institution, list the institution of authors A and C first and then the institution of author B) and for authors in private practice list the information at the end.

> *Byline:* Gary T. Jeng, MS; James R. Scott, MD; Leon F. Burmeister, PhD
>
> **Author Affiliations:** Department of Preventive Medicine, University of Iowa, Iowa City (Mr Jeng and Dr Burmeister); and Department of Obstetrics and Gynecology, University of Utah, Salt Lake City (Dr Scott).
>
> *Byline:* Daniel G. Deschler, MD; Robert Osorio, MD; Nancy L. Ascher, MD, PhD; Kelvin C. Lee, MD
>
> **Author Affiliations:** Departments of Otolaryngology–Head and Neck Surgery (Drs Deschler and Lee) and General Surgery (Drs Osorio and Ascher), University of California, San Francisco.
>
> *Byline:* Carol L. Shields, MD; Arman Mashayekhi, MD; Jacqueline Cater, PhD; Abdullah Shelil, MD; Steven Ness, MD; Anna T. Meadows, MD; Jerry A. Shields, MD
>
> **Author Affiliations:** Ocular Oncology Service, Wills Eye Hospital, Thomas Jefferson University, Philadelphia, Pennsylvania (Drs C. L. Shields, Mashayekhi, Cater, Shelil, Ness, and J. A. Shields); and Division of Oncology, The Children's Hospital of Philadelphia (Dr Meadows).
>
> *Byline:* Yves Vander Haeghen, PhD; Jean Marie Naeyaert, PhD
>
> **Author Affiliations:** Department of Dermatology, University Hospital, Ghent, Belgium.
>
> *Byline:* Mariangela Lo Guidice, BS; Marcella Neri, MD; Michele Falco, BS; Maurizio Sturnio, BS; Elisa Calzolari, MD; Daniela Di Benedetto, PhD; Marco Fichera, PhD
>
> **Author Affiliations:** Genetic Diagnostic Laboratory, Instituto di Ricovero e Cura a Carattere Scientifico (IRCCS) Oasi Maria SS, Troina, Italy (Mss Lo Guidice and Falco, Mr Sturnio, and Drs Di Benedetto and Fichera); and Department of Experimental Medicine and Diagnostics, Medical Genetics Service, University of Ferrara, Ferrara, Italy (Drs Neri and Calzolari).

Note that the authors are also grouped by their degrees or honorifics (or courtesy titles), so that in the example below, Drs Brown and Stone are listed together, followed by Mr Fingert and Ms Taylor, even though Dr Stone comes *after* Mr Fingert and Ms Taylor in the byline.

> *Byline:* Jeremiah Brown Jr, MD; John H. Fingert; Chris M. Taylor; Max Lake, MD; Val C. Sheffield, MD, PhD; Edwin M. Stone, MD, PhD
>
> **Author Affiliations:** Departments of Ophthalmology (Drs Brown and Stone, Mr Fingert, and Ms Taylor) and Pediatrics (Dr Sheffield), University of Iowa College of Medicine, Iowa City. Dr Lake is in private practice in Salina, Kansas.

If there is a single author and a single institution with which he or she is affiliated, use the singular for the sidehead:

Byline: James R. Keane, MD

Author Affiliation: Department of Neurology, University of Southern California Medical School, Los Angeles.

If an author is affiliated with different institutions or different departments at the same institution, this information should be indicated parenthetically.

Author Affiliations: Rocky Mountain Poison and Drug Center, Denver Department of Health and Hospitals (Dr Dart, Ms Stark, and Mr Fulton), and Colorado Emergency Medicine Research Center, University of Colorado Health Sciences Center (Drs Dart and Lowenstein and Ms Koziol-McLain), Denver, Colorado.

The affiliation listed, including departmental affiliation if appropriate, should reflect the author's institutional affiliation at the time the work was done. If the author has since moved, the current affiliation also should be provided.

Author Affiliations: Department of Health Policy and Management, The Johns Hopkins University Bloomberg School of Public Health, Baltimore, Maryland. Dr Lloyd is now with the Department of Emergency Medicine, St Luke's Hospital, Milwaukee, Wisconsin.

For large groups, the name of the group may be given in the byline, and the affiliation footnote may refer the reader to the end of the article, a boxed listing within the article, or another publication for a complete listing of the participants. (See also 2.2.4, Bylines and End-of-Text Signatures, Multiple Authors, Group Authors, and 2.10.6, Acknowledgment Section, List of Participants in a Group Study.)

A complete list of the members of the Human Fetal Tissue Working Group appears at the end of this article.

A complete list of the members of the Cryotherapy for Retinopathy of Prematurity Cooperative Group was published previously (*Arch Ophthalmol.* 2001;119[8]:1110-1118).

2.4 Running Foot.

Printed pages customarily carry the journal name or abbreviation, volume number, date of issue, and page number. They may also include a shortened version of the article title. When this information appears at the top of the page, it is called a running head; when it appears at the bottom of the page, it is called a running foot. These are typically added during the editing and production process, and authors are not usually required to submit such information. (See also 22.0, Typography.)

2.4.1 Name of the Publication.

Use the accepted *List of Journals Indexed for MEDLINE*[6] abbreviations of journal names (see 14.10, Abbreviations, Names of Journals) and the following forms, as applicable to the journal involved:

JAMA:	*JAMA*, December 14, 2005—Vol 294, No. 22
Archives Journals:	*Arch Pediatr Adolesc Med*/Vol 159, Dec 2005 www.archpediatrics.com

Note that journals will differ in the amount of information included in their running feet and that the style for some abbreviations (eg, the month in the *Archives* example above) may differ from that used elsewhere in the publication.

2.4.2 Title of the Article. The shortened version of the title should be kept brief but should emphasize the main point of the article (see the options suggested in the second example below, based on the desired emphasis), not just repeat the first few words of the title. Different journals have different limits (eg, approximately 45 characters and spaces in *JAMA*). No punctuation follows the running foot/header.

Title:	Taking Health Status Into Account When Setting Capitation Rates
Running Foot:	Adjusting Capitation Rates
Title:	Decline in Hospital Utilization and Cost Inflation Under Managed Care in California
Running Foot:	Decline in Hospital Utilization and Costs *or* Managed Care in California
Title:	Domestic Production vs International Immigration: Options for the US Physician Workforce
Running Foot:	Domestic vs International Physician Workforce
Title:	Neurologic Adverse Events Associated With Smallpox Vaccination in the United States, 2002-2004
Running Foot:	Smallpox Vaccination and Neurologic Events

Careful use of abbreviations may help meet space limitations.

Title:	Ventilatory Management of Acute Lung Injury and Acute Respiratory Distress Syndrome
Running Foot:	Management of Acute Lung Injury and ARDS

In some instances the editorial department, eg, Editorials, Commentary, Letters, rather than the article's title, will constitute the running head/foot.

2.5 Abstract. In this age of electronic data dissemination and retrieval, in which abstracts are typically indexed and freely available, a well-written abstract has become increasingly important in directing readers to articles of potential clinical and research interest. The abstract of a research report summarizes the main points of an article: (1) the study objective or background, (2) the study design and methods, (3) primary results, and (4) principal conclusions. For scientific studies and systematic reviews, narrative expressions, such as "X is described," "Y is discussed," "Z is also reviewed," do not add meaning and should be avoided. Results should be presented in quantitative fashion, but authors and editors should be scrupulous in verifying the accuracy of all data and numbers reported and ensuring consistency with the results published in the full article.[7]

2.5.1 Structured Abstracts. For reports of original data, systematic reviews (including meta-analyses), and clinical reviews, structured abstracts that use predetermined sideheads are recommended. Specific advice taken from *JAMA*'s Instructions for Authors,[1] adapted from Haynes et al,[8] is given below. Note that Design, Setting, and

Patients or Other Participants may be combined depending on the description. If no intervention was performed, that sideheading may be omitted. Many journals limit the number of words to 250, but some (such as *JAMA*) allow 300 for reports of original data and for systematic reviews.

Structured Abstracts for Reports of Original Data. In reports of original data, include an abstract of no more than 300 words using the following headings: Context, Objective, Design, Setting, Patients (or Participants), Interventions (include only if there are any), Main Outcome Measure(s), Results, and Conclusions. For brevity, phrases rather than complete sentences may be used. Include the following content in each section:

Context: Begin the abstract with a sentence or two explaining the clinical (or other) importance of the study question.

Objective: State the precise objective or study question addressed in the report (eg, "To determine whether . . . "). If more than 1 objective is addressed, indicate the main objective and state only key secondary objectives. If an a priori hypothesis was tested, state that hypothesis.

Design: Describe the basic design of the study. State the years of the study and the duration of follow-up. If applicable, include the name of the study (eg, the Framingham Heart Study).

Setting: Describe the study setting to assist readers to determine the applicability of the report to other circumstances, for example, general community, a primary care or referral center, private or institutional practice, or ambulatory or hospitalized care.

Patients or Other Participants: State the clinical disorders, important eligibility criteria, and key sociodemographic features of patients. Provide the numbers of participants and how they were selected (see below), including the number of otherwise eligible individuals who were approached but refused. If matching is used for comparison groups, specify the characteristics that are matched. In follow-up studies, indicate the proportion of participants who completed the study. In intervention studies, provide the number of patients withdrawn because of adverse effects. For selection procedures, use these terms, if appropriate: *random sample* (where *random* refers to a formal, randomized selection in which all eligible individuals have a fixed and usually equal chance of selection); *population-based sample; referred sample; consecutive sample; volunteer sample; convenience sample.*

Intervention(s): Describe the essential features of any interventions, including their method and duration of administration. Name the intervention by its most common clinical name, and use nonproprietary drug names.

Main Outcome Measure(s): Indicate the primary study outcome measurement(s) as planned before data collection began. If the manuscript does not report the main planned outcomes of a study, state this fact and indicate the reason. State clearly whether the hypothesis being tested was formulated during or after data collection.

Results: Provide and quantify the main outcomes of the study, including confidence intervals (eg, 95%) or *P* values. For comparative studies, express the differences between groups with confidence intervals. Explain outcomes or measurements unfamiliar to a general medical readership. Declare important measurements not presented in results. As relevant, indicate whether observers were blinded to patient groupings, particularly for subjective measurements. If differences for the major study outcome measure(s) are not significant, state the clinically important difference sought and provide the confidence interval for the difference between the groups. When risk changes or effect sizes are given, indicate absolute values. Approaches such as number needed to treat to achieve a unit of benefit are encouraged when appropriate; reporting of relative differences alone is insufficient. For studies of screening and diagnostic tests, report sensitivity, specificity, and likelihood ratio. If predictive value or accuracy is given, provide prevalence or pretest likelihood as well. For all randomized controlled trials, include the results of intention-to-treat analysis, and for all surveys include response rates.

Conclusions: Provide only conclusions of the study directly supported by the results, taking into account the limitations (eg, observational study, selected population), along with implications for clinical practice, avoiding speculation and overgeneralization. Indicate whether additional study is required before the information should be used in usual clinical settings. Give equal emphasis to positive and negative findings of equal scientific merit.

Trial Registration: For clinical trials, provide the name of the trial registry, registration number, and URL of the registry.

Structured Abstracts for Systematic Reviews (Including Meta-analyses). In manuscripts reporting the results of meta-analyses, include an abstract of no more than 300 words using the following headings: Context, Objective, Data Sources, Study Selection, Data Extraction, Data Synthesis, and Conclusions. In the text of the manuscript, include a section describing the methods used for data sources, study selection, data extraction, and data synthesis. Follow each heading with a brief description:

Context: Provide a sentence or two explaining the importance of the review question.

Objective: State the precise primary objective of the review. Indicate whether the review emphasizes factors such as cause, diagnosis, prognosis, therapy, or prevention and include information about the specific population, intervention, exposure, and tests or outcomes that are being reviewed.

Data Sources: Succinctly summarize data sources, including years searched. Include in the search the most current information possible, ideally conducting the search several months before the date of manuscript submission. Potential sources include computerized databases and published indexes, registries, abstract booklets, conference proceedings, references identified from bibliographies of pertinent articles and books, experts or research institutions active in the field, and companies or manufacturers of tests or agents being reviewed. If a bibliographic database is used, state the exact indexing terms used for article retrieval, including any constraints (for example, English language or human subjects). If abstract space does not permit this level of detail, summarize sources in the abstract including databases and years searched, and place the remainder of the information in the "Methods" section of the text.

Study Selection: Describe inclusion and exclusion criteria used to select studies for detailed review from among studies identified as relevant to the topic. Under details of selection include particular populations, interventions, outcomes, or methodological designs. Specify the method used to apply these criteria (for example, blinded review, consensus, multiple reviewers). State the proportion of initially identified studies that met selection criteria.

Data Extraction: Describe guidelines used for abstracting data and assessing data quality and validity (such as criteria for causal inference). State the method by which the guidelines were applied (eg, independent extraction by multiple observers).

Results: State the main results of the review, whether qualitative or quantitative, and outline the methods used to obtain these results. For meta-analyses, state the major outcomes that were pooled and include odds ratios or effect sizes and, if possible, sensitivity analyses. Accompany numerical results by confidence intervals, if applicable, and exact levels of statistical significance. For evaluations of screening and diagnostic tests, include sensitivity, specificity, likelihood ratios, receiver operating characteristic curves, and predictive values. For assessments of prognosis, summarize survival characteristics and related variables. State the major identified sources of variation between studies, including differences in treatment protocols, co-interventions, confounders, outcome measures, length of follow-up, and dropout rates.

Conclusions: Clearly state the conclusions and their applications (clinical or otherwise), limiting interpretation to the domain of the review.

Structured Abstracts for Clinical Reviews. For Clinical Review articles, include an abstract of no more than 250 words with the following sections: Context, Evidence Acquisition, Evidence Synthesis, and Conclusions.

Context: Include 1 or 2 sentences describing the clinical question or issue and its importance in clinical practice or public heath.

Evidence Acquisition: Describe the data sources used, including the search strategies, years searched, and other sources of material, such as subsequent reference searches of retrieved articles. Explain the methods used for quality assessment and the inclusion of identified articles.

Results: Address the major findings of the review of the clinical issue or topic in an evidence-based, objective, and balanced fashion, emphasizing the highest-quality evidence available.

Conclusions: Clearly state the conclusions to answer the questions posed if applicable, basing the conclusions on available evidence, and emphasize how clinicians should apply current knowledge.

2.5.2 **Unstructured Abstracts.** For other major manuscripts, include a conventional unstructured abstract of no more than 150 words. Abstracts are not required for opinion pieces, letters, and special features such as news articles. Consult the journal's instructions for authors for special requirements in individual publications.

2.5.3 General Guidelines. A few specific guidelines to consider in preparing either type of abstract follow:

- Consult the journal's instructions for authors.
- Follow the journal's specific sideheadings when preparing a structured abstract.
- Do not begin the abstract by repeating the title.
- Do not cite references.
- Provide absolute results for main outcome measures (eg, report incidence rates rather than reporting only relative risks). In addition, provide confidence intervals whenever possible (if not, provide *P* values) (see 20.1, Study Design and Statistics, The Manuscript: Presenting Study Design, Rationale, and Statistical Analysis).
- Include major terms and describe databases and study groups (related to the subject under discussion) in the abstract, since the abstract can be text-searched in many retrieval systems.
- Include the stated hypothesis, if applicable.
- Ensure that all concepts and data in the abstract are included in the text.
- Include the active moiety of a drug at first mention (see 15.4, Nomenclature, Drugs).
- Avoid proprietary names or manufacturers' names unless they are essential to the study (see 15.5, Nomenclature, Equipment, Devices, and Reagents).
- Spell out abbreviations at first mention.
- If an isotope is mentioned, spell out the name of the element when first used and provide the isotope number on the line (see 15.9, Nomenclature, Isotopes).
- Provide the dates of the study, or date ranges for studies and other data included in reviews.
- Verify the numbers provided in the abstract against those provided in the text and tables to ensure internal consistency.

2.6 Keywords. Some medical journals publish a short list (3-10) of keywords at the end of the abstract. These descriptors are provided by the author and are the terms the author believes represent the key topics presented in the article. These may also be used for some journals to categorize manuscripts, to help guide in the selection of peer reviewers, and to assist the journal's indexer. *JAMA* and the *Archives* Journals do not publish keywords. Articles in *JAMA* and the *Archives* Journals are indexed by professional indexers by means of, for example, Medical Subject Headings (MeSH) for indexes[9] such as *List of Journals Indexed for MEDLINE* and databases such as MEDLINE. See 13.0, Medical Indexes.

2.7 Epigraphs. Epigraphs are rarely used for research papers. On occasion an author will use an epigraph, a short quotation set at the beginning of a nonresearch article, to suggest the theme of the article. In *JAMA* and the *Archives* Journals, epigraphs are set in italics, beginning flush left, with the signature set in roman type underneath the quotation, flush right with the longest line of the quotation. If the work cited appears in the reference list, a superscript number should indicate the source. Otherwise, the title of the work should be indicated.

> *The medical profession seems to have no place for its*
> *mistakes. . . . And if the medical profession has no*
> *room for doctors' mistakes, neither does society.*
> David Hilfiker[1]

> *Gas! Gas! Quick, boys!—An ecstasy of fumbling,*
> *Fitting the clumsy helmets just in time;*
> *But someone still was yelling out and stumbling,*
> *And flound'ring like a man in fire or lime. . . .*
> Wilfred Owen, *Dulce et Decorum Est*

2.8 Parts of a Manuscript, Headings, Subheadings, and Side Headings. A consistent pattern of organization for all headings should be used for original research articles (see also 20.1, Study Design and Statistics, The Manuscript: Presenting Study Design, Rationale, and Statistical Analysis); many scientific articles follow the IMRAD pattern (introduction, methods, results, and discussion). However, not all articles will conform to a single pattern because format and section headings vary with the type of article (see 22.0, Typography).

Introduction: The introduction should provide the context for the article, the objective of the study, and should state the hypothesis or research question (purpose statement), how and why the hypothesis was developed, and why it is important. It should convince the expert that the authors know the subject and should fill in gaps for the novice. It should generally not exceed 2 or 3 paragraphs.

Methods: The "Methods" section should include, as appropriate, a detailed description of (1) study design or type of analysis and dates and period of study, as well as mention of institutional review board or ethics committee approval (informed consent; see also 5.8, Ethical and Legal Considerations, Protecting Research Participants' and Patients' Rights in Scientific Publication); (2) condition, factors, or disease studied; (3) details of sample (eg, study participants and the setting from which they were drawn, inclusion and exclusion criteria); (4) intervention(s), if any; (5) outcome measures or observations; and (6) statistical analysis. Enough information should be provided to enable an informed reader to replicate the study, or, if a methods article has already been published, that article should be cited and important points should be summarized.

Results: The results reported in the manuscript should be specific and relevant to the research hypothesis. Characteristics of the study participants should be followed by presentation of results, from the broad to the specific. The "Results" section should not include implications or weaknesses of the study, but should include validation measures if conducted as part of the study. Results should not discuss the rationale for the statistical procedures used. Data in tables and figures should not be duplicated in the text. (See 4.0, Visual Presentation of Data.)

Discussion: The "Discussion" section should be a formal consideration and critical examination of the study. The research question or hypothesis should be addressed in this section, and the results should be compared to and contrasted with the findings of other studies. *(Note:* A lengthy reiteration of the results should be avoided.) The study's limitations and the generalizability of the results should be discussed, as well as mention of unexpected findings with suggested explanations. The type of future studies needed, if appropriate, should be mentioned. This section should end with a clear, concise conclusion that does not go beyond the findings of the study. *JAMA* and the *Archives* Journals traditionally have used "Comment" rather than "Discussion" here, as the latter heading is often used for symposium proceedings or articles in which a discussion follows the presentation of a paper.

2.8.1 **Levels of Headings.** A consistent style or typeface should be used for each level of heading throughout a manuscript so that the reader may visually distinguish between primary and secondary headings.

The styles used for the various levels of headings will vary from publisher to publisher and publication to publication, even within the same publishing house. They may also vary within a single publication, from one category of article to another (see also 22.0, Typography).

Headings are often used as navigational links for online articles. Consideration should be given to appropriate online use (eg, avoidance of excessive length and citation of images and references within headings).

2.8.2 **Number of Headings.** There is no requisite number of headings. However, because headings are meant to divide a primary part into secondary parts, and so on, there should be a minimum of 2.

Headings reflect the progression of logic or the flow of thought in an article and thereby guide the reader. Headings also help break up the copy, making the article more attractive and easier to read. Headings may be used even in articles such as editorials and reviews, which usually do not follow the organization described above for research articles. (Other typographic and design elements, such as pullout quotations, bullets [•], enumerations, tabulations, figures, and tables, may also be used for these purposes [see also 22.0, Typography].)

2.8.3 Items to Avoid in Headings

- Avoid using a single abbreviation as a heading, even if the abbreviation has been expanded earlier in the text. If the abbreviation appears as the sole item in a heading, spell it out. (See 14.11, Abbreviations, Clinical, Technical, and Other Common Terms.)
- Avoid expanding abbreviations for the first time in a heading. Spell the abbreviation out in the heading if that is its first appearance and introduce the abbreviation, if appropriate, at the next appearance of the term. (See 14.11, Abbreviations, Clinical, Technical, and Other Common Terms.)
- Avoid citing figures or tables in headings. Cite them in the appropriate place in the text that follows the heading.
- Avoid citing references in headings.

2.9 **Addenda.** Addenda may be material added to an article late in the publication process or may be material that is considered supplementary to the article. (*Note:* This is distinct from supplementary Web-only material, although addenda *may* sometimes be presented as supplementary Web-only material. For that, see 2.12, Online-Only [Supplementary] Material.) The use of addenda is discouraged in *JAMA* and the *Archives* Journals. If material is added late in the publication process, well after a manuscript has been accepted for publication (eg, the addition of another case report, extended follow-up, data or information on recent legislation or other relevant event, or additional studies that bear on the present article), this is best handled by incorporating the information into the text. If there is a compelling reason to set this material apart as an addendum, this may be done by adding a final paragraph to the existing manuscript:

> ADDENDUM
>
> After the manuscript was accepted for publication, . . .

If desired, this paragraph may be set off by extra space and/or a half-column-wide centered hairline rule. Any references cited for the first time in this final paragraph or addendum should follow the numbering of the existing reference list.

Note: If substantial material (eg, new figures, new tables, several additional cases) is added after acceptance of the manuscript or if the conclusions change after acceptance, the editor must approve all such changes; additional peer review may be required.

2.10 **Acknowledgment Section.** "Acknowledgments" is the blanket term used to cover the information that follows the body of the article and precedes the references. The Acknowledgment section is considered to be a continuation of the text, so that abbreviations expanded in the text may stand without expansion here. If a footnote that would normally appear on the first page of the article (eg, the affiliation footnote) is too long to be placed on the first page, it may be placed here immediately after the acceptance date and, if applicable, the online-publication-ahead-of-print information; if the journal does not publish acceptance dates, the affiliation footnote that did not fit on the first page would be placed first in the Acknowledgment section. (*Note:* See also 2.3, Footnotes to Title Page, where some additional types of acknowledgment footnotes are discussed. Placement of these may vary among journals.) Examples of various parts of the Acknowledgment section follow, in the order used by *JAMA* and the *Archives* Journals. (See also 5.2, Legal and Ethical Considerations, Acknowledgments, Box.)

2.10.1 **Acceptance Date.** Some journals include the date of the manuscript's acceptance; others include the date of manuscript submission, the date the revision was received, and the date accepted. Examples are shown below:

> **Accepted for Publication**: December 16, 2006.
>
> **Submitted for Publication**: November 22, 2004; final revision received May 13, 2005; accepted May 23, 2005.

2.10.2 **Online Publication Ahead of Print.** If an article was published online ahead of print, the date it was published online, along with the digital object identifier (DOI) to ensure that all article versions can be identified, should follow the acceptance date footnote (or, if the journal does not publish the acceptance date, it should be placed first).

> **Published Online**: October 20, 2005 (doi:10.1001/JAMA.294.20.joc50147).

2.10.3 Affiliation Notes That Would Not Fit on Page 1. Limited space on the first page of an article may sometimes not allow the author affiliation footnote to appear on the first page. If the author affiliation footnote does not fit there, it would appear at the end of the article, after the acceptance date and the online-publication-ahead-of-print information, if applicable.

2.10.4 Correspondence Address. Contact information for the corresponding author (street address, if possible, with zip or postal code, and e-mail address, if the author wishes) is provided in a footnote. Even for a single author, the full name of the person should be included. Follow the custom of individual countries regarding the placement of the zip or postal code. *Note:* For *JAMA,* this information is provided on the first page of the print article, not in the Acknowledgment section, and the heading used is "Corresponding Author."

> **Correspondence**: John H. Alexander, MD, MS, Box 3300, Duke University Medical Center, Durham, NC 27715 (john.h.alexander@duke.edu).

> **Correspondence**: Patrick J. Gullane, MB, FRCS, University Health Network, University of Toronto, 200 Elizabeth St, Suite 8N-800, Toronto, ON M5G 2C4, Canada (patrick.gullane@uhn.on.ca).

> **Correspondence**: Christoph Kniestedt, MD, Department of Ophthalmology, Cantonal Hospital Winterthur, Brauerstrasse 15, 8400 Winterthur, Switzerland (research@kniestedt.ch).

> **Correspondence**: Mutsuhito Kikura, MD, PhD, Department of Anesthesia and Intensive Care, Hamamatsu Medical Center, 328 Tomizuka-cho, Hamamatsu 432–8580, Japan (mkikura@hotmail.com).

> **Correspondence**: N. J. Hall, MD, Department of Pediatric Surgery, Institute of Child Health, 30 Guilford St, London WC1N 1EH, England (n.hall@ich .ucl.ac.uk).

> **Correspondence**: Jacqueline C. M. Witteman, PhD, Department of Epidemiology and Biostatistics, Erasmus Medical Center, PO Box 1738, 3000 DR Rotterdam, the Netherlands (j.witteman@erasmusmc.nl).

> **Correspondence**: Kenneth F. C. Fearon, MD, University Department of Surgery, Royal Infirmary, Lauriston Place, Edinburgh EH3 9YW, Scotland.

For smaller items (eg, letters to the editor, book reviews) with signature blocks rather than bylines, and where the signature block contains only the names and degree(s) of the author(s), a shortened form of address for the corresponding author may be used: Dr Jones, Mr Thomas, etc.

> *Signature block:* Philip Lempert, MD

Correspondence: Dr Lempert, Park View Health Care Campus, 10 Brentwood Dr, Suite A, Ithaca, NY 14850 (eyechartplus@aol.com).

In *JAMA,* the signature block typically contains the author's affiliation and e-mail address:

Brian Budenholzer, MD
budenholzer.b@ghc.org
Group Health Cooperative
Spokane, Washington

To break an e-mail address in print, always break *before* a punctuation mark so that it is clear that the address includes the mark.

cheryl.iverson@jama-archives
.org

cheryl.iverson@jama
-archives.org

This is especially important with hyphens and periods. There is no need to set the e-mail address in italics or to precede it by the word *e-mail.*

2.10.5 **Author Contributions.** Editors may ask authors to describe what each author contributed, and these contributions to the work may be published at the editor's discretion. (See also 5.1.1, Legal and Ethical Considerations, Authorship Responsibility, Authorship: Definition, Criteria, Contributions, and Requirements.) An example from the *Archives of Dermatology* is shown below:

Author Contributions: *Study concept and design:* Fortes, Melchi, and Abeni. *Analysis and interpretation of data:* Fortes, Mastroeni, and Leffondré. *Drafting of the manuscript:* Fortes. *Critical revision of the manuscript for important intellectual content:* Mastroeni, Leffondré, Sampogna, Melchi, Mazzotti, Pasquini, and Abeni. *Statistical analysis:* Fortes and Mastoeni. *Obtained funding:* Pasquini and Abeni. *Study supervision:* Fortes, Melchi, and Abeni.

JAMA and some of the *Archives* Journals require authors of manuscripts reporting original research and meta-analyses to provide an access to data statement (see 5.1.1, Legal and Ethical Considerations, Authorship Responsibility, Authorship: Definition, Criteria, Contributions, and Requirements). If such a statement is provided, it is given under the sidehead "Author Contributions," before the other contributions.

Author Contributions: Dr Stolzenberg-Solomon had full access to all of the data in the study and takes responsibility for the integrity of the data and the accuracy of the data analysis.

Some journals require that at least 1 author serve as "guarantor," taking "responsibility for the integrity of the work as a whole, from inception to published article, and publish that information."[2]

Author Contributions: Yoon Kong Loke developed the original idea and the protocol, abstracted and analyzed data, wrote the manuscript, and is guarantor. Deirdre Price and Sheena Derry contributed to the development of the protocol, abstracted data, and prepared the manuscript. Jeffrey K. Aronson developed the protocol and helped with the manuscript.

2.10.6 List of Participants in a Group Study. If the study was by a group of persons, the names of the participants may be listed in the Acknowledgment section (see also 2.3.3, Footnotes to Title Page, Author Affiliations). Alternatively, the list of participants may be placed in a box wherever it best fits in the layout, or the reader can be referred to a previously published list of the group's members. See also 5.2.2, Ethical and Legal Considerations, Acknowledgments, Group and Collaborative Author Lists.)

2.10.7 Financial Disclosure. *JAMA* and the *Archives* Journals require each author to sign and submit the following financial disclosure statement: "I certify that all my affiliations with or financial involvement within the past 5 years and foreseeable future (eg, employment, consultancies, honoraria, stock ownership or options, expert testimony, grants or patents received or pending, royalties) with any organization or entity with a financial interest in or financial conflict with the subject matter or materials discussed in the manuscript are completely disclosed."[1] (See also 5.5, Legal and Ethical Considerations, Conflicts of Interest.)

Authors are expected to provide detailed information about any relevant financial interests or financial conflicts within the past 5 years and for the foreseeable future, particularly those present at the time the research was conducted and up to the time of publication, as well as other financial interests, such as relevant filed or pending patents or patent applications in preparation, that represent potential future financial gain. Although many universities and other institutions and organizations have established policies and thresholds for reporting financial interests and other conflicts of interest, *JAMA* and the *Archives* Journals require complete disclosure of all relevant financial relationships and potential financial conflicts of interest, regardless of amount or value. If authors are uncertain about what might constitute a potential financial conflict of interest, they should err on the side of full disclosure and should contact the editorial office if they have questions or concerns. In addition, authors who have no relevant financial interests are asked to provide a statement indicating that they have no financial interests related to the material in the manuscript.

For some journals, financial disclosure information is for the editorial office and is not shared with peer reviewers. Other journals, such as *JAMA* and the *Archives of Dermatology,* require authors to include all such disclosures on the title page or in the Acknowledgment section of the manuscript, or both, and these *are* shown to peer reviewers. However, for all accepted manuscripts, each author's disclosures of relevant financial interests or declarations of no relevant financial interests should be published. Decisions about whether financial information provided by authors should be published, and thereby disclosed to readers, are usually straightforward. Although editors are willing to discuss disclosure of specific financial information with authors, the policy of *JAMA* and the *Archives* Journals is one of full disclosure of all relevant financial interests.

The policy requiring disclosure of financial conflicts of interest should apply for all manuscript submissions, including letters to the editor, opinion pieces, informal essays, and book reviews.

Financial Disclosures: Dr Morrow reported having received research grant support administered via Brigham and Women's Hospital from Bayer

Healthcare Diagnostics, Beckman Coulter, Biosite, Dade Behring, Merck, and Roche Diagnostics; and having received honoraria for educational presentations from Bayer Healthcare Diagnostics, Beckman Coulter, and Dade Behring. Dr de Lemos reported receiving research grants and honoraria and consulting fees for speaking from Biosite and Roche. Dr Blazing reported receiving honoraria from Merck and Pfizer.

Financial Disclosure: Dr Neuzil reported receiving research funding from MedImmune for participation in a multicenter trial of an LAIV in 2004-2005.

Financial Disclosure: Dr Smith reported serving as an expert witness for plaintiffs in US tobacco litigation.

Note: The financial disclosure may be a disclosure of no potential financial conflicts of interest. This is not obligatory, and the choice not to include such a statement should not be misinterpreted as an indication of a conflict. However, the inclusion of a statement like that below removes any ambiguity.

Financial Disclosure: None reported.

2.10.8 Funding/Support. *JAMA* and the *Archives* Journals require each author to provide detailed information regarding all financial and material support for the research and work, including but not limited to grant support, funding sources, and provision of equipment and supplies. This is outlined in the journals' instructions for authors.

All financial and material support for the research and the work should be clearly and completely identified in the Acknowledgment section. Grant or contract numbers should be included whenever possible. The complete name of the funding institution or agency should be given.

If individual authors were the recipients of funds, their names should be listed parenthetically.

Funding/Support: This study was supported in part by grant CA34988 from the National Institutes of Health and by a teaching and research scholarship from the American College of Physicians (Dr Fischl).

Funding/Support: This study was supported by a 2000 Special Projects Award of the Ambulatory Pediatric Association (Dr Hickson).

Funding/Support: This work was supported by research grant R01 MH45757 from the National Institute of Mental Health (Dr Klein).

Funding/Support: Funding for this study was provided by Agency for Healthcare Research and Quality grant 5 U18 HS011885 and through subcontracts with the Utah Department of Health (contract 026429) and the Missouri Department of Health and Senior Services (contract AOC 02380132).

Funding/Support: This study was supported by Merck and Co and Bayer Healthcare Diagnostics Division.

Funding/Support: Alefacept was provided to the patients at no cost through a Biogen Idec patient assistance program.

2.10.9 **Role of the Sponsor.** The specific role of the funding organization or sponsor in each of the following should be specified: design and conduct of the study; collection, management, and analysis of the data; and preparation, review, and approval of the manuscript. For articles that do not include original research, "design and conduct of the study" is omitted.

> **Role of the Sponsor:** The funding organizations are public institutions and had no role in the design and conduct of the study; collection, management, and analysis of the data; or preparation, review, and approval of the manuscript. The Utah and Missouri health departments provided practical support for the focus group and survey processes, including letters of endorsement, hospital contact information, and assistance with logistic arrangements for focus group sessions.

> **Role of the Sponsor:** Staff from Merck assisted in monitoring the progress and conduct of the A to Z trial. Bayer Healthcare provided reagents for B-type natriuretic peptide testing. The sponsors were not involved in the biomarker testing, analysis, or interpretation of the data, or in preparation of the manuscript for this substudy. Medical specialists employed by the sponsors reviewed the manuscript prior to submission.

2.10.10 **Independent Statistical Analysis.** For industry-sponsored studies in which the statistical analysis was conducted only by statisticians employed by the sponsor, some journals, such as *JAMA* and several of the *Archives* Journals, require that data analysis be conducted by an independent statistician at an academic institution. If issues regarding the analysis should emerge, the academic institution provides an additional level of oversight independent of the commercial sponsor. This independent analysis should be conducted using the raw data set, and the results of that analysis should be the findings that are published in the manuscript. Some journals, such as *JAMA*, specify whether compensation was received for conducting the independent statistical analysis. (See also 5.5.5, Legal and Ethical Considerations, Conflicts of Interest, Requirements for Reporting Industry-Sponsored Studies, and Fontanarosa et al.[10])

> **Independent Statistical Analysis:** Independent statistical review of the data included in this analysis was performed by Stuart Pocock, PhD, and Duolao Wang, both of the London School of Hygiene and Tropical Medicine.

> **Independent Statistical Analysis:** The accuracy of the data analysis was independently verified by Yingbo Na, MSc, and Martin Fahy, MSc, both from the Cardiovascular Research Foundation, an affiliate of Columbia University, who received the entire raw database and replicated all the analyses that were reported in the accepted manuscript. No discrepancies were discovered. Neither Mr Na nor Mr Fahy nor the Cardiovascular Research Foundation received any funding for this independent statistical analysis.

> **Independent Statistical Analysis:** All study data were transferred from Sanofi-Aventis to the Department of Medicine at St Luke's–Roosevelt Hospital Center for independent analysis by Stanley Heshka, PhD. Statistical reanalysis of the raw data was performed by Dr Heshka. There were no discrepancies between the reanalysis and the original interpretation of the results and conclusions. In lieu of financial compensation for Dr Heshka's

time and effort in performing the statistical analysis, an unrestricted educational grant from Sanofi-Aventis was given to the Obesity Research Center at St Luke's–Roosevelt Hospital Center, New York, New York.

Independent Statistical Analysis: Christopher E. Minder, PhD, professor of medical statistics at the University of Bern, Bern, Switzerland, and Peter Jüni, MD, senior lecturer in clinical epidemiology at the University of Bern, received a complete copy of the raw data from Cordis Corporation and performed an independent statistical analysis. They received no compensation for this work and had no conflicts of interest, not receiving any type of payment, equity, or reimbursement from either of the companies manufacturing the stents compared in the trial. They confirmed that they were able to replicate the analyses of the primary angiographic and secondary clinical outcomes reported in the manuscript and that they consider the analyses to be appropriate.

Independent Statistical Analysis: All study data were transferred from Hoffman–La Roche to the Department of Statistics at the British Columbia Children's Hospital for independent reanalysis. Statistical reanalyses of the raw data were performed by Ruth Milner and Victor M. Espinosa, MSc. There were only minor discrepancies between the reanalysis and the original interpretation of the results and conclusions. When there was a discrepancy, Dr Chanoine included the results from the reanalyses performed at the British Columbia Children's Hospital.

2.10.11 Disclaimer. A footnote of disclaimer is used to separate the views of the authors from those of employers, funding agencies, organizations, or others. Editors should generally retain the author's phrasing, especially if such phrasing is required by policy of the entity mentioned.

Disclaimer: The views expressed herein are those of the authors and do not necessarily reflect the views of the US Army or the Department of Defense.

Disclaimer: The opinions expressed herein are only those of the authors. They do not represent the official views of the government of India, St Michael's Hospital, University of Toronto, or the study sponsors.

Disclaimer: Use of trade names or names of commercial sources is for information only and does not imply endorsement by the US Public Health Service or the US Department of Health and Human Services.

Disclaimer: Opinions in this article should not be interpreted as the official position of the International Committee of the Red Cross.

Disclaimer: The opinions expressed herein are those of the authors and do not necessarily reflect the views of the Indian Health Service.

If the byline of a manuscript includes the editor of the journal, a member of the editorial board of the journal, or a member of the editorial staff of the publication, the following type of disclaimer is useful.

Byline: Mehmet K. Aktas, MD; Volkan Ozduran, MD; Claire E. Pothier, MPH; Richard Lang, MD, MPH; Michael S. Lauer, MD

Disclaimer: Dr Lauer, a *JAMA* contributing editor, was not involved in the editorial evaluation or decision to publish this article.

2.10.12 Previous Presentations. The following formats are used for material that has been read or exhibited at a professional meeting. The original spelling and capitalization of the meeting name should be retained. Provide the exact date and location of the meeting.

Previous Presentation: The results of this study were presented at the British Association of Dermatologists Annual Meeting; July 8, 2004; Glasgow, Scotland.

Previous Presentation: This study was presented in part at the European Congress of Epidemiology; September 10, 2004; Porto, Portugal.

Previous Presentations: This study was presented in part at the American Society of Nephrology 35th Annual Meeting; November 1-4, 2002; Philadelphia, Pennsylvania; and at the American Transplant Congress; May 13-19, 2004; Boston, Massachusetts.

2.10.13 Additional Information (Miscellaneous Acknowledgments). Occasionally, other types of announcements are listed in the Acknowledgment section. However, permission or credit for reproduction of a figure or a table, even if modified, should be given in the figure legend or the table footnote, not in the Acknowledgment section. See 4.0, Visual Presentation of Data. Notice of supplemental Web-only material may also be given under this sidehead, as well as in the text.

Additional Information: This is report 54 in a series on chronic disease in former college students.

Additional Information: This article has been reviewed by the Publications Committee of the Collaborative Study of Depression and has its endorsement.

Additional Information: This article is dedicated to the memory of my mentor, friend, and father, Clifford C. Lardinois Sr, MD.

Additional Information: A complete list of documents surveyed is available on request from the author.

Additional Information: The original data set is available from the New York State Department of Health, Albany.

Additional Information: The *P sojae* and *P ramorum* whole-genome shotgun projects have been deposited at DDBJ/EMBL/Genbank under the project accessions AAQY00000000 and AAQX00000000, respectively.

Additional Information: These documents are also available online (http://www.library.ucsf.edu/tobacco).

Additional Information: Additional studies are available from the UK Cochrane Centre, NHS R&D Programme, Summertown Pavillion, Middleway, Oxford OX2 7LG, England (ichalmers@cochrane.co.uk).

Additional Information: eTables 1 and 2 are available at http://www.jama.com.

Additional Information: The eFigure is available at http://www.archinternmed.com.

Additional Information: This article is the first of a 3-part series. The second part will appear next month.

2.10.14 Additional Contributions. Acknowledgment of other contributions and forms of assistance (eg, statistical review, preparation of the report, performance of special tests or research, editorial or writing assistance, or clerical assistance) also should be included. When individuals are named, their given names and highest academic degrees (see 2.2.3, Bylines and End-of-Text Signatures, Degrees) are listed, and some publications, such as *JAMA,* also list their affiliations, if appropriate, and whether they received compensation for their assistance. For any individual named as providing additional contributions, the author should obtain written permission from that person indicating his or her authorization to be so named (see 5.2.1, Ethical and Legal Considerations, Acknowledgments, Acknowledging Support, Assistance, and Contributions of Those Who Are Not Authors, and 5.2.8, Acknowledgments, Permission to Name Individuals).

Additional Contributions: Robert C. Della Rocca, MD, performed the biopsy, contributed the orbital computed tomographic scan, and provided the exenteration specimen; Ramon Font, MD, confirmed the histopathologic diagnosis.

Additional Contributions: John Hewett, PhD, and Jane Johnson, MA, provided statistical support.

Additional Contributions: The photographs that constitute Figure 1 were provided by Hans-Peter M. Freihofer, MD, Department of Maxillofacial Surgery, University Hospital of Nijmegen, Nijmegen, the Netherlands.

Additional Contributions: The Branch Retinal Vein Occlusion Study Group is grateful for the contributions of the many referring ophthalmologists, without whom this study could not have been carried out, and to the study patients, whose faithfulness to the study led to conclusions that promise hope for others with branch vein occlusion.

JAMA and some of the *Archives* Journals require authors to disclose any substantial writing and editing assistance and to recognize those persons responsible for such assistance. (*JAMA* also notes whether compensation was received for such assistance.) This information should be included in the Acknowledgment section, and permission to be identified should be obtained from all named individuals (see 5.2.1, Ethical and Legal Considerations, Acknowledgments, Acknowledging Support, Assistance, and Contributions of Those Who Are Not Authors). In such cases, institutional affiliations may be included:

Additional Contributions: William Wise, PhD, Dynapharm Inc, contributed to the writing of this article; and Sarah Jewel, MA, Medical Writers Corp, helped edit the initial manuscript.

Additional Contributions: Cheryl Christensen assisted with manuscript preparation and Stephen Ordway, ELS, provided editorial assistance.

Additional Contributions: We thank Petra Macaskill, PhD (School of Public Health, Sydney, Australia), for her comments on an earlier draft and suggestions for its improvement. Dr Macaskill did not receive any compensation.

Additional Contributions: Lucia Taddio, BA, Erwin Darra, and Omar Parvez (all from The Hospital for Sick Children) provided assistance with data collection. Ms Taddio and Mr Darra received compensation from the study sponsor.

Additional Contributions: We thank Charlotte Gerczak, MLA, for her editorial input and Keita Ebisu, MS, for his aid in collecting the particulate matter data. Neither Ms Gerczak nor Mr Ebisu received any financial compensation for their work.

2.10.15 **Preferred Citation Format.** Some journals may choose to list a preferred citation format for articles to ensure correct citation. Some may use this only for references for which citation problems or questions are likely to arise (eg, manuscripts with group authors). Although this is not used for any articles published in *JAMA* and the *Archives* Journals, the format is suggested below. (See also 2.2.1, Bylines and End-of-Text Signatures, Authors' Names, and 2.2.4, Bylines and End-of-Text Signatures, Multiple Authors, Group Authors.)

Preferred Citation Format: Gould PA, Krahn AD; for the Canadian Heart Rhythm Society Working Group on Device Advisors. Complications associated with implantable cardioverter-defibrillator replacement in response to device advisories. *JAMA*. 2006;295(16):1907-1911.

2.11 Appendixes.

Appendixes. Some journals publish appendixes, at least occasionally, for material that might be considered ancillary to the content of the article itself (eg, derivation of a complex formula used in the article, a survey instrument used in a study, statistical modeling details). *JAMA* and the *Archives* Journals generally do not use appendixes. If these are worthy of publication because they contain important information, they could be considered for online-only publication (see 2.12, Online-Only [Supplementary] Material). On rare occasions, however, they serve a useful purpose for data that cannot easily be presented as a table or a figure and are too central to the article to be deposited elsewhere. In these cases, appendixes are cited in the text as a table or figure would be cited (eg, Appendix 1) and are usually placed at the end of the article, before the references. If the appendix cites references, the references would be numbered consecutively, following the last reference number in the text, and included in the article's reference list.

Information contained in appendixes is published under the imprimatur of the journal and therefore should undergo editorial evaluation and peer review and should receive the same attention to detail in the editorial and production processes as the main body of the article.

2.12 Online-Only (Supplementary) Material.

Online-Only (Supplementary) Material. Publishing online-only material permits inclusion of audio and video components. In addition, to conserve use of budgeted

Table. Manuscript Checklist Adapted From *JAMA*'s Instructions for Authors

☐ **1.** Review manuscript submission instructions on our Web-based submission and review system (http://manuscripts.jama.com).

☐ **2.** Include a cover letter as an attachment.

☐ **3.** Designate a corresponding author and provide a complete postal/mail address, telephone and fax numbers, and e-mail address.

☐ **4.** Provide first and last names, degrees, e-mail addresses, and institutional affiliations for any coauthors.

☐ **5.** On the title page, include a word count for text only, exclusive of title, abstract, references, tables, and figure legends.

☐ **6.** Provide an abstract that conforms to the required abstract format.

☐ **7.** Double-space manuscript and leave right margins unjustified (ragged).

☐ **8.** Check all references for accuracy and completeness. Put references in proper format in numerical order, making sure each is cited in sequence in the text.

☐ **9.** Include a title for each table and figure (a brief, succinct phrase, preferably no longer than 10-15 words) and explanatory legend as needed.

☐ **10.** Have each author read, complete, and sign the Authorship Form with statements of authorship responsibility, criteria, and contributions; financial disclosure; and copyright transfer. After submission, add the manuscript number to the top of each author form and send in the author forms by mail or fax to the editorial office.

☐ **11.** Indicate specific contributions from each author (see authorship checklist on Authorship Form).

☐ **12.** Include statement signed by corresponding author that written permission has been obtained from all persons named in the Acknowledgment.

☐ **13.** For reports of original data, include statement from at least 1 author that she or he "had full access to all of the data in the study and takes responsibility for the integrity of the data and the accuracy of the data analysis."

☐ **14.** Include research or project support/funding in the Acknowledgment.

☐ **15.** Also in the Acknowledgment, specify the role of the funder(s) or sponsor(s) in each of the following: design and conduct of the study; collection, management, analysis, and interpretation of the data; and preparation, review, or approval of the manuscript.

☐ **16.** Include written permission from each individual identified as a source for personal communication or unpublished data.

☐ **17.** If appropriate, include information on institutional review board/ethics committee approval or waiver and informed consent.

☐ **18.** Reprinted tables and figures are discouraged. Original material should be provided, except under extraordinary circumstances.

☐ **19.** Include informed consent forms for identifiable patient descriptions, photographs, videos, and pedigrees.

☐ **20.** For clinical trials, add the clinical trial identification number and the URL of the registration site.

print pages and yet allow interested readers access to supplementary material (eg, additional tables, figures, or references, derivation of complex equations, appendixes, detailed description of methods, large amounts of relevant but detailed data), some journals may publish Web-only material to supplement the material that appears in print. In the print article, such items should be called out by eTable 1, etc, and a note to indicate how to access this supplementary material should be published:

Additional Information: The eTable is available at http://archderm.ama-assn.org/cgi/content/full/141/12/1591/DCM50003ET1.

Additional Information: A computer simulation of a 3-year-old child falling down the stairs is available at http://archpedia.ama-assn.org/cgi/content/full/155/9/1008.

Additional Information: Supporting online material, including the "Methods" section, the references, and Figures S1 through S6, is available at http://sciencemag.org/cgi/content/full/1122771/DC1.

Whenever possible, the exact URL of the supplementary material should be provided to help the reader more easily find the content. The Web version of the article links directly to the online supplementary material.

Alternatively, such additional material may be made available at the author's Web site; however, because URLs change frequently, the first option is preferable.

It is the policy of *JAMA* and the *Archives* Journals that online-only material is published under the imprimatur of the journal and so should undergo editorial evaluation and should receive the same attention to detail in the editorial and production processes as if it were to be published in the print journal.

ACKNOWLEDGMENT

Principal author: Cheryl Iverson, MA

REFERENCES

1. *JAMA* instructions for authors. http://jama.ama-assn.org/ifora_current.dtl. Accessed December 29, 2005.
2. International Committee of Medical Journal Editors. Uniform Requirements for Manuscripts Submitted to Biomedical Journals: Writing and Editing for Biomedical Publication. http://www.icmje.org. Updated February 2006. Accessed June 15, 2006.
3. Sun X-L, Zhou J. English versions of Chinese authors' names in biomedical journals: observations and recommendations. *Sci Editor.* 2002;25(1):3-4.
4. Black B. Indexing the names of authors from Spanish- and Portuguese-speaking countries. *Sci Editor.* 2003;26(4):118-121.
5. *The Chicago Manual of Style: The Essential Guide for Writers, Editors, and Publishers.* 15th ed. Chicago, IL: University of Chicago Press; 2003:778-782.
6. National Library of Medicine. *List of Journals Indexed for MEDLINE.* Bethesda, MD: National Library of Medicine; 2005.
7. Pitkin RM, Branagan MA. Can the accuracy of abstracts be improved by providing specific instructions? a randomized controlled trial. *JAMA.* 1998;280(3):267-269.
8. Haynes RB, Mulrow CD, Huth EJ, Altman DG, Gardner MJ. More informative abstracts revisited. *Ann Intern Med.* 1990;113(1):69-76.
9. MeSH home page. http://www.nlm.nih.gov/mesh/meshhome.html. Accessed March 20, 2006.
10. Fontanarosa PB, Flanagin A, DeAngelis CD. Reporting conflicts of interest, financial aspects of research, and role of sponsors in funded studies. *JAMA.* 2005;294(1):110-111.

3 References

References serve 3 primary purposes—documentation, acknowledgment, and directing or linking the reader to additional resources. Authors may cite a reference to support their own arguments or lay the foundation for their theses (documentation); as a credit to the work of other authors (acknowledgment); or to direct the reader to more detail or additional resources (directing or linking).

References are a critical element of a manuscript and, as such, the reference list demands close scrutiny by authors, editors, peer reviewers, manuscript editors, and proofreaders. Authors bear primary responsibility for all reference citations. Editors and peer reviewers should examine manuscript references for completeness, accuracy, and relevance. Manuscript editors and proofreaders are responsible for assessing the completeness of references, for ensuring that references are presented in proper style and format, and for checking to make sure that any reference links are accurate and functional.

Much has been written about problems with bibliographic inaccuracies[1] (eg, an author's name is misspelled; the journal name is incorrect; the year of publication or the volume, issue, or page numbers are incorrect). Such errors make it difficult to retrieve the documents cited. An even more serious problem is inappropriate citation (eg, a speculative commentary is cited in a way that implies proved causality; an article's results are generalized beyond what the data support). Not only is accuracy critical for the integrity of the individual document, but because authors may sometimes rely on secondary rather than primary sources, an inaccurate citation in a document's reference list may be replicated in subsequent articles whose authors do not consult the primary source. Authors should always consult the primary source and should never cite a reference that they themselves have not read.[2-4] (See also 3.11.9, Abstracts and Other Material Taken From Another Source, and 3.13.10, Secondary Citations and Quotations [Including Press Releases].)

3.1 **Reference Style and the Uniform Requirements.** For greater uniformity in "technical requirements for manuscripts submitted to their journals," the International Committee of Medical Journal Editors, meeting in 1978 in Vancouver, British Columbia, Canada, developed the Uniform Requirements for Manuscripts Submitted to Biomedical Journals.[5] Suggested formats for bibliographic style, developed for uniformity by the US National Library of Medicine (NLM), are included in that document, which has been revised and updated several times. Editors of approximately 500 journals have agreed to receive manuscripts prepared in accordance with this uniform style. Although Uniform Requirements is intended to aid authors in the preparation of their manuscripts for publication, not to dictate publication style to journal editors, many journals have used them for developing their publication style.[5] Formatting of references that adhere exactly to the Uniform Requirements will be acceptable without challenge in manuscripts submitted to *JAMA* and the *Archives* Journals, and any necessary formatting changes will be made by the *JAMA* and *Archives* manuscript editors.

The reference style followed by *JAMA* and the *Archives* Journals is also based on recommendations of the NLM described in the *National Library of Medicine Recommended Formats for Bibliographic Citation* (hereinafter referred to as *NLM Recommended Formats*).[6] Both the Uniform Requirements and *JAMA/Archives* style represent modifications of the NLM style but follow the general principles outlined in the NLM document. Whatever reference style is followed, consistency throughout the document and throughout the publication (journal, book, Web site) is critical.

Each reference is divided with periods into bibliographic groups. (See 3.4, Minimum Acceptable Data for References, for an illustration of these for the principal types of references.) The period serves as a field delimiter, making each bibliographic group distinct and establishing a sequence of bibliographic elements in a reference. Bibliographic elements are the items within a bibliographic group. Bibliographic elements may be separated by the following punctuation marks:

- A comma: if the items are subelements of a bibliographic element or a set of closely related elements (eg, the authors' names in the reference list)
- A semicolon: if the elements in the bibliographic group are different (eg, between the publisher's name and the copyright year) or if there are multiple occurrences of logically related elements within a group; also, before volume identification data
- A colon: before the publisher's name, between the title and the subtitle, and after a connective phrase (eg, "In," "Presented at")

3.2 **Reference List.** Reference to information that is retrievable is appropriately made in the reference list. This includes but is not limited to articles published or accepted for publication in scholarly or mass-circulation print or electronic journals, magazines, or newspapers; books that have been published or accepted for publication; papers presented at professional meetings; abstracts; theses; CD-ROMs, films, videotapes, and audiofiles; package inserts or a manufacturer's documentation; monographs; official reports; databases and Web sites; legal cases; patents; and news releases.

References should be listed in numerical order at the end of the manuscript (except as specified in 3.3, References Given in Text, and 3.5, Numbering). Two references should not be combined under a single reference number.

References to material not yet accepted for publication or to personal communications (oral, written, and electronic) are not acceptable as listed references and instead should be included parenthetically in the text (see 3.3, References Given in Text; 3.15, Electronic References; and 3.13.8, Special Print Materials, Unpublished Material).

3.3 **References Given in Text.** Parenthetical citation in the text of references that meet the criteria for inclusion in a reference list should be restricted to circumstances in which reference lists would not be used, such as news articles or obituaries. Note that in the text (1) the author(s) may not be named, (2) the title may not be given, (3) the name of the journal is abbreviated only when enclosed in parentheses, and (4) inclusive page numbers are given. Some resources, such as Web URLs, may be listed in the text when it is the Web site itself that is referred to rather than content on the site.

> Wiese et al recently reported that an extract from the fruit of the prickly pear cactus had a moderate effect on reducing the symptoms of the alcohol hangover (*Arch Intern Med*. 2004;164[12]:1334-1340).
>
> The effect of an extract from the fruit of the prickly pear cactus on reducing the symptoms of the alcohol hangover was reported in a recent issue of *Archives of Internal Medicine* (2004;164[12]:1334-1340).
>
> The *Archives of Internal Medicine* article (2004;164[12]:1334-1340) on the effects of an extract of the fruit of the prickly pear cactus on reducing

symptoms of the alcohol hangover received widespread publicity (eg, *USA Today*. June 29, 2004:7D).

Physicians may wish to consult the NIH Clinical Trials Registry (http://clinicaltrials.gov).

3.4 Minimum Acceptable Data for References. To be acceptable, a reference to journals or books or Web sites must include certain minimum data. The information varies slightly for journals and books online and journals and books in print. For all of these forms, please consult the specific section in this chapter devoted to that form for more complete requirements. The summary below represents only a skeleton for quick reference.

Journals:

Print: Author(s). Article title. *Journal Name.* Year;vol(issue No.): inclusive pages.

Online: Authors(s). Article title. *Journal Name.* Year;vol(issue No.): inclusive pages. URL. Accessed [date].

Books:

Print: Author(s). *Book Title.* Edition number (if it is the second edition or above). City, State (or Country) of publisher: Publisher's name; copyright year.

Online: Author(s). *Book Title.* Edition number (if it is the second edition or above). City, State (or Country) of publisher: Publisher's name; copyright year. URL. Accessed [date].

Web Site: Author (or, if no author is available, the name of the organization responsible for the site). Title (or, if no title is available, the name of the organization responsible for the site). Name of the Web site. URL. Accessed [date].

Enough information to identify and retrieve the material should be provided. More complete data (see 3.11.1, References to Print Journals, Complete Data; 3.12.1, References to Print Books, Complete Data; 3.15, Electronic References; and 3.13.8, Special Print Materials, Unpublished Material) should be used when available.

3.5 Numbering. References should be numbered consecutively with arabic numerals in the order in which they are cited in the text. Unnumbered references, in the form of a resource or reading list, are rarely used in *JAMA* and the *Archives* Journals. When they are used, these references appear alphabetically, by the first author's last name, in a list separate from the specifically cited reference list.

3.6 Citation. Each reference should be cited in the text, tables, or figures in consecutive numerical order by means of superscript arabic numerals. It is acceptable for a reference to be cited only in a table or a figure legend and not in the text if it is in sequence with references cited in the text. For example, if Table 2 contains reference 13, which does not appear in the text, this is acceptable as long as the last reference cited (for the first time) before the first text citation of Table 2 is reference 12.

Use arabic superscript numerals *outside* periods and commas, *inside* colons and semicolons. When more than 2 references are cited at a given place in the manuscript, use hyphens to join the first and last numbers of a closed series; use commas without space to separate other parts of a multiple citation.

As reported previously,[1,3-8,19]

The derived data were as follows[3,4]:

Avoid placing a superscript reference citation immediately after a number or an abbreviated unit of measure to avoid any confusion between the superscript reference citation and an exponent.

Avoid: The 2 largest studies to date included 26[2] and 18[3] patients.

Better: The 2 largest studies to date included 26 patients[2] and 18 patients.[3]

Avoid: The largest lesion found in the first study was 10 cm.[2]

Better: The largest lesion found in the first study[2] was 10 cm.

When a multiple citation involves sufficient superscript characters to create the appearance of a "hole" in the print copy (20-25 characters, including spaces and punctuation, depending on the column width and type size), use an asterisk in the text and give the citation in a footnote at the bottom of the page (Figure).

generate information based on arriving data and trigger the action of the informed person without a preceding specific request. Passive systems require the user to recognize when advice would be useful and to make an explicit effort to start processing.[116] The following successful information interventions were analyzed:

- The provider prompt/reminder intervention was typically used to improve the provision of preventive care services through computer-generated reminders to physicians. For example, patients of physicians who received reminders on the encounter forms were significantly more likely to have a mammogram ordered.[30] Procedures frequently targeted by the provider prompt/reminder trials included cancer screening (stool occult blood,[19,40,57,64,66,90] sigmoidoscopy,[40,64] rectal examination,[19,40,64,93] mammography,[30,40,57,63,66,90,93] breast examination,[18,19,40,64,93] Papanicolaou test,* and pelvic examination[18,40,64]) and vaccinations (influenza,[29,57,62] pneumococcal,[57,90] tetanus,[66,93] and infant[86] immunizations).
- The patient prompt/reminder intervention encouraged the action of patients through the use of telephone[24,59,61,62] or mail† reminders. The main function of the computer system was usually to identify patients and trigger the use of a particular clinical procedure. For example, in a trial testing the effect of reminders on influenza vaccination, patient reminder letters led to a significant (35.1%) improvement.[59] Most trials of patient prompt/reminders focused on cancer screening compliance rates (stool occult blood,[40,64,66] sigmoidoscopy,[40,64] rectal examination,[40,64] mammography,[40,64,66] breast examination,[40,64] Papanicolaou

**References 18, 19, 40, 57, 61, 64, 74, 90, 93.*
†References 40, 59, 61, 62, 64, 66, 86, 107.

Figure. For references that occupy more than 23 characters and spaces, bottom-of-page footnotes are used. This example shows 2 such footnotes within a single column.

Note: (1) Reference numerals in such a footnote are set full size and on the line rather than as superscripts. (2) The spacing is different from that in superscript reference citations. (3) If 2 or more such bottom-of-the-page footnotes appear in a single article, use an asterisk for the first footnote, a dagger for the second such footnote, a double dagger for the third. *Note:* This is less relevant for the Web.

As reported previously,*

**References 3, 5, 7, 9, 11, 13, 21, 24-29, 31.*

Note: In tables, if a cell in the table involves citation of a reference number *and* a footnote symbol, give the reference number first, followed by a comma and the footnote symbol (eg, [3,a]) (see 4.1.3, Visual Presentation of Data, Tables, Table Components).

If the author wishes to cite different page numbers from a single reference source at different places in the text, the page numbers are included in the superscript citation and the source appears only once in the list of references. Note that the superscript may include more than 1 page number, citation of more than 1 reference, or both, and that all spaces are closed up.

These patients showed no sign of protective sphincteric adduction.[3(p21),9]

Westman[5(pp3,5),9] reported 8 cases in which vomiting occurred.

In listed references, do not use *ibid* or *op cit.*

3.7 **Authors.** Use the author's surname followed by initials without periods. In listed references, the names of all authors should be given unless there are more than 6, in which case the names of the first 3 authors are used, followed by "et al." *Note:* The NLM guidelines do not limit the number of authors listed but, for space considerations, we have elected to depart from the NLM guidelines on this point.

Note spacing and punctuation. Do not use *and* between names. Roman numerals and abbreviations for Junior (Jr) and Senior (Sr) follow author's initials. *Note:* Although NLM uses "2nd," "3rd," and "4th," *JAMA* and the *Archives* Journals prefer II, III, and IV, unless the author prefers arabic numerals.

Also, although *JAMA* and the *Archives* Journals, in bylines, make a distinction between a group of individuals writing *for* a group and a group of individuals writing *as* a group or *in addition to* (ie, *and*) a group (see 5.1.7, Legal and Ethical Considerations, Authorship Responsibility, Group and Collaborative Authorship), this distinction is not retained in the NLM database and hence in MEDLINE. If authors, in their reference lists, provide this information, the *for* or *and* will be retained, but if this information is not provided, the reference will use the individuals named and the group name, without *for* or *and.* Both styles are illustrated in the examples below. Note that the group name is preceded by a semicolon rather than a comma (to show, as noted in 3.1, Reference Style and the Uniform Requirements, that the information that follows is related to what precedes it but somehow distinct) and that articles (eg, *the*) in the group name are removed.

1 author:	Doe JF.
2 authors:	Doe JF, Roe JP III.

6 authors:	Doe JF, Roe JP III, Coe RT Jr, Loe JT Sr, Poe EA, van Voe AE.
>6 authors:	Doe JF, Roe JP III, Coe RT Jr, et al.
1 author *for* or *and* a group:	Doe JF; Laser ROP Study Group. *or* Doe JF; for Laser ROP Study Group. *or* Doe JF; and Laser ROP Study Group.
>6 authors *for* or *and* a group	Doe JF, Roe JP III, Coe RT Jr, et al; Laser ROP Study Group. *or* Doe JF, Roe JP III, Coe RT Jr, et al; for Laser ROP Study Group. *or* Doe JF, Roe JP III, Coe RT Jr, et al; and Laser ROP Study Group.

When mentioned in the text, only surnames of authors are used. For a 2-author reference, list both surnames; for references with more than 2 authors or authors and a group, include the first author's surname followed by "et al," "and associates," or "and colleagues."

> Doe[7] reported on the survey.
>
> Doe and Roe[8] reported on the survey.
>
> Doe et al[9] reported on the survey.

Note: Do not use the possessive form *et al*'s; rephrase the sentence.

> The data of Doe et al[9] support our findings.

In material that is less clinical (eg, book reviews, historical features, letters to the editor), the author's first name or honorific may be used at first mention:

> We agree with Dr Tayeb that the prevalence of domestic violence is difficult to determine.
>
> In *Growing Up Fast,* Joanna Lipper profiles 6 teenaged mothers living in Pittsfield, Massachusetts, at the turn of the 21st century.

3.8 Prefixes and Particles. Surnames that contain prefixes or particles (eg, von, de, La, van) are spelled and capitalized according to the preference of the persons named.

1. van Gylswyk NO, Roche CI.
2. Van Rosevelt RF, Bakker JC, Sinclair DM, Damen J, Van Mourik JA.
3. Al-Faquih SR.
4. Kang S, Kim KJ, Wong T-Y, et al.

3.9 Titles.

Titles. In titles of articles, books, parts of books, and other material, retain the spelling, abbreviations, and style for numbers used in the original. *Note:* Numbers that begin a title are spelled out (although exceptions are made for years; see 2.1.2, Manuscript Preparation, Titles and Subtitles, Numbers).

3.9.1 English-Language Titles

Journal Articles and Parts of Books. In English-language titles, capitalize only (1) the first letter of the first word, (2) proper names, and (3) abbreviations that are ordinarily capitalized (eg, DNA, EEG, VDRL). Do not enclose article and book chapter titles in quotation marks. However, if a book, book chapter, or article title contains quotation marks in the original, retain them as double quotation marks (unless both double and single quotation marks are used).

Books, Government Bulletins, Documents, and Pamphlets. In English-language titles, italicize the titles of books, government bulletins, documents, and pamphlets and capitalize the first letter of each major word. Do not capitalize articles, prepositions of 3 or fewer letters, coordinating conjunctions *(and, or, for, nor, but, yet)*, or the *to* in infinitives (see 2.1.6, Manuscript Preparation, Titles and Subtitles, Capitalization, for exceptions). *Do* capitalize a 2-letter verb, such as *Is*.

3.9.2 Non–English-Language Titles

Capitalization. In non–English-language titles, capitalization does not necessarily follow the same rules as in English-language titles. For example, in German titles (both articles and books), all nouns and only nouns are capitalized; typically, in French, Spanish, and Italian book titles, capitalize only the first word, proper names, and abbreviations that are capitalized in English. As with English-language books, government bulletins, documents, and pamphlets, italicize the title.

Translation. Non–English-language titles may be given as they originally appeared, without translation:

1. Richartz E, Schott KJ, Wormstall H. Psychopharmakotherapie bei Demenzerkrankungen. *Dtsch Med Wochenschr.* 2004;129(25/26):1434-1440.
2. Ohayon MM. Prevalencia y factores de riesgo de cefaleas matinales en la población general. *Arch Intern Med Ed Espanol.* 2004;1(1):41-47. Originally published, in English, in: *Arch Intern Med.* 2004;164(1):97-102.

If non–English-language titles are translated into English, bracketed indication of the original language should follow the title:

3. Miyazaki K, Murakami A, Imamura S, et al. A case of fundus albipunctatus with a retinol dehydrogenase 5 gene mutation in a child [in Japanese]. *Nippon Ganka Gakkai Zasshi.* 2001;105(8):530-534.

If both the non–English-language title and the translation are provided, both may be given, as shown below, with the non–English-language title given first, followed by the English translation, in brackets:

4. Camici M. Cancro prostático e screening con test PSA [Prostate cancer and prostate-specific antigen screening]. *Minerva Med.* 2004;95(1):25-34.

Non–English-language titles should be verified from the original when possible. Consult a dictionary in the appropriate language for accent marks, spelling, and other particulars.

Reference to the primary source is always preferable, but if the non–English-language article is not readily available or not accessible, the translated version is acceptable. The citation should always be to the version consulted.

Such words as *tome* (volume), *fascicolo* (part), *Seite* (page), *Teil* (part), *Auflage* (edition), *Abteilung* (section or part), *Band* (volume), *Heft* (number), *Beiheft* (supplement), and *Lieferung* (part or number) should be translated into English.

3.9.3 **Names of Organisms.** In all titles, follow the style recommended for capitalization and use of italics in scientific names of organisms (see 10.3.6, Capitalization, Proper Nouns, Organisms, and 15.14, Nomenclature, Organisms and Pathogens). Use roman type for genus and species names in book titles.

3.9.4 **Non-English Words and Phrases.** In all titles, follow the guidelines recommended for use of italics or roman in non-English words and phrases (see 12.1.1, Non-English Words, Phrases, and Accent Marks, Non-English Words, Phrases, and Titles, Use of Italics). For example, even if *In Vivo* or *In Vitro* were set italic in a cited title, *JAMA* and the *Archives* Journals would set these in roman type.

3.10 **Subtitles.** Style for subtitles follows that for titles (see 3.9, Titles) for spelling, abbreviations, numbers, capitalization, and use of italics, except that for journal articles the subtitle begins with a lowercase letter. A colon and space separate title and subtitle, even if a period was used in the original. Do not change an em dash to a colon. If the subtitle is numbered, as is common when articles in a series have the same title but different—numbered—subtitles, use a comma after the title, followed by a roman numeral immediately preceding the colon.

1. Klein R, Klein BEK, Moss SE, et al. The relation of retinal vessel caliber to the incidence and progression of diabetic retinopathy, XIX: the Wisconsin Epidemiologic Study of Diabetic Retinopathy. *Arch Ophthalmol.* 2004;122(1):76-83.

3.11 References to Print Journals

3.11.1 **Complete Data.** A complete print journal reference includes the following:

- Authors' surnames and initials
- Title of article and subtitle, if any
- Abbreviated name of journal
- Year
- Volume number
- Issue number

- Part or supplement number, when pertinent
- Inclusive page numbers

3.11.2 **Names of Journals.** Abbreviate and italicize names of journals. Use initial capital letters. Abbreviate according to the listing in the PubMed Journals database (see also 14.10, Abbreviations, Names of Journals). Include parenthetical designation of a city if it is included in the PubMed abbreviation, for example, *Medicine (Baltimore), Ann Urol (Paris).* Information enclosed in brackets should be retained without brackets, eg, *J Comp Physiol A* for *J Comp Physiol [A].*

If the name of a journal has changed since the time the reference was published, use the name of the journal at the time of publication. For example, the journal formerly called *Transactions of the Ophthalmological Societies of the United Kingdom* is now called *Eye.* If a citation was from the older-named journal, do not change the journal name to *Eye*; use the former title: *Trans Ophthalmol Soc U K.* When the name has not changed but the abbreviation used by PubMed has changed (eg, *Br Med J* to *BMJ*), use the abbreviation in use by PubMed at the time the reference was published (so, *Br Med J* through 1987; *BMJ* from 1988 forward). This policy will ensure that the online links to the citation will work.

3.11.3 **Page Numbers and Dates.** Do not omit digits from inclusive page numbers. The year, followed by a semicolon; the volume number and the issue number (in parentheses), followed by a colon; the initial page number, a hyphen, and the final page number, followed by a period, are set without spaces.

1. Rainier S, Thomas D, Tokarz D, et al. Myofibrillogenesis regulator 1 gene mutations cause paroxysmal dystonic choreoathetosis. *Arch Neurol.* 2004; 61(7):1025-1029.
2. Hyduk A, Croft JB, Ayala C, Zheng K, Zheng Z-J, Mensah GA. Pulmonary hypertension surveillance—United States, 1980-2002. *MMWR Surveill Summ.* 2005;54(5):1-28.

3.11.4 **Discontinuous Pagination.** For an article with discontinuous pagination, in one issue, follow the style shown in the example below:

1. Herr KA, Garand L. Assessment and measurement of pain in older adults. *Clin Geriatr Med.* 2001;17:457-478, vi.

3.11.5 **Journals Without Volume or Issue Numbers.** In references to journals that have no volume or issue numbers, use the issue date, as shown in example 1 below. If there is an issue number but no volume number, use the style shown in example 2 below.

1. Flyvholm MA, Susitaival P, Meding B, et al. Nordic occupational skin questionnaire—NOSQ-2002: Nordic questionnaire for surveying work-related skin diseases on hands and forearms and relevant exposure. *Tema-Nord.* April 2002:518.
2. Keppel K, Pamuk E, Lynch J, et al. Methodologic issues in measuring health disparities. *Vital Health Stat 2.* 2005;(141):1-16.

3.11.6 **Parts of an Issue.** If an issue has 2 or more parts, the part cited should be indicated in accordance with the following example:

1. McCormick MC, Kass B, Elixhauser A, Thompson J, Simpson L. Annual report on access to and utilization of health care for children and youth in the United States: 1999. *Pediatrics*. 2000;105(1, pt 3):219-230.

3.11.7 **Special or Theme Issue.** The *NLM Recommended Formats*[6] defines a special or theme issue as follows: "Special issues are frequently published to present the papers from conferences. . . . They may also be published to commemorate a specific event or to bring together papers on a specific subject." *JAMA* and the *Archives* Journals refer to these as *theme issues*. References to the complete contents of a special or theme issue of a journal should be cited as follows:

1. Flanagin A, Winker MA, eds. Global health. *JAMA*. 2004;291(21, theme issue):2511-2664.
2. Blodi BA, Ferris FL III, guest eds. Blindness. *Arch Ophthalmol*. 2004;122(4, theme issue):437-676.

Special or theme issues may also be published as supplements (see 3.11.8, Supplements, for the recommended style for these).

3.11.8 **Supplements.** The following example illustrates the basic format:

1. Body JJ, Greipp P, Coleman RE, et al. A phase I study of AMGN-0007, a recombinant osteoprotegerin construct, in patients with multiple myeloma or breast carcinoma related metastases. *Cancer*. 2003;97(3)(suppl):887-892.

If the supplement is numbered, and there is no issue number, use the following form:

2. McDougle CJ, Stigler KA, Posey DJ. Treatment of aggression in children and adolescents with autism and conduct disorder. *J Clin Psychiatry*. 2003; 64(suppl 4):16-25.

If the supplement is numbered, and there is an issue number, use the form below:

3. Crino L, Cappuzzo F. Present and future treatment of advanced non–small-cell lung cancer. *Semin Oncol*. 2002;29(3)(suppl 9):9-16.

When numbered supplements have several parts, denoted by "pt 1" or by letters, each supplement having independent pagination, use the following form:

4. Rosenwasser LJ. Treatment of allergic rhinitis. *Am J Med*. 2002;113(suppl 9A):17S-24S.

Note: It is common for page numbers in supplements to include letters as well as numbers (eg, 17S-24S in example 4 above). Also, example 4 has no issue number.

3.11.9 **Abstracts and Other Material Taken From Another Source.** Several types of published abstracts may be cited: (1) an abstract of a complete article taken from another publication, as in the Abstracts section of *JAMA*, (2) a rewritten abstract of a published article with an appended commentary, and (3) an abstract published in the society proceedings of a journal. (For examples of abstracts presented at meetings, published or unpublished, see 3.13.3, Special Print Materials, Serial Publications, and 3.13.8, Special Print Materials, Unpublished Material.)

Ideally, reference to any of these types of abstracts should be permitted only when the original article is not readily available (eg, non–English-language articles or papers presented at meetings but not yet published). If an abstract is published in the society proceedings section of a journal, the name of the society before which the paper was read need not be included, but see example 3 below if this information is included.

1. Abstract of a complete article taken from another publication:

    1. Elner VM, Hassan AS, Frueh BR. Graded full-thickness anterior blepharotomy for upper eyelid retraction [abstract taken from *Arch Ophthalmol.* 2004;122(1):55-60]. *Arch Facial Plast Surg.* 2004;6(4):277.

2. Rewritten abstract of a published article with an appended commentary:

    2. Bigby ME. The end of the sunscreen and melanoma controversy [abstract of Dennis LK, Beane Freeman LD, VanBeek MJ. Sunscreen use and the risk for melanoma: a quantitative review. *Ann Intern Med.* 2003;139(12):966-978]? *Arch Dermatol.* 2004;140(6):745-746.

3. Abstract of a paper published in the society proceedings of a journal:

    3. Fliesler SJ, Richards MJ, Peachey NS, Buchan B, Vaughan DK, Organisciak DT. Potentiation of retinal light damage in an animal model of Smith-Lemli-Opitz syndrome [ARVO abstract 3373]. *Invest Ophthalmol Vis Sci.* 2001;42(suppl):S627.

Note: In example 3, the abstract number is also provided; if a number is included, it is placed in brackets along with the "abstract" designation. Also, example 3 has no issue number.

3.11.10 Special Department, Feature, or Column of a Journal. When reference is made to material from a special department, feature, or column of a journal, the department should be identified only in the following cases:

1. The cited material has no byline or signature. (*Note:* This is preferable to citing Anonymous, unless "Anonymous" or something similar was actually used [see 2.2, Manuscript Preparation, Bylines and End-of-Text Signatures].)

    1. Who is responsible for adolescent health [editorial]? *Lancet.* 2004;363(9426):2009.

2. The column or department name might help the reader identify the nature of the article and is not apparent from the title itself. *Note:* In these cases, the inclusion of the department or column name is optional and should be used as needed, at the editor's discretion.

    2. Harris JC. *Dead Mother I* [Art and Images in Psychiatry]. *Arch Gen Psychiatry.* 2004;61(8):762.

    3. Gross R, Neria Y. Posttraumatic stress among survivors of bioterrorism [letter]. *JAMA.* 2004;292(5):566.

Identification of other special departments, features, or columns may not require additional notation (eg, book or journal reviews, cover stories) as their identity will be apparent from the citation itself:

4. Calfee JE, reviewer. *Nature.* 2004;429(6994):807. Review of: Goozner M. *The $800 Million Pill: The Truth Behind the Cost of New Drugs.*
5. Southgate MT. The Cover (Thomas Hart Benton, *Pussycat and Roses*). *JAMA.* 2004;292(6):661.

3.11.11 Other Material Without Named Author(s) or With Named Authors and a Group Name. Reference may be made to material that has no named author or is prepared by a committee or other group. The following forms are used:

1. Ferguson JJ, Califf RM, Antman EM, et al; SYNERGY Trial Investigators. Enoxaparin vs unfractionated heparin in high-risk patients with non-ST-segment elevation acute coronary syndromes managed with an intended early invasive strategy: primary results of the SYNERGY randomized trial. *JAMA.* 2004;292(1):45-54.
2. Eye Diseases Prevalence Research Group. Prevalence of age-related macular degeneration in the United States. *Arch Ophthalmol.* 2004;122(4):564-572.
3. Centers for Disease Control and Prevention (CDC). Prevalence of receiving multiple preventive-care services among adults with diabetes—United States, 2002-2004. *MMWR Morb Mortal Wkly Rep.* 2005;54(44):1130-1133.

References may also have bylines containing the names of individuals and the name of a group or several groups.

4. Hennis A, Wu S-Y, Nemesure B, Leske MC; Barbados Eye Studies Group. Risk factors for incident cortical and posterior subcapsular lens opacities in the Barbados Eye Studies. *Arch Ophthalmol.* 2004;122(4):525-530.
5. Taylor Z, Nolan CM, Blumberg HM; American Thoracic Society; Centers for Disease Control and Prevention; Infectious Diseases Society of America. Controlling tuberculosis in the United States: recommendations from the American Thoracic Society, CDC, and the Infectious Diseases Society of America. *MMWR Recomm Rep.* 2005;54(RR-12):1-81.

In examples 4 and 5 above, a semicolon, not a comma, precedes the group name in the author field and no articles (eg, *the*) are included with the group names.

3.11.12 Discussants. If reference citation in the text names a discussant specifically rather than the author(s), eg, "as noted by Easter,[1]" the following form is used (see also 3.13.10, Special Print Materials, Secondary Citations and Quotations [Including Press Releases]).

1. Easter DW. In discussion of: Farley DR, Greenlee SM, Larson DR, Harrington JR. Double-blind, prospective, randomized study of warmed humidified carbon dioxide insufflation vs standard carbon dioxide for patients undergoing laparoscopic cholecystectomy. *Arch Surg.* 2004;139(7):739-744.

3.11.13 Corrections. If the reference citation is to an article with a published correction, provide both the information about the article and the information about the published correction, if available, as follows.

1. Korpi A, Mantyjarvi R, Rautiainen J, et al. Detection of mouse and rat urinary aeroallergens with an improved ELISA [published correction appears in *J Allergy Clin Immnol.* 2004;113(6):1226]. *J Allergy Clin Immunol.* 2004;113(4):677-682.

3.11.14 Retractions. If the reference citation is to an article that has since been retracted, or to the retraction notice itself, use the appropriate example below. Uniform Requirements notes, "Ideally, the first author should be the same in the retraction as in the article, although under certain circumstances the editor may accept retractions by other responsible persons."[5] (See also 5.4.4, Ethical and Legal Considerations, Scientific Misconduct, Editorial Policy and Procedures for Detecting and Handling Allegations of Scientific Misconduct.)

Citing the retraction:

1. Duckmanton L, Tellier R, Richardson C, Petric M. Notice of retraction of "The novel hemagglutinin-esterase genes of human torovirus and Breda virus" [retraction of: Duckmanton L, Tellier R, Richardson C, Petric M. In: *Virus Res.* 1999;64(2):137-149]. *Virus Res.* 2001;81(1-2):167.

Citing the article retracted:

2. Duckmanton L, Tellier R, Richardson C, Petric M. The novel hemagglutinin-esterase genes of human torovirus and Breda virus [retracted in: *Virus Res.* 2001:81(1-2):167]. *Virus Res.* 1999;64(2):137-149.

3.11.15 Duplicate Publication. The following form is suggested for citation of a notice of duplicate publication. (See also 5.3, Ethical and Legal Considerations, Duplicate Publication.)

1. Mettler L. Notice of duplicate publication [duplicate publication of Mettler L, Audebert A, Lehmann-Willenbrock E, Schive K, Jacobs VR. Prospective clinical trial of SprayGel as a barrier to adhesion formation: an interim analysis. *J Am Assoc Gynecol Laparosc.* 2003;10(3):339-344]. *J Am Assoc Gynecol Laparosc.* 2004;11(1):130.

3.12 References to Print Books

3.12.1 Complete Data. A complete reference to a print book includes the following:

1. Authors' surnames and first and middle initials
2. Chapter title (when cited)
3. Surname and first and middle initials of book authors or editors (or translator, if any)
4. Title of book and subtitle, if any
5. Volume number and volume title, when there is more than 1 volume

6. Edition number (do not indicate first edition)
7. Place of publication (see 14.5, Abbreviations, Cities, States, Counties, Territories, Possessions; Provinces; Countries)
8. Name of publisher
9. Year of copyright
10. Page numbers, when specific pages are cited

3.12.2 **Reference to an Entire Book.** When referring to an entire book, rather than pages or a specific section, use the following format (see also 3.7, Authors).

1. Modlin J, Jenkins P. *Decision Analysis in Planning for a Polio Outbreak in the United States.* San Francisco, CA: Pediatric Academic Societies; 2004.
2. Adkinson N, Yunginger J, Busse W, Bochner B, Holgate S, Middleton E, eds. *Middleton's Allergy: Principles and Practice.* 6th ed. St Louis, MO: Mosby; 2003.
3. Sacks O. *Uncle Tungsten.* New York, NY: Alfred A Knopf; 2001.
4. Weedon D. *Skin Pathology.* London, England: Churchill Livingstone; 2002.
5. World Health Organization. *Injury: A Leading Cause of the Global Burden of Disease, 2000.* Geneva, Switzerland: World Health Organization; 2002.
6. Galanter M, ed. *Services Research in the Era of Managed Care.* New York, NY: Kluwer Academic/Plenum; 2001. *Recent Developments in Alcoholism;* vol 15.
7. Simon LS, Lipman AG, Jacox AK, et al. *Pain in Osteoarthritis, Rheumatoid Arthritis, and Juvenile Chronic Arthritis.* 2nd ed. Glenview, IL: American Pain Society; 2002.
8. Venables WN, Ripley BD. *Modern Applied Statistics With S.* 4th ed. New York, NY: Springer Publishing Co; 2003.

3.12.3 **References to Monographs.** References to monographs should be styled the same as references to books.

3.12.4 **Reference to a Chapter in a Book.** When citing a chapter of a book, capitalize as for a journal article title (see 3.9, Titles); do not use quotation marks. Inclusive page numbers of the chapter should be given (see also 3.12.11, Page Numbers or Chapter Number).

1. Solensky R. Drug allergy: desensitization and treatment of reactions to antibiotics and aspirin. In: Lockey P, ed. *Allergens and Allergen Immunotherapy.* 3rd ed. New York, NY: Marcel Dekker; 2004:585-606.
2. Yashiro M, Yanagawa H. Database construction for information on patients with Kawasaki disease. In: Yanagawa H, Nakamura Y, Yashiro M, Kawasaki T, eds. *Epidemiology of Kawasaki Disease: A 30-Year Achievement.* Tokyo, Japan: Shindan-to-Chiryosha; 2004:57-77.
3. Bergeron C, Lowe J. Frontotemporal degeneration: introduction. In: Dickson DW, ed. *Neurodegeneration: The Molecular Pathology of Dementia*

and Movement Disorders. Basel, Switzerland: ISN Neuropath Press; 2003: 342-348.

4. Tangarorang G, Kerins G, Besdine R. Clinical approach to the older patient: an overview. In: Cassel C, Leipzig R, Cohen H, Larson E, Meier D, eds. *Geriatric Medicine*. New York, NY: Springer-Verlag; 2003:149-162.

Note that in example 2 above, 2 of the authors of the chapter are also editors of the book. In cases like this, they are listed in both places: authors of the chapter and editors of the book. The same policy would apply if the authors of a particular chapter and the editors of the book were identical.

3.12.5 **Editors and Translators.** Names of editors, translators, translator-editors, or executive, consulting, and section editors are given as follows:

1. Plato. *The Laws*. Taylor EA, trans-ed. London, England: JM Dent & Sons Ltd; 1934:104-105.

[Plato is the author; Taylor is the translator-editor.]

2. Klaassen CD. Principles of toxicology and treatment of poisoning. In: Hardman JG, Limbird LE, eds. Gilman AG, consulting ed. *Goodman and Gilman's The Pharmacological Basis of Therapeutics*. 10th ed. New York, NY: McGraw-Hill Book Co; 2001:67-80.

[Klaassen is the author of a chapter in a book edited by Hardman and Limbird, for which Gilman was the consulting editor.]

In the following 4 examples, no authors are named. Each book has an editor or editors and is part of a series. *Note:* The name of the series, if any, is given in the final field. If the book has a number within a series, the number is also given in the final field (see example 6).

3. Villarreal FJ, ed. *Interstitial Fibrosis in Heart Failure*. New York, NY: Springer-Verlag; 2005. *Developments in Cardiovascular Medicine*.
4. Sharpe VA, ed. *Accountability: Patient Safety and Policy Reform*. Washington, DC: Georgetown University Press; 2004. *Hastings Center Studies in Ethics*.
5. Brune K, Handwerker HO, eds. *Hyperalgesia: Molecular Mechanisms and Clinical Implications*. Seattle, WA: IASP Press; 2004. *Progress in Pain Research and Management*; vol 30.
6. Balducci L, Extermann M, eds. *Biological Basis of Geriatric Oncology*. New York, NY: Springer-Verlag; 2005. Rosen ST, ed. *Cancer Treatment and Research*; vol 124.

3.12.6 **Volume Number.** Use arabic numerals for volume numbers if the work cited includes more than 1 volume, even if the publisher used roman numerals.

If the volumes have no separate titles, merely numbers, the number should be given after the general title.

1. US Department of Health and Human Services. *Understanding and Improving Health and Objectives for Improving Health*. Vol 1. 2nd ed. Washington, DC: US Dept of Health and Human Services; 2000.

If the volumes have separate titles, the title of the volume referred to should be given first, with the title of the overall series of which the volume is a part given in the final field, along with the name of the general editor and the volume number, if applicable.

2. Kleiss W, Marcus C, Wabitsch M, eds. *Obesity in Childhood and Adolescence.* Leipzig, Germany: Karger; 2004. *Pediatric and Adolescent Medicine*; vol 9.

In example 2 above, *Pediatric and Adolescent Medicine* is the name of the entire series; *Obesity in Childhood and Adolescence* is the ninth volume.

When a book title includes a volume number or other identifying number, use the title as it was published. *Note:* The volume number does not need to be repeated in its customary place after the year if it is included in the book's title.

3. *Field Manual 4-02.17: Preventive Medicine Services.* Washington, DC: US Dept of the Army; 2000.
4. US Veterans Health Administration/Department of Defense. *Clinical Practice Guidelines: Diabetes Mellitus Algorithms—Module F: Foot Care.* Washington, DC: Veterans Health Administration; 2003.

3.12.7 Edition Number. Use arabic numerals to indicate an edition, even if the publisher has used roman numerals, but do not indicate a first edition. If a subsequent edition is cited, the number should be given. Abbreviate "New revised edition" as "New rev ed"; "Revised edition" as "Rev ed"; "American edition" as "American ed"; and "British edition" as "British ed."

1. Glinoer D. Thyroid disease during pregnancy. In: Braverman LE, Utiger RE, eds. *Werner and Ingbar's The Thyroid: A Fundamental and Clinical Text.* 8th ed. Philadelphia, PA: Lippincott Williams & Wilkins; 2000:1013-1027.
2. Pratt-Johnson JA, Tilson G. *Management of Strabismus and Amblyopia.* 2nd ed. New York, NY: Thieme Medical Publishers; 2001.
3. Green M, ed. *Bright Futures: National Guidelines for Health Supervision of Infants, Children, and Adolescents.* 2nd rev ed. Arlington, VA: National Center for Education in Maternal and Child Health; 2002.

3.12.8 Place of Publication. Use the name of the city in which the publishing firm was located at the time of publication. Follow the style used by *JAMA* and the *Archives* Journals for state names, as well as names of cities outside the United States (see 14.5, Abbreviations, Cities, States, Counties, Territories, Possessions; Provinces; Countries). Do not list the state name if it is part of the publisher's name. If more than 1 location appears, use the one that appears first in the edition you consulted. A colon separates the place of publication and the name of the publisher.

1. Griffin JR, Grisham JD. *Binocular Anomalies: Diagnosis and Vision Therapy.* 4th ed. Boston, MA: Butterworth-Heinemann; 2002.
2. Dresser R. *When Science Offers Salvation: Patient Advocacy and Research Ethics.* New York, NY: Oxford University Press; 2001.

3. International Agency for Research on Cancer (IARC). *Cancer Incidence in Five Continents.* Vol 8. Lyon, France: IARC Press; 2002. IARC scientific publication 155.
4. Cavanagh PR, Boone EY, Plummer DL. *The Foot in Diabetes: A Bibliography.* College Station: Pennsylvania State University; 2000.
5. *Health, United States, 2004.* Hyattsville, MD: National Center for Health Statistics; 2004.

3.12.9 Publishers. The full name of the publisher (publisher's imprint, as shown on the title page) should be given, abbreviated in accordance with the style used by *JAMA* and the *Archives* Journals (see 14.7, Abbreviations, Business Firms) but without any punctuation. Even if the name of a publishing firm has changed, use the name that was given on the published work. The following is an example of the format for a book with a joint imprint:

1. Henderson DA, Inglesby TV, O'Toole T, eds. *Bioterrorism.* Chicago, IL: *JAMA/Archives* and AMA Press; 2002.

Consult the latest *Books in Print*[7] to verify names of publishers, listings, online bookstores, or the Library of Congress catalog.

If there is no publisher's name available, use "Publisher unknown" in the place of the publisher's location and name.

3.12.10 Year of Publication. If the book has been published but there is no year of publication available, use "date unknown" in the place of the year. Use the full year (eg, 2006), not an abbreviated form (eg, not 06 or '06).

3.12.11 Page Numbers or Chapter Number. Use arabic numerals, unless the pages referred to use roman pagination (eg, the preliminary pages of a book).

1. Lewinsohn P. Depression in adolescents. In: Gottlib IH, Hammen CL, eds. *Handbook of Depression.* New York, NY: Guilford Press; 2002:541-553.
2. Mahan MDF. Preface. In: *The Chicago Manual of Style.* 15th ed. Chicago, IL: University of Chicago Press; 2003:xi-xiii.

If a book uses separate pagination within each chapter, follow the style used in the book. Notice that in the example below, because the page numbers contain hyphens, an en dash is used to separate them, rather than the usual hyphen.

3. Kasmar AG, Climi SA, David BT. Infectious diseases. In: Sabatine MS, ed. *Pocket Medicine.* 2nd ed. Baltimore, MD: Lippincott Williams & Wilkins; 2000:6-1–6-20.

Inclusive page numbers are preferred. The chapter number may be used instead if the author does not provide the inclusive page numbers, even after being queried.

4. Dybul M, Connors M, Fauci AS. Immunology of HIV infection. In: Paul WE, ed. *Fundamental Immunology.* 5th ed. Philadelphia, PA: Lippincott Williams & Wilkins; 2003:chap 42.

3.13 Special Print Materials. Many of the special materials covered in this section may also be accessed (and cited) in an online format. To see examples of these citation formats, please consult 3.15, Electronic References. The version consulted (print or online) is the version that should be cited.

3.13.1 Newspapers. References to newspapers should include the following, in the order indicated: (1) name of author (if given), (2) title of article, (3) name of newspaper, (4) date of newspaper, (5) section (if applicable), and (6) page numbers. *Note*: Newspaper names are not abbreviated. If a city name is not part of the newspaper name, it may be added to the official name, for clarity, as with *Minneapolis* in example 1. See example 5 for how to treat an article that "jumps" from one page to a later page (see also 3.11.4, References to Print Journals, Discontinuous Pagination).

1. Wolfe W. State's mail-order drug plan launched. *Minneapolis Star Tribune*. May 14, 2004:1B.
2. Connolly C. A small win for proponents of drug importation. *Washington Post*. April 23, 2004:EO1.
3. Richer S. America's new war on drugs targets Canadian pharmacists. *Globe and Mail*. May 17, 2004:A1.
4. Goode E. Study finds jump in children taking psychiatric drugs. *New York Times*. January 14, 2003:A21.
5. Overbye D. A philanthropist of science seeks to be its next Nobel. *New York Times*. April 19, 2005:D1, D4.

3.13.2 Government or Agency Bulletins. References to bulletins published by departments or agencies of a government should include the following information, in the order indicated: (1) name of author (if given); (2) title of bulletin; (3) place of publication; (4) name of issuing bureau, agency, department, or other governmental division (note that in this position, Department should be abbreviated Dept; also note that if an author supplies US Government Printing Office as the publisher, it would be preferable to obtain the name of the issuing bureau, agency, or department, if possible); (5) date of publication; (6) page numbers, if specified; (7) publication number, if any; and (8) series number, if given.

1. Johnston LD, O'Malley PM, Bachman JG. *Monitoring the Future: National Survey Results on Adolescent Drug Use: Overview of Key Findings*. Bethesda, MD: National Institute on Drug Abuse, US Dept of Health and Human Services; 2003.
2. *Health, United States, 2004*. Hyattsville, MD: National Center for Health Statistics; 2004.
3. US Department of Health and Human Services. Maternal, infant, and child health. In: *Healthy People 2010*. 2nd ed. Washington, DC: US Dept of Health and Human Services; 2000.
4. Centers for Disease Control and Prevention. *Sexually Transmitted Disease Surveillance, 2000*. Atlanta, GA: Centers for Disease Control and Prevention, US Dept of Health and Human Services; 2001.
5. Shin HB, Bruno R. *Census 2000 Brief C2KBR-29: Language Use and English-Speaking Ability: 2000*. Washington, DC: US Census Bureau; 2003.

6. National Institutes of Health, US Department of Health and Human Services. *Strategic Plan for NIH Obesity Research: A Report to the NIH Obesity Research Task Force*. Bethesda, MD: National Institutes of Health; 2004. NIH publication 04-5493.
7. Central Bureau of Statistics. *Statistical Year Book of Nepal 2001*. Kathmandu, Nepal: Central Bureau of Statistics; 2001.
8. World Health Organization. *World Health Report 2002: Reducing Risk, Promoting Healthy Life*. Geneva, Switzerland: World Health Organization; 2002.
9. Commission for the Assistance of Refugees and United Nations High Commissioner for Refugees. *The Guatemalans: A History* [in Spanish]. Geneva, Switzerland: United Nations High Commissioner for Refugees; 2000.
10. Transitional Islamic Government of Afghanistan. *Afghanistan National Health Resources Assessment: Preliminary Results*. Kabul: Ministry of Public Health, Transitional Islamic Government of Afghanistan; 2002.
11. *The Swedish Cancer Registry: Cancer Incidence in Sweden 1998*. Stockholm, Sweden: National Board of Health and Welfare; 2001.
12. Danish National Board of Health. *Telephonic Investigation of the Sun Habits of the Danes* [in Danish]. Copenhagen, Denmark: Danish National Board of Health; 2000.

3.13.3 Serial Publications. If a monograph or report is part of a series, include the name of the series and, if applicable, the number of the publication.

1. Ministry of Health. *National AIDS Control Program*. Dar es Salaam: Ministry of Health, United Republic of Tanzania; 2001. HIV/AIDS/STI Surveillance Report 16.
2. West S, King V, Carey TS, et al. *Systems to Rate the Strength of Scientific Evidence*. Rockville, MD: Agency for Healthcare Research and Quality; 2002. Evidence Report/Technology Assessment 47.
3. US Department of Commerce. *Population Division: Income, Poverty and Health Insurance Coverage in the United States, 2003*. Washington, DC: US Bureau of the Census; 2003. Annual Social and Economic Supplement.

3.13.4 Theses and Dissertations. Titles of theses and dissertations are given in italics. References to theses should include the location of the university (or other institution), its name, and year of completion of the thesis. If the thesis has been published, it should be treated as any other book reference (see 3.12.1, References to Print Books, Complete Data).

1. Fenster SD. *Cloning and Characterization of Piccolo, a Novel Component of the Presynaptic Cytoskeletal Matrix* [dissertation]. Birmingham: University of Alabama; 2000.
2. Undeman C. *Fully Automatic Segmentation of MRI Brain Images Using Probabilistic Diffusion and a Watershed Scale-Space Approach* [mas-

ter's thesis]. Stockholm, Sweden: NADA, Royal Institute of Technology; 2001.

3.13.5 Special Collections. References to material available only in special collections of a library, as this example of a monograph written in 1757, take this form:

1. Hunter J. An account of the dissection of morbid bodies: a monograph or lecture. 1757;No. 32:30-32. Located at: Library of the Royal College of Surgeons, London, England.

3.13.6 Package Inserts. Package inserts (the printed material about the use and effects of the product contained in the package) may be cited as follows:

1. Cialis [package insert]. Indianapolis, IN: Eli Lilly & Co; 2003.
2. ZstatFlu [package insert]. Oklahoma City, OK: ZymeTx Inc; 2000.

3.13.7 Patents. Patent citations take the following form. Examples 1 and 2 and 4 and 5 are for patents that have been issued and example 3 is for a patent that is pending. See the US Patent and Trademark Office home page (http://www.uspto.gov/) or the European Patent Office home page (http://www.european-patent-office.org/index.en.php) for further details.

1. Rabiner RA, Hare BA, inventors; OmniSonics Medical Technologies Inc, assignee. Apparatus for removing plaque from blood vessels using ultrasonic energy. US patent 6,866,670. March 15, 2005.
2. Guiliano K, Kapur R, inventors; Cellomics Inc, assignee. System for cell-based screening. US patent 6,875,578. April 5, 2005.
3. Castellano TP, inventor; Pillsbury Winthrop LLP, assignee. Method and apparatus for administering a vaccine or other pharmaceutical. US patent application 20,050,070,876. September 26, 2003.
4. Morris D, Coffey MC, Thompson BG, inventors; Oncolytics Biotech Inc, assignee. Method for reducing pain using oncolytic viruses. European patent ES2239928T. October 16, 2005.
5. James RG, inventor; Australian Surgical Design, James RG, assignees. Surface preparation of an implant. European patent GB2412338. September 28, 2005.

3.13.8 Unpublished Material. References to unpublished material may include articles or abstracts that have been presented at a society meeting but not published and material accepted for publication but not published. If, during the course of the publication process, these materials are published or accepted for publication, and if the author is familiar with the later version, the most up-to-date bibliographic information should be included.

Items Presented at a Meeting but Not Yet Published. These oral or poster presentations take the following form:

1. Durbin D, Kallan M, Elliott M, Arbogast K, Cornejo R, Winston F. Risk of injury to restrained children from passenger air bags. Paper presented at:

46th Annual Meeting of the Association for the Advancement for Automotive Medicine; September 2002; Tempe, AZ.

2. Weber KJ, Lee J, Decresce R, Subhasis M, Prinz R. Intraoperative PTH monitoring in parathyroid hyperplasia requires stricter criteria for success. Paper presented at: 25th Annual American Association of Endocrine Surgeons Meeting; April 6, 2004; Charlottesville, VA.
3. Greenspan A, Eerdekens M, Mahmoud R. Is there an increased rate of cerebrovascular events among dementia patients? Poster presented at: 24th Congress of the Collegium Internationale Neuro-Psychopharmacologicum (CINP); June 20-24, 2004; Paris, France.
4. Khuri FR, Lee JJ, Lippman SM, et al. Isotretinoin effects on head and neck cancer recurrence and second primary tumors. In: Proceedings from the American Society of Clinical Oncology; May 31-June 3, 2003; Chicago, IL. Abstract 359.

Once these presentations are published, they take the form of reference to a book, journal, or other medium in which they are ultimately published, as in example 5 (see 3.12.1, References to Print Books, Complete Data):

5. Cionni RJ. Color perception in patients with UV- or blue-light-filtering IOLs. In: *Symposium on Catarct, IOL, and Refractive Surgery.* San Diego, CA: American Society of Cataract and Refractive Surgery; 2004. Abstract 337.

Material Accepted for Publication but Not Yet Published. Formats suggested for both journal articles and books, accepted for publication but not yet published, are shown below:

6. Carrau RL, Khidr A, Crawley JA, Hillson EM, Davis JK, Pashos CL. The impact of laryngopharyngeal reflux on patient-reported quality of life. *Laryngoscope.* In press.
7. Ofri D. *Incidental Findings: Lessons From My Patients in the Art of Medicine.* Boston, MA: Beacon Press. In press.

Note: Some publications require that authors verify that acceptance for publication has been granted (authors sometimes confuse *submitted* with *accepted*).[6,8] Some publishers also prefer the term *forthcoming* to *in press* because they feel that *in press* is not appropriate for electronic citations,[6,8] but *JAMA* and the *Archives* Journals use *in press* for both forms.

Material Submitted for Publication but Not Yet Accepted. In the list of references, do not include material that has been submitted for publication but has not yet been accepted. This material, with its date, should be noted in the text as "unpublished data," as follows:

> These findings have recently been corroborated (H. E. Marman, MD, unpublished data, January 2005).
>
> Similar findings have been noted by Roberts[6] and H. E. Marman, MD (unpublished data, 2005).

Numerous studies[12-20] (also H. E. Marman, MD, unpublished data, 2005) have described similar findings.

If the unpublished data referred to are those of the author, indicate this as follows:

Other data (H.E.M., unpublished data, 2005). . . .

3.13.9 Personal Communications. Do not include "personal communications" in the list of references. The following forms may be used in the text:

In a conversation with H. E. Marman, MD (August 2005). . . .

According to a letter from H. E. Marman, MD, in August 2005. . . .

Similar findings have been noted by Roberts[6] and by H. E. Marman, MD (written communication, August 2005).

According to the manufacturer (H. R. Smith, oral communication, May 2005), the drug became available in Japan in January 2004.

The author should give the date of the communication and indicate whether it was in oral or written (including e-mail) form. Highest academic degrees should also be given. If the affiliation of the person would better establish the relevance and authority of the citation, it should be included (see the example above, where H. R. Smith is identified as the drug's manufacturer).

See also 3.15.9, Electronic References, E-mail and E-mail List (Listserve) Messages.

Some journals, including *JAMA* and the *Archives* Journals, now require that the author provide written permission from the person whose unpublished data or personal communication is thus cited.[5,8] (See 5.2.8, Ethical and Legal Considerations, Acknowledgments, Permission to Name Individuals.)

3.13.10 Secondary Citations and Quotations (Including Press Releases). Reference may be made to one author's citation of, or quotation from, another's work. Distinguish between citation and quotation (ie, between work mentioned and words actually quoted). In the text, the name of the original author, rather than the secondary source, should be mentioned. (See also 3.11.12, References to Print Journals, Discussants.) As with citation of an abstract of an article rather than citation of the original document (see 3.11.9, References to Print Journals, Abstracts and Other Material Taken From Another Source), citation of the original document is preferred unless it is not readily available. Only items actually consulted should be listed. The forms for listed references are as follows:

1. Cauley JA, Lui L-Y, Ensrud KE, et al. Osteoporosis and fracture risk in women of different ethnic groups. *JAMA*. 2005;293(17):2102-2108. Cited by: Acheson LS. Bone density and the risk of fractures: should treatment thresholds vary by race [editorial]? *JAMA*. 2005;293(17):2151-2154.
2. Kato S, Sherman PM. What is new related to *Helicobacter pylori* infection in children and teenagers? *Arch Pediatr Adolesc Med*. 2005;159(5):415-421. Quoted by: Prazar G. How many pediatricians does it take to change a practice? or how to incorporate change into practice [editorial]. *Arch Pediatr Adolesc Med*. 2005;159(5):500-502.

3. Groups ask Canada to ban Web pharmacies [press release]. New York, NY: Associated Press; March 30, 2004.

3.13.11 Classical References. Classical references may deviate from the usual forms in some details. In many instances, the facts of publication are irrelevant and may be omitted. Date of publication should be given when available and pertinent.

1. Shakespeare W. *A Midsummer Night's Dream.* Act 2, scene 3, line 24.
2. Donne J. *Second Anniversary.* Verse 243.

For classical references, *The Chicago Manual of Style*[9] may be used as a guide.

3. Aristotle. *Metaphysics.* 3. 2.966b 5-8.

In biblical references, do not abbreviate the names of books. The version may be included parenthetically if the information is provided (see example 4). References to the Bible are usually included in the text.

The story begins in Genesis 3:1.

Paul admonished against succumbing to temptation (I Corinthians 10:6-13).

Occasionally they may appear as listed references at the end of the article.

4. I Corinthians 10:6-13 (RSV).

3.14 Other Media

3.14.1 Audiotapes, Videotapes, DVDs (Digital Video Disks). Occasionally, references may include citation of audiotapes, videotapes, or DVDs. The form for such references is as follows:

1. Moyers B. *On Our Own Terms: Moyers on Dying* [videotape]. New York, NY: Thirteen/WNET; 2000.
2. Ayers S. *Terrorism: Medical Response* [DVD]. Edgartown, MA: Emergency Film Group; 2002.
3. Acland RD. *Acland's DVD Atlas of Human Anatomy* [DVD]. Philadelphia, PA: Lippincott Williams & Wilkins; 2003.

Note that the place of the author may be held by the host and the place of the publisher may be held by the distributor.

For citation format for books on CD, see 3.15.2, Electronic References, Books and Books on CD-ROM, and for audio presentations available online, see 3.15.10, Electronic References, Online Conference Proceedings/Presentations.

3.14.2 Transcript of Television or Radio Broadcast. Citation of transcripts to television or radio broadcasts take the following form:

1. Mental illness in children—part 1 [transcript]. *Morning Edition.* National Public Radio. September 22, 2003.
2. Shutting out Tourette's syndrome [transcript]. *60 Minutes.* CBS television. January 17, 2005.

The Internet made a lot of things very simple.
Bibliographies aren't among them.
J. Kronholz[10]

... the basic rules of citation are still applicable
when referencing the Internet.
K. Patrias[11]

3.15 Electronic References. Electronic references have become considerably more common since the publication of the ninth edition of this manual. Internet references, rather than being something that only authors, editors, publishers, and librarians fretted about, were the subject of a front-page article in the *Wall Street Journal.*[10] Guidelines for handling electronic references are now readily available. Although the American Psychological Association[12,13] was among the first to propose such guidelines, those of the National Library of Medicine (NLM)[14] are more widely used for medical research.

Print and electronic references differ in several ways. Below are some issues to consider.

- Web sites may be evanescent, vanishing much faster than books go out of print. To address this phenomenon, the NLM "strongly recommend[s] that the user produce a print or other copy when possible for future reference."[6(piii)] Some journals recommend this to authors in their instructions.[15] Dellavalle et al[16] suggest that "the best current solution to improve access to Internet references is to require capture and submission of all Internet information at the time of manuscript consideration." In preparing a reference list, authors should check to make sure any URLs (uniform resource locators) they cite are still valid; editors should check these again. Since typographical errors render URLs invalid, validation may be required several times in the publication process. Although it is desirable to have functional links, it is to be expected that, over time, some links may break as sites cease to exist, much as books may go out of print. Any updating of URLs in an effort to "fix" a link should be done with care, ensuring that the material that was cited originally still exists on the revised link.

- Some publishers are using other less-transient identifiers instead of, or in addition to, URLs. Among these are the digital object identifier (DOI) and the PubMed identification number (PMID). The DOI may be used to identify not just individual journal articles, but any piece of content (eg, a single figure) within an article; DOIs may also be assigned to books and many other forms of intellectual content.

  The DOI has 2 elements, separated by a forward slash: the prefix and the suffix. The prefix is assigned by a DOI registration agency (an organization may have multiple prefixes) and the suffix, which follows the prefix and a forward slash, identifies the particular item. All DOIs begin with 10. For example, in the DOI in example 6 below (10.1038/nature02312), "10.1038" is the prefix and "nature02312" is the suffix. (*Note:* Some publishers use other identifiers as a part of the suffix.) The DOIs can be any length and, once assigned, are not changed. To find an article using the DOI, a reader can enter the DOI in the search box on the DOI Web site (http://dx.doi.org/) or in some journal search engines.[17] As close as possible to publication, it is advisable to check all DOIs to make sure that they resolve.

The PMID is assigned to the journal articles cited in a journal indexed by PubMed and is a part of the PubMed citation. To find an article, a reader can enter the PMID in the "search" box on the PubMed Web site (http://www.ncbi.nlm.nih.gov/PubMed/). Some journals publish the DOI with the article (see example 6 in 3.15.1, Online Journals); the PMID is usually not published but exists as a behind-the-scenes identifier.

- Web sites may be updated much more frequently than published books or journals; thus, it is critical to provide the date that the author accessed the site and, if possible, the date on which the information was updated.

- Some journals and books may be available in print and online, but these versions may not be identical: the differences may be as minor as the online correction of a typographical error discovered in the print journal, which is not formally corrected and is impossible to track (see 6.2.7, Editorial Assessment and Processing, Editorial Processing, Corrections), or as major as 2 versions of the same article, or situations in which additional material (eg, tables or figures) is available only online. Books are often adapted for the Web to enhance interactivity for readers and add features. Because of these possible differences between various versions, it is critical that authors cite the version consulted. *Note:* The cited version may not be the version of record (ie, the version that the publisher considers authoritative).

3.15.1 Online Journals. The basic format for reference to an article in an online journal is as follows:

> Author(s). Title. *Journal Name* [using National Library of Medicine abbreviations—see 14.10, Abbreviations, Names of Journals]. Year;vol(issue No.):inclusive pages. URL [provide the URL in this field; no need to use "URL:" preceding it]. Published [date]. Updated [date]. Accessed [date].

Note: Use the URL that will take the reader most directly to the article, not a long search string and not a short, more general URL (one to the publisher's home page, for example); if a URL is provided, as close as possible to publication verify that the link still works. Patrias[11] notes that NLM recommends using the location displayed in the Web browser as the URL. For a journal article, the accessed date will often be the only date available. This is especially important for journals that provide no "versioning" (eg, date posted, date updated or revised).

1. Duchin JS. Can preparedness for biological terrorism save us from pertussis? *Arch Pediatr Adolesc Med.* 2004;158(2):106-107. http://archpedi.ama-assn.org/cgi/content/full/158/2/106. Accessed June 1, 2004.

Many journals, such as *Archives of Pediatrics & Adolescent Medicine* in the example above, have parallel print and online publication, and the page numbers of the print article are included in the online citation. In this example, the date the article was posted (ie, published) was not provided and there were no updates, so only the date the article was accessed is listed. The inclusion of the URL and the date accessed, which differentiates this from the citation of the identical article in print, indicates that the online version of the article was seen and hence is appropriately cited.

In the example below, however, the article is *only* available online and has no page numbers.

2. Gore D, Haji SA, Balashanmugam A, et al. Light and electron microscopy of macular corneal dystrophy: a case study. *Digit J Ophthalmol.* 2004;10. http://www.djo.harvard.edu/site.php?url=/physicians/oa/671. Accessed December 6, 2005.

Other online-only articles without page numbers may be noted by other identifiers, eg, by e-page numbers (examples 3 and 4) or by article number (example 5).

3. Laupland KB, Davies HD, Low DE, Schwartz B, Green K; Ontario Group A Streptococcal Study Group. Invasive group A streptococcal disease in children and association with varicella-zoster virus infection. *Pediatrics.* 2000;105(5):e60. http://pediatrics.aappublications.org/cgi/content/full/105/5/e60. Accessed April 30, 2004.
4. e-Health Ethics Initiative. e-Health Code of Ethics. *J Med Internet Res.* 2000; 2(2):e9. http://www.jmir.org/2000/2/e9. Published May 24, 2000. Accessed April 29, 2004.

Examples 5 and 6 provide the DOI rather than a URL. In this case, it is not necessary to also provide the URL. When the DOI is provided, it is preferable to cite it rather than the URL. *Note:* The DOI is provided immediately after "doi:" and is set closed up to it, per convention. No accessed date is required for the DOI, making it the last item in the reference.

5. Smeeth L, Iliffe S. Community screening for visual impairment in the elderly. *Cochrane Database Syst Rev.* 2002;(2):CD001054. doi:10.1002/14651858.CD1001054.
6. Kitajima TS, Kawashima SA, Watanabe Y. The conserved kinetochore protein shugoshin protects centromeric cohesion during meiosis. *Nature.* 2004;427(6974):510-517. doi:10.1038/nature02312.

In some cases, different versions of the same article are published in print and online. The *BMJ*'s ELPS (electronic long, print short) is one example.[18] The print journal article (short version) is also made available online. *Note:* The version consulted is the version that should be cited. If the author consulted the article in the print journal, the reference would be cited like any other print journal article (see 3.11, References to Print Journals).

7. Deeks JJ, Smith LA, Bradley MD. Efficacy, tolerability, and upper gastrointestinal safety of celecoxib for treatment of osteoarthritis and rheumatoid arthritis: systematic review of randomised controlled trials. *BMJ.* 2002; 325(7365):619-623.

If the author consulted the same article online, the reference would be formatted as follows:

8. Deeks JJ, Smith LA, Bradley MD. Efficacy, tolerability, and upper gastrointestinal safety of celecoxib for treatment of osteoarthritis and rheumatoid arthritis: systematic review of randomised controlled trials [abridged].

BMJ. 2002;325(7365):619-623. http://bmj.bmjjournals.com/cgi/content/abridged/325/7365/619. Published September 21, 2002. Accessed October 21, 2002.

If the author consulted the long version of this article, available *only* online, the reference would be formatted as follows:

9. Deeks JJ, Smith LA, Bradley MD. Efficacy, tolerability, and upper gastrointestinal safety of celecoxib for treatment of osteoarthritis and rheumatoid arthritis: systematic review of randomised controlled trials. *BMJ*. 2002;325(7365):619. http://bmj.bmjjournals.com/cgi/content/full/325/7365/619. Published September 21, 2002. Accessed October 11, 2002.

Note that the online citation of the long version (example 9) differs from that of the short version (example 8) in that it does not provide inclusive page numbers but gives only the first page in the print journal. Many online journals, however, do use inclusive page numbers.

In the example below, the online article includes a video. This is mentioned in an editor's note in the print journal; in the online journal, a link to the video appears in the table of contents and as a link within the article. The citation to the print article appears as follows:

10. Bertocci GE, Pierce MC, Deemer E, Aguel F. Computer simulation of stair falls to investigate scenarios in child abuse. *Arch Pediatr Adolesc Med*. 2001;155(9):1008-1014.

The citation to the online article, containing the video, would be as follows:

11. Bertocci GE, Pierce MC, Deemer E, Aguel F. Computer simulation of stair falls to investigate scenarios in child abuse. *Arch Pediatr Adolesc Med*. 2001;155(9):1008-1014. http://archpedi.ama-assn.org/cgi/content/full/155/9/1008. Accessed February 27, 2004.

A citation to only the video in the online version would be as follows:

12. Bertocci GE, Pierce MC, Deemer E, Aguel F. Computer simulation of stair falls to investigate scenarios in child abuse [video]. *Arch Pediatr Adolesc Med*. 2001;155(9):1008-1014. http://archpedi.ama-assn.org/cgi/content/full/155/9/1008/DCI. Accessed February 27, 2004.

In the following example, the online article contains 3 tables not included in the print version. These are cited in the print article as eTable 1, eTable 2, and eTable 3; in the online journal, these appear as links within the article; and on the PDF they appear as pages e1 to e7.

13. DeWitt DE, Hirsch IB. Outpatient insulin therapy in type 1 and type 2 diabetes mellitus: scientific review. *JAMA*. 2003;289(17):2254-2264, e1-e7. http://jama.ama-assn.org/cgi/content/full/289/17/2254. Accessed December 6, 2005.

If an article is published online ahead of print publication, it may appear in 1 of 3 ways: (1) posted without editing; (2) edited and posted as it will appear in print, only ahead of the print publication (with or without print pagination); or (3) edited and posted as part of a specific issue of the journal. The first is found more often in the physical sciences (eg, physics preprint servers) than in medicine. Examples of the second (example 14) and third (example 15) are given below:

14. van der Hoek L, Pyrc K, Jebbink MF, et al. Identification of a new human coronavirus [published online ahead of print March 21, 2004]. *Nat Med.* doi:10.1038.nm1024.

In example 14, the article has not yet been paginated in the print journal and the DOI serves as the unique identifier for the article until publication. Once the article has been published in print, the full citation is provided to facilitate linking (see example 15).

15. van der Hoek L, Pyrc K, Jebbink MF, et al. Identification of a new human coronavirus [published online ahead of print March 21, 2004]. *Nat Med.* 2004;10(4):368-373. doi:10.1038.nm1024.

Example 16 is for an article not yet published in print and example 17 is for the reference once it has been published in print. *Note:* The title, byline, or other components may have changed slightly between online-only and print publication.

16. Cannon CP, Braunwald E, McCabe CH, et al; Pravastatin or Atorvastatin Evaluation and Infection Therapy—Thrombolysis in Myocardial Infarction 22 Investigators. Comparison of intensive and moderate lipid lowering with statins after acute coronary syndromes [published online ahead of print March 8, 2004]. *N Engl J Med.* doi:10.1056/NEJMoa040583.
17. Cannon CP, Braunwald E, McCabe CH, et al; Pravastatin or Atorvastatin Evaluation and Infection Therapy—Thrombolysis in Myocardial Infarction 22 Investigators. Intensive vs moderate lipid lowering with statins after acute coronary syndromes [published online ahead of print March 8, 2004]. *N Engl J Med.* 2004;350(15):1495-1504. doi:10.1056/NEJMoa040583.

Some journals allow the reader to submit an immediate online response to articles (eg, *BMJ's* Rapid Responses and *Pediatrics'* Post-publication Peer Reviews [P^{3}R]). Examples of these are below:

18. Deutsch J. Less is better [Rapid Response]. *BMJ.* http://bmj.bmjjournals.com/cgi/eletters/328/7438/0-g#51798. Published February 27, 2004. Accessed April 30, 2004.
19. Molloy EJ, Nigro K, Sandhaus L, Watson RWG, Walsh MC. Labor and stress at delivery are confounders in the evaluation of neonatal sepsis [Post-publication Peer Review]. *Pediatrics.* 2004;113(5):1173. http://pediatrics.aappublications.org/cgi/eletters/113/1173. Published May 28, 2004. Accessed June 2, 2004.

3.15.2 **Books and Books on CD-ROM.** The basic format for reference to an Internet-based book is as follows. *Note:* If the reference is to the entire book, the information about chapter title and inclusive pages is not included.

Author(s). Chapter title. In: Editor(s). *Book Title.* [Edition number, if it is the second edition or above; mention of first edition is not necessary] ed. City, State (or country) of publisher: Publisher's name; copyright year:inclusive pages. URL: [provide URL and verify that the link still works as close as possible to the time of publication]. Accessed [date].

1. Resnick NM. Geriatric medicine. In: Braunwald E, Fauci AS, Isselbacher KJ, et al, eds. *Harrison's Online*. Based on: Braunwald E, Hauser SL, Fauci AS, Kasper DL, Longo DL, Jameson JL, eds. *Harrison's Principles of Internal Medicine*. 15th ed. New York, NY: McGraw-Hill; 2001. http://www.hsls.pitt.edu/resources/documentation/harrisonsinfo.html. Accessed December 6, 2005.
2. Lunney JR, Foley KM, Smith TJ, Gelband H, eds. *Describing Death in America: What We Need to Know*. Washington, DC: National Cancer Policy Board, Institute of Medicine; 2003. http://www.nap.edu/books/0309087252/html/. Accessed December 6, 2005.

Citation of a book or monograph in CD-ROM format follows fairly closely the form used for a book or monograph (see 3.12, References to Print Books), with the key difference being the inclusion of the name of the medium in brackets after the title (eg, [CD-ROM]). Titles of books on CD-ROM follow the capitalization style of print book titles and are italicized. *Note:* If the title of the book (eg, *Cecil Textbook of Medicine on CD-ROM*) indicates the medium, no mention of the medium in brackets is necessary.

3. Alberts B, Johnson A, Lewis J, Raff M, Roberts K, Walter P. *Molecular Biology of the Cell* [CD-ROM]. 4th ed. New York, NY: Garland Science; 2002.
4. Longo DL. Immunology of aging. In: Paul WE, ed. *Fundamental Immunology* [CD-ROM]. 5th ed. Philadelphia, PA: Lippincott Williams & Wilkins; 2002;chap 33.

3.15.3 **Web Sites.** In citing data from a Web site, include the following elements, if available, in the order shown:

> Author(s), if given (often, no authors are given). Title of the specific item cited (if none is given, use the name of the organization responsible for the site[11]). Name of the Web site. URL [provide URL and verify that the link still works as close as possible to publication]. Published [date]. Updated [date]. Accessed [date].

As Patrias[11] notes, "the title page is the usual place to look for citation information in a print publication, but no standards have been adopted for the Internet for the content of what would equate to a title page." This can make constructing a reference for a Web site difficult, but as much relevant information as possible should be included.

1. International Society for Infectious Diseases. ProMED-mail Web site. http://www.promedmail.org. Accessed April 29, 2004.
2. Sullivan D. Major search engines and directories. SearchEngineWatch Web site. http://www.searchenginewatch.com/links/article.php/2156221. Updated April 28, 2004. Accessed December 6, 2005.
3. Interim guidance about avian influenza A (H5N1) for US citizens living abroad. Centers for Disease Control and Prevention Web site. http://www.cdc.gov/travel/other/avian_flu_ig_americans_abroad_032405.htm. Updated November 18, 2005. Accessed December 6, 2005.

4. Sample size calculation. Grapentine Co Inc. http://www.grapentine.com/calculator.htm. Accessed December 6, 2005.
5. Recommendations for the care and maintenance of high intensity metal halide and mercury vapor lighting in schools. National Electrical Manufacturers Association. http://www.nema.org/stds/halide-schools.cfm#download. Accessed December 6, 2005.
6. Truth and reconciliation: examining human rights violations in South Africa's health sector: submission to the Truth and Reconciliation Commission concerning the role of health professionals in gross violations of human rights. American Association for the Advancement of Science Web site. http://shr.aaas.org/trc-med/presub.htm. Published 1997. Accessed April 30, 2004.

3.15.4 **Online Newspapers.** Except for the citation of the URL and the accessed date, the format is the same as that for citing a print newspaper reference shown in 3.13.1, Special Print Materials, Newspapers.

1. Weiss R. The promise of precision prescriptions. *Washington Post.* June 24, 2000:A1. http://www.washingtonpost.com. Accessed October 10, 2001.
2. Perez-Pena R. Children in shelters hit hard by asthma. *New York Times.* March 2, 2004. http://www.nytimes.com/2004/03/02/nyregion/02asthma.html. Accessed March 2, 2004.

3.15.5 **Government/Organization Reports.** These are treated much like electronic journal and book references: use journal style for articles and book style for monographs. *Note:* As with electronic journal references, of the dates published, updated, and accessed, often only the accessed date will be available.

1. Jacob Siegel; Administration on Aging. Aging into the 21st century. http://www.aoa.gov/prof/Statistics/future_growth/aging21/aging_21.asp. Published May 31, 1996. Accessed December 6, 2005.
2. World Medical Association. Declaration of Helsinki: ethical principles for medical research involving human subjects. http://www.wma.net/e/policy/b3.htm. Updated June 10, 2002. Accessed February 26, 2004.
3. US Department of Health and Human Services. Protection of human subjects. 45 CFR §46. http://www.hhs.gov/ohrp/humansubjects/guidance/45cfr46.htm. Revised November 13, 2001. Effective December 13, 2001. Accessed February 27, 2004.
4. World Health Organization. Equitable access to essential medicines: a framework for collective action. http://whqlibdoc.who.int/hq/2004/WHO_EDM_2004.4.pdf. Published March 2004. Accessed December 6, 2005.

In the 2 examples below, the number of the working paper (example 5) and the publication number (example 6) provide information in addition to the URL and could prove helpful should the URLs change.

5. Dafney L, Gruber J. Does public insurance improve the efficiency of medical care? Medicaid expansions and child hospitalizations. http://www

.nber.org/papers/w7555. National Bureau of Economic Research working paper w7555. Published February 2000. Accessed February 26, 2004.

6. Johnson DL, O'Malley PM, Bachman JG. *Secondary School Students*. Bethesda, MD: National Institute on Drug Abuse; 2001. *Monitoring the Future: National Survey Results on Drug Use, 1975-2000;* vol 1. NIH publication 01-4924. http://www.monitoringthefuture.org/pubs/monographs/vol1_2000.pdf. Published August 2001. Accessed February 27, 2004.

3.15.6 **Software.** To cite software, use the following form:

1. *Epi Info* [computer program]. Version 3.2. Atlanta, GA: Centers for Disease Control and Prevention; 2004.
2. *Intercooled STATA* (for Windows) [computer program]. Version 7.0. College Station, TX: StataCorp; 2000.

Software need not be cited in the reference list if it is mentioned only in passing or is available without charge via the Internet (eg, shareware or freeware).

3.15.7 **Software Manual or Guide.** In citing a print software manual or guide, use the following form, which follows that for citation of a book (see 3.12.1, References to Print Books, Complete Data).

1. Bott E, Leonhard W. *Special Edition Using Microsoft Office XP*. Indianapolis, IN: Que; 2001.
2. Dean AG, Dean JA, Coulombier D, et al. *Epi Info, Version 6: A Word-Processing, Database, and Statistics Program for Public Health on IBM-Compatible Microcomputers*. Atlanta, GA: Centers for Disease Control and Prevention; 1994.
3. Dixon WJ, Brown MB, Engelman L, Jennirch RI, eds. *BMDP Statistical Software Manual*. Los Angeles: University of California Press; 1990.

3.15.8 **Databases.** In citing data from an online database, include the following elements, if applicable, in the order shown:

> Author(s). Title of the database [database online]. Publisher's location (city, state, *or*, for Canada, city, province, country, *or*, all others, city, country): publisher's name; year of publication and/or last update. URL [provide URL and verify that the link still works as close as possible to publication]. Accessed [date].

Additional notes that might be helpful or of interest to the reader (eg, date the site was updated or modified) may also be included.

1. PDQ: NCI's Comprehensive Cancer Database. Bethesda, MD: National Cancer Institute; 1996. http://www.cancer.gov/cancerinfo/pdq/cancerdatabase. Updated December 18, 2001. Accessed April 29, 2004.
2. Genew, HUGO Gene Nomenclature Committee (HGNC). Human Gene Nomenclature Database Search Engine. http://www.gene.ucl.ac.uk/cgi-bin/nomenclature/searchgenes.pl. Accessed February 27, 2004.

3. Online Mendelian Inheritance in Man, OMIM. Baltimore, MD: Johns Hopkins University Press; 2000. http://www.ncbi.nlm.nih.gov/entrez/query.fcgi?db=OMIM. Accessed December 6, 2005.

3.15.9 **E-mail and E-mail List (Listserve) Messages.** References to e-mail and e-mail list messages, like those to other forms of personal communications (see also 3.13.8, Special Print Materials, Unpublished Material), should be listed parenthetically in the text rather than in the reference list and should include the name and highest academic degree(s) of the person who sent the message and the date the message was sent. *Note:* As with all personal communications, permission should be obtained from the author.

An example of an e-mail citation, appearing in running text, is given below:

> There have been no subsequent reports of toxic reactions in the exposed groups (Joan Smith, MD, e-mail communication, March 29, 2004).

An e-mail list (listserve) message cited in running text would be cited as in the example below:

> The Editorial Committee of the World Association of Medical Editors (WAME) is preparing a statement on government embargoes and scientific exchange (Margaret A. Winker, MD, WAME listserve, February 25, 2004).

An e-mail (listserve) thread cited in running text would be cited as in the example below:

> How authors learn writing skills. WAME listserve discussion. October 19-22, 2005. http://www.wame.org/writingskills.htm. Accessed February 15, 2006.

3.15.10 **Online Conference Proceedings/Presentations.** These are treated much the same as a "presented at" reference (see 3.13.8, Special Print Materials, Unpublished Material), with the addition of the URL and the accessed date.

1. Chu H, Rosenthal M. Search engines for the World Wide Web: a comparative study and evaluation methodology. Paper presented at: American Society for Information Science 1996 Annual Conference; October 19-24, 1996; Baltimore, MD. http://www.asis.org/annual-96/electronicproceedings/chu.html. Accessed February 26, 2004.
2. Collins F. Talk presented at: National Human Research Protections Advisory Committee; April 9, 2001; Bethesda, MD. http://www.hhs.gov/ohrp/nhrpac/mtg04-01/0409mtg.txt. Accessed February 26, 2004.

The presentation in example 2 did not have a title; hence, the "title" field and the "presented at" field were combined.

3. Klausner R. Statement on fiscal year 2002 president's budget request for the National Cancer Institute before the House Subcommittee on Labor-HHS-Education Appropriations. http://cancer.gov/legis/testimony/house2002.html. Accessed February 26, 2004.

An audio presentation would be cited as follows:

4. Hormone replacement therapy [Morning Edition audio]. National Public Radio. August 5, 2002. http://www.npr.org/templates/story/story.php?storyId=1147833. Accessed March 4, 2004.

3.15.11 News Releases and Miscellaneous

1. Hopkins response to FDA observations [news release]. Baltimore, MD: Johns Hopkins Office of Communications and Public Affairs; September 7, 2001. http://www.hopkinsmedicine.org/press/2001/SEPTEMBER/010907A.htm. Accessed February 26, 2004.
2. If you want to quit for good—your doctor can help [patient brochure]. Kansas City, MO: Merrell Dow Pharmaceuticals; 1984. http://www.pmdocs.com/PDF/2023799793_9794_0.pdf. Accessed February 26, 2004.

3.15.12 Legal References. Legal references cited online contain the same basic information as legal references cited in print (3.16, US Legal References), with the addition of the URL and the accessed date.

1. US Food and Drug Administration. The Orphan Drug Act. 1983. http://www.fda.gov/orphan/oda.htm. Accessed December 6, 2005.
2. Bybee JS [Office of Legal Counsel, US Department of Justice]. Standards of conduct for interrogation under USC §§2340-2340A [memorandum for Alberto R. Gonzales, August 1, 2002]. http://news.findlaw.com/wp/docs/doj/bybee80102mem.pdf. Accessed December 6, 2005.

3.16 US Legal References. A specific style variation is used for references to legal citations. Because the system of citation used is complex, with numerous variations for different types of sources and among various jurisdictions, only a brief outline can be presented here. For more details, consult *The Bluebook: A Uniform System of Citation.*[19]

Legal references, as with other references (eg, journal, book), may also be cited as electronic references (see 3.15.12, Electronic References, Legal References).

3.16.1 Method of Citation. A legal reference may be included in the reference list in full, with a numbered citation in the text, or it may be included in the text parenthetically and not included in the reference list. In scholarly articles, a full citation in the reference list is preferred, but in a news article or book review, for example, a parenthetical citation in the text might be adequate.

Full Citation

In a leading decision on informed consent,[1] the California Supreme Court stated. . . .

In the case of *Cobbs v Grant*[1]. . . .

This reference would then appear in the reference list as follows:

1. *Cobbs v Grant,* 502 P2d1 (Cal 1972).

Parenthetical In-Text Citation

In a leading decision on informed consent (*Cobbs v Grant,* 502 P2d 1 [Cal 1972]), the California Supreme Court stated . . . .

In the case of *Cobbs v Grant* (502 P2d 1 [Cal 1972]) . . . .

3.16.2 **Citation of Cases.** The citation of a case (ie, a court opinion) generally includes, in the following order:

- The name of the case (including the *v*) in italics. To shorten the case name, use only the names of the first party on each side; omit "et al" and "the"; use only the last names of individuals
- The volume number, abbreviated name, and series number (if any) of the reporter (bound volume of collected cases)
- The page in the volume on which the case begins and, if applicable, the specific page or pages on which is discussed the point for which the case is being cited
- In parentheses, the name of the court that rendered the opinion (unless the court is identified by the name of the reporter) and the year of the decision. If the opinion is published in more than 1 reporter, the citations to each reporter (known as parallel citations) are separated by commas. Note that *v* (for *versus*), 2d (for *second*), and 3d (for *third*) are standard usage in legal citations.

1. *Canterbury v Spence*, 464 F2d 772, 775 (DC Cir 1972).

This case is published in volume 464 of the *Federal Reporter*, second series. The case begins on page 772, and the specific point for which it was cited is on page 775. The case was decided by the US Court of Appeals, District of Columbia Circuit, in 1972.

The proper reporter to cite depends on the court that wrote the opinion. Table T.2 in *The Bluebook*[19] contains a complete list of all current and former state and federal jurisdictions for the United States The 18th edition of *The Bluebook* also has many examples of non-US cases.

US Supreme Court. Cite to *US Reports* (abbreviated as US). If the case is too recent to be published there, cite to *Supreme Court Reporter* (SCt), *US Reports, Lawyer's Edition* (LEd), or *US Law Week* (USLW)—in that order. Do not include parallel citation. The format for these references includes the following, in the order specified (the punctuation is noted; where none is given after a bulleted item, none is used):

- *First party v Second party,*
- Reporter volume number
- Official reporter abbreviation
- First page of case, specific pages used
- (Year of decision).

Some examples follow:

2. *School Board of Nassau City v Arline,* 480 US 273, 287 (1987).
3. *Addington v Texas,* 441 US 418, 426 (1979).

US Court of Appeals (Formerly Known as Circuit Courts of Appeals). Cite to *Federal Reporter*, original or second series (F or F2d). These intermediate appellate-level courts hear appeals from US district courts, federal administrative agencies, and other federal trial-level courts. Circuits are referred to by number (1st Cir, 2d Cir, etc) except for the District of Columbia Circuit (DC Cir) and the Federal Circuit (Fed Cir), which hears appeals from the US Claims Court and from various customs and patent cases. Divisions are denoted by ED (Eastern Division), WD (Western Division), ND (Northern Division), and SD (Southern Division). Citations to the *Federal Reporter* must include the circuit designation in parentheses with the year of the decision. The format for these references includes the following, in the order specified (the punctuation is noted; where none is given after a bulleted item, none is used):

- *First party v second party*,
- Reporter volume number
- Official reporter abbreviation
- First page of case, specific page used
- (Deciding circuit court and year of decision).

Some examples follow:

4. *Wilcox v United States*, 387 F2d 60 (5th Cir 1967).
5. *Scoles v Mercy Health Corp*, 887 F Supp 765 (ED Pa 1994).
6. *Bradley v University of Texas M. D. Anderson Cancer Ctr*, 3 F3d 922, 924 (5th Cir 1993).
7. *Doe v Washington University*, 780 F Supp 628 (ED Mo 1991).

US District Court and Claims Courts. Cite to *Federal Supplement* (F Supp). (There is only the original series so far.) These trial-level courts are not as prolific as the appellate courts; their function is to hear the original cases rather than review them. There are more than 100 of these courts, which are referred to by geographical designations that must be included in the citation (eg, the Northern District of Illinois [ND Ill], the Central District of California [CD Cal], but District of New Jersey [D NJ], as New Jersey has only 1 federal district).

8. *Sierra Club v Froehlke*, 359 F Supp 1289 (SD Tex 1973).

State Courts. Cite to the appropriate official (ie, state-sanctioned and state-financed) reporter (if any) and the appropriate regional reporter. Most states have separate official reporters for their highest and intermediate appellate courts (eg, *Illinois Reports* and *Illinois Appellate Court Reports*), but the regional reporters include cases from both levels. Official reporters are always listed first, although an increasing number of states are no longer publishing them. The regional reporters are the *Atlantic Reporter* (A or A2d), *North Eastern Reporter* (NE or NE2d), *South Eastern Reporter* (SE or SE2d), *Southern Reporter* (So or So2d), *North Western Reporter* (NW or NW2d), *South Western Reporter* (SW or SW2d), and *Pacific Reporter* (P or P2d). If only the regional reporter citation is given, the name of the court must appear in parentheses with the year of the decision. If the opinion is from the highest court of a state (usually but not always known as the supreme court), the abbreviated state name is sufficient (except for Ohio St). The full name of the court is abbreviated (eg, Ill App, NJ Super Ct App Div, NY App Div). A third, also unofficial, reporter is published for a few states; citations solely to these reporters must include the court name (eg, *California Reporter* [Cal Rptr], *New York Supplement* [NYS or NYS2d]). The format for these references includes the following, in the order specified (the punctuation is noted; where none is given after a bulleted item, none is used).

- *First party v second party*,
- Reporter volume number
- Official state reporter abbreviation
- First page of case, specific page used
- Regional reporter and page number
- (Year of decision).

Some examples follow:

9. *People v Carpenter*, 28 Ill2d 116, 190 NE2d 738 (1963).
10. *Webb v Stone*, 445 SW2d 842 (Ky 1969).
11. *Beringer Estate v Princeton Med Ctr*, 592 A2d 1251 (NJ Super Ct Law Div 1991).
12. *Kerins v Hartley*, 21 Cal Rptr 2d 621 (1993) (*vacated* and remanded for reconsideration), 28 Cal Rptr 2d 151 (1994).
13. *Benson v Justin*, 1993 WL 515825 (Minn Ct App).

WL is Westlaw (www.westlaw.com), a legal citation database. A version of Westlaw's database also exists for countries other than the United States (eg, www.westlaw .co.uk for the United Kingdom).

When a case has been reviewed or otherwise dealt with by a higher court, the subsequent history of the case should be given in the citation. If the year is the same for both opinions, include it only at the end of the citation. The phrases indicating the subsequent history are set off by commas, italicized, and abbreviated (eg, *aff'd* [affirmed by the higher court], *rev'd* [reversed], *vacated* [made legally void, annulled], *appeal dismissed*, *cert denied* [application for a writ of certiorari, ie, a request that a court hear an appeal has been denied]).

14. *Glazer v Glazer*, 374 F2d 390 (5th Cir), *cert denied*, 389 US 831 (1967).

This opinion was written by the US Court of Appeals for the Fifth Circuit in 1967. In the same year, the US Supreme Court was asked to review the case in an application for a writ of certiorari but denied the request. This particular subsequent history is important because it indicates that the case has been taken to the highest court available and thus strengthens the case's value as precedent for future legal decisions.

3.16.3 Legislative Materials. The Library of Congress has a Web site (http://thomas.loc .gov) where legislative materials can be found.

Citation of Congressional Hearings. Include the full title of the hearing, the subcommittee (if any) and committee names, the number and session of the Congress, the date, and a short description if desired.

1. *Hearings Before the Consumer Subcommittee of the Senate Committee on Commerce*, 90th Cong, 1st Sess (1965) (testimony of William Stewart, MD, surgeon general).
2. *Discrimination on the Basis of Pregnancy, 1977: Hearings on S995 Before the Subcommittee on Labor of the Senate Committee on Human Resources*, 95th Cong, 1st Sess (1977) (statement of Ethel Walsh, vice-chairman, EEOC).

US Federal Bills and Resolutions. Legislation not yet enacted should include the name of the bill (if available), the abbreviated name of the House of Representatives (HR) or the Senate (S), the number of the bill, the number of the legislative body, the session number (if available), the section (if any), and the year of publication.[19]

3. Medical Error Reduction Act of 2000, S 2038, 106th Cong, 2nd Sess (2000).
4. Voluntary Error Reduction and Improvement in Patient Safety Act, S 2743, 106th Cong, 2nd Sess (2000).
5. Stop All Frequent Errors (SAFE) in Medicare and Medicaid Act of 2000, S 2378, 106th Cong, 2nd Sess (2000).

Numbered US Federal Reports and Documents

6. HR Rep No. 99-253, pt 1, at 54 (1985).
7. Carlton Koepge [author]. The Road to Industrial Peace, HR Doc No. 82-563 (1953).[1]

US Federal Statutes. Once a bill is enacted into law by the US Congress, it is integrated into the US Code (USC). Citations of statutes include the official name of the act, the title number (similar to a chapter number), the abbreviation of the code cited, the section number (designated by §), and the date of the code edition cited.

8. Comprehensive Environmental Response, Compensation, and Liability Act, 42 USC §9601-9675 (1988).

The above example cites sections 9601-9675 of title 42 of the US Code.

If a federal statute has not yet been codified, cite to Statutes at Large (abbreviated Stat, preceded by a volume number, and followed by a page number), if available, and the Public Law number of the statute.

9. Pub L No. 93-627, 88 Stat 2126.

The name of the statute may be added if it provides clarification.

10. Labor Management Relations (Taft-Hartley) Act §301(a), 29 USC §185a (1988).

US Federal Administrative Regulations. Federal regulations are published in the *Federal Register* and then codified in the Code of Federal Regulations. These references to the *Federal Register* are now treated as journal references (see 3.11, References to Print Journals).

11. Importation of fruits and vegetables. *Fed Regist*. 1995;60(51):14202-14209. To be codified at 7 CFR §300.

Regulations promulgated by the Internal Revenue Service retain their unique format. Temporary regulations must be denoted as such.

12. Treas Reg §1.72 (1963).
13. Temp Treas Reg §1.338 (1985).

US State Bills and Resolutions. Legislation should include the name of the bill or resolution (if available), the abbreviated name of the House of Representatives (HR) or the Senate (S), the number of the bill, the number of the legislative body, the session number, and the state abbreviation and the year of enactment.[19]

14. HR 124, 179th Leg, 1st Sess (Pa 1995).

US State Statutes. Table T.2 in *The Bluebook*[19] lists examples for each state.

15. Ill Rev Stat ch 38, §2.

This is section 2 of chapter 38 of Illinois Revised Statutes.

16. Fla Stat §202.

This is section 202 of Florida Statutes.

17. Mich Comp Laws §145.

This is section 145 of Michigan Compiled Laws.

18. Wash Rev Code §45.

This is section 45 of Revised Code of Washington.

19. Cal Corp Code §300.

This is section 300 of California Corporations Code.
Citation forms for state administrative regulations are especially diverse. Again, Table T.2 in *The Bluebook* lists the appropriate form for each state.

Services. Many legal materials, including some reports of cases and some administrative materials, are published by commercial services (eg, Commerce Clearing House), often in loose-leaf format. These services attempt to provide a comprehensive overview of rapidly changing areas of the law (eg, tax law, labor law, securities regulation) and are updated frequently, sometimes weekly. The citation should include the volume number of the service, its abbreviated title, the publisher's name (also abbreviated), the paragraph or section or page number, and the date.

20. 7 Sec Reg Guide (P-H) ¶2333 (1984).

The above example cites volume 7, paragraph 2333, of the *Securities Regulation Guide*, published by Prentice-Hall in 1984.

21. 54 Ins L Rep (CCH) 137 (1979).

This is volume 54, page 137, of *Insurance Law Reports*, published by Commerce Clearing House in 1979.

22. 4 OSH Rep (BNA) 750 (1980).

This is volume 4, page 750, of the *Occupational Safety and Health Reporter*, published by the Bureau of National Affairs in 1980.

Law Journals. Law journal references follow the same rules as medical journal references. List the author(s) (if any), the title of the article, the name of the journal, the volume number, issue number (or date, if there is no issue number), and page number(s).

23. *Doe v Westchester County Med Center, NY State Division of Human Rights. N Y Law J.* December 26, 1990;91:30.
24. Studdert DM, Thomas EJ, Zbar BIW, et al. Can the United States afford a "no-fault" system of compensation for medical injury? *Laws Contemp Probl.* 1997;60(2):1-34.

ACKNOWLEDGMENTS

Principal author: Cheryl Iverson, MA

Coleen Adamson, *JAMA,* and Margaret Mills, *JAMA* and *Archives* Journals, provided helpful research and guidance for the section on Legal References. Paul Frank, *JAMA* and *Archives* Journals, and Monica Mungle, *JAMA* and *Archives* Journals, gave careful review and comments for the section on electronic references.

REFERENCES

1. Yankauer A. The accuracy of medical journal references. *CBE Views.* April 1990;13:38-42.
2. Evans JT, Nadjari HI, Burchell SA. Quotational and reference accuracy in surgical journals: a continuing peer review problem. *JAMA.* 1990;263(10):1353-1354.
3. Shenoy BV. Peer review [letter]. *JAMA.* 1990;264(24):3142.
4. Schofield EK. Accuracy of references [letter]. *CBE Views.* June 1990;13:68.
5. International Committee of Medical Journal Editors. Uniform Requirements for Manuscripts Submitted to Biomedical Journals. http://www.icmje.org. Updated February 2006. Accessed November 29, 2006.
6. Patrias K. *National Library of Medicine Recommended Formats for Bibliographic Citation.* Bethesda, MD: National Library of Medicine, Reference Section; 1991. *Note:* References 6 and 14 in this reference list are being updated and will be available online as a single publication in late 2006, titled *Citing Medicine: The NLM Style Guide for Authors, Editors, and Publishers.*
7. *Books in Print, 2003-2004.* New Providence, NJ: RR Bowker; 2004. Also available at www.booksinprint.com.
8. Style Manual Committee, Council of Science Editors. *Scientific Style and Format: The CSE Manual for Authors, Editors, and Publishers.* 7th ed. New York, NY: Rockefeller University Press, in cooperation with the Council of Science Editors, Reston, VA; 2006.
9. *The Chicago Manual of Style: The Essential Guide for Writers, Editors, and Publishers.* 15th ed. Chicago, IL: University of Chicago Press; 2003.
10. Kronholz J. Bibliography mess: the Internet wreaks havoc with the form: how do you cite a Web page? that's a matter of debate; arguing over a period. *Wall Street Journal.* May 2, 2002:A1, A6.

11. Patrias K; for the CSE Style Manual Committee. Citations to the Internet. *Sci Editor.* 2002;25(3):90-92.
12. *Publication Manual of the American Psychological Association.* 5th ed. Washington, DC: American Psychological Association; 2001.
13. American Psychological Association Web site. http://www.apastyle.org. Accessed February 27, 2004.
14. Patrias K. *National Library of Medicine Recommended Formats for Bibliographic Citation: Supplement: Internet Formats.* Bethesda, MD: National Library of Medicine, Reference Section; 2001.
15. Manuscript Criteria and Information: *Archives of Internal Medicine.* http://archinte.ama-assn.org/ifora_current.dtl. Accessed February 26, 2004.
16. Dellavalle RP, Hester EJ, Heilig LF, et al. Going, going, gone: lost Internet references. *Science.* 2003;302(5646):787-788.
17. The Digital Object Identifier System. International DOI Foundation (IDF). http://www.doi.org/. Updated April 29, 2004. Accessed April 30, 2004.
18. Mullner M, Groves T. Making research papers in the *BMJ* accessible: we're developing ELPS and will soon publish papers shortly after acceptance. *BMJ.* 2002;325(7362):456.
19. *The Bluebook: A Uniform System of Citation.* 18th ed. Cambridge, MA: Harvard Law Review Association; 2005. Also available at www.legalbluebook.com.

4 Visual Presentation of Data

Tables and figures demonstrate relationships among data and other types of information. A well-structured table is perhaps the most efficient way to convey a large amount of data in a scientific manuscript. As text, the same information may take considerably more space; if presented in a figure, key details and precise values may be less apparent.

Text may be preferred if the information can be presented concisely (see Box). For qualitative information, text should be used if the relationships among data are simple and data are few, whereas a figure should be used if the relationships are complex. For quantitative information, a table should be used when the display of exact values is important, whereas a figure (eg, a line graph) should be used to demonstrate patterns or trends. Tables also are often preferable to graphics for small data sets and are preferred when data presentation requires many specific comparisons. Regardless of the presentation, the same data usually should not be duplicated in a table and a figure or in the text.

Priorities in the creation and publication of tables and figures are to emphasize important information efficiently and to ensure that each table and figure makes a clear point. In addition to presenting study results, tables and figures can be used to explain or amplify the methods or highlight other key points in the article. Like a paragraph, each table or figure should be cohesive and focused. To be most effective, tables and figures should present ideas and information in a logical sequence. The relationship of tables and figures to the text and to each other should be considered in manuscript preparation, editorial evaluation and peer review, manuscript editing, and article layout.

When used properly, tables and figures add variety to article layout and are visually compelling and distinct components of scientific publications. However,

Box. Guidelines for Using Text vs Tables vs Figures to Display Data

Uses of Text

Present quantitative data that can be given concisely and clearly

Describe simple relationships among data

Uses of Tables

Present large amounts of detailed quantitative information in a smaller space than would be required in the text

Demonstrate detailed item-to-item comparisons

Display many quantitative values simultaneously

Display individual data values precisely

Demonstrate complex relationships in data

Uses of Figures

Highlight patterns or trends in data

Demonstrate changes or differences over time

Display complex relationships among quantitative variables

Clarify or explain methods

Provide information to enhance understanding of complex concepts

Provide visual data to illustrate findings (eg, slides, photographs, maps)

Illustrate scientific or clinical concepts, mechanisms, or pathophysiology

authors and editors of scientific publications should avoid using tables and figures simply to break up text or to impart visual interest.

4.1 Tables.

Tables. Because of their ability to present detailed information effectively and in ways that text alone cannot, tables are an essential component of many scientific articles. Tables can summarize, organize, and condense complex or detailed data and therefore are commonly used to present study results.

The purpose of a table is to present data or information and support statements in the text. Information in the table must be accurate and consistent with that in the text in content and style. A properly designed and constructed table should be able to stand independently, without requiring explanation from the text.

4.1.1 Types of Tables

Table. A table displays information arranged in columns and rows (Example T1 and 4.1.3, Table Components) and is used most commonly to present numerical data. Each table should have a title, be numbered consecutively as referred to in the text, and be positioned as close as possible to its first mention in the text. Formal tables usually are set off from the text by horizontal rules, boxes, or white space.

Tabulation. A tabulation is a brief, in-text table that may be used to set material off from text. Tabulations require the text to explain their meaning. They are placed directly in the text, unlike a table, which cannot always be placed next to its text citation.

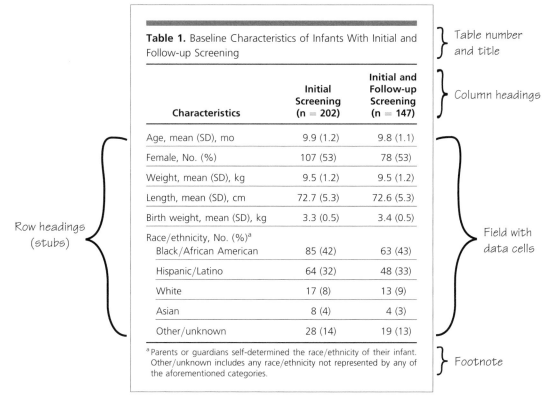

Table 1. Baseline Characteristics of Infants With Initial and Follow-up Screening

Characteristics	Initial Screening (n = 202)	Initial and Follow-up Screening (n = 147)
Age, mean (SD), mo	9.9 (1.2)	9.8 (1.1)
Female, No. (%)	107 (53)	78 (53)
Weight, mean (SD), kg	9.5 (1.2)	9.5 (1.2)
Length, mean (SD), cm	72.7 (5.3)	72.6 (5.3)
Birth weight, mean (SD), kg	3.3 (0.5)	3.4 (0.5)
Race/ethnicity, No. (%)[a]		
Black/African American	85 (42)	63 (43)
Hispanic/Latino	64 (32)	48 (33)
White	17 (8)	13 (9)
Asian	8 (4)	4 (3)
Other/unknown	28 (14)	19 (13)

[a] Parents or guardians self-determined the race/ethnicity of their infant. Other/unknown includes any race/ethnicity not represented by any of the aforementioned categories.

Example T1 Components of a table.

Tabulations usually consist of 1 or 2 columns of data; they generally should not exceed half a column in length. A tabulation is set off from text by the use of space above and below and has boldface column headings. Titles, numbering, and rules are unnecessary. The tabulation should be centered within a single typeset column and may be set in reduced type (Example T2).

younger. A history of smoking was noted in 35 patients (39%), and previous radiation exposure for a condition unrelated to MEC was reported for 10 patients (11%). Presenting symptoms are listed in the following tabulation:

Symptom	**No. (%) of Patients**
Mass in parotid region	87 (98)
Pain or tenderness	13 (15)
Facial nerve weakness	6 (7)
Skin ulceration	3 (3)
Facial twitching	1 (1)
Cervical mass separate from tumor	1 (1)
Other	5 (6)

Some patients presented with more than 1 symptom.

Example T2 In-text tabulation.

Matrix. A matrix is a tabular structure that uses numbers, short words (eg, no, yes), or symbols (eg, bullets, check marks) to depict relationships among items in columns and rows and allow comparisons among entries (Example T3).

Boxes, Sidebars, and Other Nontabular Material. Information that is complementary to the text (eg, lists) can be set off in a box or sidebar within the article (see 4.3, Nontabular Material).

4.1.2 Organizing Information in Tables.

Organizing Information in Tables. For a table to have maximum effectiveness, the information it contains must be arranged logically and clearly so that the reader can quickly understand the key point and find the specific data of interest. Information in tables should be organized into columns and rows by type and category, thereby simplifying access and display of data and information.

During the planning and creation of a table, the author should consider the primary comparisons of interest. Because the English language is read first horizontally (from left to right) and then vertically (from top to bottom), the primary comparisons should be shown horizontally across the table. Data that depict cause-and-effect or before-and-after relationships should be arranged from left to right if space allows or, alternatively, from top to bottom. Information being compared (such as numerical data) should be juxtaposed within adjacent rows or adjacent columns to facilitate comparisons among items of interest. The tables in Example T4 present the same information. Note that the second table more easily allows the reader to compare the changes over time, which is the primary outcome of interest.

Although tables frequently are used to present many quantitative values, authors should remember that tabulating all collected study data is unnecessary and actually may distract and overwhelm the reader. Data presented in a table should be pertinent and meaningful.

The length of the table should also be considered. For ease of reading and practical reasons, a table that would span horizontally or run vertically onto a second page should, if possible, be recast into 2 or more smaller tables. If this is not possible, the table may be set in smaller type. Another option is to publish the table in electronic form only, with a note in the print publication, but the same difficulty with reading large tables in print occurs online as well. In general, tables in print publications can, depending on the content, contain up to 9 or 10 columns of data (including the first column, or stub). Cells that contain words will be wider, thereby reducing the number of columns that will fit.

4.1.3 Table Components.

Table Components. Formal tables in scientific articles conventionally contain 5 major elements: title, column headings, stubs (row headings), body (data field) consisting of individual cells (data points), and footnotes (Example T1). Details pertaining to elements of style for table construction vary among publications; what follows is based on the general style of *JAMA* and the *Archives* Journals.

Title. Each table should have a brief, specific, descriptive title, usually written as a phrase rather than as a sentence, that distinguishes the table from other data displays in the article. The title should convey the topic of the table succinctly but should not provide detailed background information or summarize or interpret the results.

Tables should be numbered consecutively according to the order in which they are mentioned in the text. The word "Table" and the table number are part of the title.

Table 3. Direction of the Association Between Birth Weight and Total Blood Cholesterol and Reported Associations With Other Components of the Lipid Profile in Published Reports of Studies That Had Published Regression Coefficients

Source (Country of Study)	No. of Individuals[a]	Age as Reported in Study (Mean or Range), y	Reported Direction of Birth Weight vs Total Cholesterol Association				Associations Also Reported With				
			Inverse	None	Positive	NA	HDL-C	LDL-C	Triglycerides	ApoA	ApoB
Vestbo,[25] 1996 (Denmark)	620	48	✓								
Suzuki,[31] 2000 (Japan)	299	23	✓						✓		
IJzerman,[33] 2001 (Holland)	228	16	✓				✓	✓	✓	✓	✓
Rona,[39] 1996 (Scotland)[b]	154	9			✓						
Kesteloot,[54] 1975 (Belgium)	303	0	✓				✓				
Owen,[11] 2003 (United Kingdom)	1461	13-16	✓								
Fall,[58] 1992 (United Kingdom)	794	59-70			✓			✓			
Miura,[59] 2001 (Japan)	4951	20	✓								
Lauren,[60] 2002 (Finland)	5792	31	✓						✓		
Bavdekar,[8] 1999 (India)	477	8	✓				✓	✓	✓		
Davies,[63] 2004 (United Kingdom)	25 843	36-39	✓								

Abbreviations: ApoA, apolipoprotein A; ApoB, apolipoprotein B; HDL-C, high-density lipoprotein cholesterol; LDL-C, low-density lipoprotein cholesterol; NA, direction of association not available in the original publication.

[a] Number of individuals on whom regression coefficients in the present analyses are based, which may differ from numbers reported in the original publication.

[b] Association reported in the original publication was obtained by combining results from 5 separate studies.

Example T3 Matrix.

Table 4a. Relative Risk for Death After Onset of Heart Failure Defined by the Framingham Criteria[a]

Year	Men by Age, y			Women by Age, y		
	60	70	80	60	70	80
1979-1984	1 [Reference]	1 [Reference]	1 [Reference]	1 [Reference]	1 [Reference]	1 [Reference]
1985-1990	0.84 (0.69-1.02)	0.84 (0.73-0.97)	0.85 (0.72-1.00)	0.80 (0.63-1.03)	0.91 (0.77-1.06)	1.02 (0.90-1.15)
1991-1995	0.63 (0.50-0.80)	0.74 (0.63-0.88)	0.88 (0.75-1.04)	0.95 (0.73-1.24)	0.99 (0.83-1.18)	1.03 (0.90-1.17)
1996-2000	0.48 (0.36-0.64)	0.59 (0.49-0.71)	0.72 (0.61-0.87)	0.67 (0.48-0.92)	0.79 (0.64-0.98)	0.94 (0.82-1.09)

[a] Data are presented as relative risk (95% confidence interval).

Table 4b. Relative Risk for Death After Onset of Heart Failure Defined by the Framingham Criteria

Age, y	Relative Risk (95% Confidence Interval)			
	1979-1984	1985-1990	1991-1995	1996-2000
		Men		
60	1 [Reference]	0.84 (0.69-1.02)	0.63 (0.50-0.80)	0.48 (0.36-0.64)
70	1 [Reference]	0.84 (0.73-0.97)	0.74 (0.63-0.88)	0.59 (0.49-0.71)
80	1 [Reference]	0.85 (0.72-1.00)	0.88 (0.75-1.04)	0.72 (0.61-0.87)
		Women		
60	1 [Reference]	0.80 (0.63-1.03)	0.95 (0.73-1.24)	0.67 (0.48-0.92)
70	1 [Reference]	0.91 (0.77-1.06)	0.99 (0.83-1.18)	0.79 (0.64-0.98)
80	1 [Reference]	1.02 (0.90-1.15)	1.03 (0.90-1.17)	0.94 (0.82-1.09)

Example T4 The first table is formatted with the primary comparison—years of study—running vertically (especially evident in reading the first row across). The second table is formatted with the primary outcome running horizontally.

If the article contains only 1 table, it is referred to in the text as "Table." The capitalization style used in article titles should be followed for table titles (see 3.9, References, Titles). The following are examples of table titles:

> **Table 1.** Symptoms and Signs of Chronic Fatigue Syndrome
>
> **Table.** Relationship of Blood Pressure and Intraocular Pressure in Patients With Open-Angle Glaucoma

Column Headings. The main categories of information in the table should have separate columns. In tables for studies that have independent and dependent variables, the independent variables conventionally are displayed in the left-hand column (stub) and the dependent variables in the columns to the right. Each column should have a brief heading that identifies and applies to all items listed in that column. The stub, however, may not require a heading, particularly if the elements in the stubs are very different. If relevant, the unit of measure should be indicated in the column heading (unless it is given in the table stub) and is preceded by a comma. Column headings are set in boldface type. If necessary, column subheadings may be used. For more complex headings, braces may be used (Example T4) or additional explanatory information may be provided in the footnotes.

If all elements in a column are identical (eg, if all patients were women and a column indicated the patients' sex), this information could be provided in a footnote or in the table title and the column deleted.

In column headings, style guidelines regarding numbers (eg, use of ordinals) and abbreviations may be relaxed somewhat to save space, with abbreviations expanded in a footnote. However, when space allows spelled-out headings, expansions are preferable to abbreviations. The capitalization style used in titles should be followed (see 3.9, References, Titles).

Table Stubs (Row Headings). The left-most column of a table contains the table stubs (or row headings), which are used to label the rows of the table and apply to all items in that row. If a unit of measure is not included in the column heading, it should be included in the stub. Stubs are capitalized according to style for sentences, not titles. Therefore, if a symbol (such as %), an arabic numeral, or a lowercase Greek letter (such as β) begins the entry, the first word to follow should be capitalized. Stubs are left-justified, and indentions are used to depict hierarchical components of the stubs (Example T5). However, some publications use bold stubs or shading instead.

For a table that may be readily divided into parts to enhance clarity or for 2 closely related tables that would be better combined, cut-in headings may be considered.[1] The cut-in heading is placed above the table columns (below the column heads) and applies to all tabular material below. Cut-in headings are set boldface, are centered, and have a rule above (but not below) them (Example T6). However, cut-in headings may interfere with downward scanning and thus should be used with care.[2]

Both column headings and stubs should be consistent in style and presentation between tables in the same article.

Field. The field or body of the table presents the data. Each data entry point is contained in a cell, which is the intersection of a column and a row. Table cells may contain numerals, text, symbols, or a combination of these. Data in the field should be arranged logically so the reader can find an individual data point in the table easily. For instance, time order should be used for data collected in sequence (Example T4). Similar types of data should be grouped. Numbers that are added or averaged should be placed in the same column. Text in the field cells should be capitalized in sentence style (ie, the first word is capitalized and all that follow in the cell are lowercased).

Missing data and blank space in the table field (ie, an empty cell) may create ambiguity and should be avoided, unless an entry in a cell does not apply (eg, a column head does not apply to one of the stub items).[1] The numeral 0 should be used to indicate that the value of the data in the cell is zero. An ellipsis (. . .) may be used to indicate that no data are available for a cell or that the category of data is not

Table 5. Characteristics of Patients With Ischemic Stroke Treated With Intravenous Tissue Plasminogen Activator (tPA)[a]

Characteristics	All Patients Treated With tPA, No. (%) (n = 1658)
Age group, y	
<55	294 (17.7)
55-64	443 (26.7)
65-74	525 (31.7)
≥75	396 (23.9)
Sex	
Female	697 (42.0)
Male	961 (58.0)
Time from stroke onset to hospital admission, h	
<3	1508 (91.0)
≥3	150 (9.0)
Comorbidities	
Diabetes mellitus	395 (23.8)
Hypertension	1158 (69.8)
Previous stroke	180 (10.9)
Atrial fibrillation	496 (29.9)
Neurological signs	
Weakness/paresis	1436 (86.6)
Aphasia	777 (46.9)
Dysarthria	580 (35.0)
Disturbed level of consciousness	407 (24.6)
Hospital experience with tPA use per year	
<6	277 (16.7)
6-15	706 (42.6)
>15	675 (40.7)

[a] Analyses were restricted to patients without missing values.

Example T5 Hierarchy of stubs.

applicable for a cell. However, ellipses should not be used to denote different types of missing elements in the same table. Other designations such as NA (for "not available," "not analyzed," or "not applicable") may be used, provided their meaning is explained in a footnote (Example T7).

Blank cells may be acceptable when an entire section of the table does not contain data (Example T8).

Totals. Totals and percentages in tables should correspond to values presented in the text and abstract and should be verified for accuracy. Any discrepancies (eg, because of rounding) should be explained in a footnote.

Table 6. Trial Enrollment for Minorities vs Whites According to Cancer Type, 2000-2002

Racial/Ethnic Group	No. of Trial Participants	Enrollment Fraction, %	Odds Ratio (95% CI)	*P* Value
	All Cancers			
Total	37 635	1.7		
White	32 633	1.8	1 [Reference]	
Hispanic	1094	1.3	0.72 (0.68-0.77)	<.001
Black	3062	1.3	0.71 (0.68-0.74)	<.001
Asian/Pacific Islander	745	1.7	0.95 (0.88-1.02)	.16
American Indian/Alaskan Native	101	2.5	1.44 (1.18-1.76)	<.001
	Breast Cancer			
Total	19 893	3.2		
White	17 344	3.3	1 [Reference]	
Hispanic	635	2.4	0.71 (0.66-0.77)	<.001
Black	1393	2.5	0.74 (0.70-0.79)	<.001
Asian/Pacific Islander	465	3.1	0.95 (0.86-1.04)	.27
American Indian/Alaskan Native	56	4.5	1.37 (1.05-1.80)	.02
	Colorectal Cancer			
Total	8434	1.9		
White	7408	2.0	1 [Reference]	
Hispanic	264	1.5	0.74 (0.66-0.84)	<.001
Black	578	1.3	0.64 (0.59-0.70)	<.001
Asian/Pacific Islander	161	1.5	0.76 (0.64-0.88)	<.001
American Indian/Alaskan Native	23	2.5	1.30 (0.86-1.97)	.21

Example T6 Cut-in headings divide the table into related sections.

Boldface type for true totals (ie, those that represent sums of values in the table) should be used with discretion. Boldface should not be used to overemphasize data in the table (eg, significant odds ratios or *P* values).

Alignment of Data. Horizontal alignment (across rows) must be considered in setting tables. If the table stubs contain lines of text that exceed the width of the stub column (runover lines in the table stub) and the cell entries in that row do not, the field entries should be aligned across the first or top line of the table stub entry (Example T9). This top-line alignment of data applies to tables that have numbers, words, or both as cell entries. If some entries within the table field contain information that cannot be contained on a single line in the cell (runover lines in the table field), the table entries in that row also should be aligned across on the first line of the stub entry.

Table 7. Physical Risks From Sports in the Daily Lives of Healthy Children Older Than 6 Years[a]

	Risk per Million Instances of Participation				
Sport	**Total Injuries**	**Permanent Disability**	**Total Level IV Injuries[b]**	**Surgeries**	**Broken Bones**
Football	3800	42	500	270	910
Soccer	2400	38	300	NA	NA
Basketball	1900	58	300	160	180
Cheerleading	1700	NA	100	NA	NA
Baseball	1400	61	300	120	30
Skateboarding	800	NA	200	20	170

Abbreviation: NA, not available.

[a] Data adapted from American Sports Data Inc.[28]

[b] Those resulting in emergency department treatment, overnight hospital stay, surgery, or ongoing physical therapy and preventing participation in sports for at least 1 month.

Example T7 Use of "NA" to clarify cells with no data.

Vertical alignment within each column of a table is important for the visual presentation of data. Whenever possible, columns of data should be aligned on common elements, such as decimal points, plus or minus signs, hyphens (used in ranges), virgules, or parentheses (Example T8). If table entries consist of lengthy text, the flush-left format should be used with an indent for runover lines. If entries in a column are mixed (ie, if no common element exists or if the numbers vary greatly in magnitude), primary consideration should be given to the visual aspects of the entire table and the type of material being presented.

Rules and Shading. For *JAMA* and the *Archives* Journals, tables should be submitted without rules drawn in (as opposed to table borders, which are appropriate) or shading. If these elements are included they will have to be manually removed during the editing process (see 4.1.9, Guidelines for Preparing and Submitting Tables).

Many journals add rules and shading during the production process. For example, *JAMA* uses horizontal rules to separate rows of data (Example T8). Other journals use shading for the same purpose.

Footnotes. Footnotes may contain information about the entire table, portions of the table (eg, a column), or a discrete table entry. The order of the footnotes is determined by the placement in the table of the item to which the footnote refers. The letter for a footnote that applies to the entire table (eg, one that explains the method used to gather the data or format of data presentation) should be placed after the table title (Example T4). A footnote that applies to 1 or 2 columns or rows should be placed after the column heading(s) or stub(s) to which it refers (Example T7). A footnote that applies to a single entry in the table or to several individual entries should be placed at the end of each entry to which it applies (Example T10).

Table 8. Characteristics of Cases of Nonfatal Suicidal Behavior and Matched Controls[a]

	No. (%)				
Characteristics	**Cases (n = 555)**		**Controls (n = 2062)**		**OR (95% CI)**
Sex					
Female	363	65.4	1378	66.8	
Male	192	34.6	684	33.2	
Age, y					
10-19	68	12.3	235	11.4	
20-29	177	31.9	655	31.8	
30-39	134	24.1	514	24.9	
40-49	107	19.3	405	19.6	
50-59	48	8.7	175	8.5	
60-69	21	3.8	78	3.8	
Smoking status					
Nonsmoker	184	33.2	728	35.3	1 [Reference]
Smoker	39	7.0	211	10.2	0.72 (0.49-1.06)
Ex-smoker	27	4.9	119	5.8	0.89 (0.56-1.42)
Unknown	305	55.0	1004	48.7	1.21 (0.97-1.50)
Body mass index					
< 24	207	37.3	747	36.2	1 [Reference]
24-28	112	20.2	399	19.4	1.01 (0.77-1.32)
> 28	69	12.4	318	15.4	0.85 (0.62-1.17)
Unknown	167	30.1	598	29.0	1.03 (0.81-1.32)

Abbreviation: CI, confidence interval.

[a] Controls were matched to cases by age, sex, index date, and duration of recorded history in the UK General Practice Research Database before the index date. Odds ratios (ORs) for smoking and body mass index, which is calculated as weight in kilograms divided by height in meters squared, are conditional on the matching factors and adjusted for antidepressant drug and time since starting the antidepressant.

Example T8 Blank cells without definition. Because the footnote indicates that sex and age were matching variables, no data appear in those cells.

For both tables and figures, footnotes are indicated with superscript lowercase letters in alphabetical order (a-z). The font size of the footnote letters should be large enough to see clearly without appearing to be part of the actual data. While some publications (including, formerly, *JAMA* and the *Archives* Journals) use symbols (*, †, etc) to indicate footnotes in tables, such symbols are ordered arbitrarily and are limited in number. Use of superscript letters ensures a logical order to the entries and a much larger supply of notations (26 characters). For tables in which superscript numbers and/or letters are used to display data, care should be taken to ensure that

Table 9. Thrombosis Related to the Interval Between Symptom Onset and Surgery in Patients With Stroke

	Interval Between the Acute Cerebral Event and Carotid Endarterectomy, No. (%)				
	0-2 mo (32 Cases)	3-6 mo (18 Cases)	7-12 mo (15 Cases)	13-24 mo (13 Cases)	25-30 mo (18 Cases)
Thrombotically active plaque	32 (100)	13 (72.2)	11 (73.3)	7 (53.8)	8 (44.4)
Only organized thrombosis	0	4 (22.2)	4 (26.7)	5 (38.5)	10 (55.6)
No thrombosis	0	1 (5.6)	0	1 (7.7)	0

Example T9 Alignment of data with the first line in the stub entry.

superscript footnote letters are distinguished clearly from superscripts used for data elements (for example, see Table 15.1.2, Nomenclature, Blood Groups, Platelet Antigens, and Granulocyte Antigens, Platelet-Specific Antigens). In these situations, use of the symbol footnotes may help avoid confusion.

Footnotes are listed at the bottom of the table, each on its own line. However, to save space, tables with more than a few footnotes can run them in 2 columns (Example T10).

Footnotes may be phrases or complete sentences and should end with a period. Any operational signs, such as <, >, or =, imply a verb. For example, $P = .01$ is considered a complete sentence ("P is equal to .01.") when used as a table footnote. Footnote letters should appear before the footnote text and are followed by a space for clarity. In *JAMA* and the *Archives* Journals, the abbreviations and units of measure conversion footnotes appear first and are set off with an introductory word or phrase instead of a letter. In addition, abbreviations are expanded in alphabetical order; units of measure and applicable conversion factors are listed in a separate footnote (Example T11).

If several tables share a detailed or long footnote that explains several abbreviations or methods, this footnote may appear in the first table for which it is applicable, and a footnote in each succeeding table for which the footnote also is applicable may refer the reader to the first appearance of the detailed information:

> Study acronyms are explained in the first footnote to Table 1.

The reader also may be referred to a relevant discussion in the text by a footnote:

> See the "Statistical Analysis" section for a description of this procedure.

Several of the most common uses of footnotes include the following.

To expand abbreviations:

> Abbreviations: CI, confidence interval; OR, odds ratio.

Table 10. Baseline Values by Treatment Group

Variable	CBT With Fluoxetine	Fluoxetine Alone	CBT Alone	Placebo	Total	*P* Value
	Characteristics for Depression, Suicidality, and Functioning[a]					
No. of persons randomized	107	109	111	112	439	
Children's Depression Rating Scale-Revised Raw score[b]	60.75 (11.58)	58.96 (10.16)	59.58 (9.21)	61.11 (10.50)	60.10 (10.39)	.38
T score[c]	75.67 (6.53)	74.73 (6.74)	75.37 (6.32)	76.14 (6.11)	75.48 (6.43)	.43
Clinical Global Impressions Improvement score[d]	4.79 (0.85)	4.66 (0.85)	4.77 (0.76)	4.84 (0.84)	4.77 (0.83)	.43
Children's Global Assessment score[e]	49.95 (7.52)	49.49 (7.26)	50.01 (7.58)	49.13 (7.59)	49.64 (7.47)	.79
Reynolds Adolescent Depression total score[f]	79.91 (13.68)	77.00 (14.67)	78.83 (14.97)	81.20 (13.94)	79.24 (14.35)	.18
Suicidal Ideation Questionnaire Junior High School Version total score[g]	27.32 (24.64)	21.86 (19.22)	22.03 (21.36)	23.69 (21.66)	23.71 (21.83)	.57[h]
Current major depressive episode duration, wk	83.07 (94.00)	70.92 (94.33)	71.71 (70.14)	61.16 (67.45)	71.59 (82.35)	.28[h]
	Comorbidity at Baseline by Treatment Group[i]					
Comorbidity						
Any, No. (%)[j]	59 (55.66)	47 (43.12)	64 (58.18)	57 (51.35)	227 (52.06)	.13
Amount	0.88 (1.04)	0.83 (1.20)	0.93 (1.09)	0.90 (1.13)	0.88 (1.11)	.50
Dysthymia, No. (%)	11 (10.28)	6 (5.50)	17 (15.45)	12 (10.71)	46 (10.50)	.12
Type of disorder, No. (%)						
Anxiety	30 (28.04)	26 (23.85)	36 (32.43)	28 (25.23)	120 (27.40)	.50[h]
Disruptive behavior	23 (21.50)	25 (22.94)	27 (24.32)	28 (25.00)	103 (23.46)	.93
Obsessive-compulsive/tic	4 (3.74)	2 (1.83)	2 (1.80)	4 (3.57)	12 (2.73)	.73[k]
Substance use	3 (2.80)	3 (2.75)	1 (0.90)	0	7 (1.59)	.23[k]
Attention-deficit/hyperactivity	14 (13.08)	13 (11.93)	14 (12.61)	19 (16.96)	60 (13.67)	.70
Taking medications	4 (3.74)	3 (2.75)	4 (3.60)	10 (8.93)	21 (4.78)	.12[k]

Abbreviation: CBT, cognitive behavior therapy.

[a] Values are expressed as mean (SD) unless otherwise indicated.
[b] The range for possible scores is 17 to 113.
[c] The range for possible scores is 30 to 55.
[d] The range for possible scores is 1 to 7.
[e] The range for possible scores is 1 to 100.
[f] The range for possible scores is 30 to 120.
[g] The range for possible scores is 0 to 90.
[h] Norparametric Kruskal-Wallis test.
[i] *P* values are for the χ^2 test unless otherwise indicated.
[j] Refers to the presence of 1 or more coexisting psychiatric disorders, including dysthymia.
[k] Fisher exact test.

Example T10 When tables have many footnotes they can be presented in 2 columns instead of with a single footnote on each line.

Table 11. Distribution of Lipid and C-Reactive Protein Levels at Study Entry Among 15 632 Initially Healthy Women

	Percentile Cutoffs						
	5th	**10th**	**25th**	**50th**	**75th**	**90th**	**95th**
Cholesterol, mg/dL							
Total	149	161	181	206	234	263	283
LDL	76	85	102	124	147	171	187
HDL	32	35	41	49	59	69	77
Non-HDL	98	109	129	155	184	213	234
Apolipoprotein, mg/dL							
A-I	110	116	127	140	156	171	181
B-100	62	70	83	99	121	140	153
High-sensitivity CRP, mg/L	0.2	0.3	0.6	1.5	3.5	6.6	9.1
Ratio							
Total cholesterol to HDL cholesterol	2.6	2.8	3.4	4.1	5.2	6.2	7.0
LDL cholesterol to HDL cholesterol	1.3	1.5	1.9	2.5	3.3	4.0	4.5
Apolipoprotein B-100 to apolipoprotein A-I	0.41	0.46	0.57	0.71	0.89	1.08	1.21
Apolipoprotein B_{100} to HDL cholesterol	0.97	1.1	1.5	2.0	2.8	3.6	4.2

Abbreviations: CRP, C-reactive protein; HDL, high-density lipoprotein; LDL, low-density lipoprotein.
SI conversion factors: To convert HDL, LDL, and total cholesterol to mmol/L, multiply by 0.0259.

Example T11 Footnotes including separate entries for abbreviations (in alphabetical order) and unit of measure conversion information.

To designate reporting of numerical values:

> [a] Scores are based on a scale of 1 to 10, with 1 indicating least severe and 10, most severe.

To provide information on statistical analyses or experimental methods:

> [b] Adjusted for age, smoking status, and body mass index.

To explain a discrepancy in numerical data:

> [a] Because of rounding, percentages may not total 100.

To cite references for information used in the table. References are given as in the text and are designated with superscript arabic numbers:

> [c] Classified using *International Classification of Health Problems in Primary Care.*[45]

To acknowledge that data in the table are taken from or based on data from another source:

[a] Data from the US Census Bureau.[5]

To acknowledge credit for reproduction of a table. If the table has been reprinted or modified with permission from another source, credit should be given in a footnote:

[a] Adapted with permission from the American Medical Association.[41]

References for information in a table or figure should be numbered and listed as if this information were part of the text. For instance, if the source from which the material referred to in the table or figure is one of the references used in the text, that reference number should be used in the table or figure. If the reference pertains only to the table or figure (ie, the source is not cited elsewhere in the text), the reference should be listed and numbered according to the first mention of the table or figure in the text (see 3.6, References, Citation). All references in an article should appear in the reference list.

Note that references cited at the end of table titles are ambiguous. Instead, a footnote should be added with an explanation that it was

Adapted from . . .

Reproduced with permission from . . .

Data were derived from . . .

When both a footnote letter and reference number follow data in a table, set the reference number first followed by a comma and the letter (see also 3.6, References, Citation).

427 Patients[5,b]

4.1.4 **Units of Measure.** *JAMA* and the *Archives* Journals report laboratory values in conventional units (see 14.12, Abbreviations, Units of Measure, and 18.0, Units of Measure). In tables, units of measure, including the variability of the measurement if reported, should follow a comma in the table column heading or stub. The following are examples of stub entries with units of measure:

Age, mean (SD), y

Systolic blood pressure, mean (SD), mm Hg

Body mass index, median (IQR)

Duration of hypertension, mean (SD) [range], y

Change in rate, % (SE)

JAMA and the *Archives* Journals use a conversion footnote to indicate how to convert values to the SI or another system (Example T11).

4.1.5 **Punctuation.** As with numbers and abbreviations, rules for punctuation may be less restrictive in tables to save space (see 8.0, Punctuation). For example, slashes may be used to present dates (eg, 04/27/03 for April 27, 2003) and hyphens may be used to present ranges (eg, 60-90 for 60 to 90) (see 19.0, Numbers and Percentages). Phrases and sentences in tables may use end punctuation if required for readability (eg, if cells contain multisentence entries).

4.1.6 **Abbreviations.** Within the body of the table and in column headings, units of measure and numbers normally spelled out may be abbreviated for space considerations (see 14.12, Abbreviations, Units of Measure; 18.0, Units of Measure; and 19.0, Numbers and Percentages). However, spelled-out words should not be combined with abbreviations for units of measure. For example, "First Week" or "1st wk" or "Week 1" may be used as a column heading, but not "First wk." Abbreviations or acronyms should be explained in a footnote (see 4.1.3, Table Components, Footnotes).

4.1.7 **Numbers.** Additional digits (including zeros) should not be added, eg, after the decimal point, to provide all data entries with the same number of digits. Doing so may indicate more precise results than actually were calculated or measured. A percentage or decimal quotient should contain no more than the number of digits in the denominator. For example, the percentage for the proportion 9 of 28 should be reported as 32% (or decimal quotient 0.32), not 32.1% (or 0.321) (see 20.8, Statistics, Significant Digits and Rounding Numbers). Values reporting laboratory data should be provided and rounded, if appropriate, according to the number of digits that reflects the precision of the reported results to eliminate reporting results beyond the sensitivity of the procedure performed (see 18.4.1, Units of Measure, Use of Numerals With Units, Expressing Quantities).

Values for reporting statistical data, such as *P* values and confidence intervals, also should be presented and rounded appropriately (see 20.8, Study Design and Statistics, Significant Digits and Rounding Numbers). Although some publications[2(p512)] suggest use of specific designations for levels of significance (eg, a single asterisk in the table to denote values for entries for which $P<.05$, a dagger for $P<.01$), exact *P* values are preferred, regardless of statistical significance. In most cases, *P* values should be expressed to 2 digits to the right of the decimal point, unless the first 2 digits are zeros, in which case 3 digits to the right of the decimal place should be provided (eg, $P=.002$). *P* values less than .001 should be designated as "$P<.001$," rather than using exact values, eg, $P=.00006$. For study outcomes, individual statistically significant values should not be expressed as "$P<.05$" either in the table or in the table footnote, and nonsignificant *P* values should not be expressed as "NS" (not significant). For confidence intervals, the number of digits should correspond to the number of digits in the point estimate. For instance, for an odds ratio reported as 2.45, the 95% confidence interval should be reported as 1.32 to 4.78, not as 1.322 to 4.784.

4.1.8 **Tables That Contain Supplementary Information.** Tables that contain important supplementary information that is too extensive to be published in the journal article may be made available from other sources. These tables may be available from the author or by electronic means (eg, online database, journal Web site, CD-ROM). Supplementary tables posted on the *JAMA* and *Archives* Journals Web site undergo review and editing because they are considered part of the journal's content.

4.1.9 Guidelines for Preparing and Submitting Tables. Authors submitting tables in a scientific article should consult the publication's instructions for authors for specific requirements and preferences regarding table format. Although details about preferred table construction vary among journals, several general guidelines apply. Each table should be created by means of a table editor program in word processing software or a spreadsheet program and inserted in the electronic manuscript file. Reduced type should not be used. If a table is too large to be contained on 1 manuscript page, the table should be continued on another page with a "continued" line following the title on the subsequent page. Alternatively, if the table is large or exceedingly complex, the author should consider separating the data into 2 or more simpler tables. Tables should not be submitted on oversized paper, as a graphic image, or as photographic prints.

The following table creation instructions for authors appear on the *JAMA* Web site:

Author Instructions for Table Creation

Creating the table

Use the table editor of the word processing software to build a table. Regardless of which program is used, each piece of data needs to be contained in its own cell in the table.

Avoid creating tables using spaces or tabs. Such tables must be retyped during the editing process, creating delays and opportunities for error. Do not try to align cells with hard returns or extra spaces. Similarly, no cell should contain a hard return or tab. Although individual empty cells are acceptable in a table, be sure there are no empty columns.

Each row of data must be in a separate row of cells:

Table 1. Title

Treatment	Group A	Group B
Medical	500	510
Surgical	500	490

Note that percentages are presented in the same cell as numbers and measures of variability are in the same cell as their corresponding statistic:

Table 2. Title

Characteristics	Group A (n=50)	Group B (n=50)	Relative Risk (95% CI)
Women, No. (%)	25 (50)	20 (40)	1.25 (1.11-1.57)
Age, mean (SD), y	35 (8)	37 (7)	0.98 (0.92-1.05)

To indicate data that span more than 1 row, do not merge the cells vertically. Instead, put the data in a cell near the middle of the rows. In the example below, the final column lists the *P* value for the overall age comparison and will be bracketed to indicate the comparison:

Table 3. Title

Age, y	Blood Pressure, mm Hg	*P* Value
18-34	120/75	
35-50	110/80	.08
51-80	125/82	

Do not draw lines or rules—the table grid feature will display the outlines of each cell.

4.2 Figures. The term *figure* refers to any graphical display used to present information or data,[1] including statistical graphs, maps, algorithms, illustrations, computer-generated images, and photographs. Figures may be used to clarify or explain methods, to present evidence and quantitative results, to highlight trends and relationships among data, to clarify complex concepts, or to illustrate items or procedures. Figures should be accurate, clear, and concise.

In scientific articles, selection of a particular type of figure depends on the purpose and type of information being displayed. Some of the most common types of figures in biomedical publications are discussed herein.

4.2.1 Statistical Graphs

Line Graphs. Line graphs have 2 or 3 axes with continuous quantitative scales on which data points connected by curves demonstrate the relationship between 2 or more quantitative variables, such as changes over time. Line graphs usually are designed with the dependent variable on the vertical axis (y-axis) and the independent variable on the horizontal axis (x-axis)[3] (Example F1, Example F2).

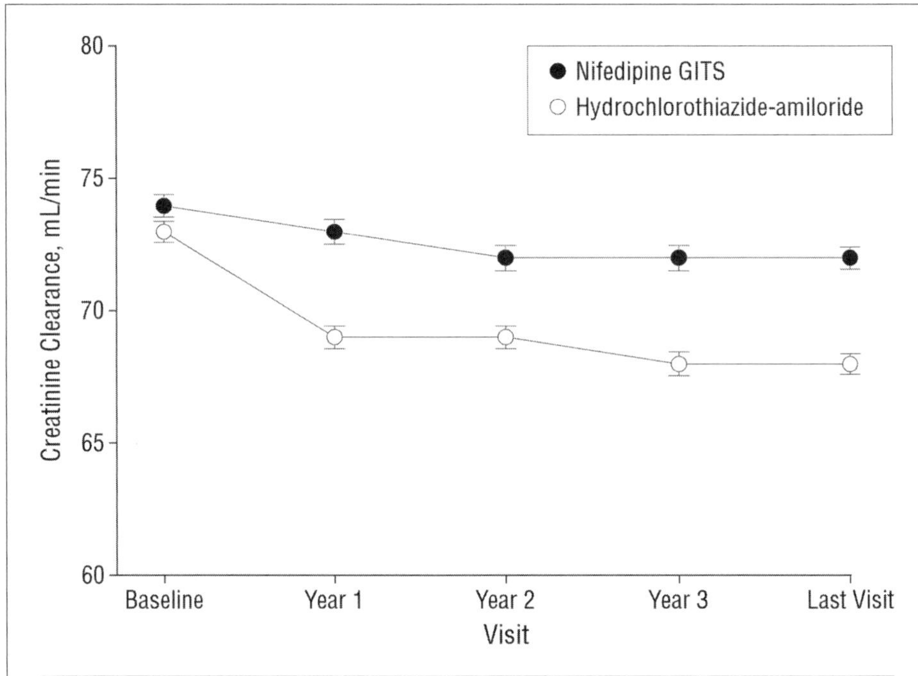

Figure 1. Creatinine clearance at baseline and at annual visits in patients treated with either nifedipine gastrointestinal therapeutic system (GITS) or hydrochlorothiazide-amiloride. Error bars indicate SD. To convert creatinine clearance to milliliters per second, multiply by 0.0167.

Example F1 Line graph with the dependent variable on the vertical axis (y-axis) and the independent variable on the horizontal axis (x-axis).

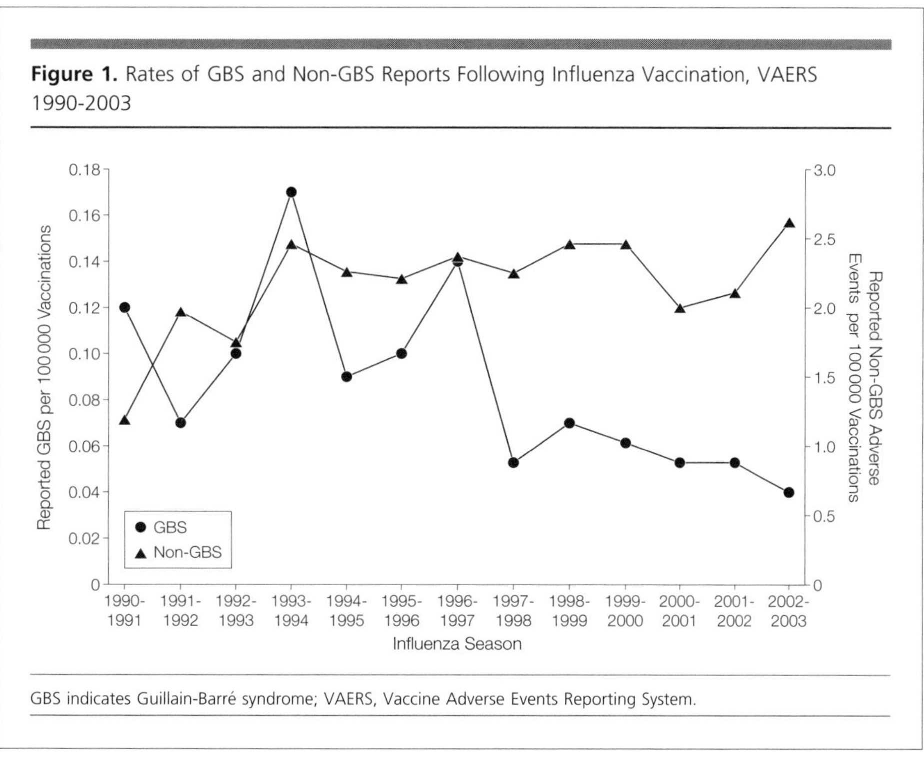

Figure 1. Rates of GBS and Non-GBS Reports Following Influenza Vaccination, VAERS 1990-2003

GBS indicates Guillain-Barré syndrome; VAERS, Vaccine Adverse Events Reporting System.

Example F2 Line graph with 3 axes to facilitate comparison of related data.

Survival Plots. Survival plots of time-to-event outcomes, such as from Kaplan-Meier analyses (see Figure 3 in 20.0, Study Design and Statistics), display the proportion of individuals, represented on the y-axis as a proportion or percentage, remaining free of or experiencing a specific outcome over time, represented on the x-axis. When the outcome of interest is relatively frequent (occurs in approximately ≥70% of the study population), event-free survival is plotted on the y-axis from 0 to 1.0 (or 0% to 100%), with the curve starting at 1.0 (100%). When the outcome is relatively infrequent (occurs in <30% of the study population), it is preferable to plot upward starting at 0 so that the curves can be seen without breaking or truncating the y-axis scale.[4] The curve should be drawn as a step function (not smoothed).

The number of individuals followed up for each time interval (number at risk) should be shown underneath the x-axis. Time-to-event estimates become less certain as the number of individuals diminishes, so consideration should be given to not displaying data when less than 20% of the study population is still in follow-up.[4] Plots should include some indication of statistical uncertainty, such as error bars on the curves at regular time points or, when time-to-event data are being compared for 2 or more groups, an overall estimate of treatment difference, such as a relative risk (with 95% confidence interval) or log-rank *P* value (Example F3).

Scatterplots. In scatterplots, individual data points are plotted according to coordinate values with continuous, quantitative x- and y-axis scales. By convention,

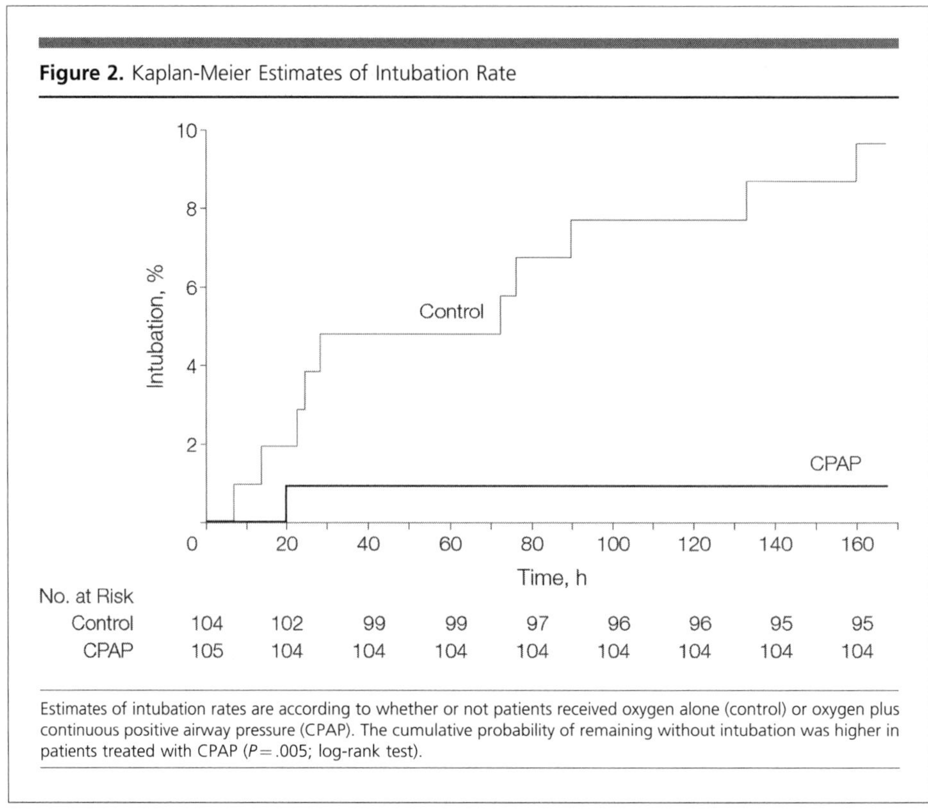

Example F3 Survival curve with the curves clearly marked by study group. The number of study participants at risk is listed under each major time point and a log-rank *P* value is included in the legend.

independent variables are plotted on the x-axis and dependent variables on the y-axis. Data markers are not connected by a curve, but a curve that is generated mathematically may be fitted to the data and summarize the relationship among the variables. The statistical method used to generate the curve and the statistic that summarizes the relationship between the dependent and independent variables, such as a correlation or regression coefficient, should be provided in the figure or legend (Example F4).

Histograms and Frequency Polygons. Histograms and frequency polygons display the distribution of data in a data set by plotting the frequency (count or percentages) of observations (y-axis) for each interval represented on the x-axis. In both histograms and frequency polygons, the y-axis must begin at 0 and should not be broken, and the x-axis is a continuous, quantitative scale. Histograms use continuous bars of equal widths determined by the x-axis intervals, where bar height represents frequency (Example F5).

Frequency polygons use data markers to represent frequency connected by a curve. Data distributions from 2 data sets that overlap can be plotted in a frequency polygon but not in a histogram (Example F6).

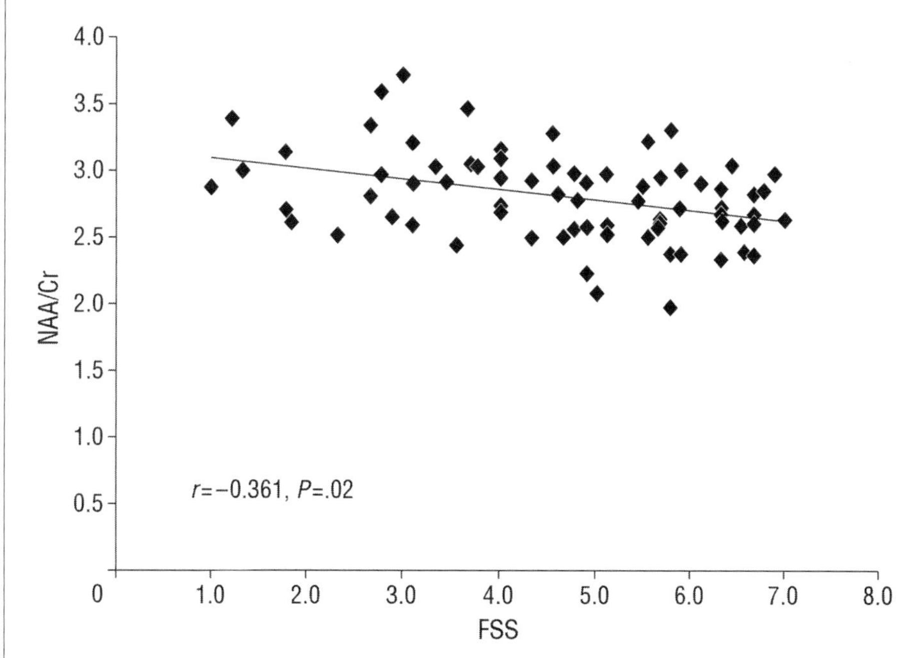

Figure 3. Scatterplot showing the relationship between Fatigue Severity Scale (FSS) score and the *N*-acetylaspartate–creatine (NAA/Cr) ratio. Solid line represents the linear regression fit across all subjects. Spearman rank correlation coefficient and Bonferroni-corrected *P* value are shown.

Example F4 Scatterplot including the regression line, correlation coefficient, and *P* value in the plot.

Bar Graphs. Bar graphs have a single axis and are used to display frequencies (counts or percentages) on the axis according to categories shown on a baseline. A bar graph is typically vertical, with frequencies shown on a vertical y-axis (Example F7), but may be horizontal (Example F8). Data in each category are represented by a bar. Bars should have the same width, be separated by a space, and be wider than the space between them. Bar lengths are proportional to frequency, the scale on the frequency axis should begin at 0, and the axis should not be broken. All bars must have a common baseline to facilitate comparison.[5] Categories of data should be presented in logical order and consistently with other figures and tables in the article. The baseline of a bar graph is not a coordinate axis and therefore should not have tick marks.

Bar graphs may be used to compare frequencies between groups. In most cases, the number of bars in a grouped bar graph should not exceed 3. Colors or tones used to designate each group should be distinct. To ensure that bars in black-and-white figures are distinguishable, a contrast in shading of at least 30% for adjacent bars is suggested. Color or shades of gray should be used instead of patterns and cross-hatching (eg, diagonal lines) on bars.

Component Bar Graph. Component bar graphs (or divided bar graphs) display the proportion of components constituting the total group, represented by the whole bar (Example F9A). Individual components are designated by distinguishing formats,

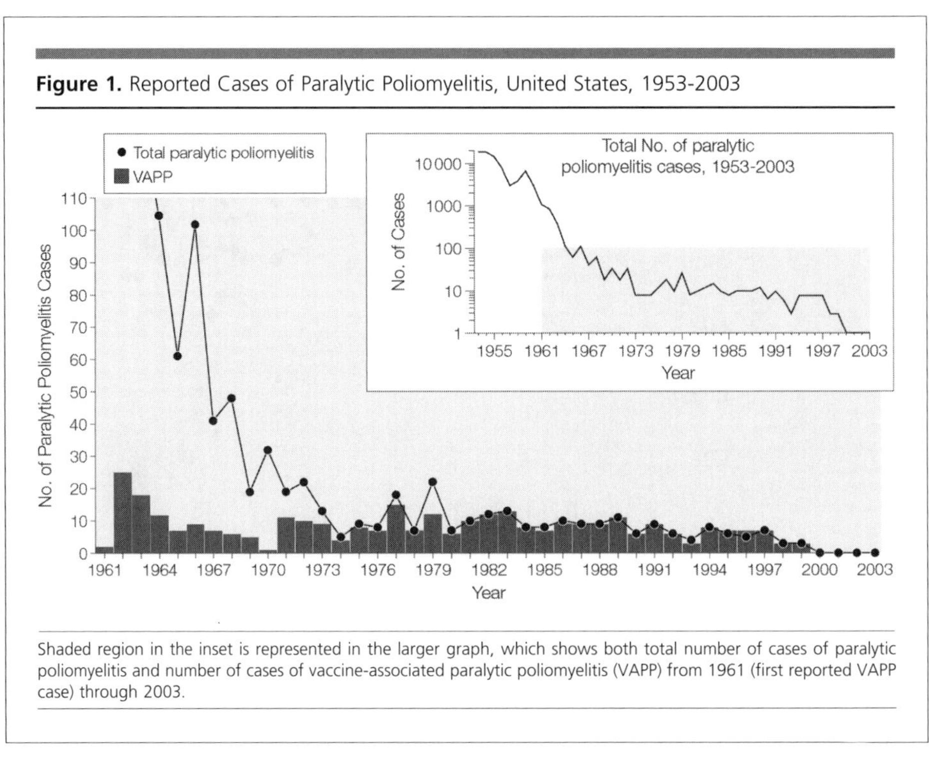
Figure 1. Reported Cases of Paralytic Poliomyelitis, United States, 1953-2003
Total paralytic poliomyelitis
VAPP
No. of Paralytic Poliomyelitis Cases
Year
Total No. of paralytic poliomyelitis cases, 1953-2003
No. of Cases
Year
Shaded region in the inset is represented in the larger graph, which shows both total number of cases of paralytic poliomyelitis and number of cases of vaccine-associated paralytic poliomyelitis (VAPP) from 1961 (first reported VAPP case) through 2003.

Example F5 Histogram showing frequencies, centered over the bar, for each time period (bar height represents number of cases). Note the use of a figure inset to show how the data fit into a larger context.

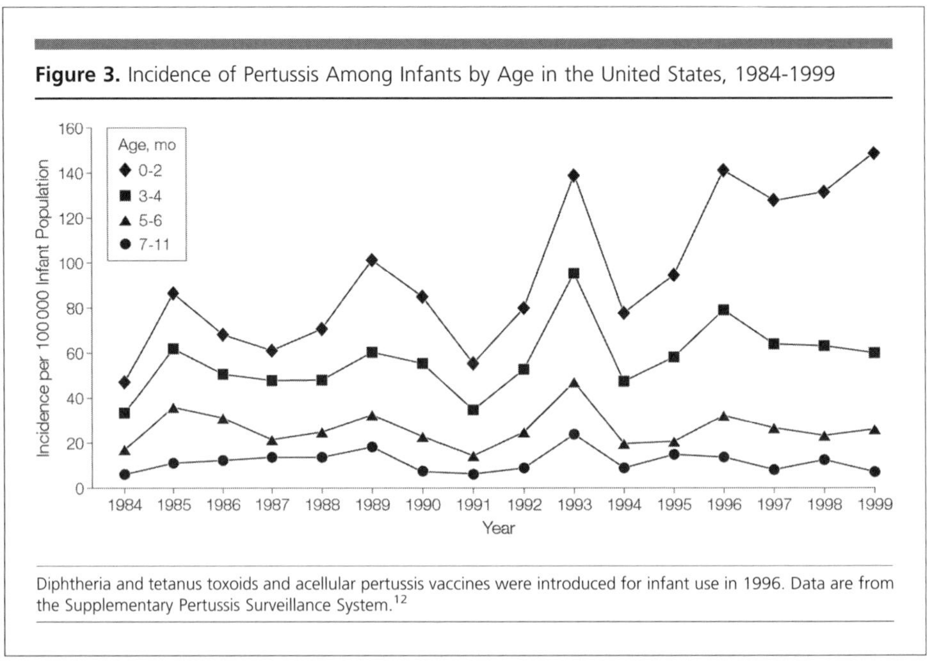
Figure 3. Incidence of Pertussis Among Infants by Age in the United States, 1984-1999
Age, mo
0-2
3-4
5-6
7-11
Incidence per 100000 Infant Population
Year
Diphtheria and tetanus toxoids and acellular pertussis vaccines were introduced for infant use in 1996. Data are from the Supplementary Pertussis Surveillance System.12

Example F6 Frequency polygons can illustrate distributions for multiple groups.

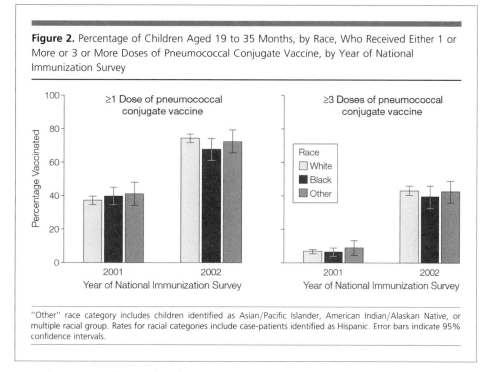

Figure 2. Percentage of Children Aged 19 to 35 Months, by Race, Who Received Either 1 or More or 3 or More Doses of Pneumococcal Conjugate Vaccine, by Year of National Immunization Survey

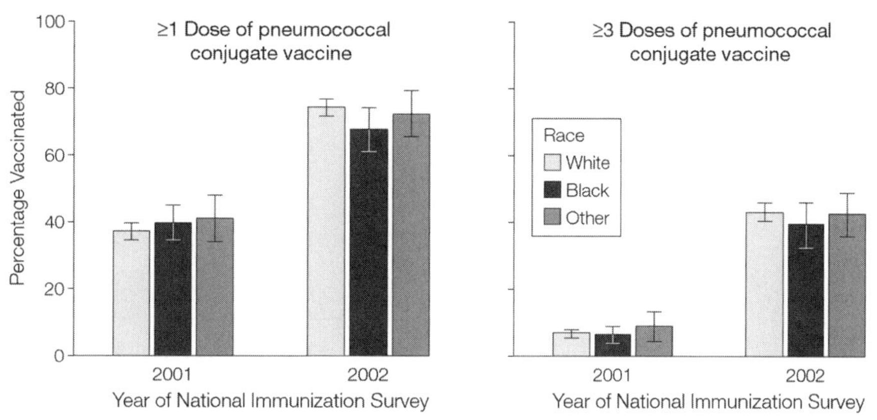

"Other" race category includes children identified as Asian/Pacific Islander, American Indian/Alaskan Native, or multiple racial group. Rates for racial categories include case-patients identified as Hispanic. Error bars indicate 95% confidence intervals.

Example F7 Vertical bar graph with shading to distinguish the 3 groups that are compared. Note that the bars are presented in the same order (white, black, other) in each grouping.

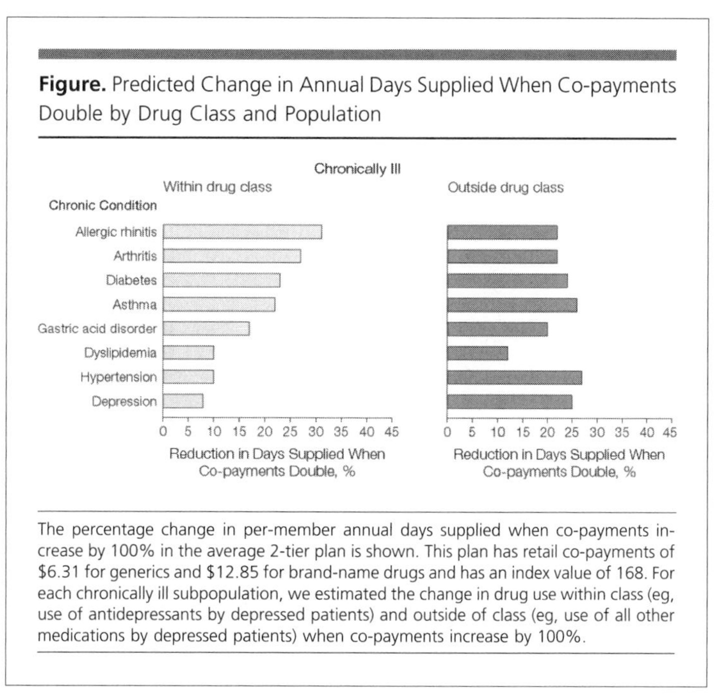

Figure. Predicted Change in Annual Days Supplied When Co-payments Double by Drug Class and Population

The percentage change in per-member annual days supplied when co-payments increase by 100% in the average 2-tier plan is shown. This plan has retail co-payments of $6.31 for generics and $12.85 for brand-name drugs and has an index value of 168. For each chronically ill subpopulation, we estimated the change in drug use within class (eg, use of antidepressants by depressed patients) and outside of class (eg, use of all other medications by depressed patients) when co-payments increase by 100%.

Example F8 Horizontal bar graph with the frequencies on the x-axis and categories on the y-axis.

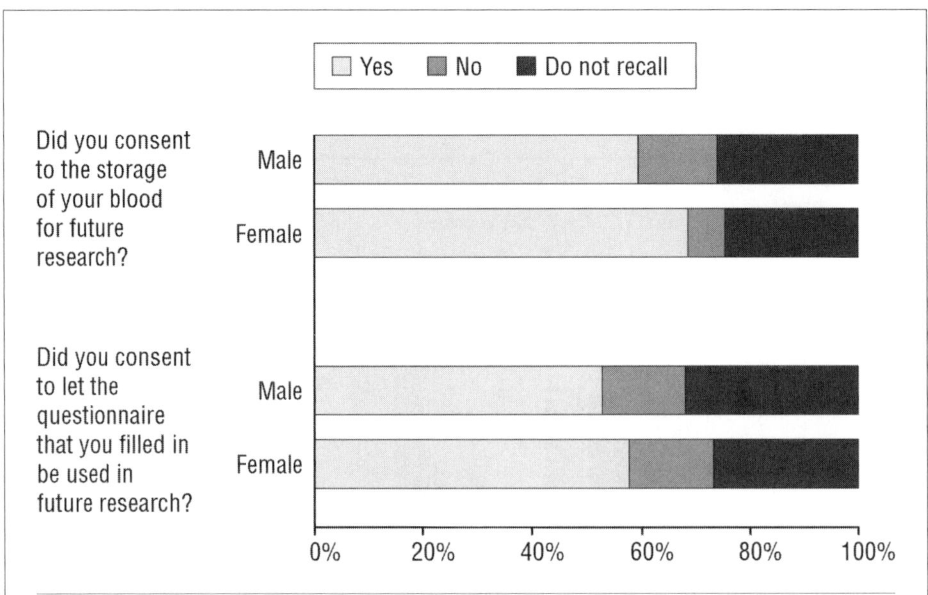

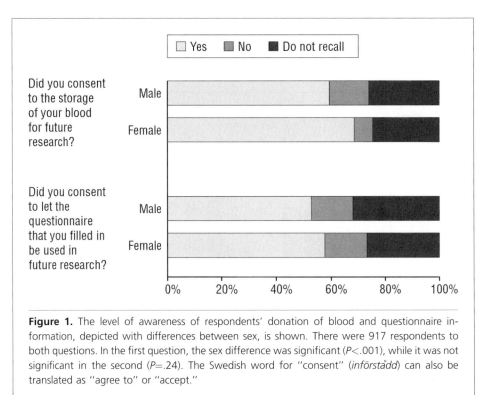

Figure 1. The level of awareness of respondents' donation of blood and questionnaire information, depicted with differences between sex, is shown. There were 917 respondents to both questions. In the first question, the sex difference was significant ($P<.001$), while it was not significant in the second ($P=.24$). The Swedish word for "consent" (*införstådd*) can also be translated as "agree to" or "accept."

Example F9A A 100% bar graph, a type of component bar graph, shows the components as part of the whole. However, the exact values are not easy to compare with one another in this format.

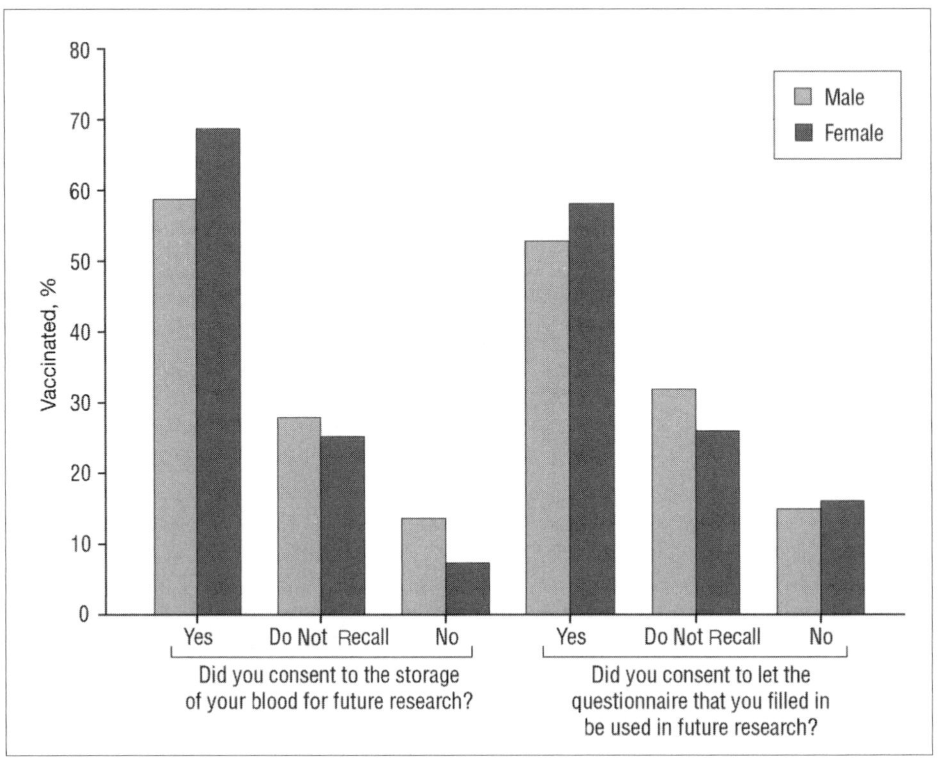

Example F9B The example in Example F9A replotted using clusters of bars.

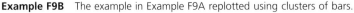

such as different shading. When possible, it is preferable to use clusters of individual bars to represent each component (Example F9B) because the only values easily interpreted in a component bar graph are the total and the end segments.[5]

Pie Chart. Like the component bar graph, pie charts compare relationships among component parts. Categories are represented by sections, with the area of the section being proportional to the relative frequency of each category. Pie charts are used commonly in publications intended for lay audiences but should be avoided in scientific publications.[6] The angular areas of the individual components of pie charts may be difficult to compare between pie charts. Usually, data depicted in pie charts can be summarized in the text or in a table.[7]

Dot (Point) Graph. Dot or point graphs display quantitative data other than counts or frequencies on a single scaled axis according to categories on a baseline (the scaled axis may be horizontal or vertical). Like that in bar graphs, the baseline does not represent a scale and therefore does not contain tick marks. Point estimates are represented by discrete data markers, preferably with error bars to designate variability (Example F10) or box and whisker symbols (Example F11). Dot or point graphs may be used to compare data between study groups, including positive and negative data values relative to a centrally located 0 baseline ("derivation graph"), paired data from

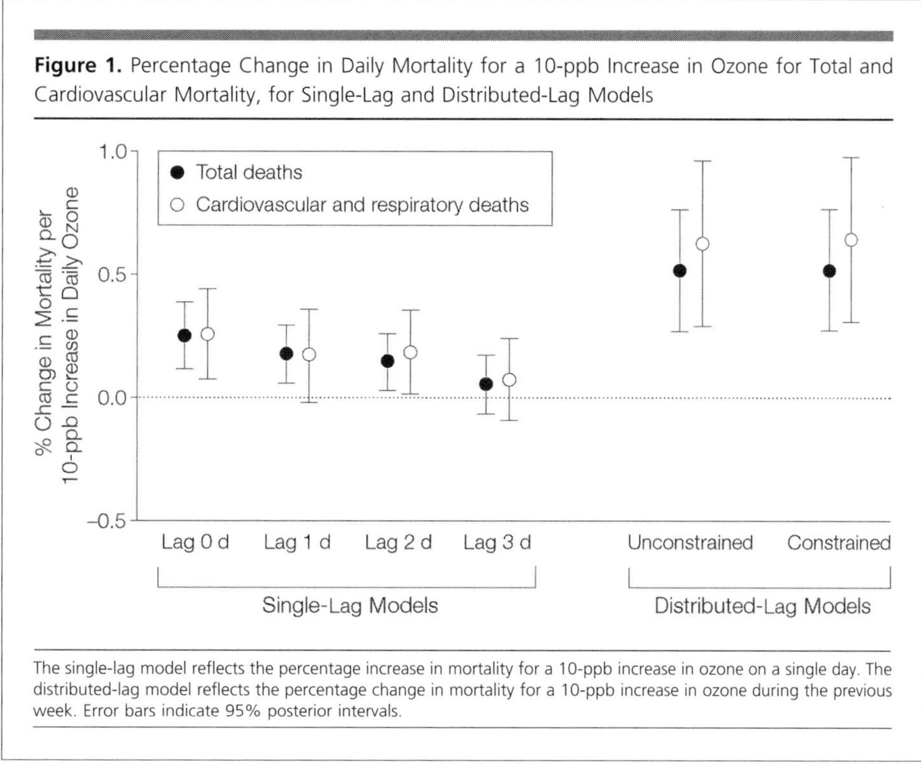
Figure 1. Percentage Change in Daily Mortality for a 10-ppb Increase in Ozone for Total and Cardiovascular Mortality, for Single-Lag and Distributed-Lag Models
% Change in Mortality per 10-ppb Increase in Daily Ozone
1.0
0.5
0.0
−0.5
Total deaths
Cardiovascular and respiratory deaths
Lag 0 d
Lag 1 d
Lag 2 d
Lag 3 d
Unconstrained
Constrained
Single-Lag Models
Distributed-Lag Models
The single-lag model reflects the percentage increase in mortality for a 10-ppb increase in ozone on a single day. The distributed-lag model reflects the percentage change in mortality for a 10-ppb increase in ozone during the previous week. Error bars indicate 95% posterior intervals.

Example F10 Point estimates plotted by category, including error bars and a marker (dotted line) of significance.

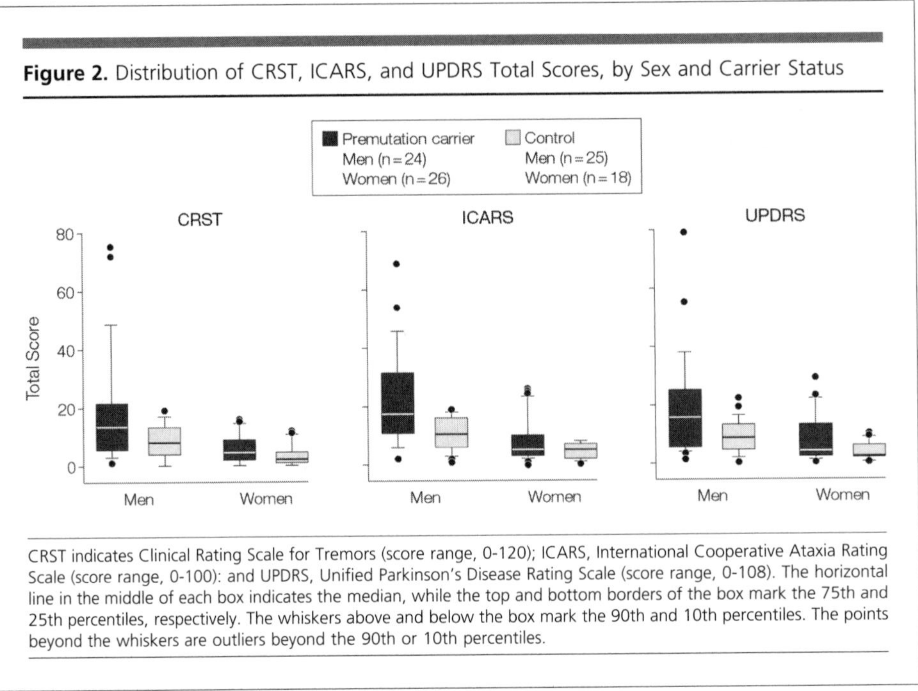
Figure 2. Distribution of CRST, ICARS, and UPDRS Total Scores, by Sex and Carrier Status
Premutation carrier
Men (n = 24)
Women (n = 26)
Control
Men (n = 25)
Women (n = 18)
CRST
ICARS
UPDRS
Total Score
80
60
40
20
0
Men
Women
Men
Women
Men
Women
CRST indicates Clinical Rating Scale for Tremors (score range, 0-120); ICARS, International Cooperative Ataxia Rating Scale (score range, 0-100): and UPDRS, Unified Parkinson's Disease Rating Scale (score range, 0-108). The horizontal line in the middle of each box indicates the median, while the top and bottom borders of the box mark the 75th and 25th percentiles, respectively. The whiskers above and below the box mark the 90th and 10th percentiles. The points beyond the whiskers are outliers beyond the 90th or 10th percentiles.

Example F11 Box and whisker plot with each element defined in the legend.

single individuals (Example F12), or pooled data in meta-analyses and other analyses that combine data from individual studies (Example F13).

4.2.2 Diagrams

Flowchart. Flowcharts demonstrate the sequence of activities, processes, events, operations, or organization of a complex procedure or an interrelated system of components. Flowcharts are useful to depict study protocol or interventions (Example

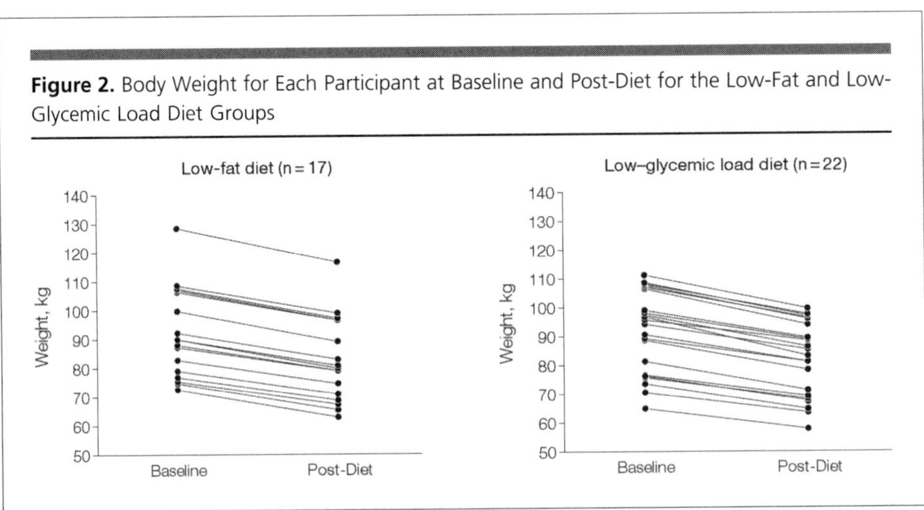
Figure 2. Body Weight for Each Participant at Baseline and Post-Diet for the Low-Fat and Low-Glycemic Load Diet Groups
Low-fat diet (n = 17)
Low–glycemic load diet (n = 22)
Weight, kg
140
130
120
110
100
90
80
70
60
50
Baseline
Post-Diet

Example F12 Individual-value graphs of weight change for each study participant.

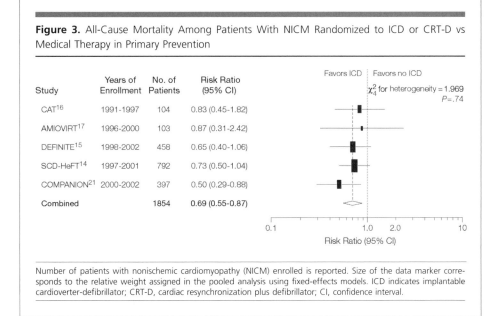

Figure 3. All-Cause Mortality Among Patients With NICM Randomized to ICD or CRT-D vs Medical Therapy in Primary Prevention

Study	Years of Enrollment	No. of Patients	Risk Ratio (95% CI)
CAT[16]	1991-1997	104	0.83 (0.45-1.82)
AMIOVIRT[17]	1996-2000	103	0.87 (0.31-2.42)
DEFINITE[15]	1998-2002	458	0.65 (0.40-1.06)
SCD-HeFT[14]	1997-2001	792	0.73 (0.50-1.04)
COMPANION[21]	2000-2002	397	0.50 (0.29-0.88)
Combined		**1854**	**0.69 (0.55-0.87)**

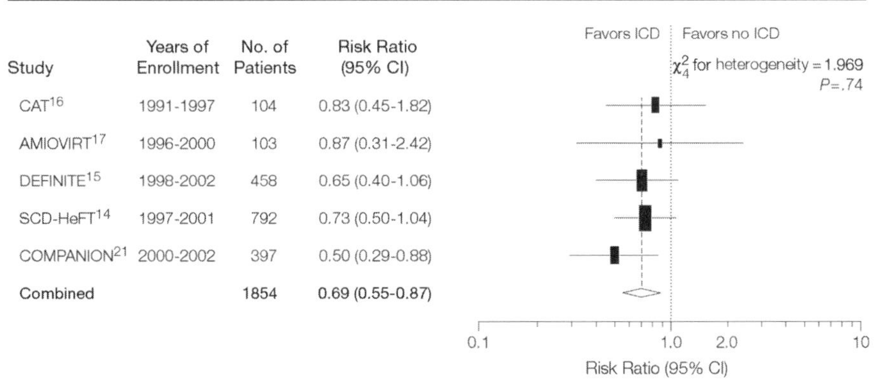

Number of patients with nonischemic cardiomyopathy (NICM) enrolled is reported. Size of the data marker corresponds to the relative weight assigned in the pooled analysis using fixed-effects models. ICD indicates implantable cardioverter-defibrillator; CRT-D, cardiac resynchronization plus defibrillator; CI, confidence interval.

Example F13 Effect sizes and pooled (combined) data in a meta-analysis, with the size of the data markers indicating the relative weight of each study. Note that the values plotted are also provided in the risk ratio column. The dotted line at 1.0 represents no effect and allows for quick visualization of the effect of each study listed. The overall χ^2 and *P* values are provided in the figure.

F14), to demonstrate participant recruitment and follow-up such as in a randomized controlled trial (CONSORT)[8] (Example F15, and Figure 1 in 20.0, Study Design and Statistics), or to show inclusions and exclusions of samples in other types of studies, such as in meta-analyses of observational studies (MOOSE),[9] meta-analyses of randomized controlled trials (QUOROM),[10] and studies of diagnostic accuracy (STARD).[11]

Decision Tree. Decision trees are analytical tools used in cost-effectiveness and decision analyses.[12] The decision tree displays the logical and temporal sequence in clinical decision making and usually progresses from left to right (Example F16). A decision node is a point in the decision tree at which several alternatives can be selected and, by convention, is designated by a square. A chance node (probability node) is a point in the decision tree at which several events, determined by chance, may occur and, by convention, is designated by a circle (see Figure 2 in 20.0, Study Design and Statistics).

Algorithm. Algorithms contain branched pathways to permit the application of carefully defined criteria in the task of identification or classification,[13] such as to aid in clinical diagnosis or treatment decisions. Standard box shapes are used to indicate various steps in the algorithm. For example, an oval begins the algorithm with the question to be answered or topic to be addressed. A diamond or hexagon shape indicates a decision box, which has at least 2 arrows leading to different paths in the algorithm. A rectangle or square indicates an action or decision box. Algorithms

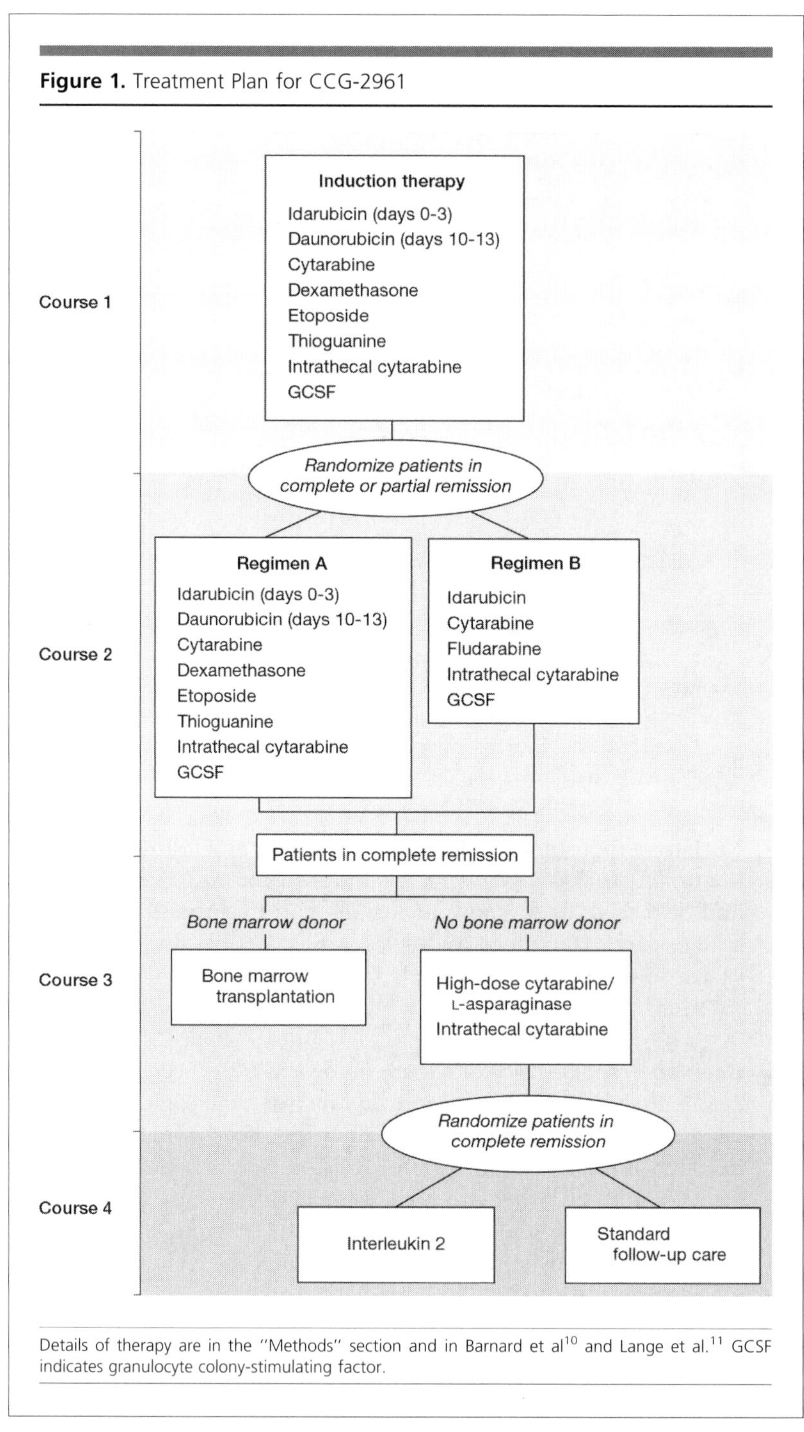

Example F14 Flowchart of a study protocol. Note the use of ovals to indicate a randomization point.

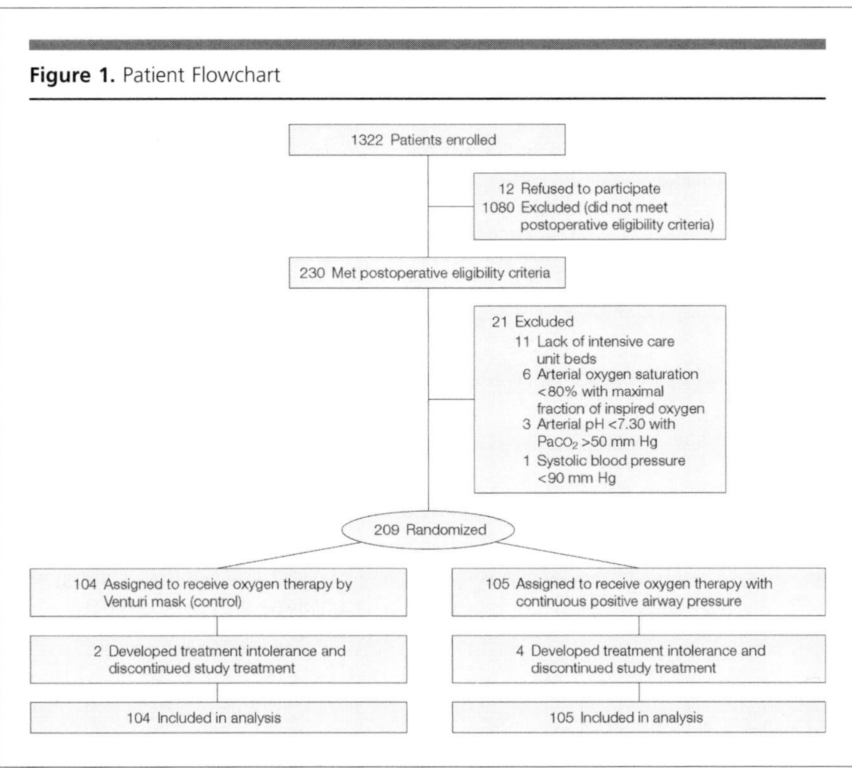

Figure 1. Patient Flowchart

Example F15 Flowchart for a randomized controlled trial using CONSORT criteria.[8]

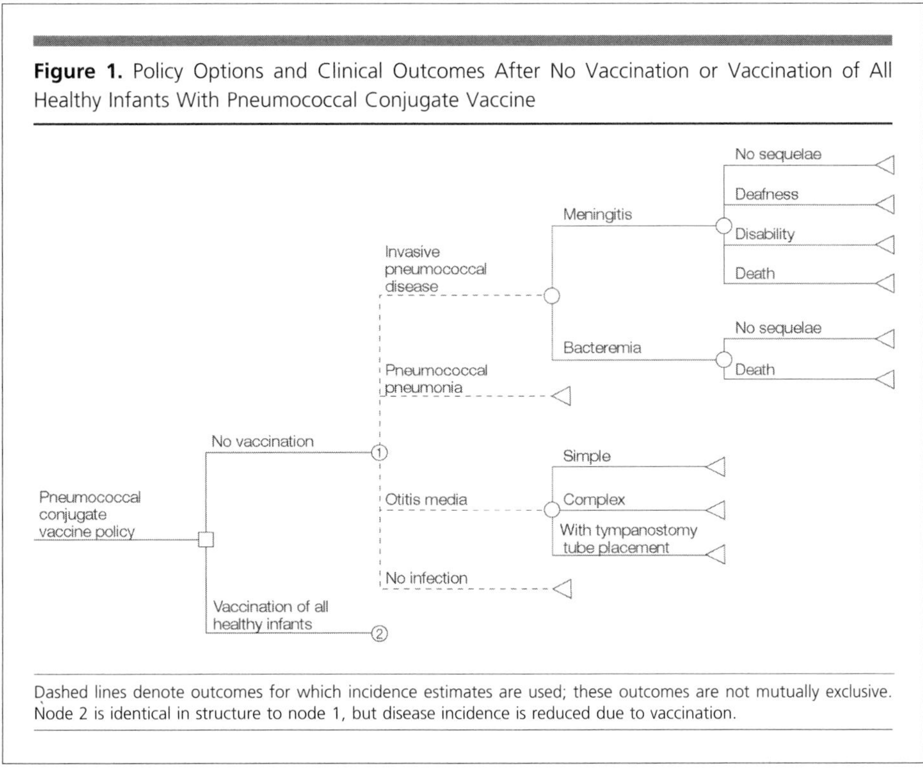

Figure 1. Policy Options and Clinical Outcomes After No Vaccination or Vaccination of All Healthy Infants With Pneumococcal Conjugate Vaccine

Dashed lines denote outcomes for which incidence estimates are used; these outcomes are not mutually exclusive. Node 2 is identical in structure to node 1, but disease incidence is reduced due to vaccination.

Example F16 Decision tree showing options and possible outcomes from left to right. Decisions are illustrated by squares and chance outcomes by circles.

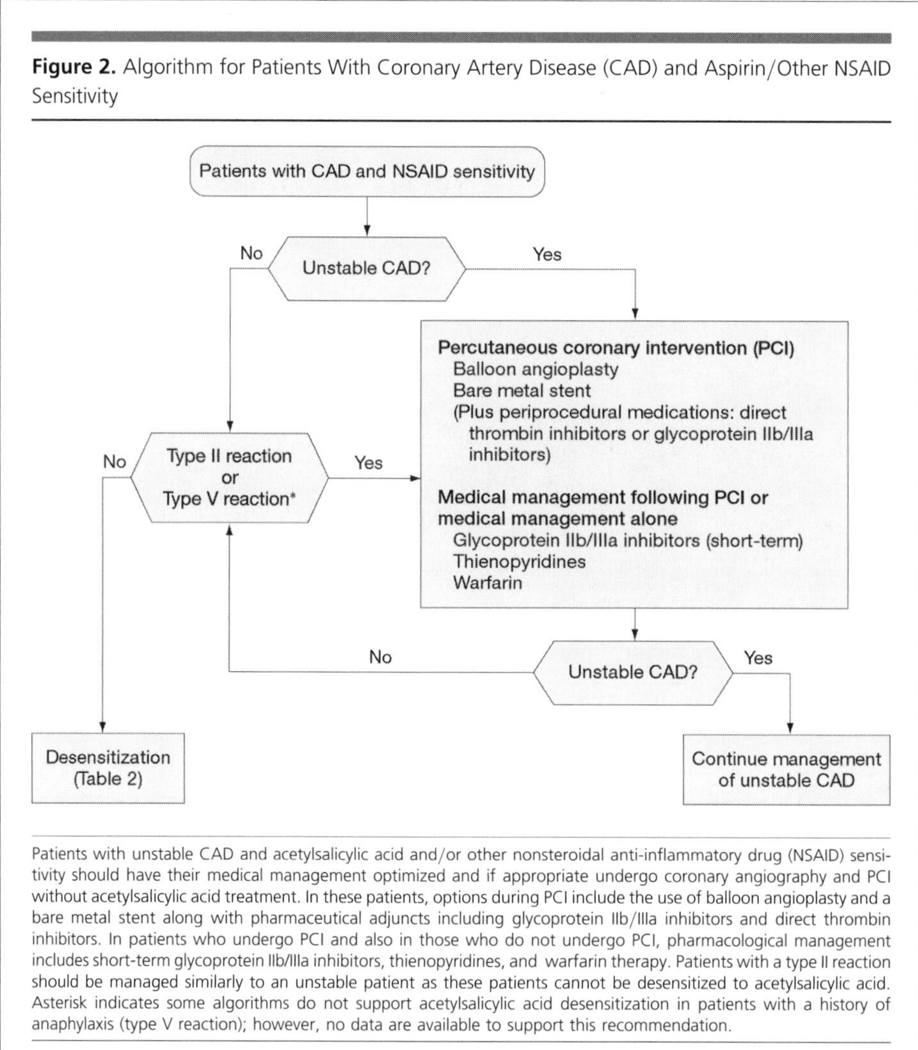

Example F17 Treatment algorithm.

use arrows to guide readers through the process, and yes and no are marked directly on the pathways (Example F17).

Pedigree. Pedigrees illustrate familial relationships and are often used in the study and description of inherited disorders. Standard symbols are used to indicate each person's sex, vital status (living or dead), and whether he or she has the condition or genetic component in question, if known. Lines drawn horizontally and vertically between symbols convey relationships, with the earliest generation at the top of the figure (Example F18) (see also 15.6.6, Nomenclature, Genetics, Pedigrees). If the sex of each person is not relevant to the discussion and there may be a concern about identifiability/confidentiality, triangles can be substituted for the standard circles and squares (see also 5.8.3, Ethical and Legal Considerations, Protecting Research

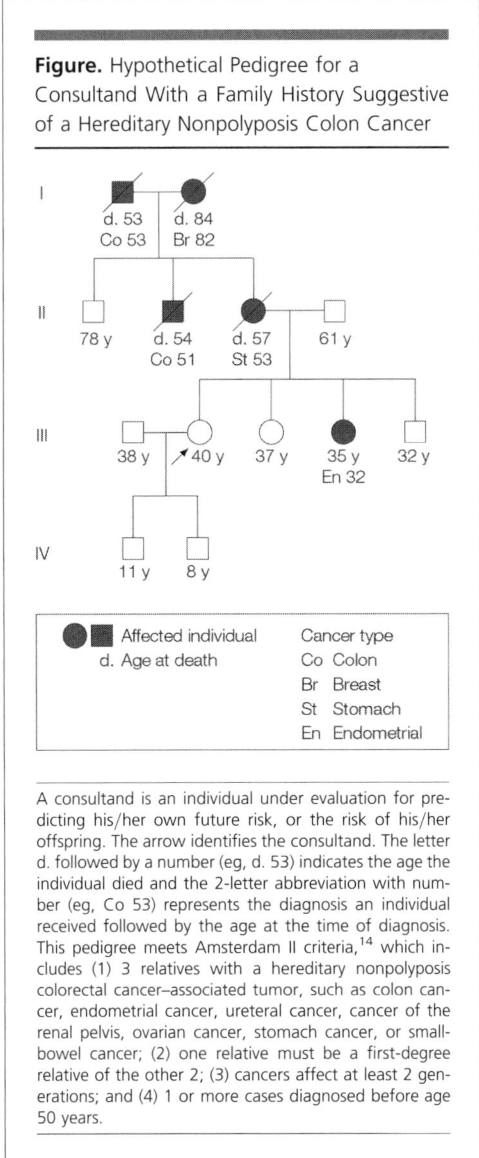
Figure. Hypothetical Pedigree for a Consultand With a Family History Suggestive of a Hereditary Nonpolyposis Colon Cancer
I
d. 53
Co 53
d. 84
Br 82
II
78 y
d. 54
Co 51
d. 57
St 53
61 y
III
38 y
40 y
37 y
35 y
En 32
32 y
IV
11 y
8 y
Affected individual
d. Age at death
Cancer type
Co Colon
Br Breast
St Stomach
En Endometrial
A consultand is an individual under evaluation for predicting his/her own future risk, or the risk of his/her offspring. The arrow identifies the consultand. The letter d. followed by a number (eg, d. 53) indicates the age the individual died and the 2-letter abbreviation with number (eg, Co 53) represents the diagnosis an individual received followed by the age at the time of diagnosis. This pedigree meets Amsterdam II criteria,14 which includes (1) 3 relatives with a hereditary nonpolyposis colorectal cancer–associated tumor, such as colon cancer, endometrial cancer, ureteral cancer, cancer of the renal pelvis, ovarian cancer, stomach cancer, or small-bowel cancer; (2) one relative must be a first-degree relative of the other 2; (3) cancers affect at least 2 generations; and (4) 1 or more cases diagnosed before age 50 years.

Example F18 Hypothetical pedigree of 4 generations, with the proband indicated by an arrow. A key inside the figure plot explains each symbol and abbreviation.

Participants' and Patients' Rights in Scientific Publications, Rights in Published Reports of Genetic Studies).

4.2.3 **Maps.** Maps are useful to demonstrate relationships or trends that involve location and distance or to illustrate study sampling methods (Example F19). Maps may be used to demonstrate geographic relationships (eg, spread of a disease). Choropleth maps depict quantitative data (eg, relative frequencies by county, state, country, province, or region), with differences in numerical data, such as rates, shown by

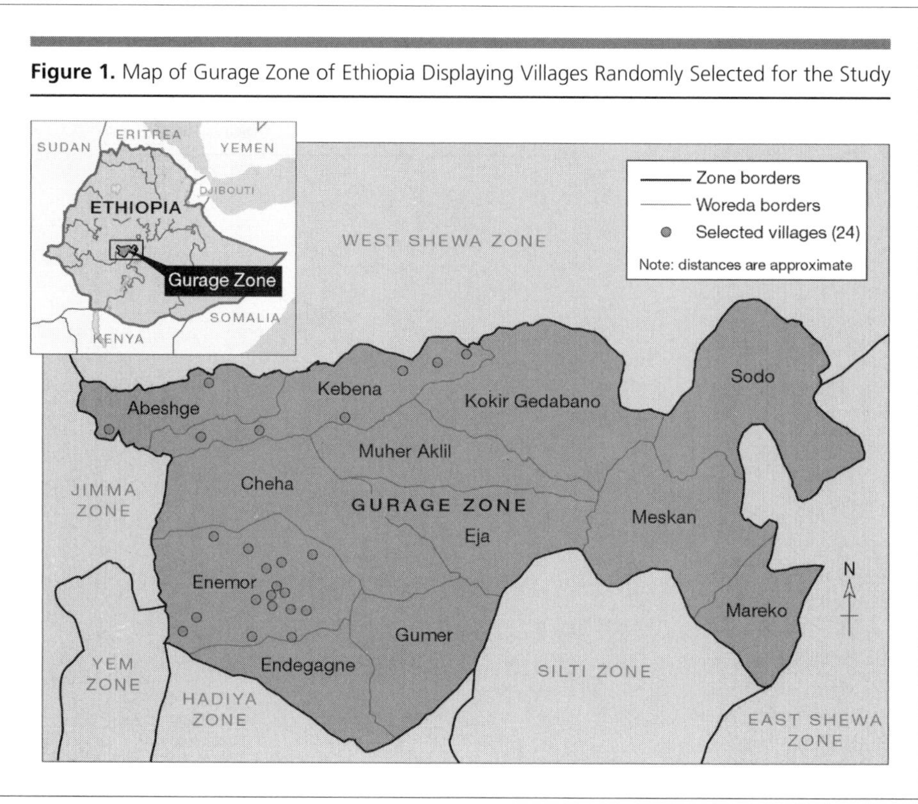

Example F19 A map to explain the locations of various study sites, including an inset to put the smaller area into geographical context.

shading or colors. Authors should verify map details to avoid misspelled or incorrect names, deleted features, distorted geographic relationships, misplaced or missing cities, and misplaced boundaries.

4.2.4 **Illustrations.** Illustrations may explain physiological mechanisms, describe clinical maneuvers and surgical techniques, and provide orientation to medical imaging. Complex interactions often are easier to convey and understand in an illustration than in text or tables (Example F20).

4.2.5 **Photographs and Clinical Imaging.** Photographs and other images in biomedical articles are used to display clinical findings, experimental results, or clinical procedures. Such figures include radiographs and those from other types of medical imaging, photomicrographs, and photographs of patients and biopsy specimens. The availability of digital imaging has provided the ability to enhance images of photographic scientific data, such as clinical images or gel electrophoresis bands.[14] Such digital manipulation may produce misleading or fraudulent images. Some publications require that authors who submit digital images also submit the original gels, while others ask authors to list image adjustments in the paper itself.[14]

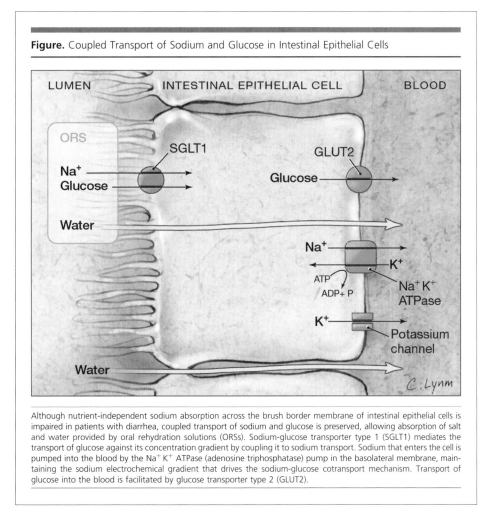

Figure. Coupled Transport of Sodium and Glucose in Intestinal Epithelial Cells

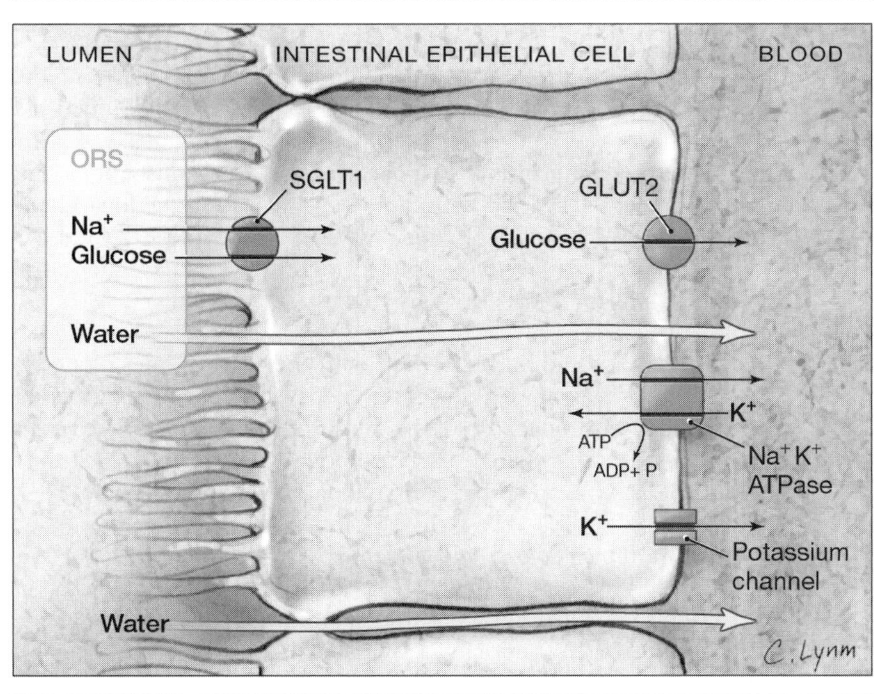

Although nutrient-independent sodium absorption across the brush border membrane of intestinal epithelial cells is impaired in patients with diarrhea, coupled transport of sodium and glucose is preserved, allowing absorption of salt and water provided by oral rehydration solutions (ORSs). Sodium-glucose transporter type 1 (SGLT1) mediates the transport of glucose against its concentration gradient by coupling it to sodium transport. Sodium that enters the cell is pumped into the blood by the $Na^+ K^+$ ATPase (adenosine triphosphatase) pump in the basolateral membrane, maintaining the sodium electrochemical gradient that drives the sodium-glucose cotransport mechanism. Transport of glucose into the blood is facilitated by glucose transporter type 2 (GLUT2).

Example F20 Illustration depicting physiological mechanisms.

4.2.6 **Components of Figures.** Clear display of data or information is the most important aspect of any figure. For figures that display quantitative information, data values may be represented by dots, lines, curves, area, length, or shading, based on the type of graph used.

Scales for Graphs. The horizontal scale (x-axis) and the vertical scale (y-axis) indicate the values of the data plotted in a graph. In most graphs, values increase from left to right (on the x-axis) and from bottom to top (on the y-axis).

Range of Values. The range of values on the axes should be slightly greater than the range of values being plotted, so that the entire data set can appear within the area defined by the axes and most of the possible range of values on the axes will be used. Ideally, the range should include 0 on both axes, if 0 is a possible value for the variable being plotted. In line graphs, if a large range of values is necessary but cannot be depicted with a continuous scale, discontinuity in the axis should be indicated with paired diagonal lines that signify a missing portion of the range (//).[15] Numerical data on 2 sides of a scale break should not be connected to avoid the implication that data on either side of the discontinuity are linear. For single-axis plots, data that exceed the limits of the axes can be indicated with an arrowhead.

Axis Scales. Divisions of the scales on the graph axes should be indicated by intervals chosen to be appropriate, simple multiples of the quantity plotted, such as multiples of 2, 5, or 10.[15] Numbers that represent the values on the axis scale are centered on their respective tick marks. For linear scales, the axis must appear linear, with equal intervals and equal spacing between tick marks. However, logarithmic scales may be useful to show proportional rates of change (Example F13) and to emphasize the change rate rather than the absolute amount of change when absolute values or baseline values for data series vary greatly.

Axis Labels. Axes should be labeled with the type of data plotted and the unit of measure used. Data may represent numerical values, percentages, or rates. For numerical data, customary units of measure and their respective abbreviations or symbols should be used (see 14.12, Abbreviations, Units of Measure). In single-axis graphs, categories should be clearly labeled along the baseline.

Symbols, Patterns, Colors, and Shading. Symbols, line styles, colors, and shading characteristics used in the figure must be explained, preferably by direct labeling of components in the figure or in a key. Alternatively, this information may be included in the legend. For a series of figures within an article, the types of symbols, line styles, colors, and shading should be used consistently. For example, if data for the intervention group and for the control group are designated as a heavy line and as a lighter line, respectively, then these same line styles should be used for similar data for these groups in subsequent figures.

When data points are plotted, symbols should be distinguished easily by shape and color or shade. For example, if 2 symbols are needed, the recommended symbols are ○ and ●,[15] although □ and ■ or △ and ▲ may be used. A combination of these symbols can be used when 3 or more symbols are required. The shading or color of the symbols can designate specific data. For instance, in all figures in an article, ○ may indicate data for the placebo group and ● for the intervention group.

In bar charts and other figures (such as maps), shading is preferable to cross-hatching and other patterns to distinguish groups. Patterns can be difficult to read both in print and online.[5] Shades should be of appropriate gradations to show contrast (eg, 10%, 40%, and 70% black).

Box and Whisker Plots. Box and whisker formatting may be useful to illustrate the nonnormal distribution of values within a group (data set). Typically, the top and bottom of the box represent the 25th and 75th percentiles, the horizontal line inside the box represents the median or mean, the whiskers are the 10th and 90th percentiles, and any outliers are shown as circles (Example F11). Because the value of each of these components may vary, it is important to define them. Mean values in box and whisker plots may be connected by curves to show trends, such as point estimates of mean values.

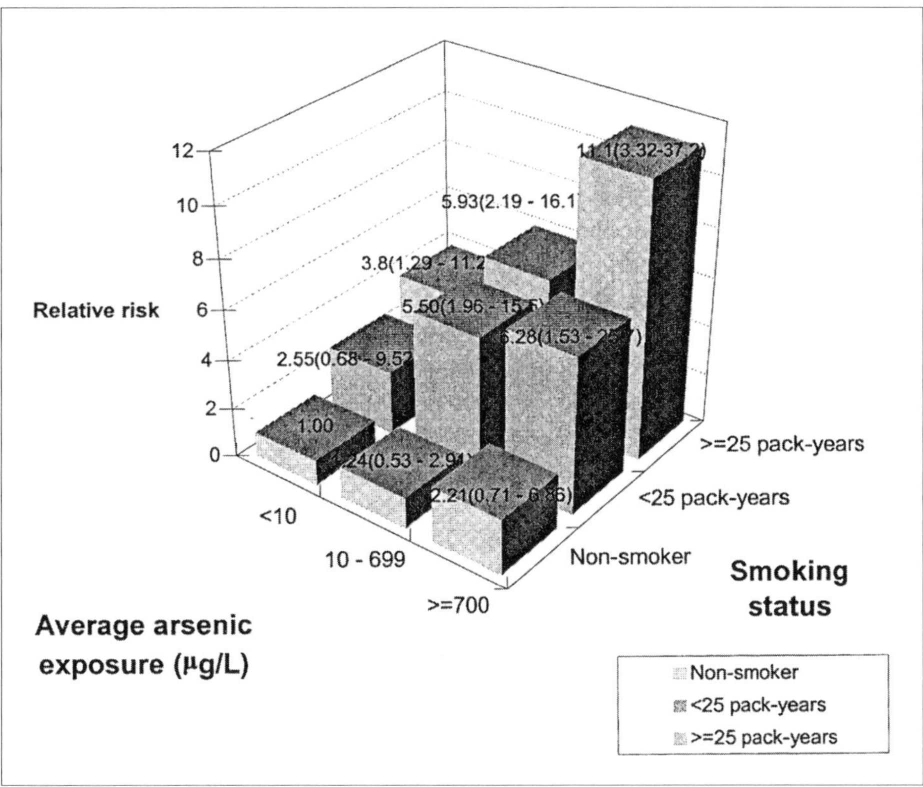

Example F21 Originally submitted 3-dimensional figure.

Error Bars. For plotted data, error bars (depicting standard deviation, standard error, range, interquartile range, or confidence intervals) are an efficient way to display variability in the data.[16] Error bars should be drawn to encompass the entire range of variability, not in just one direction (Example F7). Error bars should always be defined either in the legend or on the plot itself.

3-Dimensional Figures. In most cases, figures should not be presented in 3-dimensional format, even when data for 3 variables are being displayed. A 3-dimensional presentation is inappropriate for any figures that contain only 2 dimensions of data. Many software programs allow users to add enhancing elements to figures, but 3-dimensional display may confuse readers or distract from important graphical relationships. For instance, it may be difficult to read from the bar to the correct value on the axis. Most 3-dimensional presentations can be replotted into more straightforward graphics (Example F21, Example F22).

4.2.7 **Titles, Legends, and Labels.** Many journals, including *JAMA*, use both titles and legends to describe and clarify figures. Others, like the *Archives* Journals, combine the title and legend underneath the figure.

Title. The figure title follows the designation "Figure" numbered consecutively (ie, Figure 1, Figure 2) and does not appear in the figure itself. Articles that contain a

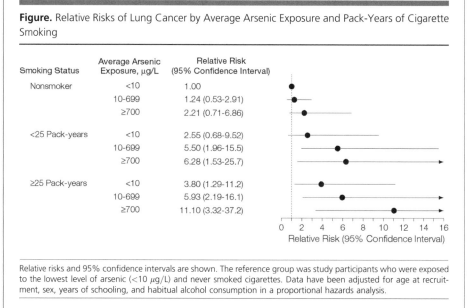

Figure. Relative Risks of Lung Cancer by Average Arsenic Exposure and Pack-Years of Cigarette Smoking

Smoking Status	Average Arsenic Exposure, μg/L	Relative Risk (95% Confidence Interval)
Nonsmoker	<10	1.00
	10-699	1.24 (0.53-2.91)
	≥700	2.21 (0.71-6.86)
<25 Pack-years	<10	2.55 (0.68-9.52)
	10-699	5.50 (1.96-15.5)
	≥700	6.28 (1.53-25.7)
≥25 Pack-years	<10	3.80 (1.29-11.2)
	10-699	5.93 (2.19-16.1)
	≥700	11.10 (3.32-37.2)

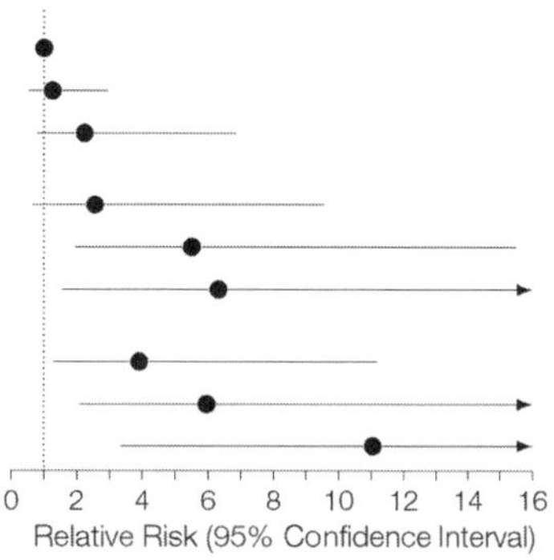

0 2 4 6 8 10 12 14 16

Relative Risk (95% Confidence Interval)

Relative risks and 95% confidence intervals are shown. The reference group was study participants who were exposed to the lowest level of arsenic (<10 μg/L) and never smoked cigarettes. Data have been adjusted for age at recruitment, sex, years of schooling, and habitual alcohol consumption in a proportional hazards analysis.

Example F22 The same data in Example F21 replotted in a point graph.

single figure use the designator "Figure" (not "Figure 1"). The title is a succinct clause or phrase that identifies the specific topic of the figure or describes what the data show. Each major word in a figure title is capitalized and follows the same rules as for article titles (see 3.9.1, References, Titles, English-Language Titles). Some publications print the figure title under the figure, in sentence style, followed immediately by the legend.

Titles of figures, including diagrams, photographs, and line drawings, generally should not begin with a phrase identifying the type of figure.

> *Avoid*: Photograph Showing Prominent Physical Signs of Familial Hypercholesterolemia
>
> *Better*: Prominent Physical Signs of Familial Hypercholesterolemia

However, a description of the type of figure may be required in certain circumstances to provide context and avoid confusion.

> **Figure** 3. Fluorescein Angiogram Showing Widespread Retinal Capillary Nonperfusion and Marked Optic Nerve Head Leakage
>
> **Figure** 4. Autoradiograph Demonstrating Loss of Heterozygosity at the 3p25 Locus in Preneoplastic Foci and Corresponding Invasive Cancer

Legend. The figure legend or caption is written in sentence format and printed below or next to the figure. The legend contains information that identifies and describes the figure, and it should provide sufficient detail to make the figure comprehensible without reference to the text. Although the recommended maximum length for figure legends is 40 words, longer legends may be necessary for figures that require more detailed explanations or for multipart figures. Figure legends should contain expansions of abbreviations and footnotes for information too cumbersome to include in the figure itself.

Composite Figures. Composite figures consist of several parts and should have a single legend that contains necessary information about each part. The legend should begin with a brief description that pertains to all of the components. Each component of the figure is then described, usually by a separate sentence beginning with the designation for the part, followed by a comma. If the parts share much of the same explanation, parenthetical mention of each part is appropriate. Such information should be clearly specified by designations corresponding to the figure components. However, the designations must be consistent in all legends.

For composite figures with 2 or more panels, capital letters (A, B, C, D, etc) should be used to label the parts of the figure. These letters should be placed in a small insert box that is positioned in the same place in each figure. The figure legend should refer to each of the figure components and the letter designators in a clear and consistent format (Example F23).

Information About Methods and Statistical Analyses. Statements regarding methodologic details are unnecessary for each figure if this information is provided in the "Methods" section of the article and the text that refers to the figure clearly indicates the source of the data. Reference to the "Methods" section or to other figures that contain this information may be appropriate. At times, brief inclusion of methodologic details in the legend may be necessary for understanding the figure.

For data that have been analyzed statistically, pertinent analyses and significance values may be included in the figure or its legend.[17] Values for data displayed in the figure (eg, mean or median values) should be indicated in the figure or in the legend. The meaning of error bars should be explained in the legend (Example F7).

Photomicrographs. Legends for photomicrographs should include details about the type of stain used and the degree of magnification. If the original illustration has been modified (enlarged or reduced), the original magnification should be noted. In figures with 2 or more parts, the stains or magnifications relevant to each individual part should be noted after its description.

> A, Histological section of the vertebral specimen showing the typical "cookie-bite" tunneling osteoclasia of the vertebral trabeculae (unstained, original magnification ×400). B, For comparison, a bone tissue section of a recent case of hyperparathyroidism demonstrates very similar defects at the trabecular surface (hematoxylin-eosin, original magnification ×400).

Electron micrograph legends may specify magnification, without information about the stain.

> *Haemophilus influenzae* microcolonies of middle ear mucosa 24 hours after inoculation (×5000).

Visual Indicators in Illustrations or Photographs. Visual indicators provided in illustrations or photographs, such as a reference bar or ruler denoting a measure of dimension (eg, length) in a photomicrograph, arrows, arrowheads, or other markers,

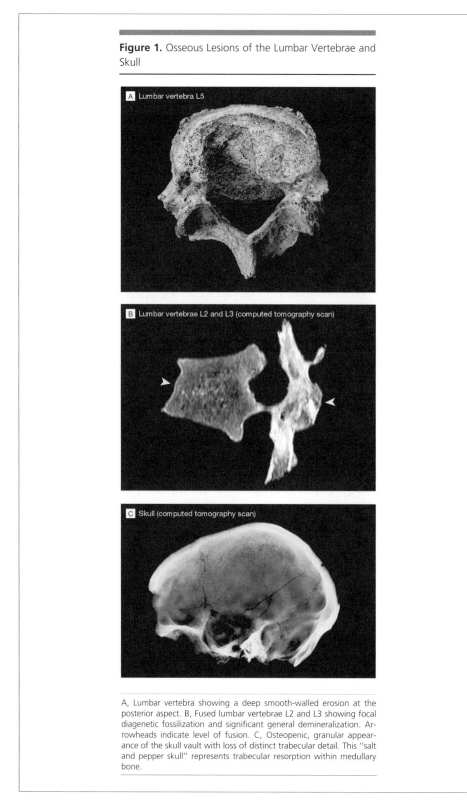

Figure 1. Osseous Lesions of the Lumbar Vertebrae and Skull

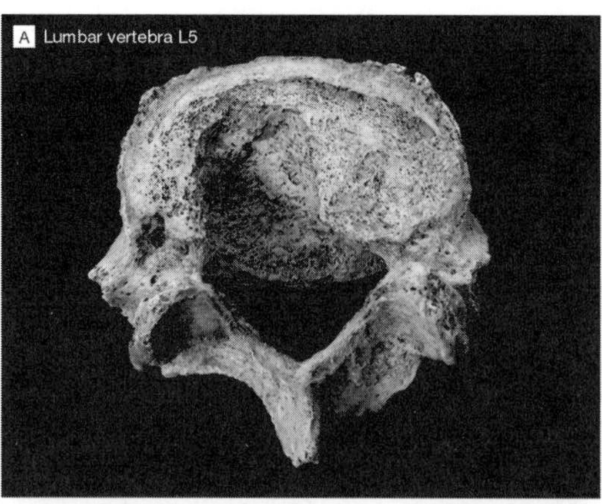

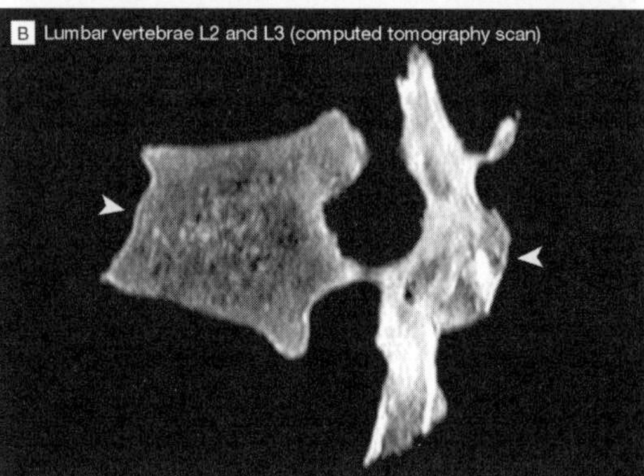

B Lumbar vertebrae L2 and L3 (computed tomography scan)

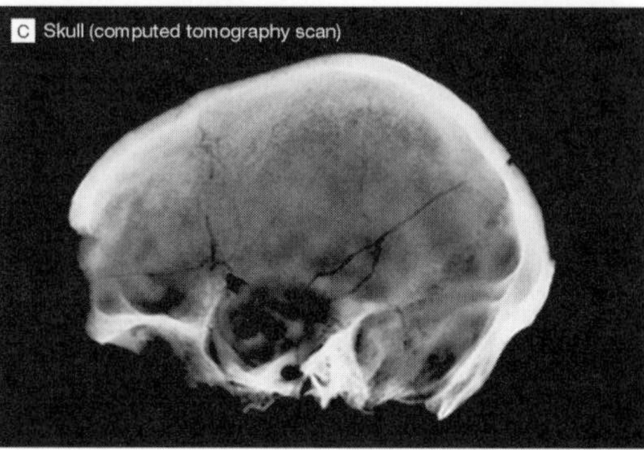

A, Lumbar vertebra showing a deep smooth-walled erosion at the posterior aspect. B, Fused lumbar vertebrae L2 and L3 showing focal diagenetic fossilization and significant general demineralization. Arrowheads indicate level of fusion. C, Osteopenic, granular appearance of the skull vault with loss of distinct trabecular detail. This "salt and pepper skull" represents trabecular resorption within medullary bone.

Example F23 Multipart figure with each panel labeled in the upper left corner and also including a brief description. Note the explanation of the arrowheads in panel B.

should be clearly defined in the figure or described in the figure legend (Example F23).

Capitalization of Labels and Other Text. Capitalization should be kept to a minimum within the body of the figure.[2] Axis labels in figures are akin to column headings in tables, so each word should be capitalized (except minor words such as prepositions of less than 4 letters). In nonaxis areas of the figure, capitalizing each major word can make comprehension difficult, especially when phrases or clauses are used. Using sentence-style capitalization is easier to read[1] and takes less space.

Abbreviations. Abbreviations in figures should be consistent with those used in the text and defined in the title or legend or in a key as part of the figure. Abbreviations may be expanded individually in the text of the legend or may be expanded collectively at the end of the legend.

> Arachidonic acid is the precursor molecule from which all eicosanoids are synthesized. Products of the cyclooxygenase 1 (COX-1) enzyme include the potent stimulator of platelet activation and aggregation thromboxane A_2, as well as prostaglandin E_2 (PGE_2).

If several illustrations share many of the same abbreviations and symbols, full explanation may be provided in the first figure legend, with subsequent reference to that legend. This practice works relatively well in print but can make understanding figures in online articles more difficult because readers may have to open separate figure files to find the legend.

4.2.8 **Placement of Figures in the Text.** In the published article, figures should be placed as close as possible to their first mention in the text. Figures should be cited in consecutive numerical order in the text, and references to figures should include their respective numbers. For example:

> Patient participation and progress through the study are shown in Figure 1.
>
> Figure 1 shows patient participation and progress through the study.
>
> Patient participation and progress through the study were monitored by the investigators (Figure 1).

Given the potential for variability in the page layout and online publication process, the text should not refer to figures by position on the page or by other designators, such as "the figure opposite," "the figure on this page," or "the figure above."

4.2.9 **Figures Reproduced or Adapted From Other Sources.** It is preferable to use original figures rather than those already published. When use of a previously published illustration, photograph, or other figure is determined necessary, written permission to reproduce it must be obtained from the copyright holder (usually the publisher). The original source should be acknowledged in the legend. If the original source in which the illustration has been published is included in the reference list, the reference may be cited in the legend, with the citation number for the reference corresponding to its first appearance in the text, tables, or figures (see 4.1.3, Table Components, Footnotes, and 3.6, References, Citation). Permission should be obtained to reproduce the material in print, online, and all licensed versions (eg, reprints). It may be necessary to include additional information to comply with specific language required by the organization (usually a publisher) granting permission to republish the figure.

Reprinted with permission from the American Academy of Pediatrics.[5]

4.2.10 Guidelines for Preparing and Submitting Figures. The preferred format for submitting figures varies among scientific journals. Authors who submit figures with a scientific manuscript should consult the instructions for authors of the publication for specific requirements. For example, some journals require all files to be submitted through a Web-based submission system, others may request e-mail attachments, and still others may prefer to receive materials in hard copy. When high-resolution graphic files are required that are too large to be sent via e-mail or a Web-based system, the images may be loaded onto a fixed medium such as a CD. The following guidelines apply for figures submitted to *JAMA* and the *Archives* Journals.

Graphs, line art, diagrams, charts, and other black-and-white figures should be submitted as an electronic file (acceptable formats include EPS, GIF, JPG, and TIF, as well as images pasted into Microsoft Word or PowerPoint as long as the vector digital file is available upon acceptance).

Photographs, photomicrographs, or radiographs (whether in color or black and white) should be submitted as high-contrast, right-reading glossy prints. Color illustrations can be submitted as color transparencies, color slides, color prints, or in a digital file (EPS, JPG, TIF) along with corresponding color prints. Transparencies should not be submitted in glass slides. If color prints are submitted, the print should be made oversized, and the negative of the print also should be provided. Polaroid-type prints and color laser prints should not be used for reproduction because the results inevitably are poor.

Providing digital files with adequate resolution is the primary key to printing high-quality images. Most digital submissions are rejected because of low resolution. The canvas size of images should be at least 5 in wide (depth is not important). Generally, digital images should have a resolution of at least 350 ppi. To ensure that color will be clinically correct, calibrated color proofs should be submitted along with the digital files. The availability of computer software for generating figures, such as statistical or graphic design programs, has simplified the creation of figures in digital format. However, the ability of publishers to use author-generated electronic files containing figures for importing, reproducing, and incorporating into production software varies considerably. Authors should consult the instructions for authors or the editorial office of the publication for information about preferred and compatible formats for submission of figures in electronic files.

Clear, sharp images are essential for accurate reproduction. Dust and scratches usually can be removed, but if details are blurred in the original, details will remain blurred in reproduction. Good exposure is another important consideration in providing the best-quality prints and transparencies. If necessary, several different exposures of the same image may be submitted, and the best candidate for image reproduction will be selected.

All figures should be numbered according to their citation order in the text. For figures submitted as hard copy, a label with the figure number, name of the first author, short form of the manuscript title, and the proper orientation (eg, "top") should be affixed to the back of the print. Writing directly on the back of the print should be avoided because it may damage the print.

Proper locations for visual indicators (eg, arrows indicating the area of interest in an illustration or photograph) should be identified clearly. This can be accomplished by providing (in addition to the required clean, unmarked copies of the illustration or photograph or copies of the 35-mm slide) an extra paper copy of the illustration or photograph with locations for indicators marked directly on the paper copy.

Titles and legends for figures should be included at the end of the text and should not appear on the illustrations.

Suggested specifications for submission of digital images have been formulated by a working group of the International Digital Enterprise Alliance. The guidelines, Digital Image Submission Criteria (DISC), are available at http://www.disc-info.org/specifications/.

Journal editors should establish clear guidelines about the acceptable amount of image manipulation (eg, cropping or contrast adjustment). The consequences of excessive image manipulation, regardless of intent, should be made clear to authors.[18]

4.2.11 **Consent for Identifiable Patients.** For photographs or videos in which an individual can be identified (either by himself/herself or by others), the author should obtain and submit a signed statement of informed consent from the identifiable person that grants permission to publish the photograph (in print, online, in video, and all licensed versions, if appropriate). Previously used measures to attempt to conceal the identity of an individual in a photograph, such as placing black bars over the person's eyes, are not effective and should not be used (see 5.8.2, Ethical and Legal Considerations, Protecting Research Participants' and Patients' Rights in Scientific Publication, Patients' Rights to Privacy and Anonymity). Individuals can be identified in photographs that show minimal body parts, usually from identifying features (eg, scars, moles, clothing). To avoid identifiability in such cases, photographs should be cropped if possible. Otherwise, permission must be obtained from the individual in the photograph.

For figures that depict genetic information, such as pedigrees or family trees, informed consent is required from all persons who can be identified. Authors should not modify the pedigree, eg, by changing the number of persons in the generation, varying the number of offspring in families, or providing inaccurate information about the sex of pedigree members, in an attempt to avoid potential identification. If knowledge of the sex of pedigree members is not essential for scientific purposes, individuals may be designated by triangles instead of circles (females) and squares (males) (see 4.2.2, Diagrams, Pedigree, and 5.8.3, Ethical and Legal Considerations, Protecting Research Participants' and Patients' Rights in Scientific Publication, Rights in Published Reports of Genetic Studies).

4.3 **Nontabular Material.** Nontabular material does not contain cells of individual data. Usually it is set off from the text by a box, rules, shading, or other elements. Sometimes the box or sidebar is cited in the text (following the citation rules for tables) and other times (eg, in news articles) it is not. Any references that appear in nontabular material should also appear in the reference list and be numbered in order of their appearance (see 4.1.3, Table Components).

4.3.1 **Boxes.** A textual table or box contains words, phrases, or sentences, often in list form. Boxes are used to emphasize key points, summarize information, and/or reduce the narrative text (Example B1).

4.3.2 **Sidebars.** Sidebars typically contain supplementary information, including related topics or lists of sources for further reading (Example B2 and Example B3).

Box 1. Modified Stepwise Analgesic Ladder

Step 1. Mild to Moderate Pain
Give patient nonsteroidal anti-inflammatory drug and/or 5 mg of oxycodone with acetaminophen, 500 mg orally (up to 8 tablets/d)

Step 2. Moderate to Severe Pain
Give patient sustained-release morphine orally. If the patient cannot tolerate morphine or oral and rectal routes are not possible, give transdermal fentanyl patch or oxycodone sustained-release orally

With additional as-needed morphine immediate-release pills or elixir orally or 5 mg of oxycodone with acetaminophen, 500 mg orally (up to 8 tablets/d), for breakthrough pain

Example B1 Box or textual table of sentences and phrases set off from the text to supplement the "Methods" section.

Avian Influenza: An Emerging Problem?

While the US Centers for Disease Control and Prevention is fairly confident it has a handle on this year's flu season, it is keeping a wary eye on avian flu activities in Asia. Avian flu is worrisome because it can cross into the human population, and the infection has proven to have a high mortality rate.

Earlier this year, an outbreak of influenza A (H5N1) occurred in Asia, with 100 million birds dying of the disease or being culled to contain its spread. Between January and March, there were 34 individuals in Thailand and Vietnam with confirmed cases of H5N1 influenza, with 23 dying. The outbreak subsided, but in June it reemerged in China, Indonesia, Thailand, and Vietnam. The first human cases from this renewed outbreak were reported August 12, with 3 individuals in Vietnam dying; a Thai man died on September 8.

Adding to the concern are reports from China of pigs becoming infected with avian flu. Because avian viruses rarely infect individuals, any jump to humans, through either birds or pigs, is a major concern because there is little or no immune protection against it. In addition, because pigs are susceptible to both avian and human influenza, health officials are worried that the pigs will serve as a "mixing vessel" where the 2 viruses can exchange genetic material and create a new influenza strain that infects humans more readily and acquires the ability to spread from person to person—setting the stage for a pandemic.

The World Health Organization and the US Centers for Disease Control and Prevention are monitoring the situation.—M.M.

Example B2 Sidebar from a news story on influenza.

For More Information

Online information is available from several organizations involved in polio eradication efforts.

Global Polio Eradication Initiative: http//www.polioeradication.org

Rotary International (Polio Plus program): http//www.rotary.org/foundation/polioplus/

US Centers for Disease Control and Prevention: http//www.cdc.gov (using the page's search function for "polio eradication" elicits links to more than 700 reports and other materials on the subject)

UNICEF (United Nations Children's Fund): http//www.unicef.org/immunization/index_polio.html

Example B3 Sidebar of sources for further reading.

ACKNOWLEDGMENTS

Principal author: Stacy Christiansen, MA

All table and figure examples in this chapter are from *JAMA* and the *Archives* Journals © American Medical Association.

Thanks to the following individuals for their contributions: Ronna Henry Siegel, MD, *JAMA*; Jessica S. Ancker, MPH, Department of Biomedical Informatics, Columbia University College of Physicians and Surgeons, New York, New York; Charl Jensen, *JAMA*; and Robert M. Golub, MD, *JAMA* and *Archives* Journals.

REFERENCES

1. Style Manual Committee, Council of Science Editors. *Scientific Style and Format: The CSE Manual for Authors, Editors, and Publishers*. 7th ed. New York, NY: Rockefeller University Press, in cooperation with the Council of Science Editors, Reston, VA; 2006.
2. *The Chicago Manual of Style*. 15th ed. Chicago, IL: University of Chicago Press; 2003.
3. Huth EJ. *Writing and Publishing in Medicine*. 3rd ed. Baltimore, MD: Williams & Wilkins; 1999.
4. Pocock SJ, Clayton TC, Altman DG. Survival plots of time-to-event outcomes in clinical trials: good practice and pitfalls. *Lancet*. 2002;359(9318):1686-1689.
5. Peterson SM. *Editing Science Graphs*. Reston, VA: Council of Biology Editors; 1999. CBE Guidelines No. 2.
6. Tufte ER. *The Visual Display of Quantitative Information*. Cheshire, CT: Graphics Press; 1983.
7. Schriger DL, Cooper RJ. Achieving graphical excellence: suggestions and methods for creating high-quality visual displays of experimental data. *Ann Emerg Med*. 2001;37(1):75-87.
8. Moher D, Schulz KF, Altman D; for the CONSORT Group. The CONSORT statement: revised recommendations for improving the quality of reports of parallel-group randomized trials. *JAMA*. 2001;285(15):1987-1991.

9. Stroup DF, Berlin JA, Morton SC, et al; for the Meta-analysis of Observational Studies in Epidemiology (MOOSE) Group. Meta-analysis of observational studies in epidemiology: a proposal for reporting. *JAMA*. 2000;283(15):2008-2012.
10. Moher D, Cook DJ, Eastwood S, Olkin I, Rennie D, Stroup DF; for the QUOROM Group. Improving the quality of reports of meta-analyses of randomised controlled trials: the QUOROM statement. *Lancet*. 1999;354(9193):1896-1900.
11. Bossuyt PM, Reitsma JB, Bruns DE, et al; for the STARD Group. Towards complete and accurate reporting of studies of diagnostic accuracy: the STARD initiative. *Clin Chem*. 2003;49(1):1-6.
12. Sox HC, Blatt MA, Higgins MC, Marton KI. *Medical Decision Making*. Boston, MA: Butterworths; 1988.
13. Hadorn DC. Use of algorithms in clinical guideline development. In: *Clinical Practice Guideline Development: Methodology Perspectives*. Rockville, MD: US Agency for Healthcare Policy and Research; 1994:93-104.
14. Pearson H. Imagine manipulation: CSI: cell biology. *Nature*. 2005;434(7036):952-953.
15. Scientific Illustration Committee of the Council of Biology Editors. *Illustrating Science: Standards for Publication*. Bethesda, MD: Council of Biology Editors; 1988.
16. Cleveland WS. *The Elements of Graphing Data*. Rev ed. Summit, NJ: Hobart Press; 1994.
17. Singer PA, Feinstein AR. Graphical display of categorical data. *J Clin Epidemiol*. 1993;46(3):231-236.
18. Rossner M. How to guard against image fraud. *Scientist*. 2006;20(3):24.

ADDITIONAL READING AND GENERAL REFERENCE

Hall GM, ed. *How to Write a Paper*. London, England: BMJ Publishing Group; 1994.

5 Ethical and Legal Considerations

If we are to live with this information explosion, let us not be terrified into dropping all our standards of the natures and ethics of scholarship and science.

Derek J. de Solla Price[1]

This chapter is intended to provide guidance to authors, editors, reviewers, and publishers in the fields of biomedicine, health, and the life sciences. The discussion focuses on ethical and legal issues involved in publication.

According to Lundberg,[2] human behavior is regulated by 3 forces: morality, ethics, and law. If personal morality does not regulate acceptable and appropriate behavior, we can rely on ethics. Ethical behavior is determined by norms, principles, guidelines, and policies. This chapter cites examples of the determinants of ethical behavior as they relate to scientific publication. If ethics do not regulate behavior, we are forced to rely on public laws. Examples of cases involving scientific publication when laws have been invoked or enforced are also provided in this chapter.

Those ethical and legal considerations and dilemmas most commonly encountered in scholarly scientific publication are the focus of this chapter. References to sources for additional guidance and information not discussed in this chapter are also provided within the text and at the end of each subsection.

ACKNOWLEDGMENT

Principal author: Annette Flanagin, RN, MA

Acknowledgments are provided at the end of each section of this chapter.

REFERENCES

1. de Solla Price DJ. Ethics of scientific publication: rules for authors and editorials may depend on something more than taste and convention. *Science.* 1964;144(3619):655-657.
2. Lundberg GD. Perspective from the editor of *JAMA, The Journal of the American Medical Association. Bull Med Libr Assoc.* 1992;80(2):110-114.

Some judge of authors' names, not works, and then
Nor praise nor blame the writings, but the men.
Alexander Pope[1]

5.1 Authorship Responsibility.

Authorship Responsibility. More than 50 years ago, Richard M. Hewitt, MD, then head of the Section of Publications at the Mayo Clinic, described the ethics of authorship in a *JAMA* article entitled "Exposition as Applied to Medicine: A Glance at the Ethics of It."[2] The following excerpts from Hewitt's article demonstrate an appreciation of the basic ethical responsibilities and obligations of authorship:

> Authorship cannot be conferred; it may be undertaken by one who will shoulder the responsibility that goes with it.
>
> The reader of a report issued by two or more authors has a right to assume that each author has some authoritative knowledge of the subject, that each contributed to the investigation, and that each labored on the report to the extent of weighing every word and quantity in it.
>
> If we would define publication of unoriginal, repetitious medical material as a violation of medical ethics, and would officially reprove it as such, the tawdry author would be silenced and the genuine one helped.
>
> The by-line, then, is not merely a credit-line. He who took some part in the investigation, be it ever so minor, is entitled to credit for what he did.... Further, the generous chap who would bestow authorship on another, perhaps without even submitting the manuscript to him, may do his colleague no favor. For the investigation is one thing, the report of it another, and, sad the day that this must be admitted: The investigation may have been excellent but the report, bad.
>
> Since all of us necessarily adopt and absorb the ideas of others, we must be scrupulous in maintaining the spirit of acknowledgment to others. Fundamentally, your integrity is at stake. Unless you make specific acknowledgment, you claim the credit for yourself for anything that you write. In general, it is better to say too much about your sources than too little.
>
> The author who paraphrases or refers to an article should have read it.

5.1.1 Authorship: Definition, Criteria, Contributions, and Requirements.

Authorship: Definition, Criteria, Contributions, and Requirements. Authorship offers significant professional and personal rewards, but these rewards are accompanied by substantial responsibility. During the 1980s, biomedical editors began requiring contributors to meet specific criteria for authorship. These criteria were first developed for medical journals under the initiative of Edward J. Huth, MD,[3] then editor of the *Annals of Internal Medicine,* who cited Hewitt's[2] work during discussions at the 1984 meeting of the International Committee of Medical Journal Editors (ICMJE). The ICMJE guidelines were first published in 1985[4] and are now part of the Uniform Requirements for Manuscripts Submitted to Biomedical Journals[5] (see also 2.0, Manuscript Preparation). These guidelines are reviewed, revised, and updated regularly, and numerous biomedical journals use them as the foundation for policies and procedures on authorship.

Authorship Definition and Criteria. According to the ICMJE guidelines, all authors should have participated sufficiently in the work to take public responsibility for the content, either all of the work or an important part of it. To take public responsibility, an author must be able to defend the content (all or an important part) and conclusions of the article if publicly challenged. Sufficient participation means that substantial contributions have been made in *each* of the following areas[5]:

1. Conception and design, or acquisition of data, or analysis and interpretation of the data,
2. Drafting the manuscript or revising it critically for important intellectual content, and
3. Approval of the version of the manuscript to be published

To justify authorship, an author must meet each of the 3 criteria. However, the term *substantial contribution* has not been adequately defined (perhaps to allow for wider application of the ICMJE criteria for authorship). As a result, the first criterion, "conception and design, or acquisition of data, or analysis and interpretation of the data," may be interpreted broadly. For example, an author of a nonresearch paper may not have analyzed data per se but may have analyzed literature, events, theories, arguments, or opinions. The following might be useful for those seeking an explanation of *substantial contribution*: a substantial contribution is an important intellectual contribution, without which the work, or an important part of the work, could not have been completed or the manuscript could not have been written and submitted for publication.

The ICMJE also notes that the following contributions, alone, are not sufficient to justify authorship[5]: "Participation solely in the acquisition of funding, or the collection of data, or general supervision of the research group is not sufficient for authorship." (See also 5.1.2, Guest and Ghost Authors.)

Author Contributions. Authors may not be aware of the ICMJE authorship criteria. To inform or remind authors of these responsibilities and to encourage appropriate authorship, many journals require authors to attest in writing how they qualify for authorship and to indicate their specific contributions to the work.[5-7] The ICMJE guidelines state, "Editors are strongly encouraged to develop and implement a contributorship policy, as well as a policy on identifying who is responsible for the integrity of the work as a whole."[5] Some journals ask authors to describe their specific contributions in an open-ended narrative format, some describe examples of various types of author contributions, and some journals provide a list of specific contributions in the form of a checklist. For example, *JAMA* and the *Archives* Journals require all authors to sign a statement of authorship responsibility based on the ICMJE guidelines and to indicate their specific contributions from a checklist based on the ICMJE authorship criteria and empiric data from studies of authorship and author contributions. This statement is required for authors of all types of manuscripts, including editorials, letters to the editor, and book reviews[8-11] (see the Box on p 130). *JAMA* and the *Archives* Journals use a single form for information about authorship responsibility, criteria, and contributions as well author's conflicts of interest disclosure, copyright transfer, and an acknowledgment statement. An updated example of this authorship form is available online in the *JAMA* Instructions for Authors at http://www.jama.com.

Some journals publish author contributions. This practice, first suggested by Rennie et al in 1997[6] and endorsed by the ICMJE[5] and the Council of Science Editors,[12] makes the specific contributions of authors transparent to editors and readers. For example, *JAMA* and the *Archives of Neurology* publish the specific contributions of each author for all articles reporting original data (eg, research and systematic reviews) in the Acknowledgment section at the end of the article (see 5.2, Acknowledgments).

According to the ICMJE, some journals also request that 1 or more authors (ie, "guarantors") be identified as those who take responsibility for the integrity of the work as a whole, from inception to published article, and publish the names of these guarantors with the article.[5]

Additional Author Requirements. Depending on the journal, authors may also be required to transfer copyright or a publication license, identify relevant conflicts of interest or to declare no such interests, identify sponsorship and the role of the sponsors in the work to be published, and attest that they had access to the data for reports of original research (see also 5.6.5, Intellectual Property: Ownership, Access, Rights, and Management, Copyright Assignment or License, and 5.5.1, Conflicts of Interest, Requirements for Authors).[13]

Access to Data Requirement. The ICMJE recommends that journals ask authors of studies funded by an entity with a proprietary or financial interest in the outcome of the study to sign a statement attesting that they had full access to the data and take responsibility for the integrity of the data and accuracy of the analysis.[5] Following this recommendation, *JAMA* requires at least 1 author who is independent of any commercial funder (eg, the principal investigator) to indicate that she or he had full access to all of the data in the study and takes responsibility for the integrity of the data and the accuracy of the data analysis for all reports containing original data (eg, research articles, systematic reviews, and meta-analyses).[13] See also 5.5.4, Conflicts of Interest, Access to Data Requirement.

Corresponding Author. Every manuscript and published article should have at least 1 author who will serve as the primary contact and correspondent for all communications about the submitted work and, if it is accepted for publication, the published article. It is not efficient for editorial offices or readers to have more than 1 formal corresponding author. However, it is helpful to provide the editorial office

Box. *JAMA* Authorship Responsibility, Criteria, and Contributions

Each author should meet all criteria below (A, B, C, and D) and should indicate general and specific contributions by reading criteria A, B, C, and D and checking the appropriate boxes.

☐ A. I certify that

- the manuscript represents original and valid work and that neither this manuscript nor one with substantially similar content under my authorship has been published or is being considered for publication elsewhere, except as described in an attachment; and
- if requested, I will provide the data or will cooperate fully in obtaining and providing the data on which the manuscript is based for examination by the editor or the editor's assignees; and
- for papers with more than 1 author, I agree to allow the corresponding author to serve as the primary correspondent with the editorial office, to review the edited typescript and proof, and to make decisions regarding release of information in the manuscript to the media, federal agencies, or both, or, if I am the only author, I will be the corresponding author and agree to serve in the roles described above.

☐ B. I have given final approval of the submitted manuscript.

C. I have participated sufficiently in the work to take public responsibility for (check 1 of 2 below)

☐ part of the content.
☐ the whole content.

D. To qualify for authorship, you must check at least 1 box for each of the 3 categories of contributions listed below.

I have made substantial contributions to the intellectual content of the paper as described below:

1. (check at least 1 of the 3 below)
   ☐ conception and design
   ☐ acquisition of data
   ☐ analysis and interpretation of data
2. (check at least 1 of 2 below)
   ☐ drafting of the manuscript
   ☐ critical revision of the manuscript for important intellectual content
3. (check at least 1 below)
   ☐ statistical analysis
   ☐ obtaining funding
   ☐ administrative, technical, or material support
   ☐ supervision
   ☐ no additional contributions
   ☐ other contributions (specify)______________________________

with contact information for coauthors in the event that the corresponding author becomes unavailable during the editorial and publication processes. For example, *JAMA* and the *Archives* Journals require a corresponding author for each submitted manuscript to serve as the primary correspondent with the editorial office and, if the paper is accepted, to review an edited typescript and proof, to make decisions regarding release of information in the manuscript to the news media and/or federal agencies, and to have his or her name published as corresponding author in the article. Corresponding authors for *JAMA* and the *Archives* Journals also sign a statement that they have identified all persons who have made substantial contributions to the work but who are not authors:

> I certify that all persons who have made substantial contributions to the work reported in this manuscript (eg, data collection, analysis, or writing or editing assistance) but who do not fulfill the authorship criteria are named with their specific contributions in an acknowledgment in the manuscript.
>
> I certify that all persons named in the Acknowledgment have provided me with written permission to be named.
>
> I certify that if an Acknowledgment section is not included, no other persons have made substantial contributions to this manuscript.

(See also 5.1.2, Guest and Ghost Authors, and 5.2, Acknowledgments.)

Deceased or Incapacitated Authors. In the case of death or incapacitation of an author during the manuscript submission and review or publication process, a family member or an individual with power of attorney can sign a journal's authorship or publication form for the deceased or incapacitated author, including the transfer of copyright or publication license, on behalf of the deceased or incapacitated author. In this event, the corresponding author can provide information on the deceased or incapacitated author's contributions (see also 2.0, Manuscript Preparation).

5.1.2 **Guest and Ghost Authors.** At least 1 author must be responsible for any part of an article crucial to its main conclusions, and everyone listed as an author must have made a substantial contribution to that specific article.[5] As described in 5.1.1, Authorship: Definition, Criteria, Contributions, and Requirements, many journals require authors to sign statements of authorship responsibility and to indicate specific contributions of all authors. In addition to improving the transparency of author responsibility, accountability, and credit, these policies may help eliminate guest authors and identify ghost authors.[14-16]

Guest (Honorary) Authors. Traditionally, supervisors, department chairs, and mentors have been given guest, or honorary, places in the byline even though they have not met all of the criteria for authorship. However, this custom is not acceptable because it devalues the meaning of authorship.[14,17] The ICMJE guidelines state specifically that "general supervision of the research group is not sufficient for authorship" and that participation solely in the "acquisition of funding, collection of data, or general supervision" does not justify authorship.[5] Such supervision and participation should be noted in the Acknowledgment (see 5.2, Acknowledgments). Guest authors have also included well-known persons in a particular field who have accepted money or other compensation to have their names attached to a manuscript that has already been researched and prepared by a ghost writer for an organization with a commercial interest in the subject of the paper.[15,18] Such practice clearly is deceitful.[14] Several studies have documented the prevalence of guest authors in biomedical journals ranging from 10% of research articles to 39% of review articles in journals that were not requesting authors to disclose their specific contributions.[9,19]

Ghost Authors. Ghost authors have participated sufficiently in the research or analysis and writing of a manuscript to take public responsibility for the work but are not named in the byline or Acknowledgment section. Studies involving journals that did not require authors to disclose specific contributions found that the prevalence of research and review articles with ghost authors ranged from 2% to 26%.[9,19] In biomedical publication, ghost authors have included employees of pharmaceutical companies (eg, researchers, managers, statisticians, epidemiologists), medical writers, marketing and public relations writers, and junior staff writing for elected or appointed officials.[15] As described elsewhere, ghost writers have been hired by firms with commercial interests to write reviews of specific subjects and their authorship is not disclosed.[14,15,17,18,20] Ghost *writers* are not necessarily ghost *authors*. For example, a writer may not have participated in the research or analysis of a study but may have been given the data and asked to draft a report for publication. If participants in the project do not meet all the criteria for authorship but have made substantial contributions to the research, writing, or editing of the manuscript, those persons should be named, with their permission, in the Acknowledgment along with their contributions and institutional affiliations, if relevant[14,21] (see 5.2, Acknowledgments). Editors and authors should not permit anyone who has participated substantially to meet authorship criteria or any nonauthor who has made other important contributions not to be appropriately identified in the byline or Acknowledgment, respectively. (See 5.2, Acknowledgments, and 5.1.6, Changes in Authorship.)

To give proper credit to medical writers and authors' editors, journal editors should require authors to identify all persons who have participated substantially in the writing or editing of the manuscript. Substantial editing or writing assistance should be disclosed to the editor at the time of manuscript submission and mentioned in the Acknowledgment.[14,21] (See 5.2, Acknowledgments.) Corresponding authors of *JAMA* and the *Archives* Journals sign a statement that all persons who have made substantial contributions to the work (eg, data collection, analysis, or writing or editing assistance) but who do not fulfill the authorship criteria are named with their specific contributions in an acknowledgment in the manuscript.

Journal editors and manuscript editors who substantially edit a manuscript to be published in a journal generally are not specifically acknowledged when their names appear in the journal's masthead or elsewhere in the journal.

5.1.3 Unsigned Editorials, Anonymous Authors, Pseudonymous Authors. The practice of publishing unsigned or anonymous editorials provides "vituperative editorialists"[22] protection from the enemies they might make when taking unpopular stands in the pages of their journals. However, without named authors and affiliations, readers lack information to judge the objectivity and credibility of the articles. Although this practice is the norm for newspaper editorial pages, it has fallen out of use in most peer-reviewed journals. One rationale for anonymity has been that editorials, signed or not, represent the official opinion of the publication or the owner of the publication. However, such anonymity distances the real author(s) from accountability. For many years, *JAMA* published unsigned editorials. However, beginning in 1960 *JAMA* began to inconsistently publish signed or initialed editorials, and since 1970 all *JAMA* editorials have been signed by their authors, including editorials written by the journal's editors. The *BMJ* began publishing signed editorials in 1981.[23] As of this writing, the *Lancet* continues to publish unsigned editorials that reflect an unstated consensus among the editors[24] (see 1.5, Types of Articles, Articles of Opinion).

Journals that publish unsigned editorials and signed scientific articles may give contradictory messages to their readers about the merits and responsibility of authorship. Authors who submit scientific papers must publicly stand by what they write, whereas unsigned editorialists can hide behind a journal's masthead. Unattributed editorials may also allow the publisher or owner of the journal and influential organizations to compromise the journal's editorial independence (see 5.10, Editorial Freedom and Integrity). Therefore, all editorials in *JAMA* and the *Archives* Journals are signed.

Occasionally, an author may request that his or her name not be used in publication. If the reason for this request is judged to be important (such as concern for personal safety or fear of political reprisal, public humiliation, or job loss), the article could be published without that author's name. However, justification for such publication is very rare and should include careful consideration of the value of the information to be published as well as the potential risks to the author. In such rare cases, the phrase "Name withheld on request" or the word "Anonymous" could be used in place of the author's name (see 2.2, Manuscript Preparation, Bylines and End-of-Text Signatures).

If anonymity is to be used, the author must still sign statements of authorship responsibility and copyright or publication license transfer (using his or her actual name), and those records must be kept confidential as part of the manuscript file (see also 5.7.1, Confidentiality, Confidentiality During Editorial Evaluation and Peer Review and After Publication). For the rare case in which withholding of an author's name is justified, the author's name should be withheld from peer reviewers as well as readers. However, both reviewers and readers should be informed that the author has requested anonymity. Citations to such articles in MEDLINE will note "No authors listed" in the author field.

Pseudonyms are inappropriate in bylines of scientific reports because they are misleading and cause problems for literature citations.

5.1.4 **Number of Authors.** The number of authors whose names appear in the byline of scientific papers increased steadily during the second half of the 20th century.[25] This increase occurred as a result of specialization, multidisciplinary collaboration, and the advent of large multicenter studies. However, authorship inflation has diluted the meaning of authorship. For example, which authors in a byline that contains more than 100 names can state that they actually wrote the paper or that they participated sufficiently to take public responsibility for the work? In response to this problem, suggestions were made in the 1980s and 1990s to limit the number of authors listed in the byline and database citations.[26,27] However, such limitations set arbitrary limits and may interfere with policies to encourage transparency of author contributions and thus are not justified. The US National Library of Medicine no longer limits the number of individual authors' names listed in an article's citation in MEDLINE.[28] For major articles, *JAMA* does not set limits on the number of authors that can be listed, as long as each author meets the journal's criteria for authorship and each author completes an authorship form indicating specific contributions. *JAMA* does limit the number of authors for an editorial or a commentary, and some *Archives* Journals continue to request justification or explanation for long lists of authors. For practical reasons (eg, space available on the first page of a print article), the names of all authors in an article with a large number of authors may be listed at the end of the article or elsewhere within an article instead of in the byline at the beginning of the article (see 5.1.7, Group and Collaborative Authorship). For online versions, all such lists are linked from the author byline.

Also for practical reasons, many journals limit the number of authors listed in reference list citations (see 3.7, References, Authors, and 5.1.7, Group and Collaborative Authorship). However, the online versions of many journal articles contain reference lists with links to original articles and to MEDLINE records in PubMed, both of which list all authors for articles published in 2000 or later.

5.1.5 **Order of Authorship.** Before proposals for identifying authors' contributions began to be implemented, proposed guides for determining order of authorship ranged from simple alphabetical listings to mathematical formulas for assessing specific levels of individual contribution levels.[29-31] However, even the most systematic calculations of contribution levels will require some measure of subjective judgment, and determination of order of authors is best done by the authors' collective assessment of each other's level of contribution. Moreover, as Rennie et al[6] have argued, attempts to provide information to readers by ordering authors in particular ways is not meaningful, especially if each author's contributions are not made public. The following may help determine order of authorship[32]:

1. Only those individuals who meet the criteria for authorship may be listed as authors (see 5.1.1, Authorship: Definition, Criteria, Contributions, and Requirements).
2. The first author has contributed the most to the work, with other authors listed in descending order according to their levels of contribution. (*Note:* Some groups of authors choose to list the most senior author last, irrespective of the relative amount of his or her contribution.)
3. Decisions about the order of authors should be made as early as possible (eg, before the manuscript is written) and reevaluated later as often as needed by consensus (see also 5.1.6, Changes in Authorship).
4. Disagreement about order should be resolved by the authors, not the editor.
5. Authors may provide a publishable footnote explaining the order of authorship, if there is a compelling reason.
6. Editors may request documentation of authors' specific contributions.

5.1.6 **Changes in Authorship.** Changes made in authorship (ie, order, addition, and deletion of authors) should be discussed and approved by all authors. Any such changes made after a manuscript has been submitted should be explained to the journal. The

BMJ's policy for alterations in authorship of papers under consideration is a useful guide for other journals:

> Any change in authors and/or contributors after initial submission must be approved by all authors. This applies to additions, deletions, change of order to the authors, or contributions being attributed differently. Any alterations must be explained to the editor. The editor may contact any of the authors and/or contributors to ascertain whether they have agreed to any alteration.[33]

5.1.7 **Group and Collaborative Authorship.** Group or collaborative authorship usually involves multicenter study investigators, members of working groups, and official or self-appointed expert boards, panels, or committees. Such group-author papers are also referred to as *collaborative*, *corporate*, and *collective author* papers. These groups can comprise hundreds of participants and often represent complex, multidisciplinary collaborations, and therefore, decisions about listing group authorship pose several problems and dilemmas for authors, editors, journals, librarians, and bibliographic databases[34-37] (see 14.9, Abbreviations, Collaborative Groups, and 2.2.4, Manuscript Preparation, Bylines and End-of-Text Signatures, Multiple Authors, Group Authors).

Large trials and studies are often best known and frequently referred to by their study name (eg, Women's Health Initiative) or by their abbreviation (eg, WHI). As a result, these groups often include the official name of the study group in an article's byline (ie, the position on an article's title page where authors are listed). However, not all members of a study group may meet authorship criteria (see 5.1.1, Authorship: Definition, Criteria, Contributions, and Requirements), and having the group name in the byline does not distinguish those members of the group who qualify for authorship from those who do not. In addition, without a single person named as author, no individual person can take responsibility and be held accountable for the work. For this reason, at least 1 individual (eg, the corresponding author or the principal investigator) should be named as corresponding author or guarantor (see also 2.0, Manuscript Preparation). To address these concerns, members of a writing team or a subgroup are often identified as the authors for large groups.

For group-author articles, providing appropriate credit and accountability for the many individuals involved—authors and nonauthors—and ensuring proper citation and online searching and retrieval of the articles are important considerations.[34,38] The guidelines that follow may help authors and editors determine who should be listed and where.

One or more authors may take responsibility for a group (as the authors or writing team). In this case, the names of individual authors are listed in the byline with a designation that these authors are writing on behalf of or *for* the group. Those members of the group who do not qualify for authorship would not be listed in the byline but may be listed in the Acknowledgment at the end of the article. In this case, the byline might read as follows:

> Jacques E. Rossouw, MBChB, MD; Garnet L. Anderson, PhD; for the Women's Health Initiative
>
> *or*
>
> Writing Group for the Women's Health Initiative

In the latter example, the writing group members are the authors for the group, and their names should be listed in the author affiliation or Acknowledgment section (with their specific contributions identified). *Note*: In these cases the formal group-author name (eg, Women's Health Initiative) should be coded in the journal's online version and in bibliographic databases so that the results of online searches for articles from this group will include articles that combine individual names or subgroup (eg, the Writing Group) with the formal group name in the byline.

The other nonauthor group members and their contributions may then be listed separately in the Acknowledgment section (see 5.2, Acknowledgments).

Some authors and groups might prefer that only the group name appear in the byline to emphasize the collaborative nature of their effort. Thus, another option is for the byline to list only the group name followed by an asterisk, which refers to a list of specific authors or a writing committee for the overall group:

Clinical Outcomes Trial Investigators*

The asterisk in the byline corresponds to another asterisk and note on the same printed page of the article or linked affiliation in the online version that identifies a list of authors who take responsibility for this article. This location of the list of authors must be clearly indicated so that readers can identify the authors and indexers of bibliographic databases can identify and properly index the names of all authors. The note might read as follows:

*__Authors/Clinical Outcomes Trial Investigators__ are John Smith, Mary Broadbent, Timothy Bowman, Jane Swanson, David Pearce, and Joan Wallace.

or

*__Authors/Writing Committee Members for the Clinical Outcomes Trial Investigators__ are listed at the end of this article.

In the second example above, the names and affiliations of all authors/writing committee members and their specific contributions may be listed at the end of the article (see 5.2.2, Acknowledgments, Group and Collaborative Author Lists). Some journals may choose to publish long lists of authors from a group in a box or separate list within the article. To ensure that authors are cited appropriately in bibliographic databases, explicit use of the term *Authors* or *Writers* is preferred.

Authorship can be attributed to an entire group, although this practice is less common than the examples given above. However, as with all articles, clear justification for all members of the group meeting all criteria and requirements for authorship must be made, and for journals that publish authors' individual contributions, all members of the group must identify their specific contributions (see 5.1.1, Authorship: Definition, Criteria, Contributions, and Requirements). In this case, the byline might read as follows:

Clinical Outcomes Trial Investigators

In cases in which every member of a large group qualifies for authorship and the group name appears in the byline, the individual members of the study group should be listed separately in the Acknowledgment section or in a clearly identified position within the article, such as a box set off by rules (as described in 2.2.4, Manuscript Preparation, Bylines and End-of-Text Signatures, Multiple Authors, Group Authors).

If the group name appears in the byline, it is recommended that at least 1 person, usually the corresponding author, be named as an individual who will coordinate questions about the article. This person can be named in the affiliation footnote as corresponding author. In this case, the byline might read

Clinical Outcomes Trial Investigators

and the affiliation footnote might read

Author Affiliations: A complete list of the authors in the Clinical Outcomes Trial Investigators appears at the end of this article.

Corresponding Author: James S. Smith, MD, Department of Neurology, University of Chicago Medical School, 555 S Main St, Chicago, IL 60615 (smithjs@umc.edu).

(See also 2.3.3, Manuscript Preparation, Footnotes to Title Page, Author Affiliations, and 2.10.4, Manuscript Preparation, Acknowledgment Section, Correspondence Address.)

Publishing the names of all authors and their specific contributions, no matter how many, with the specific article is preferred. However, a long list of investigators and affiliated centers could occupy several journal pages and may be of questionable value to readers. Yet it is important to publish the names of each author with the article, for reasons of accountability and credit and to allow proper searching and retrieval of articles by individual author names in bibliographic databases. If the identical list of authors has been published previously in a group list in an indexed and retrievable journal, the editor may choose to cite and link to that publication in an affiliation footnote or acknowledgment rather than republish the entire list (see 5.2, Acknowledgments). A journal that is simultaneously publishing 2 or more articles from the same group of authors may consider publishing the list of authors in the initial article and then citing that article in, and linking to that article from, the other related articles. Another option is to publish the list in the journal's online version of the article, as long as there is clear indication (citation and linking) of this list in the printed article. The same options apply to long lists of other collaborators who are not authors.

Study or other group participants should not be promised authorship status and a place in the byline merely for performing activities that alone do not qualify for authorship (eg, cooperating in a study, collecting data, attending a working conference, lending technical assistance). However, performing any of those activities in addition to writing or critically revising the manuscript and approving the version to be published would be sufficient to merit authorship (see 5.1.1, Authorship: Definition, Criteria, Contributions, and Requirements). Editors and authors should assess the need to publish lengthy lists of authors and other group participants on an individual basis, and journals should publish their policies about group authorship in their instructions for authors.

Citation of Articles With Group Authors. Articles with authors from a large group have been difficult to locate in bibliographic databases and have resulted in citation errors and miscalculated citation statistics.[35-37] To help resolve these problems, the following has been recommended[38]:

- Group-author articles should identify named individual authors who accept responsibility for specific articles.

- Each group-author article should clearly identify all individual authors (preferably full names, but last names and initials are acceptable) as well as the complete name of the group, whether they appear in the byline or author affiliation.
- Individual authors should be distinguished from other contributors and participants who are not authors.
- The names of individual authors and the group name should be formatted and coded for easy identifiability, searching, and retrieval of the article in print and online and in bibliographic databases. See Box in 5.2, Acknowledgments.
- Each group-author article should clearly indicate a preferred citation (eg, along with the abstract or at the end of the article).
- Search results on journal Web sites should clearly indicate a preferred citation, in addition to relevant author information.
- Citation standards for group-author papers should continue to be developed and followed by journals, bibliographic databases, and authors.

ACKNOWLEDGMENTS

Principal author: Annette Flanagin, RN, MA

I thank Drummond Rennie, MD, *JAMA*; Trevor Lane, MA, DPhil, University of Hong Kong; Catherine D. DeAngelis, MD, MPH, *JAMA* and *Archives* Journals; and C. K. Gunsalus, JD, University of Illinois, Champaign/Urbana, for reviewing and providing substantial comments to help improve this section; Daniel M. Albert, MD, MS, *Archives of Ophthalmology*; Terri S. Carter, *Archives of Surgery*; Paula Glitman, *Archives* Journals; Cindy W. Hamilton, PharmD, ELS, Hamilton House; Sheldon Kotzin, MLS, National Library of Medicine; Diana J. Mason, RN, PhD, *American Journal of Nursing*; Povl Riis, MD, University of Copenhagen; Valerie Siddall, PhD, ELS, AstraZeneca; Liz Wager, MA, Sideview; and Flo Witte, MA, ELS, AdvancMed LLC, for review and providing minor comments; and Sandra R. Schefris and Yolanda Davis, James S. Todd Memorial Library, American Medical Association, Chicago, Illinois, for bibliographic assistance.

REFERENCES

1. Pope A. *An Essay on Criticism.* 1711:part Ib, line 212.
2. Hewitt RM. Exposition as applied to medicine: a glance at the ethics of it. *JAMA.* 1954;156(5):477-479.
3. Huth EJ. Guidelines on authorship of medical papers. *Ann Intern Med.* 1986; 104(2):269-274.
4. International Committee of Medical Journal Editors. Guidelines on authorship. *BMJ.* 1985;291(6947):722.
5. International Committee of Medical Journal Editors. Uniform Requirements for Manuscripts Submitted to Biomedical Journals. http://www.icmje.org. Updated February 2006. Accessed September 2, 2006.
6. Rennie D, Yank V, Emanuel L. When authorship fails: a proposal to make contributors accountable. *JAMA.* 1997;278(7):579-585.
7. Rennie D, Flanagin A, Yank V. The contributions of authors. *JAMA.* 2000;284(1):89-91.
8. Shapiro DW, Wenger NS, Shapiro MF. The contributions of authors to multiauthored biomedical research papers. *JAMA.* 1994;271(6):438-442.

9. Flanagin A, Carey LA, Fontanarosa, PB, et al. Prevalence of articles with honorary authors and ghost authors in peer-reviewed medical journals. *JAMA*. 1998;280(3):222-224.
10. Drenth JPH. Multiple authorship: the contribution of senior authors. *JAMA*. 1998; 280(3):219-221.
11. Yank V, Rennie D. Disclosure of researcher contributions: a study of original research articles in *The Lancet*. *Ann Intern Med*. 1999;130(8):661-670.
12. Davidoff F, for the Council of Science Editors Taskforce on Authorship. Who's the author? problems with biomedical authorship, and some possible solutions. http://www.councilscienceeditors.org/publications/v23n4p111-119.pdf. February 2000. Accessed August 4, 2006.
13. DeAngelis CD, Fontanarosa PB, Flanagin A. Reporting financial conflicts of interest and relationships between investigators and research sponsors. *JAMA*. 2001;286(1):89-91.
14. Rennie D, Flanagin A. Authorship! authorship! guests, ghosts, grafters, and the two-sided coin. *JAMA*. 1994;271(6):469-471.
15. Flanagin A, Rennie D. Acknowledging ghosts. *JAMA*. 1995;273(1):73.
16. Marusic A, Bates T, Anic A, Marusic M. How the structure of contribution disclosure statements affects validity of authorship: a randomized study in a general medical journal. *Curr Med Res Opin*. 2006;22(6):1035-1044.
17. Smith J. Gift authorship: a poisoned chalice? *BMJ*. 1994;309(6967):1456-1457.
18. Brennan TA. Buying editorials. *N Engl J Med*. 1994;331(10):673-675.
19. Mowatt G, Shirran L, Grimshaw JM, et al. Prevalence of honorary and ghost authorship in Cochrane reviews. *JAMA*. 2002;287(21):2769-2771.
20. DeBakey L. Rewriting and the by-line: is the author the writer? *Surgery*. 1974;75(1): 38-48.
21. Hamilton CW, Royer MG; for the AMWA 2002 Task Force on the Contributions of Medical Writers to Scientific Publications. AMWA position statement on the contributions of medical writers to scientific publications. *AMWA J*. 2003;18(1):13-16.
22. Morgan P. *An Insider's Guide for Medical Authors and Editors*. Philadelphia, PA: ISI Press; 1986.
23. Lock S. Signed editorials. *BMJ*. 1981;283(6296):876.
24. *The Lancet*. Signed—*The Lancet*. *Lancet*. 1993;341(8836):24.
25. Fye WB. Medical authorship: traditions, trends, and tribulations. *Ann Intern Med*. 1990;113(4):317-325.
26. Burman KD. "Hanging from the masthead": reflections on authorship. *Ann Intern Med*. 1982;97(4):602-605.
27. Epstein RJ. Six authors in search of a citation: villains or victims of the Vancouver convention? *BMJ*. 1993;306(6880):765-767.
28. National Library of Medicine. MEDLINE/PubMed data element (field) descriptions. *NLM Tech Bull*. November-December 2005:347.
29. Schmidt RH. A worksheet for authorship of scientific articles. *Bull Ecol Soc Am*. 1987; 68(1):8-10.
30. Davis PJ, Gregerman RI. Parse analysis: a new method for the evaluation of investigators' bibliographies. *N Engl J Med*. 1969;281(18):989-990.
31. Chambers R, Boath E, Chambers S. The A to Z of authorship: analysis of influence of initial letter of surname of order of authorship. *BMJ*. 2001;323(7327):1460-1461.
32. Riesenberg D, Lundberg GD. The order of authorship: who's on first? *JAMA*. 1990; 264(14):1857.
33. Submitting articles to the Journal. *BMJ*. http://bmj.bmjjournals.com/advice/article_submission.shtml#author. Accessed August 1, 2006.

34. Flanagin A, Fontanarosa PB, DeAngelis CD. Authorship for research groups. *JAMA*. 2002;288(24):3166-3168.
35. Dickersin K, Scherer R, Suci EST, Gil-Montero M. Problems with indexing and citation of articles with group authorship. *JAMA*. 2002;287(21):2772-2774.
36. Errors in citation statistics. *Nature*. 2002;415(6868):101.
37. Cherfas J. With missing citations reported: *Nature* genome paper jumps. *Sci Watch*. 2002;13(1):8.
38. Flanagin A, Wrobel P, Barbour V, et al. CSE Recommendations for group-author articles in scientific journals and bibliometric databases. http://www.councilscienceeditors.org/editorial_policies/groupauthorarticles.cfm. Accessed December 28, 2006.

If you wish your merit to be known, acknowledge that of other people.

Proverb

5.2 Acknowledgments.

Acknowledgments. Acknowledgments typically are used to list grant or funding support, donors of equipment or supplies, technical assistance, and important specific contributions from individuals who do not qualify for authorship (see 2.10, Manuscript Preparation, Acknowledgment Section, and 5.1.1, Authorship Responsibility, Authorship: Definition, Criteria, Contributions, and Requirements). Sufficient space should be provided in publications, either in print or online, for acknowledgments so that authors can properly credit all important contributions.

5.2.1 Acknowledging Support, Assistance, and Contributions of Those Who Are Not Authors.

Acknowledging Support, Assistance, and Contributions of Those Who Are Not Authors. In the Acknowledgment, authors identify important sources of financial and material support and assistance and give credit to all persons who have made substantial contributions to the work but who are not authors.[1,2] Contributions commonly recognized in an acknowledgment include the following:

General advice, guidance, or supervision
Critical review of the manuscript
Critical review of study proposal, design, or methods
Data collection
Data analysis
Statistical assistance or advice
Technical assistance or advice
Research assistance or advice
Writing assistance
Editorial assistance
Bibliographic assistance
Clerical assistance
Manuscript preparation
Financial support
Material support
Grant support

Acknowledgments should identify anyone who has made substantial intellectual contributions to manuscripts but does not meet the criteria for authorship, including medical writers and author's editors[1-4] (see 5.1.2, Authorship Responsibility, Guest and Ghost Authors). For example, *JAMA* and the *Archives* Journals require the corresponding author to identify such assistance in the Acknowledgment. *JAMA* also discloses the affiliation and funding of individuals who contribute to manuscripts but who are not authors. Such disclosure is supported by the American Medical Writers Association[3] and the European Medical Writers Association[4] as it is more helpful to editors, reviewers, and readers than are vague statements about writing or editorial assistance that give no indication about financial relationships. As an example, the Acknowledgment might read as follows:

> **Additional Contribution**: We thank Joan Smart, PhD, of Medical Bibliometrics Inc, Boston, Massachusetts, who received payment from the study's sponsor, for research and editing assistance.

JAMA requires the corresponding author of all manuscripts to sign an acknowledgment statement (on the authorship form) that reads as follows:

> I certify that all persons who have made substantial contributions to the work reported in the manuscript (eg, data collection, analysis, or writing or editing assistance) but do not fulfill authorship criteria are named with their specific contributions in an acknowledgment in the manuscript.
>
> I certify that all persons named in the Acknowledgment have provided me with written permission to be named.
>
> I certify that if an Acknowledgment section is not included, no other persons have made substantial contributions to this manuscript.

Nonspecific group acknowledgments, such as "the house staff," "the nurses in the emergency department," or "patient participants" are often used to thank groups of individuals. However, if specific people are identifiable, permission to include them would be needed (see also 5.2.8, Permission to Name Individuals). Acknowledgment of unidentifiable groups, such as "the anonymous peer reviewers," is not informative, and with current policies encouraging greater transparency, acknowledging any anonymous contributions is best avoided.

5.2.2 Group and Collaborative Author Lists. A list of participants in a collaborative group may also be included in the Acknowledgment[5] (see 5.1.7, Authorship Responsibility, Group and Collaborative Authorship). However, a lengthy acknowledgment may occupy an excessive amount of journal space. Some editors have proposed limits on the length of an acknowledgment (eg, 1 column of a journal page or 600 words of reduced type),[6] but such limits seem contrary to commitments to greater transparency of the contributions to scientific publication, and journals should carefully evaluate the appropriateness of any limits on the length of acknowledgments. Yet the need to credit assistance from individuals, especially in large multicenter clinical trials, varies considerably. Thus, the editor and corresponding author should determine the length of published acknowledgments on a case-by-case basis. If it is determined that there is not sufficient space in a print publication to include a long list of collaborative participants, the list can be published online with a note indicating so in the Acknowledgment section:

> A list of study investigators and participating centers of the European Diabetes Intervention Trial is available online at http://archinte.ama-assn.org/cgi/content/full/165/22/2495.

Alternatively, if a long list of group members or collaborators has been published previously and has not changed in the interim, the list can be cited in the affiliation footnote or Acknowledgment section as follows, provided that the names of all authors are also indicated in the published article:

> A full list of investigators and participating centers of the European Diabetes Intervention Trial as of October 20, 2005, was published in the *Archives of Internal Medicine* (2005;165[22]:2488-2499).

5.2.3 **Author Contributions.** The International Committee of Medical Journal Editors (ICMJE) encourages authors and journals to disclose authors' individual contributions to the work reported in published articles.[7] Following this recommendation, a number of journals now publish lists of author contributions in the article's "Acknowledgment" section.[8] For example, *JAMA* publishes each author's contributions, as shown in the example in the Box on pages 143-144.

5.2.4 **Authors' Conflicts of Interests and Financial Disclosures.** Authors' financial disclosures should be published with articles, either on the title page or in the Acknowledgment section. *JAMA* and the *Archives* Journals include authors' financial disclosures in the Acknowledgment section at the end of the article. *JAMA* requires authors to include all potential conflicts of interest, including specific financial interests and relationships and affiliations (other than those affiliations listed in the title page of the manuscript) relevant to the subject of their manuscript in the Acknowledgment section at the time the manuscript is submitted. Authors without conflicts of interest, including specific financial interests and relationships and affiliations relevant to the subject of their manuscript, should include a statement of no such interests in the Acknowledgment section of the manuscript.[9] (See Box and 5.5.1, Conflicts of Interest, Reporting Funding and Other Support.)

5.2.5 **Access to Data Statement.** The ICMJE recommends that editors request authors of studies funded by companies or agencies with proprietary or financial interests in the study outcomes to sign a statement indicating that they had access to all of the data and can vouch for the integrity of the data analyses.[7] For example, for all reports containing original data, *JAMA* and some of the *Archives* Journals require at least 1 author (eg, the principal investigator) who is independent of any commercial funder to indicate that she or he "had full access to all of the data in the study and takes responsibility for the integrity of the data and the accuracy of the data analysis."[10,11]

JAMA publishes such an access to data statement in the Acknowledgment section. (See also 5.5.4, Conflicts of Interest, Access to Data Requirement.)

For industry-sponsored studies and any other studies in which proprietary concerns could lead to bias in the analysis, the data analysis should be conducted by an independent statistician at an academic institution, such as a medical school, academic medical center, or government research institute, that has oversight over the person conducting the analysis and that is independent of the commercial sponsor rather than only by statisticians employed by the sponsor of the research. For example, for manuscripts in which the statistical analysis was performed exclusively

Box. Hypothetical Example of an Acknowledgment Including Order of Elements

Note: Not all of the elements listed below are relevant for all manuscripts, nor are they published by all journals. Asterisk indicates items that may normally appear on page 1 of a printed article but would appear here in this order if there were not sufficient space on the first page.

For an Article With the Following Byline:
Jack Kroll, MD; Kathryn Smith, RN, PhD; Jake Otter, MPH; for the Stress Intervention Trial Investigators

Submitted for Publication: August 1, 2006; final revision received September 10, 2006; accepted September 17, 2006.
Published Online: October 20, 2006 (doi:10.1001/jama.2006.125).
***Author Affiliations:** Division of Cardiovascular Medicine, University of Florida College of Medicine, Gainesville (Dr Kroll); Department of Behavioral Science, University of Pittsburgh Medical Center, Pittsburgh, Pennsylvania (Dr Smith); Department of Psychiatry, University of Oxford, Oxford, England (Mr Otter).
***Corresponding Author**: Jack Kroll, MD, Division of Cardiovascular Medicine, University of Florida College of Medicine, 25 Main St, Gainesville, FL 32601 (krollj@ufcm.edu).
Author Contributions: As principal investigator, Dr Kroll had full access to all the data in the study and takes responsibility for the integrity of the data and the accuracy of the data analysis.
Study concept and design: Kroll, Smith, Otter
Acquisition of data: Kroll, Otter
Analysis and interpretation of data: Kroll, Smith, Otter
Drafting of the manuscript: Kroll
Critical revision of the manuscript for important intellectual content: Smith, Otter
Statistical analysis: Kroll, Smith
Obtained funding: Kroll
Administrative, technical, or material support: Kroll
Study supervision: Kroll
Financial Disclosures: Dr Kroll has received research grants from and is a paid consultant to Progen International Inc, manufacturer of the neurochemical assay used in this study, and research grants from the International Society of Stress Research. Dr Smith and Mr Otter have reported no relevant financial interests in this publication.
Funding/Support: This study was funded by Progen International Inc and the International Society of Stress Research.
Role of the Sponsor: Progen International Inc supplied the neurochemical assay used in this study and funded the study. Through Dr Kroll, Progen International Inc participated in the design and conduct of the study; in the collection, analysis, and interpretation of the data; and in the preparation of the manuscript. Progen International Inc reviewed the manuscript before submission and paid for editing assistance. The International Society of Stress Research had no role in the design and conduct of the study; in the collection, analysis,

Box. Hypothetical Example of an Acknowledgment Including Order of Elements *(cont)*

and interpretation of the data; or in the preparation of the manuscript or review of the manuscript.
Independent Statistical Analysis: Data sets were forwarded to an independent statistician, John Smythe, PhD, of the Medical Statistics Unit, Oxford University, Oxford, England. Dr Smythe, who had no involvement in the planning and conduct of the original analyses, analyzed the data and has verified that the results presented in this publication are consistent with his analysis. Dr Smythe received compensation for this analysis from Progen International Inc.
The Stress Intervention Trial Investigators: *Steering Committee:* Jeff Brown, MD, David Chillow, MD, Jane Marshall, MBBS, Lionell J. Roew, MD, Gilberto Felosa, MD, Ulrich Teich, MD, Li Wang, MD, MPH, Alexandra Zeer, PhD; *Data and Safety Monitoring Committee:* Janice Frank, MD, chair; Michelle Dickersin, MD, William Malden, MD, Adam Skowrenski, PhD, Anita Toole, MD. *Research Coordinators:* Michael Billings, MPH, Timothy Downing, PharmD, Laura Grower, RN, Kenneth Morrisey, MD, Frederic McLendon, RN, Wanda Smythe, MS, Anne Trafford, PhD.
A full list of principal investigators and participating centers has been published (*J Stress*. 2004;25[4]:42-50).
Disclaimer: The views expressed in this article are those of the authors and do not necessarily reflect the opinions of the authors' institutions.
Previous Presentation: Presented in part at the 12th International Stress Management Congress; February 15, 2005; Chicago, Illinois.
Additional Information: Online Tables 1 and 2 are available at http://www.jama.com.
Additional Contributions: We thank Joan Simpson, MS, of Write Services, who was paid by Progen International Inc for editing the manuscript. We thank the 3 patients with serious adverse events, who reviewed the submitted manuscript, for granting permission to include the details about their cases in this article.
Preferred Citation: Kroll J, Smith H, Otter J; for the Stress Intervention Trial Investigators. An intervention to reduce stress [published online ahead of print October 20, 2006]. *JAMA*. 2006;294(22):1553-1559.

by employees of the commercial sponsor, *JAMA* editors will ask the authors to have the analysis and results verified by an independent statistician at an academic institution; ask that statistician to provide a statement that he or she had access to all the data (entire raw data set, study protocol, and prespecified plan for data analysis) and has independently verified the analysis and results; and publish a notice of this independent verification in the Acknowledgment section along with information on funding for this additional analysis.[9] (See also 5.5.5, Conflicts of Interest, Requirements for Reporting Industry-Sponsored Studies.) See the examples below.

> **Independent Statistical Analysis:** The accuracy of the data analysis was independently verified by Jasmine Singh, PhD, and Frank Martin, PhD, both from the Experimental Research Foundation, an affiliate of Columbia University, who received the entire raw database and replicated all the analyses that were reported in the accepted manuscript. No discrepancies were discovered. Neither Dr Singh or Martin nor the Experimental Research Foundation received any funding for this independent analysis.

Independent Statistical Analysis: Data sets for the interim analyses were forwarded by Labyx Biometrics Inc to an independent statistician, Paul Wise, PhD, of the Medical Research Unit, University of Reading, Reading, England. Dr Wise, who had no involvement in the planning and conduct of the original analyses, conducted an independent analysis of the data and has verified that the results presented in this publication are consistent with his analysis. Dr Wise was compensated for this analysis by the sponsor of the study.

5.2.6 **Funding and Role of Sponsors.** Information about funding, sponsorship, or other financial or material support should also be clearly and completely identified in the Acknowledgment section, if not already reported in the "Methods" section.[7,9-11] For all manuscripts that are funded by commercial, governmental, or private entities, a description of the role of the sponsor(s) in the work reported and the preparation, submission, and review of the manuscript should be published as well.[9,10] For example, for all funded manuscripts, including letters to the editor, *JAMA* and some of the *Archives* Journals require the corresponding author to indicate the role of the sponsor in each of the following:

Design and conduct of the study

Collection, management, analysis, and interpretation of the data

Preparation, review, or approval of the manuscript

If the sponsor had no role in the above activities, that information should be indicated. If authors are employees of a sponsor, this information should include any role of the sponsor above and beyond the contributions of the specific sponsor-employed authors. Some journals publish this information in the "Methods" section. *JAMA* and the *Archives* Journals publish it in the Acknowledgment section (see 5.5.1, Conflicts of Interest, Requirements for Authors, and the following examples).

Role of the Sponsor: The Centers for Disease Control and Prevention had no role in the design and conduct of the study or the collection, management, analysis, and interpretation of the data; it reviewed and approved the manuscript for submission.

Role of the Sponsor: The Deutsche Krenshilfe had no role in the design and conduct of the study; the collection, management, analysis, and interpretation of the data; and the preparation, review, or approval of the manuscript. Authors who are employees of Biopharm Company participated in each of these activities. The National Institutes of Health reviewed and approved the study before funding.

Role of the Sponsor: The Medicines Co and the REPLACE-2 Steering Committee designed the trial, developed the protocol, and determined the statistical analysis plan by consensus. Data were collected through an Internet-based electronic case-report form managed by Etrials. The sponsor had no access to the database or the randomization code, which were housed at Etrials and Integrated Clinical Technologies Inc, respectively, until finalization of the database. Data management and site monitoring were performed by International HealthCare. The finalized database was electronically transferred simultaneously to the Cleveland Clinic Cardiovascular Coordinating Center and to The Medicines Co, where unblinding and statistical analyses were separately performed. All analyses for scientific publication were performed by the study statistician at the Cleveland Clinic, independently from the sponsor. Dr Lincoff wrote all drafts of the manuscript and made revisions based on the comments of the study chairman, the Steering Committee, coauthors, and the trial sponsor. The study contract specified that the sponsor had the right to review all publications prior to submission and could delay submission of such publications for up to 60 days if necessary to make new patent applications, but could not mandate any revision of the manuscript or prevent submission for publication.

5.2.7 **Acknowledgment Elements and Order of Elements.** An example of the Acknowledgment section including all possible elements as it would appear in *JAMA* or any of the *Archives* Journals is shown in the Box. In print journals, author affiliations and correspondence information typically are published on the title page (or first page) of an article. However, in some cases (eg, articles with lengthy abstracts and author bylines) and in some journals, there may not be sufficient room for all of this information and it may be published in the Acknowledgment section at the end of the article with a note indicating such on the first page of the article. Online, the author information and Acknowledgment section usually appear at the end of the article before the reference list and may be hyperlinked from the list of authors at the beginning of the article.

5.2.8 **Permission to Name Individuals.** Identification of individuals in an acknowledgment may imply their endorsement of the article's content. Thus, persons should not be listed in an acknowledgment without their knowledge and consent. For this reason, the ICMJE and *JAMA* require the corresponding author to obtain written permission from any individuals named in the Acknowledgment section and to certify in writing to the editor that such permission has been obtained.[2,6,7]

5.2.9 **Personal Communication and Credit Lines.** Following the rationale that including a person's name in an acknowledgment may imply endorsement of a manuscript's content, citing an individual's name in a personal communication citation may carry the same implication. The ICMJE recommends that authors who name an individual as a source for information in a personal communication, be it through conversation, telephone call, or a letter sent by mail, fax, or e-mail, obtain written permission from that individual to be named.[7] *JAMA* and the *Archives* Journals follow the ICMJE recommendation and require authors to forward copies of all personal communication permissions to the editorial office. The same policy might apply to identifying names in credit lines in the legends of illustrations and photographs; however, obtaining such permission from the owner of the illustration or photograph would be part of obtaining permission to include such works as required under the auspices of copyright law (see 5.6.7, Intellectual Property: Ownership, Access, Rights, and Management, Copying, Reproducing, Adapting, and Other Uses of Content).

ACKNOWLEDGMENTS

Principal author: Annette Flanagin, RN, MA

I thank C. K. Gunsalus, JD, University of Illinois; Valerie Siddall, PhD, ELS, AstraZeneca; and Liz Wager, MA, Sideview, for review and providing important suggestions for improvement of this section; the following for also providing review and minor suggestions: Daniel M. Albert, MD, MA, *Archives of Ophthalmology*; Terri S. Carter, *Archives of Surgery*; Catherine D. DeAngelis, MD, MPH, *JAMA* and *Archives* Journals; Cindy W. Hamilton, PharmD, ELS, Hamilton House; Wayne G. Hoppe, JD, *JAMA* and *Archives* Journals; Trevor Lane, MA, DPhil, University of Hong Kong; Diana J. Mason, RN, PhD, *American Journal of Nursing*; Drummond Rennie, MD, *JAMA*; Povl Riis, MD, University of Copenhagen; Cheryl Smart, MA, MBA; and Flo Witte, MA, MLS, AdvanceMed LLC; and Sandra Schefris and Yolanda Davis, James S. Todd Memorial Library, American Medical Association, Chicago, Illinois, for bibliographic assistance.

REFERENCES

1. Rennie D, Flanagin A. Authorship! authorship! guests, ghosts, grafters, and the two-sided coin. *JAMA*. 1994;271(6):469-471.
2. Flanagin A, Rennie D. Acknowledging ghosts. *JAMA*. 1995;273(1):73.
3. Hamilton CW, Royer MG; for the AMWA 2002 Task Force on the Contributions of Medical Writers to Scientific Publications. AMWA position statement on the contributions of medical writers to scientific publications. *AMWA J*. 2003;18(1):13-16.
4. Jacobs A, Wager E. EMWA guidelines on the role of medical writers in developing peer-reviewed publications. *Curr Med Res Opin*. 2005;21(2):317-321.
5. Flanagin A, Fontanarosa PB, DeAngelis CD. Authorship for research groups. *JAMA*. 2002;288(24):3166-3168.
6. Kassirer JP, Angell M. On authorship and acknowledgments. *N Engl J Med*. 1991; 325(21):1510-1512.
7. International Committee of Medical Journal Editors. Uniform Requirements for Manuscripts Submitted to Biomedical Journals. http://www.icmje.org. Updated February 2006. Accessed September 2, 2006.
8. Rennie D, Flanagin A, Yank V. The contributions of authors. *JAMA*. 2000;284(1): 89-91.
9. Fontanarosa PB, Flanagin A, DeAngelis CD. Reporting conflicts of interest, financial aspects of research, and role of sponsors in funded studies. *JAMA*. 2005;294(1): 110-111.
10. DeAngelis CD, Fontanarosa PB, Flanagin A. Reporting financial conflicts of interest and relationships between investigators and research sponsors. *JAMA*. 2001:286(1): 89-91.
11. Rosenberg RN, Aminoff M, Boller F, et al. Reporting clinical trials: full access to all of the data. *Arch Neurol*. 2002;59(1):27-28.

Wasteful publication includes dividing the results in a single study into two or more papers ("salami science"); republishing the same material in successive papers (which need not have identical format and content); and blending data from one study with additional data to extract yet another paper that could not make its way on the second set of data alone (meat extenders).

Edward J. Huth, MD[1]

5.3 Duplicate Publication. Duplicate publication is the simultaneous or subsequent reporting of essentially the same information, article, or major components of an article 2 or more times in 1 or more forms of media (either print or electronic format).[2-9] Duplicate reporting includes duplicate submission and may apply to both published and unpublished works (eg, 1 or more manuscripts not yet published but under consideration by another journal). Other terms used to describe this practice include *redundant, prior, repetitive, overlapping, related, multiple, dual, parallel, fragmented, fractionally divided*, and *topically divided* publication.[3,8,9]

Duplicate submission or publication is not necessarily unethical, but failure to disclose the existence of duplicate articles, manuscripts, or other related material to editors and readers (covert duplication) is unethical and may represent a violation of copyright law. Moreover, reports of the same data in multiple articles waste publishing resources (ie, those of editors, reviewers, and readers as well as journal pages),[1] pollute the literature, result in double counting of data or inappropriate weighting of the results of a study and thereby distort the available evidence,[2] cause problems for researchers and those who conduct systematic reviews and meta-analyses,[10,11] and may damage the reputation of authors.[12]

Duplicate publication usually involves 1 or more of the same authors, but the number of authors and order of authors may differ among the duplicate reports. Duplication occurs when there is substantial overlap in 1 or more elements of an article or manuscript. For reports of research, duplicative elements may include any or all of the following: the design, materials and methods, samples or subsamples, data, outcomes, tables, graphics and illustrative material, discussion, or conclusions. Duplication also occurs in other types of articles (eg, reviews, case reports, opinion pieces, letters to the editor, and online blogs).

A widely accepted method of quantifying the amount of overlap or duplication does not exist. Authors and editors often disagree on how to define and quantify duplication and whether duplicate articles are justified.[13] Researchers in 2 studies of duplicate publication classified an article as duplicative of another if 10% or more of the content was identical or highly similar.[7,14] Others have described levels and patterns of duplicate publication for research articles that emanate from 1 study, such as reporting identical samples and identical outcomes, identical samples and different outcomes, increasing or decreasing sample sizes and identical outcomes, and different subsamples from the same overall large study and different outcomes.[12,15] Studies have also shown that most duplicate articles are published within 1 year of the publication of the first report.[12,16]

A number of studies of duplicate publication in various fields have found that 1.4% to 28% of published articles could be classified as duplicative of other articles.[7,8,10,14,16-20] In addition, these studies have concluded that as many as 5% to 32% of duplicative articles do not include a citation or reference to the original or primary article (covert duplication).[7,10,14,18]

Following the recommendations of the International Committee of Medical Journal Editors (ICMJE),[2] a policy that prohibits or discourages duplicate publication does not preclude consideration of manuscripts that have been presented orally or in abstract or poster form at a professional meeting. This policy applies whether the presentation is made in person or via Web cast or an online meeting presentation. However, publication of complete manuscripts in proceedings of such meetings in print or online may preclude consideration for publication in a primary-source journal. News reports that cover presentations of data at scheduled professional meetings would not necessarily violate this policy, but authors should avoid distributing copies of their complete manuscripts, tables, and illustrations during such meetings. Preliminary release of information directly to the news media, usually through press conferences or news releases, may jeopardize an author's chances for publication in a primary-source journal.[21] However, exceptions are made when a government health agency determines that there is an immediate public need for such information[8,21] (see 5.13.1, Release of Information to the Public and Journal/Author Relations With the News Media, Release of Information to the Public). See Box 1 for examples of duplicate reports that may be acceptable and necessary.

5.3.1 **Secondary Publication.** Secondary publication is the subsequent republication, or simultaneous publication (sometimes called dual or parallel publication), of an article in 2 or more journals (in the same or another language) by mutual consent of the journal editors. Secondary publication can be beneficial. For example, the editors of an English-language journal and a non–English-language journal may agree to secondary publication in translated form for the benefit of audiences who speak different languages. The ICMJE approves secondary publication if all of the following conditions are met[2]:

1. The authors have received approval from the editors of both journals; the editor concerned with secondary publication must have a photocopy, reprint, or manuscript of the primary version.
2. The priority of the primary publication is respected by a publication interval of at least 1 week (unless specifically negotiated otherwise by both editors).
3. The paper for secondary publication is intended for a different group of readers; an abbreviated version could be sufficient.
4. The secondary version faithfully reflects the data and interpretations of the primary version.
5. The footnote on the title page of the secondary version informs readers, peers, and documenting agencies that the paper has been published in whole or in part and states the primary reference. A suitable footnote might read: "This article is based on a study first reported in the [title of journal, with full reference]." Permission for such secondary publication should be free of charge.
6. The title of the secondary publication should indicate that it is a secondary publication (complete republication, abridged republication, complete translation, or abridged translation) of a primary publication. Of note, the National Library of Medicine does not consider translations to be "republications" and does not cite or index translations when the original article was published in a journal that is indexed in MEDLINE.

For example, the title of a translated edition of a journal should include the journal's name and an indication of the translated edition in the title (eg, *JAMA-français*).

Box 1. Duplicate Reports That May Be Acceptable[a]

Summaries or Abstracts of Findings Reported in Conference Proceedings
Editors do not discourage authors from presenting their findings at conferences or scientific meetings, but they recommend that authors refrain from distributing complete copies of their papers, which might later appear in some form of publication without their knowledge. Previous presentation(s) should be noted in submitted manuscripts (see 2.10.12, Manuscript Preparation, Acknowledgment Section, Previous Presentations).

News Media Reports of Authors' Findings
Typically, editors do not discourage authors from reporting their findings at conferences covered by the news media, but they do discourage authors from distributing their full papers, tables, or figures, which might later appear printed in a newspaper, a newsletter, or the news section of a magazine. Editors do not discourage authors from participating in interviews with the news media after a paper has been accepted but before it is published. However, authors should remind reporters that most journals have an embargo policy that prohibits media coverage of the manuscript under consideration and the article before it is published (see also 5.13, Release of Information to the Public and Journal/Author Relations With the News Media).

Fragments or Sequential Reports of Studies
Editors make decisions about these types of duplicative research reports on a case-by-case basis. For all such papers, editors ask that authors properly reference previously reported parts of a study and send copies of these papers or articles along with their submitted manuscript.

Detailed Reports Previously Distributed to a Narrow Audience
The scope of this audience and the nature of distribution (eg, small print run, time-limited placement on closed Web site) would determine whether editors would publish a duplicative report. For all such papers, editors ask that authors properly reference all such previous publications and send copies of these along with their submitted manuscript.

Short Reports in Print and Longer, More Detailed Reports Online
Some journals publish shorter versions of articles in print and longer versions online. The existence of multiple versions of the same article should be made clear to readers and bibliographic databases.

Executive Summaries
Concise overviews or summaries of large, detailed reports or documents that are regularly updated are handled on a case-by-case basis. For all such summaries, editors ask that authors properly reference the larger, more detailed report.

Reports From Government Documents or Reports in the Public Domain
Decisions regarding republication of government documents or other reports in the public domain are based on the importance of the message, priority for the journal's readers, and availability of the information. For example, a journal may publish reports from the US Centers for Disease Control and Prevention that were initially published in the *Morbidity and Mortality Weekly Report*. The existence of multiple versions of the same report should be made clear to readers.

Translations of Reports in Another Language; Translated Articles or Same-Language Articles Republished in a Journal's International Edition
Translations are usually acceptable as long as they give proper attribution to the original publication (see 5.3.1, Secondary Publication). Translations should be faithful to the original, should not introduce any new content or authors, and should not omit any content or authors. Translators should be acknowledged.

For each of these cases, a query to the editorial office is recommended, asking whether any previous publication or release of information jeopardizes a chance for subsequent publication in a specific journal.

[a] Adapted from Blancett et al[7] with permission of Blackwell Publishing.

5.3.2 Editorial Policy for Preventing and Handling Allegations of Duplicate Publication. Covert duplicate publication violates the ethics of scientific publishing and may constitute a violation of copyright law. Editors have a duty to inform prospective authors of their policies on duplicate publication, which should be published in their instructions for authors. Reviewers should notify editors of the existence of duplicate articles discovered during their review. Authors should send copies of all duplicate or overlapping articles and manuscripts with their submitted manuscripts. Authors should also include citations to highly similar articles and any reports from the same study under their authorship in the reference list of the submitted manuscript. When in doubt about the possibility of duplication or redundancy of information in articles based on the same study or topic, authors should inform and consult the editor.

The editors of *JAMA* and the *Archives* Journals have adopted the following policies to prevent the practice of duplicate publication or minimize the risk of its occurrence:

At the time a manuscript is submitted, the author must inform the editor in the event that any part of the material (1) exists elsewhere in unpublished form (eg, large data sets or relevant data not included in the submitted manuscript); (2) is under consideration by another journal; or (3) has been or is about to be published elsewhere. In the case of a highly similar article or manuscript, the author should provide the editor with a copy of the other article(s) or manuscript(s), so that the editor can determine whether the contents are duplicative and whether such duplication affects the editorial priority of the submitted manuscript. All authors are required to sign an authorship criteria and responsibility statement, which includes the following declaration:

> Neither this manuscript nor another manuscript with substantially similar content under my authorship has been published or is being considered for publication elsewhere, except as described in an attachment, and copies of related manuscripts are provided.

In addition, many journals require authors to transfer copyright ownership or grant a publication license to the journal as a condition of publication (see 5.6.5, Intellectual Property: Ownership, Access, Rights, and Management, Copyright Assignment or License). In the case of duplicate submission, copyright or publication right is likely owned by the first journal to publish the manuscript, depending on whether copyright ownership or an exclusive publication license was transferred. Journals that require authors to grant a license (rather than transfer copyright) to publish a manuscript also expect authors to inform editors and prospective readers of any duplicative material.

In a case of suspected duplicate submission or publication, editors should first contact the corresponding author and request a written explanation. Additional actions that may be considered are described below.

Duplicate Submission. If an author submits a duplicate manuscript without notifying the editor(s), the editor should act promptly when it is discovered.[2] If duplicate submission of a manuscript is suspected before publication, the editor should notify the author and ask to see a copy of the potentially duplicative material, if not already in hand, as well as copies of any other similar articles and manuscripts, and request a written explanation. After reviewing all material, the editor will then decide whether to continue to consider or to reject the submitted manuscript. If the manuscript is rejected because of duplicate submission, this reason should be indicated clearly in the decision letter.

Duplicate Publication. If an editor suspects that duplicate publication has occurred, the editor should contact the authors and request a written explanation. If necessary, the editor (possibly with the benefit of additional expert opinion) may consult the editor of the other journal in which the material appeared. If both editors agree that duplication has occurred, the editor of the second journal to publish the article should inform the author of the intention to publish a notice of duplicate publication in a subsequent issue of the journal. It is preferable that this notice be signed by the author or be accompanied by a letter of explanation from the author, but a notice of duplicate publication should be published without the author's explanation or approval if none is forthcoming.[2] Depending on the situation, the editor may also choose to notify the author's institutional supervisor (eg, department chair, dean) to request assistance with acquisition of an appropriate letter from the author.

Notice of Duplicate Publication. The notice of duplicate publication should be published on a numbered editorial page and listed in the table of contents of the journal in a citable format to ensure that the notice will be indexed appropriately in literature databases. The notice should be labeled or titled as "Notice of Duplicate Publication" and it may be published as correspondence or as a correction or erratum. The US National Library of Medicine identifies duplicate articles in its bibliographic database by adding a publication type of "Duplicate Publication" to the record of each duplicate article and links subsequently published notices of duplicate publication to the citations of the duplicate articles.[22] It is preferable to publish an explanation from the author(s) of the duplicate article with the notice, but this is not always possible or necessary. The words *Duplicate Publication* should be included in the title of the notice, which should include complete citations to all duplicate articles (since there may be more than 1). Box 2 provides an example of such a notice (wording would depend on the circumstances in each case), and Box 3, an example of a table of contents listing. *Note:* The examples in Boxes 2 and 3 are not real and are intended to show all of the elements needed for a published notice of duplicate publication and to ensure appropriate identifiability and indexing of such notices.

All journals should develop and publish a policy on duplicate submission and publication.[6] In addition, journals should develop procedures for evaluating possible violations of such policy and actions to be taken once a violation has been determined to have occurred. This includes requesting an explanation from the author(s), and, if duplicate publication is determined to have occurred, the editor should notify the other journal(s) involved and may consider notifying the author's dean, director, or supervisor (this may be necessary if the author does not provide a satisfactory explanation), and the editor should publish a notice of duplicate publication. Some journals in a specific field (eg, pediatrics)[23] have decided to notify each other about cases of proved duplicate publication and ban the offending author(s) from publishing in their journals for a specified period.

Box 2. Hypothetical Example of a Notice of Duplicate Publication

Correction: Notice of Duplicate Publication: "Report of Multidrug-Resistant *Mycobacterium tuberculosis* Among Residents of a Long-term Care Facility" (*Infect Dis Rep.* 2004;270[12]:2004-2008)

The article "Report of Multidrug-Resistant *Mycobacterium tuberculosis* Among Residents of a Long-term Care Facility" by Anthony S. Smith, MD, published in the December 2004 issue of *Infectious Disease Reports*,[1] is virtually identical to an article by the same author, describing the same 35 cases in similar words, published in the *Journal of New Results*, September 2004.[2]

In June 2004, the author sent a signed statement of authorship responsibility stating that his manuscript had not been published and was not under consideration for publication elsewhere. He also signed a document that transferred copyright ownership in the manuscript to the publisher. Well before either publication, Dr Smith received a letter of acceptance from *Infectious Disease Reports* that included a reminder about our policy on duplicate publication.

1. Smith AS. Report of multidrug-resistant *Mycobacterium tuberculosis* among residents of a long-term care facility. *Infect Dis Rep.* 2004;270(12):2004-2008.
2. Smith AS. Multidrug-resistant tuberculosis among the elderly: an epidemiological assessment. *J New Results.* 2004;32(9):150-154.

The following response was received from Dr Smith after he was informed that the above notice would be published.—Ed.

In Reply.—I offer my sincere apologies to the readers of *Infectious Disease Reports.* I did not understand that my 2 manuscripts would be considered duplicative at the time I submitted them. I thought that since the 2 journals are read by different groups, some overlap in wording would be acceptable.

Anthony S. Smith, MD
Main University School of Medicine
Chicago, Illinois

Box 3. Hypothetical Example of a Duplicate Publication Notice Listing in a Journal's Table of Contents

ACKNOWLEDGMENTS

Principal author: Annette Flanagin, RN, MA

I thank C. K. Gunsalus, JD, University of Illinois, Champaign/Urbana; Wayne G. Hoppe, JD, *JAMA* and *Archives* Journals; and Liz Wager, MA, Sideview, for review and providing important suggestions for improvement of this section; the following for also providing review and minor suggestions: Daniel M. Albert, MD, MS, *Archives of Ophthalmology*; Terri S. Carter, *Archives of Surgery*; Catherine D. DeAngelis, MD, MPH, *JAMA* and *Archives* Journals; Paula Glitman, *Archives* Journals; Cindy W. Hamilton, PharmD, ELS, Hamilton House; Trevor Lane, MA, DPhil, University of Hong Kong; Povl Riis, MD, University of Copenhagen; Valerie Siddall, PhD, ELS, AstraZeneca; Cheryl Smart, MA, MBA; and Flo Witte, MA, ELS, AdvancMed LLC; and Sandra Schefris and Yolanda Davis, James S. Todd Memorial Library, American Medical Association, Chicago, Illinois, for bibliographic assistance.

REFERENCES

1. Huth EJ. Irresponsible authorship and wasteful publication. *Ann Intern Med*. 1986; 104(2):257-259.
2. International Committee of Medical Journal Editors. Uniform Requirements for Manuscripts Submitted to Biomedical Journals. http://www.icmje.org. Updated February 2006. Accessed September 2, 2006.
3. Broad WJ. The publishing game: getting more for less. *Science*. 1981;211(4487):1137-1139.
4. Angell M, Relman AS. Redundant publication. *N Engl J Med*. 1989;320(18):1212-1214.
5. Flanagin A, Glass RM, Lundberg GD. Electronic journals and duplicate publication: is a byte a word? *JAMA*. 1992;267(17):2374.
6. Editorial Policy Committee, Council of Biology Editors. Redundant publication. *CBE Views*. 1996;19(4):76-77.
7. Blancett SS, Flanagin A, Young RK. Duplicate publication in the nursing literature. *Image J Nurs Sch*. 1995;27(1):51-56.
8. Huston P, Moher D. Redundancy, disaggregation, and the integrity of medical research. *Lancet*. 1996;347(9007):1024-1026.
9. Susser M, Yankauer A. Prior, duplicate, repetitive, fragmented, and redundant publication and editorial decisions. *Am J Public Health*. 1993;83(6):792-793.
10. von Elm E, Poglia G, Walder B, Tramèr MR. Different patterns of duplicate publication: an analysis of articles used in systematic reviews. *JAMA*. 2003;291(8):974-980.
11. Tramer MR, Reynolds DJ, Moore RA, McQuay HJ. Impact of covert duplicate publication on meta-analysis: a case study. *BMJ*. 1997;315(7109):635-640.
12. DeAngelis CD. Duplicate publication, multiple problems. *JAMA*. 2004;292(14):1745-1746.
13. Yank V, Barnes D. Consensus and contention regarding redundant publications in clinical research: cross-sectional survey of editors and authors. *J Med Ethics*. 2003; 29(2):109-114.
14. Bailey BJ. Duplicate publication in the field of otolaryngology–head and neck surgery. *Otolaryngol Head Neck Surg*. 2002;126(3):211-216.
15. Melander H, Ahlqvist-Rastad J, Meijer G, Beermann B. Evidence b(i)ased medicine—selective reporting from studies sponsored by pharmaceutical industry: review of studies in new drug applications. *BMJ*. 2003;326(7400):1171-1173.

16. Rosenthal EL, Masdon JL, Buckman C, Hawn M. Duplicate publications in the otolaryngology literature. *Laryngoscope*. 2003;113(5):772-774.
17. Waldron T. Is duplicate publishing on the increase? *BMJ*. 1992;304(6833):1029.
18. Barnard H, Overbeke JA. Duplicate publication of original articles in and from the *Nederlands Tijdschrift voor Geneeskunde*. *Ned Tijdschr Geneeskd*. 1993;137(12): 593-597.
19. Mojon-Azzi SM, Jiang X, Wagner U, Mojon DS. Redundant publications in scientific ophthalmology journals: the tip of the iceberg? *Ophthalmology*. 2004;111(5):853-866.
20. Gwilym SE, Swan MC, Giele H. One in 13 "original" articles in the *Journal of Bone and Joint Surgery* are duplicate or fragmented publications. *J Bone Joint Surg Br*. 2004; 86(5):743-745.
21. Fontanarosa PB, Flanagin A, DeAngelis CD. The Journal's policy regarding release of information to the public. *JAMA*. 2000;284(22):2929-2931.
22. US National Library of Medicine. Fact sheet: errata, retraction, duplicate publication, comment, update and patient summary policy for MEDLINE. http://www.nlm.nih.gov/pubs/factsheets/errata.html. Accessed September 2, 2006.
23. Bier DM, Fulginiti VA, Garfunkel JM, et al. Duplicate publication and related problems *Pediatrics*. 1990;86(6):997-998.

We should ignore whining about the supposedly awful pressures of "publish or perish" when we have little credible evidence on what motivates misconduct, nor on what motivates the conduct of honest, equally stressed colleagues. Laziness, desire for fame, greed, and an inability to distinguish right from wrong are just as likely to be at the root of the problem.

Drummond Rennie[1]

5.4 Scientific Misconduct.

Scientific Misconduct. In scientific publication, the phrase *scientific misconduct* (specifically termed *research misconduct* by US government regulations and commonly known as *fraud*) has both ethical and legal connotations for authors and editors. A few studies (with limited methodologies) have estimated the prevalence of scientists who have participated in scientific misconduct to range from 1% to 2%.[2-4] In a 2002 survey[5] of a random sample of scientists funded by the US National Institutes of Health, 3247 participating scientists reported engaging in a number of unethical behaviors, including falsifying research data (0.3%), using another's ideas without permission or credit (1.4%), and inadequate record keeping related to research projects (27.5%). Although inadequate record keeping is not a form of misconduct in itself, it could permit misconduct to occur and make investigations of misconduct difficult to conduct. Legal determinations of scientific misconduct in biomedical publication are uncommon, although, when discovered, such misconduct results in serious questions about the validity of scientific research and the credibility of authors and journals. Proven cases of misconduct in the published literature as well as allegations and concerns that do not result in an official finding of misconduct raise important ethical questions and impose duties on authors and editors to protect and correct the literature.

Over the years, various definitions of scientific misconduct have been suggested by US government agencies and academic institutions, especially after highly publicized incidents of fraudulent research in the United States in the mid-1970s and early 1980s.[6-8] In 1989, the US Public Health Service released the following definition of scientific misconduct: "fabrication, falsification, plagiarism, or other practices that seriously deviate from those that are commonly accepted within the scientific community for proposing, conducting, or reporting research."[9] This definition was considered a practical tool for recognizing and dealing with allegations of scientific misconduct during the manuscript submission, review, and publication processes.[10] However, controversy grew over various interpretations of the definition (eg, how narrow or broad should the definition be? does the definition address intent or levels of seriousness of offense? can the definition stand up in court? can the definition serve multiple sciences?).

In the wake of this controversy, the US Public Health Service appointed a Commission on Research Integrity in 1993. One of the charges of the commission was to develop a better definition of scientific misconduct. In 1995, the commission released a detailed report that included a recommendation that the definition be amended to include offenses that constitute research misconduct: misappropriation, interference, and misrepresentation.[11] This definition replaced the word *plagiarism* with the broader term *misappropriation*; replaced the words *fabrication* and *falsification* with the term *misrepresentation*; and added the term *interference* to address instances "in which a person's research is seriously compromised by the intentional and unauthorized taking, sequestering, or damaging of property he or she used in the conduct of research."[11] In this context, *property* included apparatus, reagents, biologic materials, writings, data, and software.

The commission's definition was not adopted by the US Public Health Service for many reasons, including protests from scientists and some science groups to which the government responded that it wanted a definition that would work for all governmental departments (eg, both the US Public Health Service and the National Science Foundation, which at the time had different definitions).[10,12] In 1996, the National Science and Technology Council, a unit within the Office of Science and Technology Policy responsible for coordinating policy among multiple government research agencies, drafted a common definition, which, after review and comment, was approved and released in 2000.[13] This definition no longer contained a category of misconduct in the original 1989 definition: "other practices that seriously deviate from those that are commonly accepted within the scientific community for proposing, conducting, or reporting research."

The revised common definition was reviewed again in 2004 and reissued without substantial change in 2005 by the US Department of Health and Human Services (DHHS) (although there were other changes to correct errors and improve clarity in the overall policy).[14]

The current common definition of research misconduct from the DHHS follows[14]:

> Research misconduct is defined as fabrication, falsification, or plagiarism in proposing, performing, or reviewing research, or in reporting research results.

> Fabrication is making up data or results and recording or reporting them.
>
> Falsification is manipulating research materials, equipment, or processes, or changing or omitting data or results such that the research is not accurately represented in the research record.
>
> Plagiarism is the appropriation of another person's ideas, processes, results, or words without giving appropriate credit.
>
> Research misconduct does not include honest error or differences of opinion. A finding of research misconduct requires that:
>
> - there be a significant departure from accepted practices of the relevant research community; and
> - the misconduct be committed intentionally, or knowingly, or recklessly; and
> - the allegation be proven by a preponderance of evidence.

None of the definitions of scientific misconduct include honest error or differences in interpretation. Nor do they include or pertain to violations of human or animal experimentation requirements (5.8, Protecting Research Participants' and Patients' Rights in Scientific Publication), financial mismanagement/misconduct, or other acts covered by existing laws, such as sexual harassment, copyright, confidentiality, libel (see 5.6.3, Intellectual Property: Ownership, Access, Rights, and Management, Copyright: Definition, History, and Current Law; 5.7, Confidentiality; and 5.9, Defamation, Libel), or other concerns, such as authorship disputes, duplicate publication, self-plagiarism without indication of one's previous work, or conflicts of interest.[4-6] (See 5.1, Authorship Responsibility; 5.3, Duplicate Publication; and 5.5, Conflicts of Interest.)

The DHHS common definition of research misconduct is intended to apply to US government–funded research, and academic and research institutions that accept government funding must comply with the definition and associated regulations. However, this definition and associated regulations have become de facto rules for US academic and other research institutions and are applied to any work done by their employees or under their aegis regardless of the source of funding. These institutions often have other rules that cover "other practices that seriously deviate from those that are commonly accepted within the scientific community for proposing, conducting, or reporting research."[9]

5.4.1 **Misrepresentation: Fabrication, Falsification, and Omission.** Fabrication, falsification, and omission are forms of misrepresentation in scientific publication. Fabrication includes stating or presenting a falsehood and making up data, results, or "facts" that do not exist. Falsification includes manipulation of materials or processes, changing data or results, or altering the graphic display of data or digital images in a manner that results in misrepresentation (see also 5.4.3, Inappropriate Manipulation of Digital Images). Omission is the act of deliberately not reporting certain information for a desired outcome. Data fabrication, falsification, and omission occur when an investigator or author creates, alters, manipulates, selects, or presents selected or fails to report selected information for a desired outcome that distorts the interpretation of the original data, the research record, or the truth.[11-14]

5.4.2 **Misappropriation: Plagiarism and Breaches of Confidentiality.** Misappropriation in scientific publication includes plagiarism and breaches of confidentiality during the privileged review of a manuscript.[11-15] (See also 5.7.1, Confidentiality, Confidentiality During Editorial Evaluation and Peer Review and After Publication.) In plagiarism, an author documents or reports ideas, words, data, or graphics, whether published or unpublished, of another as his or her own and without giving appropriate credit.[11] Plagiarism of published work violates standards of honesty and collegial trust and may also violate copyright law (if the violation is shown to be legally actionable) (see 5.6.7, Intellectual Property: Ownership, Access, Rights, and Management, Copying, Reproducing, Adapting, and Other Uses of Content).

Four common kinds of plagiarism have been identified[16]:

1. Direct plagiarism: Verbatim lifting of passages without enclosing the borrowed material in quotation marks and crediting the original author.
2. Mosaic: Borrowing the ideas and opinions from an original source and a few verbatim words or phrases without crediting the original author. In this case, the plagiarist intertwines his or her own ideas and opinions with those of the original author, creating a "confused, plagiarized mass."
3. Paraphrase: Restating a phrase or passage, providing the same meaning but in a different form without attribution to the original author.
4. Insufficient acknowledgment: Noting the original source of only part of what is borrowed or failing to cite the source material in a way that allows the reader to know what is original and what is borrowed.

The common characteristic of these kinds of plagiarism is the failure to attribute words, ideas, or findings to their true authors, whether or not the original work has been published. Such failure to acknowledge a source properly may on occasion be caused by careless note taking or ignorance of the canons of research and authorship. The best defense against allegations of plagiarism is careful note taking, record keeping, and documentation of all data observed and sources used. Those who review manuscripts that are similar to their own unpublished work may be especially at risk for charges of plagiarism. Reviewers who foresee such a potential conflict of interest should consider returning the manuscript to the editor without reviewing it. This recommendation may be stipulated in the letter that accompanies each manuscript sent for review (see 5.5.6, Conflicts of Interest, Requirements for Peer Reviewers, and 6.0, Editorial Assessment and Processing). Some have reported that the Internet and subsequent rapid and widespread dissemination of findings and publications has resulted in an increase in plagiarism; however, the same technology as well as antiplagiarism software may now give editors and publishers better tools to detect plagiarism in submitted papers.[17,18]

5.4.3 **Inappropriate Manipulation of Digital Images.** Image processing software, such as Adobe Photoshop, has made it relatively easy for authors to manipulate images to highlight a specific outcome or feature by cropping or by adjusting color, brightness, or contrast. These same applications can be used by journal staff to screen digital images for evidence of inappropriate manipulation and fraudulent manipulation.[19,20] Some enhancements to figures, such as cropping or adjusting color of the entire image, may be appropriate if such manipulations do not alter the interpretation of the original data or omit or obscure important data. However, any manipulation that results in a change in how the original data will be interpreted or that selectively reports, omits, or obscures important data (such as adding or altering a data element or adjusting tone or compression of an image to make it appear as a uniquely different image) is considered scientific misconduct.[19,20] Authors should indicate any changes or enhancements that have been made to digital images in the legend that accompanies the image. (See also 4.2.10, Visual Presentation of Data, Figures, Guidelines for Preparing and Submitting Figures.) These same principles apply to images included in video files.

Journals should have policies and procedures in place for screening of digital images.[19,20] If resources are limited, screening can be limited to those images that are included in papers that have been accepted for publication. The *Journal of Cell Biology* has the following policy and guidelines for authors that are a good model for other journals[21]:

> No specific feature within an image may be enhanced, obscured, moved, removed, or introduced. The grouping of images from different parts of the same gel, or from different gels, fields, or exposures must be made explicit by the arrangement of the figure (ie, using dividing lines) and in the text of the figure legend. If dividing lines are not included, they will be added by our production department, and this may result in production delays. Adjustments of brightness, contrast, or color balance are acceptable if they are applied to the whole image and as long as they do not obscure, eliminate, or misrepresent any information present in the original, including backgrounds. Without any background information, it is not possible to see exactly how much of the original gel is actually shown. Non-linear adjustments (eg, changes to gamma settings) must be disclosed in the figure legend. All digital images in manuscripts accepted for publication will be scrutinized by our production department for any indication of improper manipulation. Questions raised by the production department will be referred to the Editors, who will request the original data from the authors for comparison to the prepared figures. If the original data cannot be produced, the acceptance of the manuscript may be revoked. Cases of deliberate misrepresentation of data will result in revocation of acceptance, and will be reported to the corresponding author's home institution or funding agency. [Reproduced with permission of *Journal of Cell Biology*.]

During a 3-year period of screening images in all manuscripts accepted for publication, the *Journal of Cell Biology* had to revoke acceptance of 1% of papers after detecting "fraudulent image manipulation that affected interpretation of the data."[19] In addition, 25% of the accepted manuscripts had at least 1 figure that had to be remade because of inappropriate manipulation that did not affect the interpretation of the data but that violated the above guidelines.

5.4.4 Editorial Policy and Procedures for Detecting and Handling Allegations of Scientific Misconduct. Detection of scientific misconduct in publishing is often the result of the alertness of coworkers and/or other authors of the same manuscript, and much less commonly by editors, peer reviewers, or readers.

If an allegation of scientific misconduct is made in relation to a manuscript under consideration or published, the editor has a duty to ensure confidential and timely pursuit of that allegation. According to the International Committee of Medical Journal Editors (ICMJE),[22] "If substantial doubts arise about the honesty and integrity of work, either submitted or published, it is the editor's responsibility to ensure that the question is appropriately pursued," but the editor is not responsible for conducting the investigation. This recommendation is supported by the World Association of Medical Editors, the Council of Science Editors, and the UK Committee on Publication Ethics.[23-25] A study published in 2004 that reviewed the policies of 122 leading biomedical journals (selected from those journals with the highest impact factors) found that 21 journals (18%) had a retraction policy for their journals and 76 journals reported having no policy on issuing retractions.[26] Editors have a duty to develop and follow a policy on handling allegations of scientific misconduct and retractions. The recommendations in this section are intended to help editors with such policies.

An editor's first step after receiving an allegation of falsified, fabricated, or plagiarized work published in her or his journal is to consider contacting the corresponding author, depending on the circumstances, to request an explanation while maintaining confidentiality. This initial contact can be made by telephone or brief letter marked confidential. (See also 5.7.2, Confidentiality, Confidentiality in Allegations of Scientific Misconduct.) If the explanation received from the author is satisfactory, and if guilt is admitted, the editor should request a letter of formal retraction from the author (preferably signed by the author and all coauthors); the editor should also notify the author's institution and inform the author of this notification. If the explanation allays any concerns about misconduct, the editor may need to publish some form of correction or clarification or otherwise inform the person making the allegation that no misconduct has occurred. If the explanation received is not satisfactory or leads to additional concerns, or if no explanation is received, the editor should contact the author's institutional authority to request a formal investigation and should notify the author of this plan.

The responsibility to conduct an investigation lies with an authority at the author's institution where the work was done (eg, dean, president, or ethical conduct/research integrity officer), with the funding agency, or with a national agency charged to investigate such allegations, such as the US Office of Research Integrity, the UK Medical Research Council, or the Danish Committees on Scientific Dishonesty. Many countries do not have such national agencies to investigate allegations of scientific misconduct or enforce regulations. In such cases, the journal editor must pursue an author's local institution for an appropriate response.[27] Editors should expect a prompt acknowledgment of their notification of an allegation of misconduct. The acknowledgment should include a plan for the inquiry or investigation into the matter and a timeline that specifies when the editor will be informed of the outcome. The editor cannot conduct the investigation because he or she does not have the appropriate institutional access or an employment relationship with the author or other relationship such as that between the author and a governmental funding agency. If the editor does not receive a satisfactory or timely reply (eg, within 2 months) from the investigational authority, the editor should consider contacting the authority again to request follow-up information. (Note that the DHHS 2005 policy recommends that institutions complete their initial inquiry to determine whether an official investigation is warranted within 60 days of its initiation unless circumstances clearly warrant a longer period.[14])

The editor should take great care to maintain confidentiality during any communication about the allegation. However, the editor needs to identify the person or persons about whom the allegation is made when contacting the relevant institutional, funding, or governmental authority to request an investigation. This is best done by a telephone call or a brief formal letter marked confidential. During such investigations, editors should avoid including details of the cases in e-mails that can be widely circulated and should avoid posting details, even if rendered anonymous, in e-mail lists or blogs (see also 5.7.2, Confidentiality, Confidentiality in Allegations of Scientific Misconduct).

5.4.5 Retractions, Expressions of Concern. After receiving confirmation from the author or authors and/or a report from the author's institution or other agency indicating that fabrication, falsification, or plagiarism has occurred, the journal should promptly publish a retraction. Preferably this retraction will be a signed letter from the corresponding author and all coauthors. If none of the authors will agree to publish a signed retraction, the editor may request such a retraction from the investigating institution, or the editor may issue a retraction on behalf of the journal. In each case, the editor should inform the author(s) and institutional authority of the plan to publish a retraction. See Boxes 1 and 2 (pp. 163-165) for examples of retraction notices.

A retraction should include a complete citation to the original article and should indicate the reason for retracting the original article. The retraction, whether a formal letter or notice, should be labeled as a "Retraction," be listed in the table of contents, and be published in a prominent section of the journal on a numbered page in print versions and in a citable format in online versions so that it can be identified easily by indexers and included in bibliographic databases (see also 3.11.14, References, References to Print Journal, Retractions). The US National Library of Medicine will index the retraction as long as it clearly states that an article in question is being retracted or withdrawn, whether in whole or in part, and is signed by an author, the author's legal counsel or institutional representative, or the journal editor.[28] Online versions of journals and bibliographic databases should provide reciprocal links to and from the notice of retraction and the retracted article. Retractions should be made freely available and accessible on a journal's Web site (ie, readers should not have to pay an access fee to see the retraction notice).[27] A retracted article should be properly labeled or watermarked as retracted in online versions of journals and should not be removed from the online journal or archive. Such labeling may include the words "Retracted Article" or "This Article Has Been Retracted" placed prominently at the top of the online article and on each page of a PDF file of the article. These labels can be hyperlinked to the published retraction.

If an author of a fraudulent article, or any institutional authority, refuses to submit an explanation for publication as a retraction, the editor can leverage the authority and influence of his or her position and that of the journal to compel an appropriate response, keeping in mind the journal's obligation to publish a retraction.[27,29] If, however, the editor is unable to receive a satisfactory or timely response from an author or the investigating authority on the merit of the allegation, the editor may publish an "expression of concern" to alert readers, librarians, and the scientific community that there are concerns that an article may include fabricated, falsified, or plagiarized work, and follow this later with a formal retraction. This notice of concern should follow the same publication format as recommended for notices of retraction. If evidence of misconduct is sufficient and the editor cannot obtain a retraction letter from the author and is awaiting the results of an official investigation, the editor may choose to publish an expression of concern and follow this with a formal retraction once the institution has completed its investigation.

The validity of other work published in the journal by the offending authors should also be questioned. The ICMJE recommends that editors ask institutions to provide assurance of the validity of earlier work published in their journals or to retract those as well. If this is not done, editors may chose to publish a notice or expression of concern stating that the validity of such previously published work is uncertain.[22]

Box 1 shows examples of retraction notices from authors, an institution, and an editor and a listing in the table of contents. Examples of recent retractions in the literature are shown in Box 2. Some authors may not want to explain the reason for the retraction in a forthright manner. Editors should work with authors or their institutional authority to make these notices as accurate as possible. In some cases, publishing an author's evasive or incomplete statement might be better than publishing nothing from the author; in such a case, the journal can also publish an explanatory note from the author's institutional authority or the editor.

When an article is retracted, the original article should not be physically removed from a journal's Web site or other online archival publication. However, it should be made clear to all users of online archival material that the article has been retracted and should not be used or cited. This requirement includes clear labeling of retracted articles and 2-way linking between retraction notices and the original articles. The National Library of Medicine does not remove the citation of a retracted article; the citation is updated to indicate that the article has been retracted, and links between the original citation and the citation to the retraction notice are added.[28]

Retractions may also be used for articles that are seriously and pervasively flawed because of honest error that is not a result of fabrication, falsification, or plagiarism. However, retraction of an article because of serious and pervasive errors should be used cautiously. Indeed, Sox and Rennie[27] have called for retractions to be reserved solely for cases of scientific misconduct. Retractions should never be used for typical errors; in these cases, a correction is appropriate (see also 5.11.9, Editorial Responsibilities, Roles, Procedures, and Policies, Corrections [Errata]). A study of 395 articles retracted during the years 1982 through 2002 found that 107 (27%) reflected scientific misconduct and 244 (62%) represented unintentional errors (another 44 [11%] represented other issues or provided no information about the reasons for the retractions).[30] The National Library of Medicine cites examples of such serious and pervasive errors as "conclusions based on faulty logic or computation" and data obtained after inadvertent contamination of cell lines or through poor instrumentation.[28] If the errors in an article are substantial and pervasive (eg, incorrect data throughout the text, tables, and figures), the journal may choose to publish a retraction notice from the original authors as well as a replacement article.[31] In this case, online versions of journals and bibliographic databases should provide reciprocal links to and from the notice of retraction, the retracted article, and the replacement article, and the retracted article should be labeled as retracted.

Box 1. Examples of Hypothetical Published Retraction Notices

Retraction Notices From Authors

Notice of Retraction: Falsification of Data in "Effects of Low-Fat Diet on Risk of Breast Cancer" (*J Med Res.* 2005;242[1]:135-139)

To the Editor.—We write to retract the article "Effects of Low-Fat Diet on Risk of Breast Cancer,"[1] published in the January 3, 2005, issue of the *Journal of Medical Research*. Two participants in the low-fat diet group were intentionally misclassified as not having breast cancer by one of us (J.S.). Had the reporting of these 2 cases not been falsified, our multivariate analysis would not have shown statistically significant results. We regret any problems our article and actions may have caused and we retract it from the literature.

John Smith
Jane Doe
Medical University
Chicago, Illinois

1. Smith J, Doe J. Effects of low-fat diet on risk of breast cancer. *J Med Res.* 2005;242(1):135-139.

Notice of Retraction: Plagiarism in "Effects of Low-Fat Diet on Risk of Breast Cancer" (*J Med Res.* 2005;242[1]:135-139)

To the Editor.—We regret that the first 3 paragraphs in the "Discussion" section of our article, "Effects of Low-Fat Diet on Risk of Breast Cancer,"[1] published in the January 3, 2005, issue of the *Journal of Medical Research*, were taken from another source without proper attribution. We should have cited the following article as the original source of the information contained in those paragraphs: Scott RB. Low-fat diets and cancer risk. *J Med Nutr Diet.* 2002; 20(8):1450-1455. We regret any problems our article[1] may have caused and we retract it from the literature.

John Smith
Jane Doe
Medical University
Chicago, Illinois

1. Smith J, Doe J. Effects of low-fat diet on risk of breast cancer. *J Med Res.* 2005;242(1):135-139.

Retraction Notice From Institution

Notice of Retraction: Falsification of Data in "Effects of Low-Fat Diet on Risk of Breast Cancer" (*J Med Res.* 2005;242[1]:135-139)

To the Editor.—An official investigation conducted by the Research Integrity Review Panel of Medical University of the data reported by John Smith and Jane Doe in the article "Effects of Low-Fat Diet on Risk of Breast Cancer,"[1] published in the January 3, 2005, issue of the *Journal of Medical Research*, has confirmed falsification in the reporting. Two subjects in the low-fat diet group were intentionally misclassified as not having breast cancer by one of the authors (J.S.).

Box 1. Examples of Hypothetical Published Retraction Notices *(cont)*

As a result, we retract this article from the literature. The review panel's investigation did not reveal any additional research misconduct in either author's previously published works.

Joan Brown
Dean
Medical University
Chicago, Illinois

1. Smith J, Doe J. Effects of low-fat diet on risk of breast cancer. *J Med Res.* 2005;242(1):135-139.

Retraction Notice From Journal Editor

Notice of Retraction: Falsification of Data in "Effects of Low-Fat Diet on Risk of Breast Cancer" (*J Med Res.* 2005;242[1]:135-139)

We have received confirmation from the Research Integrity Review Panel of Medical University that data reported by John Smith and Jane Doe in the article "Effects of Low-Fat Diet on Risk of Breast Cancer,"[1] published in the January 3, 2005, issue of the *Journal of Medical Research*, were falsified. Two subjects in the low-fat diet group were intentionally misclassified as not having breast cancer by one of the authors (J.S.). As a result, we retract this article from the literature. The review panel's investigation did not reveal any additional research misconduct in either author's previously published works.

Mary Frank
Editor, *Journal of Medical Research*

1. Smith J, Doe J. Effects of low-fat diet on risk of breast cancer. *J Med Res.* 2005;242(1):135-139.

Expression of Concern From Journal Editor

Notice of Retraction: Falsification of Data in "Effects of Low-Fat Diet on Risk of Breast Cancer" (*J Med Res.* 2005;242[1]:135-139)

In the January 3, 2005, issue of the *Journal of Medical Research*, we published "Effects of Low-Fat Diet on Risk of Breast Cancer,"[1] by John Smith and Jane Doe. On March 15, 2005, we received information that cast serious doubt on the validity of several cases that were reported in Tables 1 and 2 and that prompted us to alert the author and the author's institution and to request a formal investigation. An interim report from the Medical University's Research Integrity Review Panel, received on April 10, 2005, indicates that "data were falsified for two participants in this study" and that a formal investigation is under way. We have requested formal retractions from the authors and a final report from the university's review panel, including information about the validity of the author's previous publication in the *Journal of Medical Research*. In the interim, we publish this expression of concern to alert our readers to the serious concerns

Box 1. Examples of Hypothetical Published Retraction Notices *(cont)*

raised about the validity of the data, interpretations, and conclusions of the article published in January 2005.[1]

Mary Frank
Editor, *Journal of Medical Research*

1. Smith J, Doe J. Effects of low-fat diet on risk of breast cancer. *J Med Res.* 2005;242(1):135-139.

Listing of a Retraction Notice in the Table of Contents

Box 2. Citations of Published Retraction Notices and Expressions of Concern

Retraction Notices From Authors

Poehlman ET. Notice of retraction: final resolution. *Ann Intern Med.* 2005; 142(9):798.

Poehlman ET. Retraction of Poehlman et al. *Journal of Applied Physiology* 76:2281-2287, 1994. *J Appl Physiol.* 2005;99(2):779.

Note: In the following 2 retractions, the coauthors signed the retraction, but the offending author of the retracted article did not.

Cooper PK, Nouspikel T, Clarkson SG. Retraction of Cooper et al, *Science* 275(5302):990-993. *Science.* 2005;308(5729):1740.

Warloe T, Aamdal S, Reith A, Bryne M. Retraction of: Diagnostics and treatment of early stages of oral cancer. *Tidsskr Nor Laegeforen.* 2006;126(17):2287.

Retraction Notices From Editors

Sox H. Notice of retraction. *Ann Intern Med.* 2005;139(8):702.

Horton R. Retraction—Non-steroidal anti-inflammatory drugs and the risk of oral cancer: a nested case-control study. *Lancet.* 2006;367(9508):382.

Expressions of Concern From Editors

Curfman GD, Morrissey S, Drazen JM. Expression of concern: Sudbo J et al. DNA content as a prognostic marker in patients with oral leukoplakia. *N Engl J Med* 2001;344:1270-8 and Sudbo J et al. The influence of resection and aneuploidy on mortality in oral leukoplakia. *N Engl J Med.* 2004;350:1405-1413. *N Engl J Med.* 2006;354(6):638.

Kennedy D. Editorial expression of concern. *Science.* 2006;311(5757):36.

5.4.6 **Allegations Involving Unresolved Questions of Scientific Misconduct.** Cases may arise in which an allegation requires the journal editor to have access to the data on which the manuscript or article in question was based. *JAMA's* authorship statement includes the following language:

> If requested, I shall produce the data on which the manuscript is based for examination by the editors or their assignees.

For discussion of reasonable time limits for which authors should keep their data, see 5.6.1, Intellectual Property: Ownership, Access, Rights, and Management, Ownership and Control of Data.

If an author refuses a request for access to the original data, or if the author or the author's institution refuses to comply with the journal's request for information about the allegation, the journal and its editor may be left in a precarious situation. The ICMJE recommends that journals publish an expression of concern detailing the unresolved questions regarding an act of scientific misconduct in their publications (see also 5.4.5, Retractions, Expressions of Concern).[22]

5.4.7 **Allegations Involving Manuscripts Under Editorial Consideration.** In the case of a manuscript under consideration that is not yet published in which fabrication, falsification, or plagiarism is suspected, the editor should ask the corresponding author for a written explanation. If an explanation is not provided or is unsatisfactory, the editor should contact the author's institutional authority (ie, dean, director, ethical conduct/research integrity officer) or governmental agency with jurisdiction to investigate allegations of scientific misconduct to request an investigation. In all such communications with authors and institutional authorities, the editor should take care to maintain confidentiality and should follow the same procedures described in 5.4.4, Editorial Policy and Procedures for Detecting and Handling Allegations of Scientific Misconduct. If the author's explanation or institutional investigation demonstrates that the misconduct did not occur, the editor should continue to consider the manuscript on its own merits. If the author's explanation or a formal investigation demonstrates misconduct, the editor should promptly reject the paper. However, the US Office of Research Integrity advises that rejecting and returning to an author a manuscript associated with suspected or confirmed misconduct without confronting the possible misconduct issues is inappropriate because it may result in the work being published elsewhere.[29]

ACKNOWLEDGMENTS

Principal author: Annette Flanagin, RN, MA

I thank Catherine D. DeAngelis, MD, MPH, *JAMA* and *Archives* Journals; C. K. Gunsalus, JD, University of Illinois, Champaign/Urbana; and Drummond Rennie, MD, *JAMA*, for reviewing and providing substantial comments for improvement of the manuscript; the following for reviewing and providing minor comments: Terri S. Carter, *Archives of Surgery*; Cindy W. Hamilton, PharmD, ELS, Hamilton House; Trevor Lane, MA, DPhil, University of Hong Kong; Diana J. Mason, RN, PhD, *American Journal of Nursing*; Povl Riis, MD, University of Copenhagen; Roger N. Rosenberg, MD, *Archives of Neurology*; Cheryl Smart, MA, MBA; Valerie Siddall, PhD, ELS, AstraZeneca; and Flo Witte, MA, ELS, AdvancMed LLC; and Sandra Schefris and Yolanda Davis, James S. Todd Memorial Library, American Medical Association, Chicago, Illinois, for bibliographic assistance.

REFERENCES

1. Rennie D. Dealing with research misconduct in the United Kingdom: an American perspective on research integrity. *BMJ*. 1998;316(7146):1726-1728.
2. Swazey JP, Anderson MS, Louis KS. Ethical problems in academic research. *Am Sci*. 1993;81(6):542-553.
3. Ranstam J, Buyse M, George SL; for the ISCB Subcommittee on Fraud. Fraud in medical research: an international survey of biostatisticians. *Control Clin Trials*. 2000;21(5):415-427.
4. Geggie D. A survey of newly appointed consultants' attitudes towards research fraud. *Med Ethics*. 2001;27(5):344-346.
5. Martinson BC, Anderson MS, de Vries R. Scientists behaving badly. *Nature*. 2005; 435(7043):737-738.
6. Relman AS. Lessons from the Darsee affair. *N Engl J Med*. 1983;308(23):1415-1417.
7. Knox R. The Harvard fraud case: where does the problem lie? *JAMA*. 1983;249(14): 1797-1799, 1802-1807.
8. Rennie D, Gunsalus CK. Scientific misconduct: new definition, procedures, and office—perhaps a new leaf. *JAMA*. 1993;269(7):915-917.
9. US Department of Health and Human Services, Public Health Service. Responsibilities of awardee and applicant institutions for dealing with and reporting possible misconduct in science: final rule. *Fed Regist*. 1989;54(151):32446.
10. National Academy of Sciences. *Responsible Science: Ensuring the Integrity of the Research Process*. Washington, DC: National Academy Press; 1992.
11. Commission on Research Integrity. *Integrity and Misconduct in Research*. Washington, DC: Office of Research Integrity; 1995.
12. Committee on Assessing Integrity in Research Elements, Institute of Medicine. *Integrity in Scientific Research: Creating an Environment That Promotes Responsible Conduct*. Washington, DC: National Academy Press; 2002.
13. OSTP. Federal policy on research misconduct. *Fed Regist*. 2000;65(6):76260-76264.
14. US Department of Health and Human Services. Public health service policies on research misconduct; final rule. *Fed Regist*. 2005;70(94):28386.
15. Marshall E. Suit alleges misuse of peer review. *Science*. 1995;270(5244):1912.
16. Northwestern University. How to avoid plagiarism. http://www.northwestern.edu /uacc/plagiar.html. Accessed September 23, 2006.
17. Giles J. Taking on the cheats. *Nature*. 2005;435(7040):258-259.
18. Eysenbach G. Report of a case of cyberplagiarism—and reflections on detecting and preventing academic misconduct using the Internet. *J Med Internet Res*. 2001;2(1): article e4.
19. Rossner M. How to guard against image fraud. *Scientist*. 2006;20(3):24. http:// www.the-scientist.com/2006/3/1/24/1. Accessed September 9, 2006.
20. Rossner M, Yamada K. What's in a picture? the temptation of image manipulation. *J Cell Biol*. 2004;166(1):11-15.
21. *JCB* instructions to authors: image acquisition and manipulation. http://www.jcb.org /misc/ifora.shtml#image_aquisition. Updated September 6, 2006. Accessed September 26, 2006.
22. International Committee of Medical Journal Editors. Uniform Requirements for Manuscripts Submitted to Biomedical Journals. http://www.icmje.org. Updated February 2006. Accessed September 9, 2006.

23. World Association of Medical Editors. WAME recommendations on publication ethics policies for medical journals. http://www.wame.org/resources/publication-ethics-policies-for-medical-journals. Accessed December 28, 2006.
24. Council of Science Editors. CSE's white paper on promoting integrity in scientific journal publications. http://www.councilscienceeditors.org/editorial_policies/white_paper.cfm. September 13, 2006. Accessed December 28, 2006.
25. Committee on Publication Ethics. A code of conduct for editors of biomedical journals. http://www.publicationethics.org.uk/guidelines/code. Updated November 29, 2004. Accessed September 9, 2006.
26. MC Atlas. Retraction policies of high-impact biomedical journals. *J Med Libr Assoc.* 2004;92(2):242-250.
27. Sox HC, Rennie D. Research misconduct, retraction, and cleansing the medical literature: lessons from the Poehlman case. *Ann Intern Med.* 2006;144(8):609-613.
28. National Library of Medicine. Fact sheet: errata, retraction, duplicate publication, comment, update and patient summary policy for MEDLINE. http://www.nlm.nih.gov/pubs/factsheets/errata.html. Accessed September 9, 2006.
29. Office of Research Integrity, Office of Public Health and Sciences, US Department of Health and Human Services. Managing allegations of scientific misconduct: a guidance document for editors. http://ori.dhhs.gov/documents/masm_2000.pdf. January 2000. Accessed September 23, 2006.
30. Druss BG, Bressi S, Marcus SC. Retractions in the research literature: misconduct or mistakes? Paper presented at: Fifth International Congress on Peer Review and Biomedical Publication; September 16, 2005; Chicago, IL. http://www.ama-assn.org/public/peer/abstracts.html#scientific. Accessed January 15, 2006.
31. Fontanarosa PB, DeAngelis CD. Correcting the literature—retraction and republication. *JAMA.* 2005;293(20):2536.

Of all the causes which conspire to blind
Man's erring judgment, and misguide the mind,
What the weak head with strongest bias rules,
Is pride, the never-failing vice of fools.

Alexander Pope[1]

5.5 Conflicts of Interest.

Conflicts of Interest. A conflict of interest occurs when an individual's objectivity is potentially, but not necessarily, compromised by a desire for prominence, professional advancement, financial gain, or a successful outcome. Conflicts of interest that arise from personal or financial relationships, academic competition, and intellectual passion are not uncommon in science. In biomedical publication, a conflict of interest may exist when an author (or the author's institution, employer, or funder) has financial or other relationships that could influence (or bias) the author's decisions, work, or manuscript.[2-4] However, much concern has been directed toward the financial interests of researchers and authors, perhaps because such interests are the easiest to measure, and because of the complex relationships between them and the funders of their work.[5-11] In addition, concerns have increased about author biases associated with financial ties to industry[6] and pressures from commercial funders that result in delayed or suppressed publication.[5,10]

Journal editors strive to ensure that information published in their journals is as balanced, objective, and evidence-based as possible. Because of the difficulty in distinguishing the difference between an actual conflict of interest and a perceived conflict,[12] many biomedical journals require authors to disclose all relevant, potential conflicts of interest.[2-4] Financial interests may include but are not limited to employment, consultancies, stock ownership, honoraria, expert testimony, royalties, patents (filed, pending, or registered), grants, and material or financial support from industry, government, or private agencies. Nonfinancial interests include personal or professional relationships, affiliations, knowledge, or beliefs that might affect objectivity.

Many potential biases may be detected during the editorial assessment and peer review of a manuscript (eg, problems with a study's methods and analysis, inappropriate interpretation of results, unbalanced selection or citation of the literature, unjustified emphasis or overly enthusiastic language, and conclusions that go beyond a study's results) or are obvious from the author's affiliation or area of expertise. However, financially motivated biases are less easily detected. Therefore, in the 1980s biomedical journals began to require authors to disclose any financial interests in the subject of their manuscript.[13,14] During the next 20 years, authors typically included information about financial support from grant and funding agencies in their submitted manuscripts, primarily because the funding agencies require them to do so, but it was less common for authors to disclose other financial interests, unless such information had been specifically requested.

Until recently, many journals did not have conflict of interest policies. A 1997 study of 1396 high-impact biomedical and science journals identified only 181 journals (13%) with conflict of interest policies; those journals with policies were overrepresented by medical journals.[15] A study conducted in 2005 of the 7 highest-impact, peer-reviewed journals in 12 different scientific disciplines showed a higher prevalence of journals that reported having conflict of interest policies (80%), although only 33% made these policies publicly available (eg, in their instructions for authors). All of the top-ranked general medical and multidisciplinary science journals had such policies, but journals in other scientific disciplines were less likely to have such policies and/or to publish them in their instructions for authors.[16]

Many biomedical journals, including *JAMA* and the *Archives* Journals, require disclosure of financial interest from everyone involved in the editorial process: authors, reviewers, editorial board members, and editors. The International Committee of Medical Journal Editors (ICMJE),[2] the Council of Science Editors (CSE),[17] and the World Association of Medical Editors (WAME)[18] support this policy. Many journals also require individuals (such as editorial and publishing employees and full-time and part-time editors) who have access to material during the review and publication processes to comply with policies on conflicts of interest. The CSE has a framework (recommendations and a list of questions) to help journals develop and review current policies on conflicts of interest.[19]

Different journals and publishers have various conflict of interest policies and procedures (eg, some request disclosures, some require disclosures, and some exclude authors, reviewers, and editors with conflicts of interest from participation in the publication process).[16] Journals also define *relevant* conflicts of interest in different terms; they may have a broad interpretation of conflicts of interest to include financial and nonfinancial conflicts or may focus only on financial interests, and for financial interests, they may define relevance in terms of monetary amounts or lengths of time. The following discussion addresses policies in general as recommended by the ICMJE,[2] CSE,[17] and WAME[18] and provides specific examples of policies, procedures, and terms as used by *JAMA* and the *Archives* Journals.

5.5.1 Requirements for Authors.

Requirements for Authors. Authors should disclose all relevant conflicts of interest in their work at the time of manuscript submission either in the manuscript (if so required by the journal) or in a cover letter to the editor or on the journal's disclosure form (if the journal uses one). Journals should define conflicts of interest and the types of disclosures required (eg, all types of conflicts of interest or only financial interests). For example, *JAMA* requires all relevant financial disclosures of each author and coauthor to be included in the Acknowledgment section of the manuscript and to be noted in the "Financial Disclosure" section of the authorship form that each author is required to complete and sign.[20] The *Archives of Dermatology* requires authors to indicate their conflicts of interest, both financial and nonfinancial, on the manuscript's title page.[21] Both journals describe these policies in their instructions for authors and in the online manuscript submission forms. Since these disclosures are part of the manuscript, peer reviewers will see these when they review for *JAMA* and the *Archives of Dermatology*.

Some journals require authors to provide disclosure statements in a cover letter or journal disclosure form and do not share these disclosures with peer reviewers, unless the journal routinely shares author correspondence and submission forms with peer reviewers. Whether a journal requires complete disclosure of financial conflicts of interest or both financial and nonfinancial conflicts of interest and whether the disclosures are to be nonconfidential and included in the manuscript or confidential and listed only in documents and communications not shared with peer reviewers, these policies should be made clear to all prospective authors and reviewers and be publicly available in easily accessible instructions for authors. However, if a manuscript is accepted, whether the journal's disclosure policy is nonconfidential or confidential during the review process, the author's relevant conflicts of interest should be published.

JAMA and the *Archives* Journals also require all authors to report detailed information regarding all financial and material support for the research and work, including but not limited to grant support, funding sources, and provision of equipment and supplies (see also 5.5.2, Reporting Funding and Other Support). For *JAMA*, each author also is required to sign and submit the following financial disclosure statement in the authorship form:

> I certify that all my affiliations or financial involvement, within the past 5 years and foreseeable future (eg, employment, consultancies, honoraria, stock ownership or options, expert testimony, grants or patents received or pending, royalties) with any organization or entity with a financial interest in or financial conflict with the subject matter or materials discussed in the manuscript are completely disclosed in the Acknowledgment section of The manuscript.

JAMA authors are expected to provide detailed information about any relevant financial interests or financial conflicts within the past 5 years and for the foreseeable future, particularly those present at the time the research was conducted and up to the time of publication, as well as other financial interests, such as relevant filed or pending patents or patent applications in preparation, that represent potential future financial gain.[4] This includes financial involvement with a product or service that is in direct competition with a product or service described in the manuscript. Although many universities and other institutions and organizations have established policies and thresholds for reporting financial interests and other conflicts of interest, *JAMA* and the *Archives* Journals require complete disclosure of all relevant financial relationships and potential financial conflicts of interest, regardless of amount or value. If authors are uncertain about what might constitute a potential financial conflict of interest, they should err on the side of full disclosure and should contact the editorial office if they have questions or concerns. In addition, authors who have no relevant financial interests are asked to provide a statement indicating that they have no financial interests related to the material in the manuscript and to include this information in the Acknowledgment section of the submitted manuscript.[3,4,20]

The ICMJE recommends that editors publish authors' conflict of interest statements if they believe that the information will help readers.[2] Decisions about whether financial information provided by authors should be published, and thereby disclosed to readers, are usually straightforward. For example, authors of a manuscript about hypertension should report all financial relationships they have with all manufacturers of products used in the management of hypertension, not only those relationships with companies whose specific products are mentioned in the manuscript. If authors are uncertain about what constitutes a relevant financial interest or relationship, and whether or not the journal would deem a specific conflict of interest relevant, they should contact the editorial office.

Although editors are willing to discuss disclosure of specific financial information with authors, *JAMA* and the *Archives* Journals require complete disclosure of all relevant financial interests at the time of manuscript submission, and each author's disclosure of relevant financial interests or declaration of no relevant financial interests will be published in the Acknowledgment section of the article.[3,4]

A journal's conflict of interest policies should apply to all manuscript submissions, including reports of research, reviews, opinion pieces (eg, editorials), letters to the editor, and book reviews.

Some journals might not accept manuscripts from authors with financial interest in the subject of the manuscript. For example, editors of some journals prefer that authors of some types of articles, such as editorials, commentaries, and reviews, not have relevant financial interests in the subject matter.[22,23] Unlike scientific reports, editorials and nonsystematic reviews contain no primary data and offer an evaluation of a topic from a selection and interpretation of the literature; hence, they are more susceptible to bias, which accompanying financial disclosures do not obviate. Authors of opinion pieces and review articles are expected to provide an expert, unbiased, and authoritative perspective, which they may not be able to do if they have financial ties to products or services mentioned in the manuscript or are otherwise related (eg, within the same area, category, or topic). However, such policies may be overly restrictive and may limit the journal's ability to publish articles from some qualified authors. Journals with concerns about the financial interests of authors of opinion pieces and review articles must balance the risk of publishing potentially biased discussion and comment against excluding potentially valuable contributions to the literature, which in some fields may be the only expert contribution available. The key is for the editor to ensure that the editorial or review is as balanced, objective, and evidence-based as possible. If, after review and careful consideration, the editor believes the work is biased and that the author is unable or unwilling to revise the manuscript to eliminate such bias and prospective readers would be misled, the editor should not accept the manuscript for publication. *JAMA*'s policy recognizes that conflicts of interest are common, and in some cases perhaps even helpful (for example, from a knowledgeable and critical reviewer with an opposing viewpoint). This policy favors complete disclosure from all authors over a ban of authors with conflicts of interest. However, when inviting an author to write an editorial to comment on a paper to be published, the editors will ask the prospective author to disclose any relevant financial interests and consider this information carefully, in light of the potential for harm from bias vs benefit from expertise, before confirming that the author is the best available person to write the editorial.

Information about relevant financial interest can be published in the "Acknowledgment" section at the end of the article (after the list of author contributions and before information about grants and financial or material support) or on the title page of the article near the author's affiliation. (See also 2.10.7, Manuscript Preparation, Acknowledgment Section, Financial Disclosure, and 5.2, Acknowledgments.)

The following example shows placement in the Acknowledgment section:

> **Author Contributions:** As principal investigator, Dr Jones had full access to all the data in the study and takes responsibility for the integrity of the data and the accuracy of the data analysis.
>
> *Study concept and design:* Jones, Jacques, Smith, Brown
>
> *Acquisition of data:* Jones, Smith, Brown
>
> *Analysis and interpretation of data:* Jones, Jacques, Smith, Brown
>
> *Drafting of the manuscript:* Jones
>
> *Critical revision of the manuscript for important intellectual content:* Jacques, Smith, Brown
>
> *Statistical analysis:* Jacques
>
> *Obtained funding*: Jones
>
> *Study supervision*: Brown
>
> **Financial Disclosures:** Dr Jones has served as a paid consultant to Wyler Laboratories. Dr Jacques owns stock in Wyler Laboratories. Drs Smith and Brown reported no financial interests.
>
> [*Or:* **Financial Disclosures:** None reported.]
>
> **Funding/Support:** This study was funded in part by Wyler Laboratories.

The following example shows placement in the author affiliation footnote:

> **Author Affiliations:** Department of Cardiology, Ambrose University Hospital, Boston, Massachusetts (Drs Jones and Smith), and Wyler Laboratories, Geneva, Switzerland (Dr Jacques and Mr Dube).
>
> **Financial Disclosures:** Dr Jones has served as a paid consultant to Wyler Laboratories. Dr Jacques owns stock in Wyler Laboratories. Drs Smith and Brown reported no financial interests.
>
> **Corresponding Author:** John J. Jones, MD, Department of Cardiology, Ambrose University Hospital, 444 N State St, Boston, MA 01022 (jonesj@ambroseuniv.edu)

5.5.2 **Reporting Funding and Other Support.** In addition to individual financial conflicts of interest, authors should report all financial and material support for the work reported in the manuscript. This includes, but is not limited to, grant support and funding, provision of equipment and supplies, and other paid contributions.[2,3] All financial and material support should be indicated in the Acknowledgment section of the manuscript, along with detailed information on the roles of each funding source or sponsor (see also 5.2.6, Acknowledgments, Funding and Role of Sponsors). In addition, all individuals who provided other important paid contributions should be identified, with their names and affiliations listed in the Acknowledgment section of the manuscript, or as authors if they meet the full criteria for authorship. These contributions include the work of employed or compensated writers, editors, statisticians, epidemiologists, and others involved with manuscript preparation, data management, and analyses.[4] Acknowledgment of such contributions should be specific and may include information on funding. For example, *JAMA* requires authors to include information about each nonauthor contributor's role/contribution, academic degree(s), affiliation, and indication if compensation was received for each person named in the Acknowledgment section (see also, 5.2.1, Acknowledgments, Acknowledging Support, Assistance, and Contributions of Those Who Are Not Authors).

5.5.3 **Reporting the Role of the Sponsor.** In the interest of full disclosure, the ICMJE recommends that authors report how sponsors/funders have participated in the work reported in a specific manuscript.[2,24] Journals should require authors to indicate the role of the sponsor/funding organization in each of the following: "design and conduct of the study; collection, management, analysis, and interpretation of the data; and preparation, review, or approval of the manuscript." If the sponsor or funder had no such role, this should be stated. This information may be included in the "Methods" or Acknowledgment section of the manuscript[2] (see also 5.2.6, Acknowledgments, Funding and Role of Sponsors). Authors should not agree to allow sponsors with a proprietary or financial interest in the outcome of a study or review article to control the author's rights to publication, although review of such manuscripts by the funding agency is typically permitted as long as such review does not impose an unacceptable delay or suppression.[2,5,10,24] According to the ICMJE, if a sponsor or funder with a proprietary interest in a manuscript has "asserted control over the authors' right to publish," editors should decline consideration of the manuscript.[2]

5.5.4 **Access to Data Requirement.** For all reports, regardless of funding source, containing original data (research and systematic reviews), at least 1 named author should indicate that she or he "had full access to all of the data in the study and takes responsibility for the integrity of the data and the accuracy of the data analysis"[2-4] (see also 5.1.1, Authorship Responsibility, Authorship: Definition, Criteria, Contributions, and Requirements). This responsibility can vest with the principal investigator, the corresponding author, or the article's guarantor. While in some research groups, particularly small ones, all authors may have access to all of the data, it is usually not meaningful to state generically that all authors had such access.

5.5.5 **Requirements for Reporting Industry-Sponsored Studies.** Biases are potentially introduced when sponsors are directly involved in research.[2,5,6,8,10,24] As a result, for industry-sponsored studies, *JAMA* and the *Archives* Journals require an access to data statement to be provided by an investigator who is not employed by any funding source with a proprietary interest in the outcome of the study.[4] In addition, *JAMA* will not accept for publication an industry-sponsored study in which the data analysis has been conducted solely by statisticians employed by the company sponsoring the research. For these studies, an additional analysis of the data (entire raw data set, study protocol, and prespecified plan for data analysis) must be conducted by an independent statistician at an academic institution, such as a medical school, academic medical center, or government research institute, that has oversight over the person conducting the analysis who is independent of the commercial sponsor.[4] This provides the editor with an authority who does not have financial interest in the findings (eg, the independent statistician's department chair or dean) to contact if there are concerns about the analysis or any allegations of misconduct that the sponsor cannot or will not address for proprietary reasons. *JAMA* publishes the results of such analysis, along with the name and academic institution of the independent statistician and whether compensation or funding was received for conducting the analyses, in the Acknowledgment section (see 2.10, Manuscript Preparation, Acknowledgment Section, and 5.2, Acknowledgments).

5.5.6 Requirements for Peer Reviewers. Following the recommendations of the ICMJE, CSE, and WAME, reviewers should disclose conflicts of interest in reviewing specific manuscripts and disqualify themselves from a specific review if necessary.[2,17,18] Reviewers should never use information obtained from an unpublished manuscript to further their own interests. Following the same rationale applied to authors, the ICMJE also recommends that reviewers state explicitly if they have no relevant conflicts of interest to disclose.[2]

JAMA includes the following instructions regarding conflicts of interest in the letter sent requesting an individual to review a manuscript:

> While most conflicts of interest are not disqualifying, if you perceive that you have a disqualifying interest, either financial or otherwise, please contact the reviewing editor immediately (if possible, with the names of alternative reviewers). This will not affect your reviewer status.

Not all conflicts of interest are necessarily disqualifying, and in some cases the reviewer with the most expertise may also have conflicts of interest. For example, if a potential conflict of interest exists (financial or otherwise), but the editor and reviewer agree that the reviewer can provide an objective assessment, *JAMA* may request the reviewer to disclose the specific conflict and provide the review. Other journals may choose to exclude any reviewer with a conflict of interest from participating in the review process. A journal's policy on conflicts of interest for peer reviewers should be communicated to the reviewer when the review is requested.

The online review system used by *JAMA* and the *Archives* Journals also contains a field in the reviewer recommendation form that requires reviewers to disclose conflicts of interest or state that they have no relevant conflicts of interest before submitting their reviews. This information is kept confidential and is not revealed to authors or other reviewers.

Many journals, including *JAMA* and the *Archives* Journals, will consider authors' requests not to send papers to specific reviewers. The ICMJE recommends that authors who wish to exclude specific reviewers explain the reasons for such requests at the time of manuscript submission.[2] (See also 6.1.4, Editorial Assessment and

Processing, Editorial Assessment, Selection of Reviewers, and 5.11, Editorial Responsibilities, Roles, Procedures, and Policies.)

5.5.7 **Requirements for Editors and Editorial Board Members.** Editors may also have their objectivity influenced or biased by conflicts of interest.[25-29] As a result, the ICMJE, CSE, and WAME recommend that editors follow policies on conflicts of interest that require disclosure of all relevant conflicts of interest (financial and nonfinancial) and also that they not participate in the review of or decisions on any manuscripts in which they may have a conflict of interest.[2,17,18] Editors and journal editorial board members should never use information obtained during the review process for personal or professional gain. Editors and editorial board members should refrain from making any decisions or recommendations about manuscripts in which they have a personal, professional, or financial interest. Editors should also consider how to handle manuscripts from an author who is from the same institution as the editor and how to handle their own research and review articles. In the event that an editor works alone and has a conflict of interest with a particular manuscript, he or she should assign that manuscript to a guest editor or a member of the editorial board and should not take part in the review and editorial decision of such manuscripts. *JAMA* publishes a disclaimer with any articles that have an author who is also a decision-making editor for the journal to inform readers that the author-editor was not involved in the review or editorial decision.

> **Disclaimer:** Dr Brown, the journal's deputy editor, was not involved in the editorial review or decision to publish this article.

Editorials and announcements about journal policies written by journal editors are exempt from such procedures, but it may be prudent for editors to ask other editors or editorial board members to review and comment on these types of manuscripts (see 5.11, Editorial Responsibilities, Roles, Procedures, and Policies).

JAMA editors sign the following conflict of interest statement annually, which is kept confidential in the editorial office.

> I agree that I will disqualify myself from reviewing, editing, or participating in editorial decisions about any *JAMA* and the *Archives* Journals submission that deals with a matter in which either I or a member of my immediate family has direct financial interest or a competing financial interest (eg, employment, consultancies, stock ownership, honoraria, patents, patent applications, royalties, grants, or compensated expert testimony). I also agree that I will promptly disclose in writing to the editor in chief of *JAMA* all potentially conflicting financial or other relevant conflicting interests pertaining to *JAMA* and the *Archives* Journals.
>
> I agree that I will not use any confidential information obtained from my activities with *JAMA* and the *Archives* Journals to further my own or others' financial interests.

JAMA editorial board members also complete and sign the following conflict of interest and financial disclosure statement, which is kept confidential in the editorial office.

> I agree that I will promptly disclose all potentially conflicting financial and other relevant interests pertaining to *JAMA* during the course of my service as

a member of the *JAMA* Editorial Board (attach or describe below any current potential conflicts of interest). Financial interests to be disclosed can include, but are not limited to: honoraria, employment, stock ownership or options, patents, patent applications, grants, royalties, consultancies, expert witness activities, large gifts, or paid travel and accommodations.

I agree that I will not disclose or use any confidential information obtained from my activities with *JAMA* for my profit or advantage or that of anyone else, whether or not I remain a member of the *JAMA* Editorial Board.

5.5.8 Handling Failure to Disclose Financial Interest

For Authors of Manuscripts Not Yet Published. In the event that an undisclosed financial interest on the part of an author is brought to the editor's attention (usually during the review process), the editor should remind the author of the journal's policy and ask the author if he or she has anything to disclose. The author's reply may affect the editorial decision on whether to publish the manuscript.

Box. Hypothetical Example of a Notice of Financial Interest and Listing in the Journal's Table of Contents

Correction: Notice of Failure to Disclose Financial Interest: "Effective Vaccine Strategies for Pertussis" (*J Med.* 2004;27[5]:440-441)
To the Editor.—I regret that at the time I submitted my manuscript, "Effective Vaccine Strategies for Pertussis,"[1] published in the March 17, 2004, issue of the *Journal of Medicine*, I failed to disclose that I have served as a paid expert witness in several diphtheria-pertussis-tetanus vaccine injury–related lawsuits. I had signed the journal's financial disclosure statement, but I did not realize that expert testimony was considered a potential conflict of interest. I do not believe that my involvement in those legal proceedings biased me in any way, and I believe the statements made in my article are both credible and objective.

V. W. Brazen, MD
Virginia State University
Arlington

1. Brazen VW. Effective vaccine strategies for pertussis. *J Med.* 2004;27(5): 440-441.

Listing in Table of Contents

Correction **1520**
Notice of Failure to Disclose Financial Interest:
"Effective Vaccine Strategies for Pertussis" (*J Med.* 2004;27[5]:440-441)
V. W. Brazen

For Authors of Published Articles. If an editor receives information (usually from a reader) alleging that an author has not disclosed a financial interest in the subject of an article that has been published, the editor should contact the author and ask for an explanation. If the author admits that he or she failed to disclose the existence of a financial interest in the subject of the article, and if that author had previously submitted a signed financial disclosure statement that did not disclose that financial interest, the editor should request a written explanation from the author and publish it as a notice of financial disclosure in the correspondence column or elsewhere in the journal, clearly labeled as a correction (see Box).

As in the case of other types of allegations of wrongdoing (eg, scientific misconduct), editors are not responsible for investigating unresolved allegations of financial interest in an article or manuscript. That responsibility lies with the author's institution, the funding agency, or other appropriate authority. If the editor deems the author's reply to the allegation inappropriate or incomplete, the editor may need to break confidentiality and inform the author's supervisor (eg, dean, integrity officer, department chair, director) or representative of the funding agency. For example, *JAMA*'s editor contacted the deans of 2 medical schools in 2006 to request a full investigation of authors' failures to comply with *JAMA*'s conflict of interest disclosure requirements.[11]

Some journals have discussed banning authors who deliberately violate a journal's stated policy on disclosure of conflicts of interest for a period of time (1-2 years).[28] However, such policies are journal specific.

For Reviewers, Editors, and Editorial Board Members. The discovery of an undisclosed conflict of interest on the part of peer reviewers may result in the journal not asking that reviewer to consult again. Failure to disclose relevant conflicts of interest on the part of editors or editorial board members is grounds for dismissal.

ACKNOWLEDGMENTS

Principal author: Annette Flanagin, RN, MA

I thank C. K. Gunsalus, JD, University of Illinois, Champaign/Urbana; Catherine D. DeAngelis, MD, MPH, *JAMA* and *Archives* Journals; and Liz Wager, MA, Sideview, for reviewing and providing important comments to improve the manuscript; the following for reviewing and providing minor comments: Jessica S. Ancker, MPH, Columbia University College of Physicians and Surgeons; Robert M. Golub, MD, *JAMA*; Wayne G. Hoppe, JD, *JAMA* and *Archives* Journals; Diana J. Mason, RN, PhD, *American Journal of Nursing*; Povl Riis, MD, University of Copenhagen; and Valerie Siddall, PhD, ELS, AstraZeneca; and Sandra Schefris and Yolanda Davis, James S. Todd Memorial Library, American Medical Association, Chicago, Illinois, for bibliographic assistance.

REFERENCES

1. Pope A. *An Essay on Criticism*. 1711:part II, lines 1-4.
2. International Committee of Medical Journal Editors. Uniform Requirements for Manuscripts Submitted to Biomedical Journals. http://www.icmje.org. Updated February 2006. Accessed September 2, 2006.
3. DeAngelis CD, Fontanarosa PB, Flanagin A. Reporting financial conflicts of interest and relationships between investigators and research sponsors. *JAMA*. 2001;286(1):89-91.
4. Fontanarosa PB, Flanagin A, DeAngelis CD. Reporting conflicts of interest, financial aspects of research, and role of sponsors in funded studies. *JAMA*. 2005;294(1):110-111.

5. Blumenthal D, Causino N, Campbell E, Louis KS. Relationships between academic institutions and industry in the life sciences—an industry survey. *N Engl J Med.* 1996;334(6):368-373.
6. Stelfox HT, Chua G, O'Rourke K, Detsky AS. Conflict of interest in the debate over calcium-channel antagonists. *N Engl J Med.* 1998;338(2):101-106.
7. Boyd EA, Bero LA. Assessing faculty financial relationships with industry: a case study. *JAMA.* 2000;284(17):2209-2214.
8. Bekelman JE, Li Y, Gross CP. Scope and impact of financial conflicts of interest in biomedical research: a systematic review. *JAMA.* 2003;289(4):454-465.
9. Flanagin A. Conflict of interest. In: Jones AH, McLellan F, eds. *Ethical Issues in Biomedical Publication.* Baltimore, MD: Johns Hopkins University Press; 2000:137-165.
10. Rennie D. Thyroid storm. *JAMA.* 1997;277(15):1238-1243.
11. DeAngelis CD. The influence of money on medical science. *JAMA.* 2006;296(8):996-998.
12. Friedman PJ. The troublesome semantics of conflict of interest. *Ethics Behav.* 1992; 2(4):245-251.
13. Relman AS. Dealing with conflicts of interest. *N Engl J Med.* 1984;310(18):1182-1183.
14. Knoll E, Lundberg GD. New instructions for authors. *JAMA.* 1985;254(1):97-98.
15. Krimsky S, Rothenberg LS. Conflict of interest policies in science and medical journals: editorial practices and author disclosures. *Sci Eng Ethics.* 2001;7(2):205-218.
16. Ancker J, Flanagin A. A comparison of conflict of interest policies at peer-reviewed journals in multiple scientific disciplines. *Sci Eng Ethics.* In press.
17. Council of Science Editors. CSE's white paper on promoting integrity in scientific journal publications. http://www.councilscienceeditors.org/editorial_policies/white_paper.cfm. September 13, 2006. Accessed January 5, 2007.
18. World Association of Medical Editors. WAME recommendations on publication ethics policies for medical journals. http://www.wame.org/resources/publication-ethics-policies-for-medical-journals. Accessed December 29, 2006.
19. Council of Science Editors. Guidance for journals developing or revising policies on conflict of interest, disclosure, or competing financial interests. http://www.councilscienceeditors.org/events/retreat_paper_2005-02.pdf. February 2005. Accessed September 2, 2006.
20. Flanagin A, Fontanarosa PB, DeAngelis CD. Update on *JAMA*'s conflict of interest policy. *JAMA.* 2006;296(2):220-221.
21. Instructions for authors. *Arch Dermatol.* 2006;142(1). archderm.ama-assn.org/misc/ifora.dtl. Accessed January 20, 2006.
22. Publishing commentary by authors with potential conflicts of interest: when, why, and how. *Ann Intern Med.* 2004;141(1):73-74.
23. James A, Horton R. *The Lancet's* policy on conflicts of interest. *Lancet.* 2003; 361(9351):8-9.
24. Davidoff F, DeAngelis CD, Drazen JM, et al. Sponsorship, authorship, and accountability. *JAMA.* 2001;286(10):1232-1234.
25. A medical editor's resignation. *JAMA.* 1893;21(16):582.
26. Hoey J. When editors publish in their own journals. *CMAJ.* 1999;161(11):1412-1413.
27. Watson G, Watson M, Chapman S, Byrne F. Environmental tobacco smoke research published in the journal *Indoor and Built Environment* and associations with the tobacco industry. *Lancet.* 2005;365(9461):804-809.

28. Wright IC. Conflict of interest and the *British Journal of Psychiatry*. *Br J Psychiatry*. January 2002;180:82-83.
29. Pincock S. Journal editor quits in conflict scandal. *Scientist*. http://www.the-scientist.com/news/display/24445/#24969. August 28, 2006. Accessed October 21. 2006.

[Will copyright survive the new technologies?] That question is about as bootless as asking whether politics will survive democracy. The real question is what steps it will take to ensure that the promised new era of information and entertainment survives copyright. History offers a clue.

Paul Goldstein[1]

5.6 Intellectual Property: Ownership, Access, Rights, and Management.

Intellectual property is a legal term for that which results from the creative efforts of the mind (intellectual) and that which can be owned, possessed, and subject to competing claims (property).[2] Three legal doctrines governing intellectual property are relevant for authors, editors, and publishers in biomedical publishing: copyright (the law protecting authorship and publication), patent (the law protecting invention and technology), and trademark (the law protecting words and symbols used to identify goods and services in the marketplace).[1] This section focuses primarily on intellectual property and copyright law.

5.6.1 Ownership and Control of Data.

Conceptual application of the term *property* to scientific knowledge is not new, but advances in science and technology and economic factors have fueled disputes and concerns over ownership, control, and access to original data.[1-7] Data used in biomedical research, increasingly complex, now include large data sets, software, algorithms, and metadata (data that provide information or characteristics about other data). With the exception of commercially owned information, scientific data are viewed as a public good, allowing others to benefit from knowledge of and access to the information without decreasing the benefit received by the individual who originally developed the data.[8] Ideally, scientific data would become a public good, regardless of the source of funding.[9] The US National Institutes of Health (NIH) policy on data sharing states that "data should be made as widely and freely available as possible while safeguarding the privacy of participants and protecting confidential and proprietary data."[10] However, personal, professional, financial, and proprietary interests can often interfere with the altruistic goals of data sharing.[5,6,11-13]

Ownership of Data. For purposes herein, *data* include but are not limited to written and digital laboratory notes, documents, research and project records, experimental materials (eg, reagents, cultures), descriptions of collections of biological specimens (eg, cells, tissue, genetic material), descriptions of methods and processes, patient or research participant records and measurements, results of bibliometric and other database searches, illustrative material and graphics, analyses, surveys, questionnaires, responses, data sets (eg, protein or DNA sequences, microassay or molecular structure data), databases, metadata (data that describe or characterize other data), software, and algorithms. The NIH policy defines *final research data* as "recorded factual material commonly accepted in the scientific community as necessary to document, support, and validate research findings," which might include raw data and derived variables.[10] The NIH definition does not include summary statistics; rather, it pertains to the data on which summary statistics are based. In scientific research, 3 primary arenas exist for ownership of data: the government, the commercial sector, and academic or private institutions or foundations. Although an infrequent occurrence, when data are developed by a scientist without a relationship to a government agency, a commercial entity, or an academic institution, the data are owned by that scientist.

Any information produced by an office or employee of the US federal government in the course of his or her employment is owned by the government.[14] The Freedom of Information Act (FOIA), enacted in 1966, is intended to ensure public access to government-owned information (except trade secrets, financial data, national defense information, and personnel or medical records protected under the Privacy Act).[2,15] Access to documents with such data that are otherwise unavailable may be obtained through an FOIA request.

Data produced by employees in the commercial sector (eg, a pharmaceutical, device, or biotechnology company, health insurance company, or for-profit hospital or managed care organization) are most often governed by the legal relationship between the employee and the commercial employer, granting all rights of data ownership and control to the employer. However, if the data have been used to secure a government grant or contract, such data may be obtained by an outside party through an FOIA request or by a court-ordered subpoena.[3,15]

According to guidelines established by Harvard University in 1988 and subsequently adopted by other US academic institutions, data developed by employees of academic institutions are owned by the institutions.[16] This policy allows access to data by university scientists and allows departing scientists to take copies of data with them, but the original data remain at the institution.

Data Sharing and Length of Storage. The notion that data should be shared with others for review, criticism, and replication is a fundamental tenet of the scientific enterprise. Sharing research data encourages scientific inquiry, permits reanalyses, promotes new research, facilitates education and training of new researchers, permits creation of new data sets when data from multiples sources are combined, and helps maintain the integrity of the scientific record.[2,4,10] Yet the practice of data sharing has varied widely, and it was not until relatively recently that guidelines for data sharing were developed.[4,7,10]

Although data sharing is essential for research, costs and risks may result in restrictions on access to certain data imposed by the owner or initial investigator. Potential costs and risks to the owner or initial investigator include technical and financial obstacles for data storage, reproduction, and transmission; loss of academic or financial reward or commercial profit; unwarranted or unwanted criticism; risk of future discovery or exploitation by a competitor; the discovery of error or fraud; and breaches of confidentiality. The discovery of error or fraud and breaches of confidentiality have important relevance in scientific publishing. Discovery of error or fraud, if corrected or retracted in the literature, is clearly beneficial, and for research involving humans, epidemiologic and statistical procedures are available to maintain confidentiality for individual study participants[9,17-19] (see also 5.4, Scientific

Misconduct, and 5.8, Protecting Research Participants' and Patients' Rights in Scientific Publication). A number of research sponsors and governmental agencies have developed policies to encourage data sharing. For example, in 2003, the NIH began requiring investigators to include a plan for data sharing in all grant applications requesting $500 000 or more in direct costs.[10] The Wellcome Trust encourages its funded investigators to release data to the public from large-scale biological research projects, such as the International Human Genome Sequencing Consortium.[20]

A number of proposals prescribe the minimum optimal time to keep data (for example, 2-7 years). However, there is no universally accepted standard for data retention by academic and research institutions. For example, the NIH requires its funded scientists to keep data for a minimum of 3 years after the closeout of a grant or contract agreement and recognizes that an investigator's academic institution may have additional policies regarding the required retention period for data.[10] The NIH also gives the right of data management, including the decision to publish, to the principal investigator.[10]

Data Sharing, Deposit, Access Requirements of Journals. In 1985, the US Committee on National Statistics, which is part of the National Research Council (NRC),[17] released a report on data sharing that continues to serve as a useful guide for authors and editors. Among the committee's recommendations, the following have specific relevance for scientific publication.

> Data sharing should be a regular practice.
>
> Initial investigators should share their data by the time of the publication of initial major results of analyses of the data except in compelling circumstances, and they should share data relevant to public policy quickly and as widely as possible.
>
> Investigators should keep data available for a reasonable period after publication of results from analyses of the data.
>
> Subsequent analysts who request data from others should bear the associated incremental costs and they should endeavor to keep the burdens of data sharing to a minimum. They should explicitly acknowledge the contribution of the initial investigators in all subsequent publications.
>
> Journal editors should require authors to provide access to data during the peer review process.
>
> Journals should give more emphasis to reports of secondary analyses and to replications.
>
> Journals should require full credit and appropriate citations to original data collections in reports based on secondary analyses.
>
> Journals should strongly encourage authors to make detailed data accessible to other researchers (although some may view this as outside the purview of a journal's responsibilities).

Similar to policies on data sharing and storage for academic and research institutions, policies for scientific journals are highly variable and not always available. In 2002, a US NRC review of 56 of the most frequently cited life science and medical journals reported that 39% had policies on data sharing and 45% had no stated policy.[4] Of the 18 medical journals in this review, only 22% had policies on data sharing. To address the lack of standard policies for data sharing among scientific journals and recognizing that no standards are expected given the diversity of disciplines in the life sciences, the NRC recommends the following[4]:

> Scientific journals should clearly and prominently state (in their instructions for authors and on their Web sites) their policies for distribution of publication-related materials, data, and other information.
>
> Policies for sharing materials should include requirements for depositing materials in an appropriate repository.
>
> Policies for data sharing should include requirements for deposition of complex data sets in appropriate databases and for the sharing of software and algorithms integral to the finding being reported.
>
> The policies should also clearly state the consequences for authors who do not adhere to the policies and the procedure for registering complaints about noncompliance.

The NRC also has proposed a set of principles that may be useful to journals developing policies on data sharing[4]:

> Authors should include in their publications data, algorithms, or other information that is central or integral to the publication—that is, whatever is necessary to support the major claims of the paper and would enable one skilled in the art to verify or replicate the claims.
>
> If central or integral information cannot be included in the publication for practical reasons (for example, because a data set is too large), it should be made freely (without restriction of its use for research purposes and at no cost) and readily accessible through other means (for example, online). Moreover, when necessary to enable further research, integral information should be made available in a form that enables it to be manipulated, analyzed, and combined with other scientific data.
>
> If publicly accessible repositories for data have been agreed on by a community of researchers and are in general use, the relevant data should be deposited in one of these repositories by the time of publication.
>
> Authors of scientific publications should anticipate which materials integral to their publications are likely to be requested and should state in the "Materials and Methods" section or elsewhere how to obtain them.
>
> If material integral to a publication is patented, the provider of the material should make the material available under a license for research use.

A number of scientific journals (eg, *Science, Nature*) require authors to submit large data sets (eg, protein or DNA sequences, microrray or molecular structure data) to approved, accessible databases and to provide accession numbers as a condition of publication. It is appropriate for authors and journals to include links to public repositories for such data in the Acknowledgment sections of articles (see also 2.10.13,

Manuscript Preparation, Acknowledgment Section, Additional Information [Miscellaneous Acknowledgments]).

Some journals have other conditions of publication that require authors to deposit specific information about their research in a public repository or archive, although this is not data sharing per se. For example, following the recommendations of the International Committee of Medical Journal Editors (ICMJE),[21] biomedical journals that publish clinical trials require authors to have registered their trials in approved, publicly accessible trial registries and to provide registration identifiers as a condition of publication (see also 2.5.1, Manuscript Preparation, Abstract, Structured Abstracts, and 20.4, Study Design and Statistics, Meta-analysis). In addition, a number of funders require authors to post articles describing the results of their funded research in publicly available archives (see also 5.6.2, Open-Access Publication and Scientific Journals).

Some journals require authors to provide data available on request for examination by the editors or peer reviewers (see 5.4, Scientific Misconduct). For example, *JAMA* requires all authors to sign the following as part of their authorship responsibility statement:

> If requested, I shall produce the data on which the manuscript is based for examination by the editors or their assignees.

In addition, for reports containing original data (eg, research articles, systematic reviews, and meta-analyses), *JAMA* requires at least 1 author who is independent of any commercial funder (eg, the principal investigator) to indicate that she or he "had full access to all the data in the study and takes responsibility for the integrity of the data and the accuracy of the data analysis." (See also 5.5.4, Conflicts of Interest, Access to Data Requirement.)

Manuscripts Based on the Same Data. On occasion, an editor may receive 2 or more manuscripts based on the same data (with concordant or contradictory interpretations and conclusions). If the authors of these manuscripts are not collaborators and the data are publicly available, the editor should consider each manuscript on its own merit (perhaps asking reviewers to examine the manuscripts simultaneously). Authors should attempt to resolve disputes over contradictory interpretations of the same data before submitting manuscripts to journals. When more than 1 manuscript is submitted by current or former coworkers or collaborators who disagree on the analysis and interpretation of the same unpublished data, the recipient editors are faced with a difficult dilemma.[21] The ICMJE has stated that, since peer review will not necessarily resolve the discrepant interpretations or conclusions, editors should decline to consider competing manuscripts from coworkers until the dispute is resolved by the authors or the institution where the work was done.[21] Arguments against publishing both papers include that doing so could confuse readers and waste journal pages. However, publishing the competing manuscripts with an explanatory editorial may allow readers to see and understand both sides of the dispute. Alternatively, publishing the paper deemed of higher quality could result in biasing the literature and postponing publication of legitimate research.

Record Retention Policies for Journals. Journals should develop and implement consistent policies for retention of records and data related to the content that they publish. Legal documents (eg, copyright transfers, licenses, and permissions) should be kept indefinitely. All other records should be kept for a consistent period. For example, *JAMA* and the *Archives* Journals keep print and online copies of rejected manuscripts, correspondence, and reviewer comments up to 1 year to permit consideration of appeals of decisions. Print and digital copies of accepted manuscripts and related correspondence and reviews are kept for 3 years. Journals also should develop consistent policies for the retention of online metadata associated with manuscript submissions, authors, and peer reviewers. (See also, 5.7.3, Confidentiality, Confidentiality in Legal Petitions and Claims for Privileged Information.)

5.6.2 **Open-Access Publication and Scientific Journals.** The open-access movement began in the late 1990s following the proliferation of online journals available via the Internet (versions of print journals and journals published only online), the inability of declining library budgets to keep pace with increases in the numbers of journals and rising subscription prices, and demands to reduce the information gap between developed and developing countries.[22-25] Broadly defined, *open access* is the free and unrestricted online availability of content. (In the context of biomedical publication, this refers primarily to research articles.) Strictly applied, open-access publishing means that users can freely read, download, copy, distribute, print, search, or link to full text of articles provided that authors are properly acknowledged and cited.[26] There are 2 types of open access: self-archiving and open-access publishing.

Self-archiving is the deposition of content in an open archive, sometimes before formal publication. Archives may be subject based, such as the physics preprint ArXiv, which was launched in 1991, or PubMedCentral, which focuses on biomedical and life sciences. In addition, a growing number of institutions, such as universities, have archives or institutional repositories. The Massachusetts Institute of Technology's DSpace and the University of California's eScholarship Repository are among the first and best-known examples of such archiving initiatives. Concerns have been expressed that self-archiving may pose problems for version and quality control (eg, users may not understand the difference between an article that has not undergone peer review, revision, and editing and one that has undergone such measures to improve quality) and that usage of self-archived versions of articles will result in declining use of published versions of articles and journals, or even the demise of journals.[27-29]

In *open-access publishing*, all or part of a journal is freely open to unrestricted use. The funding model for open-access publishing requires author, institution, or funding agency payments, and/or a subsidy from the owner or publisher, and/or external grants. This is commonly referred to as an "author pays" publishing model (or "funder pays" in the event the research funder sets aside monies explicitly for such use). This financial model differs from the traditional journal publishing model, in which publication and sustainability of the publishing enterprise are based on revenue from paid subscriptions, advertising, licensing, royalties, reprints, and other forms of revenue.

Although a few journals were published in an open-access model before the 1990s, the majority began publication under that model after the year 2000, when BioMed Central launched a series of open-access journals that were peer reviewed but did not undergo editorial revision and editing.[23] In 2006, BioMed Central journals' article processing fees charged to authors ranged from $615 to $1775 per published article.[30] In addition, individual organizations, such as universities, may purchase a membership at a significantly greater collective fee, allowing their author-employees or affiliated authors to publish in BioMed Central journals without having to pay the initial author publication fees.

In 2003, the Public Library of Science (PLoS) launched its first in a series of open-access journals with an initial $9 million grant from the Moore Foundation.[31] The PLoS journals are peer reviewed and do provide editorial revision and editing. In addition to grants, journal operations are funded by an author-pays model: in 2003 the author fee was $1500 to publish an article; in 2006 the fee was raised to $2500. Other journals experimenting with author-pay models had publication or processing fees that ranged from $500 to $3500 in 2006, with most ranging from $2000 to $3000.[29] According to the Lund University Directory of Open Access Journals, in 2006 there were 2345 strictly interpreted open-access, peer-reviewed scientific and scholarly journals; 326 of these were health science journals, including 206 in medicine.[32]

Supporters of complete open-access publishing cite the benefits of widespread dissemination of research: universal access, enhanced global collaboration, improved visibility of researchers' work, and the belief that open-access articles will be cited more frequently than restricted-access articles.[26,31,33-35] Opponents express concern about the quality of literature published in a system that may favor those who pay, fairness of the author-pays model for researchers with limited funds (eg, those in developing countries or who lack access to funding from government agencies or industry), and the risks to the financial stability of journals with business models based on more diversified, traditional sources of revenue and to their owners.[27-29]

Coupled with the open-access movement in 2005, funding agencies (eg, NIH and the Wellcome Trust) began requesting or requiring funded investigators to permit articles describing results of their funded research to be posted on publicly accessible archives (such as PubMedCentral) in 2005.[34,35] Negotiations between these agencies and publishers resulted in another form of open access: delayed open access. In this model, which has been in wide use by scientific and biomedical publishers (especially those owned by not-for-profit professional socities) for several years, content is made freely available after a defined interval of time, such as 6 months, 1 year, or 2 years. The interval, which may be influenced by the frequency of journal publication, is intended to protect subscription, licensing, advertising, and other traditional forms of journal revenue.

A number of journals are experimenting with types of open access (eg, permitting self-archiving on authors' individual or institutional archives, open access for only some content, delayed open access, open access if author pays publication or processing fees, or giving authors a choice of free delayed access or immediate access if they choose to pay a publication fee). Open-access publishing models are evolving, and debate continues over which models might be sustainable in the long term. Each model has advantages and disadvantages. A combination of models may be the most appropriate for journals seeking to balance the advantages of open access with the financial requirements of sustainable publication and ongoing maintenance of a journal's Web site.

In addition, journals are developing and experimenting with different publication licenses in lieu of standard copyright transfers to permit various access and usage rights. According to the Association of Learned and Professional Scholarly Publishers (ALPSP), 61% of surveyed publishers required authors to transfer copyright for publication in 2005 (down from 81% in 2003); 17% required a publication license from authors; 21% initially requested copyright transfer but accepted a license; and 3% did not require any formal agreement.[36] (See also 5.6.5, Copyright Assignment or License.)

5.6.3 Copyright: Definition, History, and Current Law. *Copyright* is a term used to describe the legal right of authors to control the communication and reproduction of their original works of authorship.[1,14] Thus, copyright law provides for the protection of rights of parties involved in the creation and dissemination of intellectual property. While a variety of people and entities derive benefits from copyright laws (authors, publishers, editors, composers, artists, and the producers of television and radio programs, films, sound recordings, video, computer programs, and software), few thoroughly understand the law and its basic applications. This section discusses current copyright laws and applications in scientific publishing. Copyright laws, scope, and protections vary by country (see also 5.6.12, International Copyright Protection). The discussion in this section addresses US copyright law except where specifically indicated. This section is intended to explain copyright law as it applies to scientific publication; it is not intended to serve as legal advice. A media lawyer should be consulted for any specific concerns about rights, protections, infringements, or remedies.

Copyright is a form of legal protection provided to the author of published and unpublished original works.[14(§102,§104),37] The author, or anyone to whom the author transfers copyright, is the owner of copyright in the work. Current law gives the owner of copyright the following exclusive rights:

- To reproduce the work in copies
- To prepare derivative works based on the copyrighted work
- To distribute, perform, or display the work publicly

A copyrightable work must be fixed in a tangible medium of expression and includes the following[14(§102),38]:

- Literary works (which includes computer software and works produced in digital formats)
- Musical works
- Dramatic works
- Pantomimes and choreographic works
- Pictorial, graphic, and sculptural works
- Motion pictures and other audiovisual works
- Sound recordings
- Architectural works

The following are not protected by copyright, although they may be covered by patent and trademark laws[14(§102),37] (see 5.6.15, Patents, and 5.6.16, Trademark):

- Works not fixed in tangible form of expression (eg, speeches or performances that have not been written or recorded)
- Titles
- Names
- Short phrases

- Slogans
- Familiar symbols or designs
- Mere variation of typographic ornamentation, lettering, or coloring
- Mere listings of ingredients or contents
- Ideas, procedures, methods, systems, processes, concepts, principles, discoveries, and devices, as distinguished from a description, explanation, or illustration (although ideas or procedures may not be protected by copyright, the written or published expression of ideas and procedures may be subject to copyright protection)
- Works consisting entirely of information that is common property and containing no original authorship (eg, calendars, height and weight charts, rulers, and lists or tables taken from public documents or other common sources)

Some of the more common provisions of US copyright law as well as problems encountered by scientific authors, editors, and publishers are discussed in sections 5.6.4 through 5.6.11.

History of Copyright Law. Copyright law evolved after Gutenberg's movable type reduced the cost and labor required to make copies of written and printed works.[1,38,39] During the early 18th century, copyright became the mediator between the author or publisher and the marketplace. In 1710, England created the Statute of Anne, the first copyright act, which addressed exact copies only. Article 1, section 8, of the US Constitution, enacted in 1798, serves as the foundation for US copyright law.[40] Since then, the US law has undergone a number of updates and general revisions in response to innovations and changes in technology, to broaden the definition and scope of copyright law, and to address mechanisms for protection among different countries. In 1790, the United States created the first copyright law to cover magazines and books, but again, this was only for exact copies. During the 19th century, copyright law was extended to translations, works made for hire, music, dramatic compositions, photography, and works of art. During the 20th century, copyright law was extended to cover motion pictures, performance and recording of nondramatic literary works, sound recordings, computer programs, and architectural works. The US Copyright Act of 1909 added formal requirements to ensure protection, such as use of copyright notice, official registration, and renewal of copyright terms.[40]

US Copyright Act of 1976. Before 1978, 2 systems of copyright coexisted in the United States. Common law copyright, regulated by individual states, protected works from creation until publication, and a separate federal law protected works from publication until 28 years thereafter (with an option for a 1-time renewal of the 28-year term).[37] The Copyright Act of 1976, which became effective January 1, 1978, contained the first major revisions of US copyright law in almost 70 years. This act, reversing many of the formalities required by the 1909 act, remains in force today. Thus, for all works created after 1978, current law automatically provides protection to the creator of the work at the time it is created, whether written, typewritten, or entered into a computer; whether or not the work is published; and whether or not the work bears a copyright notice. In addition, the 1976 act changed the terms of copyright duration, with most terms equaling the life of the author plus 50 years. In

1998, the term of copyright protection for most works was extended to the life of the author plus 70 years[40] (see 5.6.4, Types of Works and Copyright Duration in the United States).

International Conventions and Treaties. In 1886, the Berne Convention was created by 10 European nations to protect copyright across national boundaries. The United States did not sign on to the Berne Convention until 1989.[40] The Universal Copyright Convention was adopted in 1952 as an alternative for countries that disagreed with some aspects of the Berne Convention. A number of conventions and treaties adopted in the 1990s address copyright as it has been affected by new economic, social, cultural, and technological developments and by new international rules, including the Trade-Related Aspects of Intellectal Property Rights (TRIPS), World Intellectual Property Organization (WIPO) Copyright and Performances and Phonograms Treaty, and the WIPO Copyright Treaty.[40,41] For more details, see 5.6.12, International Copyright Protection.

Copyright and New Technology. Throughout the 20th century, technological advances have challenged copyright law: photographs, motion pictures, radio, television, photocopying, cable television, computers, databases, new media, and the Internet.[1,39,42] The most recent challenge began in the 1990s with the increase of electronic publishing and new media. Although copyright law was designed to be technology neutral, it applied only to tangible copies and to the physical distribution of these copies. Although early users of the Internet sent e-mail messages and posted information on electronic mailing lists and bulletin boards without much concern for ownership and copyright of their communications, editors and publishers grew concerned about maintaining the integrity, quality, and ownership of their intellectual property once content was easily and widely digitized, published, and transmitted electronically.

In 1998, the US Digital Millennium Copyright Act (DMCA) was enacted to extend copyright protection to works created in a digital medium.[14] Interpreting the DMCA, Hart[42] notes that "works created in digital media are considered 'fixed' if they can be perceived, reproduced, or otherwise communicated for more than a transitory period, including the fixation on a computer disc or in a computer's random access memory." Among its major provisions, the DMCA implements the WIPO treaties, limits certain liability of online providers that adhere to specific requirements, limits liability of libraries and archives, prohibits the circumvention of technological barriers to block unauthorized access to content (anticircumvention), establishes penalties for such circumvention, addresses works now available through new technologies such as distance education and Web casts, and preserves existing rights of copyright owners.[14,36,42]

Since its enactment, the DMCA has addressed concerns about copyright protection and infringement in electronic publishing. However, continuing rapid advances in technology predict future changes in copyright law, requiring the publishing community to be alert to such changes for the foreseeable future.

5.6.4 Types of Works and Copyright Duration in the United States. The length of copyright protection in the United States depends on several factors: when the work was created (key dates are before or after January 1, 1978), the number of authors, and the type of work (eg, work made for hire or owned by the federal government).[43] See the Table for examples of types of works, conditions, and terms of copyright protection.[43]

Works Created After 1978. To be protected by copyright law, a work must be original. For works created by a single author, copyright belongs to that author from the instant of its creation and for 70 years after the author's death.[14(§302)] Copyright in works published on or after January 1, 1978, is protected for a term that covers the author's life plus 70 years after the author's death.[14,43,44] See the Table for details on other conditions and terms and see also "Joint Works" and "Works Made for Hire" below.

Works Created Before 1978. Several different rules apply to works created before 1978 and depend on whether the work was published, previous copyright duration terms, and whether the copyright has been renewed (Table).[43,44] Unpublished works created before 1978 are protected for the life of the author plus 70 years. Works published between 1923 and 1977 are protected for 95 years after date of publication provided that a copyright notice was published and appropriate renewals were made[43-45] (see also 5.6.6, Copyright Notice and Registration). Works that were published before 1923 are now in the public domain.[43]

Joint Works. A joint work is a work prepared by 2 or more authors with the intention that their contributions be merged into inseparable or interdependent parts of a unitary whole. For such works, the 70-year term begins after the death of the last surviving author.[14(§302)]

Works Made for Hire. Works created by an individual who is paid by another specifically for such work are covered by a particular provision of the copyright statute. In these cases, the law recognizes the employer or the party contracting for the work as the owner of the copyright in the work. Works made for hire generally fall into 2 categories.[14(§101),46] The first category is a work prepared by an employee within the scope of his or her employment duties, such as a journal editorial written by an editor who is employed by or otherwise contracted to work as an editor by the journal's owner. The second category comprises certain specially ordered or commissioned works. Examples include a news story written by a freelance journalist or an index prepared by an individual under contract. In these cases, although a written copyright assignment is not necessary, the parties must sign a written agreement before the work is produced specifying that the work is to be a work made for hire. Copyright duration for works made for hire is 95 years from the year of first publication or 120 years from the date of the work's creation, whichever is shorter.[14(§302)]

Works Created by Anonymous and Pseudonymous Authors. The same terms of copyright duration that apply to works made for hire apply to works published by anonymous or pseudonymous authors—95 years from the year of first publication or 120 years from the date the work was created, whichever is shorter. If 1 or more authors' names are disclosed and registered with the US Copyright Office before the 95-year or 120-year term expires, the term changes to 70 years after the last surviving author's death.[14(§302),44]

Works in the Public Domain or Created by the US Government. A work is in the public domain if it has failed to meet the requirements of copyright protection or its copyright protection has expired. Works in the public domain may be used freely by anyone without permission. US works published before 1923 are now in the public

Table. Copyright Term and the Public Domain in the United States[a]

Unpublished Works		
Type of Work	**Copyright Term**	**What Was in Public Domain as of January 1, 2006**[b]
Unpublished works	Life of the author plus 70 years	Works from authors who died before 1936
Unpublished anonymous and pseudonymous works, and works made for hire	120 years from date of creation	Works created before 1886
Unpublished works created before 1978 that were published after 1977 but before 2003	Life of the author plus 70 years or December 31, 2047, whichever is greater	Nothing; the soonest the works can enter the public domain is January 1, 2048
Unpublished works created before 1978 that were published after December 31, 2002	Life of the author plus 70 years	Works of authors who died before 1935
Unpublished works when the death date of the author is not known[c]	120 years from date of creation[d]	Works created before 1886[d]

Published Works		
Date of Publication[e]	**Conditions**[f]	**Copyright Term**[b]
Before 1923	None	In the public domain
1923 through 1977	Published without a copyright notice	In the public domain
1978 to March 1, 1989	Published without notice, and without subsequent registration	In the public domain
1978 to March 1, 1989	Published without notice, but with subsequent registration	70 Years after the death of author, or if work for hire, the shorter of 95 years from publication or 120 years from creation[b]
1923 through 1963	Published with notice but copyright was not renewed[g]	In the public domain
1923 through 1963	Published with notice and copyright was renewed[g]	95 Years after publication date[b]
1964 through 1977	Published with notice	95 Years after publication date[b]
1978 to March 1, 1989	Published with notice	70 Years after death of author, or if work for hire, the shorter of 95 years from publication or 120 years from creation[b]
After March 1, 1989	None	70 Years after death of author, or if work for hire, the shorter of 95 years from publication or 120 years from creation[b]

[a] This table was adapted and reproduced with permission from Hirtle.[43] It was first published in Hirtle PB. Recent changes to the copyright law: copyright term extension. *Archival Outlook.* January/February 1999. This version is current as of January 2006. The most recent version is found at http://www.copyright.cornell.edu/training/Hirtle_Public_Domain.htm.

The table is based in part on Gasaway LN. When US works pass into the public domain, http://www.unc.edu/~unclng/public-d.htm, and similar tables found in Malaro MC. *A Legal Primer on Managing Museum Collections.* Washington, DC: Smithsonian

Table. Copyright Term and the Public Domain in the United States[a] *(cont)*

Institution Press; 1998:155-156. A useful copyright duration chart by Mary Minow, organized by year, is found at http://www.librarylaw.com/DigitizationTable.htm. See also Library of Congress, Copyright Office, *Circular 15a, Duration of Copyright: Provisions of the Law Dealing With the Length of Copyright Protection*.[44]

[b] All terms of copyright run through the end of the calendar year in which they would otherwise expire, so a work enters the public domain on the first of the year following the expiration of its copyright term. For example, a book published on March 15, 1923, will enter the public domain on January 1, 2019, not March 16, 2018 (1923 + 95 = 2018).

[c] Unpublished works when the death date of the author is not known may still be copyrighted, but certification from the Copyright Office that it has no record to indicate whether the person is living or died less than 70 years before is a complete defense to any action for infringement. See 17 USC § 302(e).

[d] Presumption as to the author's death requires a certified report from the Copyright Office that its records disclose nothing to indicate that the author of the work is living or died less than 70 years before.

[e] "Publication" was not explicitly defined in the Copyright Law before 1976, but the 1909 act indirectly indicated that publication was when copies of the first authorized edition were placed on sale, sold, or publicly distributed by the proprietor of the copyright or under his authority.

[f] Not all published works are copyrighted. Works prepared by an officer or employee of the US government as part of that person's official duties receive no copyright protection in the United States. For much of the 20th century, certain formalities had to be followed to secure copyright protection. For example, some books had to be printed in the United States to receive copyright protection, and failure to deposit copies of works with the Register of Copyright could result in the loss of copyright. The requirements that copies include a formal notice of copyright and that the copyright be renewed after 28 years were the most common conditions and are specified in the table.

[g] A 1961 Copyright Office study found that fewer than 15% of all registered copyrights were renewed. For books, the figure was even lower: 7%. See Ringer B. Study No. 31: renewal of copyright. In: *Copyright Law Revision: Studies Prepared for the Subcommittee on Patents, Trademarks, and Copyrights of the Committee on the Judiciary, United States Senate, Eighty-sixth Congress, First [-Second] Session*. Washington, DC: US Government Printing Office; 1961:220. A good guide to investigating the copyright and renewal status of published work is Demas S, Brogdon JL. Determining copyright status for preservation and access: defining reasonable effort. *Library Resources and Technical Services* 1997;41(4):323-334. See also Library of Congress, Copyright Office. *Circular 22: How to Investigate the Copyright Status of a Work.* Washington, DC: Library of Congress, Copyright Office; 2004. http://www.copyright.gov/circs/circ22.html.

domain.[43] In 2006, the Project Gutenberg Web site included more than 19 000 books that were in the public domain.[47] Works created by US federal government employees in the course of their employment are also in the public domain[14(§105)] (see 5.6.1, Ownership and Control of Data, and 5.6.5, Copyright Assignment or License, Exception—US Federal Government Works). However, works produced by state and local governments are subject to copyright protection.

Works created by other national governments are subject to the copyright laws of their respective countries and perhaps the Berne Convention, WIPO Copyright Treaties, or other international treaties (see 5.6.12, International Copyright Protection).

Collective Works. A *collective work* comprises a number of independent contributions (usually from many authors), which constitute separate and independent works in themselves, and are assembled into a collective whole. Examples of collective works include journals, magazines, multiauthored textbooks, and encyclopedias.[14(§101)] Copyright in the independent contributions is separate from copyright in the collective work as a whole and initially belongs to the individual authors until they transfer copyright to the owner of the collective work, usually a publisher. Publishers that require authors of collective works (such as authors of a journal article) to transfer copyright should require such transfer from each author, not just the corresponding author. Editors of collective works may also be required to transfer copyright assignment or a publication license if their contributions are not already covered under work for hire or other employment agreements. Thus, both the individual articles (independent works) and the journal (collective work) can be protected by copyright.

Compilations and Derivative Works. According to US copyright law, *compilations* are works "formed by the collection and assembling of preexisting materials or data that are selected, coordinated, and arranged in such a way that the resulting work as a whole constitutes original work of authorship."[14(§101)] Examples of compilations include a compendium of previously published articles on a specific theme or topic or a collection of abstracts. The basis for protection of a compilation is the judgment required to select and arrange the material.[38] In this context, the 1991 Supreme Court ruling in *Feist Publications v Rural Telephone Service Co* is worth noting.[48] In that case, a regional telephone company used a local telephone company's directory without its permission. The local company sued for copyright infringement and lost. The court held that the "data" in the directory (collections of public telephone numbers) had no substantial originality or creativity and that comprehensive collections of data arranged in conventional formats do not merit copyright protection.[48]

Derivative works are those based on 1 or more preexisting works, such as an abridgment, condensation, or republication in a different format, language, or media.[14(§101)] Examples of compilations and derivative works include revised editions of books or translated articles that are republished individually or collected with others in an international edition.

Scientific journal publishers typically request that authors transfer broad rights to their work in the form of either a copyright transfer or exclusive license, or a nonexclusive license that includes rights to produce compilations and derivative works. Such publishers often receive royalties from the distribution and sale of compilations and derivative works. In addition, publishers who own copyright or have exclusive licenses in individual articles are legally able to address misuse or piracy of such works.

Revised Editions. A revised edition of a previously copyrighted work may be regarded as a separately copyrighted work if there is substantial original new work in the new edition. *The Chicago Manual of Style* defines *substantial* as change that occurs in 1 or more of the essential elements of the work: text, introduction, notes, appendixes, or tables and illustrations (if they are integral to the work).[45(p10)] Thus, a new foreword or preface, the addition of a few references, or corrections to the original text do not constitute a revised edition, but they may be included in subsequent printings with an explanation on the copyright notice page. For example, this edition of the *AMA Manual of Style* constitutes a major revision resulting in a new copyrighted work. For revised editions, any unaltered material retained in a subsequent edition remains protected under the original copyright, and copyright applicable to the new material does not extend the duration of copyright in the old material.

The Chicago Manual of Style recommends that publishers use standard language to designate specific editions: 2nd edition, 3rd edition, 4th edition, and so on.[45] If the new edition is simply printed in a different format, eg, in paperback or in a different language through a licensing agreement, the status can be designated as "Paperback edition 2005" or "French-language edition" (see 3.12.7, References, References to Print Books, Edition Number).

Some publishers list the various dates of revisions on the copyright page as a record of publishing history. The publishing history follows the copyright notice. For example, this manual has had 9 previous editions:

2007, *AMA Manual of Style: A Guide for Authors and Editors*, 10th ed (Iverson et al)

1998, *American Medical Association Manual of Style: A Guide for Authors and Editors,* 9th ed (Iverson et al)

1989, *American Medical Association Manual of Style,* 8th ed (Iverson et al)

1981, *Manual for Authors & Editors,* 7th ed (Barclay et al)

1976, *Stylebook/Editorial Manual of the AMA,* 6th ed (Barclay)

1971, *Stylebook/Editorial Manual of the AMA,* 5th ed (Hussey)

1966, *Stylebook and Editorial Manual,* 4th ed (Talbott)

1965, *Stylebook and Editorial Manual,* 3rd ed (Talbott)

1963, *Stylebook and Editorial Manual,* 2nd ed (Talbott)

1962, *Style Book* (Talbott)

5.6.5 **Copyright Assignment or License.** Typically, copyright of a work vests initially with the author of the work. As copyright owner, an author may transfer rights to a publisher by copyright assignment, exclusive license, or nonexclusive license.[39,45] A broadly worded exclusive license may provide much of the same rights to publishers as would a copyright transfer agreement. Thus, an owner of an exclusive assignment (through either copyright transfer or broadly worded exclusive license) may produce derivative works and sublicense specific rights to others. Some publishers permit authors to retain certain rights to their works, even when assigning copyright or granting an exclusive license (such as making copies for educational purposes, posting a copy on a personal or institutional Web site, or depositing a copy in an institutional or other repository to comply with research funding requirements). Examples of a model copyright transfer and license for publication are available from the ALPSP.[49] (*Note:* The ALPSP models include provisions for moral rights, which may not be covered for authors and journals under jurisdiction of US copyright law.) A nonexclusive license for publication permits a publisher certain rights to publish and disseminate work, but the copyright remains with the author who retains control over access, use, and distribution. Some open-access journals rely on nonexclusive licenses to publish such as those created by Creative Commons (http://creativecommons.org) and Science Commons (http://sciencecommons.org).

Publishers that have copyright or exclusive publication licenses may also grant others nonexclusive secondary-use licenses to use, reproduce, or disseminate content. A nonexclusive licensee may have a one-time right to reproduce a work in a specified manner (eg, permission to reprint or translate and distribute a specific article) (see 5.6.7, Copying, Reproducing, Adapting, and Other Uses of Content, and 5.6.10, Standards for Commercial Reprints and E-prints).

Publishers that make substantial investments in their products typically seek exclusive assignments from authors of written works.[39,45] However, few visual artists or professional photographers will agree to such terms and more commonly grant nonexclusive rights to publishers who want to include their works. In addition, some institutions encourage or require authors to transfer nonexclusive or conditional rights of their work to publishers (see also "Exception—Institutional Owners of Copyright"). In such cases, a publisher must request permission from each author before republishing the work in any derivative format, and this could include the right to publish the article on the journal's Web site. Journals that accept such limited conditional licenses need to be sure that they obtain licenses that cover all subsidiary rights that the publisher may want to exercise or sublicense (eg, online and licensed versions, reprints, e-prints, collections, and archival copies as well as versions in multiple languages and multiple types of media). Increasing demands by authors and their institutions and the increasing complexity of publishing models portend much future debate among authors, institutions, and publishers with regard to copyright assignments, licenses, and publication (see also 5.6.2, Open-Access Publication and Scientific Journals).

Common arguments in favor of copyright transfer from authors to publishers include the following:

- The publisher must have the opportunity to publish or license the publication of the work in other forms to recoup or justify the expenses associated with the editorial and peer review, editing and quality assurance, publication, distribution, and maintenance of the original work.
- The publisher, with business and legal expertise and resources, is better able to distribute and maintain the work in print and online, protect it from misuse and piracy, and take advantage of new technologies and media.
- The publisher is better equipped to invest in the work and take the risk that the work may not be successful.
- The publisher serves the author's interest in self-promotion and professional advancement.

Common arguments favoring author's retention of copyright include the following:

- Authors who retain ownership of their works and distribute their works themselves, through their institutions or libraries or other means, can help to limit the increasing subscription costs of scientific journals.
- Authors deserve to receive financial reward from both the original publication and any subsequent republication or dissemination.
- Authors' retention of copyright meets the traditional need for identification of intellectual ownership.
- New technology enables misuse and theft of intellectual property and obviates the ability of publishers to protect copyright, perhaps rendering copyright obsolete.

Written Assignment of Copyright or License. As a condition of considering a work for publication, most publishers of scientific journals require authors to transfer copyright or an exclusive publication license in the event that the work is published. This requires authors to sign a specific license indicating the transfer of copyright or a license to the publisher. Since the transfer of copyright may not actually occur until the work is published, editors may choose to consider manuscripts submitted without a statement of copyright transfer or publication license from the author and then ask for it if a revision is requested or the manuscript is to be accepted. However, to simplify the submission process, *JAMA* and the *Archives* Journals request authors to submit a statement of copyright assignment when they submit their manuscripts. This statement is included in an authorship form that all authors must sign. In addition, each author must affirm that the work submitted is original and has not been previously published (see also 5.3, Duplicate Publication). These journals also require authors to identify their specific contributions to the work and to disclose conflicts of interest at the same time and on the same authorship form (see also 5.1.1, Authorship Responsibility, Authorship: Definition, Criteria, Contributions, and Requirements, and 5.5.1, Conflicts of Interest, Requirements for Authors; a copy of this form is available online in the *JAMA* instructions for authors at http://www.jama.com). In the event that the work is published by *JAMA* or an *Archives* Journal, the author agrees to transfer copyright to the American Medical Association (the owner of these journals). If the work is not published, the copyright remains with the author. *JAMA* and the *Archives* Journals require all authors (including each coauthor) who are not US federal government employees to sign the following copyright transfer statement:

> **Copyright Transfer.** In consideration of the action of the American Medical Association (AMA) in reviewing and editing this submission (manuscript, tables, figures, audio, video, and other supplemental files submitted for publication), I hereby transfer, assign, or otherwise convey all copyright ownership, including any and all rights incidental thereto, exclusively to the AMA, in the event that such work is published by the AMA.

Assignment by Coauthors. The authors of a joint work are co-owners of copyright in the work. To transfer copyright or grant a publication license in a joint work, the copyright assignment or license must be signed by each of the authors.

Exception—US Federal Government Works. Because copyright does not vest in works created by the US federal government, no assignment from the author is necessary.[14(§105)] However, journals should obtain a signed statement from each author contributing to a work as a federal government employee. What constitutes a work of a government employee as part of the person's official duties is not always clear, but generally, the application of the federal employee exception is determined by the nature of the author rather than the nature of the work or its funding. *JAMA* and the *Archives* Journals require all authors who contribute to a work as part of their duties as an employee of the US federal government to sign the following:

> **Federal Employment:** I was an employee of the US federal government when this work was conducted and prepared for publication; therefore, it is not protected by the Copyright Act, and copyright ownership cannot be transferred.

When some authors of a joint work contibuted as employees of the US federal government and other authors did not, each government-employed author must sign the federal employment statement and all other authors must sign the standard copyright transfer agreement.

Works created by authors of other national governments may be subject to the copyright laws of their respective countries.

Exception—Institutional Owners of Copyright. On occasion, a manuscript from an author or authors from a single institution may be submitted with a copyright transfer or publication license and signed on behalf of the institution, rather than by the individual authors. The institution presumably has a written agreement with the authors, following the work-for-hire provision of the copyright law, that all work done while the authors are employees of the institution is owned by the institution. Accordingly a representative of the institution may transfer copyright or grant a publication license (see 5.6.4, Types of Works and Copyright Duration in the United States, Works Made for Hire).

Scientific journals should be cautious about accepting limits on copyright transfers or licenses from institutions or commercial entities that could remove the journal's ability and authority to approve subseqent uses of a journal article, and the journal's imprimatur of that article, for commerical or promotional purposes. Journals also need to avoid the possibility of commercial use of a work in a manner deemed unsuitable by the journal. For these reasons, *JAMA* and the *Archives* Journals do not accept any restrictions on the transfer of copyright, and all requests for reuse of a journal article must be submitted to the permissions department for review and approval.

5.6.6 **Copyright Notice and Registration.** Although use of a copyright notice is not required under copyright law, the US Copyright Office strongly recommends use of such a notice.[37] A copyright notice for all visual copies of a work should contain the following 3 elements[14(§401)]:

The word "Copyright," or abbreviation "Copr," or the symbol ©,
The year of first publication of the work, and
The name of the copyright owner

Example: Copyright 2007 American Medical Association

Note: For *JAMA* and the *Archives* Journals, the wording above includes the name of the owner of the journals (American Medical Association), not the name of the journal. It is recommended that all copyright notices be placed in such a "manner and location as to give reasonable notice of the claim of copyright."[14(§401),37] The wording and placement of copyright notices applies equally to print and online works.

The year in the copyright notice should be the year of publication. Journal home pages and other main pages of journal Web sites should change the year of copyright notice at the beginning of each year, but back-issue content should retain the copyright year for the original year of publication.

According to the US Copyright Office, "registration is a legal formality intended to make a public record of the basic facts of a particular copyright."[37] Registration is not required for copyright protection, and failure to register a work does not affect the copyright owner's rights in that property. However, registration does offer several benefits: it establishes a public record of the copyright claim and is a prerequisite to bringing suit for copyright infringement in US courts.[37] Registration requires a completed application form, filing fee, and the deposition of copies of the work (usually

2 copies of printed materials or the submission of identifying material for electronic publications).[45] Registration is best made within 3 months of publication.[37,45] Registration filing fees vary for single original works, serials (including journals, periodicals, newspapers, annuals, and proceedings), visual and performing arts, sound recordings, and copyright renewals and are available online from the US Copyright Office at http://www.copyright.gov.

5.6.7 **Copying, Reproducing, Adapting, and Other Uses of Content.** To copy or reproduce an entire work without authorization from the copyright owner constitutes copyright infringement. However, a reasonable type and amount of copying of a copyrighted work is permitted under the fair use provisions of US copyright law.[14(§107)]

Fair Use. What constitutes fair use of copyrighted material in a given case depends on the following 4 factors[14(§107)]:

1. Purpose and character of the use, including whether such use is of a commercial nature or is for nonprofit educational purposes
2. Nature of the copyrighted work
3. Amount and substantiality of the portion used in relation to the copyrighted work as a whole
4. Effect of the use on the potential market for or value of the copyrighted work

Although each of these factors may provide a safe haven for use of copyrighted works without permission from the owner, the fourth factor, the market value of the original work, has been considered important by the courts in copyright infringement cases.

Fair use purposes include "criticism, comment, news reporting, teaching, scholarship, or research."[14(§107)] This allows authors to quote, copy, or reproduce small amounts of text or graphic material. Appropriate credit should always be given to the original source. In the case of a direct quote, quotation marks or setting off the quoted material, with an appropriate reference or footnote to the original source, is required (see 5.4.2, Scientific Misconduct, Misappropriation: Plagiarism and Breaches of Confidentiality).

Text. The amount of text subject to fair use is determined by its proportion of the whole, but this proportion is not measurable by word length. Contrary to popular belief, there are no specific numbers of words or lines or amount of content that may be taken without permission. The so-called 300-word rule has been cited erroneously to justify quoting passages of text without permission. This erroneous assertion probably originated with the custom of sending out review copies of books and allowing reviewers to quote passages of 300 words or less in a published review.[50] In 1985, the *Nation* magazine lost a landmark suit for copyright infringement after publishing a 300-word excerpt from then-President Gerald Ford's 200 000-word unpublished memoirs, which were to be published as a book by Harper & Row (*Harper & Row Publishers, Inc v Nation Enterprises*).[51] In this case, the trial court ruled that the excerpt "was essentially the heart of the book."[51] *The Chicago Manual of Style* recommends that a quote never extend more than a "few contiguous paragraphs" and that quotes, even if interrupted by original text, should not "overshadow the quoter's own material."[45] The length quoted should never be such that it would diminish the potential market for or value of the original work.

Tables, Graphs, and Illustrations. Fair use of tabular and graphic material and illustrations is more difficult to assess. Although 1 or 2 lines of information from a table might be used without permission, reprinting the entire table without permission is inappropiate and could result in a claim of copyright infringement. The same applies to graphs and illustrations. *JAMA* and the *Archives* Journals require all authors to obtain permission to adapt a part of or reprint an entire table, graph, or illustration that has been previously published. Unrestricted permission is needed to reproduce this material in all "print, online, and licensed versions" of the journal. Online readers of *JAMA* and the *Archives* Journals may download copies of tables, graphs, and illustrations as PowerPoint slides for use in teaching. Citation to the original publication is indicated on each downloaded slide.

Photographs and Works of Art. Photographs and works of art protected by copyright may not be reproduced, enhanced, or altered without permission of the copyright owner, who may be the photographer or artist, a museum or gallery, an academic institution, a commercial entity, or a previous publisher. For example, *JAMA* obtains permission from owners of copyrights of works of art, typically museums and galleries, to reproduce works of art on the cover of *JAMA*. In this case, *JAMA* receives a nonexclusive 1-time right to reproduce the art on the journal's cover in print and online; often the permission for online use is a separate permission (see also "Digital Images and Other Works" later in this section). This does not permit reuse of the cover of a specific issue of *JAMA* in other works or promotional material without obtaining permission for such secondary use from the owner of the work of art included on that issue's cover.

Unpublished Works. Authors should not rely on the fair use provision to justify quoting from unpublished manuscripts and letters.[45,50] In several cases, the US courts have taken a conservative view toward use of extensive quotations and paraphrasing from unpublished works without permission, making it difficult to justify such use. In *J. D. Salinger v Random House, Inc*,[52] the Second Court of Appeals ruled that inclusion of extensive quotes from Salinger's unpublished letters in Hamilton's unauthorized biography of Salinger was improper. In a subsequent case, *New Era Publications International, ApS v Henry Holt and Company, Inc*,[53] the trial court ruled that quotation from unpublished work was not fair use "even if necessary to document serious character defects of an important public figure." For terms and conditions of copyright protection for unpublished works, see the Table.

Correspondence and Reviews Regarding Manuscripts and the Editorial Process. All correspondence regarding a manuscript and the editorial process is considered unpublished and thus should not be used without knowledge of the owner of the correspondence. In the case of a letter, the letter writer is the owner. In the case of a manuscript review, the peer reviewer is the owner, unless the reviewer was contracted under a work-for-hire provision. Thus, authors and journals have no legal right to publish extensive quotes or paraphrases of reviews without the reviewer's consent (see 5.7.1, Confidentiality, Confidentiality During Editorial Evaluation and Peer Review and After Publication) or of letters, not submitted for publication, without the letter writer's permission (see "Quotes and Paraphrases From Oral and Written Communications," below). In addition, to date, the courts have not allowed attempts to gain access to confidential peer review records or confidential information about manuscripts that are not published or not included in published articles (see 5.7.1, Confidentiality, Confidentiality During Editorial Evaluation and Peer Review and After Publication).

Quotes and Paraphrases From Oral and Written Communications. Many journals accept citations to personal communications (ie, oral and written communications). Court decisions regarding use of unpublished works[52,53] indicate that written communication, such as a letter or a memorandum (whether handwritten, typed, printed, or in digital format), if unpublished, may require permission from the letter or memo writer to be cited in a published work. Unless recorded, an oral communication, such as a personal or telephone conversation, cannot be copyrighted. However, authors should obtain written permission from the sources of quotations that are cited as oral and written communications in their manuscripts and should provide a copy of all such permissions to the journal[21] (see also 3.13.9, References, Special Print Materials, Personal Communications).

Works in the Public Domain. Works in the public domain (which are not protected by copyright) may be quoted from freely, with proper credit given to the original source. Examples of works in the public domain include those funded completely by the US government and those works on which the copyright term has expired (see also "Works in the Public Domain or Created by the US Government" in 5.6.4, Types of Works and Copyright Duration in the United States). Other examples are available from Project Gutenberg.[47]

Abstracts. One widely debated application of fair use is the reproduction of abstracts of journal articles in other publications or databases. It can be argued that abstracts, especially structured abstracts, represent the whole work. As a result, any secondary publication or commercial use of abstracts of journal articles as derivative works in print or online without permission of the copyright owner may be considered copyright infringement.

Digital Images and Other Works. Fair use considerations apply equally to reproductions of copyrighted material published in digital format. That is, what is considered fair use in the print domain is likewise fair use in the electronic world. Copyright infringement is a violation of the law—whether the infringed work is photocopied, printed, or copied electronically (see also discussion of the US Digital Millennium Copyright Act in 5.6.3, Copyright: Definition, History, and Current Law). Thus, digital works (eg, digitally produced or reproduced photographs, slides, radiographs, scans, chromatographs, and audio and video files) are protected under copyright law and require permission from the copyright owner to be reproduced in a publication.

With high-performance computer technology, digital images can be manipulated to enhance communication. However, digital adjustments could also be used to bias findings or to deceive. Journals should have guidelines for submission (including recommended file formats and sizes for editorial review and publication), enhancement, and publication of digital images, audio, and video that require authors to identify the software used as well as a record of how the original work was obtained and whether it was altered or manipulated.[54,55] Some journals have defined acceptable alterations (such as cropping) and proposed the use of standards for color, brightness, and scale. Others have developed mechanisms to identify inappropriate manipulation[54,55] (see also 5.4.3, Scientific Misconduct, Inappropriate Manipulation of Digital Images).

Linking and Framing. Linking is a fundamental feature of any electronic publication. Many online versions of articles contain hypertext links within the article (eg, to and from citations to references, tables, and figures) and links external to the article (eg, to other articles or resources). Such linking is generally considered appropriate use. However, deep linking into a particular internal page of a Web site, especially if it permits circumvention of access restrictions or barriers, may be considered an unlawful use of the linked-to material.[42(p96)] Framing is the enclosure and display of another's content within a frame that has the branding and navigation of the framing site. Such framing may be argued to be the creation of a derivative work, which, if done without permission, will likely be regarded as an infringement.[42(p98)]

Fair Use Exclusions. If a portion of a copyrighted work is to be used in a subsequent work and such use is not fair use, written permission must be obtained from the copyright owner (see 5.6.9, Permissions for Reuse). Examples of such portions include text, tables, graphs, illustrations, or photographs. It is never permissible to use an entire article unless permission to do so is obtained in writing or the article is not protected by copyright. If there is doubt about the copyright status of a particular work, an inquiry should be directed to the author, publisher, or national copyright office. In all cases, the material should carry a proper credit line and, if applicable, copyright notice:

Data Adapted From Table and Used in Subsequent Article

Table 1 is adapted with permission from Bax M, Tydeman C, Flodmark O. Clinical and MRI correlates of cerebral palsy: the European Cerebral Palsy Study. *JAMA*. 2006;296(13):1602-1608. Copyright 2006 American Medical Association.

Reprinting Entire Article

Reprinted with permission from *JAMA* (2006;296[13]:1602-1608). Copyright 2006 American Medical Association.

5.6.8 Publishing Transcripts of Discussions, Symposia, and Conferences.

When symposium papers are published, transcripts of discussion (which consist of questions or comments posed to the presenters of papers and the presenters' responses) may accompany them and are printed at the end of the article in a separate section entitled "Discussion." Journals should require named discussants to sign the same copyright transfer or publication license that authors are required to sign. Publishing discussions from online bulletin boards, "chat rooms," or electronic mailing lists requires permission from individual discussants and the online service provider. An example of a copyright transfer statement for discussants follows:

Copyright Transfer. In consideration of the action of the [name of publisher] in reviewing and editing the transcript or text of my discussion, I hereby transfer, assign, or otherwise convey all copyright ownership, including any and all rights incidental thereto, exclusively to the [name of publisher] in the event that such work is published by the [name of publisher].

5.6.9 **Permissions for Reuse.** The copyright owner has the right to attach conditions to giving permission for reuse whether in print or electronic format, such as requiring proper credit and copyright notice. The copyright owner may refuse permission altogether. Permission is usually granted by most publishers without charge, or with a small processing fee, to use portions (text, figures, or tables) of articles or other works, when such use will not result in commercial gain. To expedite review of permission requests, requestors should include the following information in each request:

- Title and complete citation of the original work
- Indication of the portion of the work to be reused, if not the entire work
- Information about the secondary use or publication in which the work will appear (including commercial or noncommercial use, method of dissemination, and intended audience)
- Scope of reuse rights (eg, nonexclusive, worldwide, all languages, print, online, and licensed versions)

Some journals may provide authors with instructions and a form for obtaining rights for reproducing or adapting material that is owned by others. See the sample form used by the *Archives of Dermatology* in Box 1.

5.6.10 **Standards for Commercial Reprints and E-prints.** Pharmaceutical and device companies, institutions, and other organizations may purchase nonexclusive rights to reproduce scientific articles as reprints, or provide access to these as e-prints, as single articles or collections of articles, to help market their products. A *reprint* is the republication of an article or collection of articles in which the content is unchanged from the original publication (except perhaps for the inclusion of postpublication corrections). An *e-print* is a digital reproduction of or an online link to an article or collection of articles, usually PDF files(s). (See also 5.12.7, Advertisements, Advertorials, Sponsorship, Supplements, Reprints, and E-prints; Reprints and E-prints.) These sponsored materials often are produced and distributed by custom publishing companies and marketing agencies. To ensure the quality of these reprints and e-prints and to protect the integrity of the scientific journals that originally published the articles, the publishers and editors of *JAMA* and the *Archives* Journals have developed standards for sponsored reprints and e-prints (Box 2).[56]

5.6.11 **Standards for Licensed International Editions.** A publisher may license others to publish international editions of its scientific journals. For example, agreements between the AMA (owner of *JAMA* and the *Archives* Journals) and international licensees give these publishers the right to publish and disseminate collections of articles from *JAMA* or the *Archives* Journals in specific markets (countries or regions)

Box 1. Request for Permission to Reproduce or Adapt Copyright-Protected Material for Publication in *Archives of Dermatology*

To____________________________________ Date______________________

Name of Copyright Owner, Publisher, or Other

I (we) request permission to reproduce or adapt the material specified below in *Archives of Dermatology*. Citation to the original publication or appropriate credit will be published. A grant of permission form is included for your use.

Requestor's Contact Information (Please Print)

Name ____________________________ Title____________________________

Organization ____

Mailing Address ____

City ________ State/Province ________ Zip/Postal Code ________ Country ________

Telephone ____________ Fax _______________ E-mail ______________________

Source Citation of Material to Be Used (Please Print)

For Journals: Author(s), article title, journal, year of publication, volume number, issue number, and inclusive pages.

For Books: Author(s) or editor(s), book title, place of publication, publisher, year of copyright, and inclusive pages.

____

____

Description of Material: Specify figure or table number(s) or description of text and page number(s).

____

How the Content Is to Be Used (Please Print)

Archives of Dermatology Manuscript Number (if known)________________________

Corresponding Author:____

Title of Article____

Terms of Use: Use in print, online, and licensed versions of *Archives of Dermatology;* includes nonexclusive rights, unrestricted time, in all languages.

Note: We cannot accept permissions that restrict use to one-time only or to English-language only.

____

Grant of Permission: Please complete and return this to the requestor listed above.

I/we hold copyright to the material specified above and grant permission for its use in association with the designated *Archives of Dermatology* article in print, online, and licensed versions of *Archives of Dermatology* according to the terms listed above.

For previously published content, citation to the original publication will accompany the content.

For unpublished content, copyright credit should read as follows (please print): __________

____

____ Date______________________

Signature of Copyright Owner or Designate

____

Print Name of Copyright Owner or Designate

Box 2. *JAMA* and *Archives* Journals Standards for Reprints and E-prints Purchased by Organizations

Fundamental Principles

The guiding principle in all *JAMA* and *Archives* Journals publishing endeavors is that physicians and others receiving any scientific materials produced by *JAMA* and the *Archives* Journals are assured that the information

- is as accurate and reliable as possible at the time,
- has undergone the journal's rigorous editorial peer review,
- has been prepared with the highest degree of professionalism throughout,
- provides information that ultimately is intended to be of benefit to individual patients and to the public at large.

To be considered for support of a *JAMA* and *Archives* Journals reprint, e-print, or republication product, the supporting organization must work within and abide by these standards. In addition, the organization must present the content in a way that maintains the integrity of the original *JAMA* and *Archives* Journal article and does not imply endorsement of a product or influence by an organization.

Responsibility for Editorial Content

The *JAMA* and *Archives* Journals editor in chief has absolute and total control over the scientific and editorial content of any *JAMA* and *Archives* Journals product at all times. The *JAMA* and *Archives* Journals editor in chief (or designee) has complete authority to oversee, review, and accept or reject any reprint, e-print, or republication request or project at any point in the process.

Ownership of Copyright

Materials published in *JAMA* and the *Archives* Journals, including translations, are owned and copyrighted by the American Medical Association (AMA). Materials under AMA copyright remain the property of the AMA and may not be reproduced without permission from the publisher.

Content

All editorial content from *JAMA* and the *Archives* Journals must be reproduced verbatim for a reprint or e-print and should incorporate any published corrections to the original content (with a notation that the article has been corrected) or should append the correction to the end of the article. Preprints (reprints or e-prints delivered prior to publication) are not available. Articles published online ahead of print may be purchased as e-prints or reprints provided that they meet the criteria listed above.

Article Reprints (Paper Format)

Description

Paper reprints of a single *JAMA* or *Archives* Journal article or multiple articles from the same issue that are linked in the original publication by an editorial notation within the articles (eg, an article and a related editorial from the same issue).

Box 2. *JAMA* and *Archives* Journals Standards for Reprints and E-prints Purchased by Organizations *(cont)*

Policy and Procedures

1. All potential article reprints are subject to approval by the *JAMA* and *Archives* Journals publishing project manager and the editorial project manager.
2. With only rare exceptions and approvals, reprints must include a front cover that includes the following:
   - Name/logo of journal
   - Title of article, complete list of authors, and issue date
   - The word "Reprint" or its translation at the top of the cover

   No other content is permitted on front cover.
3. Reprints must include the following information in the running footer of the article:
   - Footer will be the same as the original printed footer with the addition of the words, "Reprinted from [Journal Name]" and copyright information.
   - If the article has been corrected since its original publication, the footer will contain the words "Reprinted with corrections from [Journal Name]" and copyright information.
4. Prescribing information or disclaimers required or approved by a government regulatory body (eg, US Food and Drug Administration) may be included subject to approval by the *JAMA* and *Archives* Journals publishing project manager and the editorial project manager. When prescribing information is included, the printed product will consist of the article, followed by a buffer page, and then by the prescribing information. The buffer page will include a statement similar to the following:

   "This reprint is provided courtesy of [company name], which has a financial interest in the product/topic discussed in this article. The following FDA-approved labeling has been provided by [company name]. *JAMA* and the *Archives* Journals and the AMA do not assume responsibility for the content of the following information."

   Note: The above statement is only permitted on the buffer page for approved prescribing information.
5. Reprint holders including all materials contained in the holder, cover letters, or other materials printed as part of, attached to, or surrounding a reprint must be reviewed and approved by the *JAMA* and *Archives* Journals publishing project manager and editorial project manager.
6. No promotional material may be included with or attached to the reprint.

Web and Other Electronic Formats (E-prints)

Description

JAMA and *Archives* Journals e-prints are either a specific number of accesses to existing article PDF hosted at the *JAMA* and *Archives* Journals Web sites or

Box 2. *JAMA* and *Archives* Journals Standards for Reprints and E-prints Purchased by Organizations *(cont)*

electronic PDF reprints of *JAMA* and *Archives* Journals articles. Either must be accessed from a Web page or e-mail message that has been approved by the *JAMA* and *Archives* Journals editor in chief or designee. *JAMA* and *Archives* Journals e-prints allow a purchasing organization to offer defined audiences access to the electronic full-text version of a *JAMA* or *Archives* Journals article. Two models are currently available: access to the PDF that resides on the *JAMA* and *Archives* Journals Web sites (PDF-based e-print) and rights-protected PDF-based e-print.

Policy and Procedures

JAMA or *Archives* Journals e-prints may be purchased by organizations under the conditions outlined in the "Fundamental Principles" section and the following product-specific conditions:

1. All potential e-print requests as well as the Web page or e-mail message that includes the link to the article are subject to approval by the *JAMA* or *Archives* Journals publishing project manager and the editorial project manager. The potential e-print must adhere to the following criteria:
   - The PDF content of the article will not be altered.
   - The Web page or e-mail message must not describe or interpret the article.
   - The link to the article(s) must be separate from any marketing or other nonjournal content (ie, separate header stating "Journal Resources" or similar title).
   - The link must consist of the full citation to the article (ie, authors, title, and journal name, year, volume, issue, pages, or digital object identifier [DOI]).
   - The sponsor of the Web site or e-mail message must be clearly displayed.
   - After approval, the link and the information surrounding the link must not change without prior approval of the publishing and editorial project managers.
2. Following editorial approval, the publishing project manager will grant access to the electronic article.

PDF-Based E-print

Access to existing PDF residing on the *JAMA* and *Archives* Journals Web sites

Purchasing organizations wishing to link to a *JAMA* or *Archives* Journals article PDF may purchase access to that PDF for a specific number of accesses or length of time, provided that the above stipulations are met and that the page from which the article would link is provided for review. Such a page may be a Web page or an e-mail message, but either must be reviewed and approved by the editorial project manager.

Purchase of an e-print is contingent on approval of the linking page by the *JAMA* and *Archives* Journals publishing project manager and editorial project manager.

Box 2. *JAMA* and *Archives* Journals Standards for Reprints and E-prints Purchased by Organizations *(cont)*

The publishing project manager will establish password-free access from the supporting company linking page to the e-print URL and will maintain this link for the duration of the agreement.

Rights-Protected PDF-Based E-print
Access to a PDF that does not reside on the *JAMA* and *Archives* Journals Web sites

This e-print is a rights-protected PDF of the article(s) that is similar in appearance to a paper reprint. Rights protection will define aspects such as the number of copies a user may print, e-mail, or download/open.

Rights-protected PDF-based e-prints will include the cover page and running footer requirements described in the paper format reprint section of these standards.

Prescribing information or disclaimers required or approved by a government regulatory body (eg, FDA) may be included with a PDF e-print subject to approval by the *JAMA* and *Archives* Journals publishing project manager and the editorial project manager. When prescribing information is included, a buffer page with disclaimer information (described in "Article Reprints") will be required.

The company Web site and specific page and/or e-mail from which the rights-protected PDF e-print will link must be reviewed by the *JAMA* and *Archives* Journals project manager and editorial project manager for compliance with these standards and appropriate presentation.

The e-print will be produced and delivered by the publishing project manager.

and in specific languages. To ensure the quality of these editions, the following standards are recommended:

- Copyright in the international edition and all translated articles is owned by the original publisher.
- Each issue must contain a minimum number of pages or amount of content.
- Articles republished from the original journal must account for a minimum of 50% of each issue's total pages or content. The remaining 50% of total pages/content may include local editorial material and local commercial content (eg, advertisements).
- The licensed publisher will appoint an editorial director (whose appointment will be approved by the editor of the original journal) to select articles from the original edition to be republished in the international edition and review the quality of translations.
- Each republished article must include a complete citation to the original article (ie, journal, year, volume and issue numbers, inclusive page numbers) and complete original titles, author bylines, and author affiliations.
- Abridgments or changes to content, other than translation, are not permitted.

- Content should be republished within a minimum amount of time (eg, 6 months from date of original publication)
- International editions may include local editorial material that cannot constitute more than 50% of total pages/content. Local editorial includes the cover (if the original journal cover is not used), masthead, table of contents, editorial indexes, brief news reports, summaries of conferences, meeting calendars, announcements, commentaries, editorials, letters, and explanations of original articles.
- Local editorial does not include (1) any original clinical or scientific articles (ie, quantitative or qualitative research reports or analyses, case descriptions, clinical or product reviews, product or therapeutic comparisons, scientific abstracts) or (2) any articles previously published by other journals.
- All authors of all local editorial should have their complete names, academic degrees or credentials, and affiliations published with each article.
- For online publications, translated articles should link to the original article.
- Journals with advertising must have multiple advertisements and may not be sponsored by one commercial entity or interest.
- Advertisements may not appear adjacent to editorial content on the same topic.
- Commercial content shall not be presented to appear as editorial content. Appearance, artwork, and format shall be of such a nature as to avoid confusion with the editorial content of the publication.

See also 5.12, Advertisements, Advertorials, Sponsorship, Supplements, Reprints, and E-prints.

5.6.12 **International Copyright Protection.** There is no international copyright law.[57] Copyright law, scope, protections, and remedies are governed by individual nations and treaties between them. Thus, copyright laws do not automatically protect an author's work throughout the world.[58] However, most countries offer protection to works from other nations.[57] For a detailed discussion of the copyright laws of individual countries, consult WIPO (which is under the auspices of the United Nations) in Geneva, Switzerland. See 5.6.14, Copyright Resources, for contact information for WIPO.

The Berne Convention for the Protection of Literary and Artistic Works (commonly known as the Berne Convention)[59] was originally signed by 10 European countries in 1886 in Berne, Switzerland, to protect copyright across their national borders.[40,58] Today, the Berne Convention is administered by WIPO. For many years, the United States declined to sign the Berne Convention because of its lack of formality and its minimalist approach. For example, the Berne Convention does not require the use of a copyright notice, which was in conflict with prior US copyright law. To accommodate the US need for a minimum set of standards, the Universal Copyright Convention (UCC) was created by the United Nations Educational, Scientific, and Cultural Organization (UNESCO) in 1952. Under the UCC, works created in the United States could have multilateral protection without forfeiting the prior US requirement for copyright notice.[40]

After amending its copyright law by eliminating the requirement for copyright notice, the United States signed the Berne Convention in 1989. Most industrialized nations and many developing countries subscribe to this convention, and there are special provisions for developing countries that wish to make use of them.[58] As of 2006, 162 nations had signed the Berne Convention.[58,59] The Berne Convention has no formal requirements. However, each signatory country agrees to protect the copyright in works created in other member countries. Although the United States no longer mandates the use of copyright notice, the US Copyright Office still encourages voluntary use (see 5.6.6, Copyright Notice and Registration). The significance of the UCC is now largely historical after the adoption of the Trade-Related Aspects of Intellectal Property Rights (TRIPS) agreement and other international agreements in the 1990s, including WIPO's Copyright and Performances and Phonograms Treaty and the WIPO Copyright Treaty.[40] The WIPO Copyright Treaties, adopted in 1996, provide additional protections for works created in other member countries and address issues and questions raised by new economic, social, cultural, and technological developments as well as new international rules.[41]

5.6.13 **Moral Rights.** Moral rights, first introduced by the French as *droit moral*, is a doctrine of copyright law intended to protect individual creators' noneconomic investments in their work and the personality of the creator as it relates to the work regardless of copyright ownership or transfer.[38(§26.01),58] Two moral rights that are most often recognized are the right to attribution and right to integrity (ie, right to prevent destruction or mutilation of work).[38(§26.01)] This doctrine is endorsed by most member countries of the Berne Convention. Although the United States is a member of the Berne Convention, US law does not provide for moral rights, except for certain visual works of art to protect them from mutilation or misattribution through the Visual Artists Rights Act of 1990.[14(§106A)] Creators of other works in the United States are provided limited moral rights protection under other federal laws (such as the Lanham Act), state laws, or contracts that include specific provisions for moral rights.[38(§26.01)] Under interpretations of relevant US laws as well as any applicable contract provisions, US editors and publishers may not give authorship credit to someone who has not written the work and may not credit an author of a written work without the author's permission (see 5.1.2, Authorship Responsibility, Guest and Ghost Authors). In the United States, courts have also held that mutilation of a work (distortion or substantial alteration of the work without consent of the author) may result in a violation of the Lanham Act.[38(§26.03B)] However, authors are not similarly protected against unauthorized changes made during editing, proofreading, and typesetting of their work.[38(§26.03C)] Because of the ease of manipulation and distortion of electronic works, concerns about moral rights in the context of electronic publishing are increasing in the United States and may portend changes in this area of law in the future.[38(§26.03E)]

5.6.14 **Copyright Resources.** Additional information about copyright law may be obtained from several sources. For a detailed legal account, consult *Perle and Williams on Publishing Law*[38] or *Nimmer on Copyright*[39] (although these resources are expensive and may be best consulted via a library that has these in its holdings). Other useful texts include *The Chicago Manual of Style* chapter "Rights and Permissions"[45] and *Law of the Web: A Field Guide to Internet Publishing*.[42] Specific information, useful guides, and forms may be obtained free of charge from the US Copyright Office[14,37,40,44,46,57,58]:

US Copyright Office
Library of Congress
101 Independence Ave SE
Washington, DC 20559-6000
Telephone: (202) 707-3000
www.copyright.gov

Additional useful information can also be obtained from the following:

Association of American Publishers (AAP)
50 F St NW
Washington, DC 20001-1530
Telephone: (202) 247-3375
Fax: (202) 347-3690
www.publishers.org

Association of Learned and Professional Society Publishers (ALPSP)
South House
The Street
Clapham, Worthing BN13 3UU, West Sussex, United Kingdom
Telephone: 44 1903 871 686
Fax: 44 1903 871 457
www.alpsp.org/default.htm

World Intellectual Property Organization (WIPO)
34, chemin des Colombettes
PO Box 18
CH-1211 Geneva 20, Switzerland
Telephone: 41 22 338 91 11
Fax: 41 22 733 54 28
www.wipo.int

5.6.15 **Patents.** Patent law protects invention and technology. A patent is a grant of property right by the government to protect a newly created idea on the basis of its technical and legal merit.[60] In biomedicine, patents are commonly applied for and approved for new products, such as pharmaceuticals, reagents, assays, devices, and equipment and less commonly for procedures and methods. Patent law is intended to encourage discovery and investment in research of new technology by rewarding an inventor with a monopoly on the right to market the new product for a specified period. This law restricts other parties from manufacturing, selling, or using the new product without the patent holder's permission for 20 years.[60]

In the United States, patents are awarded by the US Patent and Trademark Office (USPTO). For more details, instructions, and copies of patent forms, contact the USPTO:

US Patent and Trademark Office
Department of Commerce
Washington, DC 20231
Telephone: (703) 308-4357 or (800) 786-9199
Fax: (703) 305-7786
E-mail: usptoinfo@uspto.gov
www.uspto.gov

As with copyright, there is no international patent law or protection; patents are protected by individual countries. In some regions, a regional patent office (eg, the European Patent Office or the African Regional Intellectual Property Organization) accepts and grants patent applications in the member states of that region. Detailed information about international treaties on patents is available from WIPO (for contact information, see 5.6.14, Copyright Resources).

Controversy over claims for patents of naturally occurring substances, medical and surgical methods, and even genetically altered cells and gene fragments has appeared in the scientific literature.[61-63] Desires for profit and primacy of discovery have been motives causing delay or suppression of the publication of important medical information.[5,6,64] For this reason, editors should request that authors disclose information about patents, including ownership and upcoming and pending applications for patent grants, that are related to the work included in their submitted manuscripts in their financial disclosures to journals (see 5.5, Conflicts of Interest).

5.6.16 **Trademark.** Trademark and unfair-competition laws are designed to prevent a competitor from selling goods or services under the auspices of another. Trademark law, not copyright law, protects trademarks, service marks, and trade names.[65] *Trademarks* are legally registered words, names, symbols, sounds, or colors or any combination of these items that are used to identify and distinguish goods from those goods manufactured and sold by others and to indicate the source or origin of the goods (eg, brand names).[65] Examples of commonly recognized trademarks include *Time* magazine, NBC, and Coca-Cola. A *service mark* is the same as a trademark except that it is used to distinguish services, not goods, of a specific provider.[65] Examples of service marks include McDonald's (restaurant services), AT&T (telecommunications services), and Amazon.com (Internet services). The terms *trademark* and *mark* are often used to refer to both trademarks and service marks.[65] *Trade names* are the names given by manufacturers or businesses to specific products or services. For example, Procardia is the trade name (or proprietary name) for the drug nifedipine (see also 15.4.3, Nomenclature, Drugs, Proprietary Names). Trade names are not legally protected in the same manner as are trademarks. Trademark law provides legal protection for titles, logos, fictional characters, pseudonyms, and unique groupings of words, symbols, or graphics.[38,50,65] Whereas copyright law protects an authored work, trademark law protects the words and symbols used in the marketing of that work.

Trademarks are classified into 5 categories in order of their increasing distinctiveness: generic, descriptive, suggestive, arbitrary, and fanciful.[38] Suggestive, arbitrary, and fanciful marks are more likely to receive trademark protection than are generic or descriptive marks.[38] An example of an arbitrary mark (a common word that has no specific connection to its product) is the *Nova* television series; an example of a fanciful mark (created solely for use as a trademark) is Kodak.[38] To receive trademark status, a mark must be distinctive (ie, not similar to other marks) and not generic or merely descriptive of a category of products. For example, trademark status was not awarded to *World Book* or *Farmers Almanac* because both were considered "merely descriptive of the contents of each publication,"[50] and *Software News* magazine was not considered protectable because it referred to a class of products of which the magazine is a member (ie, it was generic).[38] For additional information, contact the USPTO (contact information available in 5.6.15, Patents).

Titles. Book titles are rarely protected under trademark law because of judicial reluctance to protect titles that are used only once.[38(§25.03)] A few exceptions to this norm have occurred with book titles that have engendered common secondary meanings, ie, become widely recognized and associated with the name of the author or publisher (eg, *Gone With the Wind*).[50] The title of a series of creative works (eg, book series, journals, magazines, newspapers, television series, or software) may more easily receive trademark protection than can the title of a single creative work.[38(§25.03),50] Thus, *JAMA* is a trademarked title. However, in the biomedical sciences it is often difficult to trademark journal titles that are generic and may not be distingishable from the science or field the journal serves, such as the *Archives of Neurology* or *Neurology*.

Logos. Logos, designs, or symbols may also receive trademark protection if they distinguish particular goods or services and identify the source of those goods and services.[38(§25.05)] Examples of such logos include the Bantam publishing house rooster and Apple computer's apple. A background design, apart from the words imposed on it, can be protected by trademark if it is of a distinctive quality and functions to identify the source of a good.[38(§25.05)]

Fictional Characters and Pseudonyms. Fictional characters may be protected by trademark if they achieve secondary meaning and are widely recognized (eg, Mickey Mouse). Similarly, a pseudonym can be given trademark status.[38]

Trade Dress. Trade dress is the visual or physical appearance of a product or its packaging, which, if distinct from that of other similar products, may be protected under trademark law (eg, the Coca Cola bottle or the label on Campbell's soup). Trade dress includes graphic elements and design, typography, shape, and color. For example, the designs, including the borders, of the covers of the *National Geographic* and *Time* magazine have been awarded trademark status.[38(§25.07),50]

Application and Registration for Trademark Protection. In the United States, application for a trademark registration can be made under both federal and state laws. A legal expert should be consulted for information about registering trademarks in other countries. However, registering a trademark is not sufficient; actual use of the trademark in a given market ensures protection (ie, the longer the actual use of the trademark, the stronger the legal protection).[38,50] Typically, the rights to a trademark belong to the first user in a specific geographic market.

Trademark protection is also governed by the national laws of individual countries and international treaties, such as the TRIPS agreement. In the United States, an application to register a trademark must be filed with the USPTO.[65] Applying for trademark protection is more complicated than applying for copyright protection. The USPTO requires a formal application to be submitted (preferably electronically), along with a drawing of the mark, samples of the mark as it has been used, and a filing fee.[65] The USPTO conducts a formal review of the application, which may take several months. The office may deny the request for registration if the mark is judged to be generic, merely descriptive, or similar to another registered mark (or a mark for which another application is under review). Registration may also be denied if the mark is not used or intended for use in interstate or international commerce. If the application is approved internally by the USPTO, a notice is published in the *Official Gazette* to make the application publicly known. During the 30 days following the *Official Gazette* notice, any third party can file a formal opposition to the application.[65]

If the application is approved, the USPTO will issue a certificate of registration if the mark is in use. If the mark is not yet in use, the applicant is required to file a statement describing the mark's intended use and has 6 months to use the mark in commerce and submit a statement of such use or request a 6-month extension to file a statement of use.[65]

Trademark Symbols. Once registered, the mark is entitled to carry the trademark symbol ®. Only those marks that are officially registered by the USPTO can use the official symbol ®. Marks that are under review may use the symbol ™ or ℠, but these do not have legal significance.[65]

Duration of Trademark Protection. A US trademark registration extends for 10 years and may be extended indefinitely provided the owner continues to use the mark on or in connection with the applicable goods and/or services and files all required documentation with the USPTO at the appropriate times. For example, between the fifth and sixth years of the initial term and in the ninth year of every 10-year period thereafter, additional forms must be filed with the USPTO to ensure legal protection.[65]

Loss of Trademark Rights and Antidilution Law. A mark can lose its legal protection if the owner discontinues using it (termed *trademark abandonment*), if the owner does not file a statement that the trademark is still in use between the fifth and sixth years of the initial term, or if the owner does not renew the registration by the end of each 10-year registration period.[65] Trademark protection may also be forfeited if a mark becomes too generic or no longer identifies goods or services with a particular source (ie, the mark becomes "diluted"). In legal terms, *trademark dilution* is "the lessening of the capacity of a famous mark to identify and distinguish goods and services."[38(§25.02),66] For example, *Webster's* is no longer a registered trademark because the name lost its ability to identify a specific publisher of dictionaries, and "Zipper" used to be a trademark for "slide fastener."

A mark used in multiple contexts by different product owners or service providers may diminish the ability of a given mark to serve as unique identifier of that product or service.[38(§25.02)] Such dilution of unique trademark status is known as *blurring*. A trademark may also be diluted by *tarnishment,* when a well-known trademark is improperly associated with an inferior or offensive product or service.[38(§25.02)] The following factors may be considered in judging such dilution of unique trademark status of one mark by another[38(§25.02)]:

- Similarity of marks
- Similarity of the products covered by the marks
- Sophistication of consumers
- Predatory intent
- Renown of the senior mark
- Renown of the junior mark

For this reason, owners of trademarks will often send letters to editors and publishers objecting to misuse of their trademarks in publication. Such demands are intended to keep trademarks from being diluted by common use. For example, authors and editors should not use trademark names as generic verbs, nouns, or modifiers (eg, use "photocopied" rather than "xeroxed").

Use of Trademarked Names in Publication. Under the US Federal Trademark Dilution Act,[66] restricted use of trademark names applies mainly to commercial use of trademarks, not to editorial use in publication. For example, a photography magazine may not use the word "Kodak®" as part of its cover design and a computer manufacturer may not place the word "Kodak®" on the front of a computer. However, an author or editor may include the word "Kodak"—without the trademark symbol—in an article about cameras and film development without risking trademark infringement.

The symbol ®, or letters TM or SM, should not be used in scientific journal articles or references, but the initial letter of a trademarked word should be capitalized.

On occasion, a trademark owner will request that its trademark or trade name appear in all capital letters or a combination of capital and lowercase letters often with the trademark symbol. Authors and editors are not required by law to follow such requests. It is preferable to use an initial capital letter followed by all lowercase letters (eg, Xerox, Kodak) unless the trademark name is an abbreviation (eg, IBM, *JAMA*) or uses an intercapped construction (eg, PubMed, iTunes) (see also 10.8, Capitalization, "Intercapped" Compounds; 14.0, Abbreviations; and 15.4.3, Nomenclature, Drugs, Proprietary Names). Online databases, if trademarked, can be listed in all capital letters (eg, MEDLINE, EMBASE, CINAHL).

International Trademark Protection. Like copyright law, there is no international trademark law, and trademark protections are offered by different jurisdictions in different countries. However, WIPO (www.wipo.org) administers the Madrid System for the International Registration of Marks, which offers a route to trademark protection in multiple countries by filing a single application. Information is also available from the International Trademark Association (www.inta.org).

Trademark Protection Online. A new use of trademark has emerged in the context of the Internet. *Domain names* are Internet addresses that point to a specific Web site, usually a home page. They are usually easily remembered names that are linked to numeric Internet protocol addresses, such as uspto.gov or harvard.edu.[38(§25.09)] Domain names include top-level domain (TLD) names (eg, ".com," ".org," ".edu") and second-level names (eg, "jama" in jama.com or "nih" in nih.gov). A domain name is not automatically entitled to protection once registered; like other trademarks, it must be used in connection with the Web site located at that address.[42]

Since 1998, the Internet Corporation for Assigned Names and Numbers (ICANN) has been responsible for managing the domain name system.[67] Domain names can be registered by many different companies (known as "registrars") that are authorized by ICANN. Domain name registrars have different terms for renewal of domain name registration, ranging from 1- to 10-year increments.[67] At this writing, ICANN registrars manage the following TLD names: .aero, .biz, .cat, .com, .coop, .info, .jobs, .mobi, .museum, .name, .net, .org, .pro, .tel, and .travel. ICANN does not accredit registrars for TLDs that are restricted to specific entities and purposes, such as ".edu" for educational institutions, ".gov" for US government agencies, and ".mil" for US military sites. Country code TLDs may be obtained from host country agencies in accordance with rules determined by the Internet Assigned Numbers Authority (IANA).[42]

Disputes over ownership and rights to use domain names are considered under the principles of trademark infringement and dilution, with some specific additions to address cybersquatting and typosquatting.[38(§25.09),42] *Cybersquatting* is "the act of obtaining a trademark associated domain name with the aim of selling it to the trademark owner or otherwise benefiting from the association with the mark."[38(§25.09)] *Typosquatting* is "the registration of a domain name that is similar to another's for the purpose of capitalizing on typos that may lead the user to the squatter's Web site rather than the site the user intends to locate."[38(§25.09)] In 1999, the Anticybersquatting Consumer Protection Act was enacted to address these problems of misuse of domain names.[42]

To make a successful claim against use of a specific domain name, the following must be demonstrated[38(§25.09)]:

- the domain name is identical or confusingly similar to a trademark or service mark in which the complainant has rights,
- the registrant has no rights or legitimate interests in respect to the domain name, and
- the domain name has been registered and is being used in bad faith.

For more information on applying for and managing domain names and remedies for misuse of domain names, consult ICANN or WIPO (contact information for WIPO is available in 5.6.14, Copyright Resources).

Internet Corporation for Assigned Names and Numbers (ICANN)
www.icann.org

4676 Admiralty Way, Suite 330
Marina del Rey, CA 90292-6601
Telephone: (310) 823-9358
Fax: (310) 823-8649

or

6 Rond Point Schuman
Bt 5
Brussels B-1040, Belgium
Telephone: 32 2 234 7872
Fax: 32 2 234 7848

ACKNOWLEDGMENTS

Principal author: Annette Flanagin, RN, MA

I thank the following for reviewing and providing substantive comments to help improve the manuscript: Wayne G. Hoppe, JD, *JAMA* and *Archives* Journals; Maggie Mills, *JAMA* and *Archives* Journals; Cheryl Smart, MA, MBA; Michael T. Clark, American Medical Association Periodic Publishing and Business; Catherine D. DeAngelis,

MD, MPH, *JAMA* and *Archives* Journals; and Trevor Lane, MA, DPhil, University of Hong Kong.

REFERENCES

1. Goldstein P. *Copyright's Highway: From Gutenberg to the Celestial Jukebox*. Rev ed. Stanford, CA: Stanford University Press; 2003.
2. Nelkin D. *Science as Intellectual Property: Who Controls Scientific Research?* New York, NY: Macmillan Publishing Co; 1984.
3. Mishkin B. Urgently needed: policies on access to data by erstwhile collaborators. *Science*. 1995;270(5238):927-928.
4. Committee on Responsibilities of Authorship on the Biological Sciences, National Research Council. *Sharing Publication-Related Data and Materials: Responsibilities of Authorship in the Life Sciences*. Washington, DC: National Academy of Sciences; 2003.
5. Blumenthal D, Campbell EG, Anderson MS, Causino N, Louis KS. Withholding research results in academic life science. *JAMA*. 1997;277(15):1224-1228.
6. Campbell EG, Clarridge BR, Gokhall M, et al. Data withholding in academic genetics: evidence from a national survey. *JAMA*. 2002;287(4):473-480.
7. Arzberger P, Schroeder P, Beaulieu A, et al. Science and government: an international framework to promote access to data. *Science*. 2004;303(5665):1777-1778.
8. Straf ML. Who owns what in research data? In: Bailar JC III, Angell M, Boots S, et al, eds. *Ethics and Policy in Scientific Publication*. Chicago, IL: Council of Biology Editors Inc; 1990:130-137.
9. Fienberg SE. Sharing statistical data in the biomedical and health sciences: ethical, institutional, legal, and professional dimensions. *Annu Rev Public Health*. 1994;15: 1-18.
10. National Institutes of Health Office of Extramural Research. NIH data sharing policy and implementation guidance. http://grants.nih.gov/grants/policy/data_sharing/data_sharing_guidance.htm. Updated March 5, 2003. Accessed August 6, 2006.
11. Kondro W. Drug company experts advised staff to withhold data about SSRI use in children. *CMAJ*. 2004;170(5):783.
12. Whittington CJ, Kendall T, Fonagy P, Cottrell D, Cotgrove A, Boddington E. Selective serotonin reuptake inhibitors in childhood depression: systematic review of published versus unpublished data. *Lancet*. 2004;363(9418):1341-1345.
13. Rennie D. Trial registration: a great idea switches from ignored to irresistible. *JAMA*. 2004;292(11):1359-1362.
14. US Copyright Office, Library of Congress. *Circular 92: Copyright Law of the United States*. June 2003. http://www.copyright.gov/title17. Accessed August 25, 2006.
15. US Department of Justice. *Department of Justice Freedom of Information Act Reference Guide*. May 2006. http://www.usdoj.gov/04foia/referenceguidemay99.htm#intro. Accessed August 6, 2006.
16. National Academy of Sciences. *Responsible Science: Ensuring the Integrity of the Research Process*. Vol 2. Washington, DC: National Academy Press; 1993:127-128.
17. Fienberg SE, Martin ME, Straf ML. *Sharing Research Data*. Washington, DC: National Academy Press; 1985.
18. Duncan DT, Pearson RB. Enhancing access to microdata while protecting confidentiality: prospects for the future. *Stat Sci*. 1991;6(3):219-239.
19. Fienberg SE. Conflict between the needs for access to statistical information and demands for confidentiality. *J Off Stat*. 1994;10(2):115-132.

20. *Sharing Data From Large-scale Biological Research Projects: A System of Tripartite Responsibility*. London, England: Wellcome Trust; 2003. http://www.wellcome.ac.uk/assets/wtd003207.pdf. Accessed August 26, 2006.
21. International Committee of Medical Journal Editors. Uniform Requirements for Manuscripts Submitted to Biomedical Journals. http://www.icmje.org. Updated February 2006. Accessed August 26, 2006.
22. Tenopir C, King D. Trends in scientific scholarly publishing in the United States. *J Sch Publishing*. 1997;28(3):135-170.
23. Clark MT. Open sesame? increasing access to medical literature. *Pediatrics*. 2004;114(1):265-268.
24. Gibbs WW. Lost science in the Third World. *Sci Am*. 1995;273(3):76-83.
25. Horton R. North and South: bridging the information gap. *Lancet*. 2000;355(9222):2231-2236.
26. Budapest Open Access Initiative. http://www.soros.org/openaccess. Accessed August 6, 2006.
27. Frank M. Access to the scientific literature—a difficult balance. *N Engl J Med*. 2006;354(15):1552-1555.
28. ALPSP. Response to the Gowers Review from the Association of Learned and Professional Society Publishers (ALPSP). http://www.alpsp.org/news/GowersReview-response.pdf. Accessed August 6, 2006.
29. Ware M. Scientific publishing in transition: an overview of current developments. http://www.alpsp.org/news/STM-ALPSPwhitepaper.pdf. September 2006. Accessed October 7, 2006.
30. BioMed Central. Frequently asked questions about BioMed Central's article processing charges. http://www.biomedcentral.com/info/about/apcfaq. Accessed October 7, 2006.
31. PLoS Journals. http://www.plos.org/journals/index.html. Accessed August 20, 2006.
32. Lund University Directory of Open Access Journals. http://www.doaj.org. Accessed August 6, 2006.
33. Definition of open access publishing: Bethesda statement on open access publishing. http://www.earlham.edu/~peters/fos/bethesda.htm#definition. Released June 20, 2003. Accessed August 20, 2006.
34. National Institutes of Health. Final NIH public access policy implementation. http://publicaccess.nih.gov/publicaccess_imp.htm. Accessed August 8, 2006.
35. Wellcome Trust. Wellcome Trust position statement in support of open and unrestricted access to published research. http://www.wellcome.ac.uk/doc_wtd002766.html. Updated February 9, 2006. Accessed August 8, 2006.
36. Cox J, Cox L. *Scholarly Publishing Practice: Academic Journal Publishers' Policies and Practices in Online Publishing*. Worthing, West Sussex, United Kingdom: Association of Learned and Professional Society Publishers; 2006. Executive Summary also available at http://www.alpsp.org/publications/SPP2summary.pdf. Accessed October 7, 2006.
37. US Copyright Office, Library of Congress. *Circular 1: Copyright Office Basics*. http://www.copyright.gov/circs.circ1.html. Revised July 2006. Accessed August 20, 2006.
38. Fischer MA, Perle EG, Williams JT. *Perle and Williams on Publishing Law*. 3rd ed. Englewood Cliffs, NJ: Aspen Law & Business; 2006.
39. Nimmer D. *Nimmer on Copyright*. Vol 1-10. New York, NY: Matthew Bender & Co Inc; 2002.

40. US Copyright Office, Library of Congress. *Circular 1a: United States Copyright Office: A Brief Introduction and History*. http://www.copyright.gov/circs/circ1a.html. Revised January 2005. Accessed August 20, 2006.
41. World Intellectual Property Organization. WIPO Copyright Treaty. http://www.wipo.int/treaties/en/ip/wct/trtdocs_wo033.html. Adopted December 20, 1996. Accessed August 25, 2006.
42. Hart JD. *Law of the Web: A Field Guide to Internet Publishing*. Denver, CO: Bradford Publishing Co; 2003.
43. Hirtle PB. Copyright term and the public domain in the United States: 1 January 2006. http://www.copyright.cornell.edu/training/Hirtle_Public_Domain.htm. Accessed October 2, 2006.
44. US Copyright Office, Library of Congress. *Circular 15a: Duration of Copyright: Provisions of the Law Dealing With the Length of Copyright Protection*. December 2004. http://www.copyright.gov/circs/circ15a.html#duration. Accessed August 20, 2004.
45. *The Chicago Manual of Style*. 15th ed. Chicago, IL: University of Chicago Press; 2003.
46. US Copyright Office, Library of Congress. *Circular 9: Works Made for Hire Under the 1976 Copyright Act*. 2004. http://www.copyright.gov/circs/circ09.pdf. Accessed August 20, 2006.
47. Project Gutenberg. http://www.gutenberg.org. Modified August 26, 2006. Accessed August 26, 2006.
48. *Feist Publications Inc v Rural Tel Ser Co Inc*, 499 US 340 (1991).
49. Association of Learned and Professional Society Publishers. ALPSP guidelines. http://www.alpsp.org/htp_grantli.htm. Accessed August 6, 2006.
50. Kirsch J. *Kirsch's Handbook of Publishing Law*. Venice, CA: Acrobat Books; 1995.
51. *Harper & Row Publishers, Inc v Nation Enterprises*, 471 US 539 (1985).
52. *J. D. Salinger v Random House, Inc*, 811 F2d 90 (2d Cir 1987).
53. *New Era Publications International, ApS v Henry Holt and Company, Inc*, 695F Supp 1493, 1524-1525 (SD NY 1988).
54. Rossner M. How to guard against image fraud. *Scientist*. 2006;20(3):24. http://www.the-scientist.com/2006/3/1/24/1. Accessed September 9, 2006.
55. Rossner M, Yamada K. What's in a picture? the temptation of image manipulation. *J Cell Biol*. 2004;166(1):11-15.
56. *JAMA* and *Archives* Journals Standards for Scientific Journal Reprints, E-prints, and Republished Articles Purchased by Organizations. Chicago, IL: American Medical Association; 2006.
57. US Copyright Office, Library of Congress. International copyright. FL100. http://www.copyright.gov/fls/fl100.html. Revised July 2006. Accessed August 25, 2006.
58. US Copyright Office, Library of Congress. *Circular 38a: International Copyright Relations of the United States*. http://www.copyright.gov/circs/circ38a.html#. Revised June 2004. Accessed August 25, 2006.
59. World Intellectual Property Organization. Berne Convention for the Protection of Literary and Artistic Works. http://www.wipo.int/treaties/en/ip/berne/trtdocs_wo001.html. Accessed August 25, 2006.
60. US Patent and Trademark Office. General information concerning patents. http://www.uspto.gov/web/offices/pac/doc/general/index.html. Revised January 2005. Accessed August 25, 2006.
61. Patenting nature now. *Nature*. 1995;377(6545):89-90.
62. Deftos LJ. *Harvard v Canada*: the myc mouse that still squeaks in the maze of biopatent law. *Acad Med*. 2001;76(7):684-692.

63. Gitter DM. International conflicts over patenting human DNA sequences in the United States and the European Union: an argument for compulsory licensing and a fair-use exemption. *N Y Univ Law Rev.* 2001;76(6):1623-1691
64. Marshall E. Dispute slows paper on "remarkable" vaccine. *Science.* 1995;268(5218): 1712-1715.
65. US Patent and Trademark Office. Basic facts about trademarks. http://www.uspto.gov/main/trademarks.htm. Modified May 25, 2006. Accessed August 25, 2006.
66. Federal Trademark Dilution Act of 1996. Pub L No. 104-98, 109 Stat 985 (January 16, 1996). Codified at 15 USC 1125.
67. Internet Corporation for Assigned Names and Numbers. http://www.icann.org. Modified August 21, 2006. Accessed August 26, 2006.

Confidentiality promises are widely recognized as an ethical obligation, regardless of the legal duty accompanying them . . . maintenance of confidentiality promises fall within editorial discretion.
Jeffrey A. Richards[1]

5.7 **Confidentiality.**

The author-editor relationship is an alliance founded on the ethical rule of confidentiality. Confidentiality occurs when a person discloses information to another with the understanding that the information will not be divulged to others without permission.[2] In the context of scientific publication, this rule provides primarily for authors' rights to have the information they submit to a journal, whether in manuscript form or in communications to the editorial office, kept confidential and a concomitant duty of editors and reviewers to maintain their obligations to ensure that any information concerning a submitted manuscript is kept confidential. This compact between author and editor preserves the integrity of the scientific review and publication process. Under this compact, confidentiality may be breached only in rare circumstances, and all such breaches must be handled with care (see additional discussion in 5.7.1, Confidentiality During Editorial Evaluation and Peer Review and After Publication).

5.7.1 **Confidentiality During Editorial Evaluation and Peer Review and After Publication.**

Strict confidentiality regarding the review and evaluation of submitted manuscripts and all relevant correspondence and other forms of communication is essential to the integrity of the editorial process (see 6.1, Editorial Assessment and Processing, Editorial Assessment). Authors must feel free to submit manuscripts that contain their unique ideas and information that may affect their reputations or careers or that may be proprietary. Thus, editors and reviewers have an ethical duty to keep information about a manuscript confidential, and authors have a right to expect that confidentiality will be maintained.[3-7] Policies supporting the confidential nature of the peer review and editorial processes are well described by the International Committee of Medical Journal Editors,[3] the Council of Science Editors,[4] the World Association of Medical Editors,[5] and the UK Committee on Publication Ethics.[6] The very existence of a submission should not be revealed (by either confirmation or denial) to anyone other than the editors, editorial staff, peer reviewers, and necessary publishing staff (ie, those essential to producing the journal but not others such as sales and marketing staff), unless and until the manuscript is released for publication (see also 5.13, Release of Information to the Public and Journal/Author Relations With the News Media). In addition, editors should refrain from discussing any aspect of the peer review process of a particular manuscript or any unpublished manuscripts with anyone except authors, reviewers, and editorial staff. Even after publication, information and communications about a manuscript, its review (including reviewers' comments), or the editorial process should not be made public without consent of the author, editor, or reviewer (see also "Record Retention Policies for Journals" in 5.6.1, Intellectual Property: Ownership, Access, Rights, and Management: Ownership and Control of Data, and 5.6.7, Intellectual Property: Ownership, Access, Rights, and Management, Copying, Reproducing, Adapting, and Other Uses of Content).

To maintain confidentiality, editors should deny requests or demands for confidential information during editorial evaluation, during peer review, and after publication from any third party, including readers, authors of other manuscripts, owners of the journal, publishing staff other than those essential to producing the journal in print/online, news media, advertisers, governmental agencies, academic institutions, commercial entities, and representatives of those seeking information for use in actual or threatened legal proceedings (see 5.7.3, Confidentiality in Legal Petitions and Claims for Privileged Information). Exceptions to this policy may be made in specific circumstances provided that disclosures are limited and that anyone else given access to confidential information agrees to keep the information confidential. Examples of exceptions include the following:

- A prospective author who is invited by an editor to write an editorial commenting on a paper that has not yet been published (*Note:* such authors should be reminded about the confidential nature of the unpublished paper and not to consult anyone about the paper without prior approval of the editor, including the author of the unpublished paper)
- A governmental agency representative consulted by the editor or author on a matter considered a public health emergency or a matter that by regulation requires notification (eg, serious adverse drug event)
- An attorney who is asked to advise an editor if legal concerns are raised or who represents the journal in legal proceedings
- An institutional or funding authority requested by the editor to investigate an allegation of scientific misconduct related to a manuscript under consideration or a published article (for additional information, see 5.7.2, Confidentiality in Allegations of Scientific Misconduct, and 5.4.4, Scientific Misconduct, Editorial Policy and Procedures for Detecting and Handling Allegations of Scientific Misconduct)
- An author's violation of public journal policy, such as prohibition of covert duplicate publication or failure to disclose conflicts of interest (see also 5.3.2, Duplicate Publication, Editorial Policy for Preventing and Handling Allegations of Duplicate Publication, and 5.5.8, Conflict of Interest, Handling Failure to Disclose Financial Interest)
- An author's refusal to address an editor's questions about serious ethical concerns, such as whether research participants provided appropriate informed consent or whether a study was appropriately reviewed and approved, or waived for approval, by an independent ethics committee (see also "Reports of Unethical

Studies" in 5.8.1, Protecting Research Participants' and Patients' Rights in Scientific Publication, Ethical Review of Studies and Informed Consent)

Journals do not own or have licenses to unpublished works (because copyright and publication licenses are typically transferred in the event of publication); thus, editors should not keep print or electronic copies of rejected manuscripts. Copies should be returned to the author or destroyed. However, a journal may choose to keep a copy of a rejected manuscript for a predetermined, limited period if it has a policy that allows for author appeals of editorial decisions (see also "Record Retention Policies for Journals" in 5.6.1, Intellectual Property: Ownership, Access, Rights, and Management, Ownership and Control of Data). Similarly, reviewers should not keep copies of the manuscripts they are asked to assess. Reviewers should destroy any print and digital copies of manuscripts they have reviewed. Reviewers should not use others' manuscripts as teaching tools or in journal club discussions because doing so would violate confidentiality.

Journals should publish details about the confidential nature of the editorial, peer review, and publication processes in their instructions for authors, and editors should inform all reviewers of the confidential nature of peer review in correspondence to and instructions for reviewers[3] (see 5.11, Editorial Responsibilities, Roles, Procedures, and Policies).

Requirements During a Blinded (Masked) Peer Review Process. Journals should inform reviewers in explicit terms what they mean by "confidentiality," "confidential information," and "privileged information" (ie, that not subject to disclosure).[8] Journals should also inform reviewers and authors if the review process is single-blinded (ie, only the reviewers' identities are not disclosed), double-blinded (ie, both the reviewers' and the authors' identities are blinded), or open (ie, all author and reviewer identities are disclosed to all). For a detailed discussion of the various mechanisms of peer review (eg, single-blinded, double-blinded, open), see 6.1, Editorial Assessment and Processing, Editorial Assessment. *JAMA* and the *Archives* Journals and many other medical and scientific journals use a single-blind review process.

Peer reviewers should receive instructions reminding them to maintain confidentiality when they are invited to review and also after they agree to review (see, for example, the instructions in the Box and also 6.1, Editorial Assessment and Processing, Editorial Assessment). Reviewers should be instructed not to keep copies of manuscripts they have reviewed and to refrain from discussing the information in the manuscript with others. Reviewers should never contact authors directly to discuss their review without explicit permission from the editor.

In some circumstances, a reviewer may wish to enlist the aid of a colleague to assist with the review. Some journals prohibit such consultation, and other journals require that editorial permission be sought in advance of the consultation. If a reviewer is uncertain of a journal's policy, the reviewer should contact the editorial office. For example, *JAMA* informs reviewers that they may enlist the aid of colleagues to assist with the review as long as confidentiality is maintained and all other review policies (such as those pertaining to conflicts of interest) are followed. *JAMA* reviewers are required to inform editors if such consultation has occurred.

After an initial editorial decision (eg, rejection or revision) has been made about a reviewed paper, *JAMA* provides the corresponding author with copies of the unnamed reviewers' comments. *JAMA* reviewers are also asked to provide confidential

Box. Examples of Instructions to Peer Reviewers

Instructions for Reviewers About Maintaining Confidentiality Included in Initial E-mail Requesting Peer Review
We consider this request and the information in this e-mail to be strictly confidential. Please do not forward this e-mail to others and please delete or destroy any copies of this e-mail.

Instructions Given to Peer Reviewer Concerning Confidentiality After Reviewer Has Agreed to Conduct Review
We consider this manuscript and your review of it to be strictly confidential. Any use or distribution of the confidential information in this manuscript for any reason beyond performing this review is prohibited. If you download any electronic files or print out copies, please delete and/or destroy these documents once you have completed your review. If you need to consult a colleague to help with the review, be sure to inform her or him that the information is confidential and indicate such consultation has occurred and include that reviewer's name in your review.

Reviewers' identities are not revealed to authors or to other reviewers. Reviewers should not contact the authors. If you have any questions about this manuscript or the review process, please contact the editor.

comments to the editor, which include recommendations of acceptance, revision, or rejection; these reviewer-specific recommendations generally are not shared with the authors. However, comments directed to the editor may be summarized or excerpted and included in a letter to the author if necessary.

To provide reviewers with constructive feedback, journal editors should send to reviewers copies of other unnamed reviewers' comments.[3] Editors should inform reviewers how their reviews will be used and who will have access to the reviews and to the identities of the reviewers (see 6.1, Editorial Assessment and Processing, Editorial Assessment). In blinded peer review, reviewers have a right to expect that their identities will be protected. Thus, names and identifiers (eg, e-mail addresses, fax numbers, and initials or names) should be removed from reviewers' comments before they are disseminated to the authors or other reviewers.

Occasionally an editor may choose not to send a reviewer's comments to the author, for example, when comments are considered libelous or hypercritical. Similarly, an editor may choose to remove or mask any unhelpful or derogatory comments from an otherwise valuable review.

Signed Reviews. Occasionally, reviewers will intentionally identify themselves in their reviews or sign their reviews, even though they know the journal's peer review process is blinded. Although such identification might imply that the reviewer has waived the right to anonymity, it does not relieve the editor or the reviewer of the duty to maintain confidentiality. If the editor of a journal with a blind review process wishes to disclose the identity of a reviewer who has signed a review, the editor should first contact the reviewer to verify that the reviewer actually intended for her or his identity to be revealed. The editor should remind the reviewer and the author that any communication about the manuscript should occur through the editorial office. If the editor does not want to disclose any reviewer identities, the editor may inform the reviewer that her/his identity or signature will be removed from the review.

Disclosure of Reviewer Identities During Open Review and With Publication. Some journals, such as the *BMJ*, have an open review process that encourages reviewers to identify themselves to the authors and other reviewers.[9,10] Other journals, such as those published by BioMed Central, also publish signed comments from the reviewers with accepted papers.[11] Here again, authors and reviewers should be informed of policies regarding open review and publication of reviewer comments and identities and be reminded that all communications about the peer review and editorial process should be directed to the editor and editorial staff. Journals should clearly describe such policies in instructions for authors and reviewers and in relevant correspondence to authors and reviewers.

Acknowledging and Crediting Reviewers. An author may want to credit the help of peer reviewers in an acknowledgment. Public acknowledgment of anonymous reviewers is not necessary or informative. However, some journals will honor authors' requests to thank anonymous reviewers.

Many journals also publish the names of individuals who reviewed for the journal during the previous year to thank them publicly. Journals can notify reviewers of this plan in their instructions for reviewers or in relevant correspondence.

Rarely, an editor may receive a request from an author, who has made substantial suggestions for a complete revision, to include a peer reviewer as a coauthor. If the author's request appears justified, the editor should contact the reviewer to discuss the author's request and, if appropriate, the author and the reviewer should communicate directly. If such an arrangement is to occur, the request must be made early in the process (ie, before the major revision or complete rewrite) and the reviewer would then need to participate fully in the revision and to meet authorship criteria (see also 5.1.1, Authorship Responsibility, Authorship: Definition, Criteria, Contributions, and Requirements). Such a scenario is unlikely to occur with reports of original research.

5.7.2 **Confidentiality in Allegations of Scientific Misconduct.** Allegations of scientific misconduct (fabrication, falsification, and plagiarism) must be considered carefully vis-à-vis rules of confidentiality. In cases of credible allegations of such misconduct, an editor may need to disclose specific confidential information in a very controlled and limited manner.[3] For example, after a credible allegation of scientific misconduct, an editor may need to contact an author's or a reviewer's relevant institutional, funding, or governmental authority (eg, an academic president, dean, or ethics/integrity officer) to request a formal investigation. In this situation, the editor will need to identify the person about whom the allegation was made. This is best done by a telephone call or a brief formal letter marked confidential. During such investigations, editors should avoid including details of such cases in e-mails that can be widely circulated and should avoid posting details, even if rendered anonymous, in e-mail lists or blogs. For more details on how an editor should handle such an allegation, see 5.4.4, Scientific Misconduct, Editorial Policy and Procedures for Detecting and Handling Allegations of Scientific Misconduct.

5.7.3 **Confidentiality in Legal Petitions and Claims for Privileged Information.** A number of cases in US law have served as the foundation for or have directly supported the confidential nature of the editorial and peer review process.

In 1972, the US Supreme Court ruled in *Branzburg v Hayes* that a reporter could be forced to testify if, during the course of news gathering, the reporter became a witness to a crime.[12] However, the court also noted that individual states could create their own standards with regard to a journalistic privilege (ie, a right) to keep sources of information confidential, allowing lower courts in subsequent rulings to support such privilege. With this understanding, many states have enacted legislation that protects the press from mandatory disclosure of sources, work product, and information.[13,14] These state "shield laws" vary in scope but may offer qualified privilege to reporters to protect confidential information in legal settings unless it can be established that (1) the information sought is relevant and/or material, (2) it is unavailable by other means or through other sources, and (3) a compelling need exists for the information.[13] However, recent challenges to journalists' privilege to keep sources of information confidential are of concern.

After the 1993 US Supreme Court ruling in *Daubert v Merrell Dow Pharmaceuticals, Inc*,[15] concerns arose that attempts to breach the confidential nature of the editorial process would increase through subpoenas for journal records.[16] In this case, the court identified standards required for admissibility of scientific expert testimony. These standards include, among others, whether the evidence on which the expert opinion is based has been peer reviewed and published, and they have been applied to limit admissibility of unreliable junk science as evidence in specific cases.

In 1994, a legal precedent was set regarding confidentiality and protection from attempts to invade the confidential and privileged nature of the editorial process.[17] In *Cukier v American Medical Association,* an author whose manuscript had been rejected by *JAMA* sued to compel the journal to disclose the identity of those persons responsible for allegedly defamatory statements made to the editors concerning the author's financial interest.[17] Citing the confidential nature of the peer review process, the editors refused to disclose the source of this information. The Circuit Court of Cook County, Illinois, ruled that the editors were not required to disclose this information on the basis of the Illinois Reporter's Privilege Act,[18] which provides that members of the news media (in this case, journal editors) cannot be compelled to disclose sources unless the information cannot be obtained elsewhere and such disclosure is essential to the protection of the public interest. This decision was affirmed by the Illinois Appellate Court, and the Illinois Supreme Court declined to hear the case.

Other cases that have supported the confidential nature of the peer review process include *Henke v US Department of Commerce and the National Science Foundation*[19] and *Cistrom Biotechnology Inc v Immunex Corp.*[20]

With the case law supporting journals in resisting attempts to obtain confidential information via litigation and quashing subpoenas, journals, editors, and publishers can rely on legal precedents and principles to help them maintain confidentiality of the peer review and editorial process. Parrish and Bruns[21] have summarized the reasons journals should resist complying with subpoenas that intrude on such confidentiality as follows:

- Violation of confidentiality obligations for one case may make it more difficult to defend future intrusions, may result in perceived breach of trust that could damage a journal's reputation among authors and peer reviewers involved in a specific case as well as other current and prospective authors and reviewers, and may result in an author or reviewer suing the journal for breach of confidentiality.

- Compliance with a subpoena disrupts the journal's activities and processes and consumes the journal's time and resources.
- Substantial costs can be incurred in responding to a subpoena, collecting documents, and providing depositions.
- A subpoena may be used as a means of harassment to prevent an author or a journal from publishing.

If a journal receives a subpoena or request from an attorney for confidential information, the editor should consult the publisher, the journal's attorney, or both. The disclosure of confidential information to an attorney in this context would be protected under attorney-client privilege.[22] However, it is important to limit disclosure of such information to the publisher (eg, protecting the names of authors or reviewers). According to Parrish and Bruns,[21] in general, subpoenas are broad; therefore, editors may object to the scope and burden of having to respond to such a request. If negotiation with a party who served the subpoena must occur, editors and their legal representatives should request a narrowing of scope of the subpoena, a redaction of all irrelevant confidential information, the destruction or return of all surrendered documents containing any confidential information, and a limit on who can view any confidential information. In addition, the journal may seek indemnification from the authors or reviewers if they sue the journal for violation of confidentiality. Parrish and Bruns recommend that if such negotiations fail or do not protect the journal properly, the journal can file a legal motion to quash the subpoena.[21]

5.7.4 Confidentiality in Selecting Editors and Editorial Board Members. When editors or editorial board members are interviewed and evaluated for a prospective position with a journal, all participants in the selection process should be reminded that all discussions should remain confidential. In some cases, a signed statement of confidentiality may be requested of members of search/interview committees. Without assurance of such confidentiality, professional reputations and the journal's relationship with influential academic and political leaders may be jeopardized[23] (see 5.11.10, Editorial Responsibilities, Roles, Procedures, and Policies, Role of the Editorial Board).

ACKNOWLEDGMENTS

Principal author: Annette Flanagin, RN, MA

I thank C. K. Gunsalus, JD, University of Illinois, Urbana/Champaign; Wayne G. Hoppe, JD, *JAMA* and *Archives* Journals; and Debra Parrish, JD, Parrish Law Offices, for reviewing and providing substantial comments to improve this section; the following for review and providing minor comments: Terri S. Carter, *Archives of Surgery*; Catherine D. DeAngelis, MD, MPH, *JAMA* and *Archives* Journals; Cindy W. Hamilton, PharmD, ELS, Hamilton House; Trevor Lane, MA, DPhil, University of Hong Kong; Diana J. Mason, RN, PhD, *American Journal of Nursing*; Povl Riis, MD, University of Copenhagen; Valerie Siddall, PhD, ELS, AstraZeneca; Cheryl Smart, MBA; and Flo Witte, MA, ELS, AdvancMed LLC; and Sandra R. Schefris and Yolanda

Davis, James S. Todd Memorial Library, American Medical Association, Chicago, Illinois, for bibliographic assistance.

REFERENCES

1. Richards JA. Note: confidentially speaking: protecting the press from liability for broken confidential promises. *Washington Law Rev.* 1992;67:501.
2. Beauchamp TL, Childress JF. *Principles of Biomedical Ethics.* 5th ed. New York, NY: Oxford University Press; 2001.
3. International Committee of Medical Journal Editors. Uniform Requirements for Manuscripts Submitted to Biomedical Journals: Writing and Editing for Biomedical Publication. http://www.icmje.org. Updated February 2006. Accessed September 9, 2006.
4. Council of Science Editors. CSE's white paper on promoting integrity in scientific journal publications. http://www.councilofscienceeditors.org/editorial_policies/white_paper.cfm. Accessed January 3, 2007.
5. World Association of Medical Editors. WAME recommendations on publication ethics policies for medical journals. http://www.wame.org/resources/publication-ethics-policies-for-medical-journals. Accessed September 9, 2006.
6. Committee on Publication Ethics. A code of conduct for editors of biomedical journals. http://www.publicationethics.org.uk/guidelines/code. Accessed September 9, 2006.
7. Cummings P, Rivara FP. Reviewing manuscripts for *Archives of Pediatrics & Adolescent Medicine. Arch Pediatr Adolesc Med.* 2002;156(1):11-13.
8. Marshall E. Suit alleges misuse of peer review. *Science.* 1995;270(5244):1912-1914.
9. Smith R. Opening up *BMJ* peer review: a beginning that should lead to complete transparency. *BMJ.* 1999;318(7175):4-5.
10. Godlee F. Making reviewers visible: openness, accountability, and credit. *JAMA.* 2002;287(21):2762-2765.
11. BMC Medicine. Instructions for *BMC Medicine* authors. http://www.biomedcentral.com/bmcmed/ifora. Accessed September 9, 2006.
12. *Branzburg v Hayes*, 408 US 665 (1972).
13. Lening C, Cohen H. Journalists' Privilege to Withhold Information in Judicial and Other Proceedings: State Shield Statutes. CRS Report for Congress. Order Code RL32806. http://fpc.state.gov/documents/organization/44110.pdf. March 8, 2005. Accessed November 2, 2005.
14. Kenworthy B. *Branzburg v. Hayes*, reporters' privilege & circuit courts. First Amendment Center. http://www.firstamendmentcenter.org. July 12, 2005. Accessed November 2, 2005.
15. *Daubert v Merrell Dow Pharmaceuticals, Inc*, 113 S Ct 27866 (1993).
16. Gold JA, Zaremski MJ, Lev ER, Shefrin DH. *Daubert v Merrell Dow:* the Supreme Court tackles scientific evidence in the courtroom. *JAMA.* 1993;270(24):2964-2967.
17. *Cukier v American Medical Association,* 630 NE 2d 1198 (Ill App 1 Dist 1994).
18. Reporter's Privilege. Chapter 7835, Illinois Complied Statutes, Act 5, Article VIII, Part 9, Sections 901-909. 735 ILCS 5/8-901 to 909.
19. *Henke v US Department of Commerce and the National Science Foundation,* 83 F3d 1445 (US App 1996).
20. Peer review and the courts. *Nature.* 1996;384(6604):1.
21. Parrish DM, Bruns DE. US legal principles and confidentiality of the peer review process. *JAMA.* 2002;287(21):2839-2841.

22. Gifis SH. *Law Dictionary*. 5th ed. Hauppauge, NY: Barrons Educational Series Inc; 2003.
23. Bishop CT. *How to Edit a Scientific Journal*. Philadelphia, PA: ISI Press; 1984.

The right of the research subject to safeguard his or her integrity must always be respected. Every precaution should be taken to respect the privacy of the subject and to minimize the impact of the study on the subject's physical and mental integrity and on the personality of the subject.

World Medical Association[1]

5.8 Protecting Research Participants' and Patients' Rights in Scientific Publication.

Contemporary rules for protecting the rights of individuals (namely, research participants and patients) in scientific publication have their foundations in doctrines developed during the mid-20th century: the Nuremberg Code,[2] the World Medical Association's Declaration of Geneva,[3] and the World Medical Association's Declaration of Helsinki,[1] as well as the 1979 US Belmont Report.[4] Today, protection of such rights is governed by national and international guidelines and requirements.[5-13] Biomedical editors and authors have a specific ethical duty to follow the principles outlined in these doctrines (namely, autonomy, beneficence, and justice)[4,11] as well as to honor individuals' rights to privacy when making decisions about publishing studies that involve human experimentation and articles about patients who might be identifiable.[14-16] In addition, privacy doctrines and laws in many countries protect an individual's right to privacy.[7-9,11] A legal claim for invasion of privacy (eg, publishing identifying details about or a photograph of an individual without his or her permission) could be brought against a journal for publishing otherwise truthful statements about an individual.[17] Privacy law differs from defamation law in that truth may not be used as a defense for invasion of privacy (see 5.9, Defamation, Libel).

5.8.1 Ethical Review of Studies and Informed Consent.

To protect the safety and dignity of individuals who participate in research, academic institutions and grant agencies require that any study involving human participants be reviewed and approved by an institutional review board (IRB) or independent ethics review committee. (*Note:* When referring to individuals who participate in studies, the word *participant* is preferred to *subject* [see 11.1, Correct and Preferred Usage, Correct and Preferred Usage of Common Words and Phrases]. However, a number of guidelines and regulations cited herein refer to human "subjects.")

The US National Institutes of Health (NIH) defines *research* as "any systematic investigation designed to develop or contribute to generalizable knowledge" and a *human subject* as "a living individual about whom an investigator obtains either (1) data through interaction or intervention with the individual, or (2) identifiable private information."[6] The NIH considers the following to be components of research not involving human participants: samples from deceased individuals; samples collected for diagnostic purposes only; samples or data that are available from commercial or public repositories or registries; established cell lines that are publicly available; and self-sustaining, cell-free derivative preparations (eg, viral isolates, cloned DNA or RNA).

The NIH also identifies 6 categories of research involving human participants that may be exempt from IRB review and approval provided the study does not expose participants to physical, social, or psychological risks and does not permit identifiability of individual living participants.[5,6] These categories are study or collection of publicly available existing records, surveys, interviews, use of educational tests, observations of public behavior, and some types of research involving taste testing of food.[5,6]

In addition, the nature and purpose of all procedures and their attendant possible risks must be fully explained to potential participants in advance, and participants must fully comprehend the nature of the participation and voluntarily agree to such participation. Research protocols for studies involving human participants typically address the following minimum set of protections: risks to all participants, experimental procedures, anticipated benefits to participants (if any), anticipated number of participants, proposed consent document and process to be used, and appropriate additional safeguards if the study is to include vulnerable participants (eg, children, incapacitated adults).[4,5]

Journal Policies and Procedures. In accordance with these requirements, journals should require authors of manuscripts that report studies involving human participants to state explicitly in the "Methods" section of the manuscript that an appropriate independent ethics committee or IRB approved the study protocol or project or determined that the investigation was exempt from such approval and why. The name of the ethics committee(s) or IRB(s) should be specified in the "Methods" section. If the study protocol was approved by several ethics committees/IRBs, as would be expected in a multicenter study, it is appropriate to note that review and approval were conducted by the ethics committees/IRBs of all participating centers/institutions.

Journals should also require authors to indicate in the "Methods" section that informed consent was obtained from all adult participants and from parents or legal guardians for minors or incapacitated adults and how such consent was obtained (ie, written or oral). If an IRB or ethics committee waived the requirement for informed consent, the author should explain the reason for such waiver.

Ethical approval for research involving animals and relevant animal-handling protocols should be reviewed and approved by independent animal care and use committees as required by national regulations, such as the NIH's Office of Laboratory Animal Welfare requirements.[18] Such review and approval or waiver should be adequately described in the "Methods" section of all manuscripts reporting research involving animals.

Although numerous regulations and international documents require compliance with these procedures, and groups such as the International Committee of Medical Journal Editors (ICMJE),[14] World Association of Medical Editors,[15] and UK Committee on Publication Ethics[16] support these requirements, authors and journals continue to fail to properly report information on ethics committee review and approval and informed consent.[19-22] As recommended by the ICMJE,[14] specific guidelines regarding documentation of formal ethical review and informed consent should be included in a journal's instructions for authors.

Additional Regulations and Principles. US biomedical investigators who are subject to jurisdiction of an IRB or formal ethics review committee should follow the principles described in the Belmont Report[4] and the US Department of Health and Human

Services Regulations for the Protection of Human Subjects.[5] Investigators outside the United States who are not subject to jurisdiction of an institutional ethics review committee should rely on and cite their relevant national regulations[11]; regional guidelines, such as the Council of Europe's Convention on Human Rights in Biomedicine[12]; or international guidelines, such as the Council for International Organizations of Medical Science's International Ethical Guidelines for Biomedical Research Involving Human Subjects,[10] the Universal Declaration on Bioethics and Human Rights,[13] or the Declaration of Helsinki.[1] In addition to requiring researchers to have the protocol describing the study reviewed by a "specially appointed committee independent of the investigator and sponsor," and to obtain study participants' "freely given informed consent, preferably in writing," the Declaration of Helsinki specifies that reports of experimentation not in accordance with the basic principles described in the Declaration "should not be published."[1]

For studies conducted in a specific country by investigators from another country, regulations from both the local (host) country and the investigator's home (sponsoring) country should be followed, and both IRB/ethics committees that reviewed and approved the study should be cited in the "Methods" section of the manuscript.[10,13,23,24] For studies conducted in multiple countries, relevant regulations of all host countries and any home/sponsoring countries and/or the Declaration of Helsinki[1] or the Universal Declaration on Bioethics and Human Rights[13] should be followed, and all IRB/ethics committees that reviewed and approved the study should be cited in the "Methods" section. In all multinational, multicultural studies, attention should be given to the ethical requirements for protecting the interests of the research participants, namely, acquiring informed consent, avoiding harm, attending to needs, and obligations when the study is completed.[24] Each of these considerations should be addressed in the "Methods" section of the manuscript.

Reports of Unethical Studies. The past publication of unethical research does not justify this continued practice. In a 1966 pioneering article on ethics and clinical research, Beecher[25] identified 50 unethical studies involving human participants that were published in medical journals. Beecher concluded that "an experiment should be ethical at its inception and is not made ethical by publication" and that "failure to obtain publication would discourage unethical experimentation."[25] If the author of a report of an experimental investigation that involves humans or animals does not report in a submitted manuscript that formal ethics review and informed consent from human participants were obtained or appropriately considered and waived, the editor should ask the author why this information was not reported. The author may have neglected to report this information because of inadvertent omission or a misunderstanding. For example, an author may fail to report this information because ethics review was considered unnecessary (such as in a retrospective audit of publicly available data), or an informed consent requirement was formally waived by an IRB, or a manuscript contains a secondary analysis and the information about IRB approval and/or informed consent was reported in the primary publication.

All manuscripts, including those reporting studies in which IRB approval and/or informed consent requirements were deemed unnecessary, formally waived, or previously reported, should include details about how the ethical requirements were met or why these requirements were considered unnecessary or waived.

Even when a study has been approved by an ethics committee or IRB, the ethics of the reported research may be questioned by reviewers and editors. In such cases, editors are obliged to ask the authors to clarify the situation and respond to any concerns. Unless the authors can provide satisfactory responses and reassurance, editors may choose to reject the manuscript in question.

If an author refuses to address serious concerns about such ethical requirements, the editor may need to notify the author's institutional or funding authority (see also 5.7.2, Confidentiality, Confidentiality in Allegations of Scientific Misconduct, and 5.4, Scientific Misconduct).

Publication of an investigation that raises ethical dilemmas may be warranted if such publication would encourage professional and public debate and reform. Such publication should be accompanied by an editor's note or an editorial describing the ethical issues and concerns. Research that violates established ethical principles should not be published.

5.8.2 **Patients' Rights to Privacy and Anonymity.** *Privacy* is a state or condition of limited access to matters of a personal nature, including but not limited to personal information, as well as an individual's right to control such access.[26] When individuals grant others some form of access to themselves (eg, during a patient-clinician encounter), the individuals are exercising their right to privacy, but they are not waiving this right. Thus, a loss of privacy depends on the kinds or amount of access, who has access, through what means, and to which aspect of a person.[26] Historically, medical journals have taken steps to protect patients' rights to privacy and anonymity, including the deletion of patients' names, initials, and assigned numbers from case reports; removal of identifying information from radiographs, digital images, and laboratory slides; and the deletion of identifying details from descriptions of patients or study participants in published articles. Until the late 1980s, placing black bars over the eyes of patients in photographs was accepted as a way to protect the identities of patients. However, journals began to discontinue this practice when it became apparent that bars across eyes do not protect identities.[14,27-30] Photographs with bars placed over the eyes of patients should not be used in publication.

Case descriptions and case reports serve as important contributions to the medical literature and make up a substantial portion of some journal content, especially in some specialties. Traditionally, such reports have included specific details about patients. However, as Pitkin and Scott[31] note, "The degree of detail and specificity is sometimes sufficient to permit identification, and at the same time, it is often much greater than necessary for any message the author means to convey." Only those details essential for understanding and interpreting a specific case report or case series should be provided. In most instances, the description can be more general than specific to ensure anonymity, without loss of meaning. For example, Pitkin and Scott[31] suggest that "a 34-year-old para 2-0-0-2 black woman at 23 weeks' gestation" can be described as "a multiparous woman in midgestation." Although the degree of specificity needed will depend on the context of what is being reported, specific ages, race/ethnicity, and other sociodemographic details should be presented only if clinically or scientifically relevant and important.

Patients have occasionally recognized descriptions of themselves in medical articles without accompanying photographs and even after "superfluous social details" have been removed.[28] To protect a patient's right to privacy, nonessential identifying data (eg, sex, age, occupation) generally should be removed from a manuscript, unless clinically or epidemiologically important. However, omitting certain details may be problematic.[29,30] For example, omitting a patient's occupation from a case report might seem reasonable at first, but this information may be needed later during an occupational exposure assessment or an epidemiologic investigation. More important, authors and editors should not alter or falsify details in case descriptions to secure anonymity because doing so may introduce false or inaccurate data into the medical literature.[22] For example, changing the city in which the patient lived may seem innocuous, until another investigator subsequently cites the case report and the erroneous city in an epidemiologic analysis of locations of disease outbreaks.

Several cases have occurred in which patients who had not consented to publication of their personal details in medical journals were recognized by themselves or others in specific articles or subsequent news coverage.[28,32,33] The ICMJE and a number of medical journals have strengthened their rules for protecting patients' rights to privacy by adding a specific requirement for informed consent from any potentially identifiable patient.[14,29-31,34]

Therefore, when detailed case descriptions or photographs of faces or identifiable body parts are included in a manuscript that might permit any patient to be identified, authors should obtain written permission from the identifiable patients (or legally authorized representatives) to publish the information and should send a copy of the permission to the journal. The same applies to video files submitted for publication. Such consent should include an opportunity for the patient to read the manuscript to be submitted for publication or waive the right to do so. Nonspecific institutional consent forms that do not include a provision for a patient to review the information to be published or waive that right are not acceptable. An example of the patient permission form used by *JAMA* and the *Archives* Journals appears in the Box.

For manuscripts accepted for publication, when informed consent from identifiable patient(s) has been obtained, journals should indicate that such consent was obtained, either in the "Methods" section, if appropriate, or in the Acknowledgment section at the end of the article.

> **Methods:** This investigation was approved by the medical center's institutional review board. The 12 patients in this case series provided written informed consent for the investigation. In addition, each patient was given an opportunity to review the manuscript and consented to its publication.
>
> **Acknowledgment:** We are grateful to the 2 patients who graciously provided permission after reviewing the manuscript to publish this information for the medical community.

Some editors and authors have commented that obtaining consent from identifiable patients is too burdensome.[35-38] Asking those who so argue to consider that the identifiable person could be themselves or a close relative might help convey the rationale for this requirement. Others have argued that the process of obtaining such consent may be disturbing to the patient or the patient's family members.[35] However, subsequent discovery of unauthorized publication of a patient's information that results in identification or unwanted publicity would be even more disturbing[32,34] and may also violate national privacy laws such as the US Health Insurance Portability and Accountability Act (HIPAA).[7,8] Moreover, the publication of unauthorized identifiable patient information could result in legal claims related to invasion of privacy, allegations of professional misconduct, or criminal penalties.[7,8,17,32]

Box. *JAMA* and *Archives* Journals Patient Permission Form

Consent for Publication of Identifying Material in *JAMA/Archives* Journals

I give my permission for the following material to appear in the print, online, and licensed versions of *JAMA/Archives* Journals and for *JAMA/Archives* Journals to grant permission to third parties to reproduce this material.

Title or subject of article, photograph, or video:______________________________

____

I understand that my name will not be published but that complete anonymity cannot be guaranteed.

Please check the appropriate box below after reading each statement.

☐ I have read the manuscript or a general description of what the manuscript contains and reviewed all photographs, illustrations, or video files in which I am included that will be published.

or

☐ I have been offered the opportunity to read the manuscript and to see all photographs, illustrations, or video files in which I am included, but I waive my right to do so.

Signed______________________________ Date____________________

Print name______________________________

If you are granting permission for another person, what is your relationship to that person?____

At *JAMA*, whether a manuscript contains identifiable patient information is determined on a case-by-case basis. In most cases, potentially identifiable data are removed from the manuscript. However, if such details are required, the editors will assess the risk of identifiability after considering the type and amount of detail that is needed, circumstances surrounding the clinical situation or investigation, and, if applicable, relevant identifiable information contained in previously published reports involving the same patient(s) or news reports that have resulted in publicity.[34] (*Note:* Previous publication or news coverage does not eliminate a patient's right to privacy and does not negate the need for patient permission.) If the editors determine that the information could result in recognition—even if only by the patient—they will ask the author to delete identifiable details and material. This can be done with most manuscripts. However, if "deidentification" is not possible, the editors will ask the author to obtain consent from the patient, which includes offering the patient the opportunity to read the submitted manuscript. In this case, if the patient cannot be located or refuses to consent to publication, the manuscript will not be published.

5.8.3 **Rights in Published Reports of Genetic Studies.** The rules for ethical approval of studies and for obtaining informed consent also apply to genetic studies of family pedigrees and population-based samples. However, obtaining written informed consent from all members of a large pedigree (many of whom may be deceased or unaware of the collection of family data) may be difficult or impossible. Proposals for obtaining some form of group consent and for avoiding the publication of information about identifiable family members who will not give their permission have been considered. All such studies must be reviewed by an independent ethics review committee or IRB, and if the individual members of the family or population-based sample are considered to be "human subjects" and identifiable, informed consent may be required; otherwise a waiver may be granted.[39,40] (See also 5.8.1, Ethical Review of Studies and Informed Consent.) The "Methods" section of all reports of genetic studies should include statements about ethics committee/IRB review and approval or waiver and information about informed consent procedures or waivers.

As with reports of other types of studies, nonessential identifying information should be removed from reports of genetic studies. However, data should not be altered in an attempt to protect the identities of individuals or family members, although relevant information may be masked. For example, in pedigree charts, triangles can be used instead of squares and circles if the sex of family members is not essential to the report (eg, if the disease is known not to be sex-linked), or sections of pedigrees may be excluded from pedigree charts or not described in detail if appropriate consent could not be obtained as long as such omissions are noted. (See also "Pedigree" in 4.2.2, Visual Presentation of Data, Figures, Diagrams, and 15.6.6, Nomenclature, Genetics, Pedigrees.)

5.8.4 **Patients' Rights in Essays and News Reports in Biomedical Journals.** In essays and news stories in biomedical journals, descriptions and photographs of individuals are often included. However, if these descriptions or photographs depict patients or anyone in an actual patient-clinician encounter who is identifiable, the authors or writers should be asked to "deidentify" those patients. Identifying details may be omitted but may not be altered or falsified. If patients cannot be deidentified, their written informed consent must be obtained. (See Box.) Fictionalized cases and reports generally should not be presented except in rare cases and unless this is made clear to readers (eg, a hypothetical case to explain a clinical scenario or a fictional essay in which it is made clear to the readers that it is fictional). In news stories, third-party photographs should not be used if they include identifiable patients, unless consent for publication has been obtained. Appropriately credited stock or staged photographs depicting patients or simulating a patient-clinician encounter are acceptable.

ACKNOWLEDGMENTS

Principal author: Annette Flanagin, RN, MA

I thank Catherine D. DeAngelis, MD, MPH, *JAMA* and *Archives* Journals, and Povl Riis, MD, University of Copenhagen, for reviewing and providing important suggestions to improve the manuscript; the following for reviewing and providing minor comments: Terri S. Carter, *Archives of Surgery*; C. K. Gunsalus, JD, University of Illinois, Champaign/Urbana; Trevor Lane, MA, DPhil, University of Hong Kong;

Diana J. Mason, RN, PhD, *American Journal of Nursing*; Cheryl Smart, MBA; and Flo Witte, MA, ELS, AdvancMed LLC; and Sandra R. Schefris and Yolanda Davis, James S. Todd Memorial Library, American Medical Association, Chicago, Illinois, for bibliographic assistance.

REFERENCES

1. World Medical Association. Declaration of Helsinki: ethical principles for medical research involving human subjects. http://www.wma.net/e/policy/b3.htm. Updated 2004. Accessed October 25, 2005.
2. The Nuremberg Code. *JAMA*. 1996;276(20):1691.
3. World Medical Association. Declaration of Geneva. http://www.wma.net/e/policy/c8.htm. Updated May 2005. Accessed October 25, 2005.
4. National Commission for the Protection of Human Subjects of Biomedical and Behavioral Research. The Belmont Report: ethical principles and guidelines for the protection of human subjects of research. April 18, 1979. http://ohsr.od.nih.gov/guidelines/belmont.html. Accessed September 9, 2006.
5. US Department of Health and Human Services. Regulations for the Protection of Human Subjects (45 CFR 46). http://www.hhs.gov/ohrp/humansubjects/guidance/45cfr46.htm. Revised June 23, 2005. Accessed October 25, 2005.
6. National Institutes of Health. Guidelines for the conduct of research involving human subjects at the National Institutes of Health. http://ohsr.od.nih.gov/guidelines/graybook.html. August 2004. Accessed October 25, 2005.
7. US Department of Health and Human Services. Office for Civil Rights—HIPAA: medical privacy—national standards to protect the privacy of personal health information. http://www.hhs.gov/ocr/hipaa. Accessed September 9, 2006.
8. Office for Civil Rights. Standards for privacy of individually identifiable health information; final rule. August 14, 2002. 45 CFR parts 160 and 164.
9. UK General Medical Council. Publishing case studies. Confidentiality: protecting and providing information. http://www.gmc-uk.org/guidance/library/confidentiality_faq.asp. Accessed September 9, 2006.
10. Council for International Organizations of Medical Science. International ethical guidelines for biomedical research involving human subjects. http://www.cioms.ch/guidelines_nov_2002_blurb.htm. 2002. Accessed November 3, 2005.
11. Office for Human Research Protections, US Department of Health and Human Services. *International Compilation of Human Subject Research Protections*. 2nd ed. October 1, 2005. http://www.hhs.gov/ohrp/international/HSPCompilation.pdf. Accessed November 3, 2005.
12. Council of Europe. Additional Protocol to the Convention on Human Rights and Biomedicine, Concerning Biomedical Research. Strasbourg, France. http://www.Conventions.coe.int/treaty/en/Treaties/Html/195.htm. January 25, 2005. Accessed January 8, 2007.
13. UNESCO. Universal Declaration on Bioethics and Human Rights. Paris, France: UNESCO. 2005. http://unesdoc.unesco.org/images/0014/001461/146180E.pdf. Accessed September 9, 2006.
14. International Committee of Medical Journal Editors. Uniform Requirements for Manuscripts Submitted to Biomedical Journals: Writing and Editing for Biomedical Publication. http://www.icmje.org. Updated February 2006. Accessed September 9, 2006.

15. World Association of Medical Editors. WAME recommendations on publication of ethics policies for medical journals. http://www.wame.org/resources/publication-ethics-policies-for-medical-journals. Accessed January 5, 2007.
16. Committee on Publication Ethics. A code of conduct for editors of biomedical journals. http://www.publicationethics.org.uk/guidelines/code. Accessed September 9, 2006.
17. Kirsch J. *Kirsch's Handbook of Publishing Law*. 2nd ed. Los Angeles, CA: Acrobat Books; 1995.
18. National Institutes of Health, Office of Laboratory Animal Welfare. Public Health Services policy on humane care and use of laboratory animals. http://grants.nih.gov/grants/olaw/references/phspol.htm. Amended August 2002. Accessed November 13, 2005.
19. Yank V, Rennie D. Reporting of informed consent and ethics committee approval in clinical trials. *JAMA*. 2002;287(21):2835-2838.
20. Weil E, Nelson RM, Ross LF. Are research standards satisfied in pediatric journal publications? *Pediatrics*. 2002;110(2, pt 1):364-370.
21. Myles PS, Tan N. Reporting of ethical approval and informed consent in clinical research in leading anesthesia journals. *Anesthesiology*. 2003;99(5):1209-1213.
22. Botkin JR, McMahon WM, Smith KR, Nash JE. Privacy and confidentiality in the publication of pedigrees: a survey of investigators and biomedical journals. *JAMA*. 1998;279(22):1808-1812.
23. Kent DM, Mwamburi DM, Bennish ML, Kupelnick B, Ioannidis JPA. Clinical trials in sub-Saharan Africa and established standards of care: a systematic review of HIV, tuberculosis, and malaria trials. *JAMA*. 2004;292(2):237-242.
24. Aagaard-Hansen J, Johansen MV, Riis P. Research ethical challenges in cross-disciplinary and cross-cultural health research: the diversity of codes. *Dan Med Bull*. 2004;51(1):117-120.
25. Beecher HK. Ethics and clinical research. *N Engl J Med*. 1966;274(24):1354-1360.
26. Beauchamp TL, Childress JF. *Principles of Biomedical Ethics*. 5th ed. New York, NY: Oxford University Press; 2001.
27. Slue WE Jr. Unmasking the Lone Ranger. *N Engl J Med*. 1989;321(8):550-551.
28. Riis P, Nylenna M. Patients have a right to privacy and anonymity in medical publication. *JAMA*. 1991;265(20):2720.
29. Nylenna M, Riis P. Identification of patients in medical publications: need for informed consent. *BMJ*. 1991;302(6786):1182.
30. Smith J. Keeping confidence in published papers: do more to protect patient's rights to anonymity. *BMJ*. 1991;302(6786):1168.
31. Pitkin RM, Scott JR. Privacy and publication. *Obstet Gynecol*. 2001;98(2):198.
32. Court C. GMC finds doctors not guilty in consent case. *BMJ*. 1995;311(7015):1245-1246.
33. Borg GJ. More about parkinsonism after taking ecstasy. *N Engl J Med*. 1999;341(18):1400-1401.
34. Fontanarosa PB, Glass RM. Informed consent for publication. *JAMA*. 1997;278(8):682-683.
35. Snider DE. Patient consent for publication and the health of the public. *JAMA*. 1997;278(8):624-626.
36. Clever LH. Obtain informed consent before publishing information about patients. *JAMA*. 1997;278(8):628-629.
37. Tierney E. Consent for publication of a case report. *Anaesthesia*. 2004;59(8):822.

38. Ghai B, Saxena AK. Patient's consent for publication. *Anaesthesia*. 2005;60(3):289.
39. Botkin JR. Protecting the privacy of family members in survey and pedigree research. *JAMA*. 2001;285(2):207-211.
40. Beskow LM, Burke W, Merz JF et al. Informed consent for population-based research involving genetics. *JAMA*. 2001;286(18):2315-2321.

Truth is generally the best vindication against slander.

Abraham Lincoln[1]

5.9 Defamation, Libel.

Defamation, Libel. *Defamation* is the act of harming another's reputation by libel or slander and thereby exposing that person to public hatred, contempt, ridicule, or financial loss.[2-7] *Libel* is false and negligent or malicious publication involving words, pictures, or signs.[2,6] Technically and historically, libel has differed from slander in that slander was defined as defamation by oral expressions or gestures and libel was defined as defamation in print. With both libel and slander, resulting liability depends on a third party reading or hearing the defamatory words. With the advent of modern forms of communication, the distinction between these terms has become blurred because of the mix of print, audio, and video content in multiple forms of media.[3(§5.01),6(p131)]

Truth is considered a defense against libel in most cases.[3(§5.09)] However, the context of the alleged libelous communication, effect of the communication on the so-called average reader, intentions and actions of the author/writer, editor, and publisher, and location of the publication can each influence liability.[3,4,6,7] For example, a statement may be truthful in isolation, but coupled with other statements or placed in a different context, the same statement could result in an overall false impression, which could result in defamation.[3(§5.09)] On the other hand, a statement with minor inaccuracies or omission of inconsequential details could still be considered "substantially true" and thus not be determined to be defamatory.[3(§5.09)] In US courts, most libel cases are difficult for plaintiffs to win. This is not necessarily the case in other countries. For example, the United Kingdom is known for libel laws that are more favorable to plaintiffs.[8] Libel law is complex, and it is difficult for an author, editor, or publisher to know with certainty whether the text of a specific manuscript could be defended successfully in a libel suit.[4(p152)] Editors and publishers should consult lawyers with expertise in media law when concerned about risks of libel and should also carry liability insurance that covers claims for libel (see also 5.9.7, Defense Against Libel, and 5.9.8, Minimizing the Risk of Libel).

In the United States, libel law generally requires courts to balance 2 competing values: freedom of expression vs protection of personal reputation.[9] Freedom of expression has its foundation in the First Amendment of the US Constitution, and this freedom has been largely assured in instances involving public officials governed by US law since a landmark Supreme Court decision in 1964.[10] In *New York Times Co v Sullivan*,[10] an elected official in Alabama sued the *New York Times* for publishing an advertisement that included statements, some of which were inaccurate, about police actions against students who participated in a civil rights demonstration; the elected official had supervisory responsibility over the police force about which the statements were made. After a series of decisions on this case in which it was demonstrated that some of the published statements were false, the US Supreme Court determined that a public official could not recover damages for publication of a false statement relating to his or her official conduct unless it is proven that the defendant published the statement knowing it was false or with reckless disregard of whether it was false (ie, actual malice). This decision established important protections for the press against libel claims based on First Amendment protections to ensure that debate on public issues remains "uninhibited, robust, and wide open,"[6(p131),10] but more recent decisions in US courts have not always resulted in such favorable protections for the press.[3,7]

Libel threats and suits have been used to silence those with opposing viewpoints and censor the free flow of information. Lawsuits, referred to as SLAPP suits (the acronym for *strategic lawsuit against public participation*), have been used in an attempt to intimidate those who wish to publish criticism or information that could expose wrongdoing on the part of a particular industry or corporation. Even if the suit is groundless and the plaintiff eventually loses the case, a protracted and expensive legal battle may be damaging to an author, editor, publisher, or journal. For example, in 1984, Immuno AG, a multinational pharmaceutical company based in Austria, brought a $4 million libel suit against an unpaid editor of the *Journal of Medical Primatology*, Jan Moor-Jankowski, and the journal's publisher.[11] The lawsuit followed publication of a letter from an author who raised questions about Immuno's plans to conduct hepatitis research in Sierra Leone, West Africa, using chimpanzees caught in the wild. Prior to publication of the letter, Moor-Jankowski had sent the letter to Immuno AG for review and requested comments and a reply to be published along with the letter. The company rejected the opportunity to reply and threatened litigation. Moor-Jankowski suggested that Immuno AG contact the author for further information, but after no response was received from the company, the *Journal of Medical Primatology* published the letter. After extensive and costly legal proceedings (the publisher was uninsured), the Appellate Division of the Supreme Court of New York ruled that the statements contained in the letter were either opinion or factual statements that Immuno AG had failed to prove false. Immuno petitioned for hearing by the US Supreme Court, but that petition was denied in 1991.[12]

Publication is an essential element for a legal action of libel.[3(§5.02)] In this context, *publication* means that the alleged libelous communication was transmitted to a third party who read, saw, or heard the alleged libelous communication.[3(§5.02)]

Courts have distinguished between those who publish third-party information (ie, publishers) and those who provide facilities to third parties to transmit information (ie, online service providers). Editors and publishers of scientific journals, whether publishing information in print, online, or in both media, generally review, edit, and control the information that is transmitted and delivered, while online service providers may not provide such oversight and control of third-party postings.[6(p132)] In *Stratton Oakmont, Inc v Prodigy Services Co*,[13] the court held that even an online service provider could be held liable for a subscriber's defamatory statement because the online service provider exercised "sufficient control over its computer bulletin boards to render it a publisher with the same responsibilities as a newspaper." Thus, scientific journals are more vulnerable to libel suits than are online service providers because of the editorial control their editors typically exercise.

A publication is considered defamatory when it includes each of the following[3-7]:

- A substantially false statement concerning another
- Publication to a third party (*Note:* there are exceptions here, such as in publication of testimony made during judicial or legislative proceedings; see also 5.9.6, Republication and News Reporting)
- Fault amounting to at least "negligence" if involving a private individual (ie, failing to meet the minimum standards that a reasonable person would have been expected to meet in researching, fact checking, writing, reviewing, and publishing the statement) or "actual malice" if involving a public figure (ie, publishing with knowledge that the statement is false or with reckless disregard for the truth of the statement)

5.9.1 **Living Persons and Existing Entities.** A statement generally cannot be libelous unless it is "of and concerning" a living person or existing entity (eg, corporation, institution, or organization).[2,3,7] According to a 1992 case, *Gugliuzza v KCMC, Inc,* "once a person is dead, there is not extant reputation to injure or for the law to protect."[14] Even when the living person or entity is not named in the statement, if the person's or corporation's identity can be determined from other published facts, a case for libel can be made.[4(p150)]

5.9.2 **Public and Private Figures.** A public figure is a person who assumes a role of prominence in society, such as an elected official, a celebrity, or an infamous criminal. In cases of alleged libel, public figures are afforded less legal protection than private individuals.[3,7] In a 1964 case, *New York Times Co v Sullivan,*[10] the US Supreme Court determined that for a public official to prove defamation, the official must demonstrate that the alleged defamatory statement was made with "actual malice" (ie, with knowledge that the statement was false or with disregard for the truth of the statement) (see also 5.9, Defamation, Libel). A private figure is defined in the negative: someone who is not a public figure.[7] In contrast, a private individual need not prove malice, only negligence, to be successful in a libel suit.[3,4,6,7]

In legal settings, biomedical authors or researchers who publish might be considered "limited-purpose" public figures, for example, if they publish articles in an attempt to influence a matter of substantial public interest, a governmental agency decision, or legislation.[3(§5.05),7] In some cases, an author who publishes might be considered a limited-purpose public figure among the community represented by the readers of a specific publication (eg, journal, bulletin board, chat room).[6,15,16]

Answers to the following questions may aid in determining public figure status of an individual and vulnerability to a claim of defamation when a personal statement about an individual is published[3,4,7]:

- Is the person described someone who has assumed a role of prominence or notoriety?
- Does the content of the statement pertain to a matter of public controversy or public concern?
- If the statement refers to a public figure, does it contain references to the individual's public figure status (eg, the individual's job performance or public behavior)?

- If the statement refers to a public figure, will the connection between such references and the individual's public status be evident to a reasonable reader?
- If the reference is peripheral to the person's public figure status or responsibilities, does it involve nonrelevant, highly intimate, or embarrassing facts?

5.9.3 **Groups of Individuals.** Defamatory statements about groups of individuals are usually not legally actionable if the group is so large that no individual can be identified in the statements.[3,4] For example, broad statements about specific groups (eg, physicians) or entities (eg, the pharmaceutical industry) are not at risk for libel actions because no single individual or company is identifiable.

5.9.4 **Statements of Opinion.** Statements that contain pure opinion (ie, purely subjective judgment without assertion of fact) are not legally actionable because opinions cannot be proven true or false.[3(§5.08),5,17] However, an opinion that includes, asserts, or implies facts that are false and defamatory could result in liability.[18] As noted previously, publication of an expression of opinion about a public figure may be protected under the "fair comment" doctrine (see also 5.9.2, Public and Private Figures).[4,7] Fischer et al[3(§5.08)] offer the following questions to help distinguish statements of fact from statements of opinion:

- Can the statement be proved true or false?
- Are the facts on which the opinion is based fully disclosed to the reader?
- If not, are the facts on which the opinion is based obvious to a reasonable reader or readily available to the reader from other sources?
- Are both the disclosed and undisclosed facts on which the opinion is based substantially true?
- Does the context of the opinion suggest to a reasonable reader that it represents opinion and not fact?
- Have the statements that contain opinions been published in a manner that informs readers that they deal with opinion, commentary, or criticism (eg, a clearly identified editorial or opinion page)?

5.9.3 ***Editorials, Letters, and Reviews.*** In some publications, such as newspapers and popular magazines, editorials, correspondence, and critical reviews tend to alert the reader that the content is opinion. This is not always the case for scientific journals. No matter where the material is published, malicious criticism of an individual or entity could be considered defamatory, especially if it is demonstrated that such criticism was not based on facts.[7,18] However, criticism of a public figure or public institution or commercial entity may not be actionable if such criticism is scholarly and supported by evidence and documentation. Similarly, scholarly criticism of an individual's research, theory, opinion, or previous publication that is supported by evidence and documentation may not be actionable for libel.[15,16] In any case, editors and publishers should be cautious about statements critical of individuals or commercial entities made in editorials, letters, and reviews. Use of such phrases as "in my opinion" or "I believe" will not shield an author against an action for libel.[7] Whenever possible, authors of letters, editorials, and reviews in biomedical publications should support opinions, assertions, and interpretations with documentation and/or formal references, and editors/publishers should review all such material and require authors to provide appropriate documentation and references. Editors and publishers should consider obtaining legal review of material being considered for publication that contains potentially libelous statements. In addition, publishers should have liability insurance that covers the costs of defending against suits for libel. (See also 5.9.7, Defense Against Libel, and 5.9.8, Minimizing the Risk of Libel.)

Book Reviews. For reviews of books and other media (eg, CDs, videos, journals, and Web sites), well-documented critical comments about the book, media, or the work of an author, producer, editor, or publisher are generally acceptable, but critical comments about the author, producer, editor, or publisher should be avoided. In *Moldea v New York Times Co,*[19] the author of a book that received a disparaging review in the *New York Times* sued the paper for libel after trying and failing to get the *New York Times* to publish his rebuttal letter. The book review included a number of critical comments, including a statement that the book contained "too much sloppy journalism to trust the bulk of this book's 512 pages."[9] This comment was supported with specific examples of misspellings and allegations of mischaracterization of events.[9] After an initial decision in favor of the *New York Times,* an appeal that favored the author's claim, and an unusual reversal by the appeals court, the libel suit was dismissed. The final decision in this case reaffirmed impunity from libel suits for opinion pieces and provided a "workable test for analyzing allegedly defamatory statements of opinion"[9] (see the beginning of this section).

5.9.5 **Works of Fiction.** Fictional accounts are not actionable for defamation unless a reasonable reader believes that the story is depicting factual events and can identify the person bringing suit in the story.[3-7] Humor, satire, and parody may be exempt from defamation suits as long as they are clearly works of fiction.[3,7]

5.9.6 **Republication and News Reporting.** A publisher can be held liable for republishing a defamatory statement. For example, if a publisher reprinted a defamatory statement about a public figure knowing that the statement was false, the publisher could be held liable. Similarly, if the republished false statement was about a private figure, the publisher could be held liable for defamation even if the statement was published without knowledge of its falsity (ie, through negligence). Under the privilege of "fair reporting," an author can repeat a previously published defamatory statement if it is part of official proceedings (eg, a congressional debate or press conference) as long as the account is fair and accurate.[4,7] Under the privilege of "neutral reporting," an author may repeat a previously published defamatory statement as long as the second account is a neutral or balanced report of a public controversy or matter of legitimate public concern (see also 5.9.4, Statements of Opinion). Publishers, editors, and writers who rely on confidential sources for potentially defamatory statements are at increasing risk for libel action. For example, in the United States, shield laws, intended to protect news reporters from being legally forced to reveal identities of sources, vary by state, and their application has been challenged in a number of recent cases.[3(§5.09)]

5.9.7 **Defense Against Libel.** In the United States, truth is a defense against claims of libel in most cases (see also 5.9, Defamation, Libel). Aside from consideration of truth of damaging statements, some jurisdictions also consider whether damaging statements were made with intent to harm.[3§(5.09),4] As a result, editors should query authors about any statements that criticize or imply criticism of individuals or corporate entities and ask the authors to provide evidence or documentation to support such statements. If an editor is concerned about the risk vs benefit of publishing such statements, obtaining a legal review as part of the process of peer review is recommended. The legal review should be performed by an attorney with experience in media law. Even though legal review may result in delay and several requests for revision, it may help protect the editor and publisher from a libel claim. In addition, offering those criticized an opportunity to review the material before publication, if deemed appropriate by the editor, or to respond to the criticism after publication may reduce the risk of a successful claim.

Threats of litigation and fear of libel suits have kept some editors from meeting their ethical duties to authors, readers, and the public. For example, during the 1980s a number of medical journals declined to reprint retractions of articles by 2 separate researchers, Robert Slutsky and Stephen Breuning (even though the articles had been proven to be fraudulent and even after Breuning's federal indictment), because of fear that the journals would be liable for publishing statements impugning the work of Slutsky and Breuning.[20] Such defensive editorial practices should be avoided because they may impair the integrity of the journal and allow fraudulent research to continue to be read and cited. For example, allowing Slutsky and Breuning's fraudulent articles to remain in the literature without retraction was an injustice to the readers of those articles.[21] Biomedical editors and publishers should follow the statement on retractions from the International Committee of Medical Journal Editors[22] (see 5.4.4, Scientific Misconduct, Editorial Policy for Detecting and Handling Allegations of Scientific Misconduct).

Another case in biomedical publication involving a claim against the *Journal of Alcohol Studies* demonstrates the need for an editor's awareness of the risks of libel and the need for legal review of potentially defamatory material before acceptance for publication.[23] In this case, an author sued the *Journal of Alcohol Studies* claiming breach of contract after the journal did not publish an "accepted" manuscript. The editor had determined the manuscript to be libelous after acceptance but before publication. The journal decided to publish the manuscript following an agreement with the plaintiff/author that he would drop his lawsuit. The editor said he had no choice in light of the mounting legal fees. Ironically, a libel suit was never filed after publication of the article because the person about whom the potentially libelous statements were made believed that readers could determine that the statements made about him were not truthful.[23]

5.9.8 **Minimizing the Risk of Libel.** The suggestions in this section are offered to help authors, editors, and publishers reduce the risk of libel in biomedical publication. All statements of fact about individuals or commercial entities should be supported or documented and verified to be accurate in the context in which they were and are made. Similarly, statements of opinion should be supported, or based on documented facts, and should not be malicious. In addition, authors should disclose any conflicts of interest or concerns about the potential reactions of those criticized to the editor so that the editor and author work together to ensure responsible publication (see also 5.5,

Conflicts of Interest). Editors should consider offering those who are criticized in a submitted manuscript an opportunity to review the material of concern before publication, or to respond to the criticism after publication, or both. In addition, editors should consult experienced media attorneys when necessary, and publishers should have insurance covering claims for libel. None of these suggestions will ensure that a lawsuit—even if frivolous or groundless—will not be made, but they should help editors, authors, and publishers avoid situations in which such claims have merit.

5.9.9 **Demands to Correct, Retract, or Remove Libelous Information.** Demands to correct or retract allegedly libelous material should be handled carefully. Removal of libelous information in print is not possible, and the standard course of action has been to print corrections or retractions in an expeditious and prominent manner.[6,7] Online archives, which are considered part of the original publication in the United States (but not in other countries), may be corrected, edited, or removed, and continued posting of defamatory material in an online archive may increase the risk of liability for the author, editor, and publisher.[6] However, demands to remove libelous material must be carefully balanced against the need to preserve the integrity of the scientific record, and correction and retraction are always preferred over removal of content.[24,25] Editors should consider consulting a lawyer with expertise in media law to determine the best course of action.

If an allegation of defamation or threat to take legal action because of alleged defamation is determined to be frivolous or groundless, the editor should inform the person making the allegation that there is no merit to the allegation/threat and no further action should be taken. If the allegation is considered to have merit, the editor may wish to consider publishing a letter from the person or representative of the entity criticized and ask the author to provide for publication a letter of explanation or apology; or the editor may choose to publish a correction or a retraction. In each case, reciprocal linking should be established between any published letters, correction, or retraction and the original article. In rare and truly extraordinary circumstances, the editor may choose to remove or obscure the libelous material from an article or other online posting provided that a brief explanation of why the material has been removed or obscured is included and is made easily accessible. If the libelous material is so inextricably embedded in the context of an article that it cannot be partially removed or obscured, an entire article may need to be removed from the online archive provided that the bibliographic citation to the article remains intact and a brief explanation of why the article has been removed is included with or linked from the citation. In each of these cases, correction or retraction is highly preferred to changing or removal of content.[24,25]

In addition, republication (eg, reprints, e-prints, book collections) of articles containing defamatory material must be avoided, as these are not part of the original publication and republication of known libelous material may result in additional liability and damage claims.[6]

5.9.10 **Other Liability Concerns.** There are other sources of legal problems for publishers and editors that are beyond the scope of this manual. *Perle and Williams on Publishing Law*[3] and *Law of the Web: A Field Guide to Internet Publishing*[6] are good resources for information that address many of these problems, including issues related to copyright, patent, and trademark (see 5.6, Intellectual Property: Ownership, Access, Rights, and Management), privacy (see 5.8, Protecting Research Participants' and Patients' Rights in

Scientific Publication), advertising and liability (see 5.12, Advertisements, Advertorials, Sponsorship, Supplements, Reprints, and E-prints), circulation audits, subscription list fraud, taxation and accounting issues, and employment issues.

ACKNOWLEDGMENTS

Principal author: Annette Flanagin, RN, MA

I thank Wayne G. Hoppe, JD, and Maggie Mills, *JAMA* and *Archives* Journals, for reviewing and providing important suggestions for improvement of the manuscript; the following for reviewing and providing minor comments: Catherine D. DeAngelis, MD, MPH, *JAMA* and *Archives* Journals; Diana J. Mason, RN, PhD, *American Journal of Nursing*; and Povl Riis, MD, University of Copenhagen; and Sandra R. Schefris and Yolanda Davis, James S. Todd Memorial Library, American Medical Association, Chicago, Illinois, for bibliographic assistance.

REFERENCES

1. Lincoln A. Letter to Secretary Stanton, refusing to dismiss Postmaster General Montgomery Blair, July 18, 1864. In: Bartlett J. *Familiar Quotations*. 15th ed. Boston, MA: Little Brown & Co Inc; 1980:523.
2. Gifis SH. *Law Dictionary*. 5th ed. Hauppauge, NY: Barrons Educational Services Inc; 2003.
3. Fischer MA, Perle EG, Williams JT. *Perle and Williams on Publishing Law*. 3rd ed. Vol 1. New York, NY: Aspen Publishers; 2005.
4. Kirsch J. *Kirsch's Handbook of Publishing Law*. Los Angeles, CA: Acrobat Books; 1995.
5. Stubbs SE, Boyce WJ. The risks of libel in medical publishing. *Ann Allergy*. 1994;72(2):101-103.
6. Hart JD. *Law of the Web: A Field Guide to Internet Publishing*. Denver, CO: Bradford Publishing Co; 2003.
7. *AP Stylebook 2005*. New York, NY: Associated Press; 2005. http://www.apstylebook.com. Accessed December 1, 2005.
8. Chepesiuk R. Libel tourism chills investigative journalism: fear of libel suits deters some publishers from publishing books in Britain. *IPI Global Journalist*. http://www.globaljournalist.org/magazine/2004-2/libel-tourism.html. Second quarter 2004. Accessed January 21, 2006.
9. Hershey J. Casenote: if you can't say something nice, can you say anything at all? *Moldea v New York Times Co* and the importance of context in First Amendment law. 67 U Colo L Rev 705 (Summer 1996).
10. *New York Times Co v Sullivan,* 376 US 254, 280 (1964).
11. *Immuno AG v Moor-Jankowski,* 74 NY 2d 548, 556 (1989).
12. *Immuno AG v Moor-Jankowski,* 77 NY 2d 235 (1991).
13. *Stratton Oakmont, Inc v Prodigy Services Co,* No. 31063/94, NY Sup Ct (1995).
14. *Gugliuzza v KCMC, Inc,* 606 So2d 790, 20 Media La Rptr 1866 (La 1992).
15. Swartz BE. Defamation law: implications for medical authors. *Plast Reconstr Surg*. 2003;111(1):498-499.
16. *Ezrailson v Rohrich*, 09-01-038-CV, 17 TLCS 1075 (2001).
17. *Gertz v Robert Welch Inc*, 418 US 323, 347 (1974).
18. *Milkovich v Lorain Journal Co*, 497 US 1 (1990).
19. *Moldea v New York Times Co,* 793 F Supp 335, 337 (DDC 1992); *Moldea I, supra* note 12; *Moldea II, supra* note 12.

20. LaFollette MC. *Stealing Into Print: Fraud, Plagiarism, and Misconduct in Scientific Publishing*. Los Angeles: University of California Press; 1992.
21. Whitely WP, Rennie D, Hafner AW. The scientific community's response to evidence of fraudulent publication; the Robert Slutsky case. *JAMA*. 1994;272(2):170-173.
22. International Committee of Medical Journal Editors. Uniform Requirements for Manuscripts Submitted to Biomedical Journals: Writing and Editing for Biomedical Publication. http://www.icmje.org. Updated February 2006. Accessed September 10, 2006.
23. MacDonald KA. Rutgers journal forced to publish paper despite threats of libel suit. *Chronicle Higher Educ*. September 13, 1989:A5.
24. International Association of Scientific, Technical, and Medical Publishers. Preservation of the objective record of science: an STM guideline. http://www.stm-assoc.org/documents-statements-public-co. March 2006. Accessed September 10, 2006.
25. International Federation of Library Associations and Institutions. IFLA/IPA Joint Statement on Removal of Articles From Databases. http://www.ifla.org/VI/4/admin/joint-ifla_ipa-statementJuly2006.htm. Accessed October 27, 2006.

The freedom of the press is one of the greatest bulwarks of liberty.

George Mason[1]

5.10 Editorial Freedom and Integrity.

Editorial Freedom and Integrity. *Editorial freedom* implies a range of independence, from complete absence of external restraint and coercion to merely a sense of not being unduly hampered or frustrated.[2] *Integrity* is the state of honesty, credibility, incorruptibility, and accountability.[2] A biomedical journal has editorial integrity if it adheres to these values, but different journals have different levels of editorial freedom. The First Amendment of the US Constitution affirms several freedoms, including the freedom of the press.[3] Thus, communication through the US press or other media is a right that should not be interfered with by the government, other institutions, or individuals.[4] Many countries guarantee similar freedoms of the press.[5] Freedom of the press is a foundation for editorial independence, "which is the distinct right of the editor to publish any material that passes defined criteria for quality and that fits within the mission of the publication, without suffering undue interference from others."[6]

A journal's editorial independence must be balanced against the need for appropriate authority, responsibility, and accountability as well as trust between the editor and the journal's many stakeholders: readers, authors, reviewers, publishers, owners, subscribers, advertisers, and others[6] (see also 5.11, Editorial Responsibilities, Roles, Procedures, and Policies). The level of editorial freedom differs among different biomedical journals, from maximum independence for those peer-reviewed journals in which the editor has complete authority and responsibility for the journal, its content (including all editorial and advertising content), reuse of its content, and use of the journal name/logo, to no independence for those journals that are not peer reviewed and in which all authority and responsibility rests completely with others (eg, publishers or owners). Journals that are published primarily to serve business, political, or other concerns of their owners are known as "house organs."[2] For some biomedical journals and editors, the level of editorial freedom may be best described as somewhere between complete editorial independence and no independence. Furthermore, editorial freedom may be assumed to exist by an editor, and the journal's readers, until and unless a major conflict occurs. A 1999 survey of the editors of 33 peer-reviewed medical journals owned by professional societies (10 journals represented in the International Committee of Medical Journal Editors and a random sample of 23 specialty journals with high impact factors) found that 23 (70%) of the 33 editors reported that they had complete editorial freedom, and the remainder reported that they had a high level of freedom.[7] However, many of these editors reported having received at least some pressure in recent years over editorial content from the professional society's leadership (42%), senior staff (30%), or rank-and-file members (39%).[7]

There are numerous examples of editors and journals battling incursions from interpersonal, social, political, and economic forces. Editors have been dismissed from their posts and journals have ceased publication after a mere "stroke of the editorial pen."[8] In one case, the *Irish Medical Journal* was voted out of existence in 1987 after the editor published an editorial against physician strikes that angered some influential members of the Irish Medical Organisation.[8,9]

During the last 10 years, editors of several leading general medical journals have been unwillingly removed from their positions after publishing articles that were considered inappropriate by various external forces (eg, owners, publishers) and for having disagreements with owners or publishers about the editor's level of autonomy and authority over the journal's content and the journal's name and brand (eg, logo).[10-26] In each of these cases, long-term struggles between the editors and the owners of the journals resulted in loss of trust between the parties, and because of a lack of effective protective oversight and governance and apparent lack of an effective system for conflict resolution, precipitate decisions to remove the editors resulted in widespread criticism of the owners and threats to the integrity and continued existence of the journals. (See 5.10.1, Maintaining Editorial Freedom: Cases of Editorial Interference and the Rationale for Mission, Trust, and Effective Oversight and Governance.)

An earlier example of a medical editor credited for his struggles to maintain editorial freedom is Hugh Clegg, editor of the *BMJ* from 1944 to 1965. In 1956, Clegg wrote an unsigned editorial entitled "The Gold-headed Cane," in which he castigated the president of the Royal College of Physicians for taking office for the seventh successive year. He also admonished the college for its failure to recognize the modern welfare state and its lack of attention to postgraduate medical education.[4,27] With much difficulty, Clegg kept his editorial position and freedom and purposely published a reply from the president that rebutted all of Clegg's criticisms. Clegg believed that medical editors are the protectors of the conscience of the profession, and he is well known for his assertion that editors who maintain this ideal will often find themselves in trouble. This trouble may come in the form of incursions into editorial freedom, which editors must be able to defend.

Editors of biomedical journals that have editorial freedom must have complete authority for determining all editorial content of their publications.[6,28-33] (*Note:* Unless otherwise dictated by a journal's specific mission, this may not be the case for journals that are house organs or that have minimal editorial freedom.) While many stakeholders may offer useful input and advice, editorial decisions must be free from restraint or interference from the publication's owner, publisher, advertisers, sponsors, subscribers, authors, editorial board or publication committee members, reviewers, and readers. Owners, publishers, boards, and publication committees may have the right to select, hire, evaluate, and dismiss the editor, but they should not interfere with day-to-day editorial decisions and policies.[6,15,29,30,33]

Without a clear delineation of editorial freedom and the authority to maintain it, an editor might not be able to ensure the integrity of the publication. Thus, owners, publishers, and editors must have a clear and mutually understood definition of the editor's level of editorial freedom, authority, responsibility, and accountability.[6,30] Editors of journals with complete editorial freedom should not comply with external pressure from any party—including owners, publishers, advertisers, sponsors, authors, reviewers, and readers—that may compromise their autonomy or their journal's integrity.[29,30] Examples of such inappropriate pressures include, but are not limited to, the following:

- Pressure from an owner or a politically powerful or motivated individual or group on the editor to avoid publishing certain types of articles or to publish a specific article
- Pressure or requirement of an editor by a publisher or owner to modify or suppress specific content before publication
- Demand from an owner or publisher to censor or remove published content deemed controversial or contrary to the owner's position or that of an another organization or entity allied with owner
- Demand from an owner or publisher or external person or organization to have access to confidential editorial or peer review records (see also 5.7.1, Confidentiality, Confidentiality During Editorial Evaluation and Peer Review and After Publication)
- Demand from an author or group of authors to bypass the journal's standard editorial and peer review processes and publish their manuscript without review or revision (eg, a society demanding acceptance and publication without review or revision of its meeting abstracts, proceedings, or papers)
- Attempt by an author or peer reviewer to have an editorial decision reversed by threatening the journal's editor or owner
- The use or repurposing of the journal's content or name by the publisher without the editor's consent or in a manner that could harm the journal's integrity
- Request by an advertiser to insert an advertisement next to an article about or related to the advertised product or a threat to withdraw advertising support because of publication of a specific article (see also 5.12, Advertisements, Advertorials, and Sponsored Supplements)
- An advertiser or publisher's attempt to publish an advertisement or sponsored content disguised as editorial content (advertorial) (see also 5.12, Advertisements, Advertorials, Sponsorship, Supplements, Reprints, and E-prints)
- A publisher demanding information about accepted or pending editorial content in advance of publication to sell that information to advertisers/sponsors or for other commercial purposes

- A sponsor attempting to exert influence over editorial decisions or selecting specific content for publication (eg, sponsored supplements) (see also 5.12, Advertisements, Advertorials, Sponsorship, Supplements, Reprints, and E-prints)
- A publisher demanding publication of an advertisement that the editor deems inappropriate (see 5.12, Advertisements, Advertorials, Sponsorship, Supplements, Reprints, and E-prints)
- Request from a company to an editor to purchase reprints of an article under consideration but not yet accepted for publication
- Demands by a commercial entity or governmental agency to publish or censor specific content
- Compliance with governmental or other external policy to not consider manuscripts from authors based on their nationality, ethnicity, race, political beliefs, or religion (see 5.11, Editorial Responsibilities, Roles, Procedures, and Policies)
- Pressure from a news organization or journalist to publish information about a journal article before the news embargo is lifted (see also 5.13.3, Release of Information to the Public and Journal/Author Relations With the News Media, Embargo)

Editors may need to educate and remind the journal's various stakeholders about the fundamentals of editorial freedom and its direct relation to the publication's integrity.

5.10.1 **Maintaining Editorial Freedom: Cases of Editorial Interference and the Rationale for Mission, Trust, and Effective Oversight and Governance.** Interference with editorial freedom has affected several prominent medical journals and has been well documented in the biomedical literature and the press. However, many other cases of such interference have not been made public or are discussed only anecdotally, privately, or via restricted electronic mailing lists. The experiences of *JAMA*, the *New England Journal of Medicine*, and the *Canadian Medical Association Journal* (*CMAJ*) are presented here for the following reasons: there is sufficient literature documenting the relevant events; effective protective oversight mechanisms and governance plans were lacking or insufficient at the time; and the mechanisms for protection of editorial freedom that were developed as a result of these events are informative and may be helpful for other journals, editors, publishers, and owners.

***The Case of* JAMA.** Since 1982, George D. Lundberg, MD, had served as editor in chief of *JAMA,* a weekly, peer-reviewed, general medical journal, and the *Archives* specialty journals that are owned and published by the American Medical Association (AMA). *JAMA* had operated under a set of goals and objectives that were developed by Lundberg and the journal's editorial staff and that were approved by the journal's editorial board and AMA management.[34] These goals and objectives had protected the editor on several occasions from external pressures to restrict the journal's editorial freedom, and in 1993 the AMA House of Delegates (the policy-setting and governing body of the association) passed a resolution reaffirming editorial independence for all of its scientific journals.[35] Although *JAMA* had a defined mission that included editorial freedom that had been publicly supported by its owner, it did not have sufficient oversight and a governance plan in place to help promote a trust

Box 1. Editorial Governance Plan for *JAMA*[38,39]

1. There will be a seven (7) member Journal Oversight Committee (JOC). This committee will function and be recognized not only as a system to evaluate the Editor in Chief but also as a buffer between the Editor in Chief and AMA management and a system to foster objective consideration of the inevitable issues that arise between a journal and its parent body.
2. The JOC will prepare an annual evaluation of the Editor in Chief, which will be reported to the AMA executive vice president (EVP) and to the Board of Trustees of the AMA. The Committee will have the charge to evaluate the performance of the Editor in Chief on the basis of objective criteria, and deliver that evaluation on an annual basis to the EVP and Board of Trustees of the AMA. The JOC will be responsible for determining the criteria for evaluation of the Editor in Chief. These criteria will be established in writing and made available to each member of the JOC, the *JAMA* Editorial Board, the Editor in Chief, and the EVP and approved by the Board of Trustees of the AMA. The *JAMA* Editorial Board will be solicited for input to the evaluation process by the Committee. Correspondence about the performance of the Editor in Chief or *JAMA* received from constituent groups will be shared with the Committee. The Editor in Chief will be offered a 5-year contract. If the Editor in Chief is dismissed during the term of the employment contract, other than for cause, the contract will be paid in full. Should such dismissal occur in year 5 of the contract, the minimum payment to the Editor in Chief shall be 12 months' salary.
3. The JOC will be charged, in addition, with reviewing and, if necessary, making additional recommendations to the AMA EVP and Board concerning governance and structural reforms necessary to ensure the AMA Journals' editorial independence. For this purpose the Editor in Chief and Vice President for Publishing will serve as advisors to the committee. This function will be ongoing.
4. The 7 members of the JOC will include 1 member of AMA senior management, 1 member from outside the AMA with publishing business experience, and 5 members representing the scientific, editorial, peer-reviewer, contributor, and medical communities. The Committee members shall serve 3-year staggered terms. A Committee member may serve no more than 2 terms.
5. No member of the JOC may be an AMA employee except for the member from AMA Senior Management. No AMA employee may be Chair of the committee, who shall be elected by the JOC.
6. Nominations for the first set of JOC members will be forwarded to the AMA Board by the Editor Search Committee, which will also recommend the initial term of each member.
7. JOC members are to be selected by the AMA Board only from a list of recommended persons submitted by the JOC. Three names per position will

Box 1. Editorial Governance Plan for *JAMA*[38,39] *(cont)*

be recommended by the JOC. In the event that the Board selects none of the three, additional names would be recommended by the JOC, as necessary. Members of the JOC can only be appointed or removed by a two-thirds supermajority vote of the AMA Board of Trustees in the exercise of its oversight function.

8. Any proposal to dismiss the Editor in Chief for any reason shall be brought before the JOC for evaluation and a formal vote. The recommendations and views of the JOC shall be presented to the AMA Board along with the recommendation and views of the EVP. A supermajority (two-thirds) vote of the AMA Board would be required for dismissal of the Editor in Chief.
9. The Editor in Chief will continue to report to the EVP only for business and financial operations. The Editor in Chief will not report to management for any aspect of the editorial content of *JAMA* or the *Archives* Journals or other AMA publications under his/her jurisdiction. Editorial independence of the Editor in Chief will be absolutely protected and respected by AMA management. In order to exercise its evaluative functions, the JOC will have full access to financial information including revenue and expense statements, budgets, and actual results. In order to have access to this proprietary information, each member of the JOC who receives it will execute the AMA's standard Confidentiality and Conflict of Interest Agreements.
10. The Editor in Chief will have total responsibility for the editorial content of *JAMA* and responsibility for the performance of the *Archives* Editors and other AMA publications under his/her jurisdiction. AMA management recognizes and fully accepts the necessity of editorial independence for the Editor in Chief at all times.

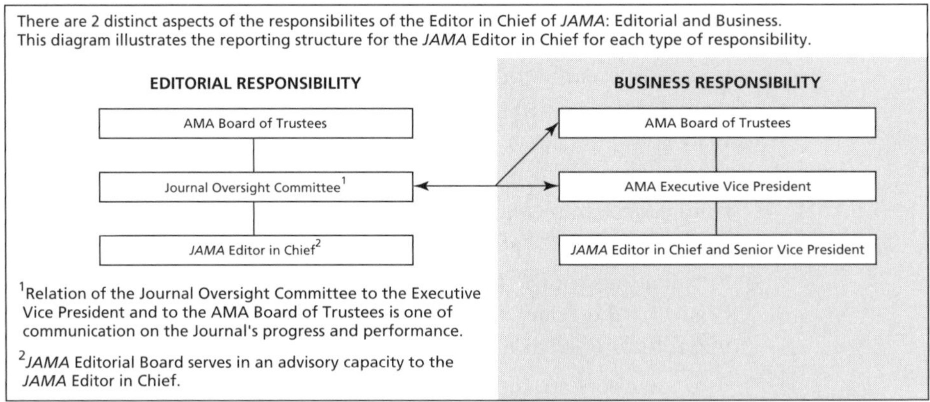

Figure. Reporting structure for *JAMA*'s Editor in Chief. Reprinted from *JAMA*. 2004;291(1):109.[39]

2000, Jeffrey M. Drazen, MD, was appointed editor in chief, and it was reported that the editorial freedoms negotiated previously by Angell would remain.[40]

***The Case of the* Canadian Medical Association Journal (CMAJ).** Since 1996, John Hoey, MD, had served as editor in chief of the *CMAJ*, a weekly, peer-reviewed general medical journal owned by the Canadian Medical Association. In 2006, the CMA abruptly fired Hoey and the journal's senior deputy editor, Anne Marie Todkill.[25,26] Initial public reasons from the publisher and CMA leadership for the dismissals were to "freshen" the *CMAJ* and because of "irreconcilable differences" between the editor in chief and the CMA, but no specific differences were cited.[25,26] While the CMA denied that the decisions had anything to do with editorial independence, Hoey, other editors, editorial board members, and members of the journal's oversight committee have all described several examples of censorship and interference with the *CMAJ* by CMA leaders and executives dating back to 2001 or earlier.[25,26,41-43]

In 2001, *CMAJ* published an editorial supporting medical use of marijuana, which contradicted the CMA's position and for which the CMA's general counsel complained to Hoey.[25] In 2002, the *CMAJ* published an editorial criticizing Quebec physicians for not properly staffing an emergency department after a patient with a myocardial infarction died while being transported from an emergency department that had closed at midnight to a second open emergency department.[25] Members of the CMA board called the editorial irresponsible, and the CMA president called for the editorial to be retracted. The *CMAJ* editorial board responded that the CMA was threatening the *CMAJ*'s editorial independence.[25,42] Following these incidents, a journal oversight committee was established in 2002. However, the oversight committee's roles and functions were unclear and interpreted differently by the CMA leadership, the editor in chief, and even the chair of the committee.[25]

In late 2004, the CMA had reorganized its publishing services and placed the ownership and direction of the *CMAJ* under a subsidiary, CMA Holdings Inc.[44] This change reduced the editor in chief's contact with the CMA and increased his interactions with the holding company and publisher, whose primary objective was profit.[41,43] However, this change did not decrease the CMA's attempts to influence the editorial direction and decisions of the journal. In late 2005 and early 2006, 2 other incidents of interference and censorship by CMA leadership and executives occurred.[25,26,41] In one case, a *CMAJ* news story reported on the difficulty Canadian women had in obtaining nonprescription emergency contraception (Plan B) from Canadian pharmacists. Apparently, the Canadian Pharmacists Association complained to the CMA's chief executive officer and objected to *CMAJ*'s plan to run this news story after one of the *CMAJ* reporters interviewed an executive with the association. The CMA's chief executive officer took the objections to the *CMAJ* publisher, who told Hoey not to run the news story. Faced with what was thought to be an unreasonable demand and to avoid a crisis, the editors and reporters then modified the news story to address some of the objections and a revised article was published.[25,26,41] An unsigned editorial was subsequently published in the *CMAJ* to alert readers to the incident of editorial interference and to "set in motion a process to ensure the future editorial independence of the journal."[45]

The second case of such interference involved a *CMAJ* news story that was critical of a Canadian public health official. The news story was published in the online version of *CMAJ* on February 7, 2006, and was subsequently removed from the Web site.[41] On February 20, Hoey and Todkill were fired, and 2 days later, a revised version of the original story was posted online that was less critical of the health official and more supportive of and beneficial to the CMA.[41]

During this time, Hoey had lost confidence in the journal's oversight committee and asked an ad hoc committee to review these events.[25,26] The ad hoc committee faulted the editors for modifying the news story on Plan B before it was published and for failing to follow the appropriate channel for conflicts (ie, the journal's oversight committee).[41] However, the ad hoc committee found more serious fault with the CMA for "blatant interference with the publication of a legitimate report" and concluded that the "*CMAJ*'s editorial autonomy is to an important degree illusory."[41]

Following the abrupt dismissals of Hoey and Todkill, the remaining editors, led by acting editor Stephen Choi, MD, published an editorial in protest of the firings.[46] Choi and colleagues drafted a proposal that included editorial independence for the *CMAJ* and aimed to ensure that the CMA and the publisher would not make decisions about editorial content.[25] The CMA did not agree to the proposal, and Choi and another editor resigned.[25] Other editors and most of the editorial board also resigned, and there were calls from academic leaders not to send papers or serve as peer reviewers for the journal.[24,47,48] The journal's former editor in chief, Bruce P. Squires, MD, was asked to serve as acting editor, but under pressure from editors of other journals, he too was unable to serve unless the CMA would agree to the journal's editorial independence.[25]

Like the events at *JAMA* and the *New England Journal of Medicine*, the abrupt firing of *CMAJ*'s editors and the refusal of the CMA to recognize the journal's editorial independence resulted in widespread news coverage of the conflicts, and a number of other leading journals published articles in support of the *CMAJ* editors.[22,23,25,49] In the wake of such criticism, in March 2006 the CMA announced the establishment of a panel to assess the journal's governance and management and agreed to an interim plan granting the editor in chief total responsibility for editorial content. With this plan in place, Noni MacDonald, MD, agreed to serve as interim editor and Squires agreed to serve as editor emeritus. The *CMAJ* governance review panel released its final report on July 14, 2006.[44] The report contained 25 recommendations, all of which were accepted by the CMA.[50-52] The recommendations included the following:

- Assurance that the editor in chief would have editorial independence
- Amendment of the *CMAJ*'s mission statement to enshrine the "principle of editorial integrity, independent of any special interests"
- Confirmation that the CMA has no right to alter any editorial content, but should be given the same advance notice of potentially controversial content that is given to the news media (see also 5.13.3, Release of Information to the Public and Journal/Author Relations With the News Media, Embargo)
- Proposal that the CMA take back direct ownership of the *CMAJ* from its for-profit holding company
- Proposal that the *CMAJ* editor in chief have separate and discrete reporting structures for editorial and business matters (ie, the editor in chief has access to the CMA Board of Directors if needed to defend or explain editorial positions or other concerns that cannot be resolved through administrative mechanisms such as the journal's oversight committee; and the editor in chief reports directly to an officer

of the CMA rather than to the publisher about the journal's business matters, and the publisher reports to the same officer)

- A recommendation for a reconstituted journal oversight committee that permits it to more effectively help resolve potential disputes between the journal's owner, publisher, and editor in chief

For more details on the makeup and responsibilities of the *CMAJ*'s oversight committee and the panel's other recommendations, see the *CMAJ* Governance Review Panel's final report.[44] In January 2007, Paul C. Hébert, MD, was appointed editor in chief of the *CMAJ* with assurance of the journal's independence as outlined in the *CMAJ* Governance Review Panel's report.[53]

5.10.2 Ensuring a Trust Relationship Between Journal Editors, Publishers, and Owners. As described by Davies and Rennie,[6] the relationship between editors and publishers/owners is interdependent and must be based on mutual trust. However, there are bound to be uncertainties, concerns, and occasional conflicts that could threaten the trust relationship.[6] To maintain trust, a formal agreement between the editor and owner should specify each party's expectations and the mission of the journal (for example, see *JAMA*'s governance plan[38,39] and Key and Critical Objectives[54] reproduced in Box 2). If these expectations are not formalized in a governance plan or other document, are not mutually understood, or are intentionally disregarded (as happened in the cases described above), either party (but usually the owner) "may seek new (and possibly costly) mechanisms of accountability, reassurance, and control,"[6] which would result in loss of trust and potentially serious damage to the integrity, credibility, and reputation of both the journal and the owner.

Uncertainty, concerns, and disputes are best resolved informally through reciprocally open communication between the editor and publisher/owner and by maintaining a trust relationship. However, formal procedures for conflict resolution must be in place in the event that a dispute cannot be resolved informally.[6] These procedures should rely on the journal's mission and objectives to direct the assessment of the dispute, should require measured consideration of the facts involved (with appropriate evidence), and should not result in hasty decisions that do not consider the outcomes of such decisions for the editor, owner, and journal (see, for example, *JAMA*'s governance plan). In the cases described in the previous section, the continued existence of each journal was suddenly and severely put at risk because there was no effective, independent mechanism to help achieve resolution of conflict, or, if resolution proved impossible, allow time for an orderly and dignified change of editors. Such an orderly system and buffer and, if all else fails, such an orderly transition best serves the interests of journals, owners, publishers, and editors.[6]

The following recommendations, many of which are supported by the International Committee of Medical Journal Editors,[29] World Association of Medical Editors,[30] Council of Science Editors,[31] and UK Committee on Publication Ethics,[32] may help editors, publishers, and owners develop policies for maintaining editorial freedom for their publications. Such policies should be regularly reviewed and made publicly available to the extent possible. For example, an individual editor's contract would not be made public, but a general description of the editor's level of authority, responsibility, and accountability can be published along with the journal's mission

Box 2. *JAMA*'s Key and Critical Objectives[54]

Key Objective

To promote the science and art of medicine and the betterment of the public health.

Critical Objectives

1. To maintain the highest standards of editorial integrity independent of any special interests
2. To publish original, important, well-documented, peer-reviewed articles on a diverse range of medical topics
3. To provide physicians with continuing education in basic and clinical science to support informed clinical decisions
4. To enable physicians to remain informed in multiple areas of medicine, including developments in fields other than their own
5. To improve health and health care internationally by elevating the quality of medical care, disease prevention, and research
6. To foster responsible and balanced debate on issues that affect medicine and health care
7. To anticipate important issues and trends in medicine and health care
8. To inform readers about nonclinical aspects of medicine and public health, including the political, philosophic, ethical, legal, environmental, economic, historical, and cultural
9. To recognize that, in addition to these specific objectives, the journal has a social responsibility to improve the total human condition and to promote the integrity of science
10. To achieve the highest level of ethical medical journalism and to produce a publication that is timely, credible, and enjoyable to read

in an editorial, on the journal's masthead, or elsewhere (eg, see the governance plans for *JAMA*[38,39] and the *CMAJ*[44]). These recommendations are offered to help journals protect against threats to editorial freedom and integrity, but even if all of these recommendations are followed, they will not provide absolute immunity from such threats.

Complete editorial freedom is recommended for all peer-reviewed biomedical journals because it ensures the highest level of editorial quality, credibility, and integrity. However, it is recognized that not all journals operate under complete editorial freedom, and achieving all of the elements necessary for complete independence may not be possible or desirable for some journals. Thus, these recommendations are provided for peer-reviewed journals with complete editorial freedom (highly preferred) and those journals with limited editorial freedom.

- The editor should have a written contract or job description that clearly defines the editor's duties, rights, level of authority, responsibility, accountability, term of appointment, relationship to the publication's owner, reporting relationship, oversight and governance plan, objective criteria for evaluating the performance of the editor and journal, rights if removed from the position before term expiration, and procedures for conflict resolution. An explicit and mutually accepted definition of the editor's authority, responsibility, and accountability before the editor accepts the position will enable the editor to make an informed decision about accepting the position. Editors should carefully consider the ramifications of signing any nondisclosure agreements that would prevent them from speaking publicly if unwillingly removed from their positions.

- A governance plan should be in place that defines oversight and evaluation policies and procedures for the editor, conflict resolution mechanisms for the editor and owner of the journal, and the level of editorial freedom provided the editor and the journal. This plan should be published or otherwise made publicly available.
- Ideally, as in journals with complete editorial freedom, the editor should have direct access to the highest level of management in the organization or company that owns the publication. If this is not possible, as in journals with limited editorial freedom, the editor's line of authority and reporting relationship should be specified in a formal agreement.
- All journals should have a published and easily accessible mission statement that clearly defines the journal's goals and objectives; for journals with editorial freedom, the mission statement should include explicit reference to editorial freedom. The mission statement should serve as guide for the editorial direction of the journal and should be relied on by the editor, editorial board, and members of the oversight or governance body when conflicts or disputes arise; it should be reviewed regularly by the editor and editorial board.
- An independent editorial oversight committee may help the editor establish and maintain the specified level of editorial freedom and resolve conflicts. To be independent, this committee's chair should not be a representative of the owner's employed, appointed, or elected leadership, and representation of the owner's employed, appointed, or elected leadership on the oversight committee should be limited (ideally to a single individual), or at most should have fewer voting positions on the committee than would constitute a majority. While this may require a different appointment procedure for some societies, the importance of an independent oversight committee for helping to maintain the journal's integrity and manage contentious conflicts cannot be overstated. *Note:* An oversight committee differs from an editorial board, which serves to advise the editor on editorial content and policies (see 5.11.10, Editorial Responsibilities, Roles, Procedures, and Policies, Role of the Editorial Board).
- In journals with complete editorial freedom, editors should have complete authority to hire, evaluate, and dismiss all editorial staff as well as the authority to appoint, evaluate, and dismiss editorial board members and peer reviewers (see 5.11, Editorial Responsibilities, Roles, Procedures, and Policies). If this arrangement is not possible for all editorial staff (eg, manuscript editors or other editorial staff employed, provided, or outsourced by the publisher), editors should at a minimum be able to review and evaluate their performance. For journals with limited editorial freedom in which the owner may make recommendations about editorial board members or

peer reviewers, the editor should have final authority to approve their appointment, evaluate their performance, and terminate their appointment.

- The editor should have the opportunity to interview and comment on candidates for a new publisher being considered during the editor's term. The publisher should have the opportunity to interview and comment on candidates for a new editor being considered by the journal owner and/or search committee. For society-owned journals using outside publishers, editors should be involved in the selection and performance review of the publisher and other external commercial companies or vendors (eg, advertising, marketing, and research agencies; printers; suppliers of editorial systems; and online vendors/hosts) as well as decisions to renew or terminate publishing agreements.
- In journals with complete editorial freedom, editors should have complete authority over use and reuse of the name, logo, and content of the journal in print, online, and other media. Content includes editorial content, covers, mastheads, design, formatting, online features and linking, and approval of advertising and sponsorship. While the editor must not be involved in the business (ie, selling) of advertisements and sponsorship, the editor should have authority over policies on appropriate types of advertisements and their placement and over policies on sponsorship activities (see also 5.12, Advertisements, Advertorials, Sponsorship, Supplements, Reprints, and E-prints). At a minimum, for journals with limited editorial freedom, the editor's level of authority and responsibility for content should be specified in a governance plan, contract, or other formal document.
- Owners and publishers should not interfere in the evaluation, review, selection, or editing of editorial content that is under the authority of the editor. For journals with complete editorial freedom, this pertains to all content. All changes and corrections made to content during production and publishing and after publication should be reviewed and approved by the editor or the editorial team reporting to the editor and production staff involved in producing the content, but not the journal's owner, publisher, or sales and marketing staff.
- Editors and owners should establish mutually understood policies and procedures that guard against the influence of external commercial and political interests as well as personal self-interest on editorial decisions (see also 5.5, Conflicts of Interest).
- Editors should be accountable for their editorial decisions, which should be based on the validity and credibility of the content and its relevance and importance to readers, not the commercial success of the journal or political interests of owners or other groups. Editors' decisions and communications with stakeholders should be based on competence, fairness, confidentiality, expeditiousness, and courtesy (see also 5.11, Editorial Responsibilities, Roles, Procedures, and Policies). However, editors need to understand the requirements for financial management and viability of their journals and should publish content that attracts readers, authors, peer reviewers, subscribers, advertisers, and other stakeholders. *Note:* This does not mean that stakeholders should determine specific editorial content to publish or not to publish. For journals to maintain editorial freedom and integrity, editors should be free to express critical but responsible views without fear of retribution,

even if these views are controversial or conflict with the commercial goals of the publisher or the policies, positions, or objectives of the owner or external forces.

- For journals with complete editorial freedom, the journal should publish a statement about its editorial independence and a prominently placed disclaimer that identifies and separates a publication's owner and sponsor from the editorial staff and content. For example, *JAMA* regularly publishes its objectives[53] (which include "to maintain the highest standards of editorial integrity independent of any special interests") and a statement that it is editorially independent of its owner and publisher, and 2 disclaimers that differentiate the journal from its owner. The following appears in the Table of Contents of each issue:

  > All articles published, including editorials, letters, and book reviews, represent the opinions of the authors and do not reflect the official policy of the American Medical Association or the institutions with which the author is affiliated, unless this is clearly specified.

  In addition, the following notice appears on the editorial opinion page:

  > Editorials represent the opinions of the authors and *JAMA* and not those of the American Medical Association.

  For journals that have limited or no editorial authority over specific types or sections of content (eg, pages reserved for the owning society/association or other content stipulated to be out of the editor's control), authority and responsibility for such content should be made clear to readers.

- Owners have the right to hire and fire editors. However, except for provisions contractually stipulated (eg, term limits or contract expiration), owners should dismiss editors only for substantial reasons that are incompatible with a position of trust, such as editorial mismanagement, scientific misconduct, fiscal malfeasance, undisclosed conflicts of interest that result in biased editorial decisions, unsupported changes to the long-term editorial direction or stated mission of the journal, criminal behavior, or specific activities that violate terms of a formal agreement.

- Editors should inform editorial board members, advisory committee members, owners, publishers, and editorial and publishing staff of the journal's policies on editorial freedom.

- Editors should publish articles on editorial freedom when appropriate and should alert readers and the wider international community to major transgressions against editorial freedom.

ACKNOWLEDGMENTS

Principal author: Annette Flanagin, RN, MA

I thank the following for reviewing and providing substantial comments to improve the manuscript: Catherine D. DeAngelis, MD, MPH, *JAMA* and *Archives* Journals; John Hoey, MD; and Drummond Rennie, MD, *JAMA*; and the following for reviewing and providing minor comments: Michael Callaham, MD, University of California, San Francisco; Terri S. Carter, *Archives of Surgery*; Wayne G. Hoppe, JD, *JAMA* and *Archives* Journals; Trevor Lane, MA, DPhil, University of Hong Kong; and June Robinson, MD, *Archives of Dermatology*.

REFERENCES

1. Mason G. *Virginia Bill of Rights*. Article 12. June 12, 1776.
2. *Merriam-Webster OnLine*. http://www.m-w.com. Accessed February 26, 2006.
3. The US Constitution Online. http://www.usconstitution.net/const.html#Am1. Accessed February 26, 2006.
4. Edwards RB, Erde EL. Freedom and coercion. In: Reich TW, ed. *Encyclopedia of Bioethics*. Vol 2. New York, NY: Macmillan Publishing Co; 1995:883.
5. Reporters Without Borders. Worldwide Press Freedom Index. http://www.rsf.org/rubrique.php3?id_rubrique=554. Accessed February 26, 2006.
6. Davies HTO, Rennie D. Independence, governance, and trust: redefining the relationship between *JAMA* and the AMA. *JAMA*. 1999;281(24):2344-2346.
7. Davis RM, Mullner M. Editorial independence at medical journals owned by professional associations: a survey of editors. *Sci Eng Ethics*. 2002;8(4):513-528.
8. Death of a journal. *Lancet*. 1987;2(8573):1442.
9. O'Brien E. Closure of the *Irish Medical Journal*. *Ir Med J*. 1987;80(5):247-248.
10. Goldsmith MF. George D. Lundberg ousted as *JAMA* editor. *JAMA*. 1999;281(5):403.
11. Tanne JH. *JAMA*'s editor fired over sex article. *BMJ*. 1999;318(7178):213.
12. Smith R. The firing of brother George. *BMJ*. 1999;318(7178):210.
13. Horton R. The sacking of *JAMA*. *Lancet*. 1999;353(9149):252-253.
14. Davidoff F. The making and unmaking of a journal. *Ann Intern Med*. 1999;130(9):774-775.
15. Kassirer JP. Editorial independence. *N Engl J Med*. 1999;340(21):1671-1672.
16. *JAMA* Editors, AMA *Archives* Journals Editors, *JAMA* Editorial Board Members. *JAMA* and editorial independence. *JAMA*. 1999;281(5):460.
17. Horton R. An unwilling exit from the *NEJM*. *Lancet*. 1999;354(9176):358.
18. Kassirer JP. Goodbye, for now. *N Engl J Med*. 1999;341(9):686.
19. Kassirer JP. The departure of Jerome P. Kassirer. *N Engl J Med*. 1999;341(17):1313.
20. Angell M. The Journal and its owner—resolving the crisis. *N Engl J Med*. 1999;341(10):752.
21. Bloom FE. Scruples or squabbles? *Science*. 1999;285(5431):1207.
22. Sacking of *CMAJ* editors is deeply troubling. *Lancet*. 2006;367(9512):704.
23. Spurgeon D. Owner fails to guarantee editorial independence. *BMJ*. 2006;332(7541):565.
24. Spurgeon D. CMA draws criticism for sacking editors. *BMJ*. 2006;332(7540):503.
25. Shuchman M, Redelmeier DA. Politics and independence—the collapse of the *Canadian Medical Association Journal*. *N Engl J Med*. 2006;354(13):1337-1339.
26. Hoey J. Editorial independence and the *Canadian Medical Association Journal*. *N Engl J Med*. 2006;354(19)1982-1983.
27. The gold-headed cane. *BMJ*. 1956;1(4970):791-793.
28. Booth CC. The *British Medical Journal* and the twentieth-century consultant. In: Bynum WF, Lock S, Porter R, eds. *Medical Journals and Medical Knowledge*. New York, NY: Routledge Chapman Hall Inc; 1992:259-260.
29. International Committee of Medical Journal Editors. Uniform Requirements for Manuscripts Submitted to Biomedical Journals. http://www.icmje.org. Updated February 2006. Accessed February 26, 2006.
30. World Association of Medical Editors. The relationship between journal editors-in-chief and owners (formerly titled Editorial independence). http://www.wame.org

/resources/policies#independence. Modified version posted May 15, 2006. Accessed January 5, 2007.

31. Council of Science Editors. Relations between editors and publishers, sponsoring societies, or journal owners. http://www.councilscienceeditors.org/editorial_policies/white_paper.cfm. Accessed January 5, 2007.
32. Committee on Publication Ethics. A code of conduct for editors of biomedical journals. http://www.publicationethics.org.uk/guidelines/code. Accessed February 26, 2006.
33. Smith R. Editorial independence and the *BMJ*. *BMJ*. 2004;329(7205):272.
34. Lundberg GD. Goals for The Journal. *JAMA*. 1982;248(5):553.
35. Lundberg GD. House of Delegates reaffirms editorial independence for AMA's scientific journals. *JAMA*. 1993;270(10):1248-1249.
36. Kassirer J. Should medical journals try to influence political debates? *N Engl J Med*. 1999;340(6):466-467.
37. Rosenberg RN, Anderson ER Jr. Editorial governance of the *Journal of the American Medical Association*: a report. *JAMA*. 1999;281(23):2239-2240.
38. Editorial governance for *JAMA*. *JAMA* 1999;281(23):2240-2242.
39. DeAngelis CD, Maves MD. Update of the Editorial Governance Plan for *JAMA*. *JAMA*. 2004;291(1):109.
40. Johannes L. *New England Journal of Medicine* appoints Drazen as editor in chief. *Wall Street Journal*. May 12, 2000;1.
41. Kassirer JP, Davidoff F, O'Hara K, Redelmeier DA. Editorial autonomy of *CMAJ*. *CMAJ*. 2006;174(7):945-950.
42. Armstrong PW, Cashman NR, Cook DJ, et al. A letter from *CMAJ*'s editorial board to the CMA. *CMAJ*. 2002;167(11):1230.
43. Kuehn BM. *CMAJ* governance overhauled: firings, resignations, compromised independence cited. *JAMA*. 2006;296(11):1337-1338.
44. *CMAJ* Governance Review Panel: final report. http://www.cmaj.ca/pdfs/GovernanceReviewPanel.pdf. July 14, 2006. Accessed January 5, 2007.
45. The editorial autonomy of *CMAJ* [published online ahead of print December 12, 2005]. *CMAJ*. 2006;174(1):9. doi:10.1503/cmaj.051608.
46. Choi S, Flegel K, Kendall C. A catalyst for change. *CMAJ*. 2006;174(7):901, 903
47. Spurgeon D. Most of *CMAJ* editorial board resigns. *BMJ*. 2006;332:687.
48. Webster P. Canadian researchers respond to *CMAJ* crisis. *Lancet*. 2006;367(9517):1133-1134.
49. Ncayiyana DJ. Journal ownership versus editorial independence tug-o'-war. *S Afr Med J*. 2006;96(6):470-471.
50. *CMAJ*. *CMAJ* and editorial autonomy. *CMAJ*. 2006;175(4):339.
51. MacDonald N, Squires B, Hawkins D. Editorial independence for *CMAJ*: signposts along the road. *CMAJ*. 2006;175(5):453.
52. Sullivan P. CMA accepts all recommendations from panel reviewing *CMAJ*'s structure. http://www.cma.ca/index.cfm?ci_id/=10035299&la_id=I. July 14, 2006. Accessed October 14, 2006.
53. Hébert PC. A new year and new opportunities. *CMAJ*. 2007;176(1):9.
54. *JAMA*'s key and critical objectives. http://jama.ama-assn.org/misc/aboutjama.dtl. Accessed March 11, 2006.

I believe the editor is the primary source for ethical responsibility among professional publications.
George D. Lundberg, MD[1]

5.11 Editorial Responsibilities, Roles, Procedures, and Policies.

Editorial Responsibilities, Roles, Procedures, and Policies. Coupled with the autonomy and authority that come with editorial freedom are responsibility and accountability (see also 5.10, Editorial Freedom and Integrity).[2-5] Editors are responsible for determining the journal's content, ensuring the quality of the journal, directing editorial staff and board members, developing and maintaining procedures, and creating and enforcing policies that allow the publication to meet its mission and goals effectively, efficiently, and ethically and in a fiscally responsible manner.[2-7] This section focuses primarily on decision-making editors (ie, editors in chief and other editors, such as deputy, associate, assistant, contributing, section, and guest editors) who make decisions to review, reject, request revision of, and accept content for publication.

5.11.1 The Editor's Responsibilities.

The Editor's Responsibilities. An editor's primary responsibilities are to inform and educate readers and to maintain the quality and integrity of the journal.[2,3] Thus, editors are obliged to make rational and consistent editorial decisions, select papers for publication that are appropriate for their readers, ensure that the content of their journal is of high quality, and maintain standards to ensure the journal's integrity[2,3,8-10] (see also 5.10, Editorial Freedom and Integrity). The editor's duty to readers often outweighs obligations to others with vested interest in the publication and may require actions that may not appear fair or suitable to authors, reviewers, owners, publishers, advertisers, or other stakeholders.

Editors' roles may be major public positions with broad, ethically based, professional and social responsibility (eg, editors in chief of major medical or scientific journals),[2-4,7,8] whereas other editors' responsibilities are more limited (eg, other decision-making editors), more focused (eg, assistant editors or section editors), or procedural or technical (eg, manuscript editors, managing editors, production editors). These responsibilities, regardless of their scope, should be clearly delineated in the editor's position description and supported by the publication's editorial mission statement (see 5.10, Editorial Freedom and Integrity).

Bishop,[10] Morgan,[11] and Riis[12] have identified 5 additional requisites of an editor: competence, fairness, confidentiality, expeditiousness, and courtesy (described in greater detail below).

Competence. Editors must possess a general scientific knowledge of the fields covered in their publications and be skilled in the arts of writing, editing, critical assessment, negotiation, and diplomacy. In addition, editors should consider joining professional societies in their respective scientific fields as well as professional organizations for editors (eg, Council of Science Editors, European Association of Science Editors, World Association of Medical Editors, American Medical Writers Association, European Medical Writers Association [see 25.11, Resources, Professional Scientific Writing, Editing, and Communications Organizations and Groups]). These societies have Web sites, and publications, policy statements and other resources, conferences, and courses and workshops for new editors. Editors who publish original research, or reviews or interpretations of research, should be familiar with the scientific methods used, including the general principles of statistics.[12] Editors should also rely on the expertise of others (eg, editorial board members, peer reviewers, statistical consultants, legal advisers) for advice and guidance, with the recognition that the editor has the ultimate authority for all editorial decisions. A competent editor will make rational editorial decisions, within a reasonable period of time, and communicate these decisions to authors in a clear and consistent manner.[2,4,8,10-12] A competent editor (whether editor in chief or manuscript editor) will also be skilled in the art of rhetoric[13] to recognize the tools of linguistic persuasion and identify and remove hyperbole, inconsistent arguments, and unsupported assertions and conclusions from manuscripts. Finally, as Bishop[10] suggests, a sense of humor should not be regarded as a trivial characteristic for an editor, as a bit of humor can often avoid, or at least soften, potential conflicts between editors and authors, reviewers, owners, publishers, other stakeholders, and other editors.

Fairness. Editors must act impartially and honestly.[4,9,12] Because editors are human, they cannot avoid the influence of all biases. Using peer review and consulting other editors during the editorial process may help control some personal biases.[8] Editors of peer-reviewed journals are responsible for maintaining the integrity of the peer review process, for developing policies regarding the peer review process, and for ensuring that editorial staff are properly trained in the procedures involved.[2,4] Editors should document factors relevant to editorial decisions and maintain records of decisions and reviewers' recommendations and comments for a defined period so they will be prepared to deal with appeals or complaints. (See also "Record Retention Policies for Journals" in 5.6.1, Intellectual Property: Ownership, Access, Rights, and Management, Ownership and Control of Data.)

Appeals. Journals should develop and maintain policies for handling appeals of decisions.[2,3,5] The *Lancet* has published a useful review of its appeals policy and procedures.[14] In 1996, the *Lancet* established an independent editorial ombudsman who is assigned to review unresolved allegations of editorial mismanagement.[15] This individual may also be called on to handle appeals of editorial decisions not considered satisfactorily resolved by the journal's initial response. The ombudsman publishes annual reports summarizing these disputes and their resolutions.[16] In resolving disputes, editors should consider all sides of an issue and avoid favoritism toward friends and colleagues or allowing editorial decisions to be influenced by powerful or threatening external forces (see 5.10, Editorial Freedom and Integrity). *Note:* Editors and journals should not keep copies of rejected manuscripts for longer than necessary to deal with appropriate appeals of decisions, and journals should have record-retention policies to direct how long decision letters and reviewer recommendations and comments should be kept (see also "Record Retention Policies for Journals" in 5.6.1, Intellectual Property: Ownership, Access, Rights, and Management, Ownership and Control of Data, and 5.11.5, Editorial Responsibility for Rejection).

Conflicts of Interest. Editors should not have financial interests in any entity that might influence editorial evaluations and decisions[2,3,8] (see 5.5, Conflicts of Interest). Editors with other types of conflicts of interest with a specific manuscript or author that could impair objective decision making should recuse themselves from involvement with such papers and should delegate responsibility of the review and decision of such papers to another editor or editorial board member.[2,3] For example, the *Archives of General Psychiatry* does not permit an editor who collaborates with an author or who is employed by the same institution as an author to make decisions about that author's manuscript; the review and decision-making authority is delegated to an editorial board member without such a relationship.[17] Some journals will not consider manuscripts from authors who also serve as editors for the journal (clearly, this does not apply to editorials). Other journals will consider such submissions, but reviews of and decisions about manuscripts for which an editor is an author or coauthor are managed independently by another editor who has complete decision-making authority (including the ability to reject a manuscript in which the editor in chief is an author). For example, the *Archives of Pediatrics & Adolescent Medicine* delegates the review and decision of such papers to an associate editor and an editorial board member,[18] and the *New England Journal of Medicine* has an independent editor at large who is assigned to handle all original research papers that are submitted by editors.[19]

Confidentiality. Editors must ensure that information about a submitted manuscript is not disclosed to anyone outside the editorial office, other than the peer reviewers and authors invited to write an editorial commenting on an accepted but not yet published manuscript (see 5.7, Confidentiality).[2,4] Editors should create and maintain policies about confidentiality and ensure that all current and new staff (editorial and production), reviewers, and editorial board members are sufficiently educated about the journal's principles of confidentiality. The following statement may be useful when handling inquiries about manuscripts under consideration or previously rejected:

> We can neither confirm nor deny the existence of any manuscript unless and until such manuscript is published.

Editors should also establish policies and procedures to handle breaches of confidentiality by authors, peer reviewers, and editorial staff (see 5.7, Confidentiality).

Expeditiousness. Although the length of time it takes to evaluate a manuscript depends on many factors (eg, number of submitted manuscripts, resources of the editorial office, time allocated for peer review, and availability of efficient submission and review systems, such as Web-based systems), an author has a right to expect to receive a decision within a reasonable time.[11,12] Journals should publish an audit or otherwise make available to prospective authors turnaround times for manuscript decisions, peer review, and publication.[2] See, for example, the annual audit published by *JAMA*[20] and 5.11.12, Editorial Audits and Research. If the review and evaluation are delayed significantly beyond the journal's standard turnaround times for any reason, notifying the author of the reason for the delay is appropriate. Authors have a right to contact the editorial office to inquire about the status of their manuscripts. Many journals that use Web-based manuscript submission and review systems offer authors the opportunity to check the progress of their submission online.

Editors should plan to accept papers with knowledge of the number of accepted manuscripts awaiting publication, the approximate number of pages and/or articles that can be published during a year, and the resources available to publish additional material online, if applicable. Morgan[11] has commented that a journal that accepts more papers than it can publish within the time span observed by other journals in the same field is suppressing, not disseminating, information.

On occasion, an editor will receive a request from an author or a suggestion from a reviewer to expedite publication of a specific manuscript. The quickened pace of scientific discovery and heightened competition among scientists and journals have fostered an increase in requests for rapid review and publication, and technologic advances have facilitated the ability to do so.[21] A number of journals have procedures for fast-track consideration. For example, *JAMA* has a procedure for expedited peer review and editorial consideration of manuscripts of high-quality evidence (usually randomized controlled trials) that have immediate clinical and/or public health importance.[22] Some biomedical journals routinely publish accepted papers online ahead of print publication. Such online ahead of print publication should include appropriate procedures for editorial review, editing, and proofing before posting, as well as for proper identification of any versions (eg, online ahead of print version vs print version). This is especially important for journals that publish information that can affect clinical decisions and patient care. For journals that do not routinely publish all content online ahead of print, a policy should be developed to allow for rapid consideration and early online publication of appropriate accepted manuscripts (eg, those with important and urgent implications for public health) that does not compromise the peer-review and editorial decision processes or the integrity of the journal and that does not result in the premature publication of an incomplete or inaccurate article (see also 5.13, Release of Information to the Public and Journal/Author Relations With the News Media).

Courtesy. More than a mere extension of etiquette and convention, editorial politeness requires editors and all editorial staff to deal with authors and reviewers in a respectful, fair, professional, and courteous manner.[10-12] Diplomacy, tact, empathy, and negotiation skills will help editors maintain positive relationships with authors, even those whose work the editor rejects.

Note: Sections 5.11.2 through 5.11.7 focus on the editor's responsibility for manuscript processing, assessment, and decisions (see also 6.0, Editorial Assessment and Processing).

5.11.2 Acknowledging Manuscript Receipt. Journals should send a notice to authors to acknowledge receipt of their manuscripts and provide names and contact information of relevant editorial staff. For journals with Web-based manuscript submission systems, acknowledgment letters may be sent automatically, usually after an author has viewed the submission and confirmed that it is complete.

5.11.3 Editorial Responsibility for Manuscript Assessment. The editor should establish and maintain procedures and policies for appropriate editorial assessment and decisions to accept, request revision of, and reject mansucripts (see also 6.0, Editorial Assessment and Processing).[4] The editor also establishes whether such decisions will be made unilaterally or by other editors (eg, deputy, associate, assistant, contributing, section, or guest editor) or in collaboration. Factors used to determine decisions should be made available to authors and reviewers. For example, *JAMA* editors use the following general criteria to evaluate manuscripts: material is original, writing is clear, study methods are appropriate, data are valid, conclusions are reasonable and supported by the data, information is important, and topic has general medical interest.[22] Through instructions for authors and reviewer forms, *JAMA* authors and reviewers are informed that these basic criteria are used to assess a paper's eligibility for publication.

Depending on the nature of a journal's editorial resources and the number of manuscripts received, the editor may rely on a triage system to evaluate all manuscripts before peer review. Not all manuscripts will be appropriate for the journal, and after an initial assessment the editor may decide to reject some papers without sending them for external peer review. For example, *JAMA* editors reject more than 50% of the approximately 6000 major manuscripts received annually without obtaining external peer review.[20] In such cases, the editor's duty to provide a detailed review to the author of each paper is outweighed by the duty to reviewers (by not requesting their time to review a manuscript that has no chance of publication), to owners (by not consuming resources needlessly), and to other authors who have submitted papers to the journal (by maintaining efficient processes) (see also 6.0, Editorial Assessment and Processing). In addition, the author may be best served by a prompt notification of a decision indicating rejection if the manuscript is unlikely to make it through the journal's review process and be considered for acceptance, thereby allowing the author to submit the manuscript to another journal without additional delay.

For manuscripts determined to be eligible for external review and additional consideration, all components of the submission should receive proper review and editorial assessment; this includes the manuscript text, tables, figures, and references, as well as relevant supplementary materials, documents, and video and audio files.

5.11.4 **Editorial Responsibility for Peer Review.** Decisions about manuscripts are made by editors, not peer reviewers. Reviewers offer valuable advice, serve as consultants to the editor, and may make recommendations about a paper's suitability for publication, but all editorial decisions should be made by the editors. Editors are obliged to be courteous to peer reviewers, provide them with guidance and explicit instructions, assign only those papers that are appropriate to specific reviewers (in terms of reviewer expertise and interest), maintain confidentiality if using blind or anonymous review, provide reviewers with sufficient time to conduct their review, and avoid overworking them.[2,4] Editors should ask reviewers in advance whether they are available for and interested in reviewing a specific manuscript, unless they have a prior agreement to assign manuscripts to reviewers without advanced consent.

Many journals publish lists of reviewers' names to acknowledge, credit, and thank them publicly for their work. Some journals offer qualifying reviewers continuing education credit, a letter of commendation that can be shared with supervisors or promotion committees, or subscriptions to the journal. Few journals offer financial compensation to peer reviewers, except perhaps those who may review a substantial number of papers or perform specialized reviews (eg, statistics). Editors should provide feedback to reviewers, such as notifying reviewers of the manuscript's final disposition, sharing copies of other reviewer comments of the same manuscript, and providing regular assessments of the quality of the reviewer's work.[2,4]

Editors should not share a specific review of a manuscript with anyone outside the editorial office, other than the authors and other reviewers, unless the journal operates an open peer-review system that includes publication of reviewer recommendations and comments and reviewers are informed of this in advance. Editors should develop a specific policy regarding who has access to copies of a review, and this policy should be clearly communicated to all persons involved in the review process (see 6.0, Editorial Assessment and Processing, and 5.7.1, Confidentiality, Confidentiality During Editorial Evaluation and Peer Review and After Publication).

Many journals develop databases of reviewers, including their addresses and affiliations, areas of expertise, turnaround times, and quality ratings for each manuscript review. Editors and publishers are obliged not to make secondary use of the information in the database without the prior consent of the reviewers and should never exploit it for personal use, benefit, or profit (eg, selling a list of peer reviewers' names and contact information for promotional purposes).

5.11.5 **Editorial Responsibility for Rejection.** Rejecting manuscripts may be one of the most important responsibilities of an editor. By rejecting papers appropriately, an editor sets standards and defines the editorial content for the journal.[11] Decisions to reject a manuscript may be based on a wide range of factors, such as lack of originality, lack of importance or relevance to the journal's readers, poor writing, flawed methods, scientific weakness, invalid data, biased interpretations and/or conclusions, timeliness, or the specific publishing priorities of the journal.[4] A rejection letter must be carefully worded to avoid offending the author and should express regret for the outcome, but also must not raise false hopes about the merits of an unsuitable paper. Many editors avoid use of the word *rejection* in any letters, opting instead for phrases such as "we are unable to accept" or "your paper is not acceptable for publication." However, editors should be certain that the intent of a letter of rejection is clear. If the letter sounds too much like a request for revision, the author may subsequently resubmit an irrevocably flawed manuscript; or worse, the author may resubmit a rejected manuscript, essentially unchanged, with the hope that the editor will not notice.[11]

An editor should determine on a case-by-case basis whether a standard rejection letter (form letter) or an individualized letter explaining the specific deficiencies of the manuscript should be sent to the author. Some editors argue that for a paper rejected for "reasons of editorial choice (usually without outside editorial peer review), the editor has no obligation to give the author any explanation beyond the statement that the manuscript was not considered appropriate."[8] Other editors suggest that all authors be provided a specific reason for rejection of their manuscript.[4] However, a standardized (form) rejection letter that includes an explanation for rejection based on editorial priority (especially for large journals that receive large numbers of submissions and/or that have very low acceptance rates) or that is accompanied by copies of detailed reviewer comments is sufficient for many papers that are rejected.

Editors should develop specific policies for the rejection process, including how to handle previously rejected manuscripts resubmitted with an appeal for reconsideration (see also the "Appeals" section under "Fairness" in 5.11.1, The Editor's Responsibilities).[2,4] If the author's appeal provides reasonable justification, the editor should carefully consider the appeal (see also 6.1.8, Editorial Assessment and Processing, Editorial Assessment, Appealing a Rejection).

Once a common act of courtesy, the practice of returning all copies of rejected manuscripts has become obsolete. However, original illustrations, photographs, slides, and other artwork should be returned if requested by the author, as should any manuscripts an author specifically requests be returned. Because journals do not own unpublished works (ie, copyright is typically transferred in the event of publication), journal offices should not keep print or electronic copies of rejected manuscripts for any period longer than that required to deal with appeals of decisions; they should be destroyed or deleted. See also "Record Retention Policies for Journals" in

5.6.1, Ownership and Control of Data, and 5.6.5, Copyright Assignment or License, both in 5.6, Intellectual Property: Ownership, Access, Rights, and Management.

5.11.6 **Editorial Responsibility for Revision.** The editor's impartial focus on improving a manuscript faciliates the process of revision. According to Morgan,[11] "in letters requesting revision the editor should use an impersonal tone in criticizing." All such communication is best if the tone is objective and constructive. Editors should clearly communicate to authors what is expected in a revision; it may be helpful for editors to request that authors submit revised manuscripts with changes, additions, and deletions indicated and a cover letter itemizing the changes made in response to the editor's and reviewers' comments and suggestions.

Editors are obligated to use sound editorial reasoning in requesting a revision. Editors must be skilled in arbitrating reviewer disagreements and reconciling contradictory recommendations, which may result from reviewers having diverse backgrounds, different expectations of the journal, and variable levels of expertise, diligence, or interest in the subject of the manuscript.[11] Authors object to receiving inconsistent or contradictory comments from reviewers and editors and may object to new and different criticisms of the revised manuscript submitted in response to the initial review. Although editors can never be certain that new issues will not surface at the time of resubmission, they are obliged to evaluate all reviewer comments, address any inconsistencies or unreasonable criticisms, censor any inappropriate criticisms, and guide authors in preparing their revisions.[4,8] Editors who make decisons about publication should never relegate themselves to the role of manuscript traffic controllers by simply passing on reviewer comments without direction for the revision or by permitting reviewers' recommendations to serve as the editor's decision.

Some editors feel uncomfortable asking an author to revise a manuscript if there is a possibility that the revision will not be published. However, a revision may be needed to permit an author to provide missing data or information or to more clearly describe the study or work being reported so that the editor can properly evaluate the manuscript. The revision may also expose an important weakness, limitation, or flaw that was not apparent in the original submission and that necessitates a decision to reject. Alternatively, a revision may introduce new issues or concerns or simply may not be satisfactory. In each of these cases, the editor's responsibility to readers outweighs any obligation to publish the author's revised manuscript. Editors should develop specific policies regarding requests for revisions, and the revision letter should state explicitly whether the author should or should not expect publication of a satisfactorily revised manuscript.[4] For example, *JAMA* editors include language similar to the following in their revision letters:

> If you decide to revise your paper along these lines, there is no guarantee that it will be accepted for publication. That decision will be based on our editorial priorities at the time, the quality of your revision, and perhaps additional peer review.

The rejection of a revised manuscript is probably best handled with a personal letter tactfully explaining why the revision was not acceptable. Although editors may need to ask for multiple revisions of a paper, such requests should include a detailed explanation to the authors. In most cases, these efforts serve to give the authors the best chance for their paper to reach a level of quality that is appropriate for acceptance and publication.

5.11.7 Editorial Responsibility for Acceptance

Acceptance. Editors should follow consistent procedures to evaluate papers and make decisions regarding acceptance (see 5.11.3, Editorial Responsibility for Manuscript Assessment). Editors should inform authors of acceptance of their manuscripts in a letter that describes the subsequent process of publication, including substantive editing and any remaining queries; editing of the manuscript, tables, and figures for accuracy, consistency, clarity, style, grammar, and formatting; and what material the author will be expected to review and approve before publication. Editors may also provide an approximate timetable for the publication process. If authors are given an expected date of publication, they should be informed of the likelihood of the date changing. The acceptance letter should also remind authors of any policies regarding duplicate publication, disclosure of conflicts of interest, and restrictions on prepublication release of information to the public or the news media (see also 5.3, Duplicate Publication; 5.5, Conflicts of Interest; and 5.13, Release of Information to the Public and Journal/Author Relations With the News Media).

Authors should avoid making substantial changes to the manuscript after acceptance, unless correcting an error, answering an editor's request for missing information, responding to an editor's or a proofreader's query, or providing an essential update. Likewise, editors should review manuscripts before acceptance and avoid asking authors for substantial changes after final acceptance.

If circumstances (eg, an unanticipated decrease in the number of pages allotted for publication or clustering of certain papers for a special issue) cause a delay in publishing an accepted manuscript beyond the typical time between acceptance and publication, editors should inform the corresponding author of the reason for the delay.

Editors should not reverse decisions to accept papers after the authors have been notified unless serious problems are subsequently identified with the content of the manuscript (eg, flawed methods, inconsistent or invalid data, allegations of misconduct) or the author has failed to meet the journal's publication requirements (eg, transfer of copyright, disclosure of duplicate submissions or publications, disclosure of conflicts of interest).[5] An example of editorial discourtesy in handling accepted manuscripts occurred when an editor "unaccepted" a paper that his journal had accepted unconditionally 20 months earlier. The reason provided to the authors for this change of decision was that the journal's inventory of accepted papers had grown too large.[23] However, if a new editor inherits from the journal's previous editor a large inventory of accepted manuscripts deemed outdated or inappropriate, the new editor may have to find ways to deal with these papers appropriately. In such a case, the editor may request a one-time or temporary increase in journal pages from the publisher. If this is not a viable option, for financial or other reasons, the editor may choose to contact the authors of accepted manuscripts that have not yet been scheduled for publication and explain that too many papers had been accepted to be able to publish them in a reasonable period. The editor may offer the authors options to withdraw their manuscript and send it to another journal, reduce the length of their manuscript to allow it and others to be published in the limited number of pages allocated to the print journal, or publish their manuscript online only. However, any decisions not to publish previously accepted papers should be made carefully and perhaps with the consultation of the journal's editorial board or legal adviser.

Provisional Acceptance. Some editors will grant authors a "provisional acceptance," offering to publish their papers if certain conditions or minor requirements are met. Some journals use provisional or conditional acceptance for revision requests when they are fairly certain that the revision will be accepted for publication. However, use of a provisional acceptance as a request for revision can cause problems if the revised manuscript is not suitable for publication. To avoid such problems, provisional acceptance decision letters should clearly communicate that acceptance is contingent on specific conditions that are clearly described for the author. If a new editorial policy requires a new condition for publication to be met by authors who submitted papers before the policy took effect, a provisional acceptance can be used to permit these papers to move forward without unnecessary delay.

5.11.8 Correspondence (Letters to the Editor). A biomedical journal should provide a forum for readers and authors to participate in postpublication peer review and scientific dialogue and to exchange important information, especially with regard to articles published in the journal.[2,3,24] A common forum for such exchange is the correspondence, or letters to the editor, column (see also 1.6, Types of Articles, Correspondence). Such letters become part of the published record and, like articles, are indexed by bibliographic databases. In the correspondence column, journal readers have the opportunity to offer relevant comments, query authors, and provide objective and scholarly criticism of published articles. Authors of articles to which the letters pertain should always be given the opportunity to respond. Whenever possible, the letter author's comments and criticisms and the author's reply should be published in the same issue to enable readers to evaluate the arguments presented. If an author chooses not to submit a reply for publication, the journal may publish a statement indicating that the author declined to comment. Follow-up or later work that clarifies or amplifies a previous publication (other than a correction of an error or omission or retraction of fraud) may also be considered for publication as a letter[4] (see also, 5.11.9, Corrections [Errata], and 5.4, Scientific Misconduct)

Editors should establish policies and procedures for processing and evaluating letters just as they have done for handling manuscripts, and these should be published in the journal's instructions for authors or as part of the regular correspondence column. Like authors of manuscripts, authors of letters are expected to follow the same policies and procedures for authorship responsibility, disclosure of duplicate publication and submissions, disclosure of conflicts of interest, copyright or publication license transfer, research ethics, and protection of patients' rights to privacy in publication.

Journals prefer to publish letters that objectively comment on or critically assess previously published articles, offer scholarly opinion or commentary on journal content or the journal itself, or include important announcements or other information relevant to the journal's readers (although journals may have separate sections for announcements, meetings, and events). Letters that merely praise authors, the editor, or the journal rarely provide any meaningful or useful information. Likewise, ad hominem attacks should not be published.[24] Some journals also publish short reports (eg, less than 500 words) of original research, technical comments, or novel case reports in the correspondence column. These reports should be handled as regular manuscripts, with peer review and revision, as necessary.

Many journals set limits on the length of letters that will be considered for publication (eg, 500 words or less and no more than 5 references). Some journals will publish small tables or figures in letters, space permitting. To maintain timeliness, some journals also set a limit on the amount of time in which a letter sent in response to a published article must be received. For example, *JAMA* and the *Archives* Journals generally allow readers 4 weeks to submit a letter in response to a published article. Journals with time limits may allow exceptions for important letters that are submitted after the recommended deadline, especially for letters that identify important errors. Journals with space and time limits have been criticized for stifling post-publication scientific exchange and debate,[25,26] but such criticism does not recognize the resource limitations of journals and their editorial and production staff or the practical concerns associated with gathering all relevant submitted letters on a specific article and sending them to the author for a reply and publishing these in a timely manner. Some journals have addressed this criticism by permitting online-only correspondence to be posted without such restrictions on length and timeliness. In 1998, the *BMJ* began an experiment with an unrestricted policy for online-only letters that included no limitations on length, timeliness, or number of online postings.[27] By 2002, the 20 000 online letters represented one-third of the journal's total online content.[28] After posting the 50 000th online-only letter in 2005, the *BMJ* recognized that the quality of some of these responses was low and commented that "the bores are threatening to take over. Some respondents feel the urge to opine on any given topic, and pile in early and often, despite having little of interest to say."[29] As a result, the *BMJ* added a maximum length requirement and raised the bar for acceptance of online-only letters for those that contribute "substantially to the topic under discussion."[29]

Typically, a submitted letter undergoes an initial assessment, at which point it may be rejected, revised, or accepted. Some letters may be sent for peer review or accepted without external peer review. Letters on the same topic or in response to the same article should be grouped, sent to the author of the original article for reply (if necessary), and published in the same issue under one general title. Journals should cross-reference, and reciprocally link online, the original article and related letters to allow readers to identify and read the original articles and all related letters. Authors of letters accepted for publication should sign statements of authorship responsibility, financial disclosure, and copyright or publication license transfer. Journals may edit accepted letters for content, length, clarity, grammar, style, and format. Authors should approve changes that alter the substance or tone of a letter or response.[24]

For journals that publish rapid-response sections for online-only letters, these postings should be reviewed to verify that they meet the journal's guidelines and requirements for such postings, to determine that they contribute substantially to the previous publication and/or the discussion under way, and to check for libel, error, and gratuitousness. If accepted, these postings require minimal editing. The *Archives of Pediatrics & Adolescent Medicine* and other *Archives* Journals that publish online-only letters under a Readers Reply section include the following instructions[30]:

> **Instructions**: Only replies that have **not** been published or posted elsewhere should be submitted. Replies will be selected for posting by the editors; those that are selected may be edited. By submitting this Readers Reply, you attest to being the sole author. You transfer copyright to AMA if your Reply is posted on the *JAMA & Archives* Journals Web site. Indicate any financial disclosures (eg, employment, consultancies, honoraria, stock ownership or

> options, expert testimony, grants received, patents received or pending, or royalties relevant to the topic discussed) in the text field. If you have none, indicate "No relevant financial interests" in the text field. This information may be posted with your response.

However, these online-only letters may not be indexed by bibliographic databases, and whether they fulfill the need for an official record of postpublication peer review is subject to debate.[29]

5.11.9 Corrections (Errata). Journals should publish corrections (or errata) following errors or important omissions made by authors or introduced by editors, manuscript editors, production staff, or printers.[2,4,24] According to the International Committee of Medical Journal Editors, journal editors have a duty to publish corrections in a timely manner[24]; however, the age of the original article in which the error was made should not be used as a reason not to publish a correction. Corrections to print publications should be published on a numbered editorial page and listed in the journal's table of contents. It is preferable to publish corrections in a consistent place in the journal, such as at the end of the correspondence column. If this is not possible or if corrections are routinely published in available white space in print versions of journals, these should still be listed on the journal's table of contents. If easily identified, corrections will then be included in literature databases, such as MEDLINE, and appended to online citations to the original article that contains the error.[31] Corrections made to online-only content and publications should also be properly labeled and identified (eg, listed in the online table of contents) and reciprocally linked to the original content. On occasion, an error may be so serious (eg, error in drug dosage) or important to the author (eg, misspelling of author's name) to warrant immediate correction online. In this case, it should be made clear in the online article that a correction has been made, and a print correction should follow.

In online publications and versions of print journals, corrections should reciprocally link to and from the original article. Corrections should also be appended to all derivative publications (eg, reprints). If major errors are corrected in derivative publications, a note should be included indicating that a correction has been made and/or linking to a correction.

Corrections (or errata) should not be used for retractions of fraudulent articles resulting from fabrication, falsification, or plagiarism (see also 5.4.5, Scientific Misconduct, Retractions, Expressions of Concern).

5.11.10 Role of the Editorial Board. Editorial boards comprise leaders and experts in the subject area(s) represented by a journal. Editorial board members provide various functions, including representation of the journal and outreach to the community of readers and authors served by the journal; advising the editor on policies, editorial content, and editorial direction of the journal; serving as peer reviewers; writing and recruiting manuscripts; and/or assisting the editor on editorial decisions (ie, handling manuscripts with which the editor has a conflict, serving as guest editor, or serving as section editor or editor for specific types of manuscripts). Some journals use editorial board members as decision-making editors who conduct initial triage of the quality and suitability of manuscripts or assign papers to peer reviewers. Journals without independent oversight committees may wish to position the editorial board with the ability to help maintain the editorial freedom and integrity of the editor and journal (see also 5.10, Editorial Freedom and Integrity). Editorial boards should be working, functional boards, with specific roles, responsibilities, direction, a clear reporting relationship, and term limits.[10,32] While nonworking figurehead boards may help the image or marketing of a journal, they will not provide reliable and consistent advice and assistance to the editor.

An editorial board should be independent of the publisher, owner, or other external forces, and the journal's editor in chief should serve as the chair of the editorial board. Editorial board members should be selected and appointed by the journal's editor, not the publisher or the owner.[10] However, if the editor has an agreement with the publisher or owner that permits an external group (eg, professional society that owns or has a formal relationship with the journal) to nominate board members, the editor should have the final authority to appoint these individuals and to review their performance, and the number of editorial board members identified by the owner or an external group should be limited to a minority of the total board membership. Editors should maintain confidentiality and fairness when making decisions to renew or not renew a specific board member's appointment.

Editors should develop, review, and update as necessary an editorial board member position description that clearly lists roles, responsibilities, requirements, and term limits. For example, see the position description for an editorial board member for *JAMA* (Box 1).

A conflict of interest policy should also be established for editorial board members (see also 5.5.7, Conflicts of Interest, Requirements for Editors and Editorial

Box 1. Editorial Board Member Position Description

1. Attends annual meeting of the editorial board.
2. Permits name to be placed on masthead of the journal.
3. Reports to the editor in chief and serves as a source of editorial advice.
4. Serves as peer reviewer and consultant, reviewing manuscripts promptly and thoroughly.
5. Represents the journal to peers in member's scientific, clinical, and academic disciplines.
6. Assists in recruiting authors, manuscripts, and reviewers for the journal.
7. Writes editorials, commentaries, and other articles as requested.
8. Reviews each issue of the journal and provides feedback to the editor in chief.
9. Makes the comments and impressions of colleagues regarding the journal available to the editor in chief.
10. Promotes readership of the journal by calling it to the attention of colleagues and using it in educational settings, as appropriate.
11. Is appointed for 2-year terms, with a general tenure of 10 years.
12. Does not serve as editor or editorial board member of a competing journal.
13. Discloses all relevant financial conflicts of interest to the editor in chief annually.
14. Performs other duties as requested.

Board Members). Editorial board members should disclose all relevant conflicts of interest (financial and nonfinancial) to the editor; they should not participate in the review of or decisions on any manuscripts in which they may have a conflict of interest; and they should never use information obtained during the review process, editorial consultation, or an editorial board meeting for personal or professional gain. Editorial board members may be asked to serve multiple journals; this may pose a conflict of interest, especially for journals that represent a small community or the same field or specialty. The following questions, developed by the *Archives of Ophthalmology,* may help editorial board members and editors decide whether positions with 2 journals pose a conflict of interest: Are both journals competing for the same readership, subject matter, and authors? Are the editorial positions and responsibilities similar? Can the editorial board member meet this journal's requirements as listed in the position description?

Journal editors should hold regular meetings of the editorial board at least annually[10] or, if resources are limited, conduct regular meetings via conference call and/or the Web. In any case, the editor should communicate frequently with the editorial board members, ensure that board members understand their responsibilities and terms, and review the performance of each board member on a regular basis and before renewing a term.

5.11.11 Disclosure of Editorial Practices, Procedures, and Policies. Underlying the ethics of editorial responsibility is the need for disclosure of editorial procedures and policies to authors, reviewers, and readers. Typically, these are listed, and explained as necessary, in the publication's instructions for authors, which should be published and readily available on the journal's Web site (if published online). Items that should be considered for inclusion in a biomedical journal's instructions for authors are listed in Box 2.

When an important editorial policy is first created or undergoes a major revision, it should be announced to prospective authors, reviewers, and readers. The easiest way to accomplish this is to publish an editorial note or an editorial. Editors should also draw attention to major changes in policy and procedures in the journal's instructions for authors and correspondence with authors.

Editors should also ensure that all individuals responsible for contributing to the publication are properly identified, typically in the masthead (eg, editorial and publishing staff, editorial board members, advisers, oversight bodies or publication committees, and owners). Other items that should be disclosed include any sources of financial support or other sponsorship that supports the publication.

5.11.12 Editorial Audits and Research. Many journals conduct internal assessments, audits, and research into various aspects of the editorial process. For example, a journal may produce monthly or annual reports from its database of manuscripts, authors, and peer reviewers to track inventory, workflow, and efficiency metrics.[2] Trends from these reports can help editors determine the number and types of papers to accept for publication, assess staffing needs, track reviewer performance, and determine when to institute corrective action. For example, *JAMA* publishes an annual editorial audit that includes the number of manuscripts received the previous year, acceptance rates, and the turnaround time for manuscripts that are reviewed, accepted or

Box 2. Items That Should Be Considered for Inclusion in a Biomedical Journal's Instructions for Authors

Information About the Journal

- Name, address, telephone and fax numbers, e-mail address, and URLs (uniform resource locators) of the journal's Web site and online submission system (if available)
- Journal's mission, goals, and objectives
- Policies and procedures on editorial assessment, review, and processing (eg, turnaround times for reviews and decisions, type of peer review process, acknowledging receipt of submissions, editing and review of accepted manuscripts)
- Types of manuscripts suitable for submission

Requirements for Manuscript Submission

- Name, address, telephone and fax numbers, and e-mail address of corresponding author; list of all coauthors with their relevant academic degrees and institutional affiliations
- Methods and requirements for submitting manuscripts, tables, and figures; cover letters; and supplementary materials, including audio or video files if acceptable (ie, via Web site, e-mail, or other means)
- If accepting submissions by mail, number of copies of manuscripts, tables, and artwork required
- Style and format of manuscript text, tables, figures, references, abstracts, and supplementary material
- Specific requirements for categories of manuscripts (eg, reports of original research, reviews, letters, editorials, or journal-specific features)
- Manuscript submission checklist

Requirements for Manuscript Consideration and Publication

- Policies on authorship, contributions of authors, access to data, and acknowledging assistance
- Policy on submission of duplicate or redundant manuscripts
- Policy on disclosure of conflicts of interest
- Policy on disclosure of funding and the role of the sponsor
- Policies for deposition of data in public repositories and registration of clinical trials
- For experimental investigations involving human or animal subjects, policy on approval by ethics committee or institutional review board and informed consent or appropriate animal care and use
- Policy on including identifiable descriptions or photographs of patients
- Policies on obtaining permission for reprinting or adapting previously published material
- Policies on transfer of copyright or publication license and open access
- Payment responsibility for open access journals with author-pay models or journals with other forms of publication (page or color) charges

rejected, and published.[20] The *Archives* Journals publish dates of acceptance with each article.

In addition, some journals systematically analyze information from submitted manuscripts as part of research to improve the quality of the editorial or peer review processes. All identifying information should remain confidential during such assessments, and any research conducted should not interfere with the review process or the ultimate editorial decision. For example, *JAMA*'s instructions for authors inform prospective authors that information related to their submissions may be subject to such analysis and that confidentiality will be maintained. If a research project involves change in the journal's usual review process (eg, random assignment to a different review procedure), authors should be informed and given the opportunity to choose whether they want their manuscripts to be included in the study. Their decision to participate or not should not adversely affect the editorial consideration of their manuscript in any way.

5.11.13 **Editorial Quality Review.** A final editorial procedure that should be a part of every journal's operation is quality review. After publication, editorial and production staff and advisers should review each issue for content errors (which, if detected, should be considered for publication as corrections), problems in presentation and format, and general appearance. All editorial and publishing staff should have the opportunity to participate in the quality review process, and all errors, problems, and suggestions for improvement should be communicated to the editor as well as those directly involved in editing and producing the publication.

ACKNOWLEDGMENTS

Principal author: Annette Flanagin, RN, MA

I thank the following for reviewing and providing helpful comments on this manuscript: Catherine D. DeAngelis, MD, MPH, *JAMA* and *Archives* Journals; C. K. Gunsalus, JD, University of Illinois, Urbana/Champaign; and Terri S. Carter, *Archives of Surgery*.

REFERENCES

1. Lundberg GD. Perspective from the editor of *JAMA, The Journal of the American Medical Association*. *Bull Med Libr Assoc*. 1992;80(2):110-114.
2. Council of Science Editors. Editor roles and responsibilities. In: CSE's white paper on promoting integrity in scientific journal publications. http://www.councilscienceeditors.org/services/draft_approved.cfm. September 13, 2006. Accessed January 5, 2007.
3. World Association of Medical Editors. WAME recommendations on publication ethics policies for medical journals. http://www.wame.org/resources/publication-ethics-policies-for-medical-journals. Accessed January 5, 2007.
4. Utiger RD; for the Education Committee, World Association of Medical Editors. A syllabus for prospective and newly appointed editors. http://www.wame.org/resources/editor-s-syllabus. Posted October 26, 2001. Accessed January 5, 2007.
5. Committee on Publication Ethics. A code of conduct for editors of biomedical journals. http://www.publicationethics.org.uk/guidelines/code. Accessed April 10, 2006.
6. Behlmer GK. Ernest Hart and the social thrust of Victorian medicine. *BMJ*. 1990; 301(6754):711-713.

7. Lundberg GD. The social responsibility of medical journal editing. *J Gen Intern Med.* 1987;2(6):415-419.
8. Relman AS. Publishing biomedical research: role and responsibilities. *Hastings Cent Rep.* May/June 1990:23-27.
9. Schiedermayer DL, Siegler M. Believing what you read: responsibilities of medical authors and editors. *Arch Intern Med.* 1986;146(10):2043-2044.
10. Bishop CT. *How to Edit a Scientific Journal.* Philadelphia, PA: ISI Press; 1984.
11. Morgan P. *An Insider's Guide for Medical Authors and Editors.* Philadelphia, PA: ISI Press; 1986.
12. Riis P. The ethics of scientific publication. In: European Association of Editors. *Science Editors' Handbook.* West Clandon, United Kingdom: EASE; January 1994. Reissued June 2003.
13. Horton R. The rhetoric of research. *BMJ.* 1995;310(6985):985-987.
14. Sperschneider T, Kleinert S, Horton R. Appealing to editors? *Lancet.* 2003;361(9373): 1926.
15. Horton R. The *Lancet*'s ombudsman. *Lancet* 1996;348(9019):6.
16. Carter R. Ombudsman's eighth report. *Lancet* 2004;364(9432):402.
17. Instructions for authors. *Arch Gen Psychiatry.* http://archpsyc.ama-assn.org/misc/ifora.dtl. Updated November 2006. Accessed January 5, 2007.
18. Instructions for authors. *Arch Pediatr Adolesc Med.* http://archpedi.ama-assn.org/misc/ifora.dtl. Accessed April 22, 2006.
19. Curfman GD, Drazen JM. Too close to call. *N Engl J Med.* 2001;345(11):832.
20. DeAngelis CD, Fontanarosa PB. Thank you, *JAMA* peer reviewers and authors. *JAMA.* 2006;295(10):1171-1172.
21. Roberts L. The rush to publish. *Science.* 1991;251(4991):260-263.
22. Instructions for authors. *JAMA.* http://jama.ama-assn.org/mic/ifora.dtl. Accessed January 3, 2007.
23. Chusid MJ, Casper JT, Camitta BM. Editors have ethical responsibilities, too. *N Engl J Med.* 1984;311(15):990-991.
24. International Committee of Medical Journal Editors. Uniform Requirements for Manuscripts Submitted to Biomedical Journals. http://www.icmje.org. Updated February 2006. Accessed April 10, 2006.
25. Altman DG. Poor-quality medical research: what can journals do? *JAMA.* 2002; 287(21):2765-2767.
26. Altman DG. Unjustified restrictions on letters to the editor. *PLoS Med.* May 2005; 2(5):e126.
27. Crossan L. Letters to the editor: the new order. *BMJ.* 1998;316(7142):1406-1410.
28. Delamothe T, Smith R. Twenty thousand conversations. *BMJ.* 2002;324(7347):1171-1172.
29. Davies S. Revitalising rapid responses: we're raising the bar for publication. *BMJ.* 2005;330(7503):1284.
30. Readers Reply submission instructions. *Arch Pediatr Adolesc Med.* http://archpedi.ama-assn.org/cgi/eletter-submit/160/4/402. Accessed April 22, 2006.
31. National Library of Medicine. Fact sheets: errata, retraction, duplicate publication, comment, update and patient summary policy for MEDLINE. January 21, 2005. http://www.nlm.nih.gov/pubs/factsheets/errata.html. Accessed April 22, 2006.
32. Marcovitch H, Williamson A. 1.1.3: Editorial boards. In: European Association of Editors. *Science Editors' Handbook.* West Clandon, United Kingdom: EASE; June 2003.

The uncertain romance between scholarly journals and the drug industry has long been like a marriage of convenience between partners who became friends ultimately, not because they were very fond of each other originally, but because they needed each other.

Robert H. Moser, MD[1]

5.12 **Advertisements, Advertorials, Sponsorship, Supplements, Reprints, and E-prints.** Commercial activities, such as advertising, sponsorship, reprints, and e-prints provide a major source of revenue for many scientific publications. With this revenue, publications can offset some of the costs of journal operations, production, and distribution; may be able to set lower subscription rates than would otherwise be possible; and can serve as a source of income for the journal's owner. Thus, editors and readers often consider advertising an unfortunate necessity. A cynic might say that generating revenue is the ultimate goal of advertisers, publishers, and editors—advertisers want to sell more products, publishers want to increase journal revenue, and editors want their journals to remain financially viable and sustainable. However, editors have a larger ethical responsibility to their readers, who must be able to rely on the editor to ensure that the journal's integrity remains intact and that the information contained in the publication is valid and objective. This includes ensuring that advertising does not influence editorial decisions or content and having policies and procedures in place that prevent such influence.

Thus, editors should have ultimate responsibility for all content published in their journals, including advertisements and sponsored content (see also 5.10, Editorial Freedom and Integrity, and 5.11, Editorial Responsibilities, Roles, Procedures, and Policies). The International Committee of Medical Journal Editors (ICMJE) recommends that editors "have full and final authority for approving advertisements and enforcing advertising policy."[2] The American Society of Magazine Editors (ASME) recommends that "every effort must be made to show all advertising pages, sections and their placement to the editor far enough in advance to allow for necessary changes" and to permit the editor to monitor compliance with advertising guidelines.[3] However, some editors may not be able to review and approve specific ads because of limited resources (personnel and time). Nevertheless, all editors should be involved in the development, enforcement, and evaluation of formal advertising policies for print and online versions of their journals. For example, principles for advertising in print and online are developed jointly by editorial and publishing staff for *JAMA* and the *Archives* Journals.[4] These principles are used by both publishing and editorial staff to determine the suitability of advertising. Although editorial and publishing staff regularly review and discuss these policies and their applicability in specific situations, the *JAMA* and *Archives* Journals editor in chief has final authority over all advertisements.

According to the ICMJE, advertising must not be allowed to influence editorial decisions.[2] All editorial decisions must be based solely on the quality and suitability of the editorial content and should not be influenced by potential revenue, or loss of revenue, from advertising, sponsorship, sales of reprints/e-prints, or related commercial activities, or the influence of ad sales and marketing representatives. This policy is also supported by the World Association of Medical Editors[5] and the UK Committee on Publication Ethics.[6] Complete separation of the roles and functions that determine editorial decisions and advertising sales is critical. Thus, editorial staff must not be involved in the promotion or sale of any advertisements, and the publishing staff who sell ads and sponsorship (including reprints) should not be permitted access to editorial content until it is published. Editors should have policies and procedures in place to address reader and online user complaints, assessment of such complaints, and appropriate remedy or action. The ICMJE recommends that editors consider publishing letters that raise important concerns about advertising content, in the same way that they publish critical letters about articles,[2] including asking the advertiser to submit a reply.

5.12.1 **Advertisements.** Advertisements appear in print and online journals, e-mail alerts, other online information products and services, and other types of media (such as podcasts and blogs). For biomedical publications, advertisements typically include the following:

- Advertisements that promote professional or trade-related products (primarily pharmaceuticals and medical equipment in biomedical publications), services, educational opportunities or products, or announcements (see also 5.12.3, Advertorials). These are typically called *display advertisements* in print; online, they may include banners, pop-up windows, or text-based ads (such as in e-mail alerts or other online communications of information) (see also 5.12.6, Advertising and Sponsorship in Online Publications).

- Display advertisements that promote products and services not specifically related to a profession or trade (such as an ad for an automobile or an airline in a medical journal).

- Classified or recruitment advertisements (listings of employment opportunities, educational courses, workshops, announcements, or other services).

In most cases, advertisers pay to place advertisements for their products and services in publications. Those advertisements for which a publisher does not typically charge a fee include public service announcements, ads for nonprofit organizations or charities, and "house ads," which promote a product or service provided by the owner of the publication.

Important considerations for editors and publishers are whether paid advertisements and sponsorship invite potential infringements on editorial independence and whether they represent important revenue opportunities for journals in increasingly competitive markets.[7,8] The keys to maintaining editorial integrity are to achieve a balance between these seemingly opposing forces, to maintain a recognizable separation between the functions and decisions of editorial and advertising departments, and to have consistent and publicly available policies on advertising and sponsorship.[2,9]

Although the primary function of most journals is to educate and inform in a neutral manner and that of advertisements is to educate and inform in a promotional manner, advertisers and editors share a common goal—to influence the behavior of readers.[10] Obvious differences between editorial text and advertising copy exist. In biomedical publication, editorial material typically comprises text composed in a consistent scholarly format with data-based tables and figures, whereas advertisements typically contain bold, colorful statements and eye-catching graphics. Scholarly editorial material is generally intended to be objective, whereas advertisements are generally intended to be preferential, selective, and persuasive. Problems arise when the means to achieve the common goal—of influencing behavior—fall outside expected norms or violate specific regulations and standards.

In many countries, advertisers must meet specific criteria established by national regulatory agencies. For example, drug ads are required to follow the regulations of the Food and Drug Administration in the United States,[11] the Association of the British Pharmaceutical Industry in the United Kingdom,[12] and the Pharmaceutical Advertising Advisory Board in Canada.[13] The International Federation of Pharmaceutical Manufacturers Associations has regularly updated guidelines for pharmaceutical marketing practices that may be helpful for countries without well-defined regulations.[14] However, each of these regulatory agencies has been criticized for not enforcing its regulations.[15,16]

5.12.2 Criteria for Advertisements Directed to Physicians and Other Health Care Professionals. The editorial and publishing staff of *JAMA* and the *Archives* Journals have developed general eligibility requirements and guidelines for advertising copy to ensure that advertisements published in these journals are appropriate (see Tables 1 and 2).[4] The ASME also has developed a guide for print-based advertisements.[3]

The following criteria for print pharmaceutical ads are adapted from the guidelines prepared by the World Health Organization[17] and the International Federation of Pharmaceutical Manufacturers Associations[14]:

1. Advertising text should be presented legibly.
2. Pharmaceutical ads in print journals must include the following (in online ads, this information may be included on a Web site to which the ad links):
   - Name of the product, typically the trade (brand) name
   - The active ingredients, using either the international nonproprietary names or the approved generic name of the drug
   - Name and address of the manufacturer or distributor
   - Date of production of the advertisement
   - Abbreviated prescribing information, which should include an approved indication or indications for use together with the dosage and method of use and a succinct statement of the contraindications, precautions, and adverse effects
   - For a "reminder" advertisement (a "short advertisement containing no more than the name of the product and a simple statement of indications to designate the therapeutic category of the product"[5]), the abbreviated prescribing information may be omitted. (See also 5.12.3, Advertorials.)
3. When published studies are cited in promotional material, standard retrievable references with complete bibliographic information should be included (see also 3.0, References). Information in advertisements and other promotional material, such as excerpts from the medical literature or quotations from personal communications, must not change or distort the intended meaning of the author(s) or the significance of the relevant work or

Table 1. Eligibility Requirements to Advertise in Journals Published by the American Medical Association (AMA)[a]

1. The AMA, in its sole discretion, reserves the right to decline any submitted advertisement or to discontinue publication of any advertisement previously accepted.
2. Products or services eligible for advertising in the scientific publications shall be germane to and useful in (*a*) the practice of medicine, (*b*) medical education, or (*c*) health care delivery, and should be commercially available.
3. In addition to the above, products and services that are offered by responsible advertisers and that are of interest to physicians, other health professionals, and consumers are also eligible for advertising.
4. Pharmaceutical products for which approval of a new drug application by the Food and Drug Administration (FDA) is a prerequisite for marketing must comply with FDA regulations regarding advertising and promotion.
5. Institutional advertising germane to the practice of medicine and public service messages of interest to physicians may be considered for inclusion in all AMA publications.
6. Alcoholic beverages and tobacco products may not be advertised.
7. **Equipment, Instruments, and Devices:** The AMA determines the eligibility of advertising for products intended for preventive, diagnostic, or therapeutic purposes. Complete scientific and technical data concerning the product's safety, operation, and usefulness may be required. These data may be either published or unpublished. Samples of equipment, devices, or instruments should not be submitted. The AMA reserves the right to decline advertising for any product that is involved in litigation with a governmental agency with respect to claims made in the marketing of the product.
8. **Food Products:**
   A. General-purpose foods, such as bread, meats, fruits, and vegetables, are eligible.
   B. Special-purpose foods (eg, foods for carbohydrate-restricted diets and other therapeutic diets) are eligible when their uses are supported by acceptable data.
   C. Dietary programs: Only diet programs prescribed and controlled by physicians are eligible.
9. **Dietary Supplements:** Advertisements for nutritional supplements and vitamin preparations are not eligible unless the safety and efficacy of the product have been reviewed and approved by the FDA for a disease claim.
10. **Books:** A book may be requested for review to determine its eligibility.
11. **Insurance Coverage:** Claims made in advertisements for insurance coverage must conform with the following specific criteria:
    A. Claims relating to policy benefits, losses covered, or premiums must be complete and truthful.
    B. Claims made shall include full disclosure of exclusions and limitations affecting the basic provisions of policy.
    C. Claims incorporating quoted testimonials must meet the same standards as other claims.
    D. Each advertisement for insurance products and services must include a statement indicating either the states in which the products or services are available or the states in which the products or services are not available.
12. **CME Programs:** Advertisements for continuing medical education (CME) programs are not eligible unless the CME sponsor is accredited by the Accreditation Council for Continuing Medical Education and is an accredited medical school (or hospital affiliated with such a school), a state or county medical society, a national medical specialty society, or other organization affiliated with the American Board of Medical Specialties member boards.
13. **Miscellaneous Products and Services:** Products or services not in the above classifications may be eligible for advertising if they satisfy the general principles governing eligibility for advertising in AMA publications.

[a] These guidelines are intended for advertisements for US-based companies, products, and services. See references 12 to 14 for examples of relevant guidelines for other countries.

Table 2. Guidelines for Advertising Copy in Journals Published by the American Medical Association (AMA)

1. The advertisement should clearly identify the advertiser of the product or services offered. In the case of drug advertisements, the full generic name of each active ingredient shall appear. [This requirement applies to print ads; for online ads, the active ingredient may appear on the company or manufacturer's Web site to which the ad links.]
2. Layout, artwork, and format shall be such as to be readily distinguishable from editorial content and to avoid confusion with the editorial content of the publication. The word *Advertisement* may be required.
3. Unfair comparisons or unwarranted disparagements of a competitor's products or services will not be allowed.
4. Advertisements will not be acceptable if they conflict with the Principles of Medical Ethics of the American Medical Association or the advertising guidelines in *Current Opinions of the Council on Ethical and Judicial Affairs of the American Medical Association.*
5. It is the responsibility of the manufacturer to comply with the laws and regulations applicable to marketing and sale of its products. Acceptance of advertising in AMA publications should not be construed as a guarantee that the manufacturer complies with such laws and regulations.
6. Advertisements may not be deceptive or misleading.
7. Advertisements will not be accepted if they are offensive in either text or artwork, or contain attacks of a personal, racial, sexual, or religious nature, or are demeaning or discriminating toward an individual or group on the basis of age, sex, race, ethnicity, religion, physical appearance, or disability.

study. Prepublication peer review and editorial evaluation of articles help to reduce problems associated with misleading or inappropriate information from published articles, but ads do not typically undergo the same level of evaluation before publication. Several studies have documented problems with advertisements in medical journals, including promotional statements not being accurately supported by references, references cited to support promotional statements that are not retrievable (eg, "data on file"), and numerical distortion of data presented in tables and graphs.[18-22] Thus, some editors have instituted formal review processes to assess the validity of claims made in ads.[23,24]

4. According to the International Federation of Pharmaceutical Manufacturers Associations,[14] the same requirements that apply to printed materials should also apply to electronic promotional materials, including audiovisuals. Specifically, in the case of pharmaceutical product–related Web sites, the identity of the pharmaceutical company and of the intended audience should be readily apparent, the content and presentation should be appropriate for the intended audience, and country-specific information should comply with local laws and regulations.[14] (See also 5.12.6, Advertising and Sponsorship in Online Publications.) Typically, an online advertisement links to a company's Web site, where the details about the prescribing information as listed above are provided.

Five issues should be addressed in any journal's policy on advertising:

1. Advertising-to-editorial content ratio
2. Advertising interspersion

3. Advertising-editorial juxtaposition (adjacency)
4. Editorial calendars
5. Appropriate advertising content

Advertising-to-Editorial Content Ratio. For print publications that have an abundance of advertising, setting an ad-editorial page ratio (ie, limiting the advertising content to no more than a certain proportion of total annual pages) may help protect the perceived integrity of the publication.[25] The ICMJE recommends that journals not be dominated by advertising and that they avoid publishing advertisements from only 1 or 2 advertisers; otherwise readers may perceive that the journal is sponsored by 1 or 2 advertisers and that these advertisers have influenced the editor and the editorial content.[2] For print journals, compliance with relevant postal regulations in some countries may also need to be considered if the number of ad pages exceeds the number of editorial pages. The ratio of editorial to advertising on Web versions of journals should also follow these general principles.

Advertising Interspersion. Placing advertisements between articles and interleaving them within articles may attract advertisers, but such practices may also diminish the perceived credibility of the publication—especially if the ads create difficulty for the reader in reading or finding editorial content.[2,25] For scholarly biomedical journals, ads should not be interleaved within a scientific or clinical article in print or online. Many print publications group, or stack, their ads in the front and back of their journals, leaving an editorial "well" in the middle of the publication for major articles that are not interspersed with ads. Stacking ads can cause some advertisers to go elsewhere because they want their ads to be placed next to editorial material. For that reason, some journals place popular editorial features (such as news articles) in the front and back of the journal to allow for ad interspersion of those sections and maintain an ad-free editorial well for the original research and other major articles. Ads should not appear on the journal's front cover. For discussion of advertising interspersion on the Web, see also 5.12.6, Advertising and Sponsorship in Online Publications.

Advertising-Editorial Juxtaposition (Adjacency). Advertisers may request placement of their ads next to related editorial content to help promote their products. Although common in consumer publishing, this practice is discouraged by the ICMJE and the ASME.[2,3] Ad adjacency, like ad interspersion, may be an impediment to readers and may diminish the perceived integrity of a scholarly publication.[2,10] To avoid the occurrence of adjacent ads and editorial content on the same topic, even by chance, the editorial staff of *JAMA* and the *Archives* Journals review the entire makeup (imposition) of the journal after the ad deadlines have closed and before the journal is printed. If an ad is scheduled to appear adjacent to an article on the same or a closely related topic, the editors ask the production staff to move the ad or may decide to move the article. For those journals that permit online ads on pages with editorial content, ad adjacency policies should be developed that maintain the journal's editorial integrity. (See also 5.12.6, Advertising and Sponsorship in Online Publications, for additional discussion of advertising-editorial adjacency in online publications.)

Editorial Calendars. Providing advertising sales representatives with editorial calendars that include specific content scheduled for upcoming issues invites pressure for advertising-editorial adjacency and other attempts from industry to interfere with editorial decisions. The ICMJE states that advertising should not be sold on the condition that it will appear in the same issue as a particular article.[2] Journal editors and publishers can respond to industry pressure by reminding advertisers of the importance of the journal's integrity. Advertisers understand this issue, because without integrity, a publication will have few readers, and without readers, the advertiser cannot sell products. For this reason, advertising sales staff should not have access to the journal contents until after publication. However, sales staff may know about general editorial plans, such as plans for theme issues, proceedings, symposia, or sponsored supplements (see 5.12.4, Sponsored Supplements).

Appropriate Advertising Content. Appropriate ads must meet the following requirements[4,13,16,17,26]:

- No false claims
- No implied false claims
- Ability to substantiate claims
- No omissions of important facts
- No distortion of data
- Good taste (although this is difficult to define objectively)
- Clear identification of the advertiser of the product or services being offered
- Layout, artwork, and format that differ from those of the editorial content so that readers can clearly distinguish the advertising and editorial content

Biomedical journals typically publish a disclaimer statement to separate the claims made by advertisers from the views of the journals' owners. For example, the following statement appears in each issue of *JAMA*:

> ADVERTISING PRINCIPLES—Advertisements in this issue have been reviewed to comply with the principles governing advertising in *JAMA* and the *Archives* Journals. A copy of these principles is available on request and online at www.jama.com. The appearance of advertising in *JAMA* is not an AMA guarantee or endorsement of the product or the claims made for the product by the manufacturer.

5.12.3 Advertorials. An advertorial is an ad that imitates editorial content or presents content in an editorial-like format, such as using text, tables, or figures in a manner similar to the journal's editorial content. During the early 1990s, following a decline in the biomedical advertising market, advertorials became more common. The ASME developed guidelines for special advertising sections,[27] which may help a publication maintain its integrity if it publishes advertorials (see Table 3).

Companies may submit advertisements that provide information on a topic pertaining to a product the company markets (or plans to market) but that do not name any commercial product. It is essential that such ads are clearly labeled "Advertisement," have a different format from the journal's editorial content, and include

Table 3. ASME Guidelines for Special Advertising Sections[a]

1. Each page of special advertising must be clearly and conspicuously identified as a message paid for by advertisers.
2. To identify special advertising sections clearly and conspicuously:
   A. The words *advertising, advertisement,* or *special advertising section* should appear prominently at or near the top of every page of such sections containing text, in type at least equal in size and weight to the publication's normal editorial body typeface. (The word *advertorial* should not be used.)
   B. The layout, design, and type of such sections should be distinctly different from the publication's normal layout, design, and typefaces.
   C. Special advertising sections should not be slugged on the publication's cover or included in the editorial table of contents.
   D. If the sponsor or organizer of the section is not the publisher, the sponsor should be clearly identified.
3. The editors' names and titles should not appear on, or be associated with, special advertising sections, nor should the names and titles of any other staff members or of regular contributors to the publication appear or be associated with special advertising sections. The publication's name or logo should not appear as any part of the headlines or text of such sections.
4. Editors and other editorial staff members should not prepare advertising sections for their own publication, for other publications in their field, or for advertisers in the fields they cover.
5. For the publication's chief editor to have the opportunity to monitor compliance with these guidelines, material for special advertising sections should be made available to the publication's editor in ample time to review and recommend necessary changes. Monitoring would include reading the text of special advertising sections *before* publication for problems of fact, interpretation, and taste and for compliance with any relevant laws.
6. To avoid potential conflicts or overlaps with editorial content, publishers should notify editors well in advance of their plans to run special advertising sections.
7. The size and number of special advertising sections within a single issue should not be out of balance with the size and nature of the magazine.

[a] Adapted and reprinted with permission from the American Society of Magazine Editors.[27]

a prominent display of the company name and/or logo so that readers can quickly ascertain that the information is an advertisement from the company and is not part of the journal's editorial content.

5.12.4 Sponsored Supplements. Sponsored supplements are collections of articles, usually on a single topic, and are published as an extra edition or a separate section of a journal, often after a meeting or symposium. A study of 58 highly cited and read medical journals found that the number of supplements published by these journals had increased 4-fold from 1966 to 1989.[28] Forty-two percent (262 of 625) of these supplements were single-sponsored (ie, sponsored by 1 pharmaceutical company) and, compared with supplements funded by other types of sponsors, were less likely to have been formally peer reviewed and more likely to have promotional attributes, such as misleading titles, focus on a single-drug topic, and use of brand names only.[28] Because of the promotional and biased quality of such industry-sponsored supplements, *JAMA* and the *Archives* Journals will not publish them. In addition, the US National Library of Medicine will not index articles in sponsored supplements unless certain disclosure conditions are met.[29]

However, supplements can serve useful educational purposes, provided that the content is objective, balanced, independent, and scientifically rigorous.[9,30] Sponsored supplements also may provide additional revenue to publishers. Recognizing this, the ICMJE developed a set of principles to guide editors when considering the publication of sponsored supplements.[2] These principles should help avoid bias in the selection of content for inclusion in industry-sponsored publications[2]:

1. The journal editor must take full responsibility for the policies, practices, and content of supplements, including complete control of the decision to publish all portions of the supplement. Editing by the funding organization should not be permitted.

2. The journal editor must retain the authority to send supplement manuscripts for external peer review and to reject manuscripts submitted for the supplement. These conditions should be made known to authors and external supplement editors before beginning editorial work on the supplement.

3. The journal editor must approve the appointment of any external editor of the supplement and take responsibility for the work of the external editor.

4. The sources of funding for the research, publication, and the products the funding source make that are considered in the supplement should be clearly stated and prominently located in the supplement, preferably on each page. Whenever possible, funding should come from more than 1 sponsor.

5. Advertising in supplements should follow the same policies as those of the rest of the journal.

6. Journal editors must enable readers to distinguish readily between ordinary editorial pages and supplement pages.

7. Journal editors and supplement editors must not accept personal favors or personal remuneration from sponsors of supplements.

8. Secondary publication in supplements (republication of papers previously published elsewhere) should be clearly identified by the citation of the original paper. Supplements should avoid redundant or duplicate publication. Supplements should not republish research results, but the republication of guidelines or other material in the public interest might be appropriate.

9. The principles of authorship and conflict of interest disclosure should apply to supplements.

5.12.5 **Other Forms of Sponsorship.** Other forms of sponsorship include sales of bulk subscriptions to commercial entities for distribution to individuals, noncommercial sponsorship or grants to support specific editorial sections, and grants to support publication of journals in resource-poor communities. With each type of sponsorship, the funding source should be clearly indicated to recipients and readers/users, and all editorial content should be under the complete authority of the editor, should undergo the journal's usual editorial evaluation and peer review, and should not be influenced by the sponsor(s).

5.12.6 Advertising and Sponsorship in Online Publications. Online ads are not restricted by the physical limits of a printed page. For example, a user can increase the type size of the prescribing information that appears in small type in print pharmaceutical ads. Ads can rotate, expand, be animated, or pop up on a screen without the user's request. An ad for a particular drug, product, or service can be hyperlinked to the manufacturer or provider's Web site. In addition, ads can be targeted for specific users or a specific user experience. The standards for protecting editorial integrity of print publications apply to advertising in online publications and other electronic products, such as CDs, DVDs, Web sites, e-mail, audio and video casts, and online databases, especially for publications in clinical and health-related fields. For example, just as a print reader can choose to read an ad or skip over it, an online user should have the same choice; online ads should not interfere with the reading and use of editorial content and should not dominate the online content; and online ads should not appear adjacent to editorial content on the same or a closely related topic. As stated by the ASME, "While linking and other technologies can greatly enhance the user experience, the distinction between independent editorial content and paid promotional information should remain clear."[31]

Privacy Concerns. Privacy rights of online journal users and visitors must be maintained. If any specific or personal information about users is to be collected and specifically distributed or sold to third parties (such as advertisers), users should be informed in advance and given the opportunity to not have their information shared with others. Aggregate demographic information about numbers and types of users may be provided to advertisers to guide decisions about placing advertisements in specific journals in the same manner that circulation numbers are provided to advertisers and used for decisions to place print ads. This information may also be used by publishers to set advertisement rates and fees. Data on overall numbers of users, impressions (ie, number of times an advertisement has been viewed), and click rates (percentage of impressions that account for a click through to an advertiser's Web site) are acceptable to share with advertisers provided that the journal advertising policy and use of such information are made clear to users.

Guidelines for Online Advertising and Sponsorship. As the technology advances, online advertising will provide additional opportunities and ethical dilemmas for publishers and editors. Accordingly, guidelines for online advertising and sponsorship will also continue to evolve. The following guidelines, which are based on some of those developed for use in online versions of *JAMA* and the *Archives* Journals,[4] provide guidance for advertising in online publications.

Online Advertising

- Policies and procedures for online advertising should be jointly developed, reviewed, and approved by editorial and publishing staff. Similar principles should apply to print and online ad guidelines.
- Journals that have policies for editorial review and approval of print ads should apply similar policies for review and approval of online ads.
- Online advertising may appear on journal Web sites, journal-related e-mail messages (eg, e-mail alerts of new content or tables of contents that users have

registered to receive), other communications of journal information, and other media (such as podcasts).

- Online advertisements must be readily distinguishable from editorial content; ads should be labeled with the word *Advertisement* (ie, placed above or below the ad).

- Online advertisements may appear as text, fixed or rotating banners, or pop-up windows. Online advertising should not interfere with a user's ability to read, use, navigate within, search, or interact with editorial content. Users should have the ability to easily navigate away from such advertisements (eg, close a pop-up advertisement).

- Online advertisements should not be juxtaposed with, appear in line with, or appear adjacent to editorial content on the same or a closely related topic, or be linked with editorial content on the same topic. However, just as advertising may appear across from the print table of contents, ads may appear adjacent to online tables of contents or similar listings of article titles (eg, a journal or publisher's home page).

- Online advertising may appear on screen with specific types of articles as long as the separation between editorial and advertising content is made clear and juxtaposition of editorial and advertisements on the same or a closely related topic does not occur. It is preferred that such ads not appear on editorial pages of scholarly, peer-reviewed articles and be reserved for other types of articles, such as news sections.

- Logos of journals or journal owners may not appear on commercial Web sites as logos or in any other form without prior written approval.

- Advertisements may link from the journal to an off-site commercial Web site, provided that viewers are clearly informed that they are viewing an advertisement by means of the word *Advertisement* placed above, below, or in the ad. The Web site to which the ad links should be reviewed in advance. The linked page must include the following elements:

    - Company sponsoring the Web site is clearly displayed.

    - Claims on the online advertisement and the landing page of the Web site are reasonable and substantiated.

    - No registration requiring personal information is required before reaching the Web site. For journals that permit facilitation of the gathering of such personal information (eg, promotional leads), privacy policies and procedures should be followed (see also "Privacy Concerns" above).

- Non–journal-affiliated Web sites should not frame a journal's Web site content without express permission; should not prevent the viewer from returning to the journal's Web site or other previously viewed screens, such as by disabling the viewer's Back button; and should not redirect the viewer to a Web site that the viewer did not intend to visit.

- E-mail alerts and other forms of online information dissemination may have text or HTML ads embedded in the e-mail (top and/or bottom) provided that the relevant guidelines herein are followed.

- Journals should not permit their content to be used on an advertiser's site. However, journals may sell e-prints to advertisers who then link to the journal's article from the Web site. In such cases, the advertiser's Web site should not imply any relationship with the journal (see also 5.12.7, Reprints and E-prints).
- Ads should not be linked to editorial content search terms. Journal search engines should not include the ability to search content from advertisements unless the results of such searches clearly indicate the difference between editorial and advertising content. Advertisers or sponsors should not receive preferential treatment in search programs and search results.

Online Sponsorship

- Editorial content of any sponsored product (eg, online publications, CDs, DVDs, Web sites, e-mail, audio and video casts, and online databases) should be determined by the standard editorial process. The sponsor should have no influence over the editorial content of any sponsored product.
- Sponsorship policies should be clearly noted, either in text accompanying the product or on a disclosure page, and should clarify that the sponsor had no input into or influence over the content.
- All financial or material support for sponsored content should be acknowledged and clearly indicated (eg, on the home or landing page as well as on any packaging and collateral material included).
- These acknowledgments should not make any claim for any supporting company product(s). The final wording and positioning of the acknowledgment should be determined by the journal, with review and approval by the editor. The wording could be similar to "Produced by [*Journal Name*] with support from [Company Name]."
- The acknowledgment of the sponsor's support may be linked to the sponsor's Web site.
- Journal names and logos should not appear on the sponsoring company Web site without prior written approval by the journal.
- Journal search engines should not include content from sponsors unless the results of such searches clearly indicate the difference between sponsored and nonsponsored content. Sponsors should not receive preferential treatment in search programs and search results.

See also 5.12.4, Sponsored Supplements.

5.12.7 **Reprints and E-prints.** Publishers of journals may sell reprints and e-prints of journal articles as a source of revenue. Reprints and e-prints may be purchased by authors for personal use, by others for educational purposes, or by commercial entities for promotional purposes. In biomedical journal publishing, a *reprint* is the republication of an article or collection of articles in which the content is unchanged from the original publication (except perhaps for the inclusion of postpublication corrections). An *e-print* is a digital reproduction of or an online link to an article or collection of articles, usually PDF files(s). For example, publishers of *JAMA* and the

Archives Journals sell reprints to authors (at relatively low cost) as a service for authors and to the pharmaceutical industry as a source of revenue. *JAMA* and the *Archives* Journals also provide authors with complimentary access to their articles as e-prints and sell access to e-prints to commercial entities. Some journals permit authors to post e-prints of their articles (usually PDF files) on personal or other archival/institutional Web sites (see also 5.6.2, Intellectual Property: Ownership, Access, Rights, and Management, Open-Access Publication and Scientific Journals), and some journals permit commercial entities to purchase and post copies of e-prints on their Web sites. *Note:* Reprints and e-prints differ from *preprints*, which are print and online versions of articles/manuscripts made formally available to others before publication in a peer-reviewed journal.

Journals should establish and follow consistent policies and procedures on the production, sale, review/approval, and distribution/dissemination of reprints and e-prints. For an example of such standards, see those developed for *JAMA* and the *Archives* Journals in 5.6.10, Intellectual Property: Ownership, Access, Rights, and Management, Standards for Commercial Reprints and E-prints. Editorial decisions must be free of any influence from the potential for sale of reprints and e-prints, and all such sales must not be permitted to occur until after publication of the original article. Reprinted articles should not be abridged or altered by the purchaser and should not include an advertisement or the advertiser's logo or other commercial content. A publisher may incorporate or append a correction to a previously published article in a reprint/e-print as long this is noted in the reprint/e-print.

ACKNOWLEDGMENTS

Principal author: Annette Flanagin, RN, MA

I thank the following for reviewing and providing useful comments on the manuscript: Geoffrey Flick, American Medical Association, Periodic Publishing & Business; Trevor Lane, MA, DPhil, University of Hong Kong; and June Robinson, MD, *Archives of Dermatology*.

REFERENCES

1. Moser RH. Advertisements and our journal. *Ann Intern Med*. 1977;87(1):114-115.
2. International Committee of Medical Journal Editors. Uniform Requirements for Manuscripts Submitted to Biomedical Journals: Writing and Editing for Biomedical Publication. http://www.icmje.org. Updated February 2006. Accessed July 22, 2006.
3. American Society of Magazine Editors. *ASME Guidelines for Editors and Publishers*. 13th ed. New York, NY: American Society of Magazine Editors; 2006. http://www.magazine.org/Editorial/Guidelines. Accessed June 11, 2006.
4. American Medical Association. Principles governing advertising in publications of the American Medical Association. Chicago, IL: American Medical Association. http://pubs.ama-assn.org/misc/adprinciples.pdf. Revised October 2006. Accessed January 5, 2007.
5. Utiger R; for the Education Committee of the World Association of Medical Editors. A syllabus for prospective and newly appointed editors. http://www.wame.org/resources/editor-s-syllabus. Posted October 26, 2001. Accessed January 5, 2007.
6. Committee for Publication Ethics. COPE Code of Conduct for Editors. http://www.publicationethics.org.uk/reports/2005/code. Accessed July 16, 2006.

7. Fletcher RH. Adverts in medical journals: caveat lector. *Lancet.* 2003;361(9351):10-11.
8. Tsai AC. Conflicts between commercial and scientific interests in pharmaceutical advertising for medical journals. *Int J Health Serv.* 2003;33(4):751-768.
9. Callaham M. Journal policy on ethics in scientific publication. *Ann Emerg Med.* 2003;41(1):82-89.
10. Dixon T. Pharmaceutical advertising: information or influence? *Can Fam Phys.* 1993;39:1298-1300.
11. US Food and Drug Administration. Title 21: Food and Drugs. Chapter 1: Food and Drug Administration, Department of Health and Human Services. Subchapter C: Drugs: General. 21CFR 202.1. http://www.fda.gov. Revised April 1, 2005. Accessed July 16, 2006.
12. Association of the British Pharmaceutical Industry. Code of practice for the pharmaceutical industry 2006. http://www.abpi.org.uk/links/assoc/PMCPA/code06use.pdf. Accessed July 16, 2006.
13. Pharmaceutical Advertising Advisory Board. Code of advertising acceptance. http://www.paab.ca/index_en.html. Updated April 1, 2005. Accessed July 16, 2006.
14. International Federation of Pharmaceutical Manufacturers Associations. *IFPMA Code of Pharmaceutical Marketing Practices.* 2006 Rev. http://www.ifpma.org/pdf/IFPMA-TheCode-FinalVersion-30May2006-EN.pdf. Accessed June 11, 2006.
15. Kessler DA. Addressing the problem of misleading advertising. *Ann Intern Med.* 1992;116(11):950-951.
16. Lexchin J, Holbrook A. Methodologic quality and relevance of references in pharmaceutical advertisements in a Canadian medical journal. *CMAJ.* 1994;151(1):47-54.
17. World Health Organization. *Ethical Criteria for Medicinal Drug Promotion.* Geneva, Switzerland: World Health Organization; 1988.
18. Villanueva P, Peiro A, Liberos J, Immaculada P. Accuracy of pharmaceutical advertisements in medical journals. *Lancet.* 2003;361(9351):27-32.
19. Wilkes MS, Doblin BH, Shapiro MF. Pharmaceutical advertising in leading medical journals: experts' assessments. *Ann Intern Med.* 1992;116(11):912-919.
20. van Winkelen P, van Denderen JS, Vossen CY, Huizinga TW, Dekker FW. How evidence-based are advertisements in journals regarding the subspecialty of rheumatology? *Rheumatology (Oxford).* 2006;45(9):1154-1157.
21. Cooper RJ, Schriger DL. The availability of references and the sponsorship of original research cited in pharmaceutical advertisements. *CMAJ.* 2005;172(4):487-491.
22. Cooper RJ, Schriger DL, Wallace RC, Mikulich VJ, Wilkes MS. The quantity and quality of scientific graphs in pharmaceutical advertisements. *J Gen Intern Med.* 2003;18(4):294-297.
23. Pitkin RM. Advertising in medical journals. *Obstet Gynecol.* 1989;74(4):667-679.
24. Wilkes MS, Kravitz RL. Policies, practices, and attitudes of North American medical journal editors. *J Gen Intern Med.* 1995;10(8):443-450.
25. Rennie D, Bero LA. Throw it away, Sam: the controlled circulation journals. *CBE Views.* 1990;13(13):31-35.
26. Parmley WW. Has Madison Avenue become Medicine Avenue? *J Am Coll Cardiol.* 1994;23(7):1726-1727.
27. American Society of Magazine Editors. *Guidelines for Special Advertising Sections.* 8th ed. New York, NY: American Society of Magazine Editors; July 1996.
28. Bero LA, Galbraith A, Rennie D. The publication of sponsored symposiums in medical journals. *N Engl J Med.* 1992;327(16):1135-1140.

29. US National Library of Medicine. Fact sheet: response to inquiries about journal selection for indexing at NLM. http://www.nlm.nih.gov/pubs/factsheets/j_sel_faq.html. Last updated October 13, 2006. Accessed January 5, 2007.
30. Kessler DA. Drug promotion and scientific exchange: the role of the clinical investigator. *N Engl J Med.* 1991;325(3):201-203.
31. American Society of Magazine Editors. Best practices for digital media. http://www.magazine.org/Editorial/Guidelines/Best_Practices_for_Digital_Media. Accessed July 16, 2006.

Most people understand science and technology less through direct experience than through the filter of journalism. . . . Journalists are, in effect, brokers, framing social reality and shaping the public consciousness about science.

Dorothy Nelkin[1]

5.13 Release of Information to the Public and Journal/Author Relations With the News Media.

Public interest in matters of health and in news about medicine and health is substantial. A telephone survey of 1250 US adults concluded that the majority of citizens consider news coverage of science to be as important as coverage of crime, the economy, politics, sports, and entertainment.[2] Many factors affect science journalism and the communication of scientific information to the public, including poor science literacy among the public; the increase in costs for print publication and distribution; a concomitant decline in print newspaper circulation and the decline of newspaper sections dedicated to health and science; a dearth of investigative journalists trained as scientists and more coverage of science news by reporters who do not understand science; the rise of online news systems and on-demand news delivered to niche markets; news and topic-specific e-mail lists and blogs; tabloid journalism; sponsored infotainment, infomercials, and Web sites masquerading as credible and objective providers of science and health information; and the increasingly competitive nature of the businesses of news delivery and scientific journals.[3-9]

The responsible dissemination of the results of new scientific research and information to the public is critical. Unfortunately, amid the burgeoning means of conveying such information, accuracy and reliability in science news coverage in the news media are not increasing proportionately. To gain a competitive edge in the information chain, news organizations may exchange complexity, analysis, background, and perspective for immediacy and sensationalism.[10] Thus, the need for journal editors to develop and maintain viable and ethical relationships with news journalists—for all types of media—has become even more important.

Scientific journal editors have several responsibilities regarding communicating scientific information to the public and their relationship with the news media:

- Publish appropriate, accurate, reliable, timely, and accountable scientific information.
- Inform authors and journalists about journal policies regarding release of information in manuscripts under consideration or accepted prior to publication and journal

embargoes prohibiting news media coverage of articles before publication (see 5.13.1, Release of Information to the Public).

- Assist the news media to prepare accurate stories of the information about to be published by providing news releases, answering questions, facilitating equal advanced access to the journal articles in a controlled and consistent manner, and providing access to authors or other experts as needed (see 5.13.1, Release of Information to the Public).
- Evaluate the quality of news coverage of information published in the journal. For example, if a news organization has published an inaccurate report of a particular journal article, the journal editor should consider notifying the journalist and/or news editor to identify the errors in the report.[11]

Studies have documented that reporting of science, biomedicine, and health in the lay media is often inaccurate, incomplete, or without adequate context.[12-18] Journal editors and news journalists share a common obligation—to ensure that the public receives accurate information and is not misled.[11,12,19] This obligation becomes particularly important when information about risk is communicated to the public. For example, failure to describe health risks accurately and in proper perspective may be misleading, can create unnecessary concern, and may result in loss of public trust in reporters, editors, and scientists. Tensions between journalists, editors, and scientists—often driven by self-interests—can do much to confuse the public. These tensions should be recognized and mitigated,[19] and journals should seek an appropriate balance between their duties to the community of readers they serve, the integrity of the scientific literature, and public entitlement to access to important scientific information without unreasonable delay.[20]

5.13.1 Release of Information to the Public. In many ways, biomedical journals and their editors act as gatekeepers for the release of scientific information to their readers as well as to the public. However, conflicts often arise between journal editors (who have an ethical duty to ensure that the information they publish has been appropriately peer reviewed and assessed for quality) and scientists (who want to disseminate their findings as widely and quickly as possible) and between editors and news reporters (who want to deliver information about new scientific developments to their readers as quickly as possible).[19] The announcement of "scientific breakthroughs" at press conferences or through press releases before the data that support the supposed advance have been evaluated and published in a peer-reviewed journal may cause confusion for the public (who may be given misleading or inaccurate information), news media (who may give undue attention to an inaccurate or incomplete claim), journal editors (who may have a policy that discourages publication of data that have already been reported in the press), and investigators (who may forfeit their chance for publication in a reputable peer-reviewed journal by choosing to publish by press conference or through press releases).[21-23]

Journal editors have developed 2 policies to discourage premature release of information to the public. The first policy, based on the "Ingelfinger rule" (developed in 1969 by Franz Ingelfinger, MD, then editor of the *New England Journal of Medicine*), is an understanding between authors and editors that a manuscript will be considered for publication on the condition that it has not been submitted or reported elsewhere [24] (see also 5.3, Duplicate Publication). The second policy is a news embargo, which is an agreement between journalists and editors that prohibits news coverage of a journal article until it is published (see 5.13.3, Embargo). Although some authors and journalists misunderstand or disagree with the intent of the Ingelfinger rule and the news embargo,[25,26] many journals have found that both, if applied consistently and fairly, effectively serve all communities interested in disseminating quality scientific information to the public (with exceptions made in cases of urgent public need for information or to coincide with presentations at scientific meetings).

The International Committee of Medical Journal Editors (ICMJE) and the World Association of Medical Editors (WAME) recommend that journals develop and follow policies for orderly, controlled, and consistent release of information to the public, including the use of embargoes.[20,27] There are 4 general exceptions to a journal policy that precludes prepublication release of information to the public: presentation of information during scientific or clinical meetings, release of information that is determined to be of urgent public need, testimony before government agencies, and, in rare instances, release of information that is in the public domain.[22]

Presentation of Information During Scientific or Clinical Meetings. Presentation of findings during scientific or clinical meetings (via oral presentation or poster presentation) does not preclude consideration of a manuscript reporting the complete findings for publication.[20,22,27] Authors may include abstracts of their findings in print and/or online proceedings published for these meetings. However, authors should refrain from disseminating or publishing details in proceedings that are not included in the meeting abstract or presentation. Authors should not include a complete report of their findings (ie, a mansucript that they plan to submit to a journal) or distribute copies of their detailed findings or tables and figures to meeting attendees or journalists. Authors are encouraged to participate in discussion and the usual exchange with meeting attendees during their presentation. Audiocasts and videocasts of meeting presentations also do not preclude consideration of the full manuscript for publication provided these are intended for meeting participants.

Authors may also answer questions from journalists about their meeting presentations, but they should limit their discussion to explaining and clarifying the findings presented during the meeting and should not discuss any related manuscripts under consideration by a journal or accepted but not yet published. In the event that an author is presenting findings at a meeting that are also included in a manuscript that is under consideration or has been accepted by a journal but not yet published, the author should limit her or his remarks to the findings as presented at the meeting. In this case, the author should inform the editor of plans to present the work at a meeting before the meeting occurs and should discuss options with the editor (see also 5.13.3, Embargo, and 5.13.4, Suggestions for Authors Interacting With the News Media). News media coverage (based on these interactions) about manuscripts that are accepted but not yet published or that are under consideration by a journal occurring before the journal embargo is lifted and without prior approval of the editor may be grounds for rejection of the manuscript by some journals.

Authors of papers under consideration by a journal or accepted but not yet published, as well as authors' institutions and funders, should not participate in press conferences before publication of the peer-reviewed article. Thus, authors should not participate in press conferences at meetings separate from their scientific presentation unless they have prior approval from the journal to which the full paper has been submitted.

On occasion, the journal and the author may plan to publish the complete manuscript online before the article appears in print (after peer review and revision) on the same date of the presentation of the findings during a scientific meeting (eg, with a late-breaking trial that is likely to have a practice-changing effect). In these cases, news releases prepared by an author's institution or funder that summarize information to be published in a journal should be coordinated with the journal (see also 5.13.5, News Releases). Proper planning is needed among all parties (journal, author, and meeting organizer) to ensure that findings are released in an orderly manner that does not confuse journalists or the public.

Release of Information Determined to Be of Urgent Public Need. Contrary to what many authors and news reporters believe, few findings from scientific and medical research have such significant and urgently important implications for the public that the information should be released to the public before it has been peer reviewed, revised, and published in a journal (online or in print). Calling such circumstances "exceptional," the ICMJE recommends that public health authorities should make such decisions and should be responsible for disseminating such information to health professionals and the news media.[20] However, an editor may recognize the public health urgency of releasing information contained in a manuscript under consideration without prompting from the authors or relevant authorities. In such a case, the editor should ask the author to notify the appropriate authority to consider advance dissemination of the information, and this dissemination should be coordinated between the responsible authority or agency and the journal. In situations in which there is an immediate public health need for the information, there should be no delay in its release even if this release antedates publication in the print journal.[28] Journals should expedite the editorial and peer review process and speed the publication process to permit online publication as quickly as possible. If such online publication occurs before print publication of the article, care should be taken that this is conducted in an orderly and consistent manner so as not to confuse journalists and the public.

Testimony Before Government Agencies. An author's testimony before a governmental agency or institution (eg, the US Congress or Food and Drug Administration) that includes information not yet published should not preclude consideration of that information in a manuscript under consideration or subsequently submitted for publication.[22] Authors and editors should discuss whether consideration and publication of a manuscript with information relevant to such testimony can be expedited to coincide with or be published before the testimony on a case-by-case basis.

Information in the Public Domain. Reports of important information from national government or international agencies published in print and widely disseminated or published online (eg, an urgent health alert or Web posting from the US National Institutes of Health or the World Health Organization) should be considered selectively for publication in a peer-reviewed journal on a case-by-case basis.[22] In such a case, the editor needs to determine if the information would be useful to the journal's readers, there is demonstrated need for an additional report (eg, additional important details or follow-up information is available), and if the initial alert did not already include the complete report.

5.13.2 **Expedited Publication and Release of Information Early Online.** Many journals have policies to expedite the evaluation and publication of manuscripts deemed worthy of accelerated dissemination, including release of an article online ahead of its print publication.[22] Editors should use consistent and orderly policies and procedures to identify manuscripts containing such information, expedite the editorial/peer review and publication process, and, if feasible, notify and provide controlled advance access to journalists.

5.13.3 **Embargo.** A news embargo is an agreement between journals and news reporters and their organizations not to report information contained in a manuscript that has been accepted but not yet published until a specified date and time in exchange for advance access to the information. Among medical journals, the embargo system may have been initiated by Morris Fishbein, MD, editor of *JAMA* between 1924 and 1949.[29]

As an example, the standard embargo date and time for *JAMA* is 3 PM central time on the day before the journal's cover date (issue publication date). Qualified journalists are given early access to the journal online via a password-protected Web site for the news media (usually 5 days before issue publication date). During this time, the embargo is intended to provide competitive news reporters an equal amount of access and time to research and prepare their news stories. However, those news reports cannot be released until the embargo has lifted. *JAMA* is printed and mailed in advance of the cover date, so that physicians can read pertinent journal articles before they are reported in the news media and before patients begin asking them questions after reading or viewing the news coverage.[22]

The news embargo has been criticized for being overly restrictive, delaying public access to information, and serving the self-interest of journals.[25] However, the embargo system is intended to create a level playing field for journalists to prepare accurate and complete news stories and to maintain consistency in the timing of release of scientific information to the public and help prevent confusion that may result from sporadic reporting on the same study at different dates and times. According to the ICMJE, such consistency of timing helps to minimize economic chaos surrounding those articles that contain information that may influence financial markets.[20]

On occasion, a news reporter or organization may break an embargo and report on information from a peer-reviewed journal article before the embargo is lifted, either unintentionally (owing to miscommunication or misunderstanding) or intentionally, to scoop competitors.[29,30] The rare intentional embargo break is a serious breach of trust and can result in the journal applying sanctions against the reporter and the news organization. Such sanctions may include barring the reporter, and perhaps the news organization, from receiving news releases and advance access to journal content and declining requests for interviews, access to authors, or other assistance.

5.13.4 **Suggestions for Authors Interacting With the News Media.** The following recommendations are provided for interactions between authors and the news media.[12,18,20,22]

- Authors should abide by agreements with journals not to publicize their work while their manuscript describing their work is under consideration or awaiting publication by a journal. If authors have any questions about prior release of such information, they should contact the journal's editorial office.[20,22]

- Authors presenting research at clinical and scientific meetings may discuss their presentations with reporters but should refrain from distributing copies of their presentations, data, tables, or figures (see 5.3, Duplicate Publication).[20,22]

- Authors should inform editors of previous news coverage of their work at the time of manuscript submission (see 5.3, Duplicate Publication).[20]

- Authors of manuscripts under consideration by a journal or accepted but not yet published should not participate in press conferences before publication of their findings in the journal unless this is an approved exception by the journal editor and this is done in coordination with the journal.[22]

- Authors who receive telephone calls or other communications from journalists about their research or other work reported in manuscripts that are under consideration but not yet accepted by a journal may indicate that the manuscript is under consideration but should not provide details on the name of the journal if and until the manuscript is accepted. (See also 5.7.1, Confidentiality, Confidentiality During Editorial Evaluation and Peer Review and After Publication.)

- Authors should establish an understanding with a reporter before an interview about the journal's embargo policy, comments made "on and off the record," and the opportunity to review direct quotations.[12] *Note:* Authors should be cautious about making comments "off the record."

- For accepted manuscripts about to be published and those just published, authors should be as accessible to the news media as their schedules permit, keeping reporters' deadlines in mind and setting aside time to prepare for and give interviews.[12]

- During an interview, authors should avoid use of medical/scientific jargon, acronyms, and too many statistics; explain commonly used jargon and acronyms and provide easily understood statistics; avoid answering hypothetical questions; and avoid responding with "no comment" (provide an explanation for not being able to answer a specific question).[18]

- Authors should inform reporters and news organizations of errors in news stories and request published corrections if necessary.[12]

- Authors who expect to be interviewed frequently by the news media should consider having training in providing informative and accurate interviews.[12]

In addition, journal editors should inform authors of accepted manuscripts of the journal's policies regarding release of information prior to publication and relations with the news media. For example, *JAMA* reminds authors of its policies on duplicate publication and news embargoes in acceptance letters, noting that authors and the news media should not release any information about the author's accepted article until the specified embargo date and time. This embargo does not preclude authors from participating in interviews with reporters who are preparing stories; it is meant to remind authors that any news stories resulting from such interviews should not precede publication of the authors' articles in the journal.

Some journals notify authors of projected publication dates in their acceptance letters, and some journals include a notice of the publication date on the edited manuscript or page proof sent to authors for approval before publication. Editorial and publishing staff may also receive calls from authors requesting information about expected dates of publication. Staff and authors should not assume that such dates or their corresponding embargo dates are definite or final. Editors may rearrange the editorial content schedules of specific issues; thus, publication dates may change. When informing authors of the expected dates of publication for their accepted articles, editors should remind authors that these dates may change.

If authors want to coordinate news coverage of their published articles through a press conference or press release, they should first contact the journal editor to ascertain the exact date of publication. The ICMJE suggests that editors and publishers may want to help authors and representatives from their organizations coordinate press conferences and releases with the simultaneous publication of their articles.[20] Editors and publishers can also help the news media prepare accurate reports by providing news releases, answering questions, providing access to the authors and other experts, and providing advanced access to journal articles. This assistance should be contingent on agreement with and cooperation of the news media in timing their release of stories to coincide with the publication of the article. Press releases, advance copies of journals, and journal articles released online in advance should indicate the date and time of the news embargo and be restricted to qualified news journalists and agencies that agree to honor the journal's embargo policy.

5.13.5 **News Releases.** Many journals issue news releases on selected articles determined by the editors to be of interest to the public. For *JAMA* and the *Archives* Journals, experienced science writers prepare the news releases, which are reviewed by the editors to ensure accuracy and objectivity. News releases of journal content should be under the authority of the editor, not the journal's publisher or owner (see also 5.10, Editorial Freedom and Integrity).

News editors, writers, and producers receive hundreds of news releases a week. Thus, a news release must attract attention, but it also must conform to a familiar format and style (see Box). Journalists are taught to present facts accurately, but they may not know how to interpret biomedical statistics or understand the specific context of new scientific information. In news releases and news stories, research findings and statistics are often cited inaccurately or out of context to support an exaggerated medical claim.[14,15,31,32] To help prevent exaggerated or misleading claims, news releases must include accurate and clearly stated statistics[33] (see 20.1, Study Design and Statistics, The Manuscript: Presenting Study Design, Rationale, and Statistical Analysis). In addition, research findings must be placed in proper context and should include important background, summary of study methods, limitations of the methods, and information on study sponsorship and relevant conflicts of interests of authors (see 5.5, Conflicts of Interest). Care should be taken to provide balance (eg, citing a related editorial) and to avoid sensationalism (eg, use of terms

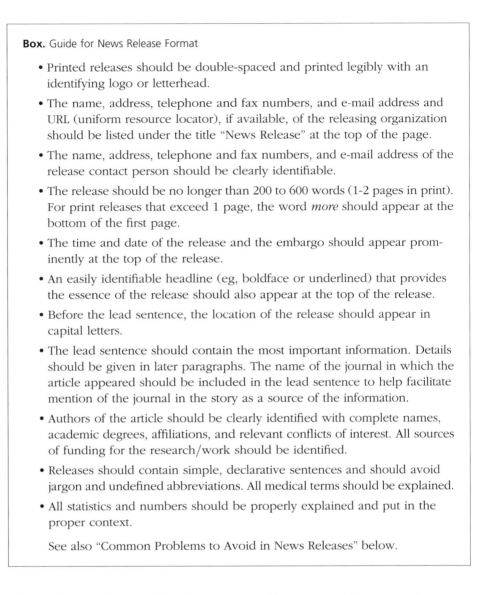

Box. Guide for News Release Format

- Printed releases should be double-spaced and printed legibly with an identifying logo or letterhead.
- The name, address, telephone and fax numbers, and e-mail address and URL (uniform resource locator), if available, of the releasing organization should be listed under the title "News Release" at the top of the page.
- The name, address, telephone and fax numbers, and e-mail address of the release contact person should be clearly identifiable.
- The release should be no longer than 200 to 600 words (1-2 pages in print). For print releases that exceed 1 page, the word *more* should appear at the bottom of the first page.
- The time and date of the release and the embargo should appear prominently at the top of the release.
- An easily identifiable headline (eg, boldface or underlined) that provides the essence of the release should also appear at the top of the release.
- Before the lead sentence, the location of the release should appear in capital letters.
- The lead sentence should contain the most important information. Details should be given in later paragraphs. The name of the journal in which the article appeared should be included in the lead sentence to help facilitate mention of the journal in the story as a source of the information.
- Authors of the article should be clearly identified with complete names, academic degrees, affiliations, and relevant conflicts of interest. All sources of funding for the research/work should be identified.
- Releases should contain simple, declarative sentences and should avoid jargon and undefined abbreviations. All medical terms should be explained.
- All statistics and numbers should be properly explained and put in the proper context.

See also "Common Problems to Avoid in News Releases" below.

like *breakthrough*). Examples of common problems to avoid in news releases are listed below:

Common Problems to Avoid in News Releases

- Unfamiliar mathematical and statistical terms and numbers that are difficult to interpret should be avoided; do not confuse association and correlation with causation.

- Results should be reported in context, including locations and dates of the study, representativeness of the sample, and limitations of the study. Risks of events should be acknowledged to be common (eg, common cold) or rare (eg, being hit by lightning).[18]

- If the results of a survey are reported, the response rate should be provided along with a caveat that the results may not be generalizable if the response rate is low.
- If a news release mentions a specific sample that was studied or a specific number of cases, whether the number is large or small, information about the size of the total population from which the sample or cases were drawn should be included.
- Statements about statistical significance should not be quoted from an article out of context or without an explanation. Reporters and readers do not necessarily know the difference between statistical significance and clinical significance. For example, quoting a statement that there was a trend toward a statistically significant association between treatment X and outcome Y may give undue importance to a treatment that has no real clinical value.
- Absolute event rates should be reported. Care should be taken to avoid confusing absolute and relative risks because relative risks are often erroneously translated to specific risks. For example, a decrease from 2.5% to 2.0% should not be reported as a 20% reduction in risk, but could be reported as a 0.5% absolute risk reduction and 20% relative risk reduction. It is also helpful to report excess or decreased risk in terms of numbers per 1000 or 10 000.
- Avoid reporting odds ratios, especially for common outcomes, which may overstate a relative risk.[18]
- If reporting the results of a study about an intervention, event rates for benefits and harms should be reported equally and in a balanced manner.[18]

Before news releases are distributed, they should be proofread and the content should be reviewed by a professional familiar with the article or report covered in the release, or by the editor.

ACKNOWLEDGMENTS

Principal author: Annette Flanagin, RN, MA

I thank Joan Stephenson, PhD, *JAMA* Medical News & Perspectives, and Jann Ingmire, *JAMA* and *Archives* Journals Media Relations, for reviewing and providing important suggestions to improve the manuscript; and the following for reviewing and providing minor comments: Terri S. Carter, *Archives of Surgery*; Catherine D. DeAngelis, MD, MPH, *JAMA* and *Archives* Journals; Robert M. Golub, MD, *JAMA*; Wayne G. Hoppe, JD, *JAMA* and *Archives* Journals; Trevor Lane, MA, DPhil, University of Hong Kong; and Povl Riis, MD, University of Copenhagen.

REFERENCES

1. Nelkin D. Journalism and science: the creative tension. In: *Health Risks and the Press*. Washington, DC: Media Institute; 1989:53-71.
2. Science news: what does the public want: a survey by Lou Harris commissioned by SIPI. *SIPIscope*. 1993;20(2):1-10.
3. Hume E. *Tabloids, Talk Radio, and the Future of News: Technology's Impact on Journalism*. Washington, DC: Annenberg Washington Program; 1995.
4. Hard times hit science sections. *SIPIscope*. 1992;20(1):1-4.
5. Ethiel N, ed. *Medicine and the Media: A Changing Relationship*. Chicago, IL: Robert R McCormick Tribune Foundation; 1995.

6. Levi R. *Medical Journalism: Exposing Fact, Fiction, Fraud.* Lund, Sweden: Studentlitteratur; 2000.
7. Schwitzer G, Mudur G, Henry D, et al. What are the roles and responsibilities of the media in disseminating health information? *PLoS Med.* 2005;2(7):e215:0576-0582.
8. Ankney RN, Moore RA, Heilman P. Newspaper coverage of medicine: a survey of editors and cardiac surgeons. *AMWA J.* 2001;16(1):23-32.
9. Erickson A, McKenna J, Romano R. Past lessons and new uses of the mass media in reducing tobacco consumption. *Public Health Rep.* 1990;105(3):239-244.
10. Garrett L. Reporting epidemics: real and unreal. Paper presented at: Institute of Medicine Annual Meeting: Emerging and Reemerging Infections; October 16, 1995; Washington, DC.
11. Freischlag J. "Wrong" surgery is rare occurrence. *USA Today.* April 26, 2006:A12.
12. Rubin R, Rogers HL Jr. *Under the Microscope: The Relationship Between Physicians and the News Media.* Nashville, TN: Freedom Forum; 1993.
13. Smith DE, Wilson AJ, Henry DA; on behalf of the Media Doctor Study Group. Monitoring the quality of medical news reporting: early experience with Media Doctor. *Med J Aust.* 2005;183(4):190-193.
14. Moynihan R, Bero L, Ross-Degnan D, et al. Coverage by the news media of the benefits and risks of medications. *N Engl J Med.* 2000;342(22):1645-1650.
15. Schwartz LM, Woloshin S. News media coverage of screening mammography for women in their 40s and tamoxifen for primary prevention of breast cancer. *JAMA.* 2002;287(23):3136-3142.
16. Voss M. Checking the pulse: midwestern reporters' opinions on their ability to report health care news. *Am J Public Health.* 2002;92(7):1158-1160.
17. Motl SE, Timpe EM, Eichner SF. Evaluation of accuracy of health studies reported in mass media. *J Am Pharm Assoc.* 2005;45(6):720-725.
18. Stamm K, Williams JW, Noel PH, Rubin R. Helping journalists get it right: a physician's guide to improving health care reporting. *J Gen Intern Med.* 2003;18(2):138-145.
19. Glass RM, Flanagin A. Communication, biomedical II. scientific publication. In: Reich WT, ed. *Encyclopedia of Bioethics.* 2nd ed. New York, NY: Macmillan Publishing Co; 1995:428-435.
20. International Committee of Medical Journal Editors. Uniform Requirements for Manuscripts Submitted to Biomedical Journals: Writing and Editing for Biomedical Publication. http://www.icmje.org. Updated February 2006. Accessed April 30, 2006.
21. Butler D. "Publication by press conference" under fire. *Nature.* 1993;366(6450):6.
22. Fontanarosa PB, Flanagin A, DeAngelis CD. THE JOURNAL's policy regarding release of information to the public. *JAMA.* 2000;284(22):2929-2931.
23. Schwartz LM, Woloshin S, Baczek L. Media coverage of scientific meetings: too much, too soon? *JAMA.* 2002;287(21):2859-2863.
24. Kassirer JP, Angell M. The Ingelfinger rule revisited. *N Engl J Med.* 1991;325(19):1371-1373.
25. Altman L. The Ingelfinger rule, embargoes, and journal peer review, part 1. *Lancet.* 1996;347(9012):1382-1386.
26. Who's responsible to whom—and for what. In: Ethiel N, ed. *Medicine and the Media: A Changing Relationship.* Chicago, IL: Robert R McCormick Tribune Foundation; 1994:16-47.
27. Utiger RD; for the Education Committee, World Association of Medical Editors. A syllabus for prospective and newly appointed editors. http://www.wame.org/resources/editor-s-syllabus. Posted October 26, 2001. Accessed January 5, 2007.

28. Lundberg GD, Glass RM, Joyce LE. Policy of AMA journals regarding release of information to the public. *JAMA*. 1991;265(3):400.
29. Stacy J. The press embargo—friend or foe? *JAMA*. 1985;254(14):1965-1966.
30. Fontanarosa PB, DeAngelis CD. The importance of the journal embargo. *JAMA*. 2002;288(6):748-750.
31. Hough GA. *News Writing*. 3rd ed. Boston, MA: Houghton Mifflin Co; 1984.
32. Cohn V, Cope L. *News and Numbers: A Guide to Reporting Statistical Claims and Controversies in Health and Related Fields*. 2nd ed. Ames, IA: Blackwell Publishing Professional; 2001.
33. Woloshin S, Schwartz LM. Press releases: translating research into news. *JAMA*. 2002;287(21):2856-2858.

6 Editorial Assessment and Processing

The principal goals of editing biomedical publications are to select, improve, and disseminate information that will advance the art and science of the discipline covered by the publication. For example, biomedical publications are a major source of information for the improvement of medical care. In addition to initial transmission to readers at the time of publication, information from journal articles is often carried by the public media. Published articles influence educators and opinion leaders, who transmit the information to many persons who do not read the original publications. Medical journal articles can also be subsequently accessed by clinicians and researchers seeking information about particular topics. Such searches are facilitated by online search engines (see 25.0, Resources) and provide the information essential to practicing evidence-based medicine,[1] in which patient-care decisions are informed by acquiring and assessing the relevant medical literature. These myriad uses of biomedical literature indicate the importance of the procedures to improve quality involved in editorial assessment and processing.

6.1 **Editorial Assessment.** The assessment process (Figure 1) consists of 2 phases: editorial review and peer review. In editorial review, editors first assess submissions for their overall quality and appropriateness for the publication's readership. Some manuscripts are rejected on the basis of this editorial "triage." Manuscripts that pass this initial step go on to the peer review phase. Peer review (see 6.1.3, Peer Review) involves evaluation by experts who are "peers" of the authors with regard to knowledge about the topic of the submission, and may also include evaluation by expert statistical reviewers (see 6.1.5, Statistical Review). The integrity of the editorial assessment process requires strict confidentiality (see 5.7.1, Ethical and Legal Considerations, Confidentiality, Confidentiality During Editorial Evaluation, Peer Review, and After Publication) and attention to possible biases and conflicts of interest.

6.1.1 **Editorial Decisions.** On the basis of evaluations by the editors and peer reviewers, submitted manuscripts are either rejected or returned to authors with suggestions for improvement through revision. Authors should realize that a request for revision does

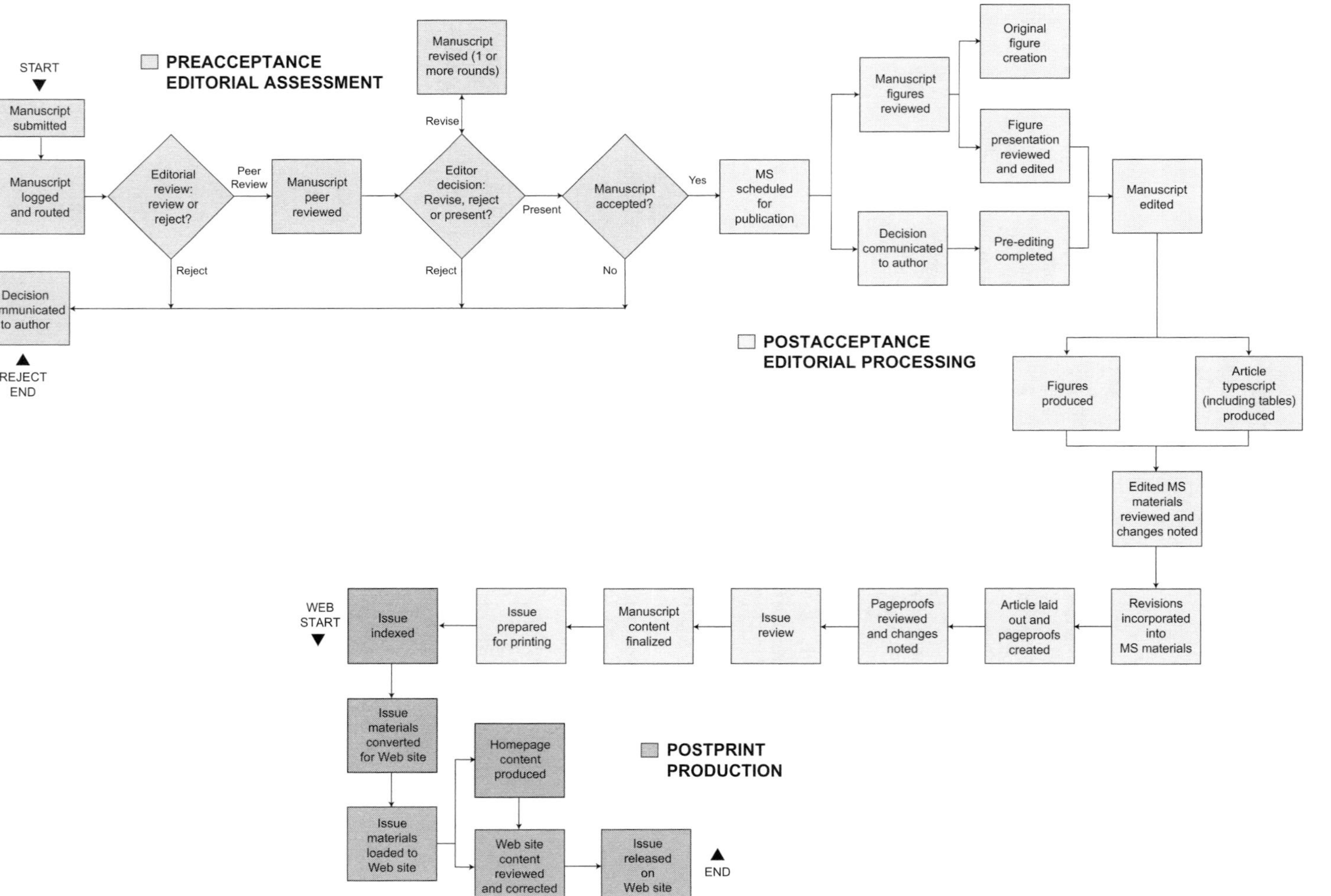

Figure 1. *JAMA* manuscript (MS) workflow: editorial assessment and processing.

not guarantee acceptance, because revised manuscripts are subject to editorial review and may also have additional peer review. Several rounds of review and revision may occur before a final decision is reached. Acceptance of manuscripts expressing viewpoints, perspectives, or opinions may be based solely on editorial review, but reports of original data and other major articles almost always undergo peer review, statistical review, and revision before acceptance for publication (see 1.0, Types of Articles). Journals with more than 1 editor may hold meetings during which submitted manuscripts and their reviews, and also revised manuscripts, are presented and discussed before decisions are reached regarding revision or acceptance for publication.

The decisions for rejection, revision, and acceptance all belong to the editor, not the peer reviewers. The term *referee*, meaning a person to whom a paper is referred for review, is sometimes used synonymously with peer reviewer. However, in the United States *referee* can be misleading because that term often implies one who has authority for decisions, particularly in sports events. In biomedical publishing, editors have that decision responsibility. Peer reviewers have an important and helpful but advisory role, essentially serving as consultants to editors.

6.1.2 **Assessment Criteria.** Two major criteria are central to the evaluation of manuscripts submitted for publication: importance and quality. *Importance* involves an assessment of whether the work

- Represents a scientific advance (recognizing that individual articles usually convey only small advances)
- Has clinical relevance (if the journal is to be read and the information used by practicing clinicians)
- Presents new information
- Will be of interest to readers

An additional component of importance is *editorial priority*, a composite judgment made by the editor regarding the value of a particular submission relative to other submissions under evaluation at the same time, weighed in the context of the articles that journal has recently published and has scheduled for publication. The reality of limited space may also be a consideration, even in the era of electronic publication. Cyberspace may appear infinite, but the attention span and patience of readers are not. Furthermore, the editorial processing requirements (see 6.2, Editorial Processing) for material to be published electronically may be very similar to those for print publication. Hence, concise submissions may be given higher priority than long ones (other factors being equal) because they take up a smaller proportion of a journal's resources and total space allotment.

Evaluation of *quality* involves an assessment of how well a paper treats its topic, including how well the topic and the methods used to deal with that topic are described. For original research reports, assessment of quality involves consideration of whether

- The design and methods are appropriate to answer the stated research questions
- The research questions and the methods used to answer them are well described and rigorously conducted
- The data analysis is appropriate

- The conclusions are supported by the results
- Patients or research participants were treated ethically (see 5.8, Ethical and Legal Considerations, Protecting Research Participants' and Patients' Rights in Scientific Publication)

The quality of the writing may be a major factor in the assessment of editorials, commentaries, and other nonresearch submissions where the elegance and impact of the writing itself may constitute major reasons for publication. For research and review articles (see 1.0, Types of Articles), writing quality (especially clarity) may affect the reactions of editors and peer reviewers even though the importance and quality of the research should be the main focus for assessment. Writing quality can be improved by manuscript editing (see 6.2.1, Manuscript Editing), but only if the research is described with sufficient clarity to permit basic understanding.

The specific nature or direction of results should not be an issue in quality assessment. If a paper addresses an important question and uses high-quality methods to answer it, the results are worth publishing no matter what they are. Publication bias that results from a tendency for investigators not to submit, or editors not to accept, papers that do not report statistically significant "positive" results should be eliminated.[2] A well-done study that shows that a particular intervention is ineffective is usually just as important as a study that reports a "positive" result.

6.1.3 **Peer Review.** Peer review was first used for biomedical publications by the Royal Societies of London and Edinburgh in the 18th century, but it evolved haphazardly and was not used consistently until after World War II.[3-5] The essence of peer review consists of asking experts "How important and how good is this paper, and how can it be improved?" (see 6.1.2, Assessment Criteria). The use of expert consultants to advise editors about the selection and improvement of papers has become a standard quality-assessment measure in biomedical publication. Yet the process and effectiveness of peer review have come under scientific scrutiny only since the 1980s.[5-9]

Experts in the topic of a paper are needed to assess importance and quality. However, peer review has been criticized for its reliance on human judgments that are subject to biases and conflicts of interest, and there have been few empirical documentations of the efficacy of the peer review process.[8-13] Empirical research on editorial peer review has begun to address some of the deficiencies in knowledge about it. See the March 9, 1990; July 13, 1994; July 15, 1998; and June 5, 2002, issues of *JAMA* for articles from the first 4 International Congresses on Peer Review in Biomedical Publication.

Peer reviewers should assess all components of a manuscript, including online-only supplementary material, and are usually asked to provide comments for the authors regarding the strengths and weaknesses of a paper, including suggestions for improvement. Reviewers also make recommendations to the editor, usually on a form provided by the journal (Figure 2), but specific criticisms and suggestions are much more valuable than summary judgments. It is remarkable that the peer review process depends largely on the efforts of peer reviewers who donate their time—sometimes large amounts of it[14]—in the interest of the quality of publications in their field. The speed and efficiency of the peer review process has been improved by the availability of electronic or Internet-based peer review systems. Using such systems, which are often combined with electronic or Internet-based manuscript submission, peer reviewers can be queried regarding their availability, receive or

JAMA

JAMA&ARCHIVES

JAMA

MANUSCRIPT HOME | AUTHOR INSTRUCTIONS | REVIEWER INSTRUCTIONS | HELP | TIPS | LOGOUT | JOURNAL HOME

Reviewer's Overall Assessment

Reviewer	
Reviewing Editor	
Date Due	
Manuscript#	
Title	
Corresponding Author	
Contributing Author	

Recommendation
Please Select — Accept as is / Accept if suitably revised / Revise and reconsider / Reject

Publication Timing:
Please Select — Routine / ASAP / Fast Track / N/A

Quality:
Please Select — Superior / Good / Fair / Poor

Priority:
Please Select — 1 (low) / 2 / 3 / 4 / 5 (high)

Consortium Manuscript?
None

Material Original?
○ Yes ○ No ○ Uncertain ○ N/A

Data Valid?
○ Yes ○ No ○ Uncertain ○ N/A

Conclusions Reasonable?
○ Yes ○ No ○ Uncertain ○ N/A

Information Important?
○ Yes ○ No ○ Uncertain ○ N/A

Writing Clear?
○ Yes ○ No ○ Uncertain ○ N/A

General Medical Interest?
○ Yes ○ No ○ Uncertain ○ N/A

Tables/Figures Appropriate?
○ Yes ○ No ○ Uncertain ○ N/A

If no, please explain how the tables/figures are inappropriate.

Editorial Needed?
○ Yes ○ No ○ Uncertain ○ N/A

If yes, please indicate if you would like to volunteer to write the Editorial or suggest someone who may be interested. (Confidential)

Confidential remarks for the Reviewing Editor:

(These remarks will **NOT** be transmitted to the author.)

Please provide your general and specific comments to the Author:

Do not reveal your name in the text of the message. This message will be sent as is to the author. You may copy/paste your text into the box above. Please do not use Greek characters.

Please disclose below your conflict(s) of interest (if any) in reviewing this manuscript. (Required)

Review Attachments

Attach author comments or supplemental files.

Browse...

After pressing the "Browse" button, select "All files (*.*)" on the pop-up's File Type menu.

Browse...

Browse...

Save As Draft | Submit Recommendation

MANUSCRIPT HOME | AUTHOR INSTRUCTIONS | REVIEWER INSTRUCTIONS | HELP | LOGOUT | JOURNAL HOME

TERMS OF SERVICE | PRIVACY POLICY

EJPress Version 4.04 by eJournalPress

© 2004 American Medical Association. All Rights Reserved.

Figure 2. *JAMA* peer reviewer comments form. N/A indicates not applicable.

download a copy of the submission for review, and send their review and recommendations electronically, eliminating the time previously required for telephone contacts and mailing or faxing of paper copies.

6.1.4 **Selection of Reviewers.** The selection of peer reviewers and the number of reviewers for a particular submission are matters of editorial judgment. Peer reviewers are usually experts who are not part of the journal staff. However, editorial staff members may serve as peer reviewers in areas of their expertise. Reviewers may be members of the journal's editorial board, or a peer review panel, or they may have no other association with the journal. The editor's knowledge of experts in a particular field often determines reviewer selection. Many journals maintain a database of reviewers indexed by areas of expertise and including information on review quality and turnaround time. A paper's reference list can be useful in indicating contributors to the literature on the same topic. A literature search by the editor can also be helpful in identifying potential reviewers.

Authors sometimes suggest names of possible reviewers and also may indicate persons they believe should not review their paper, usually because of perceived bias. Editors should consider such information, but the selection of reviewers belongs to the editor, who must use judgment in distinguishing a reviewer's valid praise or criticism from unwarranted bias for or against a particular submission. In an observational study at 10 biomedical journals,[15] reviewers suggested by authors did not differ in the quality of their reviews compared with reviewers selected by editors, but author-suggested reviewers tended to make more favorable recommendations for publication. Reviewers should disclose to the editor any conflicts of interest they may have regarding a topic or an author (see 5.5.6, Ethical and Legal Considerations, Conflicts of Interest, Requirements for Peer Reviewers).

6.1.5 **Statistical Review.** Reviewers with expertise in statistics (including the assessment of study design and research methods) are essential to evaluate the quality of original research reports. Such reviewers may serve as paid consultants to a journal. Empirical studies have shown that statistical review can be very helpful in selecting and improving scientific reports for publication.[16,17] Unfortunately, many published research articles are flawed by weaknesses in study design and methods that should have been detected by review or, far better, prevented by appropriate statistical consultation in planning the research before the manuscript was written.

6.1.6 **Concealing of Author and Reviewer Identities.** Among the unsettled issues in peer review are efforts to conceal the identities of authors (and their affiliations) from reviewers, and the question of whether the identities of reviewers should be revealed to authors. Biomedical journals commonly use a "single-blind" (single-masked) review process in which authors' identities are revealed to reviewers, but the names of reviewers are not revealed to authors (see 5.7.1, Ethical and Legal Considerations, Confidentiality, Confidentiality During Editorial Evaluation and Peer Review and After Publication). This process recognizes the difficulty of concealing author identities, makes it easier for reviewers to detect attempts at duplicate publication by the same authors, and may encourage more candid reviews because the reviewers know they are anonymous to the authors, who may be their professional colleagues.

However, this single-blind tradition is controversial. Reviewers might be influenced by the identities and reputations of authors or their affiliations and thus not judge a manuscript solely on quality and importance. Furthermore, some critics believe that authors ought to know who is evaluating their work and that reviewers should stand by their critiques by signing them, a process sometimes called "open peer review."[5,18] Journal policies vary regarding concealing or revealing author and reviewer identities, and these practices should be indicated in the instructions for authors (see 5.11.4, Ethical and Legal Considerations, Editorial Responsibilities, Roles, Procedures, and Policies, Editorial Responsibility for Peer Review). In some disciplines (eg, nursing and psychology), "double-blind" review, in which neither author nor reviewer identities are revealed, is common. Authors who submit a paper to a journal that attempts to conceal author identities should remove identifying information from all parts of the manuscript. Author names, affiliations, and acknowledgments (including funding sources) should be submitted separately.

A few empirical studies of these issues have been published. One relevant finding is that attempts to conceal author identities are often not successful due to self-references in the paper or reviewer knowledge of the authors' work. The latter is not surprising because the reviewers are experts in the authors' fields. Thus, "blind" review is often unblinded. A multijournal randomized controlled trial[19] found that masking of author identities was successful for only 68% of manuscripts overall, and that author masking tended to be less successful for reviewers with more research experience and for well-known authors, but was unrelated to a journal policy of masking.[20] Even more important, masking of author identities, whether it was successful or not, did not improve the quality of reviews as assessed by editors or authors.[19] These findings were similar to the results of trials of masking of author identities undertaken at single journals.[21-23] In a large-scale "field trial," the *Canadian Medical Association Journal* (*CMAJ*) in 1984 switched to concealing author identities but reversed this practice in 1990 after concluding that the time-consuming efforts to conceal author identities were often unsuccessful and did not improve the review process.[24]

Less empirical information is available on the effects of identifying peer reviewers to authors (open peer review) vs keeping them anonymous. A randomized trial[25] performed at the *BMJ* concluded that asking reviewers to consent to being identified to authors had no important effects on quality of reviews, recommendations regarding publication, or the time taken to review, but it increased the likelihood of reviewers declining to review. Positions in favor of open peer review are usually taken on the grounds of ethics and accountability.[5]

Whatever its problems may be, it is clear that peer review "has been indispensable for the progress of biomedical science"[26] and that no better alternative has emerged for the assessment and improvement of submissions to biomedical and scientific journals.[27] Rennie[5(p12)] has observed, "It is therefore no surprise that as the evidence of its flaws and inefficiencies accumulates, peer review, far from foundering as it hits iceberg after iceberg, shrugs them off and sails proudly on."

6.1.7 **Revision.** If an editorial decision is made to request revision of a submitted manuscript, the author should receive specific recommendations from the editor about how to improve the paper, in addition to receiving the comments of the peer reviewers. Guidance from the editor is particularly important if recommendations from the peer reviewers are discordant. The revision process is also the appropriate time for the editor to make suggestions regarding condensing the manuscript and requests for additional data or analyses, and to obtain required authorship, funding, and conflict of interest statements. Authors are usually requested to submit a list of the revisions completed and the reasons for any suggested revisions not undertaken when they return the revised manuscript. As previously noted (see 6.1.1, Editorial Decisions), the editor should make it clear that a revision will require editorial evaluation and possibly additional peer review, so no promise of acceptance for publication can be made in advance of that assessment. Unless there is a compelling reason for the revised paper to be evaluated by a new reviewer, peer review of a revision (if it is necessary in the editor's judgment) should usually be done by the original peer reviewers, who, along with the reviewing editor, are in the best position to evaluate the success of the revision process.

6.1.8 **Appealing a Rejection.** If a paper is rejected, authors occasionally ask for reconsideration, usually because they believe the reviewers or the editor have misjudged the importance and quality of the submission. This situation can be viewed in 2 different ways. On the one hand, peer review and editorial decisions are based on fallible human judgments. Mistakes can be made, so perhaps the rejected manuscript merits reconsideration. On the other hand, heeding appeals for reconsideration may fulfill the adage "The squeaky wheel gets the grease." Reconsideration of papers solely on the basis of author complaints could be unfair to authors who have equally legitimate grounds for reconsideration but who do not appeal. Thus, some journals take the position that rejections are final. Other journals reconsider rejected submissions at the discretion of the editor who made the initial decision. Such discretion usually would include consideration of whether the authors provide objective grounds for reconsideration of the original decision, particularly if they can provide new data or new analyses, as opposed to differences of opinion about editorial priority (see 6.1.2, Assessment Criteria, and 5.11.5, Ethical and Legal Considerations, Editorial Responsibilities, Rules, Procedures, and Policies, Editorial Responsibility for Rejection).

6.1.9 **Postpublication Review.** Evaluation does not end with publication. Postpublication review includes letters to the editor that identify flaws or additional implications, rapid online responses to published articles, efforts to replicate the work, and the experience of clinicians in applying the information in practice. Such evaluations are at least as important as prepublication review. Electronic journals should link from articles to the letters related to them to facilitate retrieval. Editors should also perform a quality review of each published issue of their journal, looking for problems in content and format that can be corrected or improved in subsequent issues (see 5.11.13, Ethical and Legal Considerations, Editorial Responsibilities, Rules, Procedures, and Policies, Editorial Quality Review).

6.2 **Editorial Processing.** Editorial processing refers to the processing of manuscripts after acceptance in preparation for publication (Figure 1). With the development of electronic document processing, the term *manuscript* has moved increasingly far from its handwritten origins to refer to a prepublication document, whether it happens to be a hard-copy typescript or an electronic file. Manuscript submission, peer review, editing, processing, and tracking are now commonly performed electronically. A major technical issue for many publishers is the need to efficiently process content for multiple publication outputs, such as print, Web, reprints, and personal digital assistants (PDAs). The use of electronic markup languages such as XML or

SGML to provide coding for each content element facilitates the conversions necessary for such multiple outputs.

6.2.1 **Manuscript Editing.** After acceptance for publication, a manuscript undergoes copy editing, now often referred to as *manuscript editing.*[28] Extensive editing for clarity, accuracy, and internal consistency may be necessary for some manuscripts. The manuscript editor coordinates communication between the editor, author, and production staff. Manuscript editors incorporate suggestions of the reviewing editor; correct grammar, spelling, and usage; query ambiguities and inconsistencies; verify mathematical calculations; verify reference citations; and edit to journal style. Tables, boxes, and figures are also edited for style (see 4.0, Visual Presentation of Data), accuracy, and consistency with the text. Original figures may be created by a graphics specialist in consultation with the author and reviewing editor. The manuscript editor sends the edited manuscript, including online-only content, with proposed additions and deletions clearly indicated (see 23.0, Manuscript Editing and Proofreading), as well as queries, along with a cover letter and the edited art and tables, to the reviewing editor and the author for approval. After the author responds, the manuscript editor incorporates the author's changes. Any substantive changes requested by the author (eg, inclusion of additional data or analyses, requests for addition of figures or tables) should be discussed with and approved by the reviewing editor.

6.2.2 **Composition, Page Makeup, and Web Content.** Once the author's and reviewing editor's changes have been made in the manuscript file, the document is ready to be composed, or made into pages. Before the widespread use of electronic page makeup systems, galley proofs of typeset text in long columns were produced. A layout served as the model for the page, showing breaks (if any) in the title, type sizes and spacing in the text, and placement of tables, figures, and headings. The galley proofs were then cut and pasted along with the tables and art to make page proofs.

In an electronic composition system, codes must be inserted for each element (eg, title, authors, abstract, headers) of an article according to journal style. An electronic composition operator then pulls the text, tables, and art together in the electronic composition system and arranges these elements into pages according to design and typographic specifications. These pages can be printed as page proofs, or can be sent electronically, for review and approval. For print publication, the pages can be transmitted electronically to a printer. For electronic publication, coded files are converted to an appropriate language (eg, HTML) or format (eg, PDF) for Web posting.

6.2.3 **Proofreading.** The page proofs are checked by a proofreader and by the manuscript editor. In a traditional publishing process, the proofreader checks the manuscript copy word for word against the typeset copy, alerting the manuscript editor to any discrepancies (see 23.0, Manuscript Editing and Proofreading). In an electronic processing system, the role of the proofreader has changed. The proofreader may look only for line breaks and problems that arose through improper coding (eg, space problems or incorrect font) or page makeup (eg, misplaced blocks of type or improper line justification). The manuscript editor, reviewing editor, and/or author may perform the word-for-word reading once done by a proofreader. Revised page proofs can be generated and checked again by a proofreader. Content for electronic publication should also be reviewed and compared with print content for errors and missing elements before release.

6.2.4 **Advertising.** At the same time as the manuscript editing and composition of articles for an issue are proceeding, advertisements are scheduled for specific issues, and possibly for specific positions in an issue (eg, back cover or facing the table of contents). Advertising sales and placement should be administratively separate from all editorial functions to ensure that there is no influence by an advertiser on any editorial decisions. As stated by the International Committee of Medical Journal Editors,[29] editors must have full and final authority for approving advertisements and enforcing advertising policies. Staff members responsible for issue makeup should ensure that there is no inadvertent link between advertisements and articles—for instance, that no advertisement for an antihypertension medication appears next to a research report on hypertension (see 5.12, Ethical and Legal Considerations, Advertisements, Advertorials, Sponsorship, Supplements, Reprints and e-Prints).

6.2.5 **Issue Makeup and Review.** For each journal issue, the production staff merges the editorial and the advertising material, numbers the pages, prepares the table of contents, and produces an imposition (a list that shows the sequential order of pages with placement of editorial and advertising content). The editorial content of each issue should be determined by the journal editor or managing editor, considering the balance of types of articles and thematic consistency (eg, there might be several articles on related topics). The made-up issue is reviewed by editorial and production staff, and final changes are incorporated. When final pages have been created, the electronic files can be telecommunicated to the printer. For print publication, proofs for each page may be prepared and returned to the journal for final review. When all pages have been approved, the issue is printed, bound, and mailed.

6.2.6 **Reprints.** Authors have the option to purchase reprints or e-prints of their articles. Reprints may also be sold to individuals, organizations, or companies interested in disseminating the article (see 5.6.10, Ethical and Legal Considerations, Intellectual Property: Ownership, Access, Rights, and Management, Standards for Commercial Reprints and E-prints).

6.2.7 **Corrections.** Errors are an inevitable part of the publishing process. Fortunately, authors or readers commonly call them to the journal's attention, or they are found during the internal quality-review process, and corrections can be published. In *JAMA*, corrections are printed at the end of the Letters to the Editor section and are listed in the Table of Contents. Corrections should be indexed, with a cross-reference to the original article. This will enable online database services (such as MEDLINE) to link indexed articles with published corrections (see 5.11.8, Ethical and Legal Considerations, Editorial Responsibilities, Roles, Procedures, and Policies, Correspondence [Letters to the Editor], and 5.11.9, Legal and Ethical Considerations, Editorial Responsibilities, Roles, Procedures, and Policies, Corrections [Errata]). Corrections should also be linked from the article to the correction on the journal's Web site and appended to the article PDF. If online-only corrections are made or corrections are made online before appearing in print, the change and date should be indicated in the electronic file.

6.2.8 **Index.** Indexes organized by subject and author's surname are published regularly in most medical journals. Some journals publish indexes only online and not with their print version. Indexes may be created by indexing specialists or by indexing software that searches articles for key words.

ACKNOWLEDGMENTS

Principal author: Richard M. Glass, MD

Karen Adams-Taylor, MS, *JAMA* and *Archives* Journals, reviewed the section on editorial processing. Kathy Schneider, Harmony Communications & Design, Inc, Downers Grove, Illinois, provided the figures.

REFERENCES

1. Guyatt G, Rennie D, eds. *Users' Guides to the Medical Literature: A Manual for Evidence-Based Clinical Practice.* Chicago, IL: AMA Press; 2002.
2. Chalmers TC, Frank CS, Reitman D. Minimizing the three stages of publication bias. *JAMA.* 1990;263(10):1392-1395.
3. Kronick DA. Peer review in 18th-century scientific journalism. *JAMA.* 1990;263(10): 1321-1322.
4. Burnham JC. The evolution of editorial peer review. *JAMA.* 1990;263(10):1323-1329.
5. Rennie D. Editorial peer review: its development and rationale. In: Godlee F, Jefferson T, eds. *Peer Review in Health Sciences.* London, England: BMJ Books; 1999:3-13.
6. Lock S. *A Difficult Balance: Editorial Peer Review in Medicine.* Philadelphia, PA: ISI Press; 1988.
7. Rennie D. Editorial peer review in biomedical publication: the First International Congress. *JAMA.* 1990;263(10):1317.
8. Godlee F, Jefferson T, eds. *Peer Review in Health Sciences.* London, England: BMJ Books; 1999.
9. Weller AC. *Editorial Peer Review: Its Strengths and Weaknesses.* Medford, NJ: American Society for Information Science and Technology; 2001.
10. Goodman SN, Berlin J, Fletcher SW, Fletcher RH. Manuscript quality before and after peer review and editing at *Annals of Internal Medicine. Ann Intern Med.* 1994;121(1):11-21.
11. Lock S. Does editorial peer review work? *Ann Intern Med.* 1994;121(1):60-61.
12. Pierie J-PEN, Walvoort HC, Overbeke AJPM. Readers' evaluation of effect of peer review and editing on quality of articles in the *Nederlands Tijdschrift voor Geneeskunde. Lancet.* 1996;348(9040):1480-1483.
13. Jefferson T, Alderson P, Wager E, Davidoff F. Effects of editorial peer review: a systematic review. *JAMA.* 2002;287(21):2784-2786.
14. Yankauer A. Who are the peer reviewers and how much do they review? *JAMA.* 1990;263(10):1338-1340.
15. Schroter S, Tite L, Hutchings A, Black N. Differences in review quality and recommendations for publication between peer reviewers suggested by authors or by editors. *JAMA.* 2006;295(3):314-317.
16. Altman DG, Schulz KF. Statistical peer review. In: Godlee F, Jefferson T, eds. *Peer Review in Health Sciences.* London, England: BMJ Books; 1999:157-171.
17. Altman DG. Poor-quality medical research: what can journals do? *JAMA.* 2002;287(21): 2765-2767.
18. Fabiato A. Anonymity of reviewers. *Cardiovasc Res.* 1994;28(8):1134-1139.

19. Justice AC, Cho MK, Winker MA, Berlin JA, Rennie D; and PEER Investigators. Does masking author identity improve peer review quality? a randomized controlled trial. *JAMA*. 1998;280(3):240-242.
20. Cho MK, Justice AC, Winker MA, et al. Masking author identity in peer review: what factors influence masking success? *JAMA*. 1998;280(3):243-245.
21. McNutt RA, Evans AT, Fletcher RH, Fletcher SW. The effects of blinding on the quality of peer review: a randomized trial. *JAMA*. 1990;263(10):1371-1376.
22. Yankauer A. How blind is blind review? *Am J Public Health*. 1991;81(7):843-845.
23. van Rooyen S, Godlee F, Evans S, Smith R, Black N. Effect of blinding and unmasking on the quality of peer review: a randomized trial. *JAMA*. 1998;280(3):234-237.
24. Squires B. Editor's page: blinding the reviewers. *CMAJ*. 1990;142(4):279.
25. Rooyen S, Godlee F, Evans S, Black N, Smith R. Effect of open peer review on quality of reviews and on reviewers' recommendations: a randomized trial. *BMJ*. 1999;318(7175): 23-27.
26. Kassirer JP, Campion EW. Peer review: crude and understudied, but indispensable. *JAMA*. 1994;272(2):96-97.
27. Godlee F, Jefferson T. Introduction. In: Godlee F, Jefferson T, eds. *Peer Review in Health Sciences*. London, England: BMJ Books; 1999:xi-xv.
28. Iverson C. "Copy editor" vs "manuscript editor" vs . . . : venturing onto the minefield of titles. *Sci Editor*. 2004;27(2):39-41.
29. International Committee of Medical Journal Editors. Advertising. In: Uniform Requirements for Manuscripts Submitted to Biomedical Journals: Writing and Editing for Biomedical Publication. http://www.icmje.org. Updated February 2006. Accessed December 15, 2006.

Section

2 Style

7 Grammar

The difference between the almost right word and the right word is really a large matter—it's the difference between the lightning bug and the lightning.

Mark Twain[1]

A clear understanding of grammar is basic to good writing. Many excellent grammar books provide a detailed discussion of specific principles (see 25.3, Resources, General Style and Usage). In this section, the focus is on how to avoid common grammatical and writing errors. The content of this chapter is organized from the smallest parts of speech (eg, nouns and pronouns) to larger structures (eg, sentences and paragraphs).

7.1 **Nouns.** Nouns (words that name a person, place, thing, or idea) may serve as subjects or objects.

7.1.1 **Modifiers (Noun Strings).** Although in English nouns can be used as modifiers, overuse of noun modifiers can lead to a lack of clarity. Purists may demand stricter rules on usage, but, as with the use of nouns as verbs (see 11.3, Correct and Preferred Usage, Back-formations), the process of linguistic change is inevitable, and grammatical rigor must be tempered by judgment and common sense.

Avoid	*Preferred*
diabetes patient	patient with diabetes, diabetic patient
depression episode	depressive episode, episode of depression
elderly over-the-counter drug users	elderly users of over-the-counter drugs

In *The Careful Writer*, Bernstein[2] advises the use of no more than 2 polysyllabic noun modifiers per noun for the sake of clarity. However, long noun strings are sometimes difficult to avoid. If several of the attributive nouns are read as a unit, the use of more than 2 may not compromise clarity, especially in scientific or technical communications. Thus, noun strings may be more acceptable, for the sake of brevity, if the terms have been previously defined without noun strings. Some acceptable examples appear below:

community hospital program	nicotine replacement program
physician provider organization	placebo pain medication
risk factor surveillance system	proficiency testing program
baseline CD4 cell counts	clinical research organization
sudden infant death syndrome	community outreach groups

If there is a possibility of ambiguity, hyphens may be added for clarity (large-vessel dissection) (see Temporary Compounds in 8.3.1, Punctuation, Hyphens and Dashes, Hyphen).

7.1.2 **Modifying Gerunds.** When a noun or pronoun precedes a gerund (a verb form ending in *-ing* that is used as a noun), the noun or pronoun is possessive. (See also 8.7, Punctuation, Apostrophe.)

The toxicity of the drug was not a factor in the patient's dying so suddenly.

The award recognized the researcher's planning as well as his performance.

Present participles (used adjectivally) should not be confused with gerunds. In the sentence below, the objective case (*them*) is correct.

I watched them gathering in the auditorium.

If the possessive *their* were used instead of the objective *them*, the emphasis would be on the action (*gathering*).

7.1.3 **Subject-Complement Agreement.** Subjects and complements should agree in number.

The child can take off his own shoes.

We asked trial participants to return their pill dispensers.

However, when the complement is shared by all constituents of the plural subject, it remains singular.

The authors were asked to revise their paper.

All study sites obtained approval from their institutional review board.

Investigators inserted a catheter into the study participants' pulmonary artery.

7.2 **Pronouns.** Pronouns replace nouns. In this replacement, the antecedent must be clear and the pronoun must agree with the antecedent in number and gender.

Avoid: The authors unravel the process of gathering information about diethylstilbestrol and disseminating it. [Antecedent unclear; does *it* refer to information or to diethylstilbestrol?]

Correct: The authors unravel the process of gathering and disseminating information about diethylstilbestrol.

Avoid: A questionnaire was given to each medical student and their spouses. [Disagreement of pronoun with referent in number; the referent is *each medical student* (singular), but the pronoun used is plural (*their spouses*).]

Better: A questionnaire was given to the medical students and their spouses.
or
A questionnaire was given to each medical student and his or her spouse.

Note: The possessive pronoun *its* should not be confused with the contraction *it's* (see also 8.7.2, Punctuation, Apostrophe, Possessive Pronouns).

7.2.1 **Personal Pronouns.** Care must be taken to use the correct case of personal pronouns: subjective (the pronoun is the subject of the phrase or clause) or objective (the pronoun is the object of the phrase or clause).

She was assigned to the active intervention group. (*She* is the subject.)

Collect all the samples and give them to her. (*Her* is the object.)

Your decision affects him and me. (Both *him* and *me* are objects.)

Do not substitute a reflexive pronoun, ending in *-self* or *-selves*, for a simple personal pronoun.

Avoid: George, Patricia, and myself attended the lecture.

The author replied to the editor, illustrator, and myself.

Correct: George, Patricia, and I attended the lecture.

The author replied to the editor, illustrator, and me.

7.2.2 **Relative Pronouns.** Relative pronouns (*who*, *whom*, *whose*, *that*, and *which*) introduce a qualifying clause.

Who *vs* Whom. *Who* is used as a subject and *whom* as an object. The examples below illustrate correct usage.

Give the award to whomever you prefer. [Objective case: *whomever* is the object of the verb *prefer*.]

Give the award to whoever will benefit most. [Subjective case: *whoever* is the subject of *will benefit*.]

Whom did you consult? [Objective case: *whom* is the object of *consult*.]

Who was the consultant on this case? [Subjective case: *who* is the subject of the sentence.]

He is one of the patients whom Dr Rundle is treating. [Objective case: *whom* is the object of *is treating*.]

He is one of the patients who are receiving the placebo. [Subjective case: *who* is the subject of *are receiving*.]

That *vs* Which. Relative pronouns may be used in subordinate clauses to refer to previous nouns. The word *that* introduces a restrictive clause, one that is essential to the meaning of the noun it describes. The word *which* introduces a nonrestrictive clause, one that adds more information but is not essential to the meaning. Clauses that begin with *which* are preceded by commas. Two examples of correct usage follow.

A study on the impact of depression on US labor costs was published in the 2003 *JAMA* theme issue on depression, which contains articles on a range of similar topics. [*Nonrestrictive*; there was only one theme issue on depression in 2003.]

The issue of *JAMA* that contained the article on the impact of depression on US labor costs was the 2003 depression theme issue. [*Restrictive*; there are thousands of issues of *JAMA*.]

Following are examples of ambiguous or incorrect usage that highlight this grammatical problem.

Incorrect: The high prevalence of antibodies to the 3 *Bartonella* species, which were examined in the present study, indicates that health care workers should be alert to possible infection with any of these organisms when treating intravenous drug users. [There are more than 3 species of *Bartonella*. Hence, the correct form here would be "... the 3 *Bartonella* species that were examined. . . ."]

Ambiguous: Many reports have been based on series of patients from urology practices that may not fully reflect the entire spectrum of illness. [Do the patients or the practices not fully reflect the entire spectrum of illness? Also, do the reports involve all or only some urology practices?]

Reworded: Many reports have been based on patients in urology practices, which may not fully reflect the entire spectrum of illness. [Urology practices in general do not capture the range of the disease.]

or

> Many reports have been based on data from urology practices that may not fully reflect the entire spectrum of illness. [Some particular urology practices do not capture the range of the disease, but others might.]

Note: The omission of *that* to introduce a clause may cause difficulty in comprehension.

Avoid: This morning he revealed evidence that calls the study's integrity into question has been verified.

Better: This morning he revealed that evidence that calls the study's integrity into question has been verified.

The addition of *that* after *revealed* frees the reader from backtracking to uncover the meaning of the sentence above. The use of *that* to introduce a clause is particularly helpful when the second verb appears long after the first has been introduced (above, the interval between *revealed* and *has been verified*).

7.2.3 **Indefinite Pronouns.** Indefinite pronouns refer to nonspecific persons or things. Most indefinite pronouns express the idea of quantity and share properties of collective nouns (see 7.8.5, Subject-Verb Agreement, Collective Nouns).

Pronoun-Verb Agreement. Some indefinite pronouns (eg, *each, either, neither, one, no one, everyone, someone, anybody, nobody, somebody*) always take singular verbs; some (eg, *several, few, both, many*) always take the plural; and some (eg, *some, any, none, all,* and *most*) may take either the singular or the plural, depending on the referents. In the last case, usually the best choice is to use the singular verb when the pronoun refers to a singular word and the plural verb when the pronoun refers to a plural word, even when the noun is omitted.

Singular referent: Some of her improvement is due to the increase in dosage.

Plural referent: Some of his calculations are difficult to follow.

Singular referent: Most of the manuscript was typed with a justified right-hand margin.

Plural referent: Most of the manuscripts are edited electronically.

Singular referent: Some of the manuscripts had merit, but none was of the caliber of last year's award winner.

Plural referent: None of the demographic variables examined were found to be significant risk factors.

Pronoun-Pronoun Agreement. The use of an indefinite pronoun as the antecedent of another pronoun can create confusion. Some writers try to avoid gender bias by using *their* or *he/she* with plural indefinite pronouns (eg, Everyone should cite *their* sources.). Grammatically, the use of a plural pronoun is not correct, and constructions such as *s/he* are distracting. *He* or *she* should be used consistently and the writer should keep the context in mind when making these decisions. Better still, when possible use the plural throughout[3] (eg, All authors should cite their sources.). (See also 11.10.1, Correct and Preferred Usage, Inclusive Language, Sex/Gender.)

7.3 Verbs.

7.3 **Verbs.** Verbs express an action, an occurrence, or a mode of being. They have voice, mood, and tense.

7.3.1 **Voice.** In the active voice, the subject does the acting; in the passive voice, the subject is acted on. In general, authors should use the active voice, except in instances in which the actor is unknown or the interest focuses on what is acted on (as in the following example of passive voice).

> He was shot in the abdomen and within 10 minutes was brought to the emergency department.

If the actor is mentioned in the sentence, the active voice is preferred over the passive voice.

Passive:	Data were collected from 5000 patients by physicians.
Active (better):	Physicians collected data from 5000 patients.
Passive:	The definition of bullying used in the survey was taken from previous studies.
Active (better):	The authors used previous definitions of bullying in the survey.

7.3.2 **Mood.** Verbs may have 1 of 3 moods: (1) the indicative (the most common; used for ordinary objective statements), (2) the imperative (used for requesting or commanding), and (3) the subjunctive.

Subjunctive verbs cause the most difficulty; they are used primarily for expressing a wish (I wish it were possible), a supposition (If I were to accept the position . . .), or a condition that is uncertain or contrary to fact (If that were true . . . ; If I were younger . . .). The subjunctive occurs in fairly formal situations and usually involves past (*were*) or present (*be*) forms.

Past form:	If we were to begin treatment immediately, the patient's prognosis would be excellent.
Present form:	The patient insisted that she be treated immediately.

The subjunctive is sometimes used incorrectly, eg, where matters of fact—not supposition—are discussed. In the following examples, the indicative, not the subjunctive, is correct.

> Therefore, we determined whether there had been [not the subjunctive, *were*] deviation from the prescribed regimen.

> We investigated whether the fracture had been [not the subjunctive, *were*] set incorrectly.

7.3.3 **Tense.** Tense indicates the time relation of a verb: present (*I am*), past (*I was*), future (*I will be*), present perfect (*I have been*), past perfect (*I had been*), and future perfect (*I will have been*). It is important to choose the verb that expresses the time that is intended. It is equally important to maintain consistency of tense.

The present tense is used to express a general truth, a statement of fact, or something continuingly true.

> He discovered enzymes—RNA polymerases—that directly copy [not *copied*] the messages encoded in DNA.

For this reason, the present tense is often used to refer to recently published work, indicating that it is still valid.

> Kilgallen's assay results demonstrate the highest recorded sensitivity and specificity to date.

The present perfect tense illustrates actions completed in the past but connected with the present[2] or those still ongoing. It may be used to refer to a report published in the recent past that continues to have importance.

> Kaplan and Rose have described this phenomenon.

The past tense refers to a completed action. In a biomedical article the past tense is usually used to refer to the methods and results of the study being described:

> We measured each patient's blood pressure.
>
> Group 1 had a seropositivity rate of 50%.

The past tense is also used to refer to an article published months or years ago that is now primarily of historical value. Frequently a date will be used in such a reference.[4]

> In their 1985 article, Northrup and Miller reported a high rate of mortality among children younger than 5 years.

In general, tense must be used consistently:

> *Incorrect:* There were no adverse events reported in the control group, but there are 3 in the intervention group.
>
> *Correct:* There were no adverse events reported in the control group, but there were 3 in the intervention group.

However, tense may vary within a single sentence, as dictated by context and judgment.

> We determined which medications are used most frequently by this population.

Alternatively, the past tense and the present tense may be used in the same sentence to place 2 things in temporal context:

> Although the previous report demonstrated a significant response, the follow-up study does not.

Even when tenses are mixed, however, consistency is still the rule:

> *Incorrect:* I found it difficult to accept Dr Smith's contention in chapter 3 that the new agonist has superior pharmacokinetics and was therefore more widely used.
>
> *Correct:* I found it difficult to accept Dr Smith's contention in chapter 3 that the new agonist has superior pharmacokinetics and is therefore more widely used.

7.3.4 **Double Negatives.** Two negatives used together in a sentence constitute a double negative. The use of a double negative to express a positive is acceptable, although it yields a weaker affirmative than the simpler positive and may be confusing:

> Our results are not inconsistent with the prior hypothesis.
>
> More direct incentives have produced substantial changes in behavior in the past, although not without adverse consequences.
>
> Rheumatologic symptoms were not uncommon in both groups.

However, it is not grammatically acceptable to use a double negative to emphasize the negative. In the following example, the double negative conveys the opposite of what is intended.

> The authors cannot barely contain their enthusiasm.

A double negative is best avoided in scientific writing because it often causes the reader to go back and reread the sentence to make sure of the meaning.

7.3.5 **Split Infinitives and Verb Phrases.** Although some authorities may still advise the avoidance of split infinitives, this proscription—a holdover from Latin grammar, wherein the infinitive is a single word and cannot be split—has been relaxed. In some cases, moreover, clarity is better served by the split infinitive.

> *Ambiguous:* The authors planned to promote exercising vigorously. [Is it the exercising or the promotion of exercising that is vigorous?]
>
> *Clearer:* The authors planned to vigorously promote exercising.
> *or*
> The authors planned to promote vigorous exercise.

7.3.6 **Contractions.** A contraction consists of 2 words combined by omitting 1 or more letters (eg, *can't*, *aren't*). An apostrophe shows where the omission has occurred. Contractions are usually avoided in formal writing.

7.4 **Modifiers.** A modifier describes another word or word group. Words, phrases (groups of words without a subject or predicate, usually introduced by a preposition or conjunction), and clauses (groups of words with a subject and verb within a compound or complex sentence) may all be modifiers. An adjective modifies a noun or a pronoun. An adverb modifies a verb, an adjective, another adverb, or a clause. Clauses or phrases may serve as adjectives or adverbs.

7.4.1 **Misplaced Modifiers.** Misplaced modifiers result from failure to make clear what is being modified. Illogical or ambiguous placement of a word or phrase can usually be avoided by placing the modifying word or phrase appropriately close to the word it modifies.

> *Unclear:* Dr Young treated the patients using antidepressants. [Who used the antidepressants? Ambiguity makes 2 meanings possible.]

Better: Dr Young treated the patients with antidepressants.
or
[alternative meaning]: Dr Young treated the patients who were using antidepressants.

Unclear: The patient was referred to a specialist with severe bipolar disorder. [Who had the bipolar disorder?]

Better: The patient with severe bipolar disorder was referred to a specialist.

Likewise, sometimes it is necessary for clarity to place an adverb within a verb phrase. Note the shift in meaning when the adverb is moved outside of the verb phrase.

He had just called me.

He had called just me.

Use of the word *only* as a modifier poses particular problems. It must be placed immediately before the word or phrase it modifies for the meaning to be clear. Note the different meanings achieved depending on placement in the examples below.

Only medication can ease the pain.

Medication can only ease the pain.

Medication can ease only the pain.

7.4.2 **Verbal Phrase Danglers.** A participle is a verb form used as an adjective. A dangling participle implies an actor but fails to indicate correctly who or what that actor is. The following examples of dangling participles illustrate the problem.

Avoid: Working quickly, the study was completed early by my research team. [The participle appears to refer to "the study"; however, it is the *research team* that was working quickly.]

Better: My research team worked quickly and completed the study early.
or
The study was completed early because my research team worked quickly.

Avoid: Based on our experience, educational interventions are needed to foster higher-quality end-of-life care. [Are the educational interventions based on the authors' experience? No—it is the statement about the need for higher-quality end-of-life care that is based on the authors' experience.]

Better: We have found that educational interventions are needed to foster higher-quality end-of-life care.
or
Experience has shown that educational interventions are needed to foster higher-quality end-of-life care.

A gerund is a verb form used as a noun (see 7.1.2, Nouns, Modifying Gerunds). Like the dangling participle, the dangling gerund implies an actor but does not specify who or what that actor is and sometimes may be confused with a participle modifying the wrong entity.

Avoid: Dietary therapy slows the return of hypertension after stopping long-term medical therapy. [This states that dietary therapy not only slows the return of hypertension but also stops medical therapy.]

Better: Dietary therapy slows the return of hypertension after cessation of long-term medical therapy.
or
After patients discontinue long-term medical therapy, dietary therapy slows the return of hypertension.

Avoid: Before initiating an exercise program or engaging in heavy physical labor after a myocardial infarction, a physician should review the exercise program carefully. ["A physician" is erroneously implied to be the actor, the one initiating an exercise program or engaging in heavy physical labor.]

Better: Anyone about to initiate an exercise program or engage in heavy physical labor after a myocardial infarction should consult his or her physician.

7.5 **Diction.** Diction, or word choice, is important for any writing to be understood by its intended audience. In scientific writing, concrete and specific language is preferred over the abstract and general.

Avoid: The area under study provides new evidence for a solution.

Better: Immunology provides new evidence for a solution.

Avoid: An individual with a medical degree should examine this lesion.

Better: A physician should examine this lesion.

7.5.1 **Homonyms.** Homonyms are words that sound alike but are spelled differently and have different meanings. They are easily confused, and computer spell-check programs are unable to differentiate them. Common examples include *affect/effect, accept/except, altar/alter, assistance/assistants, cite/site/sight, council/counsel, its/it's, patience/patients, peace/piece, peak/peek/pique, pleural/plural, principal/principle,* and *your/you're.* (See also 11.1, Correct and Preferred Usage, Correct and Preferred Usage of Common Words and Phrases.)

7.5.2 **Idioms, Colloquialisms, and Slang.** Some language is best avoided in material written for a professional or academic audience.

Idioms are fixed expressions that cannot be understood literally (*kick the bucket, on a roll, put up with, pay attention*). In addition, some may have multiple meanings that can be understood only in context (*pass out, stand for*). Idioms are not governed by any rules and each stands on its own. Be wary of using idioms, particularly for audiences that include readers whose first language is not English.

Colloquialisms (or casualisms[2]) are characteristic of informal, casual communication (*ain't, anyways, cold turkey, flat line, OK, shell-shocked, tax hike*).

Slang includes informal, nonstandard terms whose meanings are not readily understood by all speakers of a language. Sometimes slang words are newly coined (*bick, rinky-dink, FAQ*) and sometimes they are created by applying new meanings to existing words (*bad, cool, awesome, random, killer*).

Colloquialisms and slang should be avoided except in special situations, such as "flavorful" prose or direct quotations.

> My sense is that part of the reason why Claude is able to survive is denial. He just says, flat out, "This ain't happening."

The technical terminology specific to various disciplines is considered *jargon* and should be avoided (see 11.4, Correct and Preferred Usage, Jargon).

7.5.3 **Euphemisms.** Euphemisms (from the Greek *eu,* "good," and *pheme,* "voice") are indirect terms used to express something unpleasant. Although such language is often necessary in social situations ("He passed away."), directness is better in scientific writing ("The patient died."). (See also 11.4, Correct and Preferred Usage, Jargon.)

7.5.4 **Clichés.** Clichés are worn-out expressions (*sleep like a log, dead as a doornail, first and foremost, crystal clear*). At one time they were clever metaphors, but overuse has left them lifeless, unable to conjure in the reader's mind the original image. Avoid clichés like the plague.

7.6 Sentence Fragments.

A sentence must have at minimum a subject and a verb; it also usually contains modifiers. Sentence fragments, which lack a subject or a verb, should not be used in scientific or technical writing (except within the structured abstract; see 2.5, Manuscript Preparation, Abstract). Occasionally, writers of prose and poetry use sentence fragments intentionally, for effect.

> Her affect signaled depression. Utter depression.

In scientific writing, these fragments are likely to be unintentional and are definitely inappropriate.

Incorrect: The clinical spectrum of disease varying according to the population and age group under study.

Correct: The clinical spectrum of disease varies according to the population and age group under study.

7.7 Parallel Construction.

Parallel construction can be used to build a sentence or emphasize a point.

7.7.1 **Correlative Conjunctions.** Parallelism may rely on accepted cues (*either/or, neither/nor, not only/but also, both/and*). All elements of the parallelism that appear on one side of the coordinating conjunction should match corresponding elements on the other side.

Avoid: The compleat physician has not only mastered the science of medicine but also its art.

Correct: The compleat physician has mastered not only the science of medicine but also its art.

Better: The compleat physician has mastered both the science and the art of medicine.

Avoid: Poor drug efficacy may be caused by either lack of absorption or by increased clearance.

Correct: Poor drug efficacy may be caused either by lack of absorption or by increased clearance.

Also correct: Poor drug efficacy may be caused by either lack of absorption or increased clearance.

Avoid: Three patients either took their medication incorrectly or not at all.

Correct: Three patients took their medication either incorrectly or not at all.

Note: *Either/or* is used with only 2 comparators (use with more than 2 items is considered nonstandard).

Incorrect: This medication can be taken with either water, milk, or juice.

Correct: This medication can be taken with water, milk, or juice.

7.7.2 **Elliptical Comparisons.** The conjunction *than* often introduces an abridged expression (eg, "You are younger than I [am young])." Correct placement of *than* is important to avoid ambiguity:

Unclear: Women are more likely to take vitamins than men. [Are women more likely to consume vitamins than men are, or are women more likely to consume vitamins than they are to consume men?]

Rewritten: Women are more likely than men to take vitamins.

7.7.3 **Series or Comparisons.** Parallel construction may also present a series or make comparisons. In these usages, the elements of the series or of the comparison should be parallel structures, eg, nouns with nouns, prepositional phrases with prepositional phrases.

Avoid: Surgery, radiation therapy, and to give chemotherapy are possible therapeutic approaches.

Correct: Surgery, radiation therapy, and chemotherapy are possible therapeutic approaches.

Avoid: When an operation is designed to improve function rather than extirpation of an organ, surgical technique dictates outcome.

Correct: When an operation is designed to improve the function of an organ rather than to extirpate the organ, surgical technique dictates outcome.

Avoid: There was a long delay between the purchase of a scanner and when it started to be widely used.

Correct: There was a long delay between the purchase of a scanner and its widespread use.

Note: Avoid the use of *nor* when the first negative is expressed by *not* or *no*.

Fetuses with congenital diaphragmatic hernia who were stillborn would not have been included in this study or [not *nor*] in many previously published studies.

But: Fetuses with congenital diaphragmatic hernia who were stillborn would not have been included in this study, nor would they have been included in other trials. [*Nor* is acceptable in noncorrelative constructions containing a negative in the first element.[5]]

7.7.4 **Lists.** Parallel construction is also important in lists, whether run in or set off by bullets or some other device (see Enumerations in 8.2.2, Punctuation, Comma, Semicolon, Colon, Semicolon, and 19.5, Numbers and Percentages, Enumerations).

After completing this CME exercise, readers should be able to

- identify the causal mechanism of the disease;
- describe the most common symptoms;
- understand the limitations of pharmacologic treatment.

7.8 **Subject-Verb Agreement.** The subject and verb must agree in number; use a singular subject with a singular verb and a plural subject with a plural verb. Unfortunately, this simple rule is often violated, especially in complex sentences.

7.8.1 **Intervening Phrase.** Plural nouns take plural verbs and singular nouns take singular verbs, even if a phrase ending in a plural noun follows a singular subject or if a phrase ending in a singular noun follows a plural subject.

A review of all patients with grade 3 tumors was undertaken in the university hospital. [The subject in this sentence is *review*. Ignore all modifying prepositional phrases that follow a noun when determining verb agreement.]

Avoid: The patient, one of many study participants given access to state-of-the-art medical care from the university's clinical researchers, were followed up for more than a year. [The verb should be *was* followed up—the subject is *patient*.]

Sometimes the simplest solution is to rewrite it as 2 separate sentences:

Better: The patient was followed up for more than a year. She was one of many study participants given access to state-of-the-art medical care from the university's clinical researchers.

If the intervening phrase is introduced by *with*, *together with*, *as well as*, *along with*, *in addition to*, or similar constructions, the singular verb is preferred if the subject is singular because the intervening phrase does not affect the singularity of the subject.

The editor, as well as the reviewers, believes that this article is ready for acceptance.

The patient, together with her physician and her family, makes this decision.

The investigator, in addition to all participants, was expected to abide by the institution's safety guidelines.

In these instances, recasting the sentence may eliminate confusion.

The patient, physician, and family members make this decision together.

7.8.2 **False Singulars.** A few plural nouns are used so often in the singular that they are often paired with a singular verb.

The agenda has been set for our next meeting.

Frequently treated erroneously in this way are the plurals *bacteria, criteria, phenomena*, and *memoranda*. The distinction between singular and plural, however, should be retained; when the singular is intended, use *bacterium, criterion, phenomenon*, and *memorandum*.

Also, many now consider acceptable the use of *data* as a singular.[5] In this usage, *data* is thought of as a collective noun and, when considered as a unit rather than as the individual items of data that compose it, it takes the singular verb. However, *JAMA* and the *Archives* Journals prefer to retain the use of the plural verb with *data* in all situations.[2]

Very few data were [not *very little data was*] available to support our hypothesis.

The word *media* in the sense of communications media is becoming acceptable in this collective usage, although its use in this sense has not yet reached the acceptability that *agenda* has gained and *data* is close to gaining.[5,6] Most scientific journals retain the distinction between singular and plural.

Singular: Each news medium shapes journalism to its own constraints.

Plural: The media give much attention to the managed care debate. [Here *media* refers to all types of news coverage.]

In the sense of laboratory culture or contrast media, *medium* should be used for the singular and *media* for the plural.

7.8.3 **False Plurals.** Some nouns, by virtue of ending in a "plural" *-s* form, are mistakenly taken to be plurals even though they should be treated as singular and take a singular verb (eg, measles, mumps, mathematics, politics, genetics). (See 9.8, Plurals, False Singulars.)

7.8.4 **Parenthetical Plurals.** When *-s* or *-es* is added parenthetically to a word to express the possibility of a plural, the verb should be singular. However, in most instances it is preferable to avoid this construction and use the plural noun instead.

Acceptable: The risk factor(s) for each study participant was not always clear.

Better: The risk factors of the study participants were not always clear.

7.8.5 Collective Nouns. A collective noun is one that names more than 1 person, place, or thing. When the group is regarded as a unit, the singular verb is the appropriate choice. (See also 9.2, Plurals, Collective Nouns.)

> The couple has a practice in rural Montana. [*Couple* is considered a unit here and so takes the singular verb.]
>
> Twenty percent of her time is spent on administration. [*Twenty percent* is thought of as a unit, not as 20 individual units, and so takes the singular verb.] (See also 18.3.3, Units of Measure, Format, Style, and Punctuation, Subject-Verb Agreement.)
>
> The paramedic crew responds to these emergency calls. [*Crew* is thought of as a unit here and so takes the singular verb.]

When the individual members of the pair or group are emphasized, rather than the group as a whole, the plural verb is correct.

> The couple are both family physicians. [*Couple* is thought of as the 2 individuals who compose the couple, not as a unit, and so takes the plural verb.]
>
> Ten percent of the staff work flexible hours. [*Ten percent* is thought of as being composed of each individual staff member, not as a unit, and so takes the plural verb.]
>
> The surgical faculty were from all over the country. [*Faculty* here refers to the individual members of the faculty, rather than to the faculty as a group, and so takes the plural verb.]

The use of a phrase such as "the members of" may make this last example less jarring.

> The members of the surgical faculty were from all over the country.

7.8.6 Compound Subject. When 2 words or 2 groups of words, usually joined by *and* or *or*, are the subject of the sentence, either the singular or plural verb form may be appropriate, depending on whether the words joined are singular or plural and on the connectors used.

***Compound Subject Joined by* and.** With *and*, a plural verb is usually correct.

> The nurse and the physician are discussing my case.

A singular verb should be used if the 2 elements are thought of as a unit:

> Dilation and curettage was suggested.

or refer to the same person or thing:

> The first author and principal investigator takes responsibility for the data analysis.

***Compound Subject Joined by* or *or* nor.** With a compound subject joined by *or* or *nor*, the plural verb is correct if both elements are plural; if both elements are singular, the singular verb is correct. When one is singular and one is plural, the verb should agree with the noun closer to the verb.

Both plural:	Neither hospital staff nor family members were in the room.
Both singular:	Neither a false-positive result nor a false-negative result is definitive.
Mixed:	Neither the physicians nor the hospital was responsible for the loss.

7.8.7 **Shift in Number of Subject and Resultant Subject-Verb Disagreement.** In elliptical constructions involving the verb (ie, the second verb is omitted because it is understood), if the number of the subject changes, the construction is incorrect.

Incorrect:	Her tests were run and her chart updated.
Correct:	Her tests were run and her chart was updated.
Incorrect:	The diagnosis was made and physical therapy sessions begun.
Correct:	The diagnosis was made and physical therapy sessions were begun. *or* The diagnosis was made and physical therapy begun.

7.8.8 **Subject and Predicate Noun Differ in Number.** The predicate noun is the complement of a subject; it identifies, describes, or renames the subject. When the subject and predicate noun differ in number, follow the number of the subject in selecting the singular or plural verb form.

Incorrect:	The most significant factor that affected the study results were interhospital variations in severity of illness.
Correct:	The most significant factor that affected the study results was interhospital variations in severity of illness.

Avoid this by rephrasing:

Study results were most affected by interhospital variations in severity of illness.

7.8.9 ***Every* and *Many a.*** When *every* or *many a* is used before a word or series of words, use the singular verb form.

Many a clinician does not understand statistics. (*But, better yet:* Many clinicians do not understand statistics.)

Every issue profiles a leader in medicine.

7.8.10 ***One of Those.*** In clauses that follow *one of those*, the plural verb form is always correct.

Dr Cotter is one of those researchers who prefer the library to the laboratory.

7.8.11 ***Number.*** *The number* is singular and *a number of* is plural (see also 7.8.5, Collective Nouns).

The number that responded was surprising.

A number of respondents were concerned about adverse effects.

The same is true for *the total* and *a total of*.

7.9 **The Paragraph.** A paragraph is a cohesive group of sentences. It presents a thought or several related thoughts. Each paragraph should be long enough to stand alone but short enough to hold the reader's attention and then direct that attention to the next thought. Too many short paragraphs are jarring to the reader, whereas too many long paragraphs strain the reader's attention. Sentences within a single paragraph should use parallel structure and consistent tense as much as possible.

Transitions are words or phrases that signal a connection among ideas. Transitions build bridges between paragraphs (and between sentences) and help the text flow.[6]

To show addition: also, furthermore, in addition, moreover

To show contrast: however, yet, conversely, nevertheless, although

To show comparison: similarly, likewise

To show results: therefore, thus, as a result, consequently

To show time sequence: first (second, third, etc), later, meanwhile, subsequently, while

To summarize: hence, in summary, finally

ACKNOWLEDGMENT

Principal author: Stacy Christiansen, MA

REFERENCES

1. Platt S, ed. *Respectfully Quoted: A Dictionary of Quotations Requested From the Congressional Research Service.* Washington, DC: Library of Congress; 1989:entry 540.
2. Bernstein TM. *The Careful Writer: A Modern Guide to English Usage.* New York, NY: Free Press; 1998.
3. Crews F, Schor S, Hennessy M. *The Borzoi Handbook for Writers.* 3rd ed. New York, NY: McGraw-Hill Inc; 1993.
4. Huth EJ. *Writing and Publishing in Medicine.* 3rd ed. Baltimore, MD: Williams & Wilkins; 1999.
5. Burchfield RW. *The New Fowler's Modern English Usage.* Rev 3rd ed. Oxford, England: Oxford University Press; 2000.
6. *The American Heritage Dictionary of the English Language.* 4th ed. Boston, MA: Houghton Mifflin Co; 2000.

ADDITIONAL READINGS AND GENERAL REFERENCES

The Chicago Manual of Style: The Essential Guide for Writers, Editors, and Publishers. 15th ed. Chicago, IL: University of Chicago Press; 2003.

Copy Editor: Language News for the Publishing Professional. New York, NY: McMurry Newsletters. http://www.copyeditor.com. Accessed September 27, 2006.

Editorial Eye. Alexandria, VA: Editorial Experts Inc. http://www.eeicommunications.com/eye/. Accessed September 27, 2006.

Follett W. *Modern American Usage: A Guide*. Wensberg E, ed. New York, NY: Hill & Wang; 1998.

Gordon KE. *The Deluxe Transitive Vampire: The Ultimate Handbook of Grammar for the Innocent, the Eager, and the Doomed*. New York, NY: Pantheon Books; 1993.

Kilpatrick JJ. *The Writer's Art*. Kansas City, KS: Andrews McMeel & Parker Inc; 1985.

Merriam-Webster's Dictionary of English Usage. Springfield, MA: Merriam-Webster; 1994.

Strunk W Jr, White EB. *Elements of Style*. 3rd ed. New York, NY: Macmillan Publishing Co Inc; 1994.

Walsh B. *Lapsing Into a Comma: A Curmudgeon's Guide to the Many Things That Can Go Wrong in Print—and How to Avoid Them*. Lincolnwood, IL: Contemporary Books; 2000.

8 Punctuation

. . . after journeying through the world of punctuation, and seeing what it can do, I am all the more convinced that we should fight like tigers to preserve our punctuation and we should start now.

Lynne Truss[1]

8.1 Period, Question Mark, Exclamation Point. Periods, question marks, and exclamation points are the 3 end-of-sentence punctuation marks.

8.1.1 Period. Periods are the most common end-of-sentence punctuation marks. Use a period at the end of a declarative or imperative sentence and at the end of each table footnote and each figure legend.

> Advances in medical technology have saved many lives.
>
> Always listen carefully.

Also use a period after a rhetorical question (one not requiring an answer).

> Where, indeed, is the Osler of today.

Placement. The period precedes ending quotation marks and reference citations.

> The child is rated in 7 areas, such as "accepts responsibility" and "interacts appropriately with peers."
>
> We followed the methods of Wilkes et al.[5]

The period follows a closing apostrophe:

> Their data were inconsistent with their associates'.

Enumerations. Use a period after the arabic numeral when enumerating paragraphed items.

> The signed authorship form required by the journal included the following sections:
>
> 1. Authorship responsibility, criteria, and contributions
> 2. Data access and responsibility
> 3. Financial disclosure
> 4. Acknowledgment statement

(See also 19.5, Numbers and Percentages, Enumerations, and the Enumerations section in 8.2.2, Semicolon, for examples of ways to handle enumerations that are run into the text or that are set off with bullets.)

Decimals. Use the period as a decimal indicator. (See 19.7.1, Numbers and Percentages, Forms of Numbers, Decimals.)

> $r = 0.75$ .32 caliber
>
> 0.1% $P < .05$

Multiplication. The period in raised position indicates multiplication. (See also 18.2.2, Units of Measure, Expressing Unit Names and Symbols, Products and Quotients of Unit Symbols, and 21.6, Mathematical Composition, Expressing Multiplication and Division.)

When Not to Use a Period. *JAMA* and the *Archives* Journals do not use periods with honorifics (courtesy titles), scientific terms, and abbreviations (*exceptions*: No. for "number" and St. when it is part of a person's name, although no period is used with St in a city name, eg, St Louis, Missouri) (see 2.1, Manuscript Preparation, Titles and

Subtitles; 2.2, Manuscript Preparation, Bylines and End-of-Text Signatures; and 14.0, Abbreviations).

Dr Hussey	*JAMA*
George Hussey, MD	NIH
George R. Hussey, MD	ie
E coli	eg

8.1.2 **Question Mark.** The primary use of the question mark is to end interrogative sentences.

When did he go into private practice?

If this article were a work of the 1930s, not the 1990s, would we view it differently? And should we?

In Dates. Use the question mark to show doubt about specific data.

Hippocrates (460?-375 BCE) is often referred to as the Father of Medicine.

Placement. Place the question mark inside the end quotation mark (see 8.6.5, Quotation Marks, Placement), the closing parenthesis, or the end bracket when the question mark is part of the quoted or parenthetical material.

The patient asked her physician of 25 years, "Why are you retiring, Doctor?"

The chapter on interpretation asks the question "Can I be wrong?"

The mandate for health reform (can we agree on this?) will change practice as we know it.

In declarative sentences that contain a question, place the question mark at the end of the interrogative statement.

Why did I bother to attend this conference? she wondered.

The first section of the book, "What Medical Advances Made Open Heart Surgery Possible?" is certain to interest medical historians.

The investigators asked the question "Have you ever injected drugs?" of every study participant.

(*Note:* The question mark, like the exclamation point [see 8.1.3, Exclamation Point, Placement], is never combined with another question mark, exclamation point, period, semicolon, or comma; thus, the need for a comma is obviated in the 3 examples above. This usage is sometimes referred to as "dueling punctuation marks," and in this duel, the stronger mark wins.)

Rhetorical questions (those not requiring an answer) do not require a question mark. (See 8.1.1, Period.)

What is gained by recounting past losses when we have a chance to start afresh in our efforts to provide health care to the uninsured.

Indirect or reported speech also does not require a question mark.

> She wondered why there were no illustrations in the article.

8.1.3 **Exclamation Point.** Exclamation points indicate emotion, an outcry, or a forceful comment. Try to avoid their use except in direct quotations and in rare and special circumstances. They are not appropriate in scientific manuscripts and are more common in less formal articles, such as book reviews, editorials, and informal essays, where added emphasis may be appropriate. If they are used, limit their use to one.

> Beware!
>
> Although it may be referrred to as the gold standard, nothing is perfect!
>
> I had almost given up hope of his recovery. He was terribly sick!

Placement. When it completes the emphasized material, the exclamation point goes inside the end quotation mark, parenthesis, or bracket. (The exclamation point, like the question mark [see 8.1.2, Question Mark, Placement], is never combined with another exclamation point, question mark, period, semicolon, or comma; thus, there is no comma in the first example below.)

> "Let the reader beware!" the editor warned.
>
> The frightened child cried, "I don't want my tonsils taken out!"

Factorial. In mathematical expressions, the exclamation point is used to indicate a factorial. (See 21.6, Mathematical Composition, Expressing Multiplication and Division.)

$$5! = 5 \times 4 \times 3 \times 2 \times 1$$

8.2 **Comma, Semicolon, Colon.** Commas, semicolons, and colons can be used to indicate a break or pause in thought, to set off material, or to introduce a new but connected thought. Each has specific uses, and the strength of the break in thought determines which mark is appropriate.

8.2.1 **Comma.** Commas are the least forceful of the 3 marks. There are definite rules for using commas; however, usage is often subjective. Some writers and editors use the comma frequently to indicate what they see as a natural pause in the flow of words, but commas can be overused. The trend is to use them sparingly. Follow the accepted rules and use commas only when breaks are needed for sense or readability or to avoid confusion or misinterpretation.

Separating Groups of Words. The comma is used to separate phrases, clauses, and groups of words and to clarify the grammatical structure and the intended meaning.

Use a comma after opening dependent clauses (whether restrictive or not) or long opening adverbial phrases.

> If the infection recurs within 2 weeks, an additional course of antibiotics should be given.

When you have to pay for your own health care, does your consumption really become more efficient?

A comma is not essential if the introductory phrase is short.

In some patients midazolam produces paradoxic agitation.

Use commas to set off nonrestrictive subordinate clauses (see 7.2.2, Grammar, Pronouns, Relative Pronouns) or nonrestrictive participial phrases.

Ms Frederick, who had been waiting on hold for more than an hour, abandoned all hope of having her questions answered.

The numbness, which had been apparent for 3 days, disappeared after drug therapy.

The delegates, attaining consensus, passed the resolution.

But avoid setting a phrase off with commas where it would make the meaning ambiguous.

Avoid: Although numerous investigators have called for measures to improve sight in nursing home residents, to our knowledge, none have attempted a study of the effect of a vision restoration-rehabilitation program on function and quality in this population.

In the example above, it is not clear whether the phrase "to our knowledge" applies to what precedes it or what follows it. Removing the comma after "to our knowledge" makes the meaning clear.

Better: Although numerous investigators have called for measures to improve sight in nursing home residents, to our knowledge none have attempted a study of the effect of a vision restoration-rehabilitation program on function and quality in this population.

Use a comma to avoid ambiguous or awkward juxtaposition of words.

Outside, the ambulance siren shrieked.

Still, noting the trends and highlighting the lack of funding for achieving world health goals does not translate into more positive actions.

Use commas to set off appositives. (*Note:* Commas precede and follow the apposition.)

Two colleagues, John Smith and Perry White, worked with me on this study.

The battered-child syndrome, a clinical condition in young children who have experienced serious physical abuse, is a frequent cause of permanent injury or even death.

Series. In a simple coordinate series of 3 or more terms, separate the elements by commas. (See 7.1.1, Grammar, Nouns, Modifiers [Noun Strings].)

Each patient was asked to complete a 21-item, 7-point, self-administered questionnaire.

Use a comma before the conjunction that precedes the last term in a series to prevent ambiguity (this is often referred to as a serial comma).

> Outcomes result from a complex interaction of medical care and genetic, environmental, and behavioral factors.
>
> The physician, the nurse, and the family could not convince the patient to take his medication daily.
>
> While in the hospital, these patients required neuroleptics, maximal observation, and seclusion.

However, a series of 3 or more modifiers should not be separated by commas when the modifiers are seen as 1 term or entity:

> The patient has chronic progressive multiple sclerosis.
>
> Gray matter magnetic resonance imaging was used to predict longitudinal brain atrophy.

Judgment and common sense are required in the interpretation of this rule. If the order of the adjectives can be rearranged without loss of meaning or clarity, use the comma.

> The studies selected for inclusion were English-language, randomized, double-blind, controlled trials of newer atypical antipsychotic medications.
>
> Data from several large, multicenter, administrative databases were analyzed.

Note: When fewer than 3 modifiers are used, avoid adding a comma if the modifiers and the noun are read as one entity:

> We conducted a randomized placebo-controlled trial.
>
> Data from multicenter administrative databases were analyzed.

Names of Organizations. When an enumeration occurs in the name of a company or organization, the comma is usually omitted before the ampersand. However, follow the punctuation used by the individual firm, except in references. (See 3.12.9, References, References to Print Books, Publishers.)

Farrar, Straus & Giroux Inc	Little, Brown & Co
GlaxoSmithKline Pharmaceuticals	Mayer, Brown, Rowe & Maw
Houghton Mifflin Co	Sidley Austin Brown & Wood

***Setting Off* ie, eg, viz.** Use commas to set off *ie, eg,* and *viz* and the expanded equivalents, *that is, for example,* and *namely.*

> The use of standardized scores, eg, *z* scores, has no effect on statistical comparisons.
>
> The most important tests, that is, the white blood cell and platelet counts, were unduly delayed.

Note: If an independent clause follows these terms or their equivalents, precede the clause with a semicolon.

> Our double-blind study compared continuous with cyclic estrogen treatment; ie, estrogens for 4 weeks were compared with estrogens for 3 weeks followed by placebo for 1 week.

Separating Clauses Joined by Conjunctions. Use commas to separate main clauses joined by coordinating conjunctions (*and, but, or, nor, for*).

> Plasma lipid and lipoprotein concentrations were unchanged after low-intensity training, but high-intensity training resulted in a reduction in triglyceride levels.

> No subgroup of responders could be identified, and differences between centers were so great that no real comparison was possible.

If both clauses are short, punctuation can be omitted.

> The test may be useful or it may be harmful.

> I have read the article and I am concerned about the data collection methods.

Be careful not to confuse the coordinating conjunction used between independent clauses with a coordinating conjunction used to link a compound predicate.

> These facilities are beginning to resemble "minihospitals" and they are losing their identity as freestanding ambulatory surgery centers.

Clauses introduced by *yet* and *so* and subordinating conjunctions (eg, *while, where, after, whereas*) are preceded by a comma. (See 11.1, Correct and Preferred Usage, Correct and Preferred Usage of Common Words and Phrases.)

> He taught medical students, performed careful research, and wrote thoughtful articles, yet was denied tenure.

> The United States spends more than $1000 per capita per year on paperwork related to health care, whereas Canada spends only about $300 per capita.

> One recent study found that low literacy was associated with worse mental health, whereas another concluded that literacy was not associated with depression.

If such conjunctions appear at the beginning of a sentence, however, the comma following the conjunction may not be necessary.

> I have seen many cases of vertigo. Yet this one was particularly troubling.

Setting Off Parenthetical Expressions. Use commas to set off parenthetical words, phrases, questions, and other expressions that interrupt the continuity of a sentence, eg, *therefore, moreover, on the other hand, of course, nevertheless, after all, consequently, however*. (See 8.8.1, Ellipses, Omission Within a Sentence.)

> The real issue, after all, was how to fund the next study.

> Therefore, we were disappointed that the article did not include consideration of medical schools and their influence on the culture of medicine.

> What is needed, then, is collective empowerment of practitioners, guided by accountability to the public.

Note: In some cases, removal of the commas around parenthetical expressions changes the meaning of the sentence. In the example immediately above, *then* suggests a summing-up. Without these commas, *then* suggests time, ie, what comes next.

Setting Off Degrees and Titles. Academic degrees and titles are set off by commas when they follow the name of a person. Although it is not incorrect to set *Jr* and *Sr* off by commas when they follow the name of a person, *JAMA* and the *Archives* Journals are now deleting these commas.

> Berton Smith Jr, MD, and Priscilla Armstrong, MD, PhD, interpreted the radiographic findings in this study.

> Joyce Fredrickson-Smith, MD, PhD, vice-chancellor, attended the conference on health system reform.

Addresses. In running text and in affiliation footnotes, use commas to separate the elements in an address. Use commas after the city and before and after the state or country name. (*Note*: In US and Canadian addresses, commas are not used before the zip or the postal code.)

> This year, the editorial board meeting will be held in conjunction with the Academy meeting at the Westin Bonaventure Hotel and Suites, 404 S Figueroa St, Los Angeles, CA 90071.

> The study was conducted at The Wilmer Institute, Baltimore, Maryland, in 2004.

Dates. In dates and similar expressions of time, use commas according to the following examples. Commas are not used when the month and year are given without the day, or between a holiday and its year.

> The first issue of *JAMA* was published on Saturday, July 14, 1883.

> The patient's rhinoplasty was scheduled for August 19, 2002, at Strong Memorial Hospital, with postoperative evaluation on August 30.

> The terrorist attack in London, England, in July 2005 led to further examination of major disaster preparedness.

> The publication offices were closed on New Year's Day 2005.

Numbers. In accordance with SI convention, separate digits with a thin space, not a comma, to indicate place values beyond thousands. (See 18.4.3, Units of Measure, Use of Numerals With Units, Number Spacing.)

> 5034 12 345 615 478 9 473 209

A comma may be used to separate adjacent unrelated numerals if neither can be expressed easily in words, but it is preferable to reword the sentence or spell out 1 of the numbers.

By December 2003, 929 985 cases of AIDS had been reported in the United States.

Better: By December 2003, a total of 929 985 cases of AIDS had been reported in the United States.

Units of Measure. Do not use a comma between 2 or more measures whose units are the same dimension.

3 years 4 months 2 days old 3 lb 4 oz

Placement. The comma is placed inside quotation marks (see 8.6.5, Quotation Marks, Placement) and before superscript citation of references and footnote symbols.

As a result of the "back-to-sleep campaigns," a call has been issued for a "back-to-the-bench" campaign.

These missed opportunities have been shown to occur during office visits,[6-9] health department appointments,[10-13] and hospitalizations.[16]

To Indicate Omission. The comma is used to indicate omission or to avoid repeating a word when the sense is clear. (See 7.8.7, Grammar, Subject-Verb Agreement, Shift in Number of Subject and Resultant Subject-Verb Disagreement.)

Three patients could not be studied: in 1, duration of treatment was too short; in 2, too long.

A plus indicates present; a minus, absent.

Dialogue. Commas are often used before direct dialogue or conversation is introduced. (See also 8.2.3, Colon, Introducing Quotations or Enumerations.)

In the middle of the laboratory examination, a student asked, "Would it be OK to take a break?"

8.2.2 Semicolon.

Semicolon. Semicolons represent a more definite break in thought than commas. Generally, semicolons are used to separate 2 independent clauses. Often a comma will suffice if sentences are short; but when the main clauses are long and joined by coordinating conjunctions or conjunctive adverbs, especially if 1 of the clauses has internal punctuation, use a semicolon.

Separating Independent Clauses. Use a semicolon to separate independent clauses in a compound sentence when no connective word is used. In most instances it is equally correct to use a period and create 2 sentences.

The conditions of 52% of the patients improved greatly; 4% of the patients withdrew from the study.

However, if clauses are short and similar in form, use a comma.

Seventy grafts were patent, 5 were occluded.

Use a semicolon between main clauses joined by a conjunctive adverb (eg, *also, besides, furthermore, then, however, thus, hence, indeed, yet*) or a coordinating conjunction (*and, but, or, for, nor*) if 1 of the clauses has internal punctuation or is considerably long.

The patient's fever had subsided; however, his condition was still critical.

The word *normal* is often used loosely; indeed, it is not easily defined.

Introduction to the knowledge, skills, and attitudes relevant to safety should begin in medical and nursing school; eg, the first 2 years of medical school may be the most appropriate to learn error science and principles of leadership.

Enumerations. For clarity, use semicolons between items in a complex or lengthy enumeration within a sentence or in an enumeration that contains serial commas in at least 1 of the items listed. (In a simple series with little or no internal punctuation, even with multiword elements, use commas.)

A number of questions remain unresolved: (1) whether beverages that contain caffeine are an important factor in arrhythmogenesis; (2) whether such beverages can trigger arrhythmias de novo; and (3) whether their arrhythmogenic tendency is enhanced by the presence and extent of myocardial impairment.

The photomicrographic illustrations of the gross and microscopic features of normal skin, Spitz congenital and dysplastic nevi, lentigines, and melanoma demonstrated the complexity of pigmented lesions.

In less formal writing and where the last element of a series is also a series, commas are acceptable provided that clarity is preserved.

The statistician addressed limitations in case-control studies, cohort studies, and randomized, double-blind, controlled trials.

8.2.3 **Colon.** The colon is the strongest of the 3 marks used to indicate a decided pause or break in thought. It separates 2 main clauses in which the second clause amplifies or explains the first.

This dictum is often believed to be in the Hippocratic Oath: First, do no harm.

When Not to Use a Colon. Do not use a colon if the sentence is continuous without it.

You will need enthusiasm, organization, and a commitment to your beliefs.

Not: You will need: enthusiasm, organization, and a commitment to your beliefs.

Avoid using a colon to separate a preposition from its object or to separate a verb (including *to be* in all of its manifestations) from its object or predicate nominative.

Incorrect: The point is: do not insert the catheter at this time.

Better: The point is not to insert the catheter at this time.

Do not use a colon after *because* or forms of the verb *include.*

Introducing Quotations or Enumerations. Use a colon to introduce a formal or extended quotation. (If the sentence to follow is in quotation marks, the first word is capitalized.)

> Harold Johnson, MD, chair of the committee, summarized: "The problems we face in developing a new vaccine are numerous, but foremost is isolating the antigen."

Use a colon to introduce an enumeration, especially after anticipatory phrasing such as *thus, as follows, the following.*

> The solution included the following components: phosphate buffer, double-distilled water, and a chelating agent.
>
> Laboratory studies yielded the following values: hemoglobin, 11.9 g/dL; erythrocyte sedimentation, 104 mm/h; calcium, 16.9 mg/dL; phosphorus, 5.6 mg/dL; and creatinine, 3 mg/dL.
>
> Phytoestrogens are subdivided into 3 main classes: isoflavones, lignans, and cumestrans.

If 2 or more grammatically independent statements follow the colon, they may be treated as complete sentences separated by periods, and the initial words may or may not be capitalized.

> The following procedure has been established for updating the journal's instructions for authors: (1) Update and review the Word file. (2) Style the Word document according to guidelines and send to the electronic media staff. (3) Insert links. (4) Proofread final version. (5) Code and post on the Web.

Numbers. Use a colon to separate chapter and verse numbers in biblical references, hours and minutes in expressions of time, and the elements of ratios when they are expressed as numbers or abbreviations. For ratios expressed as words, use the word *to* rather than a colon, unless the term conventionally takes a hyphen (eg, "cost-benefit ratio"). In that case, follow the conventional usage and use a hyphen.

> The first Old Testament mention of leprosy is in Exodus 4:6.
>
> Medication was given twice a day, at 8:30 AM and at 8:30 PM.
>
> The chemicals were mixed in a 4:3 ratio.
>
> The controls and study subjects were randomized in a 2:1 ratio.
>
> The ACTH:TSH ratio was elevated when the patient was first examined.
>
> The ratio of albumin to globulin was one of the outcome measures in the study.
>
> The student to instructor ratio was 7 to 1.

References. In references, use a colon (1) between title and subtitle; (2) for periodicals, between issue number and page numbers; and (3) for books, between publisher's location and name. (See also 3.0, References.)

8.3 Hyphens and Dashes.

Hyphens and Dashes. Hyphens and dashes are internal punctuation marks used for linkage and clarity of expression.

8.3.1 Hyphen.

Hyphen. The hyphen is a connector; it may join "what is similar and also what is disjunctive. . . . it divides as well as marries."[2] The hyphen connects words, prefixes, and suffixes permanently or temporarily. Certain compound words always contain hyphens. Such hyphens are called *orthographic*. Examples are *merry-go-round, free-for-all,* and *mother-in-law*. For temporary connections, hyphens help prevent ambiguity, clarify meaning, and indicate word breaks at the end of a line.

In general, when not otherwise specified, hyphens should be used only as an aid to the reader's understanding, primarily to avoid ambiguity. For capitalization of hyphenated compounds in titles, subtitles, subheads, and table heads, see 10.2.2, Capitalization, Titles and Headings, Hyphenated Compounds.

Temporary Compounds. Hyphenate temporary compounds according to current dictionary usage and the following rules:

Hyphenate a compound that contains a noun or an adverb (except for adverbs ending in *-ly*; see below, When Not to Use Hyphens) and a participle that together serve as an adjective modifying the noun they precede. Do not use the hyphen if the compound follows the noun.

> decision-making methods (*But:* methods of decision making)
>
> most-read work in the collection (*But:* The work was the most read in the collection.)
>
> It was a placebo-controlled trial. (*But:* The trial was placebo controlled.)
>
> This is a well-edited volume. (*But:* This volume is well edited.)
>
> The rash was a treatment-related adverse event. (*But:* The adverse event was treatment related.)

Hyphenate a compound adjectival phrase when it precedes the noun it modifies but not when it follows the noun.

> side-by-side placement (*But:* placed side by side)

Hyphenate an adjective-noun compound when it precedes and modifies another noun but not when it follows the noun.

> low-quality suture material (*But:* suture material of low quality)
>
> highest-quality printing (*But:* printing of highest quality)
>
> low-density resolution (*But:* resolution of low density)
>
> low-density nerve fibers (*But:* nerve fibers of low density)
>
> high-altitude sickness (*But:* sickness at high altitude)
>
> very low-birth-weight children (*But:* children of very low birth weight)
>
> low-molecular-weight heparin (*But:* heparin of low molecular weight)
>
> very low-density lipoprotein (*But:* lipoprotein of very low density)

Note: In most instances *middle-, high-,* and *low-* adjectival compounds are hyphenated.

For compound adjectival phrases, adverb-participle compounds, and adjective-noun compounds that have become commonplace and familiar in everyday usage, hyphenate these phrases or compounds whether they precede or follow the noun they modify. (Follow *The Chicago Manual of Style*, 15th edition, to verify.)

long-term therapy
the commitment was long-term

up-to-date vaccinations
the vaccinations were up-to-date

state-of-the-art equipment
equipment that was state-of-the-art

Hyphenate a combination of 2 or more nouns used coordinately as a unit modifier when preceding the noun but not when following.

the Binet-Simon test (*But:* the test of Binet and Simon)

Beer-Lambert law (*But:* the law of Beer and Lambert)

Charcot-Marie-Tooth disease (*But:* the disease described by Charcot, Marie, and Tooth)

Hosmer-Lemeshow goodness-of-fit test (*But:* the goodness-of-fit test of Hosmer and Lemeshow)

the physician-patient relationship (*But:* the relationship between the physician and the patient)

Presentation of ratios as numbers or abbreviations is an exception to this rule. In ratios presented as numbers or abbreviations, use a colon (see 8.2.3, Colon). For ratios presented as words, use the word *to* or, if the word combination has become accepted as a single term, such as *cost-benefit analysis,* a hyphen.

Hyphenate a combination of 2 nouns of equal participation used as a single noun. (See also 8.4.1, Forward Slash [Virgule, Solidus], Used to Express Equivalence or Duality.)

William Carlos Williams was a physician-poet.

W. Somerset Maugham is considered a great physician-writer.

She is an obstetrician-gynecologist.

Provide the best health care for all, says the citizen-patient; but don't allow costs to rise, says the citizen-taxpayer.

The physician-patient may become impatient with treatment.

The study involved 1000 patient-years.

Hyphenate most compound nouns that contain a preposition. Follow the latest edition of *Merriam-Webster's Collegiate Dictionary*.

tie-in tie-up follow-up hand-me-down go-between

(*But:* onlooker, passerby, handout, workup, makeup)

Hyphenate a compound in which a number is the first element and the compound precedes the noun it modifies.

18-factor blood chemistry analysis

7-fold increase

2-way street

ninth-grade reading level

1-cm increments

Hyphenate 2 or more adjectives used coordinately or as conflicting terms whether they precede the noun or follow as a predicate adjective.

The false-positive test results were noted.
The test results were false-positive.

We performed a double-blind study.
The test we used was double-blind.

The author provided black-and-white illustrations.
The author's illustrations were black-and-white.

Hyphenate color terms in which the 2 elements are of equal weight.

blue-gray eyes

blue-black lesions (lesions were blue-black)

(*But:* bluish gray lesions)

Hyphenate compounds formed with the prefixes *all-*, *self-*, and *ex-* whether they precede or follow the noun.

self-reported intake	one's self-respect
all-powerful ruler	the patient's ex-husband

(*Note:* With the prefix *vice*, follow the latest edition of *Merriam-Webster's Collegiate Dictionary*, eg, vice-chancellor, vice-consul, *but* vice president, vice admiral.)

Hyphenate compounds made up of the suffixes *-type*, *-elect*, and *-designate*.

Hodgkin-type lymphoma	president-elect
Valsalva-type maneuver	secretary-designate
chair-elect	

Hyphenate most contemporary adjectival *cross-* compounds (consult the latest edition of *Merriam-Webster's Collegiate Dictionary* for absolute accuracy; there are exceptions, eg, crossbred, crosshatched, crossover, crossmatch, cross section).

cross-reactive	cross-discipline training
cross-contamination	cross-coherence analysis
cross-tolerance reaction	cross-reference citation

Hyphenate *adjectival* compounds with *quasi*.

quasi-legislative group	quasi-analytic model
quasi-diplomatic efforts	quasi-experimental design

Most nouns that begin with *quasi* are not hyphenated but instead are set open (eg, quasi diplomat), although some are closed up (eg, quasicrystal, quasiparticle). Follow the latest edition of *Merriam-Webster's Collegiate Dictionary*.

Hyphenate some compounds in which the first element is a possessive. Consult the latest edition of *Merriam-Webster's Collegiate Dictionary*.

bird's-eye view	bull's-eye
crow's-feet	bird's-nest filter

Hyphenate all prefixes that precede a proper noun, a capitalized word, a number, or an abbreviation.

pro-African initiatives

pre-AIDS era

post-2005 ruling

Note: There is growing recognition and acceptance of the use of a stand-alone prefix with a hyphen when an alternative unhyphenated prefix follows.

We found a need for pre- and postoperative examination.

Patients were categorized as hyper- or hypotensive.

This could be an in- or outpatient procedure.

JAMA and the *Archives* Journals choose *not* to follow this trend and instead would use the following:

We found a need for preoperative and postoperative examination.

Patients were categorized as hypertensive or hypotensive.

This could be an inpatient or outpatient procedure.

When 2 or more hyphenated compounds have a common base, omit the base in all but the last. In unhyphenated compounds written as 1 word, repeat the base.

first-, second-, and third-grade students

10- and 15-year-old boys

anterolateral and posterolateral aspects

Hyphenate compound numbers from 21 to 99 (cardinal and ordinal) when written out, as at the beginning of a sentence. (See 19.1, Numbers and Percentages, Use of Numerals.)

Thirty-six patients were examined.

Twenty-fifth through 75th percentile rankings were shown.

One hundred thirty-two people were killed in the plane crash.

Hyphenate fractions used as nouns or adjectives.

> A two-thirds majority was needed.
>
> The flask was three-fourths full.
>
> Three-fourths of the questionnaires were returned.

Clarity. Use hyphens to avoid ambiguity. If a term could be misleading without a hyphen, hyphenate it. As with the use of commas to indicate pauses, the use of the hyphen to provide clarity may be subjective. What is clear to one person may be a source of ambiguity to another. Use the following guidelines and a healthy dose of common sense.

> a small-bowel constriction (constriction of the small bowel)
> a small bowel constriction (a small constriction of the bowel)
>
> a single-specialty center (a center devoted to a single specialty)
> a single specialty center (1 center devoted to a specialty)
>
> a large-bowel resection (resection of the large bowel) (*Better:* a colon resection)
> a large bowel resection (a large resection of the bowel)
>
> a solid-organ transplantation program (a program for transplantation of solid organs)
> a solid organ transplantation program (a program for organ transplantation that is solid, ie, well established) (*Better:* a well-established transplantation program)

Use a hyphen after a prefix when the unhyphenated word would have a different meaning.

re-treat	re-formation
re-creation	un-ionized

Note: Do not hyphenate other forms of these words for which no ambiguity exists: *retreatment, recreational.*

Occasionally, a hyphen is used after a prefix or before a suffix to avoid an awkward combination of letters, such as 2 of the same vowel or 3 of the same consonant (with exceptions noted below, When Not to Use Hyphens). Follow the latest edition of *Merriam-Webster's Collegiate Dictionary* or *Dorland's* or *Stedman's* medical dictionary.

semi-independent	intra-abdominal
hull-less	bell-like
ultra-atomic	anti-inflammatory
de-emphasize	

(Some exceptions to this rule include *microorganism, cooperation, reenter* [see below, When Not to Use Hyphens].)

In complex modifying phrases that include suffixes or prefixes, hyphens and en dashes are sometimes used to avoid ambiguity. (See also 8.3.2, Dashes, En Dash.)

non-self-governing	non-English-language journals
non-group-specific blood	non-Q-wave myocardial infarction
non-brain-injured subjects	

Expressing Ranges and Dimensions. When expressing ranges or dimensions used as modifiers, use hyphens and spacing in accordance with the following examples in the left-hand column. The alternatives in the right-hand column give the expression of dimensions when not used as modifiers.

As Modifier	*Alternative*
in a 10- to 14-day period	10 to 14 days' duration
a 3×4-cm strip	a strip measuring 3×4 cm
a 5- to 10-mg dose	a dose of 5 to 10 mg
in a 5-, 10-, or 15-mg dose	in a dose of 5, 10, or 15 mg
a 3-cm-diameter tube	a tube 3 cm in diameter
5-mm-thick lesion	a lesion 5 mm thick

In the text, do not use hyphens to express ranges. (See 19.4, Numbers and Percentages, Use of Digit Spans and Hyphens.)

> The adverse events were experienced by 5% to 10% of the group.

The exceptions to this rule about ranges are for (1) ranges expressing fiscal years, academic years, life spans, or study spans and (2) ranges given in parentheses.

> We present results from the 2002-2004 Renal Study Group.
>
> The patients' median age was 56 years (range, 31-92 years).

Note that no hyphens are needed in the following cases:

> a 3 to 4 ratio
>
> a case of mild to moderate pruritus

Word Division. Use hyphens to indicate division of a word at the end of a line (follow the latest edition of *Merriam-Webster's Collegiate Dictionary* or *Stedman's* or *Dorland's* medical dictionary).

When Not to Use Hyphens. Rules also exist for when not to use hyphens.

The following common prefixes are not joined by hyphens except when they precede a proper noun, a capitalized word, or an abbreviation: *ante-, anti-, bi-, co-, contra-, counter-, de-, extra-, infra-, inter-, intra-, micro-, mid-, non-, over-, pre-, post-, pro-, pseudo-, re-, semi-, sub-, super-, supra-, trans-, tri-, ultra-, un-, under-.*

antimicrobial	nonresident
coauthor	overproduction
codirects	overrepresented
coexistence	overtreatment
coidentity	posttraumatic

coworker	preexisting
deidentify	reevaluation
interrater	repossess
midaxillary	transsacral
midbrow	ultramicrotome
multicenter	underrepresented
nonnegotiable	

Retain the hyphen if needed to avoid ambiguity or awkward spelling that could interfere with readability: co-opt, co-payment, co-twin, intra-aortic.

Retain the hyphen when the term after the prefixes *anti-*, *neo-*, *pre-*, *post-*, and mid- is a proper noun or a number (see also above, Temporary Compounds), eg, mid-1900s, mid-Atlantic crossing.

The following suffixes are joined without a hyphen, with exceptions if the clarity would be obscured (see Temporary Compounds above): *-hood, -less, -like, -wise.*

womanhood	shoeless
manhood	insulinlike
catatoniclike	probandwise concordance

Some combinations of words are commonly read together as a unit. As such combinations come into common use, the hyphen tends to be omitted without a sacrifice of clarity. Use the latest editions of *Merriam-Webster's Collegiate Dictionary* and *Dorland's* and *Stedman's* medical dictionaries as guides to common usage (eg, *broad-spectrum antibiotics* is hyphenated in *Dorland's; open heart surgery, deep venous thrombosis,* and *small cell carcinoma* are not). For terms not found in these sources, use a reader's perspective and the context as guides (eg, *JAMA* and the *Archives* Journals hyphenate *soft-tissue*, as in *soft-tissue mass,* to avoid confusion). When no confusion is likely, leave open. If there is a possibility of confusion, hyphenate. A short list of examples that can usually be presented without hyphens is given below.

amino acid levels	medical school students
birth control methods	natural killer cell
bone marrow biopsy	open heart surgery
deep venous thrombosis	peer review process
foreign body infiltrate	primary care physician
health care system	public health official
inner ear disorder	small cell carcinoma
lower extremity amputation	tertiary care center

Do not hyphenate names of disease entities used as modifiers.

basal cell carcinoma	connective tissue tumor
hyaline membrane disease	sickle cell trait
clam diggers' itch	grand mal seizures

Do not use a hyphen after an adverb that ends in *-ly* even when used in a compound modifier preceding the word modified; in these cases, ambiguity is unlikely and the hyphen can be dispensed with.

the clearly stated purpose	biologically mediated therapy
a highly developed species	previously published recommendations
clinically derived databases	clinically relevant variables

Do not hyphenate names of chemical compounds used as adjectives.

sodium chloride solution

tannic acid test

Most combinations of proper adjectives derived from geographic entities are not hyphenated when used as noun or adjective formations.

Central Americans	Pacific Rim countries
Southeast Asian countries	Central American customs
African American	Latin Americans
Mexican American	

(*But:* Scotch-Irish ancestry. Here the hyphen is used to indicate 2 countries of origin.)

Do not hyphenate Latin expressions or non-English-language phrases used in an adjectival sense. Most of these are treated as separate words; a few are joined without a hyphen. Follow the latest edition of *Merriam-Webster's Collegiate Dictionary*.

an a priori argument	an ex officio member
per diem employees	antebellum South
prima facie evidence	in vivo specimens
postmortem examination	carcinoma in situ
café au lait spots	post hoc testing

Note that when *post* is used as a combining adjectival form, as in *postmortem examination,* it is set closed up. When it is used as an adverb, as in *post hoc testing,* it is set as 2 separate words. This distinction is apparent in the examples below:

postpartum depression

depression occurring post partum

Do not hyphenate modifiers in which a letter or number is the second element.

grade A eggs

study 1 protocol

type 1 diabetes mellitus

Compound Official Titles. Hyphenate combination positions of office but not compound designations as follows:

secretary-treasurer
acting secretary
honorary chair
(*But:* past vice president, executive vice president, past president)

Special Combinations. Special combinations may or may not necessitate the use of hyphens. Consult *Stedman's, Dorland's,* and the latest edition of *Merriam-Webster's Collegiate Dictionary*. (See 15.0, Nomenclature, and 17.0, Greek Letters.)

B cell	Mann-Whitney test
graft-vs-host disease	T-shirt
T tube	face-lift
B-cell helper	prostate-specific antigen
I beam (I-shaped beam)	Z-plasty
T wave	forehead-lift
β-blocker	T square
J curve	γ-globulin
T-cell marker	*t* test
brow-lift	

8.3.2 **Dashes.** Dashes as another form of internal punctuation convey a particular meaning or emphasize and clarify a certain section of material within a sentence. Compared with parentheses, dashes may convey a less formal or more emphatic "aside."

There are 4 types of dashes that differ in length: the *em* dash, the most common; the *en* dash; the *2-em* dash; and the *3-em* dash. When preparing a manuscript, if symbols for various dashes are not available in the word-processing program, use 2 hyphens to indicate an em dash (--) and 1 for an en dash (–).

Em Dash. Em dashes are used to indicate a marked or pronounced interruption or break in thought. It is best to use this mode sparingly; do not use an em dash when another punctuation mark will suffice, for instance, the comma or the colon, or to imply *namely, that is,* or *in other words,* when an explanation follows.

> All of these factors—age, severity of symptoms, psychic preparation, and choice of anesthetic agent—determine the patient's reaction.

An em dash may be used to separate a referent from a pronoun that is the subject of an ending clause.

> Osler, Billings, Apgar—these were the physicians she tried to emulate.

En Dash. The en dash is longer than a hyphen but half the length of the em dash. The en dash shows relational distinction in a hyphenated or compound modifier, 1 element of which consists of 2 words or a hyphenated word, or when the word being modified is a compound.

Winston-Salem-oriented group	post-World War I
physician-lawyer-directed section	multiple sclerosis-like symptoms

anti-Norwalk virus
phosphotungstic acid-hematoxylin stain
decision tree-based analysis
non-small cell carcinoma

2-Em Dash. The 2-em dash is used to indicate missing letters in a word.

The study was conducted at N—— Hospital, noted for its low autopsy rate.

3-Em Dash. The 3-em dash is used to show missing words.

Each subject was asked to fill in the blank in the following statement: "I usually sleep ——— hours per day."

I admire Dr ——— too much to expose him in this anecdote.

8.4 **Forward Slash (Virgule, Solidus).** The forward slash is used to represent *per, and,* or *or* and to divide material (eg, numerator and denominator in fractions; month, day, and year in dates [only in tables and figures]; lines of poetry). It may also be used in URLs (see 2.0, Manuscript Preparation).

8.4.1 **Used to Express Equivalence or Duality.** When 2 terms are of equal weight in an expression and *and* is implied between them to express this equivalence, the forward slash can be retained.

The diagnosis and initial treatment/diagnostic planning were recorded.

If the approval process raises concerns among the researchers or the ethics committee/IRB members, the author may want to explain the resolution of these issues.

When the question of duality arises in the he/she construction, change the slash construction when the gender is to be specified; substitute the word *or* for the forward slash or, preferably, rephrase to be gender neutral.

Dr Kate Wolf and Dr Rob Cox agreed to serve on the nomenclature committee. Now I need to know whether he or she [not he/she] will lead the subcommittee on genetic nomenclature.

Better: Now I need to know which of them will lead the subcommittee.

If the sex is unspecified and does not matter, retain the slash construction.

This aspiration technique is one that any physician can master whether or not he/she has surgical expertise.

Note: The trend today is toward rephrasing such sentences and using the plural to avoid sexist language; eg, "This aspiration technique can be mastered by physicians whether or not they have surgical expertise." (See 11.10, Correct and Preferred Usage, Inclusive Language.)

Although the forward slash can be used to indicate alternative or combined states in the same person, such as Jekyll/Hyde personality, it is important that no ambiguity be introduced. If there is any likelihood of ambiguity, the sentence should be reworded.

8.4.2 Used to Mean *per*. In the "per" construction, use a forward slash only when (1) the construction involves units of measure (including time) *and* (2) at least 1 element includes a specific numerical quantity *and* (3) the element immediately adjacent on each side is either a specific numerical quantity or a unit of measure. In such cases, the units of measure should be abbreviated in accordance with 14.12, Abbreviations, Units of Measure. (See also 19.7.3, Numbers and Percentages, Forms of Numbers, Reporting Proportions and Percentages.)

The hemoglobin level was 14 g/dL.

The $CD4^+$ cell count was 200/μL.

Blood volume was 80 mL/kg of body weight.

Respirations were 60/min; pulse rate was 98/min.

The drug dosage was 30 mg/d.

Do *not* use the forward slash in a "per" construction (1) when a prepositional phrase intervenes between the 2 units of measure, (2) when no specific numerical quantity is expressed, or (3) in nontechnical expressions.

4.5 mEq of potassium per liter
(*Avoid:* 4.5 mEq/L of potassium; instead reword: a potassium concentration of 4.5 mEq/L.)

expressed in milliliters per minute

2 days per year

8.4.3 In Dates. Use the forward slash in dates only in tables and figures to save space (month/day/year) (see 4.1.5, Visual Presentation of Data, Tables, Punctuation). Avoid this presentation of dates in the text.

8.4.4 In Equations. In equations that are set on line and run into the text rather than centered and set off (see 21.3, Mathematical Composition, Stacked vs Unstacked), use the forward slash to separate numerator and denominator.

The "stacked" fraction $y = \frac{r_1+r_2}{p_1-p_2}$ is written as $y = (r_1 + r_2)/(p_1 - p_2)$.

Note that when the slash is used for this purpose, parentheses and brackets must often be added to avoid ambiguity.

8.4.5 In Ratios. Although a forward slash may be used to express a ratio (eg, the male/female [M/F] ratio was 2/1), *JAMA* and the *Archives* Journals recommend use of a colon to express ratios involving numbers or abbreviations (the Apo B:Apo A-I ratio was 2:1) and the word *to* to express ratios involving words (the male to female ratio). (See 8.2.3, Colon, Numbers.)

8.4.6 In Phonetics, Poetry. The forward slash is also used to set off phonemes and phonetic transcription and to divide run-in lines of poetry.

/d/ as in *dog*

. . . cold-breathed earth/earth of the slumbering and liquid trees/earth of the mountains misty-topped.

8.5 Parentheses and Brackets. Parentheses and brackets are internal punctuation marks used to set off material that is nonrestrictive or, as in the case of mathematical and chemical expressions, to alert the reader to the special functions occurring within.

8.5.1 Parentheses

Supplementary Expressions. Use parentheses to indicate supplementary explanations, identification, direction to the reader, or translation. (See also 8.3.2, Dashes, and 8.5.2, Brackets.)

> A known volume of fluid (100 mL) was injected.
>
> The differences were not significant ($P > .05$).
>
> One of us (B.O.G.) saw the patient in 2006.
>
> Asymmetry of the upper part of the rib cage (patient 5) and pseudarthrosis of the first and second ribs (patient 8) were incidental anomalies (Table 3).
>
> Of the 761 hospitalized patients, 171 (22.5%) were infants (younger than 1 year).
>
> In this issue of *JAMA* (p 1037), a successful transplant is reported.
>
> The 3 cusps of the aortic valve (the "Mercedes-Benz sign") were clearly shown on the echocardiogram.

If there is a close relationship between the parenthetical material and the rest of the sentence, commas are preferred to parentheses.

> The hemoglobin level, although in the normal range, was lower than expected.

If the relationship in thought after the expressions *namely* (*viz*), *that is* (*ie*), and *for example* (*eg*) is incidental, use parentheses instead of commas.

> He weighed the advice of several committee members (namely, Jones, Burke, and Easton) before making his proposal.

Punctuation Marks With Parentheses. Use no punctuation before the opening parenthesis except in enumerations (see Enumerations below).

Any punctuation mark can follow a closing parenthesis, but only the 3 end marks (the period, the question mark, and the exclamation point) may precede it when the parenthetical material interrupts the sentence. If a complete sentence is contained within parentheses, it is not necessary to have punctuation within the parentheses if it would noticeably interrupt the flow of the sentence. Note that with complete sentences, the initial letter of the first word is capitalized.

> The discussion on informed consent lasted 2 hours. (A final draft has yet to be written.) The discussion failed to resolve the question.
>
> The discussion on informed consent lasted 2 hours (a final draft has yet to be written) and did not resolve the question.

After what seemed an eternity (It took 2 hours!), the discussion on informed consent ended.

When the parenthetical material includes special punctuation, such as an exclamation point or a question mark, or several statements, terminal punctuation is placed inside the closing parenthesis.

Oscar Wilde once said (When? Where? Who knows? But I read it in a book once upon a time, hence it must be true.) that "anyone who has never written a book is very learned."[3]

Identifying Numbers or Letters. When an item identified by letter or number is referred to later by that letter or number only, enclose the letter or number in parentheses.

You then follow (3), (5), and (6) to solve the puzzle.

If the category name is used instead, parentheses may be dropped.

Steps 1, 2, and 3 must be done slowly.

Enumerations. For division of a short enumeration that is run in and indicated by numerals or lowercase italic letters, enclose the numerals or letters in parentheses. (See also 19.5, Numbers and Percentages, Enumerations.)

The patient is to bring (1) all pill bottles, (2) past medical records, and (3) our questionnaire to the first office visit.

References in Text. Use parentheses to enclose all or part of a reference given in the text. (See also 3.3, References, References Given in Text.)

Two cases of invasive zygomycosis with a fatal outcome were reported in the *Archives of Dermatology* (2005;141[10]:1211-1213).

In Legends. In legends, use parentheses to identify a case or patient and parts of a composite figure when appropriate. (See also 4.2.7, Visual Presentation of Data, Figures, Titles, Legends, and Labels.)

Figure 6. Facial paralysis on the right side (patient 3).

Figure 2. Fracture of the left femur (patient 7).

The date, if given, is similarly enclosed.

Figure 2. Fracture of the left femur (patient 7, October 23, 2004).

For photomicrographs, give the magnification and the stain, if relevant, in parentheses (see also 4.2.7, Visual Presentation of Data, Figures, Titles, Legends, and Labels).

Figure 3. Marrow aspiration 14 weeks after transplantation (Wright stain, original magnification ×600).

Trade Names. If there is a reason to provide a trade name for a drug or for equipment, enclose the trade name in parentheses immediately after the first use of the non-proprietary name in the text and in the abstract. (See also 15.4.3, Nomenclature, Drugs, Proprietary Names; and 15.5, Nomenclature, Equipment, Devices, and Reagents.)

> Treatment included oral administration of indomethacin (Indocin), 25 mg 3 times a day.

Abbreviations. If used in the text, specialized abbreviations (as specified in 14.11, Abbreviations, Clinical, Technical, and Other Common Terms) are enclosed in parentheses immediately after first mention of the term, which is spelled out in full.

Explanatory Notes. Explanatory notes, when incorporated into the text, are placed within parentheses. In such instances, terminal punctuation is used before the closing parenthesis, the sentence(s) within the parentheses being a complete thought but only parenthetical to the text.

Parenthetical Expressions Within a Parenthetical Expression. These are enclosed in brackets.

> (Antirejection therapy included parenteral antithymocyte globulin [ATGAM], at a dosage of 15 mg/kg per day.)
>
> *But:* In mathematical expressions, parentheses are placed *inside* brackets. See 8.5.2, Brackets, Within Parentheses.

Parenthetical Plurals. Parentheses are sometimes used around the letters *s* or *es* to express the possibility of a plural when singular or plural could be meant. (See also 7.8.4, Grammar, Subject-Verb Agreement, Parenthetical Plurals.)

> The name(s) of the editor(s) of the book in reference 2 is unknown.

Note: If this construction is used, the verb should be singular, because the *s* is parenthetical. In general, try to avoid this construction and use the plural noun instead or rephrase the sentence:

> We do not know the name(s) of the editor(s) of the book in reference 2.

8.5.2 Brackets

Insertions in Quotations. Brackets are used to indicate editorial interpolation within a quotation and to enclose corrections, explanations, or comments in material that is quoted. (See also 8.6.1, Quotation Marks, Quotations; 8.8.6, Ellipses, Change in Capitalization; and 8.8.7, Ellipses, Omission of Ellipses.)

> "Enough questions had arisen [these are not described] to warrant medical consultation."
>
> Thompson stated, "Because of the patient's preferences, surgery was *absolutely* contraindicated [italics added]."
>
> "The following year [1947] was a turning point."

Note: Use *sic* (Latin for "thus" or "so") in brackets to indicate an error or peculiarity in the spelling or grammar of the preceding word in the original source of the quotation. As with apologetic quotation marks (see 8.6.8, Quotation Marks, Apologetic Quotation Marks), use *sic* with discretion.

"The plural [*sic*] cavity was filled with fluid."

"Breathing of the gas is often followed by extraordinary fits of extacy [*sic*]."

Within Parentheses. Use brackets to indicate parenthetical expressions within parenthetical expressions.

A nitrogen mustard (mechlorethamine hydrochloride [Mustargen]) was one of the drugs used.

In scientific text, one often encounters complex parenthetical constructions such as consecutive parentheses and brackets within parentheses.

Her platelet count was 100 000/mm^3 (100 × 10^9/L) (reference range, 150 000 to 450 000/mm^3 [150 to 450 × 10^9/L]).

In Formulas. In mathematical formulas, parentheses are generally used for the innermost units, with parentheses changed to brackets when the formula is parenthetical. (See also 21.3, Mathematical Composition, Stacked vs Unstacked.)

$t = d(r_1 - r_2)$

The equation suggested by this phenomenon ($t = d[r_1 - r_2]$) can be applied in a variety of circumstances.

In chemical formulas, the current trend is to use only parentheses and brackets, making sure that every parenthetical or bracketed expression has an opening and closing parenthesis or bracket symbol. Consult the most recent edition of *USP Dictionary of USAN and International Drug Names* for drug formulas and *The Merck Index* for chemical compounds to verify the correct use of parentheses and brackets.

An experimental drug (9-[(2-hydroxy-1-(hydroxymethyl)ethoxymethyl)]guanine) was used to treat the cytomegalovirus retinopathy in patients with AIDS.

If the older style of parentheses, braces, and brackets has been used by the author, retain it. The notation will be readily understood by the author's intended audience.

When a parenthetical or bracketed insertion in the text contains a mathematical formula in which parentheses or brackets appear, the characters within the formula should be left as given unless that would place 2 identical punctuation symbols (eg, 2 open parentheses) immediately adjacent to each other. To avoid adjacent identical characters, change parentheses to brackets or brackets to parentheses in the formula as needed, working from inside out, starting with parentheses, to brackets, to braces.

$CV_t^2 = [CV_b^2 + (CV_a^2/NR)]/NS$

8.6 Quotation Marks. Quotation marks are used to indicate material that is taken directly from another source.

8.6.1 **Quotations.** Use quotation marks to enclose a direct quotation of no more than 4 lines from textual material or speeches (for longer material, see also 8.6.14, Quotation Marks, Block Quotations). When the quotation marks enclose conversational dialogue, there is no limit to the length that may be set in run-on format.

In all quoted material, follow the wording, spelling, and punctuation of the original exactly. The only time this rule does not apply is when the quoted material, although a complete sentence or part of a complete sentence in its original source, is now used as part of another complete sentence. In this case, the capital letter in the quoted sentence would be replaced by a lowercase letter in brackets.

Similarly, in legal material any change in initial capital letters from quoted material should be indicated by placing the change in brackets. (See 8.5.2, Brackets, Insertions in Quotations.)

To indicate an omission in quoted material, use ellipses. (See 8.8, Ellipses.)

To indicate editorial interpolation in quoted material, use brackets. (See 8.5.2, Brackets, Insertions in Quotations.) Use [*sic*] after a misspelled word or an incorrect or apparently absurd statement in quoted material to indicate that this is an accurate rendition of the original source. However, when quoting material from another era that uses now obsolete spellings, use *sic* sparingly. Do not use *sic* with an exclamation point. (*Note:* The use of *sic* is not limited to quoted material; in other instances, it means that any unusual or bizarre appearance in the preceding word is intentional, not accidental.) (See 8.5.2, Brackets, Insertions in Quotations.)

The author should always verify the quotation from the original source.

8.6.2 **Dialogue.** With conversational dialogue, enclose the opening word and the final word in quotation marks.

> "Please don't schedule the surgery for a Tuesday."
>
> "OK, if that's inconvenient for you, I won't."

8.6.3 **Titles.** Within titles (including titles of articles, references, and tables), centered heads, and run-in sideheads, use double quotation marks.

> The "Sense" of Humor

8.6.4 **Single Quotation Marks.** Use single quotation marks for quotations within quotations.

> He looked at us and said, "As my patients always told me, 'Be a good listener.'"

8.6.5 **Placement.** Place closing quotation marks outside commas and periods, inside colons and semicolons. Place question marks, dashes, and exclamation points inside quotation marks only when they are part of the quoted material. If they apply to the whole statement, place them outside the quotation marks.

> Why bother to perform autopsies at all if the main finding is invariably "edema and congestion of the viscera"?
>
> The clinician continues to ask, "Why did he die?"

"I'll lend you my stethoscope for clinic"—then she remembered the last time she had lent it and said, "On second thought, I'll be needing it myself."

(*Note:* Commas are not always needed with quoted material. For example, in the following example commas are not necessary after "said" or to set off the quoted material.)

He said he had had his "fill of it all" and was "content" to leave the meeting.

8.6.6 **Omission of Opening or Closing Quotation Marks.** The opening quotation mark should be omitted when an article beginning with a stand-up or dropped initial capital letter also begins with a quotation. It is best, however, to avoid this construction.

Doctors need some patients," a sage had said.

When excerpting long passages that consist of several paragraphs, use opening double quotation marks before each paragraph and closing quotation marks only at the end of the final paragraph. (See also 8.8, Ellipses, and 8.6.14, Block Quotations.)

8.6.7 **Coined Words, Slang.** Coined words, slang, nicknames, and words or phrases used ironically or facetiously may be enclosed in quotation marks at first mention. Thereafter, omit quotation marks. (See also 22.5.4, Typography, Specific Uses of Fonts, Italics.)

We further hope that, above all, those who have been fed only "docufiction" on this matter, as if it were truth, will cease to be misled.

Nelson Essentials of Pediatrics is not a . . . synopsis of or a companion to the *Nelson Textbook of Pediatrics,* although initially our associates dubbed it "Baby Nelson," "Half Nelson," and "Junior Nelson."[4]

It has been said that shoes and latrines are the best "medicine" for ancylostomiasis (hookworm disease).

Do not use quotation marks when emphasizing a word, when using a non-English word, when mentioning a term as a term, or when defining a term. In these instances, italics is preferred. (See also 22.5.4, Typography, Specific Uses of Fonts, Italics.)

The page number is called the *folio.*

The eye associated with the greater reduction in hitting ability when dimmed by a filter was termed the *dominant eye* for motion stereopsis.

Pulsus paradoxus is defined as an exaggeration of the physiologic inspiratory drop in systolic blood pressure.

8.6.8 **Apologetic Quotation Marks.** Quotation marks are sometimes used around words for special effect or to indicate irony. In most instances, however, they are unnecessary.

Using their own finances and being informed about the economics of the approach, some may opt for the "boutique class" of health care.

8.6.9 ***So-called.*** A word or phrase following *so-called* should not be enclosed in quotation marks.

> The so-called harm principle holds that competent adults should have freedom of action unless they pose a risk to themselves or to the community.

8.6.10 **Common Words Used in a Technical Sense.** Enclose in quotation marks a common word used in a special technical sense when the context does not make the meaning clear. (See also 8.6.11, Definition or Translation of Non–English-Language Words.)

> In many publications, "running feet" on left-hand pages face the "gutter" at the bottom of the page.
>
> "Coma vigil" (akinetic mutism) may be confused with conscious states.

8.6.11 **Definition or Translation of Non–English-Language Words.** The literal translation of a non–English-language word or phrase is usually enclosed in quotation marks if it follows the word or phrase, whereas the simple definition of the word or phrase is not. (See also 12.2, Non-English Words, Phrases, and Accent Marks, Accent Marks [Diacritics].)

> Hysterical patients may exhibit an attitude termed *la belle indifférence* ("beautiful indifference" or total unconcern) toward their condition.

8.6.12 **Titles of Works.** In the text, use quotation marks to enclose titles of short poems, essays, lectures, radio and television programs, songs, the names of electronic files, parts of published works (chapters, articles in a periodical), papers read at meetings, dissertations, theses, and parts of the same article (eg, the "Results" section). (See also 10.5, Capitalization, Types and Sections of Articles, and 22.5.4, Typography, Specific Uses of Fonts, Italics.)

8.6.13 **Indirect Discourse, Discussions.** After indirect discourse, do not use quotation marks.

> The nurse said he would be discharged today.

Do not use quotation marks with yes or no.

> His answer to the question was no.

In interview or discussion formats when the name of the speaker is set off, do not use quotation marks.

> Dr Black: Now let us review the slides of the bone marrow biopsy.
>
> Dr Smith: The first slide reveals complete absence of granulocytic precursors.

8.6.14 **Block Quotations.** If material quoted from texts or speeches is longer than 4 lines of text, the material should be set off in a block, ie, in reduced type and without the quotation marks. Paragraph indents are generally not used unless the quoted material is known to begin a paragraph. Space is often added both above and below these longer quotations.

If the block quotation appears in a section to be set in reduced type, do not reduce the type size of the quoted material further.

If another quotation appears within a block quote, use double quotation marks around the contained quotation, rather than setting off in blocks, regardless of the length.

8.7 Apostrophe

8.7.1 **To Show Possession.** Use the apostrophe to show the possessive case of proper nouns in accordance with the following examples (see also 16.2, Eponyms, Nonpossessive Form):

Jones' bones (1 person named Jones)
the Joneses' bones (2 or more people named Jones)

If a singular or plural word does not end in *s*, add *'s* to form the possessive.

a child's wants	men's concerns
women's health	everyone's answer

If a proper noun or name ends in a silent *s*, *z*, or *x*, form the possessive by adding *'s*.

Theroux's *The Mosquito Coast*
Jacqueline du Pres's recordings

8.7.2 **Possessive Pronouns.** Do not use *'s* with possessive pronouns: his, hers, ours, its, yours, theirs, whose.

The idea was hers.

Give the book its due.

Note: Do not confuse the contraction of *it is* (*it's*) with the possessive *its*, eg, "It's an excellent resource. I have not seen its equal."

8.7.3 **Possessive of Compound Terms.** Use *'s* after only the last word of a compound term.

father-in-law's health	someone else's problem
editor in chief's decision	secretary of health's ruling

8.7.4 **Joint Possession.** When joint possession is being shown with nouns, or with an organization's or business firm's name, use the possessive form only in the last word of the noun or name.

Food and Drug Administration's policy

Farrar, Straus & Giroux's books

Centers for Disease Control and Prevention's Task Force

Hammond and Horn's study

When possession is individual, each noun takes the possessive form.

We matched the infant's and mother's records.

Note: When one of the nouns takes a possessive pronoun, the other nouns take the possessive as well.

I presented the intern's and my workups.

8.7.5 Using Apostrophes to Form Plurals. Do not use an apostrophe to indicate the plural of a name. Do not use an apostrophe in the name of an organization in which the qualifying term is used as an adjective or an attributive rather than a possessive. Of course, always follow the official name.

The Chicago Cubs	state parks rangers
Veterans Affairs	musicians union
Rainbow Babies Hospital	nurses station

Use *'s* to indicate the plural of letters, signs, or symbols spoken as such, or words referred to as words when *s* alone would be confusing. Note the italics with inflectional ending in roman type for words, letters, and numbers but not for symbols and signs.

He uses too many *and*'s.

The manuscript editor was mindful of the list of *do*'s and *don't*'s.

Mind your *p*'s and *q*'s.

There are 9 +'s on the page.

His *1*'s looked like *7*'s.

Do not use an apostrophe to form the plural of an all-capital abbreviation or of numerals (including years). (See also 9.5, Plurals, Abbreviations.)

ECGs	RBCs
EEGs	a woman in her 40s
IQs	during the late 1990s
WBCs	

8.7.6 Units of Time and Money as Possessive Adjectives. With units of time (minute, hour, day, month, year, etc) used as possessive adjectives, an *'s* is added. The same holds true for monetary terms:

a day's wait	a few hours' time
an hour's delay	6 months' gestation
5 days' hard work	a dollar's worth

8.7.7 Prime. Do not use an apostrophe where a prime sign is intended. Do not use a prime sign as a symbol of measurement. (See also 15.4.4, Nomenclature, Drugs, Chemical Names.)

The methyl group was in the 5′ position.

8.8 **Ellipses.** Ellipses are 3 spaced dots (. . .) generally used to indicate omission of 1 or more words, lines, paragraphs, or data from quoted material (this omission being the *ellipsis*). Excerpts from the following paragraph will be used to demonstrate the use of ellipses.

> In *Fruit Displayed on a Stand* (cover), exhibited in 1882, Caillebotte depicts a traditional subject in a manner far removed from the traditional cornucopian flow of fruit. Instead, he shows a stark, rectangular grid lit by centers of rounded forms, brilliantly colored. Vivid oranges, reds, and purples, light greens, creamy violets, and color-flecked gold are cupped within areas of crinkly blue-white paper, the cooler shades in the center separating the hotter tones, preventing them from spilling into each other.[5]

8.8.1 **Omission Within a Sentence.** If the ellipsis occurs within a sentence, ellipses represent the omission.

> Instead, he shows a . . . grid lit by centers of rounded forms, brilliantly colored.

In some such instances, additional punctuation may be used on either side of the ellipses if it helps the sense of the sentence or better shows the omission.

> Instead, he shows a stark, rectangular grid . . . , brilliantly colored.

If the quotation *itself* contains ellipses, to make clear that the ellipses were part of the original a note to this effect should be included in brackets.

8.8.2 **Omission at the End of a Sentence or Between Complete Sentences.** If the ellipsis occurs at the end of a complete sentence, or between 2 complete sentences, ellipses follow the final punctuation mark, the final punctuation mark being set close to the word preceding it, even when this word is not the final word in that sentence in the original.

> In *Fruit Displayed on a Stand* (cover), exhibited in 1882, Caillebotte depicts a traditional subject in a manner far removed from the traditional. . . . Instead, he shows a stark, rectangular grid lit by centers of rounded forms, brilliantly colored.

8.8.3 **Grammatically Incomplete Expressions.** The sentence within which an ellipsis occurs should be a grammatically complete expression. However, ellipses and no period may be used at the end of a sentence fragment to indicate that it is purposely grammatically incomplete.

> Complete the sentence "When I retire, I plan to . . . " in 20 words or less.

8.8.4 **Omissions in Verse.** Use 1 line of em-spaced dots to indicate omission of a full line or several consecutive lines of verse.

> Sometimes you say it's smaller. Today
> . . . .
> you said it was a touch larger, and would change.
>
> Marc Straus, MD, "Autumn"

8.8.5 Omissions Between or at the Start of Paragraphs. With material in which several paragraphs are being quoted and omissions of full paragraphs occur, a period and ellipses at the end of the paragraph preceding the omitted material are sufficient to indicate this omission.

> Indeed, it is no more than the just desert of Dr Theodore Schott and his late brother to attribute to them the credit of having introduced and elaborated a method capable of restoring most cases of heart disease to a state of complete compensation, after the failure of other means, such as digitalis. . . .

If the initial word(s) or the first sentence of the paragraph being quoted is omitted, begin that paragraph with a paragraph indention and ellipses to indicate that this is not the beginning of that paragraph.

> . . . it is no more than the just desert of Dr Theodore Schott and his late brother to attribute to them the credit of having introduced and elaborated a method capable of restoring most cases of heart disease to a state of complete compensation, after the failure of other means, such as digitalis. . . .

8.8.6 Change in Capitalization. The first word after the end punctuation mark and the ellipses should use the original capitalization, particularly in legal and scholarly documents. This facilitates finding the material in the original source and avoids any change of meaning. If a change in the original capitalization is made, brackets should be used around the letter in question. (See also 8.5.2, Brackets, Insertions in Quotations, and 8.6.1, Quotation Marks, Quotations.)

> [H]e shows a stark, rectangular grid lit by centers of rounded forms, brilliantly colored.

> In the cover story, the artist is described as using "[v]ivid oranges, reds, and purples, light greens, creamy violets, and color-flecked gold" to depict "a traditional subject."

8.8.7 Omission of Ellipses. Ellipses are not necessary at the beginning and end of a quotation if the quoted material is a complete sentence from the original.

> In a 1985 *JAMA* cover story, Martha Bier wrote, "Instead, he shows a stark, rectangular grid lit by centers of rounded forms, brilliantly colored."

Omit ellipses within a quotation when the omitted words occur at the same place as a bracketed editorial insertion. (See also 8.5.2, Brackets, Insertions in Quotations.)

> "[Caillebotte] shows a stark, rectangular grid lit by centers of rounded forms, brilliantly colored."

When a quoted phrase is an incomplete sentence, readers understand that something precedes and follows; therefore, ellipses are not used.

> In *Place de L'Europe on a Rainy Day,* Caillebotte does not use "centers of rounded forms, brilliantly colored" but instead uses muted grays and purples to give the feel of the rain.

Ellipses are generally not needed when the first part of the sentence is deleted.

> Here Caillebotte "depicts a traditional subject in a manner far removed from the traditional. . . . "

8.8.8 **Ellipses in Tables.** In tables, ellipses may be used, for example, to indicate that no data were available or that a specific category of data is not applicable. (See also 4.1.3, Visual Presentation of Data, Tables, Table Components.) An explanatory footnote should always be included if it is not absolutely clear from the context what the ellipses represent.

> [a]Ellipses indicate no test performed.

ACKNOWLEDGMENT

Principal author: Cheryl Iverson, MA

REFERENCES

1. Truss L. *Eats, Shoots & Leaves: The Zero Tolerance Approach to Punctuation.* New York, NY: Gotham Books; 2003:201.
2. Shields C. Invention. In: *Dressing Up for the Carnival.* New York, NY: Penguin Putnam Inc; 2000:151.
3. Ball P. *The Unauthorized Biography of a Local Doctor: Or From Infancy Through Puberty and On to Senility.* Hagerstown, MD: Exponent Publishers; 1993.
4. Behrman R, Kleigman R. *Nelson's Essentials of Pediatrics.* Philadelphia, PA: WB Saunders; 1990.
5. Bier ML. The Cover. *JAMA.* 1985;254(8):1000.

9 Plurals

9.1 How Plurals Are Formed. The plurals of most nouns are formed by adding *-s* or *-es*.

Singular	*Plural*
book	books
church	churches
decision	decisions
disease	diseases
turnip	turnips
yurt	yurts

However, English is irregular enough that it pays to consult a dictionary for most forms.

Singular	*Plural*
woman	women
baby	babies
tooth	teeth
wolf	wolves
child	children

9.2 Collective Nouns. Collective nouns may take either singular or plural verbs, depending on whether the word refers to the group as a unit or to its members as individuals. In American English, most nouns naming a group regarded as a unit are treated as singular. (See also 7.8.5, Grammar, Subject-Verb Agreement, Collective Nouns.)

> Fifty percent of my time is spent on administration.
>
> Fifty percent of all physicians do not exercise regularly.
>
> The audience was enthralled.

This gathering is becoming noisy.

At noon today the jury delivers its verdict.

For a unit of measure, use a singular verb.

Five milliliters was injected.

Two weeks of symptoms is common.

9.3 **Latin and Greek vs English.** There is a trend toward using English plurals rather than the traditional Latin or Greek. However, in most cases the latest edition of *Merriam-Webster's Collegiate Dictionary* or *Dorland's* or *Stedman's* medical dictionary should be followed. Consistency within a manuscript is key.

Singular	*Preferred Plural*
alga	algae
amoeba	amoebas
appendix	appendixes *or* appendices [consult dictionary for specific usage]
cannula	cannulas
condyloma acuminatum	condylomata accuminata [with 2-word Latin plurals, both parts become plural]
cranium	crania
fistula	fistulas
formula	formulas
genus	genera
index	indices *or* indexes [consult dictionary for specific usage]
maxilla	maxillas
orbit	orbits
rhytid	rhytids
sequela	sequelae
vertebra	vertebrae

9.4 **Microorganisms.** When referring to the common vernacular plural of a genus, use roman lowercase letters. Consult the latest edition of *Dorland's* or *Stedman's* medical dictionary. For organisms that do not have a common plural, add the word *species* or *organisms* to the genus name to indicate a plural use (see also 15.14, Nomenclature, Organisms and Pathogens).

Genus	*Plural Noun Form*
Chlamydia	chlamydiae
Escherichia	*Escherichia* organisms
Mycobacterium	mycobacteria
Proteus	*Proteus* species
Pseudomonas	pseudomonads

Salmonella	salmonellae
Staphylococcus	staphylococci
Streptococcus	streptococci

9.5 Abbreviations. For most all-capital abbreviations, the plural is formed by adding *s*. Do not use an apostrophe before the *s*. (See also 8.7.5, Punctuation, Apostrophe, Using Apostrophes to Form Plurals.)

CIs	HMOs
EEGs	ICUs
ORs	RBCs

Note: When plural all-capital-letter abbreviations are found in an all-capital setting, such as a first-level heading, the plural *s* is still lowercase.

REFERRAL PATTERNS IN MIDWESTERN HMOs

9.6 Plurals of Symbols, Letters, Numbers, and Years. Use *'s* to indicate the plural of letters, signs, or symbols spoken as such, or for words referred to as words when *s* alone would be confusing. Note the use of italics with the inflectional ending in roman type for words, letters, and numbers but not for symbols and signs. (See also 8.7.5, Punctuation, Apostrophe, Using Apostrophes to Form Plurals.)

He uses too many *and*'s.

All of the capital *P*'s should be underlined.

Please use +'s to indicate a positive result.

Note: If the symbol can be easily expressed using words, this is preferred:

Please use plus signs to indicate positive results.

Do not use an apostrophe to form the plural of numerals (including years).

during the 1920s
a woman in her 50s

9.7 When Not to Use Plurals. Beware of "pluralizing" nouns that cannot stand on their own as plurals.

serum samples (not "sera")
urine tests (not "urines")

9.8 False Singulars. Some nouns, because they end in a "plural" form, are mistakenly taken to be plurals even though they should be treated as singular and take a singular verb (eg, measles, mumps, mathematics, genetics).

Measles is a deadly disease in underdeveloped countries.

A few nouns are usually used in the plural form; however, the distinction between plural and singular should be retained where appropriate. (See also 7.8.3, Grammar, Subject-Verb Agreement, False Plurals.)

Plural	*Singular*
data	datum
criteria	criterion
media	medium [for a specific type: *Television is a good medium for disseminating important health news.*]
phenomena	phenomenon

ACKNOWLEDGMENT

Principal author: Brenda Gregoline, ELS

10 Capitalization

10.1 **First Word of Sentences, Statements, Quotations, Titles, Subtitles, and Table Headings.** The first word of every complete sentence should be capitalized. The following should also be capitalized:

- The first word of a formal statement that follows a colon

  Our conclusions may be stated thus: More research is needed.

- The first word of a direct quotation (but see 8.6.1, Punctuation, Quotation Marks, Quotations)

  The report noted: "A candidate may be admitted after completing 2 years of medical school."

  Kurt Vonnegut put it best when he said, "Writers can treat their mental illnesses every day."

  Note: If the quotation is run into the sentence, a lowercase letter on the first word may be preferable (see 8.6.1, Punctuation, Quotation Marks, Quotations).

  The patient described her headache pain as feeling like "needles behind the eyes."

- Each major word in the title of a table (see 10.2.1, Titles and Headings, Titles of Medical Articles, and 4.1.3, Visual Presentation of Data, Tables, Table Components). In column and row headings (table stubs), only the initial word should be capitalized. If a symbol, numeral, or lowercase Greek letter begins the stub, the first word that follows should be capitalized.

10.2 Titles and Headings. Capitalize major words in titles, subtitles, and headings of publications, musical compositions, plays (stage and screen), radio and television programs, movies, paintings and other works of art, software programs, Web sites and weblogs, electronic systems, trademarks, and names of ships, airplanes, spacecraft, awards, corporations, and monuments.

Do not capitalize a coordinating conjunction, an article, or a preposition of 3 or fewer letters, except when it is the first or last word in a title or subtitle. (For more on typeface rules when referring to works of art, see 22.5.4, Typography, Specific Uses of Fonts, Italics, and 8.6.3, Punctuation, Quotation Marks, Titles.)

All My Children

the Cochrane Database

the USS *Cole*

the space shuttle *Endeavor*

The Four Seasons by Antonio Vivaldi

Lucian Freud's *Girl With a White Dog*

Golden Globe Award

Internet

the *Journal of the American Medical Association*

the *Kitty Hawk*

The Lasker Award

the Lincoln Memorial

MEDLINE

MeSH [Medical Subject Headings]

MetaFilter

the *Monitor* and the *Merrimac*

My Man Godfrey

the *New England Journal of Medicine*

Oscar

PubMed

The Sopranos

Symphony No. 8, "Symphony of a Thousand," by Gustav Mahler

the Tomb of the Unknown Soldier

Windows

WordPerfect

World Wide Web (the Web, Web site)

Note: The may be dropped from titles if the syntax of the sentence improves without it.

10.2.1 Titles of Medical Articles. Titles of articles take initial capitals when they are in the title position but not when they are in the reference position.

Title: Autonomic Response in Depersonalization Disorder

Reference: Sierra M, Senior C, Dalton J. Autonomic response in depersonalization disorder. *Arch Gen Psychiatry.* 2002;59(8):100-103.

In titles and headings, capitalize 2-letter verbs, such as *go, do, am, is, be. Note:* In infinitives, "to" is not capitalized. Do not capitalize a coordinating conjunction, article, or preposition of 3 or fewer letters, except when it is the first word in the title or subtitle.

What Is Sarcoma?

We Do Need to Treat Mild Hypertension

Where the World Will Be in the Year 2020

Defining the Role of Computed Tomography in Injuries Resulting From Blunt Abdominal Trauma

Cardiovascular Risk Factors in Patients With Type 2 Diabetes

Opportunities for Comprehensive Risk Management

In compound terms from languages other than English, capitalize all parts of the expression.

Fluorescence In Situ Hybridization in Surgical Specimens of Lung Cancer

Nephrectomy With Concomitant En Bloc Adrenalectomy

With a phrasal verb, such as "follow up," capitalize both parts in a title.

The Need to Follow Up the Patient With Esophageal Cancer

10.2.2 **Hyphenated Compounds.** In titles, subtitles, table headings, and text headings, do not capitalize the second part of a hyphenated compound in the following instances:

- If either part is a hyphenated prefix or suffix (see Temporary Compounds in 8.3.1, Punctuation, Hyphens and Dashes, Hyphen)

Nonsteroidal Anti-inflammatory Drugs

Self-referral to Psychiatrists [compound words with the prefix *self-* are considered one word]

Intra-abdominal Surgery

- If both parts together constitute a single word (consult the current edition of *Merriam-Webster's Collegiate Dictionary* or *Stedman's* or *Dorland's* medical dictionary)

Long-term Treatment of Diabetes

Follow-up Studies of Patients With Leukemia

Part-time Nursing Staff

How to Interpret X-ray Films

However, in the case of a temporary compound, in which each part of the hyphenated term carries equal weight, capitalize both words.

Cost-Benefit Analysis

Low-Level Activity

Drug-Resistant Bacteria

B-Cell Lymphoma

Obsessive-Compulsive Disorder

Age-Related Macular Degeneration

In titles, subtitles, table heads, text headings, and line art, capitalize the first letter of a word that follows a lowercase (but not a capital) Greek letter (see 17.2, Greek Letters, Capitalization After a Greek Letter), a numeral (except when an abbreviated unit of measure that never is capitalized follows), a symbol, or an italicized organic chemistry prefix such as *trans*- and *cis*-.

> Systemic Adverse Effects of Ophthalmic β-Blockers
>
> Enhancement of Δ-aminolevulinic Acid Photodynamic Therapy
>
> Effectiveness of Timolol at 10% Strength
>
> High-Dose 308-nm Excimer Laser for the Treatment of Psoriasis
>
> α_1-Antitrypsin Inhibits Overexpressed Serine Proteinases During Inflammation

Both genus and species should be capitalized in all-capital text headings.

> *HELICOBACTER PYLORI* AND THE PATIENT WITH ULCERS

However, they should be treated normally in mixed capital and lowercase headings (see 10.3.6, Proper Nouns, Organisms, and 15.14.1, Nomenclature, Organisms and Pathogens, Biological Nomenclature).

> *Helicobacter pylori* and the Patient With Ulcers

10.3 Proper Nouns.

Proper Nouns. Proper nouns are words used as names for unique individuals, events, objects, or places.

10.3.1 Geographic Names.

Geographic Names. Capitalize names of cities, towns, counties, states, countries, continents, islands, airports, peninsulas, bodies of water, mountains and mountain ranges, streets, parks, forests, canyons, dams, and regions.

the Antarctic
Arabian Gulf
the Bay Area
Central America
the 23rd Congressional District
Cook County
Dismal Swamp
El Paso
the Florida Panhandle
Grand Canyon
Hoover Dam
the Iron Curtain
the Isle of Skye
Kennedy Expressway
LaGuardia International Airport
Lake Placid
the Loop [Chicago]
Mexico City
Mississippi River
New Hampshire
New York State [*but*: the state of New York]
Oman *or* Sultanate of Oman [either is correct]
Quebec City
Saudi Arabia *or* Kingdom of Saudi Arabia [either is correct]
the Silk Route
Third World
United Kingdom
Upstate New York
the West Coast

If a common noun is capitalized in the singular, it is generally not capitalized in the plural.

Atlantic and Pacific oceans

Kennedy and Eisenhower expressways

Mississippi and Missouri rivers

Compass directions are not capitalized unless they are generally accepted terms for regions.

There is a large time difference between Europe and the Far East.

Walk east until you arrive at the lake.

There is no party like a West Coast party because a West Coast party doesn't stop.

He lives in northern Michigan.

The practice of meditation is finding followers in the Western world.

10.3.2 **Sociocultural Designations.** Capitalize names of languages, nationalities, ethnicities, political parties, religions, and religious denominations. Do not capitalize political doctrines (conservative, progressive). Do not capitalize *white* or *black* as a designation of race.

African American

an Arab man

the Berbers

the Catholic Church (*but:* a Methodist church, First Methodist Church)

English language

Ethiopian food

the French

Hispanic population

Indian American community

of Italian heritage

Latina girls

Native American

Protestant

Sanskrit

Although she has been a member of the Republican party for years, at one time she was a Democrat.

This legislation endorses the principles of democracy in our republican form of government.

10.3.3 Events, Awards, and Legislation. Capitalize the names of historical and special events, historical periods, and awards (but not common nouns that may follow the names). Capitalize the official names of awards and specific parts of laws and bills, but follow the official name (as in the lowercase *w* in Americans with Disabilities Act).

Americans with Disabilities Act	the Great Depression
Civil War	Medicare
Civil War era	Nobel Prize
Congressional Medal of Honor	Physician's Recognition Award
Declaration of Helsinki	Public Law 89-74
Equal Rights Amendment	Purple Heart
Family and Medical Leave Act of 1993	Special Olympics
French Revolution	Taste of Chicago
Geneva Convention	Title IX

10.3.4 Eponyms and Words Derived From Proper Nouns. With eponyms, capitalize the proper name but not the common nouns that follow it.

Down syndrome	Trendelenburg position
Rose-Waaler test	Wada test

Most common words derived from proper nouns are not capitalized. In general, follow the current edition of *Merriam-Webster's Collegiate Dictionary* or *Dorland's Illustrated Medical Dictionary* (for medical terms).

arabic numerals	mendelian
brussels sprouts	parkinsonism
candidiasis	roman numerals
darwinian	schistosomiasis
india ink	

Note: *JAMA* and the *Archives* Journals do not capitalize *arabic* and *roman* when referring to numerals.

10.3.5 Proprietary Names. Capitalize trademarks and proprietary names of drugs and brand names of manufactured products and equipment. Do not capitalize generic names or descriptive terms.

> The patient had swallowed 46 tablets of acetaminophen (Tylenol; Johnson & Johnson, New Brunswick, New Jersey) and was treated for acetaminophen overdose.

All references to exact brand names must be verified and include the city and state or country of the manufacturer. (See also 15.5, Nomenclature, Equipment, Devices, and Reagents.) The trademark and copyright symbols are not used in *JAMA* and *Archives* Journals style.

10.3.6 Organisms. Capitalize the formal name of a genus when used in the singular, with or without a species name. Capitalize formal genus names but not traditional plural generic designations (eg, streptococci) or derived adjectives (streptococcal) (see also 9.4, Plurals, Microorganisms). Do not capitalize the name of a species, variety, or subspecies. Do capitalize phylum, class, order, or family (see 15.14, Nomenclature, Organisms and Pathogens). For capitalization of virus names, see 15.14.3, Nomenclature, Organisms and Pathogens, Virus and Prion Nomenclature.

10.3.7 Seasons, Deities, Holidays. Do not capitalize the names of the seasons. Do capitalize the names of specific deities and manifestations.

Allah
Ganesh
God or Goddess (when used in a monotheistic sense)
the goddess Athena
the Holy Spirit
Jesus Christ
Nature
Shiva
Zeus

Capitalize recognized holidays and calendar events.

Christmas
Eid ul-Fitr
Fourth of July
Good Friday
Kwanzaa
Labor Day
New Year's Eve
Passover
Ramadan
Rosh Hashanah
Thanksgiving Day

10.3.8 Tests. The exact and complete titles of tests and subscales of tests should be capitalized. The word *test* is not usually capitalized except when it is part of the official name of the test. Always verify exact names of any tests with the author or with reference sources.

10.3.9 Official Names. Capitalize the official titles of organizations, businesses, conferences, congresses, institutions, and governmental agencies. Do not capitalize the conjunctions, articles, or prepositions of 3 or fewer letters contained within these names. For names of institutions, do not capitalize *the* unless it is part of the official title.

Chicago Board of Education
the Communist Party
Congress
Council of Science Editors
the Federal Bureau of Investigation
Harvard University
House of Representatives
the International Subcommittee on Viral Nomenclature
Knox College
Northwestern Memorial Hospital
The Ohio State University
Quaker Oats Corporation
Robert Wood Johnson Foundation

the Senate	Tufts University School of Medicine
Sigma-Aldrich Corporation	the US Navy
Supreme Court (*Note*: capitalize Court only when referring to the Supreme Court)	

But: the board of trustees, the boards of health, the company, congressional reports, a congresswoman, the federal government, the navy, US senators

Often when referring to themselves and their officers in abbreviated form, institutions and organizations use initial capitals for titles. We prefer lowercasing such generic terms. For example, *JAMA* and the *Archives* Journals use the following designations:

the American Medical Association	the association
the Board of Trustees	the board *or* the trustees
the Council on Scientific Affairs	the council
the House of Delegates	the delegates
the president of the AMA	the president

In running text, a singular form that is capitalized as part of the official name is usually not capitalized in the plural.

> She is chair of the Department of Pediatrics at the University of Illinois, Urbana.

> Funding was received from the departments of pediatrics and neurology at the University of Illinois, Urbana.

(See 2.3.3, Manuscript Preparation, Footnotes to Title Page, Author Affiliations, for an example of capitalization of department titles in an affiliation footnote.)

10.3.10 Titles and Degrees of Persons. Capitalize a person's title when it precedes the person's name but not when it follows the name.

> Committee Chair Lawrence Mandelbaum led the meeting.

> At the meeting, Lawrence Mandelbaum was named committee chair.

Capitalize academic degrees when abbreviated but not when written out.

> Irene Briggs, MA

> Irene Briggs received her master's degree from the University of Pennsylvania.

10.4 Designators.

When used as specific designations within a particular article, with or without numerals, capitalize *Table*, *Tables*, *Figure*, and *Figures*.

> summarized in Table 2

> as seen in the Table

> the middle third of the basilar artery (Figure 2)

Do not capitalize the following words, even when used as specific designators, unless used as part of a heading or title:

axis	month
case	notes
chapter	page
chromosome	paragraph
column	part
control	patient
day	phase
edition	schedule
experiment	section
factor	series
fraction	stage
grade	step
grant	stub
group	type
lead	volume
level	wave
method	week

But: Step I diet, Schedule II drug, and Axis I of the *Diagnostic and Statistical Manual of Mental Disorders, Fourth Edition*

10.5 Types and Sections of Articles. General terms used to refer to a type of article or a section within an article should be set lowercase.

His letter to the editor was published in the December issue.

The methods sections of articles are often inadequate.

However, when referring to a specific type of article, or a section within a specific article, capitalize the first letter in the words of the category or section name.

The Letters to the Editor section of *Archives of Neurology* is a favorite of mine.

See the "Methods" section for a full description of each of the groups in the study.

10.6 Acronyms and Initialisms. Do not capitalize the words from which an acronym or initialism is derived (see 14.0, Abbreviations).

prostate-specific antigen (PSA)

enzyme-linked immunosorbent assay (ELISA)

Exception: When the words that form the acronym or initialism are proper names, use capitals as described in 10.3.9, Proper Nouns, Official Names:

National Institute of Mental Health (NIMH)

When there has been a "stretch" to create a study name or the name of a writing group that makes sense, is easy to say, and somehow relates to the name of the group, but where the first letters of the major words do not match the acronym, do not use unusual capitalization to indicate how the study name was derived. Expanded study or group-authorship names use normal *JAMA* and the *Archives* Journals capitalization style.

Evaluation of Platelet IIb/IIIa Inhibitor for Stenting (EPISTENT)

Enhanced Suppression of the Platelet IIb/IIIa Receptor With Integrilin Therapy (ESPRIT)

Clopidogrel as Adjunctive Reperfusion Therapy (CLARITY)

Clopidogrel in Unstable Angina to Prevent Recurrent Events (CURE)

c7E3 Fab AntiPlatelet Therapy in Unstable Refractory Angina (CAPTURE)

10.7 **Capitalized Computer Terms.** Use initial capitals with computer commands, functions, or features.

Please do not press the Back button on your browser until we have finished processing your request.

Enter one or more search terms and click Go.

Items in the History folder will be deleted after 90 days.

The word *e-mail* takes a lowercase letter in *JAMA* and *Archives* Journals style except when it starts a sentence.

Please send e-mail messages to my work address.

E-mail submissions are preferred.

10.8 **"Intercapped" Compounds.** *JAMA* and the *Archives* Journals capitalize trade names according to the spelling of the legal trademarks, even if they begin with a lowercase letter and contain a capitalized letter.

She sold her collection of vintage hats on eBay.

Data were processed in the field on iBook computers (Apple, Cupertino, California).

Avoid starting a sentence with one of these trade names. It is almost always preferable to reword the sentence so that it begins with a word that takes an initial capital letter, while retaining the preferred spelling of the trade name.

ACKNOWLEDGMENT

Principal author: Brenda Gregoline, ELS

11 Correct and Preferred Usage

What would become of us if the deleatur *did not exist, sighed the proofreader.*

José Saramago[1]

We not infrequently are compelled to refuse publication to an article which contains valuable facts, but which is weighed down with so many imperfections as to discourage one—as does the porcupine—from closer investigation.

JAMA[2]

11.1 Correct and Preferred Usage of Common Words and Phrases. The second quote, from a 1904 editorial in *JAMA*, certainly holds true today, but of course, editors do consider manuscripts that are poorly written but are of good science, although they may feel less confident about a paper's content if the presentation is sloppy. Also, authors whose first language is not that of the journal should still be given consideration. In particular, editors should not lose the author's voice, especially in informal usage. Still, scientific writing should be as precise as possible to avoid misinterpretation. This section provides a selection of correct and preferred terms.

A note about the entries: All terms (and pairs of terms) are in alphabetical (not preferential) order.

abnormal, normal; negative, positive: Examinations and laboratory tests and studies are not in themselves abnormal, normal, negative, or positive. These adjectives apply to observations, results, or findings (see also 20.0, Study Design and Statistics). *Note:* Avoid the use of "normal" and "abnormal" to describe persons' health status.

Results of cultures and tests for microorganisms and specific reactions to tests may be negative or positive. Other tests focus on a pattern of activity rather than a single feature, and hence a range of normal and abnormal results is possible. These tests include electroencephalograms and electrocardiograms and modes of imaging such as isotopic scans, radiographic studies, and tomography.

Incorrect: The physical examination was normal.

Correct: Findings from the physical examination were normal.

Incorrect: The throat culture was negative.

Correct: The throat culture was negative for β-hemolytic streptococci.

Incorrect: The electroencephalogram was positive.

Correct: The electroencephalogram showed abnormalities in the temporal regions.

Incorrect: Serologic tests for *Treponema pallidum* hemagglutination, which were previously negative, are now positive.

Correct: Serologic test results for *Treponema pallidum* hemagglutination, which were previously negative, are now positive.

Also correct: Serologic tests for *Treponema pallidum* hemagglutination, the results of which were previously negative, showed a titer of 1:80.

See also 11.8, Laboratory Values.

Exceptions: HIV-positive men
seronegative women
negative node

abort, terminate: *Abort* means to stop a process prematurely. In pregnancy, *abortion* means the premature expulsion—spontaneous (miscarriage) or induced—from the uterus of the products of conception. A *pregnancy* may be aborted, not a fetus or a woman. The synonym *terminate*—to bring to an ending or a halt—may also be used.

accident, injury: According to the National Center for Injury Prevention and Control of the US Centers for Disease Control and Prevention, *accident* should not be used to refer to injuries from any cause. Although *accident* implies a random act that is unpredictable and unavoidable, epidemiologic studies and injury control programs indicate that injuries may be predictable and therefore preventable. The preferred terms refer either to the external cause (eg, injury from falls, injury from motor vehicle crashes, gunshot injury) or to the intentionality ("unintentional injury" for injuries resulting from acts that were not intended to cause harm and "violence" for any act in which harm was intended).[3,4]

In addition, *accident* (and *accidental*) is considered by the public health community to be imprecise. The injury-causing event can be described as noted above or with other terms, such as *crash*, *shooting*, *drowning*, *collision*, *poisoning*, or *suffocation*.

Note: Do not change *accident* if it is integral to the terminology being used, for example, an established injury classification system (eg, Fatal Accident Reporting System, *International Classification of Diseases*).

acute, chronic: These terms are most often preferred for descriptions of symptoms, conditions, or diseases; they refer to duration, not severity. Avoid the use of *acute* and *chronic* to describe patients, parts of the body, treatment, or medication.

Avoid:	chronic dialysis
	chronic heroin users
	acute administration of epinephrine
	chronic diagnosis
	chronic care
	chronic aspirin therapy
Preferred:	long-term dialysis (*also:* maintenance dialysis [query author])
	long-term heroin users
	immediate administration of epinephrine
	long-standing diagnosis of a chronic disease
	long-term care [see note below]
	long-term aspirin therapy
	chronic obstructive pulmonary disease
	acute renal failure
	chronic arthritis
	acute nephritis
Also:	acute, severe cystitis
	acute, mild pruritus

Exception: Acute abdomen is a specific medical condition.

A note on short- and long-term patient care: According to Kane and Kane,[5] "*acute care hospital* is preferred to *short-term care hospital. Long-term care* has come to include both an acute component (sometimes called *subacute care* or *postacute care*), which effectively provides the care formerly offered in hospitals, and the more traditional chronic component, which includes both medical and social services. As the name implies, subacute care has a shorter time frame and serves patients who are expected to recuperate or die, while the more chronic form provides more sustained supportive services."

adapt, adopt: To *adapt* means to modify to fit a particular circumstance or requirement. To *adopt* means to take and use as one's own.

> As evidence-based medicine continues to evolve and to adapt, it is useful to refine the discussion of what it is and what it is not.

> Australia became the first nation to formally adopt evidence-based medicine as a key feature of its health system.

adherence, compliance: Although these terms are often used as synonyms, there are differences. *Adherence* can be defined as the extent to which a patient's behavior (for example, taking medication, following a diet, modifying habits, or attending clinics) coincides with medical or health advice. Use of the term *adherence* is intended to be nonjudgmental, a statement of fact rather than of blame of the prescriber, patient, or treatment.[6] *Noncompliance* connotes a stigmatizing image of rule, enforcement, and control; dominance and submission; and deviance from expected social roles. Whether a patient chooses to adhere to a therapeutic regimen may depend on many aspects of his or her experience with the disease and the medical encounter itself.[7]

> Although incompletely characterized and understood, the association between poor adherence to drug therapy and virologic failure with resistance has been clearly established in HIV infection.

Possible exception: A patient with a severe mental illness may be required to *comply* with court-ordered therapy.

adverse effect, adverse event, adverse reaction, side effect: *Side effect* is a secondary consequence of therapy (usually drug-based) that is implemented to correct a medical condition. The term is often used incorrectly when *adverse effect, adverse event*, or *adverse reaction* is intended. Since a side effect can be either beneficial or harmful, specific terminology should be used.

> A recent study examined the incidence of serious and fatal adverse drug reactions—any harmful, unintended, or undesired effect of a drug—in hospitalized patients.

> A side effect of therapy with hydrochlorothiazide is improved bone mineral density.

affect, effect: *Affect* (a-ˈfekt), as a verb, means to have an influence on. *Effect* (i-ˈfekt), as a verb, means to bring about or to cause. The 2 words cannot be used interchangeably.

> Ingesting massive doses of ascorbic acid may affect his recovery [influence the recovery in some way].

> Ingesting massive doses of ascorbic acid may effect his recovery [produce the recovery].

Affect (ˈa-fekt), as a noun, refers to immediate expressions of emotion (in contrast to *mood*, which refers to sustained emotional states). *Affect* is often used as part of psychiatric diagnostic terminology. *Effect* (i-ˈfekt), as a noun, means result.

> The patient's general lack of affect was considered to be an effect of recent trauma.

age, aged, school-age, school-aged, teenage, teenaged: The adjectival form *aged*, not the noun *age*, should be used to designate a person's age. Similarly, *school-aged* and *teenaged* are preferred to *school-age* and *teenage*. However, a precise age or age range should be given whenever possible. See also 11.5, Age and Sex Referents.

> The patient, aged 75 years, had symptoms of cognitive decline.

Alternative form: The 75-year-old patient had symptoms of cognitive decline.

Routine screening of sexually active teenaged girls during regular physician visits is an effective way to detect *Chlamydia trachomatis.*

Note: In some expressions regarding age, it is redundant to add *of age* after the number of months or years, since it is implied in the adjectives *younger* and *older.*

Influenza vaccination is not recommended for infants younger than 6 months.

See also 11.2.1, Redundant, Expendable, and Incomparable Words and Phrases, Redundant Words.

aggravate, irritate: When an existing condition is made worse, more serious, or more severe, it is *aggravated* (also, *exacerbated*), not *irritated. Irritated* indicates reaction, often excessive (eg, inflammation), to a stimulus.

although, though: *Although* and *though* may be considered interchangeable. However, *although* is preferable as a complete conjunction, because *though* in this construction is an "abbreviation" and thus may be less appropriate for formal prose. *Though*, as an adverb, meaning "however" or "nevertheless," is correct, as are the fixed expressions "even though" and "as though."

Although the analysis was done correctly, the fundamental terms of the investigation were too narrow to be interesting.

Basal cell carcinoma of the skin and melanoma are the subjects of an extensive literature. Squamous cell carcinoma, though, remains largely unreported and unstudied.

among, between: *Among* usually pertains to general collective relations and always in a group of more than 2. *Between* pertains to the relation between 1 entity and 1 or more other entities. For instance, a treaty may be made *between* 4 powers, since each is defining a relationship with each of the others, but peace may exist *among* them.

The patients shared the library books among themselves.

Between you and me, we are certain to find the common factor among those we have examined.

analog, analogue: Use *analog* when referring to items related to computers or electronic equipment. Use *analogue* when "something similar to something else" is meant or when referring to chemical compounds. Use *visual analog scale* (not *visual analogue scale*).

apt, liable, likely: When *apt* refers to volition or a habitual tendency, it should not be used of an inanimate object. This restriction does not apply when *apt* means "suited to a purpose." *Liable* connotes the possibility of risk or disadvantage to the subject. *Likely* merely implies probability and thus is more inclusive than *apt.*

Correct: A child is apt to cry when frustrated.

Incorrect: A polyethylene catheter is less apt to kink than one made of vinyl.

Correct: The team must decide on the most apt configuration before the first incision is made.

Correct: Patients receiving immunosuppressant drugs are liable to acquire fungal infections.

Correct: The computer system is likely to crash if it is overloaded.

article, manuscript, paper, typescript: An unpublished study, report, or essay—that is, the document itself—may be referred to as a *manuscript, paper,* or *typescript.* When published, it is an *article* (also, a *study*).

The authors thank Frank J. Kobler, PhD, for statistical review of the manuscript.

Nancy MacClean assisted with manuscript preparation.

The content of this article does not necessarily reflect the views or policies of the US Department of Health and Human Services.

The article by Carrozza and Sillke addresses the therapeutic options for a 69-year-old woman with disease of the left main coronary artery.

as, because, since: *As, because,* and *since* can all be used when "for the reason that" is meant. However, in this construction, *as* should be avoided when it could be construed to mean *while.*

Ambiguous: She could not answer her page as she was examining a critically ill patient.

Better: She could not answer her page, as she was examining a critically ill patient [comma used].

Preferred: She could not answer her page because she was examining a critically ill patient.

Similarly, *since* should be avoided when it could be construed to mean "from the time of" or "from the time that."

Ambiguous: She had not been able to answer her page since she was in the clinic.

Preferred: She had not been able to answer her page because she was in the clinic.

association, relationship: *Association* is a connection between two variables in which one does not necessarily cause the other. *Relationship* implies cause and effect. See 20.9, Study Design and Statistics, Glossary of Statistical Terms.

assure, ensure, insure: These verbs are used synonymously in many contexts, but there are distinctions. *Assure* means to provide positive information to a person or persons and implies the removal of doubt and suspense (*assure* the study's participants that their test results will be held in complete confidence). *Ensure* means to make sure or certain (ensure the statistical power of the study). *Insure* means to take precaution beforehand (insure his life).

The insurance company assured workers' families that their policies ensured that workers with few assets would get a decent (ie, permanent) burial.

> By mandating that every relevant paper expressly state that an institutional review board approved the study protocol, journal editors can assure readers that the research itself was conducted ethically.[8]

attenuate, attenuation: In computed tomographic (CT) imaging, *attenuation* refers to the absorption of x-rays by the patient's body. The appearance of the patient's tissues on the CT scan is dependent on the amount of x-rays absorbed (ie, *attenuated*) by that tissue. *Low attenuation* (or hypoattenuation) refers to areas of blackness on the CT scan. *High attenuation* (or hyperattenuation) refers to areas of whiteness on the scan.

because: see *as, because, since*

because of, caused by, due to, owing to: These phrases are not synonymous, but the differences are subtle. *Due to* and *caused by* are adjectival phrases; *owing to* and *because of*, adverbial phrases. The use of *due to* in both situations can sometimes alter a sentence's meaning.

> Survivors of child abuse tend to enter abusive relationships due to intrapsychic conflicts.
>
> *Meaning:* Survivors of child abuse tend to enter abusive relationships that are caused by intrapsychic conflicts.

Because *due to* is adjectival, "intrapsychic conflicts" describes the relationships. *Caused by* could be substituted for *due to*, and the meaning would be retained. *That are* could be inserted before *due to* without changing the sentence's meaning.

> Survivors of child abuse tend to enter abusive relationships owing to intrapsychic conflicts.
>
> *Meaning:* Because of intrapsychic conflicts, survivors of child abuse tend to enter abusive relationships.

Because *owing to* is used adverbially, "intrapsychic conflicts" characterizes the entrance into abusive relationships. *Because of* could be substituted for *owing to*, and the meaning would be retained. However, if *that are* is inserted before *owing to*, the sentence's meaning changes.

Clue to usage: The phrase "coughs due to colds" is a good example of correct usage of *due to*. If "because of" sounds right, use it or "owing to." If "caused by" is intended, use it or "due to" (or possibly "attributable to" or "that result from").

between: see *among, between*

biopsy: *Biopsy* refers to the removal and examination (usually microscopically) of tissue or cells from the living body. Use of *biopsy* as a verb was previously considered to be incorrect. However, such use has become common and acceptable.

> *Acceptable:* The lung mass was biopsied.
>
> A biopsy of the lung mass was performed.
>
> Lesions believed to be malignant were biopsied.

Observations are made of the biopsy specimen, not on the biopsy itself.

Incorrect: Biopsy was normal.

Correct: The results of the biopsy were normal.

blinding, masking: The statistical term *blinding* (or *blinded review* or *assessment*) is the evaluation or categorization of an outcome in which the person assessing the outcome is unaware of the treatment assignment; blinding is used to avoid bias. The term is also used to refer to peer review, usually to represent cases in which the author's name and affiliation are concealed from the reviewer. The equivalent term *masking* (or *masked assessment*) is preferred by some investigators and journals, particularly those in ophthalmology. See also 20.9, Study Design and Statistics, Glossary of Statistical Terms.

breastfeed, nurse: When referring to human lactation, use *breastfeeding*. This term is more specific than *nursing* and prevents any confusion with the profession of nursing.

cadaver, donor: When describing the source of human organs and tissues used for transplantation, avoid *cadaver* (or *dead body*). Correct usage is *deceased donor* (or *recovered from deceased organ and tissue donors*).

When referring to a deceased person whose body is to be used for anatomical dissection, *cadaver* is correct (*cadaveric* as adjective).

can, may: Referring to one meaning of *can* and *may*, Bernstein[9] in *The Careful Writer* stated: "Whatever the interchangeability of these words in spoken or informal English, the writer who is attentive to the proprieties will preserve the traditional distinction: *can* for ability or power to do something, *may* for permission to do it."

A second meaning of *may* refers to likelihood or possibility:

Dehydration may have contributed to the early onset of shock.

The lesion may or may not resolve without treatment.

case, client, consumer, participant, patient, subject: In clinical research, a *case* is a particular instance of a disease. A *patient* is a particular person under medical care. A research *participant* (preferred to *subject*; see below) is a person with a particular characteristic or behavior, or a person who undergoes an intervention as part of a scientific investigation, usually a case-control study or randomized controlled trial. A control *participant* is a person who does not have at least some of the characteristics under study, or does not receive the intervention, but provides a basis of comparison with the case patient (see 20.0, Study Design and Statistics). In case-control studies, it is appropriate to refer to *cases*, *patients in the case group*, or *case patients*; and *controls*, *participants in the control group*, or *control patients*.

Some consider *subject* (as in *study subject*) to be impersonal, even derogatory, as if the person in the study were in a subservient role. Similarly, the use of *case* is dehumanizing when referring to a specific person. For example:

Avoid: A 63-year-old case of type 2 diabetes . . .

Preferred: A 63-year-old man with type 2 diabetes . . .

Note: Make the distinction between *person* and *patient*:

Many persons in the United States have type 2 diabetes [persons with type 2 diabetes regardless of care].

> Many patients in the United States have type 2 diabetes [only persons under medical care].

A *case* is evaluated, documented, and reported. A *patient* is examined, undergoes testing, and is treated. A *research participant* is recruited, selected, sometimes subjected to experimental conditions, and observed. (See ***diagnose, evaluate, examine, identify***; and ***follow, follow up, observe***.)

Note: In general, patients should not be referred to as *clients* or *consumers*. However, persons enrolled in substance abuse treatment programs, for example, or persons undergoing treatment at a dialysis center are sometimes referred to as *clients*. *Client* may also be used by social workers or psychologists and in some research settings where *patient* or *participant* is inappropriate. *Consumer*—one who consumes goods or services—has worked its way into the medical lexicon and may be appropriate in certain discussions. For instance, in the following example, *patient* would not fit the context:

> The Internet has become an important mass medium for consumers seeking health information and health care services online.

case-fatality rate, fatality; morbidity, morbidity rate; mortality, mortality rate: See 20.9, Study Design and Statistics, Glossary of Statistical Terms.

catatonic, manic, psychotic, schizophrenic: These adjectives refer to severe psychiatric disorders. It is inappropriate to trivialize the disorders by using these terms to describe normal variations of individual or group behavior, for which suitable descriptors are available. For example, in common trivial uses of these terms, *contradictory* can usually be substituted for *schizophrenic*; *strange*, *disorganized*, or *senseless* for *psychotic* (depending on the context); *overactive* for *manic*; and *motionless* for *catatonic*.

Note: It is dehumanizing to refer to a patient as "a schizophrenic." Use "the patient with schizophrenia" or "the schizophrenic patient." See also 11.10.4, Inclusive Language, Disabilities.

caused by: see ***because of, caused by, due to, owing to***

cesarean delivery, cesarean section: According to the American College of Obstetricians and Gynecologists, the preferred terms are *cesarean delivery* (or *cesarean birth*) or *abdominal delivery* (to differentiate it from *vaginal delivery*). *Cesarean section* is incorrect, as are the spellings *Caesarean* and *caesarean*.

chief complaint, chief concern: *Chief complaint* has been traditionally used by physicians when taking a patient's history. However, *chief concern* may be a better description because *complaint* may be construed as pejorative and confrontational.

chronic: see ***acute, chronic***

classic, classical: In most scientific writing, the adjective *classic* generally means authentic, authoritative, or typical (the *classic* symptoms of myocardial infarction include angina, dyspnea, nausea, and diaphoresis). In contrast, *classical* refers to the humanities or the fine or historical arts (the elements of *classical* architecture can be applied in radically different architectural contexts than those for which they were developed).

However, some disciplines (eg, genetics, immunology) use *classical* for specific terms:

> Classical lissencephaly may be caused by mutations of genes in chromosome bands 17p13.3 and Xq22.3-q23.
>
> The classical and alternative pathways of complement components are described in 15.8.3, Nomenclature, Immunology, Complement.
>
> The authors suggest how to present results of data analysis under each of 3 statistical paradigms: classical frequentist, information-theoretic, and Bayesian.

client: see *case, client, consumer, participant, patient, subject*

clinician, practitioner: Depending on context, these terms can be used to describe persons in the clinical practice of the health fields of medicine, nursing, psychology, dentistry, optometry, and podiatry (as well as occupational and physical therapy and veterinary medicine, for example), as distinguished from those specializing in laboratory science, research, policy, theory, or writing and editing. When referring to a particular type of clinician or practitioner, it is preferable to use the more descriptive term (eg, physician, nurse, dentist, optometrist). The plural forms of *clinician* and *practitioner* may be appropriate to refer to a group of such professionals from different fields. See also ***provider***.

compare to, compare with: One thing or person is usually compared *with* another when the aim is to examine similarities or differences in detail. An entity is compared *to* another when a single striking similarity (or dissimilarity) is observed, or when a thing of one class is likened to one of another class, without analysis (ie, one entity is comparable to another).

> Compared with patients receiving only routine medical care, patients in both active treatment groups had greater improvements from baseline in psychosocial functioning and intermediate markers of cardiovascular risk.
>
> Few medical discoveries can compare to the discovery of penicillin.

compliance: see *adherence, compliance*

compose, comprise: Although these 2 verbs are often used interchangeably, *compose* is not synonymous with *comprise. Comprise* means to be composed of or to include (the pituitary gland *comprises* the adenohypophysis and the neurohypophysis). *Compose* means to make up or be a constituent of (the adenohypophysis and the neurohypophysis *compose* the pituitary gland; the pituitary gland is *composed* of the adenohypophysis and the neurohypophysis). The phrase *comprised of* is never correct.

> The chemotherapeutic regimen is composed of several toxic ingredients.
>
> The chemotherapeutic regimen comprises several toxic ingredients.

consumer: see *case, client, consumer, participant, patient, subject*

continual, continuous: *Continual* means to recur at regular and frequent intervals. *Continuous* means to go on without pause or interruption.

The patient with emphysema coughed continually.

His labored breathing was eased by a continuous flow of oxygen through a nasal cannula.

contrast, contrast agent, contrast material, contrast medium: Distinguish between *contrast* (ie, blackness and whiteness on an image) and *contrast material* (or *contrast agent, contrast medium*) (ie, a substance administered to enhance certain structures on an image).

A suspension of barium injected into the intestine was used as the contrast agent for radiological examination.

criterion standard, gold standard: See 20.9, Study Design and Statistics, Glossary of Statistical Terms.

describe, report: Both patients and cases are *described*; only cases are *reported*. (See *case, client, consumer, participant, patient, subject; management, treatment; diagnose, evaluate, examine, identify.*)

diabetes mellitus: The types of diabetes currently recognized by the American Diabetes Association are as follows:

Older Terms	*Preferred Terms*
juvenile diabetes, juvenile-onset diabetes, insulin-dependent diabetes mellitus	type 1 diabetes mellitus
maturity-onset diabetes, adult-onset diabetes, non–insulin-dependent diabetes mellitus	type 2 diabetes mellitus
chemical diabetes, borderline diabetes, latent diabetes	impaired glucose tolerance (nondiagnostic fasting blood glucose level, glucose tolerance abnormal)
. . .	gestational diabetes mellitus

For other specific types, consult Table 1 ("Etiologic Classification of Diabetes Mellitus") in *Diabetes Care.*[10]

diagnose, evaluate, examine, identify: *Diagnose*, *evaluate*, and *identify* apply to conditions, syndromes, and diseases. Patients themselves are not diagnosed but their conditions may be diagnosed. Patients are also *examined*. Patients may be *evaluated* for the possibility of a condition (eg, The patient was evaluated for possible cardiac disease). (See also *case, client, consumer, participant, patient, subject*; and *management, treatment.*)

Incorrect: The patient was diagnosed as schizophrenic 4 years ago

Correct: The patient's schizophrenia was diagnosed 4 years ago.

die from, die of: Persons die *of*, not *from*, specific diseases or disorders.

He died of complications of disseminated intravascular coagulation.

dilate, dilation, dilatation: Acccording to the American College of Obstetricians and Gynecologists,[11] *dilate* is a verb meaning to expand or open. *Dilation* means the act of dilating. *Dilatation* means the condition of being stretched or expanded.

> The patient's cervix dilated over a period of 12 hours.
>
> The patient was treated by dilation and curettage.
>
> After 4 hours of labor, cervical dilatation was 3 cm.

disc, disk: For ophthalmologic terms, use *disc* (eg, optic disc); for other anatomical terms, use *disk* (eg, lumbar disk).

In discussions related to computers, use *disk* (eg, floppy disk, disk drive, diskette) (exceptions: *compact disc*, *videodisc*). (See also 24.0, Glossary of Publishing Terms.)

disinterested, uninterested: Although these 2 words are increasingly treated as synonyms in written and spoken language, their differences in meaning are sufficiently useful to be worth preserving. To be *disinterested* is to be unbiased or impartial; to be *uninterested* is to be unconcerned, indifferent, or inattentive. A disinterested judge is admirable; an uninterested judge is not. As with many "word pairs," context is key.

> She was uninterested in a career in basic research.
>
> He was a disinterested observer of the complex procedure.

doctor, physician: *Doctor* is a more general term than *physician* because it includes persons who hold such degrees as PhD, DDS, EdD, DVM, and PharmD. Thus, the term *physician* should be used when referring specifically to a doctor of medicine or osteopathy, ie, a person with an MD or a DO degree (also FRCP, MBBS, ScD, etc). (See also *clinician, practitioner; provider*; and 11.4, Jargon.)

donor: see *cadaver, donor*

dosage, dose: A *dose* is the quantity to be administered at one time, or the total quantity administered during a specified period. *Dosage* implies a regimen; it is the regulated administration of individual doses and is usually expressed as a quantity per unit of time.

> The usual initial dosage of furosemide for adult hypertension is 80 mg/d, typically divided into doses of 40 mg twice a day. Dosage should then be adjusted according to the patient's response.

due to: see *because of, caused by, due to, owing to*

effective, effectiveness; efficacious, efficacy: *Efficacy* and *efficacious*, used especially in pharmacology and decision analysis, have to do with the ability of a medication or intervention (procedure, regimen, service) to produce the desired or intended effect under *ideal* conditions of use. The determination of efficacy is generally based on the results of a randomized controlled trial.

Effective and *effectiveness*, however, describe a measure of the extent to which an intervention produces the effect in *average* or *routine* conditions of use, or a measure of the extent to which an intervention fulfills its objectives.

See also 20.9, Study Design and Statistics, Glossary of Statistical Terms.

eg, ie: Use *eg* (from the Latin *exempli gratia*: "for example") and *ie* (*id est*: "that is") with care.

> Persons in risk groups for endemic disease (eg, tuberculosis in immigrants or homeless persons, histoplasmosis in residents of the Mississippi and Ohio River valleys) warrant special consideration.

> With 95% power and a 2-sided significance level of 5%, the study had statistical power to detect a significant odds ratio of 0.76 (ie, a 24% reduced risk) for individuals in the highest quartile of intake.

endemic, epidemic, hyperendemic, pandemic: *Endemic* conditions or diseases are prevalent in a particular place or among a particular group of people. *Epidemic* conditions occur abruptly in a defined area and are usually temporary. A *hyperendemic* condition is one that has a high prevalence. A *pandemic* condition is one that is epidemic over a wide geographic area, even worldwide.

> Cowpox is an orthopoxvirus infection endemic in European wild rodents but with a wide host range, including human beings.

> Public health officials feared an epidemic of infectious disease after Hurricanes Katrina and Rita in 2005.

> The researchers used remote sensing and geographic information system technology to identify individual high-risk residences in Westchester County, New York, where Lyme disease has been hyperendemic since 1982.

> Internationally, between 20 million and 40 million people died in the 1918-1919 influenza pandemic.

ensure: see *assure, ensure, insure*

epidemic: see *endemic, epidemic, hyperendemic, pandemic*

erectile dysfunction, impotence: *Erectile dysfunction* is the inability to develop and maintain an erection for satisfactory sexual intercourse or activity (in the absence of an ejaculatory disorder). *Erectile dysfunction* is the preferred term rather than the less precise term *impotence*.

etc: Use *etc* (or *and so on* or *and the like*) with discretion. Such terms are often superfluous and are used simply to extend a list of examples. When, in other instances, omission would be detrimental, substitute more specific phrasing such as *and other methods* or *and other factors*. *Etc* may be used in a noninclusive listing when a complete list would be unwieldy *and* its content is obvious to the reader.

> Gelatin is made from animal ligaments, tendons, bones, etc, that have been boiled in water. It is often used in confectionery, ice cream, and other dairy products.

Note: It is redundant to add "etc" at the end of a list introduced by "include" or "including" or a list introduced by ***eg***.

ethnicity, race: These terms are not equivalent. See 11.10.2, Inclusive Language, Race/Ethnicity, for a discussion of usage.

evaluate: see *diagnose, evaluate, examine, identify*

examine: see *diagnose, evaluate, examine, identify*

fasted, fasting: These derivatives of the verb *fast* are often used in the scientific literature. *Fasting* may be a present participle (verbal adjective), as in "the fasting mouse," or a gerund (verbal noun), as in "the effects of overnight fasting." *Fasted* may be the simple past tense form of the verb, as in "patients who fasted regularly," or a past participle, as in "12 fasted rats." Either word, when associated with 1 or more auxiliary verbs, can form part of a compound verb: "she had fasted since midnight," "he had been fasting since midnight."

fatality: see *case-fatality rate, fatality; morbidity, morbidity rate; mortality, mortality rate*

fever, temperature: *Fever* is a condition in which body temperature rises above that defined as normal. It is incorrect to say a person has a temperature if "fever" is intended. Everyone has a temperature, either normal or abnormal.

Incorrect: The patient has a fever of 39.5°C.

Correct: The patient has a fever (temperature, 39.5°C).

Correct: The patient is febrile (temperature, 39.5°C).

Correct: The patient has an elevated temperature (39.5°C).

fewer, less: *Fewer* and *less* are not interchangeable. Use *fewer* for number (individual persons or things) and *less* for volume or mass (indicating degree or value).

Fewer interventions may not always mean less care.

The authors evaluated fewer than 100 studies yet still reported more support for the conventionally prescribed therapy.

Note: spent less than $1000 (*not:* spent fewer than $1000)
reported fewer data (*not:* reported less data)

film, radiograph: These 2 terms are not interchangeable. In radiography, *film* is an outdated term that refers to an image obtained when actual film is exposed to x-rays (rather than when a digital technique is used). *Film* should be reserved to refer to actual film that is exposed and then developed into a resultant image. When referring to resultant images, use the specific name of the image, eg, arteriogram, mammogram, radiograph.

follow, follow up, observe: Cases are *followed*. Patients are not *followed* but *observed*. However, either cases or patients may be *followed up* (eg, the maintenance of contact with or reexamination of a person or patient, especially after treatment). Their clinical course may be *followed*.

In a study, case or control participants may be *lost to follow-up* (eg, the investigators were unable to locate them to complete documentation on participants in the initial study groups) or *unavailable for follow-up* (eg, they could not be contacted or the investigators were unable to persuade them to complete the study).

> Patients with retained intracranial fragments have been followed up, and the sequelae of such fragments were analyzed; to date, 9 patients have been lost to follow-up.

gender, sex: *Sex* is defined as the classification of living things as male or female according to their reproductive organs and functions assigned by chromosomal complement. *Gender* refers to a person's self-representation as man or woman, or how that person is responded to by social institutions on the basis of the person's gender presentation. *Gender* is rooted in biology and shaped by environment and experience.[12]

In most instances, authors of articles in biomedical publications intend the word *sex*.

> The authors assessed whether shifts in the ratio of males to females born in 1950-1994 in Denmark and the Netherlands, defined as the *sex ratio*, constitute a sentinel health event.

> Many studies indicate that women are less likely than men to undergo cardiac procedures after an acute myocardial infarction, which has raised concerns of sexual bias in clinical care. However, no data exist about the relationship between patient sex, physician sex, and use of cardiac procedures.

> Responses to pain and pain therapies differ between men and women. Whether this difference is related to sex-based factors (physiological), gender factors (psychosocial), or both has not been determined.

See also 11.5, Age and Sex Referents.

global, international: *Global* relates to or involves the entire world; an equivalent term is *worldwide* (a global system of communication, global climate change).

> Tuberculosis is a global public health problem.

International affects 2 or more nations (international trade, international movement).

> Researchers conducted an international survey, with respondents selected from Australia, China, France, Korea, and the United States.

> *But:* global amnesia, global aphasia, global congnitive function, global pain relief, Global Assessment of Functioning Scale

glycated hemoglobin, glycosylated hemoglobin: The preferred term is *glycated hemoglobin*. *Glycohemoglobin* is also acceptable[13] (David E. Bruns, MD, e-mail communication, May 17, 2006). See also 15.10.2, Nomenclature, Molecular Medicine, Molecular Terms: Considerations and Examples.

gold standard: see *criterion standard, gold standard*

health care: Express this term as 2 words. It is not necessary to hyphenate *health care* in its adjectival form. See also 8.3, Punctuation, Hyphens and Dashes.

> health care professionals
>
> health care organizations
>
> health care insurance

historic, historical: Although their meanings overlap and they are often used interchangeably, *historic* and *historical* have different usages. *Historic* means important or influential in history (a *historic* discovery). *Historical* is concerned with the events in history (a *historical* novel).

But: A historical novel might have a historic impact.

> This historical review of pain management gives particular emphasis to the 20th century and to chronic pain and cancer pain.

hyperendemic: see *endemic, epidemic, hyperendemic, pandemic*

hyperintense, hypointense: In magnetic resonance (MR) imaging, *hyperintense* refers to areas of whiteness on an MR image. *Hypointense* refers to areas of blackness. Synonyms include *high intensity* and *low intensity* and *high signal intensity* and *low signal intensity*.

-ic, -ical: *Merriam-Webster's Collegiate*, *Stedman's*, *Dorland's*, and *American Heritage* dictionaries are resources for determining the appropriate suffix for adjectives. In some cases, the "-ical" form is more remote from the word root and may have a meaning beyond that of the "-ic" form. Although, for example, "anatomic" may be used in the same sense as "anatomical," the latter is preferred as the adjectival form. The important guideline is that the use of terms must be consistent throughout an article or chapter, and preferably throughout the entire publication. Usually the "-al" may be omitted unless its absence changes the meaning of the word. Examples of such differences in meaning include *biologic, biological*; *classic, classical*; *economic, economical*; *empiric, empirical*; *historic, historical*; *periodic, periodical*; *physiologic, physiological*.

identify: see *diagnose, evaluate, examine, identify*

ie: see *eg, ie*

immunize, inoculate, vaccinate: *Immunize* means to induce or provide immunity by giving a vaccine, toxoid, or preformed antibody. *Inoculate* means to introduce a serum, a vaccine, or an antigenic substance. *Vaccinate* refers to the act of administering a vaccine.

> To immunize the newborn infant of an HBsAg-positive woman against hepatitis B, the patient should be inoculated with both hepatitis B immunoglobin and vaccine.
>
> All participants were inoculated intranasally with influenza A/Texas/36/91(H1N1) virus.
>
> Ten vaccinia-naive participants were vaccinated with undiluted smallpox vaccine.

impaired, intoxicated: These related terms are used in the United States to define impairment in driving performance attributable to the use of alcohol or other drugs. For instance, in some jurisdictions, a blood or breath ethanol concentration of 0.08 g/dL is considered to be legal evidence of impairment for driving. By extension, some injury prevention researchers have considered this concentration of alcohol to be scientific evidence of impairment in other potentially hazardous activities. However, cognitive and other functions may be impaired at even lower concentrations of alcohol, particularly if other psychoactive drugs, including prescription drugs, have been taken. No specific blood or breath concentration of alcohol may be considered to be scientific evidence of intoxication or impairment for all persons in all settings and activities. Authors should explain, justify, and define the use of these terms, preferably in the "Methods" section of the manuscript.

imply, infer: To *imply* is to suggest or to indicate or express indirectly. To *infer* is to conclude or to draw conclusions from facts, statements, or indications.

> These results, though cross-sectional, imply that physical fitness is related to fewer coronary risk factors.
>
> Our study relied on cross-sectional data, which restricts our ability to infer the causal relations underlying the observed associations.

See also 20.9, Study Design and Statistics, Glossary of Statistical Terms *(inference).*

impotence: see *erectile dysfunction, impotence*

incidence, prevalence: See 20.9, Study Design and Statistics, Glossary of Statistical Terms.

injecting, injection drug user; intravenous: The terms *injecting drug user* and *injection drug user* are not necessarily the same as *intravenous drug user.* Injecting or injection drug users can inject drugs intravenously, intramuscularly, or subcutaneously. Do not substitute one term for the other. If *intravenous* is used, ascertain that the route of administration is through a vein. If *injecting* or *injection drug user* is used, specify the type of injection (eg, intravenous, intradermal) at first mention, unless all types are meant.

injury: see *accident, injury*

inoculate: see *immunize, inoculate, vaccinate*

in order to: *In order* can often be removed from the phrase *in order to* without changing its meaning (see also 11.2.1, Redundant, Expendable, and Incomparable Words and Phrases, Redundant Words). However, in some cases such a deletion may be awkward, change the meaning, or create a dangling infinitive.

> Our students must have the learning opportunities that they need in order to acquire not just facts but true understanding.

If "in order" is removed, the syntax is disrupted ("need to acquire" would seem to apply to "opportunities").

The sentence might be reworded as "to be able to acquire" instead of "in order to acquire."

insure: see *assure, ensure, insure*

international: see *global, international*

intoxicated: see *impaired, intoxicated*

irregardless, regardless: *Irregardless*—most likely a blend of *irrespective* and *regardless*—is incorrect, regardless of context.

irritate: see *aggravate, irritate*

less: see *fewer, less*

liable: see *apt, liable, likely*

likely: see *apt, liable, likely*

lucency, opacity: In radiography, *lucency* refers to areas of blackness on an image. *Opacity* refers to areas of whiteness.

malignancy, malignant neoplasm, malignant tumor: When referring to a specific tumor, use *malignant neoplasm* or *malignant tumor* rather than *malignancy. Malignancy* refers to the quality of being malignant.

Avoid: Pancreatic cancer is a type of malignancy that eludes early detection.

Preferred: Pancreatic cancer is a type of malignant neoplasm that eludes early detection.

management, treatment: To avoid dehumanizing usage, it is generally preferable to say that cases are *managed* and that patients are *cared for* or *treated.* However, constructions such as "the clinical management of the seriously ill patient" and "the management of patients with AIDS" are acceptable when used to refer to a general treatment protocol. *Management* is especially applicable when the care of the patient does not involve specific interventions but may include, for example, watchful waiting (eg, for prostate cancer). *Management* may also be used to refer to the monitoring or periodic evaluations of the patient.

manic: see *catatonic, manic, psychotic, schizophrenic*

manuscript: see *article, manuscript, paper, typescript*

masking: see *blinding, masking*

may: see *can, may*

militate, mitigate: These 2 words are not synonymous. *Militate* means to have weight or effect and is usually used with *against. Mitigate* means to moderate, abate, or alleviate.

The constraints of nationalism militate against state conformance with global health norms.

Tests of sprinkler systems in full-scale simulated fires indicate that such sprinklers can be expected to mitigate the risk of fatality in residential fires.

morbidity: see *case-fatality rate, fatality; morbidity, morbidity rate; mortality, mortality rate*

mortality: see *case-fatality rate, fatality; morbidity, morbidity rate; mortality, mortality rate*

negative: see *abnormal, normal; negative, positive*

normal: see *abnormal, normal; negative, positive*

nurse: see *breastfeed, nurse*

observe: see *follow, follow up, observe*

-ology: This suffix, derived from the Greek *logos*, meaning "word," "idea," or "thought," denotes *science of* or *study of*. Terms with this suffix, like *pathology*, *morphology*, *histology*, *etiology*, and *symptomatology*, are general and abstract nouns and should not be used to describe concrete physical entities.

Avoid:	The gradual decline of symptomatology paralleled the resolution of pathology as seen in serial chest films.
Preferred:	The gradual decline of symptoms paralleled the resolution of pulmonary infiltrates as seen in serial chest films.

on, upon: In scientific articles, *upon* often simply means *on* and may be changed.

opacity: see *lucency, opacity*

operate, operate on: Surgeons *operate on* a patient or *perform an operation on* a patient. Similarly, patients are not *operated* but are *operated on*.

Incorrect:	The operated group recovered quickly.
Correct:	The surgical group recovered quickly.
Also correct:	The group that underwent surgery recovered quickly.

operation, surgical procedure, surgeries, surgery: *Surgery* can mean surgical care, surgical treatment, or surgical therapy (ie, the care provided by a surgeon with the help of nurses and other personnel from the first consultation and examination, through the hospital stay, operation, and postoperative care, until the last follow-up visit is complete).

An *operation* is what occurs between the induction of and the patient's emergence from anesthesia—incision, dissection, excision, and closure—the *surgical procedure*.[14]

An operation can also be performed with the patient given local anesthesia.

Surgery is what a surgeon practices or a particular medical specialty. An *operation* is what a surgeon performs. In this context, there is no such word as *surgeries*. In the United Kingdom, *surgeries* are physicians' or dentists' offices.[15]

over, under: Correct usage of these words depends on context.

Time: Over may mean either *more than* or *during* (*for a period of*). In cases in which ambiguity might arise, *over* should be avoided and *more than* used.

Ambiguous:	The cases were followed up over 4 years.
Preferred:	The cases were followed up for more than 4 years.
Also:	The cases were followed up for 4 years.

Age: When referring to age groups, *over* and *under* should be replaced by the more precise *older than* and *younger than* (see also ***age, aged, school-age, school-aged, teenage, teenaged***).

Avoid:	All participants in the study were over 65 years old.
Preferred:	All participants in the study were older than 65 years.

Note: It is unnecessary and redundant to add *of age* after the number of years. When the terms *older* and *younger* are used, age is implied. See also 11.2.1, Redundant, Expendable, and Incomparable Words and Phrases, Redundant Words.

owing to: see *because of, caused by, due to, owing to*

pandemic: see *endemic, epidemic, hyperendemic, pandemic*

paper: see *article, manuscript, paper, typescript*

participant: see *case, client, consumer, participant, patient, subject*

patient: see *case, client, consumer, participant, patient, subject*

percent, percentage, percentage point, percentile: See 19.7.2, Numbers and Percentages, Forms of Numbers, Percentages.

physician: see *doctor, physician*

place on, put on: The phrase "to put [or to place] a patient on a drug" is jargon and should be avoided. Medications are *prescribed* or patients are *given* medications; therapy or therapeutic agents are started, administered, maintained, stopped, or discontinued.

Incorrect:	The patient with hypertension was put on hydrochlorothiazide and metoprolol.
Correct:	Hydrochlorothiazide and metoprolol were prescribed for the patient with hypertension.
Correct:	The patient with hypertension was given hydrochlorothiazide and metoprolol.
Correct:	A therapeutic regimen of hydrochlorothiazide, 25 mg/d, and metoprolol, 50 mg/d, was begun.

positive: see *abnormal, normal; negative, positive*

practitioner: see *clinician, practitioner*

prevalence: see *incidence, prevalence*

preventative, preventive: As adjectives, *preventive* and its derivative *preventative* are equal in meaning. *JAMA* and the *Archives* Journals prefer *preventive*.

prostitute, sex worker: Epidemiologic studies use the term *sex worker* (or *commercial sex worker*) to describe these persons of either sex, rather than the more derogatory *prostitute*.

provider: The term *provider* can mean a health care professional, a medical institution or organization, or a third-party payer. If the usage refers to 1 specific provider (eg, physician, hospital), use the specific name or alternative name for that provider (eg, pediatrician, tertiary care hospital, managed care organization), rather than the general term *provider*. If the term connotes several providers, it can be used to avoid repeating lists of persons or institutions; however, the term(s) should always be defined at first mention.

> Increasing pressures for cost control and the spread of managed care create an urgent, shared need for information on health care quality among all health care stakeholders: consumers, public and private purchasers, policy makers, health plans, and health care providers (eg, hospitals, physician groups, and clinics).

The phrase *nonphysician provider* should be avoided because it is similarly imprecise and can refer to numerous health care professionals licensed to provide a health care service. It is better to specify the type of professional (eg, nurse, pharmacist) or to use *health care professional* or *clinician*. If a phrase is needed to describe repeatedly and succinctly the many health care professionals who are not physicians, then *physicians and other health care professionals* may be acceptable as long as the phrase is defined at first mention. This guideline also applies to other professions (eg, nonnurses, nonpharmacists).

psychotic: see *catatonic, manic, psychotic, schizophrenic*

race: see *ethnicity, race*

radiograph: see *film, radiograph*

radiography, radiology: These 2 terms are not interchangeable. *Radiography* is an imaging technique based on x-rays passing through tissue and emerging to "hit" film on the other side. *Radiology* is the medical specialty that uses imaging to diagnose and sometimes treat disease.

regardless: see *irregardless, regardless*

regime, regimen: A *regime* is a form of government, a social system, or a period of rule. A *regimen* is a systematic schedule (involving, for example, diet, exercise, or medication) designed to improve or maintain the health of a patient.

> Resistant hypertension is defined as the failure to reach goal blood pressure in patients who are adhering to full doses of an appropriate 3-drug regimen that includes a diuretic.

relationship: see *association, relationship*

reluctant, reticent: *Reticent* is becoming more commonly seen in informal usage as an incorrect synonym for *reluctant*. *Reticent* means habitually silent or uncommunicative. *Reluctant* means unwilling or disinclined.

repeat, repeated: *Repeat* is a noun or a verb and should not be used in place of the adjective *repeated*. *Repeated* implies repetition. For precision and clarity, the exact number should be given.

Incorrect:	A repeat electrocardiogram was obtained.
Possible but misleading:	A repeated electrocardiogram was obtained.
Preferred:	A second electrocardiogram was obtained.
Preferred:	The electrocardiogram was repeated.
Preferred:	Two successive electrocardiograms showed no abnormalities.

report: see *describe, report*

respective, respectively: These words indicate a one-to-one correspondence that may not otherwise be obvious between members of 2 series. When only 1 series, or none at all, is listed, the distinction is meaningless and should not be used.

Incorrect: The 2 patients are 12 and 14 years old, respectively.

Correct: Kate and Jake are 12 and 14 years old, respectively.

Incorrect: The 2 patients' respective ages are 12 and 14 years.

Correct: The 2 patients are 12 and 14 years old.

schizophrenic: see *catatonic, manic, psychotic, schizophrenic*

school-age, school-aged: see *age, aged, school-age, school-aged, teenage, teenaged*

section, slice: Use *section* to refer to a radiological image; use *slice* to refer to a slice of tissue (eg, for histological examination).

But: frozen-section biopsy

sex: see *gender, sex*

sex worker: see *prostitute, sex worker*

side effect: see *adverse effect, adverse event, adverse reaction, side effect*

since: see *as, because, since*

subject: see *case, client, consumer, participant, patient, subject*

suffer from, suffer with: See 11.10.4, Inclusive Language, Disabilities, for a discussion of usage.

suggestive, suspicious: To be *suggestive of* is to give a suggestion or to evoke. To be *suspicious* is to tend to arouse suspicion. Thus, the 2 phrases are not synonymous, and care should be taken to avoid confusing them. A finding may be abnormal (ie, suspicious) but may not indicate a specific diagnosis (ie, suggestive).

Incorrect: The chest film was suspicious for tuberculosis.

Correct: The chest film was suggestive of tuberculosis.

Also correct: The chest film showed abnormalities suggestive of tuberculosis.

Also correct: The chest film showed a suspicious lesion, but its nature was unclear.

surgical procedure: see *operation, surgical procedure, surgeries, surgery*

survivor, victim: In scientific publications, use of the word *victim*—when describing persons who survive physical, domestic, sexual, or psychological violence or a natural disaster—should be avoided. Similarly, avoid labeling (and thus equating) people with a disability or disease as victims (eg, AIDS victim, stroke victim; see 11.10.4, Inclusive Language, Disabilities).

Victim may imply a state of helplessness.[16] Characterizing a person who has experienced abuse or other violence as a victim perpetuates the stereotype of a passive person who cannot recover from the effects of the malady. In such cases *survivor* may be more appropriate (eg, rape survivor, tsunami survivor, survivor of torture).

If a person who experienced such trauma has died, referring to him or her as *victim* may be appropriate (victim of a land mine explosion). *Victim* may also be used in the vernacular (victim of his own success).

teenage, teenaged: see *age, aged, school-age, school-aged, teenage, teenaged*

temperature: see *fever, temperature*

terminate: see *abort, terminate*

though: see *although, though*

titrate, titration: In clinical medicine as in analytical chemistry, *titrate* and *titration* refer to making a series of small adjustments in the quantity or concentration of a substance until a goal or end point is attained—a color change or precipitation in the laboratory, control of symptoms or a therapeutic blood level in the patient. Drug dosages are titrated; patients are not.

toxic, toxicity: *Toxic* means pertaining to or caused by a poison or toxin. *Toxicity* is the quality, state, or degree of being poisonous. A patient is not toxic. A patient does not have toxicity.

> Dactinomycin is a toxic antineoplastic drug of the actinomycin group.
>
> The drug had a toxic effect on the patient.
>
> The patient had a toxic reaction to the drug.
>
> The patient had a toxic appearance.
>
> The toxicity of the drug must be considered.

transplant, transplantation: *Transplant* is both a noun (typically meaning the surgical operation itself but also increasingly referring to the overall field) and a transitive verb. Use *graft* (or *allograft*, *autograft*, *xenograft*, and so on, depending on the level of precision needed) as the general noun for the organ or tissue that is transplanted, or specify which organ or tissue (eg, liver, skin), rather than continue to use the noun *transplant* in this context. *Transplantation* is traditionally the noun used to describe the overall field. Never use the plural *transplantations*.

Incorrect:	The patient was transplanted.
	The surgeon transplanted the patient.
	The patient underwent a transplantation.
	Fifteen transplantations were performed.
Correct:	The patient underwent a transplant.
	The patient received a kidney allograft.
	The transplanted intestine functioned well.
	The surgeon transplanted the deceased donor's heart into a 4-year-old girl.
	Fifteen transplants were performed.
	She performed the first successful heart-lung transplant at our center.
	Cyclosporine has been used as monotherapy in pediatric liver transplantation [also, *transplant*].

Islet transplantation [also, *transplant*] is now a clinical reality at our institution.

The researchers collected transplantation data.

For the adjectival form, use *transplant*, as well as *pretransplant* and *posttransplant* (not *pretransplantation* and *posttransplantation*).

Avoid: The transplantation coordinator described the pretransplantation and posttransplantation data from her transplantation program.

Preferred: The transplant coordinator described the pretransplant and posttransplant data from her transplant program.

treatment: see *management, treatment*

typescript: see *article, manuscript, paper, typescript*

ultrasonography, ultrasound: These terms are not interchangeable. When referring to the imaging procedure, use *ultrasonography*. *Ultrasound* refers to the actual sound waves that penetrate the body during ultrasonography.

uninterested: see *disinterested, uninterested*

upon: see *on, upon*

use, usage, utility, utilize: *Use* is almost always preferable to *utilize*, which has the specific meaning "to find a profitable or practical use for," suggesting the discovery of a new use for something. However, even where this meaning is intended, *use* would be acceptable.

During an in-flight emergency, the surgeon utilized a coat hanger as a "trocar" during insertion of a chest tube.

Some urban survivors utilized plastic garbage cans as "lifeboats" to escape flooding in the aftermath of Hurricane Katrina.

Exception: Utilization review and *utilization rate* are acceptable terminology.

Usage refers to an acceptable, customary, or habitual practice or procedure, often linguistic in nature. For the broader sense in which there is no reference to a standard of practice, *use* is the correct noun form.

The correct usage of *regime* vs *regimen* is discussed on page 401.

Who determines what is correct usage?

Some authors use the pretentious *usage* where *use* would be appropriate. As a rule of thumb, avoid *utilize* and be wary of *usage*. Use *use*.

Note: Utility—meaning fitness for some purpose, or usefulness—should never be changed to the noun *use*. Nor should the verb *employ* be routinely changed to *use*. Use *employ* to mean hire.

vaccinate: see *immunize, inoculate, vaccinate*

visual acuity, vision: *Vision* is a general term describing the overall ability of the eye and brain to perceive the environment. *Visual acuity* is a specific measurement of one aspect of the sensation of vision assessed by an examiner.

A patient describing symptoms of his or her visual sensation would be describing the overall visual performance of the eye(s) and would use the term *vision*: "My vision is improved [or worse]."

A practitioner reporting the examination findings at one specific time would describe *visual acuity* (20/30, 20/15, etc). However, the practitioner might also refer to the general visual function as *vision*: "As the vitreous hemorrhage cleared, the vision improved and visual acuity returned to 20/20." It is possible to have normal visual acuity despite marked vision impairment, eg, when the peripheral visual field is abnormal.

11.2 Redundant, Expendable, and Incomparable Words and Phrases

It's déjà vu all over again.
Yogi Berra (1925-)

11.2.1 Redundant Words.

Redundant Words. A redundancy is a term or phrase that unnecessarily repeats words or meanings. Below are some common redundancies that can usually be avoided (redundant words are *italicized*):

adequate *enough*
advance planning
aggregate *together*
brief *in duration*
combine *together*
completely full [empty]
consensus *of opinion*
contemporaneous *in age*
count [divide] *up*
covered *over*
distinguish *the difference*
each *individual* person
eliminate *altogether*
empty *out*
enter *into* (*exception:* enter into a contract)
equally as well as
estimated at *about*
fellow colleagues
fewer *in number*
filled *to capacity*
first initiated
fuse *together*
future plans
general rule
herein we describe
interval *of time*
large [small, bulky] *in size*
lift *up*
major breakthrough
near *to*
out *of* [*but:* out of bounds, out of place, out of the question, out of the jurisdiction, out of the woods]
outside *of*
oval [square, round, lenticular] *in shape*
own *personal* view
past history
period *of time*, *time* period, *point in* time
personal friend
precedes *in time*
predict *in advance*
raised *up*
reassessed *again*
red *in color*
rough [smooth] *in texture*
similar results were obtained *also* by

skin rash
soft [firm] *in consistency*
sour [sweet, bitter] *tasting*
split *up*
still continues
sum *total*
tender *to the touch*
true fact
12 noon [midnight]
2 halves
2 *out* of 12
uniformly consistent
whether *or not* [unless the intent is to give equal emphasis to the alternative]
younger [older] than 50 years *of age*

11.2.2 Expendable Words and Circumlocution. Some words and phrases can usually be omitted without affecting meaning, and omitting them often improves the readability of a sentence:

as already stated
in other words
it goes without saying
it is important [interesting] to note
it may be said that
it stands to reason that
it was found that
it was demonstrated that
needless to say
take steps to
the fact that
the field of
to be sure

Quite, *very*, and *rather* are often overused and misused and can be deleted in many instances (see also 11.1, Correct and Preferred Usage of Common Words and Phrases).

Avoid roundabout and wordy expressions:

Avoid	*Better*
in terms of	in, of, for
an increased [decreased] number of	more [fewer]
as the result of	because of
during the time that	while
at this [that] point in time	now [then]
in close proximity to	near
in regard to, with regard to	about, regarding
the majority of	most
produce an inhibitory effect on	inhibit
commented to the effect that	said, stated
draws to a close	ends
file a lawsuit against	sue
have an effect [impact] on	affect
in the vicinity of	near
in those areas where	where

carry out	perform, conduct
look after, take care of	watch, care for
fall off	decline, decrease

11.2.3 **Incomparable Words.** An adjective denoting an absolute or extreme state or quality does not logically admit of quantification or comparison. Thus, we do not, or should not, say *deadest*, *more perfect*, or *somewhat unique*. It is generally acceptable, however, to modify adjectives of this kind with adverbs such as *almost*, *apparently*, *fortunately*, *nearly*, *probably*, and *regrettably*. Listed below are words that should not be used with a comparative (*more*, *less*), superlative (*most*, *least*), or quantifying (*quite*, *slightly*, *very*) modifier.

absolute
ambiguous
complete [*but:* almost or nearly complete]
comprehensive
entire
equal
eternal
expert
fatal [*but:* almost or nearly fatal]
final
full [*but*: half full, nearly full]
infinite
omnipotent
original
perfect [*but:* almost or nearly perfect]
preferable
pregnant
supreme
total
ultimate
unanimous [*but:* almost or nearly unanimous]
unique

Note: In general, superlatives should be avoided in scientific writing.

11.3 **Back-formations.** Back-formation is the creation of a new word in the mistaken belief that it was the source of an existing word. Many back-formations are verbs, some of them derived from abstract nouns (*ambulate* from *ambulation*, *diagnose* from *diagnosis*, *dialyze* from *dialysis*) and others from agent nouns, real or supposed (*beg* from *beggar*, *peddle* from *peddler*, *scavenge* from *scavenger*). These examples of back-formations have achieved acceptance; however, many of those pertaining to medical jargon have not, including *adhese*, *cyanose*, *defervesce*, *diurese*, *lyse*, *necrose*, *pex* (from *orchidopexy*), *plege* (from *cardioplegia*), and *torse*. Medical jargon also includes many deviant singular forms of nouns derived by back-formation from plural forms (*comedone* from *comedones*, plural of *comedo*; *fomite* from *fomites*, plural of *fomes*) or supposed plural forms (*bicep*, *forcep*, *pubis*). Back-formations not recorded in dictionaries should be avoided in formal technical writing.

Back-formation: The patient was diuresed.

Preferred: The patient was given diuretics [or underwent diuresis].

Many words have found their way into medical vocabularies with unusual meanings that are not recognized even by medical dictionaries. Such writings may be characterized as medical jargon or medical slang. When these words appear in medical manuscripts or in medical conversation, they are unintelligible to other scientists, particularly those of foreign countries; they are not translatable and are the mark of the careless and uncultured person.

Morris Fishbein, MD[17]

I have laboured to refine our language to grammatical purity, and to clear it from colloquial barbarisms, licentious idioms, and irregular combinations.

Samuel Johnson (1709-1784)

11.4 Jargon.

Jargon. Words and phrases that can be understood in conversation but are vague, confusing, or depersonalizing are generally inappropriate in formal scientific writing (see also 7.5, Grammar, Diction; 11.1, Correct and Preferred Usage of Common Words and Phrases; and 20.9, Study Design and Statistics, Glossary of Statistical Terms).

Jargon	*Preferred Form*
4+ albuminuria	proteinuria (4+)
blood sugar	blood glucose
cardiac diet	diet for a patient with cardiac disease
chart	medical record
chief complaint	chief concern
congenital heart	congenital heart disease; congenital cardiac anomaly
emergency room	emergency department
exam	examination
gastrointestinal infection	gastrointestinal tract infection *or* infection of the gastrointestinal tract
genitourinary infection	genitourinary tract infection *or* infection of the genitourinary tract
heart attack	myocardial infarction
hyperglycemia of 250 mg/dL	hyperglycemia (blood glucose level of 250 mg/dL)

jugular ligation	jugular vein ligation *or* ligation of the jugular vein
lab	laboratory
labs	laboratory test results
left heart failure	left ventricular failure [preferred, but query author]; left-sided heart failure
normal range	reference range
Pap smear	Papanicolaou test
the patient failed treatment	treatment failed
preemie	premature infant
prepped	prepared
psychiatric floor	psychiatric department, service, unit, ward
respiratory infection	respiratory tract infection *or* infection of the respiratory tract
status post	after; following
surgeries	operations or surgical procedures
symptomatology	symptoms [query author]
therapy of [a disease or condition]	therapy for
treatment for [a disease or condition]	treatment of
urinary infection	urinary tract infection *or* infection of the urinary tract

The following terms and euphemisms should be changed to preferred forms:

Avoid	*Use*
expired, passed away, succumbed	died
sacrificed	killed; humanely killed [query author]

Avoid trivializing or dehumanizing disciplines or specialties. For example:

Osteopathic physician and *osteopathic medicine*, not *osteopath* and *osteopathy*

Cardiologic consultant or *cardiology consultation*, not *cardiology* [for the person]

Orthopedic surgeon, not *orthopod*

Colloquialisms, idioms, and vulgarisms should be avoided in formal scientific writing. Exceptions may be made in editorials, informal articles, and the like.

When the administration of drugs is described, *intra-articular*, *intracardiac*, *intramuscular*, *intrathecal*, *intravenous*, *intraventricular*, *intravitreal*, *oral*, *parenteral*, *rectal*, *subconjunctival*, *subcutaneous*, *sublingual*, *topical*, and *transdermal* are acceptable terms when these are the usual or intended routes of administration. Except for systemic chemotherapy, however, drugs are usually neither systemic nor local but are given for systemic or local effect.

Some topical corticosteroid ointments produce systemic effects.

Oral penicillin is often preferred to parenteral penicillin.

Intravenously injected heroin may be contaminated.

Exceptions: Local anesthetics are a class of drug. Techniques for delivering anesthesia are general, local, and regional. Certain drugs may be inhaled.

11.5 Age and Sex Referents. Use specific terminology to refer to persons' age. See also 11.10.3, Inclusive Language, Age.

Neonates or *newborns* are persons from birth to 1 month of age.

Infants are children aged 1 month to 1 year (12 months).

Children are persons aged 1 to 12 years. Sometimes, *children* may be used more broadly to encompass persons from birth to 12 years of age. These persons may also be referred to as *boys* or *girls*.

Adolescents are persons aged 13 through 17 years. They may also be referred to as *teenagers* or as *adolescent boys* or *adolescent girls*, depending on context.

Adults are persons aged 18 years and older and should be referred to as *men* or *women*. Persons 18 to 24 years of age may also be referred to as *young adults*.

Note: If the age of an individual patient is given, it may be expressed as a mixed fraction (eg, 6½ years) or as "6 years 6 months." But when age is presented as a mean, use the decimal form: 6.5 years. See also 20.0, Study Design and Statistics.

Whenever possible, a patient should be referred to as a man, woman, boy, girl, or infant, not as a male or female. Occasionally, however, a study group may comprise children and adults of both sexes. Then, the use of *male* and *female* as nouns is appropriate. *Male* and *female* are also appropriate adjectives.

11.6 Anatomy. Authors often err in referring to anatomic regions or structures as the "right heart," "left chest," "left neck," and "right brain." Generally these terms can be corrected by inserting a phrase such as "part of the" or "side of the."

right side of the heart; right atrium; right ventricle

left side of the chest; left hemithorax

left aspect of the neck

right hemisphere [query author]

ascending [not right] and descending [not left] colon

Where appropriate, use specific anatomic descriptors:

proximal jejunum   distal ureter
distal esophagus   femoral neck
distal radius

The *upper extremity* comprises the arm (extending from the shoulder to the elbow), the forearm (from the elbow to the wrist), and the hand. The *lower extremity* comprises the thigh (extending from the hip to the knee), the leg (from the knee to the ankle), and the foot. Therefore, references to upper and lower arm and upper and lower leg are often redundant or ambiguous. When such references appear in a manuscript, the author should be queried.

11.7 Clock Referents. Occasionally, reference to a locus of insertion, position, or attitude is given in terms of a clock-face orientation, as seen by the viewer (see also 19.1.3, Numbers and Percentages, Use of Numerals, Measures of Time).

Ambiguous: The foreign body was observed in the patient's left eye at 9 o'clock.

Use: The foreign body was observed in the patient's left eye at the 9-o'clock position.

Note: The terms *clockwise* and *counterclockwise* can also be confusing. The point of reference (eg, that of observer vs subject) should be specified if the usage is ambiguous.

11.8 Laboratory Values. Usually, in reports of clinical or laboratory data, the substance per se is not reported; rather, a value is given that was obtained by measuring a substance or some function or constituent of it. For example, one does not report hemoglobin but hemoglobin level. Some other correct forms are as follows:

differential white blood cell *count*

agglutination *titer*

prothrombin *time*

pulse *rate*

erythrocyte sedimentation *rate*

total serum cholesterol *value* or *level* or *concentration*

increase in antibody *level*

creatinine *level* or *clearance*

serum phosphorus *concentration*

increase in bilirubin *level*

platelet *count*

24-hour urine *output* or *volume*

antinuclear antibody *titer*

mean corpuscular *volume*

hemagglutination inhibition *titer*

high-density lipoprotein *fraction*

urinary placental growth factor *concentration*

urinary protein *excretion*

In reports of findings from clinical examinations or laboratory values, data may be enumerated without repeating *value*, *level*, etc, in accordance with the following example:

Laboratory studies disclosed the following values: alkaline phosphatase, 722 U/L; serum creatinine, 4 mg/dL; serum urea nitrogen, 148 mg/dL; γ-glutamyltransferase, 138 U/L; prothrombin time, 15.3 seconds; and partial thromboplastin time, 48.8 seconds. Immunoglobulin concentrations were normal except for IgA levels of 6.7 g/L and λ chain concentrations of 383 mg/dL.

11.9 **Articles.** The article *a* is used before the aspirate *h* (eg, *a* historic occasion) and nonvocalic *y* (eg, *a* ubiquitous organism). Abbreviations and acronyms are preceded by *a* or *an* according to the *sound* following (eg, a UN resolution, an HMO plan). (See also 14.8, Abbreviations, Agencies and Organizations.)

a hypothesis [*h* sound]	a hematocrit [*h* sound]
an ultraviolet source [*u* sound]	an honorarium [*o* sound]
a WMA report [*d* sound]	an MD degree [*e* sound]
a UV source [*y* sound]	an NIH grant [*e* sound]

Sexist language, racist language, theistic language—all are typical of the policing languages of mastery, and cannot, do not, permit new knowledge or encourage the mutual exchange of ideas.
Toni Morrison[18]

11.10 **Inclusive Language.** *JAMA* and the *Archives* Journals avoid the use of language that imparts bias against persons or groups on the basis of sex, race or ethnicity, age, physical or mental disability, or sexual orientation. The careful writer avoids generalizations and stereotypes and is specific when choosing words to describe people.

11.10.1 **Sex/Gender.** *Sex* refers to the biological characteristics of males and females. *Gender* includes more than sex and serves as a cultural indicator of a person's personal and social identity. An important consideration when referring to sex is the level of specificity required: specify sex when it is relevant. Choose sex-neutral terms that avoid bias, suit the material under discussion, and do not intrude on the reader's attention. See also 11.5, Age and Sex Referents.

Nouns

Avoid	*Preferred*
chairman, chairwoman	chair, chairperson [*but:* see note]
corpsman	medical aide, corps member (*corpsman* is used by the US Marine Corps and it may refer to either a man or a woman)
fireman	firefighter
foreman	supervisor

Avoid	*Preferred*
housewife	homemaker
layman	layperson
mailman	letter carrier, mail carrier
man, mankind	people, human beings, humans, humanity, humankind, the human race, human species [*but:* see note]
manmade	artificial, handmade, synthetic
manpower	employees, human resources, personnel, staffing, workforce
mothering	parenting, nurturing, caregiving
policeman, policewoman	police officer
spokesman, spokeswoman	spokesperson
steward, stewardess	flight attendant

Note: Use *man* or *men* when referring to a specific man or group of men, *woman* or *women* when referring to a specific woman or a group of women. Similarly, *chairman* or *spokesman* might be used if the person under discussion is a man, and *chairwoman* or *spokeswoman* if the person is a woman. Any of these might be used in an official title, eg, Dorothy J. Tillman, alderman of the Third Ward, City of Chicago (verify with the author).

Do not attempt to change all words with *man* to *person* (eg, *manhole*). If possible, choose a sex-neutral equivalent such as *sewer hole* or *utility access hole*.

Terms such as *physician*, *nurse*, and *scientist* are sex-neutral and do not require modification (eg, female physician, male nurse) unless the sex of the person or persons described is relevant to the discussion (eg, a study of only female physicians or male nurses).

> After completing her internship, the physician specialized in emergency medicine and worked at several hospitals in California; she was selected as an astronaut candidate by NASA in 2007.

Personal Pronouns. Avoid sex-specific pronouns in cases in which sex specificity is irrelevant. Do not use common-gender "pronouns" (eg, "s/he," "shem," "shim"). Reword the sentence to use a singular or plural pronoun that is not sex-specific, a neutral noun equivalent, or a change of voice; or use "he or she" ("him or her," "his or her[s]," "they or their[s]").

Avoid:	The physician and his office staff can do much to alleviate a patient's nervousness.
Preferred:	Physicians and their office staff can do much to alleviate a patient's nervousness. [plural]
	The physician and the office staff can do much to alleviate a patient's nervousness. [neutral noun equivalent]
Avoid:	Everyone must allocate their time effectively.

Preferred: One must allocate one's time effectively. [singular]
People must allocate their time effectively. [plural]
Time must be allocated effectively. [change of voice]

Note: In an effort to avoid both sex-specific pronouns and awkward sentence structure, some writers use plural pronouns with singular indefinite antecedents (eg, Everyone allocates their time [note singular verb and "their" instead of "his or her"]), particularly in informal writing. Editors of *JAMA* and the *Archives* Journals prefer that agreement in number be maintained in formal scientific writing (see also 7.8, Grammar, Subject-Verb Agreement).

Avoid: One must allocate their time.
Everyone must allocate their time.

Preferred: One must allocate one's time.
Or: One must allocate time.
Or: Everyone must allocate time.

11.10.2 Race/Ethnicity. *Race* is defined as "a category of humankind that shares certain distinctive physical traits."[19] *Ethnicity* relates to "groups of people classed according to common racial, national, tribal, religious, linguistic, or cultural origin or background."[19]

Like gender, race and ethnicity are cultural constructs, but they can have biological implications. Caution must be used when the race concept is described in health-related research. Some have argued that the race concept should be abandoned, on the basis of the scientific evidence that human races per se do not exist. Others argue for retaining the term but limiting its application to the social, as opposed to the biological, realm.

A person's genetic heritage can convey certain biological and therefore medically related predispositions (eg, cystic fibrosis in persons of Northern European descent, lactose intolerance in persons with Chinese or Japanese ancestry, Tay-Sachs disease in persons with Jewish Eastern European ancestry, sickle cell disease seen primarily in persons of West African descent).

Specifying persons' race or ethnicity can provide information about the generalizability of the results of a specific study. However, because many people in ethnically diverse countries such as the United States, Canada, and some European, South American, and Asian nations have mixed heritage, a racial or ethnic distinction should not be considered absolute, and it is often based on a person's self-designation.

JAMA and several of the *Archives* Journals indicate the following in their instructions for authors:

> If race and/or ethnicity is reported, indicate who classified individuals as to race/ethnicity, the classifications, and whether the options were defined by the investigator or the participant. Explain why race and/or ethnicity was assessed in the study. See also Winker MA. Measuring race and ethnicity: why and how? *JAMA*. 2004;292(13):1612-1614.

A manuscript's "Methods" section is a good place in which to explain how persons were classified according to race/ethnicity. Authors should explain and justify the inclusion or exclusion of certain groups. Following are some examples from manuscripts' "Methods" sections.

> METHODS
>
> **Categorization of Race/Ethnicity**
>
> Individuals were categorized on the basis of self-reported race/ethnicity. Individuals were categorized as non-Hispanic, non-Jewish white (white); Ashkenazi Jewish (Jewish); African American; Hispanic; or Asian. Because of the unique spectrum and frequency of *BRCA1* and *BRCA2* mutations that occur in Ashkenazi Jewish individuals, these persons were analyzed separately from other whites.

> METHODS
>
> **Study Participants**
>
> Race or ethnicity was self-reported by the parents of the children from a list including non-Hispanic white, non-Hispanic black, Hispanic, Asian or Pacific Islander, Native American (including Alaskan), biracial or multiracial (specify), or other (specify).

> METHODS
>
> **Participants and Measures**
>
> Participants were asked to self-identify their race with the question, "Do you consider yourself to be primarily white or Caucasian, black or African American, American Indian, Asian, Hispanic or Latino, or something else?" We combined American Indian, Asian, and other categories into "other" because of the small numbers in those categories. We considered all participants to be Hispanic regardless of whether they also identified themselves as white, black, or other.

> METHODS
>
> **Study Population**
>
> Race was determined by self-identification and for analysis was categorized as African American or non–African American. Non–African American cases were predominantly white but also included 14 women who reported their race as Native American, Hispanic, Asian American, or multiracial. Information on race was obtained because a primary goal of the study was to better understand breast cancer in African American women.

When mention of race or ethnicity is relevant to an understanding of scientific information, be sensitive to the designations that individuals or groups prefer. Be aware also that preferences may change and that individuals within a group may disagree about the most appropriate designation. For terms such as *white*, *black*, and *African American*, manuscript editors should follow author usage.

Exception: Despite the example given above, *Caucasian* is sometimes used to indicate white but is technically specific to people from the Caucasus region in Eurasia and thus should be avoided.

In the United States, the term *African American* may be preferred to *black* (note, however, that this term should be allowed only for US citizens of African descent). A hyphen is not used in either the noun or adjectival form (see also When Not to Use Hyphens in 8.3.1, Punctuation, Hyphens and Dashes, Hyphen).

In reference to persons indigenous to North America (and their descendants), *American Indian* is generally preferred to the broader term *Native American*, which is also acceptable but includes (by US government designation) Hawaiian, Samoan, Guamanian, and Alaskan natives. Whenever possible, specify the nation or peoples (eg, Navajo, Nez Perce, Iroquois, Inuit).

Hispanic and *Latino* are broad terms that may be used to designate Spanish-speaking persons as well as those descended from the Spanish-speaking people of Mexico, South and Central America, and the Caribbean. However, the terms are not interchangeable, since *Latino* is understood by some to exclude those of Mexican or Caribbean ancestry. In either case, these terms should not be used in noun form, and when possible, a more specific term (eg, Mexican, Mexican American, Latin American, Cuban, Cuban American, Puerto Rican) should be used.

Similarly, Asian persons may wish to be described according to their country or geographic area of origin, eg, Chinese, Indian, Japanese, Sri Lankan. Note that *Asian* and *Asian American* (*Chinese* and *Chinese American*, and so on) are not equivalent or interchangeable. Do not use *Oriental* or *Orientals*.

Note: Avoid using "non-" (eg, "white and nonwhite participants"), which is a nonspecific "convenience" grouping and label. Such a "category" may be oversimplified and misleading, even incorrect. Occasionally, however, one sees these categorizations used for comparison in data analysis. In such cases, the author should be queried. *Multiracial* and *people of color* are sometimes used in part to address the heterogeneous ethnic background of many people.

11.10.3 **Age.** Discrimination based on age (young or old) is *ageism*. Because the term *elderly* connotes a stereotype, avoid using it as a noun. When referring to the entire population of elderly persons, use of *the elderly* may be appropriate (as in the impact of prescription drug costs on the elderly, for example). Otherwise, terms such as *older persons, older people, elderly patients, geriatric patients, older adults, older patients, aging adults, persons 65 years and older*, or *the older population* are preferred.

Note: In studies that involve human beings, age should always be given specifically. Researchers in geriatrics may use defined terms for older age groups, eg, young-old (usually defined as 60 or 65 to 70 or so years) and old-old (80 years and older). See also 11.5, Age and Sex Referents.

Adultism is a form of ageism in which children and adolescents are discounted.[20]

11.10.4 **Disabilities.** According to the Americans with Disabilities Act (http://www.usdoj.gov/crt/ada/), "a disability exists when an individual has any physical or psychological illness that 'substantially limits' a major life activity, such as walking, learning, breathing, working, or participating in community activities."[21]

Avoid labeling (and thus equating) people with their disabilities or diseases (eg, the blind, schizophrenics, epileptics). Instead, put the person first. Avoid describing persons as *victims* or with other emotional terms that suggest helplessness (*afflicted with, suffering from, stricken with, maimed*). Avoid euphemistic descriptors such as *physically challenged* or *special*.

Avoid	*Preferred*
the disabled, the handicapped	persons with a disability
disabled child, mentally ill person, retarded person	child with a disability, person with mental illness, person with intellectual disability, person with intellectual disability (mental retardation)
diabetics	persons with diabetes, study participants in the diabetes group, diabetic patients
asthmatics	children with asthma, asthma group, asthmatic child
epileptic	person affected by epilepsy, person with epilepsy, epileptic patient
AIDS victim, stroke victim	person with AIDS, person who has had a stroke
crippled, lame, deformed	physically disabled
the deaf	deaf persons, deaf adults, deaf culture or community
confined (bound) to a wheelchair	uses a wheelchair

Avoid metaphors that may be inappropriate and insensitive (blind to the truth, deaf to the request). For similar reasons, some publications avoid the term *double-blind* when referring to a study's methodology.

Note: Some manuscripts use certain phrases many times, and changing, for example, "AIDS patients" to "persons with AIDS" at every occurrence may result in awkward and stilted text. In such cases, the adjectival form may be used.

11.10.5 **Sexual Orientation.** Sexual orientation should be indicated in a manuscript only when scientifically relevant. The term *sexual preference* should be avoided because it implies a voluntary choice of sexual orientation not supported by the scientific literature. In some contexts, reference to specific sexual behaviors (eg, *men who have sex with men*) may be more relevant than *sexual orientation*.

The nouns *lesbians* and *gay men* are preferred to the broader term *homosexuals* when referring to specific groups of women and men, respectively. Avoid using *gay* or *gays* as a noun. *Heterosexual* and *homosexual* may be used as adjectives (eg, *heterosexual men*).

A member of a heterosexual or homosexual couple may be referred to as *spouse, companion, partner*, or *life partner*. *Same-sex couple* and *same-sex marriage* are appropriate terminology.

ACKNOWLEDGMENTS

Principal author: Roxanne K. Young, ELS

Special thanks to Thomas B. Cole, MD, Contributing Editor, *JAMA*; John H. Dirckx, MD, Dayton, Ohio; Mary E. Knatterud, PhD, Department of Surgery, University of Minnesota, Twin Lakes; and Diane Berneath Lang, BS, Radiological Society of North America, Oak Brook, Illinois.

REFERENCES

1. Saramago J. *The History of the Siege of Lisbon*. Pontiero G, trans-ed. New York, NY: Harcourt Brace; 1997.
2. Why are scientists poor writers [Queries and Minor Notes]? *JAMA*. 1904;42(7):477.
3. Revised Framework of External Cause of Injury (E Code) Groupings for Presenting Injury Mortality and Morbidity Data. http://www.cdc.gov/ncipc/whatsnew/matrix1.htm. Accessed February 18, 2005.
4. Satcher D. Injury: an overlooked global health concern [From the Surgeon General]. *JAMA*. 2000;284(8):950.
5. Kane RL, Kane RA. Long-term care. *JAMA*. 1995;273(21):1690-1691.
6. McDonald HP, Garg AX, Haynes RB. Interventions to enhance patient adherence to medication prescriptions: scientific review. *JAMA*. 2002;288(22):2868-2879.
7. Chren M. Doctor's orders: rethinking compliance in dermatology [editorial]. *Arch Dermatol*. 2002;138(3):393-394.
8. Altobelli L, reporter. Ethics in medical research [annual meeting report]. *Sci Editor*. 2005;28(5):153.
9. Bernstein TM. *The Careful Writer: A Modern Guide to English Usage*. New York, NY: Free Press; 1998.
10. The Expert Committee on the Diagnosis and Classification of Diabetes Mellitus. Report of the Expert Committee on the Diagnosis and Classification of Diabetes Mellitus. *Diabetes Care*. 2003;26(suppl 1):S5-S20.
11. Publications Department, American College of Obstetricians and Gynecologists. *Publications Guidelines*. Washington, DC: American College of Obstetricians and Gynecologists; 1997:22-23.
12. Pinn VW. Sex and gender factors in medical studies: implications for health and clinical practice. *JAMA*. 2003;289(4):397-400.
13. Roth M. "Glycated hemoglobin," not "glycosylated hemoglobin." *Clin Chem*. 1983;29(11):1991.
14. Allen CA. Surgeries. *Arch Surg*. 1996;131(2):128.
15. Schur NW. *British English A to Zed*. New York, NY: Facts on File Publications; 1987.
16. Flanagin A. Re: Violence and nursing [letter]. *J Professional Nurs*. 2000;16(4):252.
17. Words and phrases. In: Fishbein M. *Medical Writing: The Technic and the Art*. Chicago, IL: American Medical Association; 1938:46.
18. Morrison T. Nobel Prize in Literature Lecture, December 7, 1993. In: Allen S, ed. *Nobel Lectures, Literature 1991-1995*. Singapore: World Scientific Publishing Co; 1997. http://nobelprize.org/literature/laureates/1993/morrison-lecture.html. Accessed February 27, 2006.
19. *Merriam-Webster's Collegiate Dictionary*. 11th ed. Springfield, MA: Merriam-Webster Inc; 2003.
20. Maggio R. *Talking About People: A Guide to Fair and Accurate Language*. Phoenix, AZ: Oryx Press; 1997.
21. Orentlicher D. Rationing and the Americans with Disabilities Act. *JAMA*. 1994;271(4):308-314.

ADDITIONAL READINGS

Burchard EG, Ziv E, Coyle N, et al. The importance of race and ethnic background in biomedical research and clinical practice. *N Engl J Med*. 2003;348(12):1170-1175.

Cooper RS, Kaufman JS, Ward R. Race and genomics. *N Engl J Med.* 2003;348(12): 1166-1170.

Indigenous: to capitalize or not. World Association of Medical Editors Web site. http://www.wame.org/indigenous.htm. Published September 2-18, 2003. Accessed April 24, 2006.

Kaplan JB, Bennett T. Use of race and ethnicity in biomedical publication. *JAMA.* 2003;289(20):2709-2716.

Leonardi M, Bickenbach J, Ustun TB, Kostanjsek N, Chatterji S; the MHADIE Consortium. The definition of disability: what is in a name? *Lancet.* 2006;368(9543):1219-1221.

Office of Management and Budget, the Executive Office of the President. Standards for the Classification of Federal Data on Race and Ethnicity. http://www.whitehouse.gov/omb/fedreg/race-ethnicity.html. Accessed April 24, 2006.

Outram SM, Ellison ETH. Improving the use of race and ethnicity in genetic research: a survey of instructions to authors in genetics journals. *Sci Editor.* 2006;29(3):78-80.

Race and ethnicity: how do we describe people? World Association of Medical Editors Web site. http://www.wame.org/describe.htm. Published January 13, 2006. Accessed April 24, 2006.

Risch N. Dissecting racial and ethnic differences. *N Engl J Med.* 2006;354(4):408-411.

Rivara FP, Finberg L. Use of the terms *race* and *ethnicity*. *Arch Pediatr Adolesc Med.* 2001;155(2):119.

Schwartz RS. Racial profiling in medical research. *N Engl J Med.* 2001;344(18):1392-1393.

Winker MA. Measuring race and ethnicity: why and how? *JAMA.* 2004;292(13):1612-1614.

12 Non-English Words, Phrases, and Accent Marks

12.1 Non-English Words, Phrases, and Titles

12.1.1 Use of Italics. Some words and phrases derived from other languages have become part of standard English usage. Those that have not should be italicized (see 22.0, Typography), and usually a definition should be given. Consult standard medical dictionaries and the most recent edition of *Merriam-Webster's Collegiate Dictionary* for guidance.

> A public health investigation revealed that the source of lead exposure was *hai ge fen* (clamshell powder), 1 of the 36 ingredients of the Chinese herbal medicine.
>
> In Vitro Susceptibility Testing of Antifungal Agents
>
> Medical information and advice abound on the Internet, but remember: *Caveat lector.*
>
> Lorenz Böhler, the son of a carpenter, eventually became the *praeceptor traumatologiae totus mundi* (teacher of traumatology in the whole world).

Non-English street addresses, names of buildings, and names of organizations should not be italicized.

> **Correspondence**: W. Wayand, MD, Allgemeines öffentliches Krankenhaus der Stadt Linz, Krankenhausstrasse 9, 4020 Linz, Austria.
>
> The Brazilian College of Surgeons (Colégio Brasileiro de Cirurgiões) was founded on July 30, 1929.

12.1.2 Translation of Titles. Non-English titles mentioned in text may be translated or not, at the author's discretion. If the original title is used, an English translation should be given parenthetically, except in cases in which the work is considered well known. Both the English translation of the title (if given) and the non-English title should be italicized for books, journals, plays, works of art, television and radio programs, long poems, films, and musical compositions.

> Stendahl's *Le rouge et le noir* (*The Red and the Black*) is required reading for all third-year students.

Tratamiento de la hipertension (*Treatment of Hypertension*)

Andreas Vesalius' 16th-century masterpiece *De Humani Corporis Fabrica* (*On the Structure of the Human Body*) marked the resurgence of anatomy as a discipline.

The rules for italicizing and translating non–English-language journal article titles are slightly different (see 3.9.2, References, Titles, Non–English-Language Titles).

12.1.3 Capitalization and Punctuation. Non-English words should be capitalized and non-English phrases punctuated according to that language's standard of correctness. Follow language dictionaries and *The Chicago Manual of Style*.

12.2 Accent Marks (Diacritics). An accent mark (diacritic), when added to a letter, indicates a phonetic value different from that of the unmarked letter. English words once spelled with accent marks (eg, cooperate, preeminent) now are written and printed without them. Consult the most recent edition of *Merriam-Webster's Collegiate Dictionary* to resolve questions about whether a word should retain its accent. In general, English words in common usage should be spelled without diacritical marks.

Accent marks should always be retained in the following instances:

- Proper names

  Dr Bönneman is a Pew Scholar in the Biomedical Sciences.

- When it is desirable to show the correct spelling in the original language

  Köln (Cologne)

- In quotations

  "Más vale pájaro en mano que cientos volando" ("a bird in the hand is worth more than a hundred flying birds") is a Spanish proverb similar to the English-language "A bird in the hand is worth two in the bush."

- In terms in which accent marks are retained in current use (consult dictionaries)

  café au lait spots

  garçon

  Möbius strip

  voilà

- To show pronunciation and syllabic emphasis

  centime (sän-tēm)

  gluteus (glutéus)

Accent marks should be clearly indicated on manuscript copy.

Accent Mark	*Example of Usage*
acute	Ménétrier
breve	Ğabdulla Tuqay
cedilla	Behçet
circumflex	Le Nôtre

dot	marlė
grave	Bibliothèque
macron	gignōskein
ring	Ångstrom
slash	København
tilde	mañana
umlaut	Henoch-Schönlein purpura
wedge	Vrapče

Some languages are not supported by commonly used word-processing programs and Web browsers. Page proofs including words in such languages should be reviewed thoroughly by a person familiar with the language, and some letters or entire words and phrases may need to be rendered online using images rather than HTML.

ACKNOWLEDGMENT

Principal author: Brenda Gregoline, ELS

13 Medical Indexes

The indexer can help save lives and can control outcomes.

L. P. Wyman[1(p28)]

Indexes are essential and highly valued components of medical textbooks and journals. Publishers should hire professional indexers conversant with medical terminology and allot sufficient time in the production schedule for a comprehensive index to be prepared. "Space limitations on indexes should not apply to medical books."[1(pviii)] Medical indexes should aim for "accuracy, thorough analysis (subheads and cross-references), completeness/comprehensiveness [and] usability."[1(p27)] A textbook index should "tie together" discussions throughout of the same or related subject, eg, an infectious disease and its pathogen.[2(p62)]

General references on indexing include *Indexing Books,*[3] the indexing chapter in *The Chicago Manual of Style,*[4] and *Indexing From A to Z,*[5] which includes a section on biomedical indexing. The American Society of Indexers Web site provides indexing resources.[6] Patton and Wyman's online guide includes information specific to biomedical indexing.[7] Biomedical indexing is covered in *Indexing Specialties: Medicine*[1] and *Indexing the Medical Sciences.*[8]

The following are some considerations specific to medical indexing.

13.1 Index Style.

The style of terms in the index must be the same as the style in the text.[4]

13.1.1 Alphabetization and Sorting.

Alphabetization in indexes begins with the first letter of the term, eg,

G period

G phase

G protein

Commas precede letters in sorting order (examples from Thomas[9]).

cold, common
cold agglutinin disease

Vibrio, noncholera
Vibrio cholerae infection

Other punctuation is ignored.[3]

Omsk hemorrhagic fever virus
O'nyong-nyong virus

For entries that are identical except for case, choose whether uppercase or lowercase will take precedence in sorting and be consistent throughout the index.[3]

abl1, 99, 106-110
Abl1, 95, 100-103

Brca1, 112
BRCA1, 54, 804-809

When an identifier in parentheses is used to clarify similar terms, the identifier may be included in sorting (follow house style).

Abl1 (mouse gene), 95, 100-103
Abl1 (mouse protein), 98-99, 106
abl1 (retroviral oncogene), 99, 106-110

BRCA1 (human gene), 54, 804-809
Brca1 (mouse gene), 112

In biomedical indexes, numeric prefixes and chemical prefixes (eg, D-, L-, keto-, *N*-), are usually ignored for purposes of alphabetization and sorting of main entries (first set of examples adapted from Thomas[9]).

dihydroxyacetone
1,25-dihydroxycholecalciferol
L-dihydroxyphenylserine

6-keto prostaglandin $F_{1\alpha}$, 119
13,14-dihydro-15-keto prostaglandin $F_{2\alpha}$, 120
prostaglandins, 98-112, 345-367

Note: A better arrangement of the latter set of entries might be as follows:

prostaglandins, 98-112, 345-367
  6-keto prostaglandin $F_{1\alpha}$, 119
  13,14-dihydro-15-keto prostaglandin $F_{2\alpha}$, 120

For terms with other prefixes, use cross-references or double-postings (see 13.2.4, Features of Indexes, Double-postings) if the text suggests that readers are likely to seek the term under the main portion of the keyword.

E-selectin. *See under* selectins
P-selectin. *See under* selectins

Terms with numbers appear in numerical order.

CD1a

CD3δ

CD4

CD6

CD8

CD10

Numbers within terms are sorted ahead of letters, eg, CX3C precedes CXC.

chemokine subfamilies, 801-858
  CC, 250, 825-830
  CX3C, 764, 820-825
  CXC, 826-840
    CXCL1, 830-832
    CXCL4, 835-839
  XC, 841-855

Numbers that are parts of formal names are alphabetized as though written out,[4] for instance, a study-group name in an author index:

Nilanont Y

903 Study Group

Nishiguchi S

For Greek letters, follow house style if specified.[8] Greek letters are usually treated as though they were spelled out, eg, β is "beta," γ is "gamma."

GABA (γ-amino butyric acid), 244, 350-366, 998

γ-amino butyric acid. *See* GABA

γ chain, 243. *See also* IgG

Alphanumeric combinations are sorted by letter (including Greek), then number (including subscripts).

α-adrenergic receptors

α_2-adrenergic receptors

β-adrenergic receptors

β_1-adrenergic receptors

In long series of Greek-letter–affixed terms that are likely to be listed together, alphabetizing according to the Greek letter and not its name spelled out in English is preferable.

IFN-α

IFN-β

IFN-λ

IFN-λ1

IFN-λ2

IFN-τ

IFN-ω

Symbols are sorted as though written out. Consider using double-postings, a separate symbol index or group,[7] cross-references, or a key to direct readers to symbol entries.

@ ("at"), in gene symbols, 495-497

χ^2 (chi-squared), 206

Formal binomial organism names (see 15.14, Nomenclature, Organisms and Pathogens) used as index entries are not separated[5]:

Staphylococcus albus
Staphylococcus aureus

Not:

Staphylococcus
  albus
  aureus

13.1.2 Consistency. A text may not be consistent in style for particular terms, eg, italics or hyphens, but the index should be stylistically consistent.[2] If no style predominates for a given term used throughout the text, the indexer should check with the editor or consult the publisher's stylebook for the form to be followed in the index. It is hoped that authors will use, and publishers will recommend, official style when that is an option (consult 15.0, Nomenclature), eg, italicizing gene symbols (*BRCA1*).

13.1.3. Letter-by-Letter vs Word-by-Word. These are 2 styles of alphabetization. Letter-by-letter considers all letters of the entire entry, ignoring spaces between words. Word-by-word sorts by the first word of an entry term, then the next word. Letter-by-letter alphabetization is commonly used by scholarly publishers[4] and is the familiar arrangement found in dictionaries and encyclopedias.[3,4] Word-by-word sorting might result in more informative groupings of terms, especially multipart terms,[3,4] but in medical indexes letter-by-letter sorting usually allows readers to locate terms equally well. Consult indexing texts for detailed descriptions of these 2 methods of sorting. The publisher may specify a sorting style. The following examples are adapted from Thomas[9]:

Letter-by-Letter	*Word-by-Word*
heart	heart
heart block	heart block
heartburn	heart disease
heart disease	heart failure
heart failure	heart murmur(s)
heart murmur(s)	heart rate

Letter-by-Letter	*Word-by-Word*
heart rate	heart sound(s)
heart sounds	heartburn
heartworm infection	heartworm infection
xanthomatosis	X chromosome
X chromosome	xanthomatosis

13.1.4 **Capitalization of Main Entries.** Although main entries have traditionally featured initial capitals to distinguish them from subentries, *The Chicago Manual of Style,* 15th edition, recommends lowercase, except when the entry term would begin with a capital, eg, proper nouns.[4] This is especially worthwhile in biomedical publications, in which capitalization may be complex and may distinguish otherwise identical terms.

AFP. *See* α-fetoprotein
Afp, 98
AFP, 103

Brca1, 112
BRCA1, 54, 804-809
breast cancer, 50-57, 110-113, 801-815

Haemophilus influenzae Rd, 998
hepatitis, 1015-1028
*Hin*dIII, 698

LPL. *See* lipoprotein lipase
LPL, 1092

Staphylococcus aureus, 1056-1077. *See also* staphylococci

13.1.5 **Abbreviations.** Include only abbreviations used in the text being indexed (ie, if a text uses only an expanded form, eg, National Institutes of Health, but never the abbreviation, do not include "NIH" in the index).

Abbreviations are listed alphabetically among other entries (examples from Thomas[9,10]).

catheterization
CAT scan. *See* computed tomography
cat-scratch disease
CEA (carcinoembryonic antigen)
cecum

ectopic ACTH syndrome, 106, 107, 109
ectopic kidney, 2226
ectopic pregnancy, 1947, **2055-2056**

Identical abbreviations are sorted by case; be consistent throughout the index, eg,

HeV, 232
HEV, 330-331

Pa_{O_2}, 464
P_{AO_2}, 251

Use cross-references and expansions with abbreviations, as in these examples (first set from Thomas[9]).

CAT scan. *See* computed tomography
computed tomography (CT, CAT scan), 2715-2716
CT. *See* computed tomography

mitral stenosis (MS), 497
MS. *See* mitral stenosis; multiple sclerosis
multiple sclerosis (MS), 503

The following example illustrates (1) a cross-reference with an abbreviated organism name and (2) use of roman cross-reference term (See) when entry terms are in italics.

E coli infection. See *Escherichia coli* infection

When an abbreviation is more familiar than the expansion, index under the abbreviation[1,2]; include the expansion in parentheses, use a cross-reference to the abbreviation from the expanded term, or both.[4] Terms in this manual for which it is specified that the abbreviation may be used without expansion (see chapter 14.0, Abbreviations, and chapter 15.0, Nomenclature) should probably be indexed under the abbreviation. However, terms expanded at first mention, as recommended in this manual, may nevertheless be more familiar in their abbreviated form. Usage in the text being indexed is a guide to which form is more familiar.

deoxyribonucleic acid. *See* DNA

DNA, 112, 334, 556-560

13.1.6 **Locators.** Locators are the citations—commonly, page numbers in print indexes—that follow the entry to indicate where the material about that entry is found. Locators may also be paragraph numbers, line numbers, section numbers, volume-page number combinations, figure identifiers in atlases,[8] hyperlinks in online indexes, etc. American Society of Indexers guidelines recommend that no more than 5 to 7 locators per term be given. When more than 7 locators accumulate under one heading (ie, 7 "undifferentiated locators"), the indexer should consider breaking them down under subheadings. This will produce a more usable index.[11]

Not:
SARS (severe acute respiratory syndrome), 18, 20, 75-79, 93,105, 117,
  145-148, 167, 187-189, 235, 280, 357, 402

Preferred:
SARS (severe acute respiratory syndrome), 75-79, 145-148
  in China, 187-189
  drug therapy for

antibiotics, 18, 20
corticosteroids, 357
interferon alfa, 402
etiology of, 93, 105, 117
quarantine for, 167, 235
in Toronto, 280

Typographic variations on locators include bold for main discussions, *t* for tables (frequently used in medical indexes), *f* for figures, and others.

eczema, 24, 275*f*, **290-295**, 294*t*

Explanatory notes are recommended when any typographic variation is used, for example, "Locators in boldface indicate main discussions. Those followed by *t* or *f* indicate tables and figures, respectively." Such notes are most useful for the reader when they appear as running headers or footers (L. P. Wyman, e-mail communication, February 19, 2004).

13.1.7 **Indented vs Run-in Style.** In indented style, main headings are followed by indented subheadings, each on its own line. In run-in style, subheadings appear continuously, not on separate lines, and are separated by commas.

Indented:
SARS (severe acute respiratory syndrome), 75-79, 145-148
in China, 187-189
drug therapy for
antibiotics, 18, 20
corticosteroids, 357
interferon alfa, 402
etiology of, 93, 105, 117
quarantine for, 167, 235
in Toronto, 280

Run-in:
SARS (severe acute respiratory syndrome), 75-79, 145-148, in China, 187-189, drug therapy for, 18, 20, 357, 402, etiology of, 93, 105, 117, quarantine for, 167, 235, in Toronto, 280

The indented style is better suited for medical indexes because complex terms in subheadings are easier to read when set on separate lines. This style is "particularly useful where sub-subentries are required. . . ."[4(18.25,p764)] Note that in the above examples, sub-subentries are used for specific drug therapies in the indented style. A mixed style—indented main entries and subentries, run-in sub-subentries—is not as well suited for medical indexes, again because of the complexity of the terms.

13.2 Features of Indexes

13.2.1 **Types of Index.** A single index is the most convenient for the reader.[4] However, separate author and subject indexes are common in biomedical publications, especially journals. Separate indexes should be "visually distinct"[4(p757)] and be distinguished typographically and by running headers or footers.[4]

13.2.2 Cross-references. Cross-references are valuable for terms that readers might seek in different alphabetic locations (last example from Thomas[10]).

cDNA. *See under* DNA

dsDNA. *See under* DNA

mtDNA. *See under* DNA

DNA, 5, 300-310, 999
  cDNA, 24, 356
  dsDNA, 24-25, 356, 900
  mtDNA, 660

DTH. *See* hypersensitivity reactions, type IV

DTH skin test, 1010-1022, 1012*f,* 1031[10]

Cross-references are also used for synonyms:

proaccelerin. *See* factor V

Stuart factor. *See* factor X

T cell. *See* T lymphocyte

In the middle example, if *Stuart factor* were used in text concerning the history of factor X, a *see also* reference might be more appropriate:

factor X, 410-425. *See also* Stuart factor

Stuart factor, 418, 563

13.2.3 Generic Cross-references. General classes, and specific members of a class, may require generic cross-references, ie, a cross-reference to a group of entries rather than to specific entries by name. The following examples are from Patton and Wyman.[7]

drugs
  antihypertensive, 483
  See also specific drugs by name

medications. *See* drugs; *specific medications*

pharmaceuticals. *See products by name*

kidney, 18-43, 586-592. *See also under* nephro- *or* renal transplantation, 551-578

13.2.4 Double-postings. Listing the same citation under 2 or more entries, known as *double-posting*, is helpful when readers might be expected to look equally frequently in more than one place.

benign prostatic hyperplasia (BPH)

BPH (benign prostatic hyperplasia)

prostatic hyperplasia, benign (BPH)

cTnC, 246

cTnC, 246
TnC, 345

[cTnC is listed in both the *c*'s and in the *t*'s.]

However, for entries that will also appear in a series of related subentries under a main heading, cross-references to the principal form of entry are preferred to double-posting.

Acceptable:

E-selectin, 550
P-selectin, 551

Selectins
  E-selectin, 550
  P-selectin, 551

Preferred:

E-selectin. *See under* selectins
P-selectin. *See under* selectins

Selectins
  E-selectin, 550
  P-selectin, 551

13.2.5 **Inversions.** An inverted form changes the order of a compound term, eg, "leukemia, B-cell." Inversions are preferred when the indexer, depending on context and the coverage of the book, believes that the reader is most likely to look up information under the keyword, eg, under "leukemia" rather than under "B-cell." Such inverted forms of entry should be cross-referenced (or double-posted) from the uninverted disease name. Avoid unnecessary inversions such as "fatigue syndrome, chronic" that break up commonly used compound terms.

13.2.6 **Subentry Levels.** Tullar[2] recommends using more main entries or first-level subentries rather than going beyond a third level of subentry, as in this example, adapted from Tullar[2]:

Not:
cancer
  treatment of
    pharmacologic
      cyclophosphamide for
        adverse effects of
          thrombocytopenia

Preferred:
cancer
  treatment of
    pharmacologic
    See also individual drugs

chemotherapy
  adverse effects of
    See also individual drugs

cyclophosphamide
  adverse effects of
    thrombocytopenia from

drug-induced disorders
  from cyclophosphamide
  thrombocytopenia

thrombocytopenia
  from cyclophosphamide
  drug-induced

Even when a main heading cites the entire page range of the discussion of a particular topic, it is useful to include subtopics as subentries so that the reader is aware that the subtopic has been covered in that discussion, as well as elsewhere in the text.[8] The following example is based on Blake et al.[8]

neurological disorders, 210-281
  diagnostic procedures, 210-224, 343-345

13.2.7 **Vocabulary Control.** An entity may be referred to by different names throughout a text. Such variation is common in multiauthor works.[3] Cross-references, double-postings, and parenthetical synonyms help the reader know that the entity sought in the index is the same entity discussed under various names. Authors and editors should use vocabulary consistently and note synonyms in the text. The indexer should consult the book author or editor and the publisher's book editor for clarification. The following example is adapted from Thomas[9]:

auditory nerve. *See* cranial nerve VIII
cranial nerves, VIII (auditory, vestibulocochlear), 781*t*, 782, 782*t*, 783*t*, 1870*t*
eighth nerve. *See* cranial nerves, VIII (auditory, vestibulocochlear)
vestibulocochlear nerve (cranial nerve VIII), 781*t*, 782, 782*t*, 783*t*, 1870*t*

Note that a reader who sought information under *vestibulocochlear nerve* would be helped by finding citations of pages discussing cranial nerve VIII. But the reader will fruitlessly skim the page for *vestibulocochlear nerve*, unless the term actually used on the page, *cranial nerve VIII*, is included in parentheses in the index entry.

The noneponymous name of a disease should be included in the index parenthetically after the eponymous index entry if the noneponymous name is used in the text[2] (see also chapter 16, Eponyms). Indexers should be cognizant of disease terms that are synonymous, are encompassing, or overlap,[2,7] eg, *nephric* and *renal*,[7] *seizures* and *epilepsy*.[2] The following example is adapted from Thomas[9]:

Crohn disease, 152-155
inflammatory bowel disease, 149-159
ulcerative colitis, 155-159

Tullar recommends, "Whenever a disorder is cited by more than one name, . . . opt for the term used in the principal discussion and cross-reference from alternate terms. Double-post folios for a single discussion rather than cross-reference."[2(p54)]

13.3 **Periodical Indexing.** Vocabulary control is of particular importance not only for indexes compiled for multiauthor texts, but also for the indexes that appear at the end of the volume year in medical journals. In general, the rules and guidelines that apply to back-of-the-book indexes also apply to journal indexes. Where, in specialty journals, nomenclature is in flux or variable, indexers should follow the style and recommendations of their publishers or editors, cross-referencing to preferred terms or forms of entry rather than double-posting. Journal indexes differ from book indexes in basing index entries largely on title and abstract information, which summarizes an article's main topics, and usually do not include entries for subject matter that is secondary or incidental within the text of the article. Locators are given as an article's beginning page or the article's page range and sometimes include issue number or date. Publishers may specify, or indexers may choose to make, general entries for the type of study ("Randomized Trial," "Review"), for the population group studied ("Child," "Men," "Women," Elderly"), and other entries for recurring article types or topics. These entries should be made consistently issue by issue throughout the volume year. If, for example, "Adverse Reactions" is established as an general index entry, it should be entered for each article examining a specific reaction regardless of whether the term *adverse reaction* appears in the title or abstract.

13.4 **Controlled Vocabulary Indexing.** In indexing journals offering broad coverage of general medicine and specialties and in indexing sets of periodicals issued by different publishers, indexers usually rely on the external authority of a controlled vocabulary. Controlled vocabularies allow indexers to resolve variances in natural language systematically. The vocabularies establish preferred terms with cross-references from alternative forms of entry. Thus, all relevant references can be gathered under a single heading. Controlled vocabularies also establish hierarchical relationships among related terms. Such hierarchies most often take the form of a thesaurus in which narrower terms are entered as subentries beneath the broader terms to which they relate. The following example is abbreviated from the National Library of Medicine's Medical Subject Headings (MeSH)[12(D:12)]:

Intercellular Signaling Peptides and Proteins
  Cytokines
    Chemokines
    Growth Substances
      Interleukins
    Interferons

In using a controlled vocabulary, entry style should follow that of the vocabulary list or thesaurus, not the text.[13] Adapting controlled vocabularies too freely for local use may result in indexing that will not be fully functional in electronic systems. Indexable terms not listed in the thesaurus (including proper nouns such as the names of people and institutions) may be added as informal identifiers either in a separate field of a database record or appropriately tagged among the controlled vocabulary terms.[13] For example, in an index based on the MeSH vocabulary, an article entitled "Effects of Bilateral Posteroventral Pallidotomy on Subjects With Parkinson Disease" may be indexed under the non-MeSH term "Pallidotomy." This term, however, should be separated from the controlled vocabulary descriptors in the index record or tagged as a local term to distinguish it from MeSH descriptors. The inclusion of local terms in this way allows for valid additional points of access without compromising the integrity of the formal vocabulary and its hierarchy.

Most indexing and abstracting services base their indexing on controlled vocabularies. Controlled vocabularies are also used among descriptive elements called meta-data, which allow digitized information to be networked in a variety of applications. MeSH is the most comprehensive controlled vocabulary in medicine and is used to index MEDLINE. Other biomedical controlled vocabularies and thesauri include The National Cancer Institute Thesaurus (http://nciterms.nci.nih.gov/NCIBrowser/Dictionary.do) and the Nursing and Allied Health Subject Headings used to index CINAHL (Cumulative Index to Nursing and Allied Health Literature) (http://www.cinahl.com/).

Even when indexing is based on the language of the text, as in back-of-the-book indexing, MeSH and specialized thesauri may be consulted along with standard medical dictionaries as sources of authority for forms of entry and cross-referencing and as general guides to the language and organization of medicine and its related fields. The MeSH is revised annually and is available both in printed volumes and online from the National Library of Medicine.[12]

A suggested reference on the subject of controlled vocabularies is *Vocabulary Control for Information Retrieval*.[14]

13.5 Online and Electronic Indexes. Although indexing services continue to index scientific literature much as in the past, few any longer compile their indexing into the printed monthly and annual cumulations such as *Index Medicus* or *Chemical Abstracts* that once sat in long rows on university library shelves. The database products that have replaced cumulated print indexes nevertheless still depend on controlled vocabulary indexing as a means of achieving acceptable degrees of relevancy in retrieving citations from among millions of abstracts. To eliminate the many marginal "hits" that result from the unmediated keyword searching of large databases, search screens typically allow users to construct their searches by selecting from thesaurus terms or employ built-in mechanisms that map natural language queries to assigned, thesaurus-based indexing terms. Taxonomies designed for the graphic interfaces of the Web have been among the more popular means of providing classified or topical access to document collections, most commonly to consumer health information. However, informal taxonomies classifying articles by topics of general interest to medical students, practitioners, and researchers have also been employed by medical publishers to supplement keyword-based search engines at their journals' Web sites. Scientific validity and consistency, rather than style, are of primary concern in both database indexing and taxonomy classification. Embedded indexing,[15,16] a process whereby the indexer embeds markers in passages of text at which index entries should point, allows index terms to be compiled into both print indexes to be included in the back of a book and electronic indexes in which hyperlinks replace page locators. Embedded indexing, usually available in desktop publishing packages, has been used mostly for technical manuals issued simultaneously in print and electronically and which may be updated frequently. Style considerations are much the same as those for traditional back-of-the-book indexes.

ACKNOWLEDGMENTS

Principal authors: Bruce McGregor and Harriet S. Meyer, MD

L. Pilar Wyman, Wyman Indexing, Annapolis, MD, reviewed this chapter and provided invaluable suggestions.

REFERENCES

1. Wyman LP, ed. *Indexing Specialties: Medicine.* Phoenix, AZ: American Society of Indexers; Medford, NJ: Information Today; 1999.
2. Tullar IC. General medicine. In: Wyman LP, ed. *Indexing Specialties: Medicine.* Phoenix, AZ: American Society of Indexers; Medford, NJ: Information Today; 1999: 47-66.
3. Mulvany NC. *Indexing Books.* 2nd ed. Chicago, IL: University of Chicago Press; 2005.
4. *The Chicago Manual of Style.* 15th ed. Chicago, IL: University of Chicago Press; 2003:755-801. Also available as *Indexes: A Chapter From* The Chicago Manual of Style, *15th ed.* Chicago, IL: University of Chicago Press; 2003.
5. Wellisch HH. *Indexing From A to Z.* 2nd ed. New York, NY: HW Wilson; 1996.
6. American Society of Indexers Web site. http://asindexing.org. Accessed April 20, 2006.
7. Patton D, Wyman LP. How to develop an index style guide. http://www.wymanindexing .com (see under "Pilar's Info," then "Pilar's Presentations"). Accessed April 20, 2006.
8. Blake D, Clarke M, McCarthy A, Morrison J. *Indexing the Medical Sciences (Society of Indexers Occasional Papers on Indexing, No. 3).* Sheffield, England: Society of Indexers; 2002.
9. Thomas S. Index. In: Beers MH, Porter RS, Jones TV, Kaplan JL, Berkwits M. *The Merck Manual of Diagnosis and Therapy.* 18th ed. Whitehouse Station, NJ: Merck Research Laboratories; 2006:2787-2991.
10. Thomas S. Index. In: Beers MH, Berkow R, eds. *The Merck Manual of Diagnosis and Therapy.* 17th ed. Whitehouse Station, NJ: Merck Research Laboratories; 1999: 2657-2833.
11. American Society of Indexers. Indexing evaluation checklist. http://www.asindexing .org/site/checklist.shtml. Updated April 7, 2006. Accessed April 20, 2006.
12. National Library of Medicine Medical Subject Headings Web site. http://www.nlm .nih.gov/mesh/meshhome.html. Accessed August 2, 2005.
13. McMaster M. Practical medical database indexing. In: Wyman LP, ed. *Indexing Specialties: Medicine.* Phoenix, AZ: American Society of Indexers; Medford, NJ: Information Today; 1999:83-91.
14. Lancaster FW. *Vocabulary Control for Information Retrieval.* 2nd ed. Arlington, VA: Information Resources Press; 1986.
15. Mauer P. Embedded indexing. In: Proceedings of 50th Annual Conference of Society for Technical Communication. 2001. http://www.stc.org/50thConf/Session_Materials /dataShow.asp?ID=230. Accessed April 20, 2006.
16. American Society of Indexers. Software tools for indexing. http://www.asindexing .org/site/software.shtml. Updated March 20, 2006. Accessed April 24, 2006.

Section

3 Terminology

14 Abbreviations

The Greeks did not use abbreviations commonly; they had no instinct for abbreviating. When they did abbreviate, it was by simple suspension (or curtailment), usually self-intelligible. The purpose was often to save numerous repetitions in one document. . . . Greek abbreviations were not standardized, but depended on the whim of the scribe.

Herbert Weir Smyth[1]

The use of acronyms and abbreviations works against clarity, and the confusion is all the greater when they vary from language to language.

Rory Watson[2]

Merriam-Webster's Collegiate Dictionary defines an abbreviation as "a shortened form of a written word or phrase used in place of the whole"[3] (eg, Dr for doctor, US for United States, dB for decibel).

An acronym is "formed from the initial letter or letters of each of the successive parts or major parts of a compound term"[3] (eg, ANCOVA for analysis of covariance). Acronyms are pronounced as words.

An initialism is "an abbreviation formed from initial letters" and pronounced either as a separate word[3] (eg, PAHO for Pan American Health Organization) or as a set of consecutive initials (eg, NSF for National Science Foundation).

Overuse of abbreviations can be confusing and ambiguous for readers—especially those whose first language is not English or those outside a specific specialty or discipline. However, since abbreviations save space, they may be acceptable to use when the original word or words are repeated numerous times.

Instructions for authors published in medical and scientific journals may include guidelines on the use of abbreviations, ranging from "limit of 4 per manuscript" to "use only approved abbreviations." Authors, editors, manuscript editors, and others involved in preparing manuscripts should use good judgment, flexibility, and common sense when considering the use of abbreviations. Abbreviations that some consider universally known may be obscure to others. Author-invented abbreviations should be avoided. See specific entries in this section and 15.0, Nomenclature, for further guidance in correct use of abbreviations.

Note: The expanded form of an abbreviation is given in lowercase letters, unless the expansion contains a proper noun, is a formal name, or begins a sentence (capitalize first word only).

Style for abbreviations used in *JAMA* and the *Archives* Journals rarely calls for the use of periods. (*But:* See 14.6, Names and Titles of Persons.)

14.1 Academic Degrees, Certifications, and Honors. The following academic degrees are abbreviated in bylines and in the text when used with the full name of a person. (See also 14.6, Names and Titles of Persons.) In some circumstances, however, use of the abbreviation alone is acceptable (eg, Katharine is a doctor of medicine and also holds a PhD in biochemistry). (See also 9.5, Plurals, Abbreviations.)

Generally, US fellowship designations (eg, FACP, FAAN, FACS) and honorary designations (eg, PhD[Hon]) are not used in bylines. In contrast, non-US designations such as the British FRCP and the Canadian FRCPC (attained through a series of qualifying examinations) should be listed in bylines.

At *JAMA* and the *Archives* Journals, for example, if an author holds both an FACP and an FRCPC, the former would be deleted.

Degrees below the master's level (eg, BA, BS) are generally not listed in bylines or elsewhere. However, if a bachelor's degree is the highest degree held, it may be listed. Exceptions are also made for specialized degrees, licenses, certifications, and credentials below the master's level in medical and health-related fields (included below). Any unusual degrees should be verified with the author.

ART	accredited record technician
BPharm	bachelor of pharmacy
BS, BCh, BC, CB, or ChB	bachelor of surgery
BSN	bachelor of science in nursing
CHES	certified health education specialist
CIH	certified industrial hygienist
CNM	certified nurse midwife
CNMT	certified nuclear medicine technologist

CO	certified orthoptist
COMT	certified ophthalmic medical technologist
CPFT	certified pulmonary function technologist
CRNA	certified registered nurse anesthetist
CRTT	certified respiratory therapy technician
CTR	certified tumor registrar
DC	doctor of chiropractic
DCh or ChD	doctor of surgery
DDS	doctor of dental surgery
DHL	doctor of humane letters
DMD	doctor of dental medicine
DME	doctor of medical education
DMSc	doctor of medical science
DNE	doctor of nursing education
DNS or DNSc	doctor of nursing science
DO or OD	doctor of optometry
DO	doctor of osteopathy
DPH or DrPH	doctor of public health; doctor of public hygiene
DPharm	doctor of pharmacy
DPM	doctor of podiatric medicine
DSW	doctor of social work
DTM&H	diploma in tropical medicine and hygiene
DTPH	diploma in tropical pediatric hygiene
DVM, DMV, or VMD	doctor of veterinary medicine
DVMS	doctor of veterinary medicine and surgery
DVS or DVSc	doctor of veterinary science
EdD	doctor of education
ELS	editor in the life sciences
EMT	emergency medical technician
EMT-P	emergency medical technician-paramedic
FCGP	fellow of the College of General Practitioners
FCPS	fellow of the College of Physicians and Surgeons
FFA	fellow of the Faculty of Anaesthetists
FFARCS	fellow of the Faculty of Anaesthetists of the Royal College of Surgeons
FNP	family nurse practitioner
FRACP	fellow of the Royal Australian College of Physicians
FRCA	fellow of the Royal College of Anesthesia

FRCGP	fellow of the Royal College of General Practitioners
FRCOG	fellow of the Royal College of Obstetricians and Gynaecologists
FRCP	fellow of the Royal College of Physicians
FRCPath	fellow of the Royal College of Pathologists
FRCPC	fellow of the Royal College of Physicians of Canada
FRCP(Glasg)	fellow of the Royal College of Physicians and Surgeons of Glasgow qua Physician
FRCPE or FRCP(Edin)	fellow of the Royal College of Physicians of Edinburgh
FRCPI or FRCP(Ire)	fellow of the Royal College of Physicians of Ireland
FRCR	fellow of the Royal College of Radiologists
FRCS	fellow of the Royal College of Surgeons
FRCSC	fellow of the Royal College of Surgeons of Canada
FRCSE or FRCS(Edin)	fellow of the Royal College of Surgeons of Edinburgh
FRCS(Glasg)	fellow of the Royal College of Physicians and Surgeons of Glasgow qua Surgeon
FRCSI or FRCS(Ire)	fellow of the Royal College of Surgeons of Ireland
FRCVS	fellow of the Royal College of Veterinary Surgeons
FRS	fellow of the Royal Society
GNP	gerontologic or geriatric nurse practitioner
JD	doctor of jurisprudence
LLB	bachelor of laws
LLD	doctor of laws
LLM	master of laws
LPN	licensed practical nurse
LVN	licensed visiting nurse; licensed vocational nurse
M(ASCP)	registered technologist in microbiology (American Society of Clinical Pathologists)
MA or AM	master of arts
MB or BM	bachelor of medicine
MBA	master of business administration
MBBS or MB,BS	bachelor of medicine, bachelor of surgery
MD or DM	doctor of medicine

MEd	master of education
MFA	master of fine arts
MHA	master of hospital administration
MLS	master of library science
MMM	master of medical management
MN	master of nursing
MPA	master of public administration
MPH	master of public health
MPharm	master of pharmacy
MPhil	master of philosophy
MPPA	master of public policy administration
MRCP	member of the Royal College of Physicians
MRCS	member of the Royal College of Surgeons
MS, MSc, or SM	master of science
MS, SM, MCh, or MSurg	master of surgery
MSN	master of science in nursing
MSPH	master of science in public health
MStat	master of statistics
MSW	master of social welfare; master of social work
MT	medical technologist
MTA	medical technical assistant
MT(ASCP)	registered medical technologist (American Society of Clinical Pathologists)
MUS	master in urban studies
ND	naturopathic doctor
NP	nurse practitioner
OT	occupational therapist
OTR	occupational therapist, registered
PA	physician assistant
PA-C	physician assistant, certified
PharmD, DP, or PD	doctor of pharmacy
PhD or DPhil	doctor of philosophy
PhG	graduate in pharmacy
PNP	pediatric nurse practitioner
PsyD	doctor of psychology
PT	physical therapist
RD	registered dietitian
RN	registered nurse

RNA	registered nurse anesthetist
RNC or RN,C	registered nurse, certified
RPFT	registered pulmonary function technologist
RPh	registered pharmacist
RPT	registered physical therapist
RRL	registered record librarian
RT	radiologic technologist; respiratory therapist
RTR	recreational therapist, registered
ScD, DSc, or DS	doctor of science
STD	doctor of systematic theology
ThD or DTh	doctor of theology

14.2 US Military Services and Titles.

JAMA and the *Archives* Journals prefer that the author's nonmilitary academic degree(s) be used in bylines, eg, Christopher Lee, MD, not Col Christopher Lee, USAF, MC. If used in the text, the abbreviation of a military service follows a name; the abbreviation of a military title (also called grade or rank) precedes a name (eg, 1LT Cornelia McNamara, AN, USAR). Military titles and abbreviations should be verified with the author (see also 2.2, Manuscript Preparation, Bylines and End-of-Text Signatures; and 2.2.3, Manuscript Preparation, Bylines and End-of-Text Signatures, Degrees).

14.2.1 US Military Services

US Army

MC, USA	Medical Corps, US Army
ANC, USA	Army Nurse Corps, US Army
SP, USA	Specialist Corps, US Army
MSC, USA	Medical Service Corps, US Army
DC, USA	Dental Corps, US Army
VC, USA	Veterinary Corps, US Army

Note: All of the preceding designations also apply to the Army National Guard (ARNG) and US Army Reserve (USAR).

US Air Force

USAF, MC	Medical Corps, US Air Force
USAF, NC	Nurse Corps, US Air Force
USAF, MSC	Medical Service Corps, US Air Force
USAF, DC	Dental Corps, US Air Force
USAF, BSC	Bio-Sciences Corps, US Air Force

Note: All of the preceding designations also apply to the Air National Guard (ANG) and US Air Force Reserve (USAFR). The US Air Force has no veterinary corps; veterinarians are in the Bio-Sciences Corps.

US Navy

MC, USN	Medical Corps, US Navy
MSC, USN	Medical Service Corps, US Navy
NC, USN	Nurse Corps, US Navy
DC, USN	Dental Corps, US Navy

Note: All of the preceding designations also apply to the US Naval Reserve (USNR).

14.2.2 US Military Officer Titles (Grades/Ranks)

US Army

General	GEN
Lieutenant General	LTG
Major General	MG
Brigadier General	BG
Colonel	COL
Lieutenant Colonel	LTC
Major	MAJ
Captain	CPT
First Lieutenant	1LT
Second Lieutenant	2LT
Chief Warrant Officer	CWO
Warrant Officer	WO

US Navy and US Coast Guard

Admiral	ADM
Vice Admiral	VADM
Rear Admiral	RADM
Captain	CAPT
Commander	CDR
Lieutenant Commander	LCDR
Lieutenant	LT
Lieutenant (Junior Grade)	LTJG
Ensign	ENS
Chief Warrant Officer	CWO

Note: All medical professionals in the US Coast Guard (except physician assistants) are commissioned officers in the US Public Health Service (PHS). US Coast Guard chief warrant officers in medicine are designated CWO(Med). This also applies to the US Coast Guard Reserve.

US Air Force and US Marine Corps

General	Gen
Lieutenant General	Lt Gen
Major General	Maj Gen
Brigadier General	Brig Gen
Colonel	Col
Lieutenant Colonel	Lt Col
Major	Maj
Captain	Capt
First Lieutenant	1st Lt
Second Lieutenant	2nd Lt

Note: The US Marine Corps does not have its own medical organization. The medical care of the US Marine Corps is provided by the US Navy.

14.3 Days of the Week, Months, Eras. Generally, days of the week and months are not abbreviated.

> The manuscript was received at *JAMA*'s editorial offices in late December 2004 and accepted for publication on January 5, 2005, after expedited peer review, revision, and discussion among the editors. Because of the importance of its topic, the article was published 3 weeks later, on Wednesday, January 26, 2005, as a *JAMA*-EXPRESS.

In tables and figures, the following 3-letter abbreviations for days of the weeks and months may be used to conserve space (see 4.1, Visual Presentation of Data, Tables; and 4.2, Visual Presentation of Data, Figures):

Monday	Mon
Tuesday	Tue
Wednesday	Wed
Thursday	Thu
Friday	Fri
Saturday	Sat
Sunday	Sun

January	Jan
February	Feb
March	Mar
April	Apr
May	May
June	Jun
July	Jul

August	Aug
September	Sep
October	Oct
November	Nov
December	Dec

Occasionally, scientific manuscripts may contain discussion of eras. Abbreviations for eras are set in small capitals with no punctuation. Numerals are used for years and words for the first through ninth centuries. The more commonly used era designations are AD (anno Domini, in the year of the Lord), BC (before Christ), CE (common era), and BCE (before the common era). CE and BCE are equivalent to AD and BC, respectively. In formal usage, the abbreviation AD precedes the year number, and BC, CE, and BCE follow it.

> William Withering was the first to report extensively, in the late 18th century, on the use of foxglove (*Digitalis purpurea*) for the treatment of dropsy (generalized edema).
>
> Hippocrates, a prominent Greek medical practitioner and teacher of the fourth century BCE, has come to personify the ideal physician.
>
> The prevalence of tuberculosis is thought to have increased greatly during the Middle Ages (roughly AD 500-1500), possibly because of the growth of towns across Europe.
>
> Cuneiform was probably invented by the Sumerians before 3000 BC.

14.4 Local Addresses. Use the following abbreviations when *complete* local addresses are given:

> The hospital was built on Eighth Street.
>
> The hospital's address is 319 W Eighth St.

In some cases, these designators may or may not be abbreviated, by convention:

Fort Saskatchewan	Ft Lauderdale
Mount St Helens	Saint Louis

Designator	*Abbreviation*
Air Force Base	AFB
Army Post Office	APO
Avenue	Ave
Boulevard	Blvd
Building	Bldg
Circle	Cir
Court	Ct
Crescent	Cres
Drive	Dr
East	E

Fleet Post Office	FPO
Fort	Ft
Highway	Hwy
Lane	Ln
Mount	Mt
North	N
Northeast	NE
Northwest	NW
Parkway	Pkwy
Place	Pl
Post Office	PO
Road	Rd
Route	Rte
Rural Free Delivery	RFD
Rural Route	RR
Saint	St or Ste (eg, Sault Ste Marie [verify])
South	S
Southeast	SE
Southwest	SW
Square	Sq
Street	St
Suite	Ste
Terrace	Terr
West	W

Do not abbreviate non-English address terms (eg, boulevard, avenue, place, rue, via, Strasse, Platz). (*Note:* The translation of such terms can be derived via the Internet.) Query author for preference of English or non-English address terms.

When the plural form of an address designator is used, do not abbreviate it (eg, Broadway and Spring streets). When a street number is not given, do not abbreviate (eg, National Hospital for Neurology and Neurosurgery, Queen Square, London WC1N 3BG, England).

Do not abbreviate *room*, *department* (except in references; see 3.13.2, References, Special Print Materials, Government or Agency Bulletins), or *division*.

Do not use periods or commas with N, S, E, W, or their combinations.

There may be exceptions to these rules. For example, "One IBM Plaza," "One Magnificent Mile," and "One Gustave L. Levy Place" are not only addresses but also proper names of buildings or office centers. In these cases it is appropriate to spell out address numbers that accompany designators such as "Place." In such cases, the editor or author should use common sense and verify unusual addresses.

Note: Use e-mail addresses exactly as given. (See also 2.10.4, Manuscript Preparation, Acknowledgment Section, Correspondence Address, and 10.3.9, Capitalization, Proper Nouns, Official Names.)

14.5 Cities, States, Counties, Territories, Possessions; Provinces; Countries. At first mention, the name of a state, territory, possession, province, or country should be spelled out when it follows the name of a city. (Because the majority of authors and readers of *JAMA* and the *Archives* Journals are from the United States, these journals do not add "United States" after the name of a US city and state. Similar rules are followed by other journals. For example, the *Lancet* does not add "United Kingdom" after the name of a UK city.)

Chicago, Illinois	Reykjavik, Iceland
Abu Dhabi, United Arab Emirates	London, England
Paris, France	London, Ontario, Canada

Names of cities, states, counties, territories, possessions, provinces, and countries should be spelled out in full when they stand alone.

Note: Be aware that the names of some cities (and other geographic entities) have changed (eg, Mumbai instead of Bombay, Chennai instead of Madras, Kolkata instead of Calcutta, Kyiv instead of Kiev). The author should be queried as to his or her preference.

Abbreviations such as "US" and "UK" may be used as modifiers (ie, only when they directly precede the word they modify) but should be expanded in all other contexts.

> The authors surveyed representative samples of urban populations in the United States and United Kingdom according to US and UK census data.

Use 2-letter abbreviations for US state and Canadian province names in addresses (with US zip codes and Canadian postal codes) and in reference lists (eg, location of book publishers) but not in the text. The US state and Canadian province names may also be abbreviated to save space in tables and figures.

> *JAMA*/*Archives* Journals Editorial Office
> 515 N State St
> Chicago, IL 60610

> Whitfield JF, Chakravarthy B. *Calcium: The Grand-Master Cell Signaler.* Ottawa, ON: NRC Research Press National Research Council Canada; 2001.

> Scott JR, Di Saia PJ, Hammond CB, Spellacy WN, eds. *Danforth's Obstetrics & Gynecology.* 8th ed. Philadelphia, PA: Lippincott Williams & Wilkins; 1999.

US State, Territory, Possession	*US Postal Service Abbreviation*
Alabama	AL
Alaska	AK
American Samoa	AS
Arizona	AZ
Arkansas	AR
California	CA
Colorado	CO

Connecticut	CT
Delaware	DE
District of Columbia	DC
Federated States of Micronesia	FM
Florida	FL
Georgia	GA
Guam	GU
Hawaii	HI
Idaho	ID
Illinois	IL
Indiana	IN
Iowa	IA
Kansas	KS
Kentucky	KY
Louisiana	LA
Maine	ME
Marshall Islands	MH
Maryland	MD
Massachusetts	MA
Michigan	MI
Minnesota	MN
Mississippi	MS
Missouri	MO
Montana	MT
Nebraska	NE
Nevada	NV
New Hampshire	NH
New Jersey	NJ
New Mexico	NM
New York	NY
North Carolina	NC
North Dakota	ND
Northern Marianas Islands	MP
Ohio	OH
Oklahoma	OK
Oregon	OR
Palau	PW
Pennsylvania	PA
Puerto Rico	PR

Rhode Island	RI
South Carolina	SC
South Dakota	SD
Tennessee	TN
Texas	TX
Utah	UT
Vermont	VT
Virginia	VA
Virgin Islands	VI
Washington	WA
West Virginia	WV
Wisconsin	WI
Wyoming	WY

Canadian city names should be followed by the province name in the text (eg, London, Ontario, Canada).

Canadian Province, Territory	*Canada Post Abbreviation*
Alberta	AB
British Columbia	BC
Manitoba	MB
New Brunswick	NB
Newfoundland and Labrador	NL
Northwest Territories	NT
Nova Scotia	NS
Nunavut	NU
Ontario	ON
Prince Edward Island	PE
Quebec	QC
Saskatchewan	SK
Yukon	YT

At first mention in the text, the name of the appropriate state or country should follow the name of a city whenever clarification of location is thought to be important for the reader, as in the following examples:

> In September 2003 Hurricane Isabel made landfall between Ocracoke and Morehead City, North Carolina.
>
> A new scientific conference created by the International AIDS Society took place in July 2001 in Buenos Aires, Argentina.

The province name may also be added for less well-known cities:

> San Miguel, Hidalgo, Mexico

If the city, state, or country is clear from the context, as in the following examples, do not include it.

> Studies were carried out at the University of Michigan Medical School, Ann Arbor [unnecessary to add "Michigan"].
>
> A cross-sectional survey assessing bicycle safety helmets was conducted in 3 Dutch primary schools in Breda, Maastricht, and Terneuzen [unnecessary to add "the Netherlands"].
>
> Illinois' Argonne National Laboratory, located about 50 km west of Chicago, supports more than 200 research programs and capabilities, ranging from analytical chemistry of long-lived radioisotopes, to x-ray beam system design, to global climate change research [unnecessary to repeat "Illinois" after "Chicago"].

Do not provide the state or country name in cases in which the entity is well known and such clarification is excessive, eg, Chicago White Sox, Philadelphia chromosome, Glasgow sign, Uppsala virus, Lyme disease, the *Boston Globe*.

Do not provide the location of an institution if it is clear that the location is not important, eg, "Using the Centers for Disease Control and Prevention criteria for AIDS . . . " or "Following the World Health Organization guidelines. . . . "

> What does it matter that she was born in Boston, or that after her parents had instilled in her the guiding principles of life, Harvard University had its turn?

In addition to the city name, provide the name of the state or country name in the author affiliation footnote and correspondence address.

> *Affiliation Footnote:*
> Department of Pediatrics, Vanderbilt University School of Medicine, Nashville, Tennessee (Dr Poehling).
>
> *Author Correspondence Address:*
> Katherine A. Poehling, MD, MPH, Department of Pediatrics, Vanderbilt University School of Medicine, AA0216 Medical Center N, Nashville, TN 37232-2504 (katherine.poehling@vanderbilt.edu).

Special Case: "New York" may refer to either the city or the state. In the former case, the state name must be added:

> New York State Psychiatric Institute, New York
>
> New York University, New York, NY

When giving the location of an institution or organization whose formal name includes a city, do not insert the state or country within the name:

Correct:	Stanford University School of Medicine in California
Also correct:	Stanford University School of Medicine, Stanford, California
Not:	Stanford University School of Medicine (California)
And not:	Stanford (California) University School of Medicine
And not:	Stanford University School of Medicine, California

The style used in the foregoing correct examples may be applied in signature bylines:

Correct: Remy I. Smith, MD
Stanford University School of Medicine
Stanford, California

Not: Remy I. Smith, MD
Stanford (California) University School of Medicine

The following are examples of address style for many countries throughout the world (see also 2.0, Manuscript Preparation, and 14.4, Local Addresses).

Andrzej Szczeklik, PhD, Allergy and Immunology Clinic, Department of Medicine, Jagellonian University School of Medicine, ul Skawinska 8, 31-0666 Krakow, Poland.

Vivek Goal, Department of Health Administration, McMurrich Bldg, 12 Queen's Park Cres W, Toronto, ON M5S 1A8, Canada.

Alain F. Broccard, MD, Division des Soins Intensifs, Départment de Médecine, BH10-92, University Hospital (CHUV), CH-1011 Lausanne, Switzerland.

N. J. Bouwmeester, MB, Department of Anaesthesiology and Paediatric Surgery, Sophia Children's Hospital, University Hospital Rotterdam, Dr Molewaterplein 60, 3015 GJ Rotterdam, the Netherlands.

Konstantinos I. Gourgoloulianis, Pulmonary Department, Medical School, University of Thessaly, 22 Papakyriazi, Larissa 41222, Greece.

Didier Blaise, MD, Unitè de Transplantation et de Thérapie Cellulare, Institut Paoli-Calmettes, 232 Bd Ste Marguerite, 13273 Marseille CEDEX 09, France.

Ruben Terg, Unidad de Hepatologia, Hospital de Gastroenterologia Bonorino Udaondo, Escuela de Medicina, Universidad del Salvador, Avenida Caseros, 2061 (1264) Buenos Aires, Argentina.

Ditlev Fossen, Department of Obstetrics and Gynecology, County Hospital of Oestfold (Sykenhuset Oestfold), 1603 Fredrikstad, Norway.

Hajime Fujimoto, MD, Third Department of Internal Medicine, Respiratory Division, Mie University School of Medicine, Edobashi 2-174, Tsu City, Mie 514-8507, Japan.

Kwang Hyun Kim, MD, Department of Otolaryngology-Head and Neck Surgery, Seoul National University, College of Medicine, 28 Tongon-Dong, Chongno-Gu, Seoul 110-744, Korea.

Colin L. Masters, MD, Department of Pathology, University of Melbourne, Parkville, Victoria, Australia 3010.

Thomas Schwarz, Division of Vascular Medicine, Department of Internal Medicine, University Hospital of Dresden Medical School, Fetscherstrasse 74, 01307 Dresden, Germany.

David M. Fergusson, Christchurch Health and Development Study, Christchurch School of Medicine, PO Box 4345, Christchurch, New Zealand.

Anand Job, Department of Otorhinolaryngology and Head and Neck Surgery, Unit 1, Christian Medical College, Vellore 632 004, India.

Neville N. Osborne, DSc, Nuffield Laboratory of Ophthalmology, Walton Street, Oxford OX2 6AW, England.

Yasemin Giles, MD, Istanbul Tip Fakültesi, Genel Cerrahi ABD, Capa, Topkapi, Istanbul, Turkey 34390.

Shurong Zheng, Department of Obstetrics and Gynecology, Peking University First Hospital, Beijing 100034, China.

Alfred Cuschieri, MD, FRSE, Department of Surgery and Molecular Oncology, Ninewells Hospital and Medical School, University of Dundee, Dundee DD1 9SY, Scotland.

J. Skordis, Department of Public Health and Policy, London School of Hygiene and Tropical Medicine, Keppel Street, London WC1E 7HT, England.

Gar-Yang Chau, MD, MPH, Division of General Surgery, Department of Surgery, Taipei Veterans General Hospital, 201 Shih-Pai Rd, Section 2, Taipei, Taiwan 11217.

Two- and three-letter ISO (International Organization for Standardization) country codes may also be used in addresses. These codes are updated regularly by the RIPE Network Coordination Centre, in coordination with the ISO 3166 Maintenance Agency, Berlin, Germany (list available at http://userpage.chemie.fu-berlin.de/diverse/doc/ISO_3166.html).

14.6 Names and Titles of Persons. Given names should not be abbreviated in the text or in bylines except by using initials, when so indicated by the author. The editor should verify the use of initials with the author. (Some publishers prefer to use initials, instead of given names.)

Do not use Chas., Geo., Jas., Wm., etc, except when such abbreviations are part of the formal name of a company or organization that regularly uses such abbreviations (see 14.7, Business Firms). When an abbreviation is part of a person's name, retain the period after the abbreviation, eg, Oliver St. John Gogarty, MD.

Initials used in the text to indicate names of persons (eg, coauthors of an article) should be followed by periods and set close within parentheses. *Note:* This is one of the few instances in which a period is used with an abbreviation.

> A method was devised to calculate familial risk (K.A.R., unpublished observations, 2006).

A person who is not an author may also be mentioned in the text, in which case the full name and academic degree are used.

> Although measurements of the various components were divided among 3 examiners (R.Z., D.O.M., and Norris T. Friedlin, MD), each examiner measured the same components at each annual session.

Senior and *Junior* are abbreviated when they are part of a person's name. The abbreviation follows the surname and is followed by a comma only when the abbreviation precedes another, such as an academic degree. (*But:* See 19.7.5, Numbers and Percentages, Forms of Numbers, Roman Numerals, and 3.7, References, Authors.) *Note:* These abbreviations are used only with the full name (*never* Dr Forsythe Jr).

> Peter M. Forsythe Jr, MD, performed his landmark research in collaboration with James Philips Sr, PhD, at the National Institutes of Health.

Names with roman numerals do not take a comma: Pope Benedict XVI, Marshall Field IV.

Many titles of persons are abbreviated but only when they precede the full name (given name or initials and surname). Spell titles out (except *Dr*, *Mrs*, etc) when (1) used before a surname alone (except in some cases as described below), (2) used at the beginning of a sentence, and (3) used after a name (in this instance, the title should not be capitalized). (*But:* See also 14.2, US Military Services and Titles.)

> Colonel Jonas
> COL Miranda Jonas, MC, USA
> Dr Jonas, colonel in the army
>
> Alderman Daley
> Ald Vi Daley
> Vi Daley, alderman of the 43rd Ward of Chicago
>
> Father Doyle
> Fr Raymond G. Doyle
> Raymond G. Doyle, SJ
>
> Governor Blagojevich
> Gov Rod Blagojevich
> Rod Blagojevich, governor of Illinois
>
> Representative McDermott
> Rep Jim McDermott
> Jim McDermott, MD, representative from the state of Washington
>
> Senator Obama
> Sen Barack Obama (D, Illinois)
> Barack Obama, US senator from Illinois
>
> Sister Monica
> Sr Monica Sobieski
> Monica Sobieski, SJC, mother superior
>
> Superintendent Smith
> Supt H. B. Smith
> Henry B. Smith, EdD, superintendent of schools
>
> the Reverend Katharine M. Burke
> the Reverend Dr Burke
> Rev Katharine M. Burke

Note: The Reverend, *Reverend*, or *Rev* is used only when the first name or initials are given with the surname. When only the surname is given, use *the Reverend Mr* (or *Ms* or *Dr*), *Mr* (or *Ms* or *Dr*), or *Father* (Roman Catholic and some Protestant denominations). Never use *the Reverend Brown*, *Reverend Brown*, or *Rev Brown*.

Exception, Heads of State: President is not abbreviated. It is capitalized when it precedes a name and is set lowercase when following a name (see also 10.3.10, Capitalization, Proper Nouns, Titles and Degrees of Persons):

President John F. Kennedy
President and Mrs Kennedy
John F. Kennedy, president of the United States
the president

The following social titles are always abbreviated when preceding a surname, with or without first name or initials: *Dr, Mr, Messrs, Mrs, Mmes, Ms,* and *Mss.* Note that in most instances, the title *Dr* should be used only after the specific academic degree has been mentioned and only with the surname.

Arthur L. Rudnick, MD, PhD, gave the opening address. At the close of the meeting, Dr Rudnick was named director of the committee on sports injuries.

14.7 **Business Firms.** In the text, use the name of a company exactly as the company uses it, but omit the period after any abbreviations used, such as *Co, Inc, Corp,* and *Ltd.* In the text, do not abbreviate these terms if the company spells them out, eg, Sandoz Pharmaceuticals Corporation. Note that in the text, periods are used with a company namesake's initials.

However, to conserve space in references, abbreviate *Company, Corporation, Brothers, Incorporated, Limited,* and *and* (using an ampersand [&]), without punctuation, even if the company expands them, and delete periods even with initials, in accordance with the following examples; and delete *The* in publishers' names. (See also 3.12.9, References, References to Print Books, Publishers; and 15.5, Nomenclature, Equipment, Devices, and Reagents.)

Text Style	*Reference Style*
Farrar, Straus & Giroux	Farrar Straus & Giroux
B. C. Decker	BC Decker
American Mensa, Ltd	American Mensa Ltd
HarperCollins Publishers	HarperCollins Publishers
The Free Press	Free Press

14.8 **Agencies and Organizations.** Many organizations (eg, academies, associations, government agencies, research institutes) are known by abbreviations or acronyms rather than by their full names. Some of these organizations have identical abbreviations (eg, AHA for both American Heart Association and American Hospital Association). Therefore, to avoid confusion, the names of all organizations should be expanded at first mention in the text and other major elements of the manuscript, with the abbreviation following immediately in parentheses, in accordance with the guidelines offered in 14.11, Clinical, Technical, and Other Common Terms.

The article *the* is often used with abbreviated forms of agencies and organizations (eg, the UN, the AMA, the FDA); however, an article is not necessary with forms pronounced as words (eg, NASA, OSHA, WAME).

The following are associations and organizations commonly cited in *JAMA* and the *Archives* Journals. This list is intended to show examples and is not all-inclusive.

Because there are other expansions of some of the abbreviations, authors and editors should verify that the expansion is correct in such instances.

AAAAI
American Academy of Allergy, Asthma, and Immunology

AAAS
American Association for the Advancement of Science

AABB
American Association of Blood Banks

AACAP
American Academy of Child and Adolescent Psychiatry

AACC
American Association of Clinical Chemists

AACIA
American Association for Clinical Immunology and Allergy

AACN
American Association of Colleges of Nursing
American Association of Critical-Care Nurses

AAD
American Academy of Dermatology

AAFP
American Academy of Family Physicians

AAFPRS
American Academy of Facial Plastic and Reconstructive Surgery

AAHSLD
Association of Academic Health Science Library Directors

AAI
American Association of Immunologists

AAMC
Association of American Medical Colleges

AAMCH
American Association of Maternal and Child Health

AAN
American Academy of Neurology
American Academy of Neuropathologists
American Academy of Nursing

AANA
American Association of Nurse Anesthetists

AANP
American Academy of Nurse Practitioners

AANS
American Association of Neurological Surgeons

AAO
American Academy of Ophthalmology

AAOHNS
American Academy of Otolaryngology-Head and Neck Surgery

AAOS
American Academy of Orthopaedic Surgeons

AAP
American Academy of Pediatrics
American Association of Pathologists

AAPA
American Academy of Physician Assistants
American Association of Pathologists' Assistants

AAPHP
American Association of Public Health Physicians

AAPM
American Academy of Pain Medicine
American Association of Physicists in Medicine

AAPMR
American Academy of Physical Medicine and Rehabilitation

AAPS
American Association of Plastic Surgeons

AARP
American Association of Retired Persons

AATM
American Academy of Tropical Medicine

AATS
American Association for Thoracic Surgery

AAUP
American Association of University Professors

AAWR
American Association for Women Radiologists

ABA
American Bar Association

ABMS
American Board of Medical Specialties

ACA
American College of Allergists
American College of Anesthetists

ACAAI
American College of Allergy, Asthma, and Immunology

ACC
American College of Cardiology

ACCME
Accreditation Council for Continuing Medical Education

ACCP
American College of Chest Physicians

ACEP
American College of Emergency Physicians

ACG
American College of Gastroenterology

ACGME
Accreditation Council for Graduate Medical Education

ACHA
American College Health Association

ACHE
American College of Hospital Executives

ACIP
Advisory Committee on Immunization Practices

ACLM
American College of Legal Medicine

ACMQ
American College of Medical Quality

ACNM
American College of Nuclear Medicine
American College of Nurse-Midwives

ACNP
American College of Nuclear Physicians

ACOEM
American College of Occupational and Environmental Medicine

ACOG
American College of Obstetricians and Gynecologists

ACP
American College of Physicians

ACPE
American College of Physician Executives

ACPM
American College of Preventive Medicine

ACR
American College of Radiology
American College of Rheumatology

ACS
American Cancer Society
American Chemical Society
American College of Surgeons

ACSM
American College of Sports Medicine

ADA
American Dental Association
American Dermatological Association
American Diabetes Association
American Dietetic Association

ADRDA
Alzheimer's Disease and Related Disorders Association

AERS
Adverse Event Reporting System
(US Food and Drug Administration)

AES
American Epilepsy Society

AFAR
American Federation for Aging Research

AFCR
American Federation for Clinical Research

AFIP
Armed Forces Institute of Pathology

AFS
American Fertility Society

AGA
American Gastroenterological Association

AGPA
American Group Practice Association

AGS
American Geriatrics Society

AHA
American Heart Association
American Hospital Association

AHRA
American Healthcare Radiology Administrators

AHRQ
Agency for Healthcare Research and Quality

AJCC
American Joint Committee on Cancer

ALA
American Library Association
American Lung Association

ALROS
American Laryngological, Rhinological and Otological Society

AMA
Aerospace Medical Association
American Management Association
American Marketing Association
American Medical Association
Australian Medical Association

AMDA
American Medical Directors Association

AMPA
American Medical Publishers' Association

AMSA
American Medical Student Association

AMSUS
Association of Military Surgeons of the United States

AMWA
American Medical Women's Association
American Medical Writers Association

ANA
American Neurological Association
American Nurses Association

ANSI
American National Standards Institute

AOA
Alpha Omega Alpha
American Orthopaedic Association
American Osteopathic Association

AOMA
American Occupational Medicine Association

AONE
American Organization of Nurse Executives

AORN
Association of Operating Room Nurses

AOS
American Otological Society

AOWHN
American Organization of Women's Health Nurses

APA
Ambulatory Pediatrics Association
American Pharmaceutical Association
American Psychiatric Association
American Psychological Association

APHA
American Public Health Association

APM
Academy of Physical Medicine

APS
American Physical Society
American Physiological Society
American Psychological Society

ARA
American Rheumatism Association

ARC
American Red Cross

ARENA
Applied Research Ethics National Association

ARRS
American Roentgen Ray Society

ARVO
Association for Research in Vision and Ophthalmology

ASA
American Society of Anesthesiologists

ASAM
American Society of Addiction Medicine

ASCN
American Society of Clinical Nutrition

ASCO
American Society of Clinical Oncology
American Society of Clinical Ophthalmology

ASCP
American Society of Clinical Pathologists
American Society of Consultant Pharmacists

ASCPT
American Society of Clinical Pharmacology and Therapeutics

ASCRS
American Society of Cataract and Refractive Surgery
American Society of Colon and Rectal Surgeons

ASDR
American Society of Diagnostic Radiology

ASDS
American Society for Dermatologic Surgery

ASG
American Society for Genetics

ASGE
American Society for Gastrointestinal Endoscopy

ASHG
American Society of Human Genetics

ASLME
American Society of Law, Medicine & Ethics

ASM
American Society for Microbiology

ASMT
American Society of Medical Technologists

ASPRS
American Society of Plastic and Reconstructive Surgeons

ASTHO
Association of State and Territorial Health Officers

ASTMH
American Society of Tropical Medicine and Hygiene

ASTRO
American Society for Therapeutic Radiology and Oncology

ASTS
American Society of Transplant Surgeons

ATA
American Thyroid Association

ATS
American Thoracic Society

AUA
American Urological Association

BMA
British Medical Association

CAP
College of American Pathologists

CDC
Centers for Disease Control and Prevention

CMA
Canadian Medical Association

CMS
Centers for Medicare & Medicaid Services

CNS
Child Neurology Society

CSE
Council of Science Editors

DHHS
Department of Health and Human Services

EASE
European Association of Science Editors

ECDC
European Centre for Disease Prevention and Control

ECFMG
Educational Commission for Foreign Medical Graduates

EEOC
Equal Employment Opportunity Commission

EIS
Epidemic Intelligence Service
(US Centers for Disease Control and Prevention)

EPA
Environmental Protection Agency

EU
European Union

FASEB
Federation of American Societies for Experimental Biology

FCC
Federal Communications Commission

FDA
Food and Drug Administration

FTC
Federal Trade Commission

GLMA
Gay and Lesbian Medical Association

GSA
Gerontological Society of America

IARC
International Agency for Research on Cancer

ICAAC
Interscience Conference on Antimicrobial Agents and Chemotherapy

ICMJE
International Committee of Medical Journal Editors

ICN
International Council of Nurses

ICRC
International Committee of the Red Cross

ICS
International College of Surgeons

IDSA
Infectious Diseases Society of America

IEEE
Institute of Electrical and Electronics Engineers

IOM
Institute of Medicine

IPPNW
International Physicians for the Prevention of Nuclear War

ISBT
International Society of Blood Transfusion

ISO
International Organization for Standardization

JCAHO
Joint Commission on Accreditation of Healthcare Organizations

MGMA
Medical Group Management Association

MLA
Medical Library Association

MRC
Medical Research Council

MSF
Médecins Sans Frontières

NAME
National Association of Medical Examiners

NAMS
North American Menopause Society

NAS
National Academy of Sciences

NASA
National Aeronautics and Space Administration

NBME
National Board of Medical Examiners

NCBI
National Center for Biotechnology Information

NCCAM
National Center for Complementary and Alternative Medicine

NCHS
National Center for Health Statistics

NCI
National Cancer Institute

NCOA
National Committee on Quality Assurance

NCRR
National Center for Research Resources

NEI
National Eye Institute

NHGRI
National Human Genome Research Institute

NHLBI
National Heart, Lung, and Blood Institute

NHO
National Hospice Organization

NIA
National Institute on Aging

NIAAA
National Institute on Alcohol Abuse and Alcoholism

NIAID
National Institute of Allergy and Infectious Diseases

NIAMS
National Institute of Arthritis and Musculoskeletal and Skin Diseases

NIBIB
National Institute of Biomedical Imaging and Bioengineering

NICHD
National Institute of Child Health and Human Development

NIDA
National Institute on Drug Abuse

NIDCD
National Institute on Deafness and Other Communication Disorders

NIDCR
National Institute of Dental and Craniofacial Research

NIDDK
National Institute of Diabetes and Digestive and Kidney Diseases

NIEHS
National Institute of Environmental Health Sciences

NIGMS
National Institute of General Medical Sciences

NIH
National Institutes of Health

NIMH
National Institute of Mental Health

NINDS
National Institute of Neurological Disorders and Stroke

NINR
National Institute of Nursing Research

NIOSH
National Institute for Occupational Safety and Health

NISO
National Information Standards Organization

NLM
National Library of Medicine

NLN
National League for Nursing

NMA
National Medical Association

NMHA
National Mental Health Association

NRC
National Research Council
Nuclear Regulatory Commission

NRMP
National Resident Matching Program

NSF
National Science Foundation

NSPB
National Society for the Prevention of Blindness

OMAR
Office of Medical Applications of Research

ONS
Oncology Nursing Society

OPRR
Office for Protection From Research Risks

ORI
Office of Research Integrity

ORWH
Office of Research on Women's Health

OSHA
Occupational Safety and Health Administration

PAHO
Pan American Health Organization

PHR
Physicians for Human Rights

PHS
Public Health Service

PSR
Physicians for Social Responsibility

PSRO
Professional Standards Review Organization

RDCRN
Rare Diseases Clinical Research Network

RPB
Research to Prevent Blindness

RSNA
Radiological Society of North America
Rehabilitation Society of North America

SAMBA
Society for Ambulatory Anesthesia

SAMHSA
Substance Abuse and Mental Health Services Administration

SCCM
Society of Critical Care Medicine

SEC
Securities and Exchange Commission

SID
Society for Investigative Dermatology

SMCAF
Society of Medical Consultants to the Armed Forces

SNM
Society of Nuclear Medicine

SSA
Social Security Administration

SSO
Society of Surgical Oncology

SSP
Society for Scholarly Publishing

STC
Society for Technical Communication

STS
Society of Thoracic Surgeons

UICC
International Union Against Cancer (Union Internationale Contre le Cancer)

UN
United Nations

UNHCR
United Nations High Commissioner for Refugees

UNICEF
United Nations Children's Fund

UNOS
United Network for Organ Sharing

USAN
United States Adopted Names [Council]

VA
Department of Veterans Affairs

WAME
World Association of Medical Editors

WFP
World Food Program

WHO
World Health Organization

WIC
Special Supplemental Nutrition for Women, Infants, and Children

WMA
World Medical Association

For more detailed listings of US and international agencies and associations, consult the current editions of *The Official American Board of Medical Specialties (ABMS) Directory of Board Certified Medical Specialists, The United States Government Manual, Federal Yellow Book, Congressional Yellow Book, Encyclopedia of Associations, Directory of European Medical Organisations, Directory of European Professional & Learned Societies, Civil Service Yearbook, The Medical Registry,* and *The World of Learning.*

There are thousands of directories of Web sites, ranging from the official (eg, US Executive Branch Web Sites at http://www.loc.gov/rr/news/fedgov.html) to commercial, private, and nonprofit (eg, http://directory.google.com/).

14.9 **Collaborative Groups.** Collaborative groups include study groups, multicenter trials, task forces, expert and ad hoc consensus groups, and periodic national and international health surveys. Such an entity's full name should be provided in addition to its abbreviation, even if it appears only once in a manuscript. Because some of these groups are often better recognized by their acronyms than by their full names, the acronym may be placed first, with the expansion in parentheses, contrary to the order usually recommended.

To save space in titles, however, the acronym may be used alone if its expansion is provided early in the manuscript, for example, in the abstract and in the text. Alternatively, the acronym might be given in the manuscript's title and the expansion in its subtitle; or, if space permits and both the expansion and the acronym convey separate and essential concepts, both could be given in the title or subtitle. The collaborative group name may be used as the byline. (See also 5.1.7, Ethical and Legal Considerations, Authorship Responsibility, Group and Collaborative Authorship; 2.2, Manuscript Preparation, Bylines and End-of-Text Signatures; and 2.10.6, Manuscript Preparation, Acknowledgment Section, List of Participants in a Group Study.)

Title:	Fluoxetine, Cognitive-Behavioral Therapy, and Their Combination for Adolescents With Depression
Subtitle:	Treatment for Adolescents With Depression Study (TADS) Randomized Controlled Trial
Byline:	Treatment for Adolescents With Depression Study (TADS) Team

Consider the manuscript's context and audience, database searches, and ease of comprehension when choosing the form in which collaborative group information is presented. Remember that many literature databases contain only the title and article citation; some, but not all, also provide the abstract.

14.10 **Names of Journals.** In reference listings, abbreviate names of journals according to the US National Library of Medicine's current Fact Sheet (Construction of National Library of Medicine title abbreviations at http://www.nlm.nih.gov/pubs/factsheets/constructitle.html). Journal names are italicized. In references, the journal-name abbreviation is followed by a period, which denotes the close of the title group of bibliographic elements.[4,5] (See also 3.11.2, References, References to Print Journals, Names of Journals.)

The following commonly referenced journals and their abbreviations are included in *Abridged Index Medicus*. *Abridged Index Medicus* is no longer published, but it is a subset limit (Core Clinical Journals) within PubMed. In this list, the article *The* has been omitted in the expanded journal titles (as in *The Journal of*...). Single-word journal titles are not abbreviated.

Academic Medicine (formerly *Journal of Medical Education,* abbreviated *J Med Educ)*
Acad Med

AJR: American Journal of Roentgenology
AJR Am J Roentgenol

American Family Physician
Am Fam Physician

American Heart Journal
Am Heart J

American Journal of Cardiology
Am J Cardiol

American Journal of Clinical Nutrition
Am J Clin Nutr

American Journal of Clinical Pathology
Am J Clin Pathol

American Journal of the Medical Sciences
Am J Med Sci

American Journal of Medicine
Am J Med

American Journal of Nursing
Am J Nurs

American Journal of Obstetrics & Gynecology
Am J Obstet Gynecol

American Journal of Ophthalmology
Am J Ophthalmol

American Journal of Pathology
Am J Pathol

American Journal of Physical Medicine & Rehabilitation/Association of Academic Physiatrists
Am J Phys Med Rehabil

American Journal of Psychiatry
Am J Psychiatry

American Journal of Public Health
Am J Public Health

American Journal of Respiratory and Critical Care Medicine
Am J Respir Crit Care Med

American Journal of Surgery
Am J Surg

American Journal of Tropical Medicine and Hygiene
Am J Trop Med Hyg

Anaesthesia
Anaesthesia

Anesthesia and Analgesia
Anesth Analg

Anesthesiology
Anesthesiology

Annals of Emergency Medicine
Ann Emerg Med

Annals of Internal Medicine
Ann Intern Med

Annals of Otology, Rhinology, & Laryngology
Ann Otol Rhinol Laryngol

Annals of Surgery
Ann Surg

Annals of Thoracic Surgery
Ann Thorac Surg

Archives of Dermatology
Arch Dermatol

Archives of Disease in Childhood
Arch Dis Child

Archives of Disease in Childhood. Fetal and Neonatal Edition
Arch Dis Child Fetal Neonatal Ed

Archives of Environmental Health
Arch Environ Health

Archives of General Psychiatry
Arch Gen Psychiatry

Archives of Internal Medicine
Arch Intern Med

Archives of Neurology
Arch Neurol

Archives of Ophthalmology
Arch Ophthalmol

Archives of Otolaryngology–Head & Neck Surgery
Arch Otolaryngol Head Neck Surg

Archives of Pathology & Laboratory Medicine
Arch Pathol Lab Med

Archives of Pediatrics & Adolescent Medicine (formerly *American Journal of Diseases of Children,* abbreviated *Am J Dis Child*)
Arch Pediatr Adolesc Med

Archives of Physical Medicine and Rehabilitation
Arch Phys Med Rehabil

Archives of Surgery
Arch Surg

Arthritis & Rheumatism
Arthritis Rheum

BJOG (continues *British Journal of Obstetrics and Gynaecology*)
BJOG

Blood
Blood

BMJ: British Medical Association (formerly *British Medical Journal,* abbreviated *Br Med J*)
BMJ

Brain; A Journal of Neurology
Brain

British Journal of Radiology
Br J Radiol

British Journal of Surgery
Br J Surg

CA: A Cancer Journal for Clinicians
CA Cancer J Clin

Cancer
Cancer

Chest
Chest

Circulation
Circulation

Clinical Orthopaedics and Related Research
Clin Orthop

Clinical Pediatrics
Clin Pediatr (Phila)

Clinical Pharmacology & Therapeutics
Clin Pharmacol Ther

CMAJ (formerly *Canadian Medical Association Journal*, abbreviated *Can Med Assoc J*)
CMAJ

Critical Care Medicine
Crit Care Med

Current Problems in Surgery
Curr Probl Surg

Diabetes
Diabetes

Digestive Diseases and Sciences
Dig Dis Sci

Disease-a-Month
Dis Mon

Endocrinology
Endocrinology

Gastroenterology
Gastroenterology

Geriatrics
Geriatrics

Gut
Gut

Heart
Heart

Heart & Lung; The Journal of Critical Care
Heart Lung

Hospitals & Health Networks/AHA (formerly *Hospitals*)
Hosp Health Netw

JAMA: The Journal of the American Medical Association
JAMA

Journal of Allergy and Clinical Immunology
J Allergy Clin Immunol

Journal of the American College of Cardiology
J Am Coll Cardiol

Journal of the American College of Surgeons (formerly *Surgery, Gynecology & Obstetrics*, abbreviated *Surg Gynecol Obstet*)
J Am Coll Surg

Journal of the American Dietetic Association
J Am Diet Assoc

Journal of Bone & Joint Surgery. American Volume
J Bone Joint Surg Am

Journal of Bone & Joint Surgery. British Volume
J Bone Joint Surg Br

Journal of Clinical Endocrinology & Metabolism
J Clin Endocrinol Metab

Journal of Clinical Investigation
J Clin Invest

Journal of Clinical Pathology
J Clin Pathol

Journal of Family Practice
J Fam Pract

Journal of Immunology
J Immunol

Journal of Infectious Diseases
J Infect Dis

Journal of Laboratory and Clinical Medicine
J Lab Clin Med

Journal of Laryngology & Otology
J Laryngol Otol

Journal of Nervous and Mental Disease
J Nerv Ment Dis

Journal of Neurosurgery
J Neurosurg

Journal of Nursing Administration
J Nurs Adm

Journal of Oral and Maxillofacial Surgery
J Oral Maxillofac Surg

Journal of Pediatrics
J Pediatr

Journal of Thoracic and Cardiovascular Surgery
J Thorac Cardiovasc Surg

Journal of Toxicology. Clinical Toxicology
J Toxicol Clin Toxicol

Journal of Trauma
J Trauma

Journal of Urology
J Urol

Journals of Gerontology. Series A, Biological Sciences and Medical Sciences
J Gerontol A Biol Sci Med Sci

Journals of Gerontology. Series B, Psychological Sciences and Social Sciences
J Gerontol B Psychol Sci Soc Sci

Lancet
Lancet

Mayo Clinic Proceedings
Mayo Clin Proc

Medical Clinics of North America
Med Clin North Am

Medical Letter on Drugs and Therapeutics
Med Lett Drugs Ther

Medicine; Analytical Reviews of General Medicine, Neurology, Psychiatry, Dermatology, and Pediatrics
Medicine (Baltimore)

Neurology
Neurology

New England Journal of Medicine
N Engl J Med

Nursing Clinics of North America
Nurs Clin North Am

Nursing Outlook
Nurs Outlook

Nursing Research
Nurs Res

Obstetrics & Gynecology
Obstet Gynecol

Orthopedic Clinics of North America
Orthop Clin North Am

Pediatric Clinics of North America
Pediatr Clin North Am

Pediatrics
Pediatrics

Physical Therapy
Phys Ther

Plastic and Reconstructive Surgery
Plast Reconstr Surg

Postgraduate Medicine
Postgrad Med

Progress in Cardiovascular Diseases
Prog Cardiovasc Dis

Public Health Reports
Public Health Rep

Radiologic Clinics of North America
Radiol Clin North Am

Radiology
Radiology

Southern Medical Journal
South Med J

Surgery
Surgery

Surgical Clinics of North America
Surg Clin North Am

Urologic Clinics of North America
Urol Clin North Am

The National Library of Medicine's (NLM's) abbreviations used in MEDLINE are based on the *American National Standard for Information Sciences—Abbreviation of Titles of Publications* (ANSI Z39.5) (1985), as well as abbreviations formulated under earlier ANSI guidelines. Use the following guide to abbreviate or not abbreviate words that may appear in journal titles. (Single-word journal titles are not abbreviated.) Note that these words are capitalized and that articles, conjunctions, prepositions, punctuation, and diacritical marks are omitted in the abbreviated title form.

The NLM's database can be searched by means of the journal title, the MEDLINE/PubMed title abbreviation, the NLM ID (NLM's unique journal identifier), the ISO (International Organization for Standardization) abbreviation, and the print and electronic International Standard Serial Numbers (pISSNs and eISSNs).

The correct abbreviations of journal titles indexed in MEDLINE can also be located through PubMed ("Journals") access.

Word	*Abbreviation or Word Used*
Abnormal	Abnorm
Abuse	Abuse
Academia	Acad
Academy	Acad
Acoustical	Acoust
Actions	Actions
Acupuncture	Acupunct
Acute	Acute
Addiction	Addict
Addictions	Addict
Additives	Addit
Administration	Adm
Adolescence	Adolescence

Adolescent	Adolesc
Advanced	Adv
Advancement	Adv
Advances	Adv
Adverse	Adverse
Aesthetic	Aesthetic
Affairs	Aff
Affective	Affective
African	Afr
Age	Age
Ageing	Ageing
Agents	Agents
Aging	Aging
Air	Air
Alabama	Ala
Alaska	Alaska
Alcohol	Alcohol
Alcoholism	Alcohol
Allergy	Allergy
Allied	Allied
America	Am
American	Am
Anaesthesia	Anaesth
Anaesthetist	Anaesthetist
Anaesthetists	Anaesth
Analgesia	Analg
Anatomical	Anat
Anatomy	Anat
Andrology	Androl
Anesthesia	Anesth
Anesthesiology	Anesthesiol
Angiology	Angiol
Angle	Angle
Animal	Anim
Ankle	Ankle
Annals	Ann
Annual	Annu
Anthropology	Anthropol
Antibiotics	Antibiot

Anticancer	Anticancer
Antigens	Antigens
Antimicrobial	Antimicrob
Antiviral	Antiviral
Apheresis	Apheresis
Appetite	Appetite
Applied	Appl
Archives	Arch
Argentina	Argent
Arizona	Ariz
Arkansas	Ark
Army	Army
Arteriosclerosis	Arterioscl
Artery	Artery
Arthritis	Arthritis
Artificial	Artif
Asian	Asian
Assessment	Assess
Association	Assoc
Asthma	Asthma
Audiology	Audiol
Audiovisual	Audiov
Auditory	Aud
Australia	Aust
Australian	Aust
Autism	Autism
Autonomic	Auton
Avian	Avian
Aviation	Aviat
Bacteriology	Bacteriol
Bangladesh	Bangladesh
Basic	Basic
Behavior	Behav
Behavioral	Behav
Behaviors	Behav
Biochemical	Biochem
Biochemistry	Biochem
Biocommunications	Biocomm
Biofeedback	Biofeedback

Biological	Biol
Biology	Biol
Biomaterials	Biomater
Biomechanical	Biomech
Biomedical	Biomed
Biometrics	Biometrics
Biophysical	Biophys
Biophysics	Biophys
Bioscience	Biosci
Biosocial	Biosoc
Biosystems	Biosystems
Biotechnological	Biotechnol
Biotechnology	Biotechnol
Birth	Birth
Blood	Blood
Bone	Bone
Brain	Brain
Brazilian	Braz
Breast	Breast
British	Br
Bulletin	Bull
Burns	Burns
Calcified	Calcif
Calcium	Calcium
Canadian	Can
Cancer	Cancer
Carbohydrate	Carbohydr
Carcinogenesis	Carcinog
Carcinogenic	Carcinog
Cardiography	Cardiogr
Cardiology	Cardiol
Cardiovascular	Cardiovasc
Care	Care
Caries	Caries
Catheterization	Cathet
Cell	Cell
Cells	Cells
Cellular	Cell
Central	Cent

Cephalalgia	Cephalalgia
Cerebral	Cereb
Ceylon	Ceylon
Chemical	Chem
Chemicals	Chem
Chemistry	Chem
Chemists	Chem
Chemotherapy	Chemother
Chest	Chest
Child	Child
Childhood	Child
Children	Child
Childs	Childs
Chinese	Chin
Chromatographic	Chromatogr
Chromatography	Chromatogr
Chronic	Chronic
Chronicle	Chron
Circulation	Circ
Circulatory	Circ
Cleft	Cleft
Cleveland	Cleve
Clinic	Clin
Clinical	Clin
Clinics	Clin
Cognition	Cogn
Collagen	Coll
College	Coll
Colon	Colon
Colorado	Colo
Communicable	Commun
Communication	Commun
Communications	Commun
Community	Community
Comparative	Comp
Complement	Complement
Comprehensive	Compr
Computerized	Comput
Computers	Comput

Connecticut	Conn
Connective	Connect
Consulting	Consult
Contact	Contact
Contaminants	Contam
Contamination	Contam
Contemporary	Contemp
Contributions	Contrib
Control	Control
Controlled	Control
Copenhagen	Copenh
Cornea	Cornea
Cornell	Cornell
Corps	Corps
Cortex	Cortex
Council	Counc
Craniofacial	Craniofac
Critical	Crit
Cryobiology	Cryobiol
Culture	Cult
Current	Curr
Currents	Curr
Cutaneous	Cutan
Cutis	Cutis
Cybernetics	Cybern
Cyclic	Cyclic
Cytogenetics	Cytogenet
Cytology	Cytol
Cytometry	Cytometry
Dairy	Dairy
Danish	Dan
Deaf	Deaf
Decision	Decis
Defects	Defects
Deficiency	Defic
Delivery	Deliv
Demography	Demogr
Dental	Dent
Dentistry	Dent

Dependencies	Dependencies
Dermatitis	Dermatitis
Dermatological	Dermatol
Dermatology	Dermatol
Dermatopathology	Dermatopathol
Detection	Detect
Development	Dev
Devices	Devices
Diabetes	Diabetes
Diagnosis	Diagn
Diagnostic	Diagn
Dialysis	Dial
Diarrhoeal	Diarrhoeal
Dietetic	Diet
Differentiation	Differ
Digestion	Digestion
Digestive	Dig
Dimensions	Dimens
Directions	Dir
Directors	Dir
Discussions	Discuss
Disease	Dis
Diseases	Dis
Disorders	Disord
Disposition	Dispos
DNA	DNA
Drug	Drug
Drugs	Drugs
Ear	Ear
Early	Early
East African	East Afr
Economic	Econ
Ecotoxicology	Ecotoxicol
Educational	Educ
Egyptian	Egypt
Electrocardiology	Electrocardiol
Electroencephalography	Electroencephalogr
Electromyography	Electromyogr
Electron	Electron

Electrotherapeutics	Electrother
Embryo	Embryo
Embryology	Embryol
Emergency	Emerg
Endocrine	Endocr
Endocrinological	Endocrinol
Endocrinology	Endocrinol
Endoscopy	Endosc
Engineering	Eng
Enteral	Enteral
Entomology	Entomol
Environmental	Environ
Enzyme	Enzyme
Enzymology	Enzymol
Epidemiologic	Epidemiol
Epidemiology	Epidemiol
Ergology	Ergol
Ergonomics	Ergonomics
Essays	Essays
Ethics	Ethics
Eugenics	Eugen
European	Eur
Evaluation	Eval
Exceptional	Except
Exercise	Exerc
Experimental	Exp
Eye	Eye
Factors	Factors
Family	Fam
Federation	Fed
Fertility	Fertil
Finnish	Finn
Fitness	Fitness
Florida	Fla
Food	Food
Foot	Foot
Forensic	Forensic
Foundation	Found

Function	Funct
Fundamental	Fundam
Gastroenterology	Gastroenterol
Gastrointestinal	Gastrointest
Gene	Gene
General	Gen
Genetic	Genet
Genetics	Genetics
Genitourinary	Genitourin
Geographical	Geogr
Georgia	Ga
Geriatric	Geriatr
Geriatrics	Geriatr
Gerontologist	Gerontologist
Gerontology	Gerontol
Group	Group
Groups	Groups
Growth	Growth
Gut	Gut
Gynaecological	Gynaecol
Gynaecology	Gynaecol
Gynecologic	Gynecol
Gynecology	Gynecol
Haematology	Haematol
Haemostasis	Haemost
Hastings Center	Hastings Cent
Hawaii	Hawaii
Head	Head
Headache	Headache
Health	Health
Hearing	Hear
Heart	Heart
Hematological	Hematol
Hematology	Hematol
Hemoglobin	Hemoglobin
Hemostasis	Hemost
Hepatology	Hepatol
Heredity	Hered
Hip	Hip

Histochemical	Histochem
Histochemistry	Histochem
Histology	Histol
Histopathology	Histopathol
History	Hist
Homosexuality	Homosex
Horizons	Horiz
Hormone	Horm
Hormones	Horm
Hospital	Hosp
Hospitals	Hospitals
Human	Hum
Humans	Hum
Hybridoma	Hybridoma
Hygiene	Hyg
Hypertension	Hypertens
Hypnosis	Hypn
Hypotheses	Hypotheses
Imaging	Imaging
Immunity	Immun
Immunoassay	Immunoassay
Immunobiology	Immunobiol
Immunogenetics	Immunogenet
Immunological	Immunol
Immunology	Immunol
Immunopharmacology	Immunopharmacol
Immunotherapy	Immunother
Implant	Implant
Including	Incl
India	India
Indian	Indian
Indiana	Indiana
Industrial	Ind
Infection	Infect
Infectious	Infect
Inflammation	Inflamm
Informatics	Inform
Information	Inf
Inherited	Inherited

Injury	Inj
Inorganic	Inorg
Inquiry	Inquiry
Institutes	Inst
Instrumentation	Instrum
Insurance	Insur
Intellectual	Intellect
Intelligence	Intell
Intensive	Intensive
Interactions	Interact
Interferon	Interferon
Internal	Intern
International	Int
Internist	Internist
Interventional	Intervent
Intervirology	Intervirol
Intraocular	Intraocul
Invasion	Invasion
Invertebrate	Invertebr
Investigation	Invest
Investigational	Investig
Investigations	Invest
Investigative	Invest
In Vitro	In Vitro
In Vivo	In Vivo
Iowa	Iowa
Irish	Ir
Isotopes	Isot
Isozymes	Isozymes
Israel	Isr
Issues	Issues
Istanbul	Istanbul
Japanese	Jpn
Joint	Joint
Journal	J
Kansas	Kans
Kentucky	Ky
Kidney	Kidney
Kinetics	Kinet

Laboratory	Lab
Language	Lang
Laparoendoscopic	Laparoendosc
Laryngology	Laryngol
Larynx	Larynx
Lasers	Lasers
Law	Law
Lectures	Lect
Legal	Leg
Leprosy	Lepr
Letters	Lett
Leukocyte	Leukoc
Leukotriene	Leukotriene
Leukotrienes	Leukotrienes
Library	Libr
Life	Life
Life-threatening	Life Threat
Lipid	Lipid
Lipids	Lipids
Literature	Lit
Louisiana	La
Lung	Lung
Lymphokine	Lymphokine
Lymphology	Lymphol
Madagascar	Madagascar
Magnesium	Magnesium
Magnetic	Magn
Main	Main
Making	Making
Malaysia	Malaysia
Management	Manage
Manipulative	Manipulative
Marital	Marital
Maritime	Marit
Maryland	Md
Mass	Mass
Mathematical	Math
Maxillofacial	Maxillofac
Measurement	Meas

Mechanisms	Mech
Media	Media
Medical	Med
Medicinal	Med
Medicine	Med
Membrane	Membr
Mental	Ment
Metabolic	Metab
Metabolism	Metab
Metastasis	Metastasis
Methods	Methods
Mexico	Mex
Michigan	Mich
Microbial	Microb
Microbiological	Microbiol
Microbiology	Microbiol
Microcirculation	Microcirc
Microscopy	Microsc
Microvascular	Microvasc
Microwave	Microw
Military	Milit
Mineral	Miner
Minnesota	Minn
Mississippi	Miss
Missouri	Mo
Modification	Modif
Molecular	Mol
Monographs	Monogr
Morphology	Morphol
Motility	Motil
Muscle	Muscle
Mutagenesis	Mutagen
Mutation	Mutat
Mycobacterial	Mycobact
Narcotics	Narc
National	Natl
Natural	Nat
Nature	Nat
Naval	Nav

Nebraska	Nebr
Neck	Neck
Neglect	Negl
Neonate	Neonate
Nephrology	Nephrol
Nephron	Nephron
Nervosa	Nerv
Nervous	Nerv
Netherlands	Neth
Neural	Neural
Neurobehavioral	Neurobehav
Neurobiology	Neurobiol
Neurochemistry	Neurochem
Neurocytology	Neurocytol
Neuroendocrinology	Neuroendocrinol
Neurogenetics	Neurogenet
Neuroimmunology	Neuroimmunol
Neurologic	Neurol
Neurological	Neurol
Neurology	Neurol
Neuropathology	Neuropathol
Neuropediatrics	Neuropediatr
Neuropeptides	Neuropeptides
Neuropharmacology	Neuropharmacol
Neurophysiology	Neurophysiol
Neuropsychobiology	Neuropsychobiol
Neuropsychology	Neuropsychol
Neuropsychopharmacology	Neuropsychopharmacol
Neuroradiology	Neuroradiol
Neuroscience	Neurosci
Neurosurgery	Neurosurg
Neurosurgical	Neurosurg
Neurotoxicology	Neurotoxicol
Neurotrauma	Neurotrauma
New	N
New England	N Engl
New Jersey	N J
New Orleans	New Orleans
New York	N Y

New Zealand	N Z
North America	North Am
North Carolina	N C
Nose	Nose
Nuclear	Nucl
Nucleotide	Nucleotide
Nurse	Nurse
Nursing	Nurs
Nutrition	Nutr
Nutritional	Nutr
Obesity	Obes
Obstetric	Obstet
Obstetrics	Obstet
Occupational	Occup
Ocular	Ocul
Official	Off
Ohio	Ohio
Oklahoma	Okla
Oncology	Oncol
Ophthalmic	Ophthalmic
Ophthalmological	Ophthalmol
Ophthalmology	Ophthalmol
Optical	Opt
Optics	Opt
Optometric	Optom
Optometry	Optom
Oral	Oral
Organization	Organ
Organs	Organs
Orthodontics	Orthod
Orthodontist	Orthod
Orthopaedic	Orthop
Orthopsychiatry	Orthopsychiatry
Orthotics	Orthot
Osaka	Osaka
Oslo	Oslo
Osteopathic	Osteopath
Otolaryngology	Otolaryngol

Otology	Otol
Otorhinolaryngology	Otorhinolaryngol
Pace	Pace
Paediatric	Paediatr
Paediatrics	Paediatr
Palate	Palate
Panama	Panama
Pan American	Pan Am
Paper	Pap
Papua New Guinea	Papua New Guinea
Parasite	Parasite
Parasitology	Parasitol
Parenteral	Parenter
Pathology	Pathol
Pediatrician	Pediatrician
Pediatrics	Pediatr
Pennsylvania	Pa
Peptide	Pept
Peptides	Pept
Perception	Perception
Perceptual	Percept
Perinatal	Perinat
Perinatology	Perinatol
Periodontal	Periodont
Periodontology	Periodontol
Personality	Pers
Perspectives	Perspect
Pharmaceutical	Pharm
Pharmacokinetics	Pharmacokinet
Pharmacology	Pharmacol
Pharmacopsychiatry	Pharmacopsychiatry
Pharmacotherapy	Pharmacother
Pharmacy	Pharm
Philosophical	Philos
Phosphorylation	Phosphorylation
Photobiology	Photobiol
Photochemistry	Photochem
Photodermatology	Photodermatol
Photography	Photogr

Physical	Phys
Physician	Physician
Physicians	Physicians
Physics	Phys
Physiological	Physiol
Physiology	Physiol
Placenta	Placenta
Planning	Plann
Plastic	Plast
Podiatric	Podiatr
Podiatry	Podiatry
Poisoning	Poisoning
Policy	Policy
Politics	Polit
Pollution	Pollut
Population	Popul
Postgraduate	Postgrad
Poultry	Poult
Practice	Pract
Practitioners	Pract
Pregnancy	Pregnancy
Prenatal	Prenat
Preparative	Prep
Prevention	Prev
Preventive	Prev
Primary	Primary
Primatology	Primatol
Proceedings	Proc
Process	Process
Processes	Processes
Products	Prod
Programs	Programs
Progress	Prog
Prostaglandin	Prostaglandin
Prostaglandins	Prostaglandins
Prostate	Prostate
Prosthetic	Prosthet
Prosthetics	Prosthet
Protein	Protein

Protozoology	Protozool
Psyche	Psyche
Psychiatric	Psychiatr
Psychiatry	Psychiatry
Psychoactive	Psychoactive
Psychoanalysis	Psychoanal
Psychoanalytic	Psychoanal
Psycholinguistic	Psycholinguist
Psychologist	Psychol
Psychology	Psychol
Psychoneuroendocrinology	Psychoneuroendocrinol
Psychopathology	Psychopathol
Psychopharmacology	Psychopharmacol
Psychophysiology	Psychophysiol
Psychosocial	Psychosoc
Psychosomatic	Psychosom
Psychosomatics	Psychosom
Psychotherapy	Psychother
Public	Public
Puerto Rico	P R
Quantitative	Quant
Quarterly	Q
Radiation	Radiat
Radiography	Radiogr
Radioisotopes	Radioisotopes
Radiologists	Radiol
Radiology	Radiol
Rational	Ration
Reactions	React
Recombinant	Recomb
Reconstructive	Reconstr
Record	Rec
Rectum	Rectum
Regional	Reg
Regulation	Regul
Regulatory	Regul
Rehabilitation	Rehabil
Renal	Renal
Report	Rep

Reports	Rep
Reproduction	Reprod
Reproductive	Reprod
Research	Res
Residue	Residue
Resonance	Reson
Respiration	Respir
Respiratory	Respir
Response	Response
Resuscitation	Resuscitation
Retardation	Retard
Retina	Retina
Review	Rev
Reviews	Rev
Rheumatic	Rheum
Rheumatism	Rheum
Rheumatology	Rheumatol
Rhinology	Rhinol
Rhode Island	R I
Safety	Safety
Scandinavian	Scand
Scanning	Scan
Schizophrenia	Schizophr
School	Sch
Science	Sci
Sciences	Sci
Scientific	Sci
Scottish	Scott
Security	Secur
Seminars	Semin
Series	Ser
Service	Serv
Sex	Sex
Sexual	Sex
Sexually	Sex
Shock	Shock
Singapore	Singapore
Skeletal	Skeletal
Sleep	Sleep

Social	Soc
Societies	Soc
Society	Soc
Sociological	Sociol
Sociology	Sociol
Somatic	Somatic
Somatosensory	Somatosens
South African	S Afr
South Carolina	S C
South Dakota	S D
Southeast	Southeast
Southern	South
Space	Space
Spectrometry	Spectrom
Speech	Speech
Spine	Spine
Sports	Sports
Stain	Stain
Standardization	Stand
Standards	Stand
Statistical	Stat
Steroid	Steroid
Steroids	Steroids
Stockholm	Stockh
Strabismus	Strabismus
Stress	Stress
Stroke	Stroke
Structure	Struct
Studies	Stud
Subcellular	Subcell
Submicroscopic	Submicrosc
Substance	Subst
Suicide	Suicide
Superior	Super
Support	Support
Surgeon	Surg
Surgeons	Surg
Surgery	Surg

Surgical	Surg
Swedish	Swed
Symposia	Symp
Symposium	Symp
System	Syst
Systems	Syst
Technical	Tech
Technology	Technol
Tennessee	Tenn
Teratogenesis	Teratogenesis
Teratology	Teratol
Thailand	Thai
Theoretical	Theor
Therapeutics	Ther
Therapies	Ther
Therapy	Ther
Thermal	Therm
Thoracic	Thorac
Thorax	Thorax
Throat	Throat
Thrombosis	Thromb
Thromboxane	Thromboxane
Thymus	Thymus
Tissue	Tissue
Today	Today
Tokyo	Tokyo
Tomography	Tomogr
Topics	Top
Total	Total
Toxicologic	Toxicol
Toxicological	Toxicol
Toxicology	Toxicol
Traditional	Tradit
Transactions	Trans
Transfer	Transfer
Transfusion	Transfusion
Transmission	Transm
Transmitted	Transm

Transplant	Transplant
Transplantation	Transplantation
Traumatic	Trauma
Tropical	Trop
Tuberculosis	Tuberc
Tumor	Tumor
Tumour	Tumour
Tunis	Tunis
Turkish	Turk
Ulster	Ulster
Ultramicroscopy	Ultramicrosc
Ultrasonic	Ultrason
Ultrasonics	Ultrasonics
Ultrasound	Ultrasound
Ultrastructural	Ultrastruct
Ultrastructure	Ultrastruct
Undersea	Undersea
Union	Union
Uremia	Uremia
Vision	Vis
Visual	Vis
Vital	Vital
Vitamin	Vitam
Vitaminology	Vitaminol
Vitamins	Vitam
Vitro	Vitro
Vivo	Vivo
Welfare	Welfare
Western	West
West Indian	West Indian
West Virginia	W Va
Wildlife	Wildl
Wisconsin	Wis
Women	Women
Women's	Womens
Zoology	Zool
Zoonoses	Zoonoses

14.11 Clinical, Technical, and Other Common Terms. This compilation of clinical, technical, and other common terms and their abbreviations is not intended to be all-encompassing but is provided as a short reference. There are many published listings of abbreviations, acronyms, and initialisms.

Many entities share the same abbreviation (eg, American Heart Association, American Hospital Association, American Historical Association, American Humanist Association, American Hyperlexia Association, American Hydrogen Association). Thus, preciseness takes precedence over abbreviating.

In addition, some abbreviations encompass more than one grammatical variant (eg, noun, adjective) of a term. For example, ECG represents both electrocardiogram and electrocardiographic. It is unnecessary to redefine the abbreviation for each variation in usage within a body of work. Similarly, terms that have singular and plural forms (eg, WBC and WBCs) are defined once, whichever form is mentioned first.

When the expanded form is possessive at first mention, the parenthetical abbreviation is also possessive at first mention:

> The National Aeronautics and Space Administration's (NASA's) Implementation Plan for Space Shuttle Return to Space and Beyond was the NASA response to the *Columbia* disaster in 2003.

Most terms should be expanded at first mention. However, considerations for which this general rule might be set aside include comprehensibility, recognition, and space, as well as avoidance of cumbersome expressions. Exceptions include using the abbreviation instead of the expansion in a long title or subtitle, a letter to the editor, or an informal essay.

Use common sense in deciding whether to abbreviate the terms in the following list and other terms. For example, if "acute respiratory distress syndrome" appears only once or twice in an article, spell it out. If the article concerns acute respiratory distress syndrome and the term is used several times, expand the term at first mention with the abbreviation immediately following in parentheses. Abbreviate it thereafter.

Note: Some terms may be known better in their abbreviated form (eg, HIPAA), and abbreviating them at first mention (with the expanded form following in parentheses) may be appropriate.

Avoid using abbreviations at the beginning of a sentence unless the expansion is cumbersome, eg, a collaborative group name or other acronym pronounced as a word (ALLHAT, AIDS, CLIA, UNICEF) (see also 14.8, Agencies and Organizations, and 14.9, Collaborative Groups).

Do not use an abbreviation as the sole term in a subheading. Also avoid introducing an abbreviation in a subheading:

> *Avoid:*
>
> **National Institutes of Health (NIH)**
> The NIH is the steward of medical and behavioral research for the United States. It is an agency under the US Department of Health and Human Services.

Preferred:

National Institutes of Health
The National Institutes of Health (NIH) is the steward of medical and behavioral research for the United States. It is an agency under the US Department of Health and Human Services.

Apply the foregoing concepts to each element of the manuscript. See also 14.0, Abbreviations, and 2.0, Manuscript Preparation, as well as specific nomenclature sections (15.0, Nomenclature), for additional guidelines for correct use of specialized terms and their abbreviations. (See also 4.0, Visual Presentation of Data.)

Note: At a 2004 National Summit on Medical Abbreviations, the Joint Commission on Accreditation of Healthcare Organizations (JCAHO) approved an official "do not use" list of abbreviations. It is important to note that this list applies to all medical orders and all medication-related documentation that are handwritten or on preprinted forms used in hospitals and other health care facilities. The JCAHO requirement does not apply to the use of abbreviations in the publication of articles in scientific journals.

However, authors and editors should be mindful of the possibility of introducing error in journal articles when using certain abbreviations and symbols. Other organizations (eg, see the Institute for Safe Medication Practices at http://www.ismp.org) have suggested the desirability of even more stringent initiatives against the use of certain abbreviations and symbols, which are designed to protect patients from potential harm.

Note: JAMA and the *Archives* Journals do not endorse any proprietary entities in this list.

Abbreviation	*Expanded Form*
AAA	abdominal aortic aneurysm
ABC	avidin-biotin complex
AC	alternating current
ACE	angiotensin-converting enzyme
ACS	acute coronary syndromes
ACTH	Use *corticotropin* (formerly adrenocorticotropic hormone)
AD	Alzheimer disease
ADH	antidiuretic hormone
ADHD	attention-deficit/hyperactivity disorder
ADL	activities of daily living (*but*: 1 ADL, 6 ADLs)
aDNA	ancient DNA
ADP	adenosine diphosphate
ADPase	adenosine diphosphatase
AED	automated external defibrillator
AF	atrial fibrillation
AFP	α-fetoprotein
AIDS*	acquired immunodeficiency syndrome

ALL	acute lymphoblastic leukemia; acute lymphocytic leukemia
allo-SCT	allogeneic stem cell transplantation
ALS	amyotrophic lateral sclerosis
ALT	alanine aminotransferase (previously SGPT)
AML	acute monocytic leukemia; acute myeloblastic leukemia; acute myelocytic leukemia
AMP	adenosine monophosphate
ANA	antinuclear antibody
ANCOVA	analysis of covariance
ANLL	acute nonlymphocytic leukemia
ANOVA	analysis of variance
AOR	adjusted odds ratio
APACHE	Acute Physiology and Chronic Health Evaluation
APB	atrial premature beat
APC	atrial premature contraction
ARC	Use *symptomatic HIV infection* (formerly AIDS-related complex)
ARDS	acute respiratory distress syndrome
ARMD	age-related macular degeneration
ARR	absolute risk reduction
ART	antiretroviral therapy
ASC	adult stem cell
ASC-US	atypical squamous cells of uncertain significance
ASD	atrial septal defect; autistic spectrum disorder
AST	aspartate aminotransferase (previously SGOT)
ATP	adenosine triphosphate
ATPase	adenosine triphosphatase
AUC	area under the curve
AUROC	area under the receiver operating characteristic curve
BAC	blood alcohol concentration
BADL	basic activities of daily living (use *activities of daily living*)
BAER	brainstem auditory evoked response
BCG	bacille Calmette-Guérin (*but*: do not expand as a drug: BCG vaccine)
BDI	Beck Depression Inventory
bid	twice a day (do not abbreviate)
BMD	bone mineral density
BMI	body mass index

BMT	bone marrow transplantation
BP	blood pressure
BPD	bronchopulmonary dysplasia
BPH	benign prostatic hyperplasia
BPRS	Brief Psychiatric Rating Scale
BSA	body surface area
BSE	bovine spongiform encephalopathy; breast self-examination
BUN	blood urea nitrogen (use *serum urea nitrogen*)
C*	complement (use with a number, eg, C1, C2, . . . C9; see 15.8.3, Nomenclature, Immunology, Complement)
c, ca	circa (do not abbreviate)
CABG	coronary artery bypass graft
CAD	coronary artery disease
CAGE	cut down, annoyed, guilty, eye opener (screening questionnaire for potential alcoholism)
CAM	complementary and alternative medicine
cAMP	cyclic adenosine monophosphate
CARS	compensatory anti-inflammatory response syndrome
CART	combination antiretroviral therapy
CBC	complete blood (add *cell*) count
CCU	cardiac care unit; critical care unit
CD*	clusters of differentiation (use with a number, eg, CD4 cell; see 15.8.2, Nomenclature, Immunology, CD Cell Markers)
CD*	compact disc
cDNA	complementary DNA
CD-ROM*	compact disc read-only memory
CEA	carcinoembryonic antigen; cost-effective analysis
CEU	continuing education unit
cf*	compare
CF	cystic fibrosis
CFS	chronic fatigue syndrome
CFT	complement fixation test
CFU	colony-forming unit
cGMP	cyclic guanosine monophosphate
CHD	coronary heart disease
CHF	congestive heart failure
CI	confidence interval
CIN	cervical intraepithelial neoplasia
CIS	carcinoma in situ

CJD	Creutzfeldt-Jakob disease
CK	creatine kinase
CK-BB	creatine kinase BB (BB designates the isozyme)
CK-MB	creatine kinase MB
CK-MM	creatine kinase MM
CL	confidence limit
CLIA	Clinical Laboratory Improvement Amendments
CME	continuing medical education (often used without expansion when describing credit hours, eg, category 1 CME credit)
CMI	cell-mediated immunity
CML	chronic myelocytic leukemia
CMV	cytomegalovirus
CNS	central nervous system
CONSORT	Consolidated Standards of Reporting Trials
COPD	chronic obstructive pulmonary disease
COX-2	cyclooxygenase 2
CPAP	continuous positive airway pressure
CPD	continuing professional development
CPK	Use *creatine kinase*
CPR	cardiopulmonary resuscitation
CPT	*Current Procedural Terminology*
CQI	continuous quality improvement
CRF	corticotropin-releasing factor
cRNA	complementary RNA
CRP	C-reactive protein
CSF	cerebrospinal fluid; colony-stimulating factor
CST*	central standard time
CT	computed tomographic; computed tomography
CUA	cost-utility analysis
CVS	chorionic villus sampling
DALY	disability-adjusted life-year
dAMP	deoxyadenosine monophosphate (deoxyadenylate)
D&C	dilation and curettage
DC	direct current
DCIS	ductal carcinoma in situ
DDD	defined daily dose
DDT*	dichlorodiphenyltrichloroethane (chlorophenothane)
DE	dose equivalent

DEV	duck embryo vaccine
DFA	direct fluorescence assay
dGMP	deoxyguanosine monophosphate (deoxyguanylate)
DIC	disseminated intravascular coagulation
DIF	direct immunofluorescence
DNA*	deoxyribonucleic acid
DNAR	do not attempt resuscitation
DNase	deoxyribonuclease
DNH	do not hospitalize
DNR	do not resuscitate
DOS*	disk operating system
DOT	directly observed therapy
DOTS	directly observed therapy, short course
dpi*	dots per inch
DRE	digital rectal examination
DRG	diagnosis related group
DS	duplex sonography
DSM-III	*Diagnostic and Statistical Manual of Mental Disorders* (Third Edition)
DSM-III-R	*Diagnostic and Statistical Manual of Mental Disorders* (Third Edition Revised)
DSM-IV	*Diagnostic and Statistical Manual of Mental Disorders* (Fourth Edition)
DSM-IV-TR	*Diagnostic and Statistical Manual of Mental Disorders* (Fourth Edition, Text Revision)
DSMB	data and safety monitoring board
DT	delirium tremens
DTaP	diphtheria and tetanus toxoids and acellular pertussis [vaccine]
DTP	diphtheria and tetanus toxoids and pertussis [vaccine]
DXA	dual-energy x-ray absorptiometry
EBM	evidence-based medicine
EBV	Epstein-Barr virus
EC	ejection click
ECA	epidemiologic catchment area
ECG	electrocardiogram; electrocardiographic
ECMO	extracorporeal membrane oxygenation
ECT	electroconvulsive therapy
ED	effective dose; emergency department
ED_{50}	median effective dose

EDTA*	ethylenediaminetetraacetic acid
EEE	eastern equine encephalomyelitis
EEG	electroencephalogram; electroencephalographic
eg*	for example (from the Latin *exempli gratia*; see 11.1, Correct and Preferred Usage, Correct and Preferred Usage of Common Words and Phrases)
EGD	esophagogastroduodenoscopy
EIA	enzyme immunoassay
ELISA	enzyme-linked immunosorbent assay
EM	electron microscope; electron microscopic; electron microscopy
EMG	electromyogram; electromyographic
EMIT	enzyme-multiplied immunoassay technique
EMS	electrical muscle stimulation; emergency medical services; eosinophilia-myalgia syndrome
EMT	emergency medical technician
ENG	electronystagmogram; electronystagmographic
EOG	electro-oculogram; electro-oculographic
ERCP	endoscopic retrograde cholangiopancreatography
ERG	electroretinogram; electroretinographic
ESBC	extended-spectrum β-lactamases
ESC	embryonic stem cell
ESR	erythrocyte sedimentation rate
ESRD	end-stage renal disease
EST*	eastern standard time
ESWL	extracorporeal shock wave lithotripsy
etc*	et cetera (and so forth) (see 11.1, Correct and Preferred Usage, Correct and Preferred Usage of Common Words and Phrases)
EVR	evoked visual response
F*	French (add *catheter*; use only with a number, eg, 12F catheter)
$FEF_{25\%-75\%}$	forced expiratory flow, midexpiratory phase (see 15.16, Nomenclature, Pulmonary, Respiratory, and Blood Gas Terminology)
FEV	forced expiratory volume
FEV_1	forced expiratory volume in the first second of expiration
F_{IO_2}	fraction of inspired oxygen
FISH	fluorescence in situ hybridization
FLAIR	fluid-attenuated inversion recovery
FSH	follicle-stimulating hormone

FTA	fluorescent treponemal antibody
FTA-ABS	fluorescent treponemal antibody absorption (add *test*)
FUO	fever of unknown origin
FVC	forced vital capacity
GABA	γ-aminobutyric acid
GAD	generalized anxiety disorder
GAF	Global Assessment of Functioning [Scale]
GB*	gigabyte
GCS	Glasgow Coma Scale
G-CSF	granulocyte colony-stimulating factor
GDP	guanosine diphosphate
GDS	Geriatric Depression Scale
GED	General Education Development
GERD	gastroesophageal reflux disease
GFR	glomerular filtration rate
GH	growth hormone
GI	gastrointestinal
GIFT	gamete intrafallopian transfer
GLC	gas-liquid chromatography
GM-CSF	granulocyte-macrophage colony-stimulating factor
GMP	guanosine monophosphate (guanylate, guanylic acid)
GMRI	gated magnetic resonance imaging
GMT	geometric mean titer
GMT*	Greenwich mean time
GnRH	gonadotropin-releasing hormone (*gonadorelin* as diagnostic agent)
GSC	germline stem cell
GU	genitourinary
GUI	graphical user interface
GVHD	graft-vs-host disease
HAART	highly active antiretroviral therapy
HALE	health-adjusted life expectancy
HAV	hepatitis A virus (see 15.14.3, Nomenclature, Organisms and Pathogens, Virus and Prion Nomenclature)
HbA_{1c}	hemoglobin A_{1c}
Hbco	carboxyhemoglobin
HBO	hyperbaric oxygen
Hbo_2	oxyhemoglobin; oxygenated hemoglobin
HbS	sickle cell hemoglobin

HBsAg	hepatitis B surface antigen (see 15.14.3, Nomenclature, Organisms and Pathogens, Virus and Prion Nomenclature)
HBSS	Hanks balanced salt solution
HBV	hepatitis B virus
hCG	human chorionic gonadotropin (do not abbreviate when used as a drug)
HCV	hepatitis C virus (see 15.14.3, Nomenclature, Organisms and Pathogens, Virus and Prion Nomenclature)
HDL	high-density lipoprotein
HDL-C	high-density lipoprotein cholesterol
HDRS	Hamilton Depression Rating Scale
hGH	human growth hormone
HHV	human herpesvirus
Hib	*Haemophilus influenzae* type b [vaccine or disease] (see 15.14.2, Nomenclature, Organisms and Pathogens, Bacteria: Additional Terminology)
HIPAA	Health Insurance Portability and Accountability Act
HIV	human immunodeficiency virus
HL	hearing level
HLA*	human leukocyte antigen (use "HLA antigen"; see 15.8.5, Nomenclature, Immunology, HLA/Major Histocompatibility Complex)
HMO	health maintenance organization
HPF	high-power field
HPLC	high-performance liquid chromatography
HPV	human papillomavirus (add hyphen to abbreviation when indicating type, eg, HPV-6)
HR	hazard ratio
HRQOL	health-related quality of life
HSC	hematopoietic stem cell
HSIL	high-grade squamous intraepithelial lesion
HSV	herpes simplex virus
HT	hormone therapy
5-HT	Use *serotonin* (also 5-hydroxytryptamine)
HTLV	human T-lymphotropic virus (use arabic numeral with specific type, eg, HTLV-1)
HTML*	hypertext markup language
http*	hypertext transfer protocol
HUS	hemolytic uremic syndrome
IADL	instrumental activities of daily living (*but*: 1 IADL, 6 IADLs)
ICD	implantable cardioverter-defibrillator

ICD-9	*International Classification of Diseases, Ninth Revision*
ICD-9-CM	*International Classification of Diseases, Ninth Revision, Clinical Modification*
ICD-10	*International Classification of Diseases, Tenth Revision*
ICD-10-CM	*International Classification of Diseases, Tenth Revision, Clinical Modification*
ICU	intensive care unit
ID	infective dose
IDU	injecting drug user; injection drug user
ie*	that is (from the Latin *id est*; see 11.1, Correct and Preferred Usage, Correct and Preferred Usage of Common Words and Phrases)
IFN	interferon (do not abbreviate when used as drug; see 15.4.13, Nomenclature, Drugs, Nomenclature for Biological Products)
Ig	immunoglobulin (abbreviate only with specification of class, eg, IgA, IgG, IgM; see 15.8.6, Nomenclature, Immunology, Immunoglobulins)
IGF-1	insulinlike growth factor 1
IL	interleukin (abbreviate only when indicating a specific protein factor, eg, IL-2) (see 15.8.4, Nomenclature, Immunology, Cytokines)
IM	intramuscular; intramuscularly
IND	investigational new drug
INR	international normalized ratio
IOP	intraocular pressure
IPA	intimate partner abuse
IPV	intimate partner violence
IQ*	intelligence quotient
IRB	institutional review board
IRMA	immunoradiometric assay
ISBN*	International Standard Book Number
ISG	immune serum globulin
ISSN*	International Standard Serial Number
ITI	intratubal insemination
ITP	idiopathic thrombocytopenic purpura
ITT	intention to treat
IUD	intrauterine device
IUGR	intrauterine growth retardation
IUI	intrauterine insemination
IV	intravenous; intravenously

IVF	in vitro fertilization
IVIG	intravenous immunoglobulin
IVP	intravenous pyelogram
JPEG*	Joint Photographic Experts Group (computer file format for digital images)
kB*	kilobyte
KUB	kidneys, ureter, bladder [plain abdominal radiograph]
LA	left atrium
LAD	left anterior descending coronary artery
LAO	left anterior oblique coronary artery
LASEK	laser epithelial keratomileusis
LASIK	laser in situ keratomileusis
LAV	lymphadenopathy-associated virus
LBW	low birth weight (*but:* low-birth-weight infant)
LCA	left coronary artery
LCR	locus control region
LCX, CX	left circumflex coronary artery
LD	lethal dose
LD_{50}	median lethal dose
LDH	lactate dehydrogenase
LDL	low-density lipoprotein
LDL-C	low-density lipoprotein cholesterol
LGA	large for gestational age
LH	luteinizing hormone
LHRH	luteinizing hormone-releasing hormone (*gonadorelin* as diagnostic agent)
LMW	low molecular weight (usually refers to low-molecular-weight heparin)
LOCF	last observation carried forward
LOD	logarithm of odds
logMAR	logarithm of the minimum angle of resolution
LOS	length of stay
LR	likelihood ratio
LSD	lysergic acid diethylamide
LSIL	low-grade squamous intraepithelial lesion
LV	left ventricle; left ventricular
LVEDV	left ventricular end-diastolic volume

LVEF	left ventricular ejection fraction
LVOT	left ventricular outflow tract
m-*	meta- (use only in chemical formulas or names)
MAOI	monoamine oxidase inhibitor
MAPC	multipotent adult progenitor cell
MB*	megabyte
MBC	minimum bactericidal concentration
MCH	mean corpuscular hemoglobin
MCHC	mean corpuscular hemoglobin concentration
MCO	managed care organization
MCV	mean corpuscular volume
MD	muscular dystrophy
MDR	multidrug-resistant
MEC	mean effective concentration
MEM	minimal essential medium
MEN	multiple endocrine neoplasia [type 1: MEN-1; type 2: MEN-2, etc]
MeSH	Medical Subject Headings [of the US National Library of Medicine]
MET	metabolic equivalent task
MGUS	monoclonal gammopathy of uncertain significance
MHC	major histocompatibility complex
MI	mitral insufficiency; myocardial infarction
MIC	minimum inhibitory concentration
MICU	medical intensive care unit
MMPI	Minnesota Multiphasic Personality Inventory
MMR	measles-mumps-rubella [vaccine]
MMSE	Mini-Mental State Examination
MODS	multiple-organ dysfunction syndrome
MOOSE	Meta-analysis of Observational Studies in Epidemiology
MPS	Mortality Probability Score
MRA	magnetic resonance angiography
MRI	magnetic resonance imaging
mRNA	messenger RNA
MRSA	methicillin-resistant *Staphylococcus aureus*
MS	mitral stenosis; multiple sclerosis
MSA	metropolitan statistical area
MSC	mesenchymal stem cell
MSET	multistage exercise test

MST*	mountain standard time
MVC	motor vehicle crash
NAD	nicotinamide adenine dinucleotide
NADP	nicotinamide adenine dinucleotide phosphate
nb*	*nota bene* (note well)
NDA	new drug application
Nd:YAG*	neodymium:yttrium-aluminum-garnet [laser]
NEC	necrotizing enterocolitis
NF	*National Formulary*
NICU	neonatal intensive care unit
NK	natural killer (add *cells*)
NMN	nicotinamide mononucleotide
NNH	number needed to harm
NNS	number needed to screen
NNT	number needed to treat
NOS	not otherwise specified
npo	nothing by mouth (do not abbreviate)
NPV	negative predictive value
NS	not significant (see 20.0, Study Design and Statistics)
NSAID	nonsteroidal anti-inflammatory drug
NSC	neural stem cell
NSTE	non-ST-segment elevation
*o-**	ortho- (use only in chemical formulas)
OC	oral contraceptive
OCD	obsessive-compulsive disorder
OD*	oculus dexter (right eye) (use only with a number, as in a refraction)
OGTT	oral glucose tolerance test
OR	odds ratio
OS*	oculus sinister (left eye) (use only with a number, as in a refraction)
OS	opening snap
OSA	obstructive sleep apnea
OU*	oculus unitas (both eyes) or oculus uterque (each eye) (use only with a number)
*p-**	para- (use only in chemical formulas or names)
PA	posteroanterior; pulmonary artery
PAC	premature atrial contraction; pulmonary artery catheter

$Pa{CO_2}$*	partial pressure of carbon dioxide, arterial (see 15.16, Nomenclature, Pulmonary, Respiratory, and Blood Gas Terminology)
$Pa{O_2}$*	partial pressure of oxygen, arterial
$PA{O_2}$	partial pressure of oxygen in the alveoli
PAD	peripheral artery disease
PAS	periodic acid-Schiff
PAT	paroxysmal atrial tachycardia
PBS	phosphate-buffered saline
PBSC	peripheral blood stem cell
PCI	percutaneous coronary intervention
$P{CO_2}$*	partial pressure of carbon dioxide
PCP	*Pneumocystis jiroveci* pneumonia (formerly *Pneumocystis carinii* pneumonia)
PCR	polymerase chain reaction
PCT	practical clinical trial; pragmatic clinical trial
PCW	pulmonary capillary wedge [pressure]
PDA	patent ductus arteriosus
PDA*	personal digital assistant
PDF*	portable document format
PDR	*Physicians' Desk Reference*
PE	pulmonary embolism
PEEP	positive end-expiratory pressure
PEG	percutaneous endoscopic gastrostomy; pneumoencephalographic; pneumoencephalography
PEP	postexposure prophylaxis
PET	positron emission tomographic; positron emission tomography
PFGE	pulsed-field gel electrophoresis
PGF	placental growth factor
pH*	negative logarithm of hydrogen ion concentration
PICC	peripherally inserted central catheter
PICU	pediatric intensive care unit
PID	pelvic inflammatory disease
PKU	phenylketonuria
PMS	premenstrual syndrome
po	orally (do not abbreviate)
$P{O_2}$*	partial pressure of oxygen
POAG	primary open-angle glaucoma
PPD	purified protein derivative (tuberculin)

PPO	preferred provider organization
PPROM	preterm premature rupture of membranes
PPV	positive predictive value
prn	as needed (do not abbreviate)
PRO	peer review organization; professional review organization
PROM	premature rupture of membranes
PSA	prostate-specific antigen
$Psqo_2$	subcutaneous tissue oxygen tension
PSRO	professional standards review organization
PST*	Pacific standard time
PSVT	paroxysmal supraventricular tachycardia
PT	physical therapy; prothrombin time
PTCA	percutaneous transluminal coronary angioplasty
PTSD	posttraumatic stress disorder
PTT	partial thromboplastin time
PUFA	polyunsaturated fatty acid
PUVA	psoralen-UV-A
PVC	premature ventricular contraction
PVR	peripheral vascular resistance; pulmonary vascular resistance
PVS	permanent vegetative state; persistent vegetative state
QA	quality assurance
QALY	quality-adjusted life-year
QC	quality control
qd	every day (do not abbreviate)
QI	quality improvement
qid	4 times a day (do not abbreviate)
qod	every other day (do not abbreviate)
QOL	quality of life
QUOROM	Quality of Reporting of Meta-analyses
RA	rheumatoid arthritis
RAM*	random access memory
RAST	radioallergosorbent test
RBC	red blood cell
RBRVS	resource-based relative value scale
RCA	right coronary artery
RCT	randomized clinical trial; randomized controlled trial
RDA	recommended daily allowance; recommended dietary allowance
RDC	Research Diagnostic Criteria

rDNA	ribosomal DNA
RDS	respiratory distress syndrome
REM	rapid eye movement
RFLP	restriction fragment length polymorphism
RFP	radiofrequency pulse
rh	recombinant human
Rh*	rhesus (of, related to, or being an Rh antibody, blood group, or factor)
rhNGF	recombinant human nerve growth factor
RIA	radioimmunoassay
RIND	reversible ischemic neurological deficit
RNA*	ribonucleic acid
RNAi	RNA interference
ROC	receiver operating characteristic [curve]
ROM*	read-only memory
ROP	retinopathy of prematurity
RPR	rapid plasma reagin
RR	relative risk; risk ratio
RSV	respiratory syncytial virus
RT-PCR	reverse transcription-polymerase chain reaction
RV	right ventricle; right ventricular
RVEF	right ventricular ejection fraction
RVOT	right ventricular outflow tract
SAD	seasonal affective disorder
SADS	Schedule for Affective Disorders and Schizophrenia
SAH	subarachnoid hemorrhage
SAPS	Simplified Acute Physiology Score
SARS	severe acute respiratory syndrome
SAS*	Statistical Analysis System
SCID	severe combined immunodeficiency; Structured Clinical Interview for *DSM* (use with *DSM* edition number)
SD	standard deviation (abbreviate only when used with a number, eg, 2 SDs; or in Mean [SD] construction in table stubs and headings)
SE	standard error (abbreviate only when used with a number; see ***SD***)
SEM	standard error of the mean (abbreviate only when used with a number; see ***SD***)
SEM	scanning electron microscope; systolic ejection murmur
SF-36	36-Item Short Form Health Survey

SGA	small for gestational age
SGML*	standardized general markup language
SGOT	Use *aspartate aminotransferase* (for serum glutamic-oxaloacetic transaminase)
SGPT	Use *alanine aminotransferase* (for serum glutamic-pyruvic transaminase)
SIADH	syndrome of inappropriate secretion of antidiuretic hormone
SICU	surgical intensive care unit
SIDS	sudden infant death syndrome
SIL	squamous intraepithelial lesion
SIP	Sickness Impact Profile
siRNA	small interfering RNA
SIRS	systemic inflammatory response syndrome
SLE	St Louis encephalitis; systemic lupus erythematosus
SNP	single-nucleotide polymorphism
SPECT	single-photon emission computed tomography
SPF	sun protection factor
SPSS*	Statistical Product and Service Solutions (formerly Statistical Package for the Social Sciences)
SSC	somatic stem cell
SSC*	standard saline citrate
SSNRI	selective serotonin-norepinephrine reuptake inhibitor
SSPE*	sodium chloride, sodium phosphate, EDTA [buffer]
SSPE	subacute sclerosing panencephalitis
SSRI	selective serotonin reuptake inhibitor
STARD	Standards for Reporting Diagnostic Accuracy
STD	sexually transmitted disease
STEMI	ST-segment elevation myocardial infarction
STI	sexually transmitted infection; structured treatment interruption
SUN	serum urea nitrogen
SVR	systemic vascular resistance
$t_{1/2}$	half-life
T_3	triiodothyronine
T_4	thyroxine
TAHBSO	total abdominal hysterectomy with bilateral salpingo-oophorectomy
TAT	Thematic Apperception Test
TB*	terabyte

TB	tuberculosis
TBI	traumatic brain injury
TBSA	total body surface area
TCA	tricyclic antidepressant
TCD_{50}	median tissue culture dose
TE	echo time
THA	total-hip arthroplasty
TI	inversion time
TIA	transient ischemic attack
TIBC	total iron-binding capacity
tid	twice a day (do not abbreviate)
TIFF*	Tag(ged) Image File Format
TLC	thin-layer chromatography; total lung capacity
TNF	tumor necrosis factor
TNM*	tumor, node, metastasis (see 15.2.2, Nomenclature, Cancer, The TNM Staging System)
tPA	tissue plasminogen activator
TPN	total parenteral nutrition
TQM	total quality management
TR	repetition time
TRH	thyrotropin-releasing hormone (*protirelin* as diagnostic agent)
tRNA	transfer RNA
TRP	tyrosine-related protein
TRUS	transrectal ultrasonography
TSH	Use *thyrotropin* (previously thyroid-stimulating hormone).
TSS	toxic shock syndrome; toxic "strep" [streptococcal] syndrome
TTP	thrombotic thrombocytopenic purpura
UHF	ultrahigh frequency
ul*	uniformly labeled (used within parentheses; see 15.9.5, Nomenclature, Isotopes, Uniform Labeling)
URI*	uniform resource identifier
URL*	uniform resource locator
URN*	uniform resource name
URTI	upper respiratory tract infection
US	ultrasonography; ultrasound
USAN	United States Adopted Names [Council]
USP	United States Pharmacopeia

USSC	unrestricted somatic stem cell
UV*	ultraviolet
UV-A*	ultraviolet A
UV-B*	ultraviolet B
UV-C*	ultraviolet C
VAIN	vaginal intraepithelial neoplasia
vCJD	variant Creutzfeldt-Jakob disease
VDRL*	Venereal Disease Research Laboratory (add *test*)
VEGF	vascular endothelial growth factor
VEP	visual evoked potential
VER	visual evoked response
VHDL	very high-density lipoprotein
VHF	very high frequency; viral hemorrhagic fever
VLBW	very low birth weight (*but*: very low-birth-weight infant)
VLDL	very low-density lipoprotein
$\dot{V}O_2$	oxygen consumption per unit time
$\dot{V}O_{2max}$	maximum oxygen consumption
VPB	ventricular premature beat
$\dot{V}/\dot{Q}$	ventilation-perfusion [ratio or scan]
vs*	versus (use *v* for legal references)
VSD	ventricular septal defect
VT	ventricular tachycardia; tidal volume
VZV	varicella zoster virus
WAIS	Wechsler Adult Intelligence Scale
WBC	white blood cell
WEE	western equine encephalomyelitis
WISC-R	Wechsler Intelligence Scale for Children
XML*	extensible markup language
YLD	years living with disability
YPLL	years of potential life lost
zip*	Zone Improvement Plan (zip code)

*This abbreviation may be used without expansion.

14.12 Units of Measure. *JAMA* and the *Archives* Journals report quantitative values in conventional units. A number of analytes, however, are dual reported in the International System of Units (SI units, Système International d'Unités), with conventional units first, followed by the SI conversion in parentheses. See 18.5, Units of Measure, Conventional Units and SI Units in *JAMA* and the *Archives* Journals.

Use the following abbreviations and symbols with a numerical quantity in accordance with guidelines in 18.0, Units of Measure. See especially 18.5, Units of Measure, Conventional Units and SI Units in *JAMA* and the *Archives* Journals; Table 2 in chapter 18, Selected Laboratory Tests, References Ranges with and Conversion Factors; and 8.4, Punctuation, Forward Slash (Virgule, Solidus). *Exception:* The following example is an acceptable format in table footnotes or figure legends:

> SI conversion factor: To convert creatinine value to mmol/L, multiply by 88.4.

Note: Do not capitalize abbreviated units of measure (unless the abbreviation itself is always capitalized or contains capital letters).

acre	acre
ampere	A
angstrom	Convert to nanometers (1 angstrom = 0.1 nm).
atmosphere, standard	atm
bar	bar
barn	b*
base pair	bp*
becquerel	Bq
billion electron volts	GeV*
Bodansky unit	BU*
British thermal unit	BTU
calorie	cal
candela	cd*
Celsius	C (Use closed up with degree symbol, eg, 40°C.)
centigram	cg
centimeter	cm
centimeters of water	cm H_2O
centimorgan	cM
centipoise	cP
coulomb	C*
counts per minute	cpm
counts per second	cps
cubic centimeter	cm^3 (Use milliliter for liquid and gas measure.)
cubic foot	cu ft
cubic inch	cu in
cubic meter	m^3
cubic micrometer	μm^3

cubic millimeter	mm^3 (Use microliter for liquid and gas measure.)
cubic yard	cu yd
curie	Ci
cycles per second	Use hertz.
dalton	Da
day	d†
decibel	dB
decigram	Convert to grams.
deciliter	dL
decimeter	Convert to meters.
diopter	D*
disintegrations per minute	dpm*
disintegrations per second	dps*
dyne	dyne
electron volt	eV
electrostatic unit	ESU*
equivalent	Eq
equivalent roentgen	equivalent roentgen
Fahrenheit	F (Use closed up with degree symbol, eg, 99°F.)
farad (electric capacitance)	F*
femtogram	fg
femtoliter	fL
femtomole	fmol
fluid ounce	fl oz
foot	ft (Convert to meters; query author.)
gas volume	gas volume
gauss	G
gigabyte	GB
grain	grain
gram	g
gravity (acceleration due to)	*g* (Use closed up to preceding number, eg, 200*g*.)
gray	Gy
henry	H*
hertz	Hz

horsepower	hp
hour	h†
immunizing unit	ImmU*
inch	in
international benzoate unit	IBU*
international unit	IU
joule	J
katal	kat*
kelvin	K
kilobase	kb*
kilobyte	kB
kilocalorie	kcal
kilocurie	kCi
kilodalton	kDa
kiloelectron volt	keV
kilogram	kg
kilohertz	kHz
kilojoule	kJ
kilometer	km
kilopascal	kPa
kilovolt	kV
kilovolt-ampere	kVA
kilovolt (constant potential)	kV(cp)*
kilovolt (peak)	kV(p)*
kilowatt	kW
King-Armstrong unit	King-Armstrong unit
knot	knot
liter	L
lumen	lumen
lux	lux
megabyte	MB
megacurie	MCi
megacycle	Mc
megahertz	MHz
megaunit	MU
megawatt	MW
meter	m

metric ton	metric ton
microampere	μA
microcurie	μCi
microfarad	μF*
microgram	μg
microliter	μL
micrometer	μm
micromicrocurie	Use picocurie.
micromicrogram	Use picogram.
micromicrometer	Use picometer.
micromolar	μM
micromole	μmol
micron	Use micrometer.
micronormal	μN
microosmole	μOsm
microunit	μU
microvolt	μV
microwatt	μW
mile	mile
miles per hour	mph
milliampere	mA
millicurie	mCi
millicuries destroyed	mCid*
milliequivalent	mEq
millifarad	mF*
milligram	mg
milligram-element	mg-el*
milli-international unit	mIU
milliliter	mL
millimeter	mm
millimeters of mercury	mm Hg
millimeters of water	mm H_2O
millimolar	mM
millimole	mmol
million electron volts	MeV
milliosmole	mOsm
millirem	mrem
milliroentgen	mR
millisecond	ms†

milliunit	mU
millivolt	mV
milliwatt	mW
minute (time)	min†
molar	M
mole	mol
month	mo†
morgan	M*
mouse unit	MU*
nanocurie	nCi
nanogram	ng
nanometer	nm
nanomolar	nM
nanomole	nmol
newton	N
normal (solution)	N
ohm	Ω
osmole	osm
ounce	oz
outflow (weight)	C*
parts per million	ppm
pascal	Pa
picocurie	pCi
picogram	pg
picometer	pm
picomolar	pM
picomole	pmol
pint	pt
pound	lb (Convert to milligrams, kilograms, or grams; query author.)
pounds per square inch	psi
prism diopter	PD, Δ*
quart	qt
rad	rad
radian	radian
rat unit	RU*
revolutions per minute	rpm

roentgen	R
roentgen equivalents human (or mammal)	rem
roentgen equivalents physical	rep
Saybolt seconds universal	SSU*
second	s†
siemen	siemen
sievert	Sv
sp g	specific gravity (Use with a number, eg, sp g 13.6.)
square centimeter	cm^2
square foot	sq ft
square inch	sq in
square meter	m^2
square millimeter	mm^2
Svedberg flotation unit	Sf*
tesla	T
torr	Use millimeters of mercury.
tuberculin unit	TU
turbidity-reducing unit	TRU*
unit	U
volt	V
volume	vol
volume per volume	vol/vol
volume percent	vol%
watt	W
week	wk†
weight	wt
weight per volume	wt/vol
weight per weight	wt/wt
yard	yd
year	y†

*Expand at first mention, with the abbreviation immediately following in parentheses. Abbreviate thereafter, except at the beginning of a sentence. (See also 18.3.4, Units of Measure, Format, Style, and Punctuation, Beginning of Sentence, Title, Subtitle.)

†Use the abbreviation only in a virgule construction and in tables and line art.

14.13 Elements and Chemicals. In general, the names of chemical elements and compounds should be expanded in the text at first mention and elsewhere in accordance with the guidelines for clinical and technical terms. (See also 15.4.4, Nomenclature, Drugs, Chemical Names; and 15.9, Nomenclature, Isotopes.) However, in some circumstances it may be helpful or necessary to provide the chemical symbols or formulas in addition to the expansion if the compound under discussion is new or relatively unknown or if no nonproprietary term exists. For example:

> 2,3,7,8-Tetrachlorodibenzo-p-dioxin (TCDD, or dioxin) is often referred to as the most toxic synthetic chemical known. [Use *TCDD* or *dioxin* thereafter; TCDD is more specific, because there is more than 1 form of dioxin.]

> 3,4-Methylenedioxymethamphetamine (MDMA, ecstasy, XTC), a synthetic analogue of 3,4-methylenedioxyamphetamine, has been the center of controversy over its potential for abuse vs its use as a psychotherapeutic agent. [Use *MDMA*, *ecstasy*, or *XTC* thereafter, depending on the article's context.]

The following format may also be used:

> Isorhodeose (chemical name, 6-deoxy-D-glucose [$CH_3(CHOH)_4CHO$]) is a sugar derived from *Cinchona officinalis*. [Use "isorhodeose" thereafter.]

Names such as "sodium lauryl sulfate" are easier to express and understand (and typeset) than "$CH_3(CH_2)_{10}CH_2OSO_3Na$." Similarly, "oxygen" and "water" do not take up much more space than "O_2" and "H_2O" and hence should remain expanded throughout a manuscript, unless specific measurements (eg, gas exchange) are under discussion.

> The venous CO_2 pressure is always greater than arterial CO_2 pressure; specifically, $P\text{VCO}_2/P\text{aCO}_2$ is greater than 1.0 except when $P\text{O}_2$ plus $P\text{CO}_2$ is measured. Nevertheless, the CO_2 levels should be carefully measured.

> Near the earth's surface, the atmosphere has a well-defined chemical composition, consisting of molecular nitrogen, molecular oxygen, and argon. It also contains small amounts of carbon dioxide and water vapor, along with trace quantities of methane, ammonia, nitrous oxide, hydrogen sulfide, helium, neon, krypton, xenon, and various other gases.

In the following example, sodium and potassium are not abbreviated.

> Repeated serum chemistry studies confirmed a serum sodium level of 140 mEq/L and a serum potassium level of 145 mEg/L.

In the text and elsewhere, the expansion of such symbols as Na^+ or Ca^{2+} can be cumbersome, since these symbols have a specific meaning for the reader. Usage should follow the context. For example, in nontechnical pieces, the flavor of the writing might be lost if, for example, the editor arbitrarily changed "CO_2" to "carbon dioxide" ("What's the patient's CO_2?").

When chemical symbols and formulas are used, they must be carefully marked for the printer, especially when chemical bonds are expressed. (See also 21.1, Mathematical Composition, Copy Marking.) Three types of chemical bonds commonly seen in organic and biochemical compounds are single, double, and triple:

> $H_3{-}CH_3 \quad H_2C{=}CH_2 \quad HC{\equiv}CH$

When deciding whether to expand or abbreviate element and chemical names, the editor and the author should consider guidelines for established terminology, the manuscript's subject matter, technical level, and audience, and the context in which the term appears.

14.14 Radioactive Isotopes. In general, the expanded terms for radioactive isotopes are used in *JAMA* and the *Archives* Journals, as described in 15.9, Nomenclature, Isotopes, with exceptions noted, for example, in radioactive pharmaceuticals and certain chemical notations. The following table lists radioactive isotopes (and their symbols) used in medical diagnosis and therapy (adapted from *The Merck Index*[6]). (See also 15.9.2, Nomenclature, Isotopes, Radiopharmaceuticals, and 15.9.3, Nomenclature, Isotopes, Radiopharmaceutical Compounds Without Approved Names.)

Name	*Symbol*
americium	Am
calcium	Ca
cesium	Cs
chromium	Cr
cobalt	Co
copper	Cu
fluorine	F
gadolinium	Gd
gallium	Ga
gold	Au
indium	In
iodine	I
iridium	Ir
iron	Fe
krypton	Kr
mercury	Hg
phosphorus	P
potassium	K
radium	Ra
radon	Rn
ruthenium	Ru
selenium	Se
sodium	Na
strontium	Sr
sulfur	S
technetium	Tc

Name	*Symbol*
thallium	Tl
xenon	Xe
ytterbium	Yb

ACKNOWLEDGMENT

Principal author: Roxanne K. Young, ELS

REFERENCES

1. Smyth HW; Messing GM, rev ed. *Greek Grammar*. Cambridge, MA: Harvard University Press; 1984:104.
2. Watson R. Presented by Kinnock N. A journalist's view of clarity at the Commission. Presented at: First Clear Writing Awards; July 12, 2001; Brussels, Belgium. http://europa.eu.int/comm/translation/en/ftfog/clear_writing_awards_watson.htm. Accessed February 11, 2004.
3. *Merriam-Webster's Collegiate Dictionary*. 11th ed. Springfield, MA: Merriam-Webster Inc; 2003.
4. Patrias K. *National Library of Medicine Recommended Formats for Bibliographic Citation*. Bethesda, MD: Reference Section, National Library of Medicine, National Institutes of Health, US Dept of Health and Human Services; 1991.
5. National Library of Medicine, National Institutes of Health. *List of Journals Indexed in Index Medicus*. Bethesda, MD: National Library of Medicine; 1996. NIH publication 96-267.
6. O'Neil MJ, Smith A, Heckelman PE, eds. *The Merck Index: Encyclopedia of Chemicals, Drugs, & Biologicals*. 13th ed. Whitehouse Station, NJ: Merck & Co Inc; 2001.

15 Nomenclature

A generally accepted and universally used system of nomenclature is an essential tool in any area of study.

Julia G. Bodmer[1]

. . . the Author of this editorial thought nomenclature was boring and went sight-seeing—a serious misjudgment, in retrospect.

H. Zola[2]

Evolution continues, in nomenclature as in the real life which cannot be discussed and hence understood without it.

Richard V. Melville[3]

I am away from my desk. . . . If you are in need of immediate nomenclature assistance, please contact . . .

Lois Maltais, Jackson Laboratory,
e-mail message

This chapter is devoted to nomenclature: systematically formulated names for specific entities.

Biological nomenclature dates back at least to the 18th century. Since the mid-20th century, many biomedical disciplines have established committees to develop and promulgate official systems of nomenclature.

Accelerating knowledge, particularly from molecular biology, necessitated the official biomedical nomenclature systems, sometimes with dramatic results. For instance, a single coagulation factor had been referred to by 14 different names.[4] An investigator deemed the official coagulation nomenclature "one of the most significant, even if only semantic, recent advances in the field."[5(p16)] The results, probably true in other disciplines as well, were that an "impenetrable confusion was cleared away, apparent disagreements were often shown to be conflicts of terminology, not of fact, and a much freer exchange of information was made possible."[5(p16)]

In microbiology, with publication of the approved list of bacterial names in 1980, the number of names of bacteria decreased by an order of magnitude, from around 30 000 to around 2000[6,7] (now nearly 7500[8]). The CD (clusters of differentiation) nomenclature is thought to have prevented mistakes in laboratory and clinical research.[9]

Those are some indications of the compelling need for systematic nomenclature, which requires the ongoing work of international groups. The development of nomenclature, however, faces challenges besides multiplicity of names. There is tradition—"the ruins of previous systems"[10(p7)]—which investigators are often reluctant to give up. When disciplines converge—for instance, when the genetics of a physiologic system are delineated—preexisting systems of nomenclature may operate in parallel, and names proliferate.[11] For instance, concerning the homologous human HLA and mouse H-2 tissue antigen systems, it has been observed:

> The situation is perhaps similar to what one might have encountered in the field of immunoglobulins had researchers working with immunoglobulins in different species not realized relatively early that the classes of heavy chains and light chains they were working with were homologous and been willing to adopt a common nomenclature. We might then have separate names in each species for IgM, IgG, IgA, kappa, lambda, and so on.[12(p578)]

A system of nomenclature may face the test of sheer numbers. The count of assigned gene symbols has increased from several hundred[13,14] to more than 23 000,[15] with more than 25 000 human genes anticipated.[16,17] The system was devised with a foresight that has allowed transition from typescript to print to online database.[18-20]

Another challenge is to remain flexible. Those who deal with nomenclature accept it as a construct[21-24] and have noted the need to reflect new knowledge.[22,25] Biomedical classification is arbitrary and "artificial," created by humans.[26,27] Nomenclature needs to "evolve with new technology rather than be restrictive as sometimes occurs when historical . . . systems are applied."[28(p12)]

Such flexibility, however, places a burden on clinicians, who must replace familiar names with new ones.[29] Often, "colorful or descriptive names,"[9(p1245)] which are more easily retained,[30] give way to more efficient terms, such as the alphanumeric epithets of many systems.

Nomenclature systems may differ markedly in approach. Stability is an overriding principle of the codes of taxonomic nomenclature, which avoid name changes.[31] For instance, the bacteriologic code has a provision that a name may be rejected "whose application is likely to lead to accidents endangering health or life or both or of serious economic consequences."[32(p43)] For example, the name *Yersinia pseudotuberculosis* subsp *pestis* for the plague bacillus was rejected and the name *Yersinia pestis* retained[32,33] because of concerns about public health hazards (owing to confusion of the name of the plague bacillus with that of the less virulent *Yersinia pseudotuberculosis*[34,35]). In contrast, currency is an overriding principle of the official human gene nomenclature, with genes renamed to reflect new knowledge. (Of the approximately 260 gene symbols in the first Catalog of Gene Markers following introduction of the current system of gene nomenclature, more than half have been renamed.[14,36]) Yet the principles of stability and currency are not mutually exclusive; for instance, the bacteriologic code requires name changes necessitated by revisions of taxonomy, and the human gene nomenclature acknowledges former names and aliases.

Nomenclature is "the means of channelling the outputs of systematic research for general consumption"[37] and aims for international scope ("'... Science should unite Nations ...'"[38(p10)]). Giangrande[39(p710)] writes that international nomenclature efforts in coagulation "provide[d] an outstanding early example of international collaboration to resolve a scientific problem. This sort of co-operation is now commonplace, but was certainly not typical in [the post–World War II] period." To facilitate worldwide access to the latest terms, large computerized databases have been created. But computerized databases require consistent use of nomenclature.[11] Unique identifiers provide a home base for terms in large databases but are not practical for referring to entities throughout published articles and textbooks[40]—hence, names.

Our purpose in the nomenclature chapter is to explain not how names should be devised (although we cite the sources of such rules) but rather which names should be used and how they should be styled. Official systems of nomenclature are not universally observed to the letter (literally or figuratively), but style that is consistent with official guidelines and within publications reduces ambiguity. Editors have the task of mediating between official systems and authors' actual usage. To that end, the goals of this chapter are to present style for terms and to explain terms in hopes that they are more easily dealt with.

In medical nomenclature the stylistic trend has been toward typographic simplicity, driven by computers. Terms lose hyphens, superscripts, subscripts, and spaces. However, such features have not been eliminated completely, either within or beyond these pages. In 1950 standardized terms in pulmonary-respiratory medicine and physiology were put forth, and typographic features impossible on a typewriter were expressly retained, seen as indispensable components of a systematic and enlightening nomenclature.[25] Computers are increasingly capable of generating unusual characters, and typographic simplification and electronic sophistication may cross paths before medical nomenclature loses its last defining flourishes.

An umbrella resource for biomedical terminology is the Unified Medical Language System (UMLS), a project of the National Library of Medicine. The UMLS is intended to provide integrated terminology (including synonyms and relationships among terms) for use in electronic applications, ie, computer systems.[41,42] A major component of the UMLS is the Metathesaurus, a comprehensive repository of biomedical terms and their relationships. The Metathesaurus is accessible online at the UMLS Knowledge Source Server, http://umlsks.nlm.nih.gov. (Complimentary registration is required.) That site offers concept and term searches that can be useful to medical authors and editors seeking explanations of particular terms, including their relationships to other terms (eg, human gene, protein, condition, and animal counterparts).[42]

ACKNOWLEDGMENTS

Principal authors: Margaret A. Winker, MD, sections 15.4, 15.5, and 15.9; Richard M. Glass, MD, section 15.15; Harriet S. Meyer, MD, remaining sections

The following individuals reviewed drafts and provided invaluable suggestions: *Blood Groups and Platelet Antigens:* Geoff Daniels, PhD, Bristol Institute for Transfusion Sciences, Bristol, England; *Cancer:* Irvin D. Fleming, MD, Methodist Healthcare, Memphis, Tennessee; *Cardiology:* Michael S. Lauer, MD, Cleveland Clinic Heart Center, Cleveland, Ohio, *JAMA/Archives* Journals, Chicago, Illinois; *Drugs:* Stephanie C. Shubat, MS, Director, USAN Program, Chicago, Illinois; David S. Cooper, MD, Sinai Hospital of Baltimore, Johns Hopkins University School of Medicine, Baltimore, Maryland, *JAMA/Archives* Journals, Chicago, Illinois (hormones and insulin); Julie A. Mares, PhD, University of Wisconsin-Madison (vitamins and related compounds); *Genetics:* Richard G. H. Cotton, PhD, DSc, University of Melbourne, Melbourne, Australia; Stylianos E. Antonarakis, MD, DSc, Centre Médical Universitaire, Genève, Switzerland; Dr Johan den Dunnen, Leiden University Medical Center, Leiden, the Netherlands, Human Genome Variation Society; Daniel W. Nebert, MD, University of Cincinnati Medical Center, Cincinnati, Ohio (nucleic acids and amino acids; human genes); Hester Mary Wain, PhD, Galton Laboratory, University College, London, England (human gene nomenclature); Boris Pasche, MD, PhD, Northwestern University Medical Center, *JAMA/Archives* Journals, Chicago, Illinois (oncogenes and tumor suppressor genes); Dr Felix Mitelman, University Hospital, Lund, Sweden (chromosomes); Lois J. Maltais, BS, The Jackson Laboratory, Bar Harbor, Maine (nonhuman genetic terms); Robin L. Bennett, MS, CGC, University of Washington Medical Center, Seattle (pedigrees); *Hemostasis:* Leon W. Hoyer, MD, Annapolis, Maryland; *Immunology:* Tristram G. Parslow, MD, PhD, Emory University, Atlanta, Georgia, Howard M. Gebel, PhD, Emory University, Atlanta, Georgia, Robert A. Bray, PhD, Emory University, Atlanta, Georgia; Steven G. E. Marsh, PhD, ARCS, Anthony Nolan Research Institute, Royal Free Hospital, London, England; *Molecular Medicine:* Boris Pasche, MD, PhD, Northwestern University Medical Center, Chicago, Illinois, *JAMA/Archives* Journals, Chicago, Illinois; Jeanette M. Smith, MD, *JAMA/Archives* Journals, Chicago, Illinois; *Neurology:* Michael J. Aminoff, MD, DSc, FRCP, University of California, San Francisco, School of Medicine; *Ophthalmology:* Neil M. Bressler, MD, Johns Hopkins Medical Institutions, Baltimore, Maryland, Daniel M. Albert, MD, University of Wisconsin Hospitals and Clinics, Madison; *Organisms and Pathogens:* Kevin C. Hazen, PhD, D(ABBM), University of Virginia, Charlottesville (biological nomenclature); *Pulmonary and Respiratory Terminology:* John B. West, MD, PhD, DSc, University of California, San Diego, La Jolla.

Cassio Lynm, *JAMA*, provided illustrations. Joanne Weiskopf, *JAMA* and *Archives* Journals, adapted illustrations. Yolanda Davis-Ellis and Sandra Schefris, James S. Todd Memorial Library, American Medical Association, Chicago, Illinois, assisted in obtaining references.

REFERENCES

1. Bodmer JG. Nomenclature 1991 foreword. *Hum Immunol.* 1991;34(1):2-3.
2. Zola H. The CD nomenclature: a brief historical summary of the CD nomenclature, why it exists and how CDs are defined. *J Biol Regul Homeost Agents.* 1999;13(4): 226-228.
3. Melville RV. *Towards Stability in the Names of Animals: A History of the International Commission on Zoological Nomenclature 1895-1995.* London, England: International Trust for Zoological Nomenclature; 1995.
4. Abe T, Alexander B, Astrup T, et al; and the International Committee for the Nomenclature of Blood Clotting Factors, Wright IS, chair. The nomenclature of blood clotting factors. *JAMA.* 1962;180(9):733-735.
5. Biggs R, ed. *Human Blood Coagulation, Hemostasis and Thrombosis.* 2nd ed. Oxford, England: Blackwell Scientific Publications; 1976:15-16.

6. Baron EJ, Weissfeld AS, Fuselier PA, Brenner DJ. Classification and identification of bacteria. In: Murray PR, ed. *Manual of Clinical Microbiology*. 6th ed. Washington, DC: ASM Press; 1995:249-264.
7. Brooks GF, Butel JS, Morse SA. *Jawetz, Melnick, and Adelberg's Medical Microbiology*. 22nd ed. New York, NY: Lange Medical Books/McGraw-Hill; 2001:40.
8. DSMZ-Deutsche Sammlung von Mikroorganismen und Zellkulturen GmBH, Braunschweig, Germany. Microorganisms: bacterial nomenclature. http://www.dsmz.de/microorganisms/main.php?contentleft_id=14. Accessed April 20, 2006.
9. Singer NG, Todd RF, Fox DA. Structures on the cell surface: update from the Fifth International Workshop on Human Leukocyte Differentiation Antigens. *Arthritis Rheum*. 1994;37(8):1245-1248.
10. Wildy P. *Classification and Nomenclature of Viruses: First Report of the International Committee on Nomenclature of Viruses*. New York, NY: S Karger AG; 1971:1-26. Melnick JL, ed. *Monographs in Virology*; vol 5.
11. Cammack R. The biochemical nomenclature committees. *IUBMB Life*. 2000;50(3):159-161.
12. Hansen TH, Carreno BM, Sachs DH. The major histocompatibility complex. In: Paul WE, ed. *Fundamental Immunology*. 3rd ed. New York, NY: Raven Press; 1993:577-628.
13. Shows TB, McAlpine PJ. The 1981 catalogue of assigned human genetic markers and report of the nomenclature committee. *Cytogenet Cell Genet*. 1982;32(1-4):221-245.
14. Evans HJ, Hamerton JL, Klinger HP, McKusick VA. *Human Gene Mapping 5: Edinburgh Conference (1979): Fifth International Workshop on Human Gene Mapping*. Basel, Switzerland: S Karger AG; 1979.
15. HUGO Gene Nomenclature Committee Web site. http://www.gene.ucl.ac.uk/nomenclature/. Updated March 29, 2006. Accessed April 20, 2006.
16. Wain HM, Bruford EA, Lovering RC, Lush MJ, Wright MW, Povey S. Guidelines for human gene nomenclature (2002). *Genomics*. 2002;79(4):464-470. Also available at http://www.gene.ucl.ac.uk/nomenclature/guidelines.html. Updated April 20, 2006. Accessed April 20, 2006.
17. Reaney R. Humans have fewer genes than previously thought. http://www.reuters.com/newsArticle.jhtml?type=topNews&storyID=6562986. Posted October 20, 2001. Accessed October 26, 2004.
18. Shows TB, Alper CA, Bootsma D, et al. International system for human gene nomenclature (1979). *Cytogenet Cell Genet*. 1979;25(1-4):96-116.
19. Ruddle FH, Kidd KK. The Human Gene Mapping Workshops in transition. *Cytogenet Cell Genet*. 1989;51(1-4):1-2.
20. Progress in nomenclature and symbols for cytogenetics and somatic-cell genetics [editorial]. *Ann Intern Med*. 1979;91(3):487-488.
21. Staley JT, Krieg NR. Bacterial classification, I: classification of procaryotic organisms: an overview. In: Krieg NR, Holt JF, eds. *Bergey's Manual of Systematic Bacteriology*. Vol 1. Baltimore, MD: Williams & Wilkins; 1984:1-4.
22. Erzinclioglu YZ, Unwin DM. The stability of zoological nomenclature [letter]. *Nature*. 1986;320(6064):687.
23. Lublin DM, Telen MJ. What is a blood group antigen [letter]? *Transfusion*. 1992;32(5):493.

24. Lublin DM, Telen MJ. More about use of the term Drb [letter]. *Transfusion.* 1993;33(2):182.
25. Pappenheimer JR, chairman; Comroe JH, Cournand A, Ferguson JKW, et al. Standardization of definitions and symbols in respiratory physiology. *Fed Proc.* 1950;9: 602-605.
26. Madias JE. Killip and Forrester classifications: should they be abandoned, kept, reevaluated, or modified? *Chest.* 2000;117(5):1223-1226.
27. Vandamme PAR. Taxonomy and classification of bacteria. In: Murray PR, Baron EJ, Jorgensen JH, Pfaller MA, Yolken RH, eds. *Manual of Clinical Microbiology.* 8th ed. Washington, DC: ASM Press; 2003:271.
28. Shows TB, McAlpine PJ, Boucheix C, et al. Guidelines for human gene nomenclature: an international system for human gene nomenclature (ISGN, HGM9). *Cytogenet Cell Genet.* 1987;46(1-4):11-28.
29. Patterson PY, Sommers HM. A proposed change in bacterial nomenclature: a rose by any other name. *J Infect Dis.* 1981;144(1):85-86.
30. Flexner CW. In praise of descriptive nomenclature [letter]. *Lancet.* 1996;347(8993):68.
31. Jeffrey C. *Biological Nomenclature.* 3rd ed. London, England: Edward Arnold; New York, NY: Routledge Chapman & Hall; 1989.
32. Lapage SP, Sneath PHA, Lessel EF, Skerman VBD, Seeliger HPR, Clark WA; Sneath PHA, ed. *International Code of Nomenclature of Bacteria and Statutes of the Bacteriology and Applied Microbiology Section of the International Union of Microbiological Societies, 1990 Revision.* Washington, DC: American Society for Microbiology; 1992.
33. Euzéby JP. List of bacterial names with standing in nomenclature—genus *Yersinia.* http://www.bacterio.cict.fr/xz/yersinia.html. Accessed April 20, 2006.
34. Williams JE. Proposal to reject the new combination *Yersinia pseudotuberculosis* subsp *pestis* for violation of the first principles of the International Code of Nomenclature of Bacteria: request for an opinion. *Int J Syst Bacteriol.* 1984;34(2):268-269.
35. Judicial Commission of the International Committee on Systematic Bacteriology. Rejection of the name *Yersinia pseudotuberculosis* subsp *pestis* (van Loghem) Bercovier et al. 1981 and conservation of the name *Yersinia pestis* (Lehmann and Neumann) van Loghem 1944 for the plague bacillus. *Int J Systemat Bacteriol.* 1985;35(4):540.
36. Searchgenes. Human Gene Nomenclature Database Search Engine. http://www.gene .ucl.ac.uk/cgi-bin/nomenclature/searchgenes.pl. Updated August 23, 2005. Accessed August 23, 2005.
37. Greuter W, Hawksworth DL. Preface. In: Greuter W, McNeill J, Farrie FR, et al. *International Code of Botanical Nomenclature (St Louis Code).* International Association for Plant Taxonomy. 2000. http://www.bgbm.org/IAPT/Nomenclature/Code /SaintLouis/0002Preface.htm. Updated February 12, 2001. Accessed April 20, 2006.
38. International Society for Microbiology founding brochure. Quoted in: Murray RGE, Holt JG. The history of *Bergey's Manual.* In: Boone DR, Castenholtz RW, eds. *Bergey's Manual of Systematic Bacteriology.* Vol 1. 2nd ed. New York, NY: Springer-Verlag; 2001:1-13.
39. Giangrande PL. Six characters in search of an author: the history of the nomenclature of coagulation factors. *Br J Haematol.* 2003;121(5):705-712.
40. Beutler E, McKusick VA, Motulsky AG, Scriver CR, Hutchinson F. Mutation nomenclature: nicknames, systematic names, and unique identifiers. *Hum Mutat.* 1996; 8(3):203-206.

41. National Library of Medicine. Unified Medical Language System. http://www.nlm.nih.gov/research/umls/about_umls.html. Published March 22, 2004. Updated July 19, 2004. Accessed April 20, 2006.
42. Bodenreider O. The Unified Medical Language System (UMLS): integrating biomedical terminology. *Nucleic Acids Res.* 2004;32(database issue):D267-D270. doi:10.1093/nar/gkh061.

[A]lthough erythrocytes have traditionally been considered relatively inert cellular containers of hemoglobin, they are in fact active in a variety of physiologic processes.

L. Calhoun and L. D. Petz[1(p1843)]

15.1 Blood Groups, Platelet Antigens, and Granulocyte Antigens

15.1.1 Blood Groups.

Blood Groups. Blood groups are characterized by erythrocyte (red blood cell) antigens with common immunologic properties (eg, group A). Blood group systems are series of such antigens encoded by a single gene or by a cluster of 2 or 3 closely linked homologous genes[1-3] (eg, ABO system).

There are about 600 recognized erythrocyte antigens.[2] The International Society of Blood Transfusion (ISBT) designates around 270 blood group antigens. Of these, around 250 belong to 1 of 29 systems.[3,4] (Other antigens remain in officially designated series or collections.) Some antigens are erythrocyte-specific; others appear widely, but specifically, on cells of other organs and tissues.

The discovery of blood group antigens was prompted by hemolytic disease of the newborn and transfusion reactions, but many antigens have since been implicated in infection and other disease processes[1,5]; whether fundamentally or incidentally is not known.[6] Erythrocytes are estimated to contain millions of antigen sites.[1]

Traditional/Popular Nomenclature.[7-10] Traditional blood group system nomenclature is typically used in medical publications. It comprises several approaches, and, therefore, sometimes the same entity (eg, a particular erythrocyte antigen) can be expressed by more than 1 term. Editors generally should follow author preference.

The principal elements named are blood group systems, antigens, phenotypes, genes, and alleles.

Blood Group Systems. The following list shows the blood group system names and symbols. (The column of derivations of names of blood group systems is provided for background interest[1,2,9,11-14] [also Geoff Daniels, PhD, written communications, May 13 and 17, 2004].)

System Name	*Symbol*	*Derivation*
ABO	ABO	Alphabetical (A and B); letter O may derive from "ohne" (German for *without*)
Chido/Rogers	Ch/Rg	Names of antibody makers

System Name	*Symbol*	*Derivation*
Colton	Co	Name of antibody maker
Cromer	Cromer	Name of antibody maker
Diego	Di	Name of antibody maker
Dombrock	Do	Name of antibody maker
Duffy	Fy	Name of antibody maker
Gerbich	Ge	Name of antibody maker
Gill	GIL	Name of antibody maker
Globoside	GLOB	Globoside synthetase
Hh	H	Concept ("heterogenetic")
I	I	Concept ("individuality")
Indian	In	Geographic
John Milton Hagen	JMH	Name of antibody maker
Kell	K	Name of antibody maker (Kelleher)
Kidd	Jk	Initials of infant child of antibody maker (K already in use)
Knops	Kn	Name of antibody maker
Kx	Kx	Association with Kell and X chromosome
Lewis	Le	Name of antibody maker
Lutheran	Lu	Name of antibody maker (actually *Lutteran*[9] or *Luteran*[13])
LW or Landsteiner/Wiener	LW	Names of investigators
MNSs	MNS	M, N: the word *immune*; S: location (Sydney, Australia)
		U (an antigen of the MNSs system): universal
Ok	OK	Family name initials (Kobutso; letters reversed because "K_o" was in use)
P	P	Alphabetical
Raph	Raph	Name of antibody maker
Rh	Rh	Rhesus monkeys (antigens were LW antigens)
Scianna	Sc	Name of antibody maker
Xg	Xg	X chromosome and location (Grand Rapids, Michigan)
Yt or Cartwright	Yt	. . .

The ISBT prefers an all-capital style for blood group system symbols[3] (see "ISBT Name and Number" in this section).

The following are examples of usage:

ABO incompatibility

A cell

type AB recipient

type O donor

Hemolytic disease of the newborn primarily occurs from incompatibilities of the Rh, ABO, or Kell blood groups.

Antigens. Antigen terms use single or dual letters, often with a qualifier that is a letter (usually superscript) or number (subscript or typeset on the line).

A, A_1, A_2, A_x, B

Cr^a

Fy^a, Fy^b

He

Jk^a, Jk^b

K, k

Kp^a, Kp^b, Ku, Js^a, Js^b

K11, K12, K13, K14, Km

Le^a, Le^b, Le^{bH}, ALe^b, BLe^b

Lu^a, Lu^b

Lu3, Lu4, Lu5, Lu6

P^1

Sc1, Sc2

Xg^a

The Rh system historically has used 3 alternative schemes: the Rh-Hr nomenclature, the CDE nomenclature, and the numerical nomenclature.[7] Terms from the first, eg, rh′, hr″, rh^x, Rh^A, are appropriate in historical discussions, but otherwise, the CDE and numerical nomenclatures are favored:

D, C, E, c, e, f

Ce, C^w, C^x . . . BARC

or

Rh1, Rh2, Rh3, Rh4, Rh5, RH6

RH7, RH8, RH9 . . . RH52

The following are examples of antigen-term usage:

anti-Jk^a alloantibody

Rh(D) incompatibility

human monoclonal anti-D antibodies

Studies using anti-Ch and anti-Rg antisera have demonstrated Ch and Rg determinants on complement component C4.

Phenotypes. In phenotypic expressions—terms that describe an individual's blood group or type—the presence or absence of an antigen is often indicated by a plus or minus sign:

Antigen: M

Phenotype: M+

M+N+S−s+ erythrocytes

M+N+S−s+ phenotype

Lowercase letters that were superscripts in the antigen terms are set on the line in parentheses in phenotypic terms.

Antigen: Lu^b

Phenotype: Lu(b+)

More than 98% of the Western population is Lu(b+).

If the numerical terminology is used for the antigen, a colon is added in the phenotype.

Antigen: Sc1

Phenotype: Sc:1

the Sc:1,−2,3 phenotype

Other sample phenotypic terms include the following:

Fy(a−b+), Fy(a+b−), Fy(a−b−)

Jk(a−b+), Jk(a+b−), Jk(a+b+)

K+k−, Kp(a−b+), Js(a−b+)

Le(a−b+), Le(a+b−), Le(a−b−)

Lu(a−b+), Lu(a+b−), Lu(a+b+)

M+N+, M+, N−, M−N+, S+s+, S+s−, S−s+

P_1, P_2, P_1^k, P_2^k

Xg(a+), Xg(a−)

the silent phenotype Le(a−b−)

A superscript w can indicate a weak reaction:

$M+^w$

$K+^w$

$Fy(a+^w)$

The ABO system is an exception: its phenotypic terms do not feature plus or minus signs; A (not A+) indicates A erythrocyte antigens; O (not A− B−) indicates the absence of A and B antigens:

Groups: O, A, B, AB, O_h, O_h^A

Subgroups: A_1, A_2, A_1B, A_2B

O_h^A individuals do not express the H determinant but do have the *A* allele.

Terms for Rh phenotypes, which do not feature plus and minus signs, are also in use:

D-positive (Rh positive)

D-negative (Rh negative)

DccE, DCce

RH:1,2,3

Rh_{null}

Absence of C, c, E, and/or e antigens is indicated with 1 or 2 minus signs[14]:

Dc−

D− −

Usage note: Terms such as O+ ("O positive"), A+, and AB− are common parlance as shorthand for blood of the ABO system and its Rh specificity. However, in scientific articles, use standard terms that specifically indicate Rh status:

O Rh-positive

O Rh+

or more specific designations of phenotype:

group B, D-negative

group A, Rh D-positive

In a blood group profile, elements from different systems may be separated by commas, as above, or, for more complex specificities, with semicolons:

The patient's blood was group B, Rh positive, D+ C+ c+ E− e+; M+ N+ S− s+; P1+; Le(a−b−); K− k+; Fy(a−b+); Jk(a+b−).[15(p846)]

Note that in phenotypic expressions commas do not appear within elements of the same blood group system:

D+ C+ c+ E− e+

Not: D+, C+, c+, E−, e+

Commas may be dispensed with between different blood group systems in brief expressions:

K+Fy(a+)

Genes. As with International Standard Gene Nomenclature (the "HUGO" recommendations; see 15.6.2, Genetics, Human Gene Nomenclature), ISBT gene terms are italicized. Traditional blood-group gene symbols often mixed uppercase and lowercase. However, symbols recommended by ISBT, like those of HUGO, use all capital letters.

The following list[3,4,9,16] shows gene symbols associated with blood group systems.

Traditional	*ISBT*	*HUGO*
ABO	*ABO*	*ABO*
Ch/Rg	*C4A, C4B*	*C4A, C4B*
Co	*AQP1*	*AQP1* (was *CO*)
Cromer	*DAF*	*CD55* (was *DAF*)
Di	*SLC4A1*	*SLC4A1*
Do	*DO*	*ART4* (was *DO*)
Fy	*FY*	*DARC* (was *FY*)
Ge	*GYPC*	*GYPC*
[GIL]	*AQP3*	*AQP3*
[Globoside]	*B3GALT3*	*B3GALT3*
Hh	*FUT1*	*FUT1*
[I]	*GCNT2*	*GCNT2*
In	*CD44*	*CD44*
Jk	*SLC14A1*	*SLC14A1*
[JMH]	*SEMA7A*	*SEMA7A*
K	*KEL*	*KEL*
Kn	*CR1*	*CR1*
Kx	*XK*	*XK*
Le	*FUT3*	*FUT3*
Lu	*LU*	*BCAM* (was *LU*)
LW	*ICAM4*	*ICAM4*
MN or *MNSs*	*GYPA, GYPB, GYPE*	*GYPA, GYPB, GYPE*
Ok	*BSG*	*BSG* (previously *OK, CD147*)
P^1	*P1*	*A4GALT*
Raph	*CD151* (was *MER2*)	*CD151*
Rh	*RHCE, RHD*	*RHCE, RHD*
Sc	*ERMAP*	*SC*
Xg	*XG, MIC2*	*XG*
Yt	*ACHE*	*ACHE*

Gene symbols expressed according to ISBT[4] or HUGO[16] are preferred to traditional symbols.

Parenthetic synonyms are helpful:

BSG (formerly *OK*)

ERMAP (also called *SC*)

The Lutheran inhibitor gene is expressed as follows:

In(Lu) [traditional]

INLU [standard]

Do not confuse *In* with the traditional Indian blood group gene symbol, *In* (recommended gene symbol: *CD44*).

Alleles. The italicized blood group symbol—*ABO, MNS, RH,* etc—is used for alleles (which are also distinguished by an asterisk and number). In the following example, compare the gene symbol and an allele term from the same blood group:

*SC*1* [allele]

ERMAP [gene symbol]

Note that qualifiers that are subscripts in antigen terms are superscripts in allelic terms, eg, A_1 antigen, A^1 allele). The following are examples of genotypic terms.

A^1O, A^1A^1, A^1B, *OO*

MN, MM, NN, MSNs

DCe/DCe (R^1R^1)

DcE/dce (R^2r)

dce/dce (rr)

D− −/D− −

Lu^aLu^a, Lu^bLu^b, Lu^aLu^b

Lele, LeLe, lele

Fy^aFy^a, Fy^bFy^b, *FyFy*

Kk, Kp^aKp^b, Js^bJs^b

Jk^aJk^a, Jk^bJk^b, Jk^aJk^b

Xg^aXg^a, Xg^aXg, *XgXg*

Xg^aY, *XgY*

For expressing alleles, the ISBT gives an option, eg, either Fy^a or *FY*1* (with appropriate superscripts and italics). Mixing the 2 styles, however (eg, *FY*A*), is not appropriate (Geoff Daniels, PhD, written communications, May 13 and 17, 2004).

ISBT Name and Number.[3,7,17,18] In the 1980s the Working Party on Terminology for Red Cell Surface Antigens of the ISBT developed an alphanumeric system of blood group notation, intended to provide "a uniform nomenclature that is both eye and machine readable and in keeping with the genetic basis of blood groups."[7(p273)] The system does not replace traditional terminology; rather, its terms correspond to traditional terms. It is also used to assign new terms as needed. In the ISBT terminology, each blood group system has a symbol, usually of 1 to 3 capital letters, and a system number of 3 digits.

System			*Antigen No. Within System*			
Name	*Symbol*	*No.*	*001*	*002*	*003*	*004*
ABO	ABO	001	A	B	A,B	A1
MNS	MNS	002	M	N	S	s
Rh	RH	004	D	C	E	c
Kx	XK	019	Kx			

Sinistral (left-hand) zeros can be dropped from system and antigen terms, and system letter symbols can be used as part of the alphanumeric term. The following, for instance, are all acceptable for blood type AB:

AB

ABO:1,2,3

001:1,2,3

The following are acceptable terms for the antigen A,B:

A,B

ABO3

001003

Authors may use ISBT terms in parentheses following traditional terms:

AB (1.3)

D (RH1)

Le^a (007001)

The patient's red blood cells were negative for Cromer blood system antigens Cr^a (CROM1) and Tc^a (CROM2).

In notations that use plus and minus signs to express presence and absence of particular antigens, phenotypic expressions in the numerical notation use a colon and numbers in place of letters, as in these examples:

LE:−1,2 [for Le(a−b+)]

FY:1,−2 [for FY(a+b−)]

Genotypic expressions are italicized:

FY 1/2 or *FY*1/2* (for Fy^aFy^b)

Tables of blood group systems, symbols, antigens, and ISBT numbers are available at the ISBT Committee on Terminology for Red Cell Surface Antigens Web site.[4]

15.1.2 **Platelet-Specific Antigens.** The current system of human platelet antigen (HPA) nomenclature, adopted in 1990, is overseen by the Platelet Nomenclature Committee of the ISBT and the International Society on Thrombosis and Haemostasis.[19-21] As with blood groups, there are platelet antigen systems and specific antigens within those systems. The HPA nomenclature pertains to "all protein alloantigens expressed on the platelet membrane, except those coded by genes of the major histocompatibility complex (MHC)."[21(p241)] (See 15.8.5, Immunology, HLA/Major Histocompatibility Complex.) Currently, there are 6 HPA systems: HPA-1, HPA-2, HPA-3, HPA-4, HPA-5, and HPA-15.[21]

Complete tables of HPA terms are available at the IPD-HPA Database, http://www.ebi.ac.uk/ipd/hpa/.[21] Sample terms include the following:

Antigen system:	HPA-1
Associated glycoprotein:	GpIIIa
CD designation of glycoprotein:	CD61

Former names:	Zw, P1A
Antigens:	HPA-1a
	HPA-1b
Former antigen names:	Zw^a, $P1^{A1}$
	Zw^b, $P1^{A2}$
Gene:	*ITGB3*
Alleles:	*ITGB3*001*
	*ITGB3*002*
Epitopes:	HPA-1a
	HPA-1b
Locuslink ID:	3690
Ref_Seq:	NM_000212
Swiss-Prot:	ITB3_Human
Nucleotide change:	176T>C

For CD (clusters of differentiation) nomenclature, see 15.8.7, Immunology, Lymphocytes. For gene and allele nomenclature, see 15.6.2, Genetics, Human Gene Nomenclature. For database identifiers and nucleotide nomenclature, see 15.6.1 Genetics, Nucleic Acids and Amino Acids.

15.1.3 **Granulocyte Antigens.** The Granulocyte Antigen Working Party of the ISBT has formulated rules for well-defined human neutrophil antigens (HNAs),[22] as presented in the following tabulation, although at this writing they have not met with universal acceptance.[23,24]

Antigen System	*Antigen*	*Former Name*	*Alleles*
HNA-1	HNA-1a	NA1	*FCGR3B*1*
	HNA-1b	NA2	*FCGR3B*2*
	HNA-1c	SH	*FCGR3B*3*
HNA-2	HNA-2a	NB1	*CD177*1*
HNA-3	HNA-3a	5b	
HNA-4	HNA-4a	$Mart^a$	*CD11B*1*
HNA-5	HNA-5a	Ond^a	*CD11A*1*

See also 15.8.6, Immunology, Immunoglobulins, for Fc receptor terminology and 15.8.7, Immunology, Lymphocytes, for CD terminology.

REFERENCES

1. Calhoun L, Petz LD. Erythrocyte antigens and antibodies. In: Beutler E, Lichtman MA, Coller BS, Kipps TJ, Seligsohn U, eds. *Williams Hematology*. 6th ed. New York, NY: McGraw-Hill; 2001:1843-1857.
2. Schenkel-Brunner H. *Human Blood Groups: Chemical and Biochemical Basis of Antigen Specificity*. 2nd ed. New York, NY: Springer-Verlag; 2000.

3. Daniels GL, Fletcher A, Garratty G, et al. Blood group terminology 2004: from the International Society of Blood Transfusion Committee on Terminology for Red Cell Surface Antigens. *Vox Sang.* 2004;87(4):304-316.
4. International Society for Blood Transfusion Committee on Terminology for Red Cell Surface Antigens Web site. http://blood.co.uk/IBGRL/ISBT%20Pages/ISBT%20Terminology%20Pages/Terminology%20Home%20Page.htm. Accessed September 9, 2006.
5. Dzieczkowski JS, Anderson KC. Transfusion biology and therapy. In: Kasper DL, Braunwald E, Fauci AS, Hauser SL, Longo DL, Jameson JL, eds. *Harrison's Principles of Internal Medicine.* 16th ed. New York, NY: McGraw-Hill; 2005:662-667.
6. Webert KE, Chan HHW, Smith JW, Heddle NM, Kelton JG. Red cell, platelet, and white cell antigens. In: Greer JP, Foerster J, Lukens JN, Rodgers GM, Paraskevas F, Glader B, eds. *Wintrobe's Clinical Hematology.* 11th ed. Philadelphia, PA: Lippincott Williams & Wilkins; 2004:791-829.
7. Daniels GL, Anstee DJ, Cartron JP, et al. Blood group terminology 1995: ISBT Working Party on Terminology for Red Cell Surface Antigens. *Vox Sang.* 1995;69(3):265-279.
8. Issitt PD, Crookston MC. Blood group terminology: current conventions. *Transfusion.* 1984;24(1):2-7.
9. Garratty G, Dzik W, Issitt PD, Lublin DM, Reid ME, Zelinski T. Terminology for blood group antigens and genes—historical origins and guidelines in the new millennium. *Transfusion.* 2000;40(4):477-489.
10. Lewis M, Anstee DJ, Bird GWG, et al. Blood group terminology 1990: the ISBT Working Party on Terminology for Red Cell Surface Antigens. *Vox Sang.* 1990;58(2):152-169.
11. Daniels GL, Anstee DJ, Cartron JP, et al. Reports and guidelines: International Society of Blood Transfusion working party on terminology for red cell surface antigens. *Vox Sang.* 2001;80(3):193-196.
12. Daniels GL, Cartron JP, Fletcher A, et al. International Society of Blood Transfusion Committee on Terminology for Red Cell Surface Antigens: Vancouver Report. *Vox Sang.* 2003;84(3):244-247.
13. Serum, cells, and rare fluid exchange: ISBT human blood group systems. http://jove.prohosting.com/~scarfex/blood/groups.html. Accessed September 9, 2006.
14. Avent ND, Reid ME. The Rh blood group system: a review. *Blood.* 2000;95(2):375-387.
15. Whitsett CF, Hare VW, Oxendine SM, Pierce JA. Autologous and allogeneic red cell survival studies in the presence of autoanti-AnWj. *Transfusion.* 1993;33(10):845-847.
16. Searchgenes. HUGO Gene Nomenclature Committee. http://www.gene.ucl.ac.uk/cgi-bin/nomenclature/searchgenes.pl. Accessed February 15, 2005.
17. Issitt PD, Moulds JJ. Blood group terminology suitable for use in electronic data processing equipment. *Transfusion.* 1992;32(7):677-682.
18. Daniels GL, Anstee DJ, Cartron JP, et al. Terminology for red cell surface antigens: ISBT Working Party Oslo Report. *Vox Sang.* 1999;77(1):52-57.
19. Metcalfe P, Watkins NA, Ouwehand WH, et al. Nomenclature of human platelet antigens. *Vox Sang.* 2003;85(3):240-245.
20. von dem Borne AEG, Décary F. ICSH/ISBT Working Party on Platelet Serology: nomenclature of platelet-specific antigens. *Vox Sang.* 1990;58(2):176.
21. European Bioinformatics Institute. IPD-HPA Database. http://www.ebi.ac.uk/ipd/hpa/. Accessed September 15, 2006.

22. Bux J. Nomenclature of granulocyte alloantigens: ISBT Working Party on Platelet and Granulocyte Serology, Granulocyte Antigen Working Party: International Society of Blood Transfusion. *Transfusion*. 1999;39(6):662-663.
23. Lalezari P. Nomenclature of neutrophil-specific antigens. *Transfusion*. 2002;42(11):1396-1397.
24. Stroncek D, Bux J. Is it time to standardize granulocyte alloantigen nomenclature? *Transfusion*. 2002;42(4):393-395.

15.2 Cancer

15.2.1 Cancer Stage. Cancer stages are expressed with the use of capital roman numerals:

stage I
stage II
stage III
stage IV

The term "stage 0" usually indicates carcinoma in situ.

Histologic grades are expressed with arabic numerals, eg, grade 2.

Letter and numerical suffixes, usually set on the line, may be added to subdivide individual cancer stages, as in the following examples:

stage 0a
stage 0is
stage IA
stage IE
stage IB2
stage IIIE+S
stage IVA
stage IVB

(E indicates extralymphatic spread; S, splenic involvement [as seen in Hodgkin disease]; "is," in situ.)

15.2.2 The TNM Staging System. The TNM staging system[1-9] is an internationally standardized system for the staging of cancer and is in its seventh decade of continuing formulation. The TNM classification is put forth by the American Joint Committee on Cancer (AJCC) and the International Union Against Cancer (UICC; http://www.uicc.org).[1] The AJCC's *Cancer Staging Manual*[2] and the UICC's *TNM Classification of Malignant Tumours*[3] present the stages of cancer as defined by TNM classifications. The TNM definitions and stage groupings are based on prognostic outcome. Information about TNM may be accessed at the UICC Web site, http://www.uicc.org/index.php?id=508. The TNM symbols follow.

- T: tumor (indicates size, extent, or depth of penetration of the primary tumor). T is followed by numerical or other suffixes set on the line, eg:

  TX: primary tumor cannot be assessed

  T0: no evidence of a primary tumor

Tis: in situ carcinoma

T1, T2, T3, T4: increasing size, extent, or other characteristics of the primary tumor

Note: The number following T does not refer to an absolute size. For example, for one type of tumor, T1 may indicate size of 2 cm or less, for another, a depth (or thickness) of 0.75 mm or less, and for another, tumor confinement within the underlying mucosa.

- N: node (indicates the absence or presence and extent of regional lymph node involvement)

  NX: regional lymph nodes cannot be assessed

  N0: no regional lymph node metastasis

  N1, N2, N3: increasing metastatic involvement of regional lymph nodes according to criteria that vary for different anatomic sites
- M: metastasis (indicates absence or presence of distant metastasis)

  MX: extent of metastasis cannot be determined

  M0: no metastasis

  M1: distant metastasis
- Site of metastasis may be indicated with parenthetic 3-letter abbreviations:

ADR	adrenals
BRA	brain
HEP	hepatic
LYM	lymph nodes
MAR	bone marrow
OSS	osseous
OTH	others
PER	peritoneum
PLE	pleura
PUL	pulmonary
SKI	skin
Example:	M1(PUL)

The TNM System and Cancer Staging. Various combinations of the T, N, and M categories are used to define cancer stages (consult the AJCC or UICC manuals for specifics). For example, a TNM stage grouping that defines stage I for many types of cancer is

T1N0M0

The combinations that define individual stages differ among anatomic sites, for example:

lung cancer, stage IIA: T1N1M0

pancreatic cancer, stage IIA: T3N0M0

More than one combination of the T, N, and M categories may constitute the definition of a single stage: eg, in a given cancer, stage III may be defined as T1N1M0 *or* T2N1M0 *or* T3N0M0 *or* T3N1M0.

Optional Descriptors. Additional descriptors, although not part of the TNM staging system, may be used as adjuncts to the T, N, and M categories for defining the extent of disease; these are indicated by capital letters as follows:

certainty factor (C-factor)	C1, C2, C3, C4, C5
histopathologic grading	GX, G1, G2, G3, G4
lymphatic vessel invasion	LX, L0, L1
residual tumor	RX, R0, R1, R2
venous invasion	VX, V0, V1, V2

C-factor terms may be used together with T, N, and M categories, eg, T3C2, N2C1, M0C2 (example from Sobin and Wittekind[3(p15)]).

Lowercase prefixes to the T, N, M, and other symbols may be used to indicate the mode of determining criteria for tumor description and staging or other attributes; these are as follows:

a	autopsy
c	clinical
p	pathologic
r	recurrent tumor
y	classification during or after multimodality treatment

Examples: cTNM, pT3

The T, N, M, and other symbols used in cancer staging may be followed by suffixes in addition to the common X, 0, and numerals, which further specify qualities such as size, invasiveness, and extent of metastasis, eg:

Ta	T2a	M1a	N1a	pN1a	pN0
Tis	T2(m)	M2a	N2a	pN1mi	pN0(i)
T1b	T2(5)		N2b	pN0(sn)	pN0(i+)
T1c	T3a		N2c	pN3c	pN0(mol)
T1a1					pN0(mol+)

(m indicates multiple primary tumors at a single site; mi, micrometastasis; sn, sentinel node status; i, isolated tumor cells; mol, isolated tumor cells demonstrated by nonmorphologic [eg, molecular] techniques.)

Examples of such combined terms are

pN0(i)(sn)

pT2cN1cM0

Usage. Terms such as "stage I cancer," "TNM staging system," and "T1N1M0" are widely recognized and may be used in articles without expansion. However, authors should specify the clinical and/or pathologic criteria that define any stage (optionally but preferably citing the staging system of the AJCC or UICC manuals).

Use terms as follows (see also 11.1, Correct and Preferred Usage, Correct and Preferred Usage of Common Words and Phrases [Case, Client, Consumer, Patient, Subject]):

Correct	*Incorrect*
T category	T stage
N category	N stage
M category	M stage
stage III cancer, patient with stage III cancer	stage III patient
N1 lesions	N1 patients
patients with T1N0M0 tumor, T1N0M0 tumors, T1N0M0 cases	T1N0M0 patients
TXN0M0 classification	

For some sites, the histologic grade has been integrated into the staging system.

Other Staging Systems and the TNM System. The AJCC-UICC TNM classification and stage grouping is not the only system used for staging cancer, and equivalency of the same stage number among different systems cannot be assumed. However, 2 cancer staging systems, the FIGO (International Federation of Gynecology and Obstetrics; http://www.figo.org) staging system for gynecologic cancers[10,11] and the Dukes stage system for colon and rectal cancers,[12,13] have virtual equivalence with the AJCC-UICC stage. The AJCC-UICC system contains subsets of TNM classifications within stage groups that provide greater prognostic precision within each stage for colorectal cancer than does the Dukes system.[12,13]

FIGO stages are expressed similarly to TNM stages:

stage I	stage IA	stage IA1	stage IB	stage IB1	stage IC
stage II	stage IIA	stage IA2	stage IIB	stage IB2	stage IIC
stage III	stage IIIA		stage IIIB		stage IIIC
stage IV	stage IVA		stage IVB		

Dukes stages are expressed with letters:

Dukes A	*or*	Dukes stage A
Dukes B	*or*	Dukes stage B
Dukes C	*or*	Dukes stage C
Dukes D	*or*	Dukes stage D

15.2.3 Bethesda System. The Bethesda System for Reporting Cervical Cytology, dating to 1988, is a standardized, systematic means of reporting Papanicolaou test results.[14] Resources are the published handbook (the "blue book")[14] and the Web site (http://www.cytopathology.org/NIH).[15]

Expand the following abbreviations at first mention. Punctuate as shown:

Expansion	*Abbreviation*
adenocarcinoma in situ of endocervix	AIS
American Society for Colposcopy and Cervical Pathology	ASCCP
American Society of Cytopathology	ASC
ASCUS/LSIL Triage Study	ALTS
atypical glandular cells	AGCs
atypical squamous cells	ASCs
atypical squamous cells, cannot exclude high-grade squamous intraepithelial lesion	ASC-H
atypical squamous cells of undetermined significance	ASC-US
Bethesda Interobserver Reproducibility Project	BIRP
carcinoma in situ	CIS
cervical intraepithelial neoplasia	CIN
conventional preparation	CP
endocervical/transformation zone	EC/TZ
high-grade squamous intraepithelial lesion	HSIL
human papillomavirus	HPV
intrauterine device *or* intrauterine contraceptive device	IUD
liquid-based preparation	LBP
loop electrosurgical excision procedure	LEEP
last menstrual period	LMP
lower uterine segment	LUS
low-grade squamous intraepithelial lesion	LSIL
malignant mixed mesodermal tumor	MMMT
National Cancer Institute, Bethesda, Maryland	NCI
negative for intraepithelial lesion or malignancy	NILM
not otherwise specified	NOS
nuclear to cytoplasmic ratio	N:C
small cell undifferentiated carcinoma	SCUC
squamous intraepithelial lesion	SIL
the Bethesda System	TBS
transitional cell carcinoma	TCC
transformation zone	T zone
vaginal intraepithelial neoplasia	VAIN

In the following examples, unexpanded abbreviations are assumed to have been previously defined in the text:

> Low-grade squamous intraepithelial lesions (LSILs) have been described as a benign cytologic consequence of active human papillomavirus (HPV) replication. Several studies have reported that certain behavioral and biological risks exist for LSIL, suggesting that HPV alone is not sufficient for the development of LSIL.
>
> AIS (CP)
>
> ASC-H (CP)
>
> exfoliated endometrial cells (liquid-based preparation [LBP])
>
> atrophy (LBP)
>
> glandular cells post hysterectomy (CP)

Grades are expressed as follows:

> CIN 1, CIN 2, CIN 3
> VAIN 1, VAIN 2, VAIN 3

15.2.4 **Multiple Endocrine Neoplasia.** Abbreviations for types of multiple endocrine neoplasia (MEN) feature arabic numerals and a space, as follows:

> MEN 1
> MEN 2
> MEN 2A
> MEN 2B
> MEN 3

Gene terms are italicized with spaces closed up (see 15.6.2, Genetics, Human Gene Nomenclature):

> *MEN1*

15.2.5 **Molecular Cancer Terminology.** See also 15.10, Molecular Medicine. The style for the cell cycle is as follows:

Phase	*Expansion or Derivation*
G_1	growth 1 *or* gap 1
S	synthesis (of DNA)
G_2	growth 2 *or* gap 2
M	mitosis
G_0	quiescent state
R point	restriction point

Miscellaneous molecular terms are styled as shown in the following tabulation. (See also 15.6.3, Genetics, Oncogenes and Tumor Suppressor Genes.)

Protein	*Derivation*	*Variant Examples*	*Associated Genes*
actinin	α-actinin		*ACTN1, ACTN2, ACTN3*
Bcl	B-cell lymphoma	bcl-2	*BCL2*
CAK	cyclin-activating enzyme (= cyclinH/CDK7)	bcl-X	*BCLX*
catenin		β_1-catenin	*CTNNB1*
cdc2	cell division cycle		*CDC2*
CDK	cyclin-dependent kinase	cdk2	*CDK2*
CDKI	CDK inhibitor		
cyclin/CDK complex		cyclin B/CDK1, cyclinD/CDK4/CDK6	
G protein	GTP-binding regulatory protein		
INK4	inhibitors of CDK4	$p16^{Ink4}$ (p16)	*CDKN2A*
p21			*CDKN1A*
p53			*TP53*
Rb protein	retinoblastoma protein		*RB1*
TGF	tumor (or transforming) growth factor		TGF-β
tumor necrosis factor (TNF)			*TNF*

Note: Gene terms follow standard gene nomenclature style (see 15.6.2, Genetics, Human Gene Nomenclature).

REFERENCES

1. International Union Against Cancer/Union International Contre le Cancer Web site. http://www.uicc.org. Accessed March 14, 2006.
2. Greene FL, Page DL, Fleming ID, et al; for the American Joint Committee on Cancer, eds. *Cancer Staging Manual.* 6th ed. New York, NY: Springer; 2002.
3. Sobin LH, Wittekind C; for the International Union Against Cancer [UICC], eds. *TNM Classification of Malignant Tumours.* 6th ed. New York, NY: Wiley-Liss; 2002.
4. Wittekind C, Henson DE, Hutter RVP, Sobin LH, eds. *TNM Supplement: A Commentary on Uniform Use.* New York, NY: Wiley-Liss; 2001.
5. Gospodarowicz MK, Henson DE, Hutter RVP, O'Sullivan B, Sobin LH, Wittekind C, eds. *Prognostic Factors in Cancer.* 2nd ed. New York, NY: Wiley-Liss; 2001.
6. Sobin LH. TNM: principles, history, and relation to other prognostic factors. *Cancer.* 2001;91(suppl):1589-1592.
7. Sobin LH. Frequently asked questions regarding the application of the TNM classification. *Cancer.* 1999;85(6):1405-1406.

8. Gospodarowicz MK, Miller D, Groome PA, Greene FL, Logan PA, Sobin LH; for the UICC TNM Project. The process for continuous improvement of the TNM classification. *Cancer*. 2004:100(1):1-5.
9. Sobin LH. TNM: evolution and relation to other prognostic factors. *Semin Surg Oncol*. 2003;21(1):3-7.
10. Benedet JL, Bender H, Johnes H III, Pecorelli S; for the FIGO Committee on Gynecologic Oncology. FIGO staging classifications and clinical practice guidelines in the management of gynecologic cancers. *Int J Gynaecol Obstet*. 2000;70(2):209-262.
11. International Federation of Gynecology and Obstetrics Web site. http://www.figo.org. Accessed March 14, 2006.
12. Hutter RVP, Sobin LH. A universal staging system for cancer of the colon and rectum: let there be light. *Arch Pathol Lab Med*. 1986;110(5):367-368.
13. Winawer SJ, Fletcher RH, Miller L, et al. Colorectal cancer screening: clinical guidelines and rationale. *Gastroenterology*. 1997;112(2):594-642.
14. Solomon D, Nayar R, eds. *The Bethesda System for Reporting Cervical Cytology: Definitions, Criteria, and Explanatory Notes*. 2nd ed. New York, NY: Springer-Verlag; 2004.
15. 2001 Terminology. NCI Bethesda System 2001. http://bethesda2001.cancer.gov/terminology.html. Accessed March 14, 2006.

15.3 Cardiology.

Cardiology. Several areas of cardiology use simple letter terms and alphanumeric terms that need not be expanded at first mention.

15.3.1 Electrocardiographic Terms.

Electrocardiographic Terms. International standardization of electrocardiographic nomenclature dates back to the mid-20th century.[1-4]

The preferred abbreviation for electrocardiogram and electrocardiographic in *JAMA* and the *Archives* Journals is ECG, not EKG. In the following examples of ECG terms note the use of capitals, lowercase letters, subscripts, and hyphens.

Leads. Leads (recording electrodes) are designated as follows:

Types of Leads	*Names*
Standard (bipolar) leads	I, II, III
Augmented limb leads/unipolar extremity leads (a, augmented; V, voltage; R, right arm; L, left arm; F, foot)	aVR, aVL, aVF
Inverted aVR lead	−aVR
(Unipolar) precordial (chest) leads	V_1, V_2, V_3, V_4, V_5, V_6, V_7, V_8, V_9
Right precordial leads	V_1R, V_2R, V_3R, V_4R, V_5R, V_6R
Modified chest lead using V_1	MCL_1

Example: The abnormality appeared in leads V_3 through V_6 [*not* V_3-V_6 or $V_{3\text{-}6}$].

Deflections. The main deflections of the ECG (see Figure 1) are named in alphabetical sequence (P, Q, R, S, T, U), a usage that dates back to the inventor, Willem Einthoven.[2] Other deflections use initial letters of the entity being described.

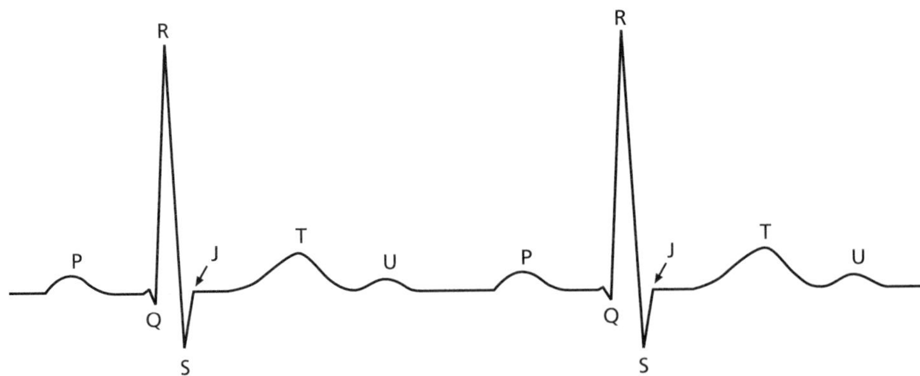

Figure 1. Electrocardiographic deflections (schematic).

As a guide, hyphens usually do not link deflection terms in the same PQRSTU complex (eg, QT) but do link deflections in different waves (eg, R-R), with the exception of ST-T. The following are examples of terms descriptive of deflections and patterns in ECG tracings:

delta wave (preferred over Δ wave)

F wave (atrial flutter wave)

f wave (atrial fibrillation wave)

J point, J junction (junction of QRS complex and ST segment; do not confuse with the J curve in hypertension)

J-ST axis, vector

P wave, axis, etc

PR interval, segment, etc (*not* P-R)

Q wave, q wave

qR complex

QR-type complex

QRS complex, configuration, axis, duration, etc

qrs complex, etc

QRS-T complex

QS wave, qs wave

QT interval, prolongation, etc (*not* Q-T)

QTc (corrected QT interval)

R wave, r wave, R′ wave, r′ wave

R-on-T

R-R interval

rS, RS, Rs complex, configuration, etc

R/S (ratio)

rSR′ pattern

S wave, s wave

S′ wave, s′ wave

ST segment, depression, axis, etc (*not* S-T)

ST-segment abnormality

ST-T segment, elevation, changes, axis, etc (*not* S-T-T)

T wave, axis, etc

Ta wave (atrial repolarization)

TQ segment

U wave

When terms such as the foregoing are used as modifiers, use a hyphen before the modifying noun (see also 8.3, Punctuation, Hyphens and Dashes).

P-wave duration

Q-wave irregularity

non–Q-wave myocardial infarction

ST-segment depression (*not* S-T)

The following symbols are used in connection with paced ECGs:

A	atrial stimulus
V	ventricular stimulus
AV	interval from atrial stimulus to succeeding ventricular stimulus
AR	interval from atrial stimulus to conducted spontaneous ventricular depolarization
PV	interval from spontaneous atrial depolarization to succeeding "atrial-synchronous" ventricular stimulus

Capital letters are used to describe generic ECG deflections.

Improper paper speed will spuriously alter the QRS configuration. [*not* qrs configuration]

In reference to an individual ECG tracing, or in descriptions of some specific ECG patterns, capitals may indicate larger waves and lowercase letters smaller waves; in practice, this most often applies to the Q, R, and S waves.

Pathologic Q waves occur in myocardial infarction.

The q wave in aVF and the Rr′ pattern in lead V_3 in this patient's ECG were considered normal findings.

An rSR′ complex in the anterior chest leads and qRs in the left chest leads may indicate right bundle-branch block.

Lead and tracing terms may be combined to describe pattern and location together.

Term	*Explanation*
R_I	R wave in lead I
RaVL	R wave in aVL
S_{III}	S wave in lead III

Term	*Explanation*
$_{R}V_3$	R wave in V_3
$S_1Q_3T_3$ pattern	Prominence of S wave in lead I, Q wave in lead III, and T-wave inversion in lead III
$SV_1 + RV_5$	Sum of voltages of S wave in V_1 and R wave in V_5

The P axis, QRS axis, ST axis, and T axis are specified with a plus or minus sign followed by the number of degrees in arabic numerals, eg, +60°, −30°.

15.3.2 Electrograms. Electrogram (EGM) terms pertain to invasive electrophysiologic recording of cardiac impulse conduction. Expand them at first mention.

Term	*Expansion*
AH interval	atrial-His interval
His	His potential
HV interval	His-ventricular interval

15.3.3 Heart Sounds. The 4 heart sounds and 4 components are commonly abbreviated in discussions of cardiac auscultatory findings; numerical subscripts are used.

S_1 first heart sound

M_1 mitral valve component

T_1 tricuspid valve component

S_2 second heart sound

A_2 aortic valve component

P_2 pulmonic valve component

S_3 third heart sound

S_4 fourth heart sound

Examples:

The presence of an audible S_3 was consistent with the patient's ventricular aneurysm.

An audible S_4 may be due to a variety of cardiac and systemic conditions.

Sound names may be written out in full when discussed generically.

Third heart sounds are suggestive of congestive heart failure, but an S_3 gallop may be a normal finding in children and young adults.

or:

The S_3 is suggestive of congestive heart failure, but an S_3 gallop may be a normal finding in children and young adults.

For plurals, follow the term with "sounds" or another noun.

S_3 sounds [not S_3s] may be normal or pathologic.

S_3 gallops may be a normal finding in children and young adults.

15.3.4 Murmurs. Murmurs are graded from soft (lower grade) to loud (higher grade). Murmur grades are written in arabic numerals. Systolic murmurs may be graded from 1 to 6 (see Freeman and Levine[5]) and diastolic murmurs from 1 to 4. Murmurs may also be presented by means of a virgule construction. Examples:

grade 2 systolic murmur

grade 1 diastolic murmur

grade 4/6 systolic murmur

grade 2/4 diastolic murmur

The patient had a grade 3 systolic murmur radiating to the axilla consistent with the diagnosis of mitral valve regurgitation.

15.3.5 Jugular Venous Pulse. The jugular venous pulse contours are expressed with italic single letters and roman words:

a wave (atrial)

x descent

z point

c wave

x′ descent

v wave (ventricular)

y descent (*or y* trough)

h wave

Examples:

prominent *a* wave

giant *a* wave

steep *x* descent

increased *v* wave

abrupt *y* descent

15.3.6 Echocardiography. The names of major echocardiographic methods are listed below. Expand any abbreviations at first mention, unless otherwise indicated.

Name	*Common Abbreviation*
2-dimensional echocardiography	2DE
3-dimensional echocardiography	3DE
4-dimensional echocardiography	4DE
adenosine stress echocardiography	
color Doppler echocardiography	
color flow Doppler echocardiography	
continuous-wave Doppler echocardiography	CW Doppler
contrast echocardiography	

Name	*Common Abbreviation*
dipyridamole stress echocardiography	
dobutamine stress echocardiography	
Doppler echocardiography	
Doppler flow imaging	
exercise echocardiography	
intravascular ultrasonography	IVUS
pharmacologic stress echocardiography	
pulsed Doppler echocardiography	
spectral Doppler echocardiography	
stress echocardiography	
transesophageal echocardiography	TEE

The following commonly used echocardiographic indexes should also be expanded at first mention but are included here for reference:

Term	*Expansion*
AVA	aortic valve area
EF	ejection fraction
EPSS	E point septal separation
FAC	fractional area change
FS	fractional shortening
IVS, IVST	interventricular septal thickness
LVID	left ventricular internal dimension
MVA	mitral valve area
PHT	pressure half-time
PW, PWT	posterior wall thickness
RVID	right ventricular internal dimension
SAM	systolic anterior motion of the mitral valve
d or ed	end diastole
s or es	end systole

Terms are combined as in the following examples:

IVSd

IVSs

LVIDd

LVIDed

LVIDes

LVIDs

LVPWd

LVPWs

RVIDd

Ejection fraction is expressed as a percentage, eg, 60% (see also 19.0, Numbers and Percentages).

15.3.7 **Pacemaker Codes.** The capabilities and operation of cardiac pacemakers are described by 3- to 5-letter codes.[6,7]

> DDIR pacing
>
> VVI pacemaker

The code system for antibradycardia pacemakers endorsed by the North American Society of Pacing and Electrophysiology and the British Pacing and Electrophysiology Group is known as the NASPE/BPEG Generic Code or NBG Code. Although the code need not be expanded when mentioned in passing, it is good practice to describe pacing modes in prose at first mention, eg, "dual-chamber, adaptive-rate (DDDR) pacing." The NBG Code was revised in 2001 to apply to antibradycardia, adaptive-rate, and multisite pacing.[8,9]

In Table 1, positions I through V refer to the first through fifth letters of the NBG Code. The character for "None" is the letter O, not the numeral 0. In practice, the first 3 positions are always given; the fourth and fifth are added when necessary to provide additional information.

Table 1. Revised NASPE/BPEG Generic Code for Antibradycardia Pacing[a]

Position	I	II	III	IV	V
Category	**Chamber(s) Paced**	**Chamber(s) Sensed**	**Response to Sensing**	**Rate Modulation**	**Multisite Pacing**
	O = none	O = none	O = none	O = none	O = none
	A = atrium	A = atrium	T = triggered	R = rate modulation	A = atrium
	V = ventricle	V = ventricle	I = inhibited		V = ventricle
	D = dual (A + V)	D = dual (A + V)	D = dual (T + I)		D = dual (A + V)
Manufacturers' designation only	S = single (A or V)	S = single (A or V)			

[a] Reprinted, with permission, from Bernstein et al.[8]

Note: The principal changes from the previous (1987) code are the dropping of classifications from position IV (P, simple programmatic; M, multiprogrammable; C, communicating) and additions to position V (shown in the table) and deletions from position V (P, pacing; S, shock). Position V, which formerly applied to antitachyarrhythmia functions, now applies to multisite pacing.

15.3.8 **Implanted Cardioverter/Defibrillators.** A similar code, known as the NASPE/BPEG Defibrillator Code or NBD Code,[10] exists for implanted cardioverter/defibrillators (ICDs), as defined in Table 2.

Table 2. Defibrillator Code[a]

Position I (Shock Chamber)	Position II (Antitachycardia Pacing Chamber)	Position III (Tachycardia Detection)	Position IV (Antibradycardia Pacing Chamber)
O = none	O = none	E = electrocardiogram	O = none
A = atrium	A = atrium	H = hemodynamic	A = atrium
V = ventricle	V = ventricle		V = ventricle
D = dual (A + V)	D = dual (A + V)		D = dual (A + V)

[a] Reprinted from Bernstein et al[10] by permission of Blackwell Publishing.

Examples are as follows:

DDH defibrillator

VOEO defibrillator

There is also a Short Form of the NBD Code intended only for use in conversation:

ICD-B: ICD with antibradycardia pacing as well as shock

ICD-T: ICD with antitachycardia pacing as well as shock and antibradycardia pacing

ICD-S: ICD with shock capability only

The foregoing terms can each represent a variety of devices; for instance, ICD-S could indicate VO, VOE, VOEO, DOH, or DOHV. The same devices may also be represented by more than 1 term, eg, ICD-B may also represent VO and VOE, among other devices. Therefore, only the Long Form is used in writing. As in the case of the NBG Code, at first mention of an ICD it is good practice to include a prose description as well as the NBD Code designation.

For maximum conciseness and completeness in ICD labeling and record keeping, the first 3 positions of the NBD Code are given, followed after a hyphen by the first 4 positions of the NBG Code. Thus, "VAE-DDDR" refers to an ICD providing ventricular shock, atrial antitachycardia pacing, EGM sensing for tachycardia detection, and dual-chamber, adaptive-rate antibradycardia pacing.

15.3.9 **Pacemaker-Lead Code.** The NASPE/BPEG Pacemaker-Lead Code (NBL Code) is as follows:

I (Electrode Configuration)	*II (Fixation Mechanism)*	*III (Insulation Material)*	*IV (Drug Elution)*
U = unipolar	A = active	P = polyurethane	S = steroid
B = bipolar	P = passive	S = silicone rubber	N = nonsteroid
M = multipolar	O = none	D = dual (P+S)	O = none

(Reprinted from Bernstein and Parsonnet[11] by permission of Blackwell Publishing.)

Typically, all 4 positions are mentioned, eg, UPSO, BAPS.

15.3.10 Heart Disease Classifications. Several classifications pertaining to heart disease are in use:

Classification	*Applies to*	*Classes*	*Example*
Braunwald[12]	Unstable angina	I-III	Braunwald class I
		IA-IIIC	Braunwald class IIIB
Canadian Cardiovascular Society (CCS)[13,14]	Exertional angina	I-IV	CCS class II
Forrester[15-17]	Cardiac function after myocardial infarction	I-IV	Forrester class I
Killip[17-19]	Cardiac status after myocardial infarction	I-IV	Killip class I heart failure
New York Heart Association (NYHA)[20]	Cardiac disease and functional capacity	I-IV	NYHA class I

The classes are assessed in various ways, for instance, by physical examination (Killip), hemodynamic measurement (Forrester), and patient history (NYHA). The detailed meanings of each class are beyond the scope of this book, but several style points may be noted:

- Severity increases from lower to higher numbers and letters.
- There is no automatic correspondence between classes (eg, Killip class I is not equivalent to NYHA class I).
- The numerals are designators and are not quantitative or semiquantitative. Therefore, roman numerals are appropriate.

Avoid:	Forrester class >2
Acceptable equivalents:	Forrester class above II
	class greater than Forrester II
	Forrester classes III and IV

- Authors should describe their classification criteria, for instance:

> Killip class on admission was determined as the following: patients in class I were free of rales and a third heart sound; patients in class II had rales up to 50% of each lung field regardless of the presence of the third heart sound . . . (adapted from Neskovic et al[21]).

> We suggest that cases of unstable angina class IIIB now be subdivided into troponin-positive and troponin-negative subgroups . . . (adapted from Hamm and Braunwald[22[p120]]).

15.3.11 Coronary Artery Angiographic Classifications. Guidelines are available for nomenclature of coronary artery segments,[23] used in coronary artery catheterization and thrombolysis in myocardial infarction flow (TIMI flow).

The TIMI flow is expressed as grade 0, grade 1, grade 2, or grade 3, from lowest flow (or severest lesion) to highest flow.[23]

15.3.12 Cellular and Molecular Cardiology.[24-26] See also 15.10, Molecular Medicine.

Cardiac Muscle. These descriptive terms do not require expansion:

Term	*Derivation*
A band	actin-myosin overlap
H band	Hensen (discoverer)
M line	mesophragma
T tubules	tubulus transversus
Z line	*Zückung* (German: "contraction")

Expand these terms at first mention:

Term	*Expansion*	*Derivation*
TnC	troponin C	binds calcium
TnI	troponin I	inhibits actin-myosin interactions
TnT	troponin T	binds to tropomyosin
cTnC	troponin C, cardiac form	
cTnI	troponin I, cardiac form	
cTnT	troponin T, cardiac form	

Miscellaneous Cellular and Molecular Terms. If an expansion is given, use at first mention. Otherwise, terms may be used without expansion.

Term	*Expansion*	*Derivation/Explanation*
athero-ELAM	endothelial leukocyte adhesion molecule involved in atherosclerosis	
CK-MB	creatine kinase, myocardial	
NOS	nitric oxide synthase	
NOS1		Named in order of discovery, also nNOS (neuronal NOS)
NOS2		Also iNOS (inducible NOS)
NOS3		Also eNOS, ecNOS (endothelial constitutive isoform of NOS)
P cell		Nodal cells of the sinus node
tPA	tissue plasminogen activator	

Expand the following lipoproteins and related terms at first mention:

Term	*Expansion*	*Note*
acyl CoA	acyl coenzyme A	
HDL	high-density lipoprotein	
HDL_1	HDL variant	

Term	*Expansion*	*Note*
HDL_2	HDL subfraction 2	
HDL_3	HDL subfraction 3	
HDL-C	HDL cholesterol	
HDL-R	HDL receptor	
HMG CoA	3-hydroxy-3-methylglutaryl coenzyme A	
IDL	intermediate-density lipoprotein	
IDL-C	IDL cholesterol	
IDL-R	IDL receptor	
LDL	low-density lipoprotein	
LDL-C	LDL cholesterol	
LDL-R	LDL receptor	
LPL	lipoprotein lipase gene	See also 15.6.2, Genetics, Human Gene Nomenclature
LPL_{188}	mutation in *LPL* at codon 188	See also 15.6.1, Genetics, Nucleic Acids and Amino Acids
$\mathrm{LPL}_{\mathrm{Asn29Ser}}$	substitution in LPL of serine at asparagine residue 29	
LP-X	lipoprotein X	
LRP_1	LDL-R–related protein	
LRP_2	LDL-R–related protein 2	
VHDL	very high-density lipoprotein	
VLDL-C	VLDL cholesterol	
VLDL-R	VLDL receptor	

Expand *apo* as *apolipoprotein* at first mention of terms such as the following:

apo AI	apo B_{48}	apo CI	apo D	apo E	apo J
apo AII	apo B_{100}	apo CII	apo E2		
apo AIII	apo CIII	apo E3			
apo AIV					
apo(a)					
apo $\mathrm{AI}_{\mathrm{Milano}}$					
apo $\mathrm{AI}_{\mathrm{Arg173Cys}}$					

REFERENCES

1. Barnes AR, Pardee HEB, White PD, Wilson FN, Wolferth CC; for the Committee of the American Heart Association for the Standardization of Precordial Leads. Standardization of precordial leads: supplementary report. *Am Heart J*. 1938;15:235-239.

2. Barnes AR, Katz LN, Levine SA, Pardee HEB, White PD, Wilson FN. Report of the Committee of the American Heart Association on the Standardization of Electrocardiographic Nomenclature. *Am Heart J.* 1943;25:528-534.
3. Barnes AR, Pardee HEB, White PD, Wilson FN, Wolferth CC. Second supplementary report by the Committee of the American Heart Association for the Standardization of Precordial Leads. *Am Heart J.* 1943;25:535-538.
4. Wilson FN, Kossmann CE, Burch GE, et al. Recommendations for standardization of electrocardiographic and vectorcardiographic leads. *Circulation.* 1954;10:564-573.
5. Freeman AR, Levine SA. The clinical significance of the systolic murmur: a study of 1000 consecutive "non-cardiac" cases. *Ann Intern Med.* 1933:6(11):1371-1385.
6. Bernstein AD, Camm AJ, Fletcher RD, et al. The NASPE/BPEG Generic Pacemaker Code for antibradyarrhythmia and adaptive-rate pacing and antitachyarrhythmia devices. *Pacing Clin Electrophysiol.* 1987;10(4):794-799.
7. Parsonnet V, Furman S, Smyth NPD. Implantable cardiac pacemakers status report and resource guideline: Pacemaker Study Group. *Circulation.* 1974;50(4):A21-A35.
8. Bernstein AD, Daubert J-C, Fletcher RD, et al. The revised NASPE/BPEG generic code for antibradycardia, adaptive-rate, and multisite pacing. *PACE.* 2002;25(2):260-264.
9. Bernstein AD, Camm AJ, Furman S, Parsonnet V. The NASPE/BPEG codes: use, misuse, and evolution. *Pacing Clin Electrophysiol.* 2001;24(5):787-788.
10. Bernstein AD, Camm AJ, Fisher JD, et al. North American Society of Pacing and Electrophysiology Policy Statement: the NASPE/BPEG defibrillator code. *Pacing Clin Electrophysiol.* 1993;16(9):1776-1780.
11. Bernstein AD, Parsonnet V. The NASPE/BPEG pacemaker-lead code (NBL Code). *Pacing Clin Electrophysiol.* 1996;19(11):1535-1536.
12. Braunwald E. Unstable angina: a classification. *Circulation.* 1989;80(2):410-414.
13. Campeau L. Grading of angina pectoris [letter]. *Circulation.* 1976;54(3):522-523.
14. Campeau L. The Canadian Cardiovascular Society grading of angina pectoris revisited 30 years later. *Can J Cardiol.* 2002;18(4):371-379.
15. Forrester JS, Diamond G, Chatterjee K, Swan HJC. Medical therapy of acute myocardial infarction by application of hemodynamic subsets (first of two parts). *N Engl J Med.* 1976;295(24):1356-1362.
16. Forrester JS, Diamond GA, Swan HJC. Correlative classification of clinical and hemodynamic function after acute myocardial infarction. *Am J Cardiol.* 1977;39(2):137-145.
17. Madias JE. Killip and Forrester classifications: should they be abandoned, kept, reevaluated, or modified [comment]? *Chest.* 2000;117(5):1223-1226.
18. Killip T, Kimball JT. Treatment of myocardial infarction in a coronary care unit: a two year experience with 250 patients. *Am J Cardiol.* 1967;20(4):457-464.
19. Werns SW, Bates ER. The enduring value of Killip classification. *Am Heart J.* 1999;137(2):213-215.
20. Criteria Committee of the New York Heart Association. *Nomenclature and Criteria for Diagnosis of Diseases of the Heart and Blood Vessels.* 9th ed. Boston, MA: Little Brown & Co; 1994:254.

21. Neskovic AN, Otasevic P, Bojic M, Popovic AD. Association of Killip class on admission and left ventricular dilatation after myocardial infarction: a closer look into an old clinical classification. *Am Heart J.* 1999;137(2):361-367.
22. Hamm CW, Braunwald E. A classification of unstable angina revisited. *Circulation.* 2000;102(1):118-122.
23. Scanlon PJ, Faxon DP, Audet AM, et al. ACC/AHA guidelines for coronary angiography: a report of the American College of Cardiology/American Heart Association Task Force on Practice Guidelines (Committee on Coronary Angiography). *J Am Coll Cardiol.* 1999;33(6):1756-1824.
24. Jameson JL, ed. *Principles of Molecular Medicine.* Totowa, NJ: Humana Press; 1998.
25. Braunwald E, Zipes DP, Libby P, eds. *Heart Disease: A Textbook of Cardiovascular Medicine.* 6th ed. Philadelphia, PA: WB Saunders Co; 2001.
26. Zipes DP, Libby P, Bonow RO, Braunwald E. *Braunwald's Heart Disease: A Textbook of Cardiovascular Medicine.* 7th ed. Philadelphia, PA: Elsevier Saunders; 2005.

15.4 Drugs. Physicians and other health care professionals, patients, researchers, manufacturers, and the public may refer to drugs by several names, including the nonproprietary name (often referred to as the generic name) and at least 1 proprietary (brand) or trademark name selected by the manufacturer of the drug. Other drug identifiers include chemical names, trivial (unofficial) names, and code designations.[1(pp12-15)] However, only 1 drug name, the nonproprietary name, is regulated internationally to ensure consistent usage and no duplication with other drugs. Once a drug has been assigned a nonproprietary name, the nonproprietary name should always be used to refer to the drug. (See 15.4.2, Nonproprietary Names.)

The nonproprietary name is established through nomenclature agencies, such as the United States Adopted Names (USAN) Council (http://www.ama-assn.org/ama/pub/category/2956.html), which work with the World Health Organization (WHO) to establish a single nonproprietary name. According to the WHO, "the existence of an international nomenclature for pharmaceutical substances, in the form of INN [international nonproprietary name], is important for the clear identification, safe prescription and dispensing of medicines to patients and for communication and exchange of information among health professionals and scientists worldwide."[2] The nonproprietary names of drugs that are to be marketed within the United States must be approved by the USAN Council. The nomenclature rules provided in 15.4.13, Nomenclature for Biological Products, are established by the USAN Council.

The pharmaceutical naming system of the WHO has been in operation since 1953. When a drug is being considered for possible approval, the sponsoring manufacturer must file an INN application with the WHO's Essential Drugs and Medicines team of Quality Safety and Medicines Policy (QSM), or with one of the drug nomenclature councils such as USAN or Japanese Adopted Names (JAN). The British Approved Names (BAN) and Dénominations Communes Françaises (DCF) Councils have now been superceded by the European Union, which does not have a separate council but requires that the INN be used for drugs marketed within the European Union. These organizations work in conjunction with the WHO to approve a nonproprietary name identical to the INN.[3] Manufacturers in countries without a nomenclature agency can request an INN from the WHO directly or apply in a country that has a nomenclature agency.[1(p13)]

15.4.1 **The Drug Development and Approval Process.** This brief summary of the drug development process is provided to help define the origins of different names used to identify drugs.

Drugs intended for clinical use undergo several phases of development before they can be considered for human use. Animal studies are performed initially to assess pharmacologic and toxicologic effects. While clinical studies are being conducted, animal studies may continue to assess effects on reproduction, teratogenicity, and carcinogenicity.[4(p63)]

To perform clinical studies in the United States, the developer or manufacturer must obtain an investigational new drug (IND) approval from the US Food and Drug Administration (FDA).[4(p59)] Once an IND application has been filed, the company must apply to USAN for a nonproprietary name. Until a nonproprietary name has been approved, the developers of a drug may refer to it by the code name. The code designation is usually alphanumeric, with letters to refer to the institution or manufacturer that assigns the code designation for the drug and numbers to refer to the chemical compound.[1(pp13-14)]

Drug developers must adhere to the Declaration of Helsinki and obtain institutional review board approval and patient informed consent to perform drug studies in humans. Phase 1 studies generally are conducted in healthy volunteers to assess safety, biological effects, metabolism, kinetics, and drug interactions.[4(p60)] Phase 2 studies usually are conducted to establish the therapeutic efficacy of a drug for its proposed indication and to study dose range, kinetics, and metabolism.[4(p60)] Phase 3 trials typically are randomized controlled trials that assess a drug's safety and efficacy in a large sample of patients (generally 2000 to 3000).[4(p61)] The patients selected have the condition(s) for which the drug is thought to be effective and for which the manufacturer wishes to obtain approval. The 3 phases of clinical testing take from 2 to 10 years (average, 5.6 years).[4(p60)] The FDA reviews drugs for approval in less than 1 year and performs expedited reviews for drugs for life-threatening illnesses.[4(p59)]

In the United States, a drug cannot be marketed or prescribed (other than for specific exceptions) until it has been approved by the FDA. The FDA approves *labeling* for the drug for specific indications for which the FDA believes sufficient evidence of effectiveness has been provided. Approved labeling defines the indications for which the drug can be *marketed*. The FDA does not approve indications for which a drug may be *prescribed*, since a company may not study all possible conditions for which a drug may be effective. In what is known as *off-label prescribing*, physicians may prescribe a marketed drug for indications for which it does not have FDA approval for labeling or marketing. The approved labeling is included in drug packaging, marketing materials, and the *Physicians' Desk Reference*.[5]

Because the number of patients tested before a drug is approved is insufficient to identify rare adverse events, some countries require physicians to report adverse events experienced by their patients, and some manufacturers may be required to systematically monitor drug adverse events after approval in a process known as *postmarketing surveillance*. Physicians and other health care professionals in the United States should report adverse drug events to the voluntary reporting system MEDWATCH (http://www.fda.gov/medwatch) or to the pharmaceutical manufacturer, which is obligated to file reports with the FDA. The United Kingdom, Canada, New Zealand, Denmark, and Sweden have legally mandated adverse event reporting systems.[4(p62)] In addition, the WHO maintains the WHO Collaborating Centre for International Drug Monitoring in Uppsala, Sweden.[6]

15.4.2 Nonproprietary Names. The INN identifies a specific pharmaceutical substance or active pharmaceutical ingredient. The INN is in the public domain and can be used without restriction. It is sometimes referred to colloquially as the *generic name.*[3] However, the terms *generic* and *nonproprietary* are not synonymous. Generic drugs are nontrademarked formulations of a drug that can be manufactured once a drug is no longer under patent restrictions. Generic drugs should be referred to by their nonproprietary name, just as are proprietary drugs.

The INN reflects the chemistry, pharmacologic action, and therapeutic use through its stem. Herbals (see 15.4.15, Herbals and Dietary Supplements), homeopathic products, mixtures, drugs in common use for decades (eg, morphine, codeine), and those with trivial chemical names (eg, acetic acid) do not receive INNs. The committees involved in reviewing and selecting INNs agree to a name that is then published as a proposed INN. During a 4-month comment period, any person can comment on or object to the proposed INN. If no objection is raised, the name is published as a recommended INN. New INNs are published in *WHO Drug Information* in English, French, and Spanish (http://www.who.int/druginformation). A cumulative INN list is published, which also includes INNs in Russian. More than 7000 INNs have been designated as of 2004; 120 to 150 are added each year.[2]

Stems. In addition to having a distinct sound and spelling to avoid confusion with other names, the INN includes a "stem" that designates the drug as a member of a family of related drugs, indicating that the drug has similar pharmacologic properties.[2]

The stem is usually a suffix common to a particular drug class that is incorporated into new drug names to indicate a chemical and/or pharmacologic relationship to older drugs.[7] For example:

> H_2-receptor antagonists: cimetidine, ranitidine, lupitidine (*-tidine* is the stem)
>
> Tyrosine kinase inhibitors: canertinib, imatinib, mubritinib (*-tinib* is the stem)
>
> β-Blockers: propranolol, timolol, atenolol (*-olol* is the stem)
>
> Combined α- and β-blockers: labetalol, medroxalol (*-alol* is the stem)

For some classes of drugs, the position of the stem varies within the drug name. For the group of antiviral drugs (not necessarily having common pharmacologic properties), the stem may be *vir-*, *-vir-*, or *-vir*:

> ganciclovir, enviradene, viroxime, alvircept, delavirdine

Approved stems are provided on the USAN Web site[7] and in the *USP Dictionary.*[1(pp1226-1232)]

The goal of the WHO INN system is to have a single INN for each drug used throughout the world. However, if the substance was in existence before the coordination of nomenclature by WHO, nonproprietary names may differ between countries. For example, *acetaminophen* is the USAN for the same drug that has the BAN and DCF name *paracetamol.* The USAN *albuterol* has a JAN of *salbutamol* (not to be confused with *salmeterol*, a longer-acting β-adrenergic agonist).[1(p44)] Some other names are more similar, such as *cyclobarbitone* (BAN) and *cyclobarbitol* (USAN). For these few drugs for which nonproprietary names differ by country, the nonproprietary name used depends on the primary audience, although the European Union has required that nonproprietary names that differ from the INN will be phased out over time. In cases in which international recognition is essential (such as adverse drug reactions), both names should be given at first mention.

> Acetaminophen (paracetamol) was recommended as an initial treatment for pain in the practice guidelines.

The existence of more than 1 nonproprietary name is also important when performing searches on drugs in journals or databases; all nonproprietary names for a particular drug should be used for a complete search. The *USP Dictionary*[1] lists the INN and nonproprietary names by nomenclature agency, if they differ.

Orphan Drugs. Drugs that may be used to treat relatively rare diseases but that otherwise are believed to have limited marketability are termed *orphan drugs*.[8] When a drug is designated an orphan drug by the FDA, the name it receives is not necessarily the name it will receive if it is approved for marketing.[1(p13)] A listing of orphan drugs is available at http://www.fda.gov/orphan.

Changes in Nonproprietary Names. Nonproprietary names may be changed if they are believed to be confusing or could result in medication errors, or if they are proven to infringe on trademark. For example, the antineoplastic compound mithramycin became plicamycin to avoid confusing mithramycin with the similar-sounding antineoplastic mitomycin and its proprietary name Mutamycin. The nomenclature committees have procedures for applying to change the nonproprietary name. (USAN's procedure is available at http://www.ama-assn.org/ama/pub/category/9916.html.)

15.4.3 Proprietary Names. The manufacturer's name for a drug (or other product) is called a *proprietary name* or *brand name*.[1(p15)] Proprietary names use initial capitals, with a few exceptions (eg, pHisoHex). *JAMA* and the *Archives* Journals do not use the trademark symbol (™) or the registered trademark symbol (®) because capitalization indicates the proprietary nature of the name (see also 5.6.16, Legal and Ethical Considerations, Intellectual Property: Ownership, Access, Rights, and Management, Trademark). The International Trademark Association has information about specific trademarks and may be reached at http://www.inta.org/ or International Trademark Association, 1133 Avenue of the Americas, New York, NY 10036.

Proprietary names for drugs often differ between countries (for example, nifedipine initially was marketed as Procardia in the United States and Adalat in Europe). Most US proprietary names are listed in the *Physicians' Desk Reference*[5] and *USP Dictionary*[1] and are cross-referenced to their USAN name. Unlike the nonproprietary name, the proprietary name does not undergo a coordinated international effort to provide consistent naming. One example is the proprietary name Bextra, which is the brand name for both valdecoxib (a cyclooxygenase 2 inhibitor type of nonsteroidal anti-inflammatory drug) in the United States and bucindolol (a β-blocker not approved in the United States) in Europe.[9] Even when the same brand name does not refer to different drugs in different countries, a drug is often marketed under different brand names in different countries. Therefore, because the medical literature is read internationally and confusion about the intended drug could lead to patient harm, the nonproprietary name should always be used and the proprietary name should almost never be used in the medical literature.

The exceptions to this rule are reports of adverse events that might be unique to a specific product formulation, or comparison of a generic formulation of a drug with the drug that was first approved. When both the nonproprietary and proprietary names are used in text, the nonproprietary name should appear first, with the proprietary name capitalized and in parentheses. Because proprietary drugs and manufacturers are listed in the *Physicians' Desk Reference* and other sources, the manufacturer does not need to be listed after the proprietary name.

> The lot of penicillin G potassium (Pentids) was inspected and found to meet the industry production standards.

Proprietary names may be used in questionnaires when the individuals responding may be unfamiliar with the nonproprietary name or when the specific proprietary product is important; in these cases the exact wording of the question should be maintained, but the nonproprietary name should still be provided.

> Parents were asked, "Have you ever given your child Tylenol [acetaminophen, paracetamol] or products containing Tylenol?"

Herbals and "natural" products generally do not have INNs. Whenever possible, the nonproprietary name (as listed in the *USP Dictionary* or the *PDR for Nonprescription Drugs and Dietary Supplements*, for example) should be used. For some proprietary formulations that comprise a blend of ingredients, however, the proprietary name may be the only way to refer to the formulation. (See also 15.4.15, Herbals and Dietary Supplements.)

> The authors used mass spectrometry to analyze samples from a bottle of Niagra Actra-R_x and a bottle of Actra-R_x (Body Basics) for the presence of sildenafil.

15.4.4 Chemical Names.

Chemical Names. The chemical name describes a drug in terms of its chemical structure.[1(p9)] Chemical names are provided in the American Chemical Society's *Chemical Abstracts* (information available at http://www.cas.org/PRINTED/printca.html) and can be listed in 1 of 2 ways; the first reflects the way in which *Chemical Abstracts* indexes inverted chemical names:

> hydrazinecarboxyimidamide, 2-[-(2,6-dichlorophenoxy)ethyl]-, sulfate, (2:1)

The second is the uninverted form:

> 2-[-(2,6-dichlorophenoxy)ethyl] hydrazinecarboxyimidamide sulfate, (2:1)

Both forms follow the recommendations of the International Union of Pure and Applied Chemistry and the International Union of Biochemistry and Molecular Biology. Each chemical is also designated a registry number with the Chemical Abstract Society (information available at http://www.cas.org/EO/regsys.html#q2). This number is included in the *USP Dictionary*[1] listing for the drug. Chemical names and registry numbers are rarely used in medical publications, and nonproprietary names are preferred.[1(pp13-15)]

15.4.5 Code Designations. A code designation is a temporary designation assigned to a product by the institution or manufacturer and may be used to refer to a drug under development before a nonproprietary name has been assigned. Codes may be numeric, alphabetic, or alphanumeric; letters in alphanumeric codes designate the institution or manufacturer assigning the code designation of the drug, and are followed by numbers to designate the chemical compound.[1(p15)]

Once a nonproprietary name has been assigned, code designations become obsolete and are rarely used in medical publications. If both the code and the nonproprietary name are provided, such as in discussion of the history of a drug, the nonproprietary name should be used preferentially and the code name may be added in parentheses.

> Mifepristone (formerly known as RU 486) was approved by FDA on September 28, 2000.
>
> Zidovudine (BW A509U) first became known as azidothymidine (commonly known as AZT) during testing and eventually was marketed as Retrovir.

15.4.6 Trivial Names. Drugs occasionally become known by an unofficial trivial name. The trivial name should be used in biomedical publications only to reproduce the exact language used as part of a study (eg, in a questionnaire), for historical reasons, or rarely when readers may be unfamiliar with the nonproprietary name. When reproducing the exact language used in a study, the nonpropietary name should be provided in brackets after the term used in the study.

> The participants were asked, "Have you ever taken AZT [zidovudine] or ddI [didanosine]?" Participants who said they had taken zidovudine or didanosine were classified as having had prior exposure to antiretroviral agents.

When names other than the nonproprietary name are used for historical reasons or because readers are unfamiliar with the nonproprietary name, the nonproprietary name should be used preferentially and the alternative name provided in parentheses.

> Semustine (NSC-95441) has been referred to in the scientific literature by its trivial name, methyl-CCNU, a contraction of its chemical name 1-(2-chloroethyl)-3-(4-methylcyclohexyl)-1-nitrosourea.

15.4.7 Drugs With Inactive Components. Drugs often contain a pharmacologically inactive component, eg, a base, salt, or ester, that is not responsible for the drug's mechanism of action but lends stability or other properties to the drug. Drugs with both an active and inactive component generally require a 2-part name that provides the active and inactive portion of the drug. Inorganic salts and simple organic acids are named in the order cation-anion (eg, sodium chloride, magnesium citrate). For more complex organic compounds, the active component is named first (eg, oxacillin sodium).[1(p1224)]

Pharmacologically inactive components are generally salts, esters, and complexes. Sodium, potassium, chloride, hydrochloride, sulfate, mesylate, and fumarate are common components of salts.

acyclovir sodium

midazolam hydrochloride

benztropine mesylate

morphine sulfate

Quaternary ammonium salts usually are designated by a 2-part name and have the suffix *-ium* on the first word of the name.

atracurium besylate

alcuronium chloride

octonium bromide

Salts and esters are frequently designated by the ending *-ate*. Three-word names are used for compounds that are both salts and esters.

clomegestone acetate [ester]

hydrocortisone valerate [ester]

testosterone cypionate [ester]

methylprednisolone sodium phosphate [salt and ester]

roxatidine acetate hydrochloride [ester and salt]

If more than one pharmacologically inactive molecule interacts with the pharmacologically active component, the number of molecules is reflected in the name. If the number is not designated, the number of molecules is assumed to be 1.[1(p1224)]

balsalazide disodium [2 sodium molecules]

gusperimus trihydrochloride [3 hydrochloride molecules]

besipirdine hydrochloride [1 hydrochloride molecule]

Complexes of 2 or more components may include a term ending in *-ex* to indicate a complex.

bisacodyl tannex

nicotine polacrilex

codeine polystirex

Chemical names are often too complex for general use. In such cases, shorter nonproprietary names may be created. For example, for the drug erythromycin acistrate, *acistrate* refers to the 2′-acetate (ester) and octadecanoate (salt). For the drug erythromycin estolate, *estolate* refers to the double salt propanoate and dodecyl sulfate.[1(pp1224-1225)]

In the past, some INNs included inactive components as part of their name (eg, levothyroxine sodium). The WHO modified this policy so that the INN refers to only the active component of the drug (oxacillin, ibufenac). The name that includes the salt (oxacillin sodium, ibufenac sodium) is referred to as the *modified INN* (INNM). However, for drugs originally named for the full entity, such as levothyroxine sodium, the shorter (active entity only) name, eg, levothyroxine, is considered the INNM.[2]

When a drug is referred to as a general category, the INN for the drug can be used without providing the inactive moiety.

> The β-blockers most selective for β-1 activity are bisoprolol and metoprolol; acebutolol, carvedilol, and nebivolol are somewhat selective. All lose their selectivity when given at higher doses.

However, if a specific drug is discussed for a specific use, particularly when more than one formulation is available, the inactive moiety should be included with the drug name.

> The patient was administered erythromycin ethylsuccinate, 400 mg by mouth every 6 hours.

The inactive component should not be used when referring to an organism's sensitivity to an antibiotic or to allergic reactions to drugs.

> The strain of *Streptococcus pneumoniae* isolated by the laboratory was highly resistant to penicillin.
>
> The patient's plasma lithium level at 8 AM was 2.0 mEq/L.
>
> The woman developed urticaria after taking erythromycin.

The inactive component may also be used with the proprietary name (see 15.4.3, Proprietary Names).

> Hydralazine hydrochloride was marketed as Apresoline Hydrochloride.

If both the nonproprietary name and the proprietary name are provided together, the inactive component is given only once.

> The patient had been taking hydralazine (Apresoline) hydrochloride in the 1980s but developed an urticarial papular rash.

15.4.8 **Stereoisomers.** Some chemical compounds may occur in more than 1 optical orientation, referred to as stereoisomers, and they may have very different biological effects, such that most biological activity is exerted by 1 stereoisomer. Stereoisomers are designated as *levorotatory* or *dextrorotatory*; a mixture of the 1 is *racemic*. In addition, chemical compounds may have different biological chirality (determined by mass spectrometry), referred to as *enantiomers*.[10(pp13-14)] Enantiomers are designated as R(−) or S(+). Nonproprietary names for new chemical entities do not usually specify the stereoisometric form of the molecule. For example, carnitine and ibuprofen are racemic mixtures, remoxipride is a levo isomer, and butopamine is a dextro isomer. If a subsequent drug is another isometric form of the same chemical, a prefix may be used to designate the stereoisomer.[1(p1226)]

For the racemate, *rac*- or *race*- is added to the compound (eg, racepinephrine). For the levorotatory form, the "S" isomer uses the *lev*- or *levo*- prefix (eg, levamisole, levdobutamine), whereas the "R" isomer uses the *ar*- prefix. For the dextrorotatory form, the "S" isomer uses the *es*- prefix, whereas the "R" isomer uses the *dex*- or *dextro*- prefix (eg, dexibuprofen, dextroamphetamine, dexamisole).

15.4.9 **Combination Products.** For combination products (mixtures), the names of the active ingredients should be provided. The proprietary name of the combination may be given in parentheses if necessary to clarify the product to which the article refers.

pseudoephedrine hydrochloride and triprolidine hydrochloride (Actifed)

povidone and hydroxyethylcellulose (Adsorbotear)

If the list of active ingredients is too long to use when referring to the combination product, the active ingredients should be listed at first mention and either an abbreviation or the proprietary name used thereafter.

The patient reported having taken several doses of Vanex HD, a liquid suspension of hydrocodone bitartrate, 10 mg, phenylephrine hydrochloride, 30 mg, and chlorpheniramine maleate, 12 mg, per 30 mL, the previous day.

The patient had been administered an artificial tear product containing 0.42% hydroxyethylcellulose and 1.67% povidone (Adsorbotear).

Only the active ingredients must be listed. However, in some circumstances it may be necessary to include all ingredients, including preservatives, if sensitivity to an ingredient may be important.

The patient had complained of red, itching eyes after using an artificial tear product containing hydroxyethylcellulose and povidone with edetate disodium and thimerosal as preservatives (Adsorbotear).

The USP may provide a pharmacy equivalent name (PEN)[1(p13)] to refer to a combination product, such as co-triamterzide for the combination of triamterene and hydrochlorothiazide. However, PEN terms are not official USP titles and should be used only if they are familiar and clear to readers. Because co-triamterzide is unlikely to be familiar to most readers, the following approach can be used:

Participants were given a capsule containing a combination of 25 mg of hydrochlorothiazide and 50 mg of triamterene each day at 8 AM. Those not able to tolerate hydrochlorothiazide-triamterene were given 50 mg of metoprolol at 8 AM.

Trimethoprim-sulfamethoxazole (80 mg of trimethoprim and 400 mg of sulfamethoxazole) administered once daily effectively prevented reinfection in 93% of patients.

15.4.10 Drug Preparation Names That Include a Percentage. Some drug names, such as those used in topical preparations, include the percentage of active drug contained in the preparation. In these cases the percentage should be listed after the drug name.

The patient was treated with adalapalene gel, 1%.

Metronidazole lotion, 0.75%, was applied twice a day.

15.4.11 Multiple-Drug Regimens. Regimens that include multiple drugs may be referred to by an abbreviation after the nonproprietary names of the drugs have been provided at first mention (see also 15.4.12, Drug Abbreviations, and 14.11, Abbreviations, Clinical, Technical and Other Common Terms). Drug regimens used in oncology frequently are referred to by abbreviations of combinations of antineoplastic agents, but often the abbreviations are not derived from the INNs. For example, the letter *O* in MOPP is derived from Oncovin, the proprietary name for vincristine sulfate, and the *A* in ABVD is derived from Adriamycin, the proprietary name for doxorubicin hydrochloride. When the abbreviation is expanded the proprietary names may be provided after the nonproprietary names to clarify the origin of the abbreviation.

> The MOPP (methotrexate, vincristine sulfate [Oncovin], prednisone, and procarbazine hydrochloride) regimen for advanced Hodgkin disease was compared with MOPP alternating with ABVD (doxorubicin hydrochloride [Adriamycin], bleomycin sulfate, vinblastine sulfate, and dacarbazine).

15.4.12 **Drug Abbreviations.** Some drugs have commonly used abbreviations, such as INH for isoniazid and TMP for trimethoprim. However, abbreviations may be used inconsistently or confused with other terms or be unfamiliar to some readers. Because of the potential for harm from erroneous interpretation of abbreviated drug names, abbreviations should not be used except in rare instances (eg, trimethoprim-sulfamethoxazole may not fit in a table heading and may need to be abbreviated, eg, TMP-SMX; in that case the expansion should be provided in a table footnote).

15.4.13 **Nomenclature for Biological Products.** Several categories of drugs are identical to or derived from biological products. Some hormones given as drugs, for example, require special mention because the drug name differs from the name used for the endogenous substance (please note that this is not a comprehensive list of such drugs). Other categories of biologicals are derived from specific guidelines developed by USAN, outlined below.

Using the appropriate name can help clarify that the substance referred to is a drug, although for less familiar drug names it may be necessary to include the endogenous hormone name in parentheses to clarify the action of the drug for readers. (For more information on appropriate abbreviations for hormones, see 14.11, Abbreviations, Clinical, Technical, and Other Common Terms.) The following information is based on the *USP Dictionary*.[1(pp1225-1232)]

Hypothalamic Hormones. The suffix *-relin* denotes hypothalamic peptide hormones that stimulate release of pituitary hormones and the suffix *-relix* denotes hormones that inhibit release.

Native Substance	*Diagnostic/Therapeutic Agent*
thyrotropin-releasing hormone (TRH)	protirelin
luteinizing hormone-releasing hormone (LHRH) (or gonadotropin-releasing hormone [GnRH])	buserelin acetate, gonadorelin acetate (or hydrochloride), histrelin, lutrelin acetate, nafarelin acetate
growth hormone-releasing factor (GHRF)	somatorelin
growth hormone release-inhibiting factor (somatostatin, GHRIF)	detirelix acetate

Example:

After venipuncture, protirelin (synthetic thyrotropin-releasing hormone) was injected.

Growth Hormone. The *som-* prefix is used for growth hormone derivatives.

Native Substance	*Diagnostic/Therapeutic Agent*
growth hormone	somatrem (methionyl human growth hormone)
	somidobove, sometribove, somagrebove (bovine somatotropin derivatives)
	somalapor, somenopor, sometripor, somfasepor (bovine somatotropin derivatives)

Thyroid Hormones. Abbreviations for thyroxine and triiodothyronine are provided in parentheses and may be used after the name is expanded at first mention.

Description	*Therapeutic Agent INN*
levorotatory thyroxine (T_4)	levothyroxine sodium
triiodothyronine (T_3)	liothyronine sodium
dextrorotatory triiodothyronine	dextrothyroxine sodium
mixture of liothyronine and levothyroxine sodium	liotrix sodium

Insulin. Insulin terminology can be a source of clinically important confusion, particularly with regard to insulin concentrations and types. Insulin concentrations are as follows (not necessary to expand at first mention):

U100 contains 100 U of insulin per milliliter (the most commonly used concentration).

U40 contains 40 U of insulin per milliliter.

U500 contains 500 U of insulin per milliliter.

Insulin types include those that may be administered intravenously, subcutaneously, or intramuscularly (injections) and those that may be administered only subcutaneously or intramuscularly (suspensions). Another form of insulin may be inhaled.

Insulin is prepared with the use of recombinant DNA technology (referred to as human insulin, since the source is human DNA) or as a synthetic modification of porcine insulin. Proprietary names are provided below because they are often used to refer to the potentially confusing various types of insulin preparations. For clarity and conciseness, use of proprietary terms in addition to the nonproprietary terms may be necessary in some cases. The following lists are not comprehensive but are intended to provide examples of the nonproprietary names that should be used and their corresponding proprietary names.

Injections

Preferred Term	*Proprietary Name*
human insulin injection	Humulin
insulin lispro injection	Humalog
insulin aspart injection	Novolog
insulin glargine injection	Lantus

Suspensions

Preferred Term	*Proprietary Name*
insulin zinc suspension, prompt	Semilente
insulin zinc suspension	Lente
human insulin extended zinc suspension	Ultralente
insulin isophane suspension	NPH [neutral protamine Hagedorn]*

*NPH is the single exception to expressing drugs as abbreviations and can be used in its abbreviated form.

Insulin is available in combinations of injections and suspensions:

Preferred Term	*Proprietary Name*
70% human isophane suspension/30% human insulin injection	Humulin 70/30
70% insulin aspart protamine suspension/30% insulin aspart injection	Novolog Mix 70/30
75% insulin lispro protamine suspension/25% insulin lispro injection	Humalog Mix 75/25
50% insulin isophane suspension/50% human insulin injection	Humulin 50/50

Interferons. Interferon is defined as "the class name for a family of species-specific proteins (or glycoproteins) produced according to information encoded by species of interferon genes and exert complex antineoplastic, antiviral, and immunomodulating effects."[1(p1225)] (See also 15.8, Immunology.)

The 3 main types used for therapy are as follows:

interferon alfa (formerly leukocyte or lymphoblastoid interferon) [The *f* is used rather than *ph* to avoid the confusing *ph* in international usage.]

interferon beta (formerly fibroblast interferon)

interferon gamma (formerly immune interferon)

Subcategories are designated by a numeral and a lowercase letter. The lowercase letter after the number differentiates one manufacturer's interferon from another's. Examples of pure interferons are as follows:

interferon alfa-2a

interferon alfa-2b

interferon beta-1a

interferon beta-1b

interferon gamma-la

For naturally occurring mixtures of interferons, a lowercase *n* precedes the numeral:

interferon alfa-n1

interferon alfa-n2

Interleukins. There are 12 interleukin derivatives. All except interleukin 3 end in *-kin* (eg, aldesleukin). Interleukin 3 is designated by the *-plestim* stem (eg, daniplestim) and is a pleiotropic colony-stimulating factor (see also Colony-Stimulating Factors).

Stem	*Interleukin*
-nakin	interleukin 1 derivatives
-onakin	interleukin 1a derivatives
-benakin	interleukin 1b derivatives
-leukin	interleukin 2 derivatives
-trakin	interleukin 4 derivatives
-penkin	interleukin 5 derivatives
-exakin	interleukin 6 derivatives
-eptakin	interleukin 7 derivatives
-octakin	interleukin 8 derivatives
-nonakin	interleukin 9 derivatives
-decakin	interleukin 10 derivatives
-elvekin	interleukin 11 derivatives
-dodekin	interleukin 12 derivatives

Colony-Stimulating Factors. Therapeutic recombinant colony-stimulating factors are named according to the following guidelines[1(p1225)] (see also 15.8, Immunology).

The suffix *-grastim* is used for granulocyte colony-stimulating factors (G-CSFs):

lenograstim

filgrastim

The suffix *-gramostim* is used for granulocyte-macrophage colony-stimulating factors (GM-CSFs):

molgramostim

regramostim

sargramostim

The suffix *-mostim* is used for macrophage colony-stimulating factors (M-CSF):

mirimostim

The suffix *-plestim* is used for interleukin 3 (IL-3) factors, which are classified as pleiotropic colony-stimulating factors:

muplestim

daniplestim

The suffix *-distim* is used for conjugates of 2 types of colony-stimulating factors:

milodistim

The suffix *-cestim* is used for stem cell–stimulating factors:

ancestim

Erythropoietins. The word *epoetin* is used to describe erythropoietin preparations that have an amino acid sequence that is identical to the endogenous cytokine. The words *alfa*, *beta*, and *gamma* are added to designate preparations with different composition and carbohydrate moieties.[1(p1225)]

epoetin alfa

epoetin beta

epoetin gamma

Monoclonal Antibodies. Therapeutic monoclonal antibodies and fragments are designated by the suffix *-mab*. Monoclonal antibodies are derived from animals as well as from humans and the nomenclature is based on the source of the antibody (mouse, rat, hamster, primate, or human) and the disease target or antibody subclass. Some examples of monoclonal antibodies are abciximab, daclximab, and satumomab.[1(p1225-1226)]

The following letters are used to identify the source of the monoclonal antibody:

u	human
e	hamster
o	mouse
i	primate
a	rat
xi	chimera
zu	humanized

These identifiers precede the *-mab* suffix stem, for example:

-umab	human
-omab	mouse
-ximab	chimera
-zumab	humanized

The general disease state subclass is also incorporated into the name by use of a code syllable.

-vir-	viral
-bac-	bacterial
-lim-	immune
-les-	infectious lesions
-cir-	cardiovascular

Monoclonal antibodies used to treat particular tumors are incorporated into the name using the following syllables.

-col-	colon
-mel-	melanoma
-mar-	mammary
-got-	testicular
-gov-	ovarian
-pr (o)-	prostate
-tum-	miscellaneous

Key elements are combined in the following sequence: the letters representing the target disease state, the source of the product, and the monoclonal root *-mab* used as a suffix (eg, bi*ciromab*, sa*tumomab*). When a target or disease stem is combined with the source stem for chimeric monoclonal antibody, the last consonant of the target/disease syllable is dropped to facilitate pronunciation:

Target	*Source*	*-mab Stem*	*USAN*
-cir-	*-xi*	*-mab*	abciximab
-lim-	*-zu*	*-mab*	daclizumab

Radiolabeled or Conjugated Products. Some products are radiolabeled or conjugated to other chemicals such as toxins. Such conjugates are identified by a separate, second word or other chemical designation. For monoclonal antibodies conjugated to a toxin, the "*-tox*" stem indicates the toxin (eg, zolimomab *aritox*, in which the designation *aritox* was selected to identify ricin A-chain). For radiolabeled products, the isotope, element symbol, and isotope number precede the monoclonal antibody.[1(p1226)] (See also 15.9.2, Isotopes, Radiopharmaceuticals.)

technetium Tc 99m biciromab

indium In 111 altumomab pentetate

A separate term is also used to designate a linker or chelator that conjugates the monoclonal antibody to a toxin or isotope, or for pegylated (having polyethylene glycol, or PEG, attached) monoclonal antibodies.[1(p1226)]

telimomab aritox

enlimomab pegol

15.4.14 Vitamins and Related Compounds.

Vitamins and Related Compounds. The familiar letter names of most vitamins generally refer to the substances as found in food and in vivo. With the exception of vitamins A, E, and B complex, the INNs for vitamins given therapeutically differ from their in vivo names. (To enhance clarity for readers, the equivalent vitamin name may also be provided.) Various types of carotenoids (alpha- and beta-carotene and beta-cryptoxanthin) may be converted to vitamin A within the body, so the specific agent that is administered should be provided. The native form of vitamin A is most often supplied as retinol acetate. Other forms of vitamin A may be administered topically (such as retinoic acid). Vitamin E refers to a group of tocopherol compounds, and the specific chemical names should be provided (eg, alpha-tocopherol, gamma-tocopherol, delta-tocopherol, or mixed tocopherols). The specific stereoisomers and whether the product is natural or synthetic should be provided where relevant (eg, DL-alpha tocopherol acetate). For vitamin B complex, the specific components included in the B complex should be provided. (For additional information see the Institute of Medicine texts listed under "Additional Readings and General References" at the end of this section.) The following are examples of USAN drug names equivalent to their vitamin names[1(p930)]:

Native Vitamin	*Drug Name*
vitamin B_1	thiamine hydrochloride
vitamin B_1 mononitrate	thiamine mononitrate
vitamin B_2	riboflavin
vitamin B_6	pyridoxine hydrochloride
vitamin B_8	adenosine phosphate
vitamin B_{12}	cyanocobalamin
vitamin C	ascorbic acid
vitamin D	cholecalciferol
vitamin D_1	dihydrotachysterol
vitamin D_2	ergocalciferol
vitamin G	riboflavin
vitamin K_1	phytonadione
vitamin K_2	menaquinone
vitamin P_4	troxerutin

15.4.15 **Herbals and Dietary Supplements.** Herbals and dietary supplements do not receive INNs, and they are not regulated as drugs in many countries, including the United States (as mandated by the Dietary Supplement Health and Education Act, passed in 1994[10]).

In the United States, Congress has defined a dietary supplement as

> a product taken by mouth that contains a "dietary ingredient" intended to supplement the diet. The "dietary ingredients" in these products may include: vitamins, minerals, herbs or other botanicals, amino acids, and substances such as enzymes, organ tissues, glandulars, and metabolites. Dietary supplements can also be extracts or concentrates, and may be found in many forms such as tablets, capsules, softgels, gelcaps, liquids, or powders. They can also be in other forms, such as a bar, but if they are, information on their label must not represent the product as a conventional food or a sole item of a meal or diet. Whatever their form may be, [Dietary Supplement Health and

> Education Act] places dietary supplements in a special category under the general umbrella of "foods," not drugs, and requires that every supplement be labeled a dietary supplement.[10,11]

Components of dietary supplements may be pharmacologically active, so accurate and specific nomenclature is essential. As noted above, dietary supplements are often mixtures of several ingredients, and quantities of each may be proprietary. Such a mixture makes standard nomenclature policy difficult to establish. Whenever possible, a nonproprietary name should be used to refer to a dietary supplement. However, if the dietary supplement is a mixture of many components, either an abbreviation derived from the components or the proprietary name must be used. (See also 15.4.9, Combination Products.)

> Metabolife 356 (Metabolife International Inc, San Diego, California) is a dietary supplement containing 19 labeled ingredients including ephedra and caffeine (hereinafter abbreviated as DSEC).

The *USP Dictionary*,[1] *Physicians' Desk Reference for Nonprescription Drugs and Dietary Supplements*,[12] *Physicians' Desk Reference for Herbal Medicines*,[13] and *The Complete German Commission E Monographs: Therapeutic Guide to Herbal Medicines*[14] are useful resources for naming herbals and dietary supplements. If these resources do not provide the necessary information, the Web can be helpful in identifying substances as well, although of course the accuracy of the source should be considered.

Herbal medicines generally can be named according to their botanical genus and species, although the lack of regulation in some countries again makes consistent nomenclature a challenge. A review of regulation of herbal medicines worldwide has been completed by the WHO.[15] Particularly in countries where botanicals are not regulated, the specific herbal and manufacturer, wherever relevant, should be included, since different manufacturing techniques result in different biological activity. According to WHO,

> It is not unusual for a common name to be used for two or more different species. Unless the names of herbal plants follow an international system of plant nomenclature, the potential for confusion when exchanging information is enormous. The information attached to a name is thus crucial. As an example, because common names are often used, heliotrope (*Heliotropium europaeum*)—containing potent hepatotoxins—is often confused with garden heliotrope (*Valeriana officinalis*), which is used as a sedative and muscle relaxant. Identification of the herbal preparation by the Latin binomial system, in addition to the common name, is therefore essential.[16]

Thus, whenever possible, herbals derived from a specific plant should be named according to the botanical name (eg, *Ginkgo biloba*, *Echinacea purpurea*) to ensure that the correct entity is identified. When the plant itself is referred to, the genus and species may be abbreviated after being spelled out at first mention:

> The main pharmacologic substances with immunostimulant activity in experimental and clinical studies are purified polysaccharides that can be extracted only in small quantity from pressed *Echinacea purpurea*.

> Given our laboratory findings, the symptoms we have described may be attributed to an overdose of *Illicium verum,* contamination with *Illicium anisatum,* or a combination of both.
>
> One day prior to taking *Ginkgo biloba* or placebo and again at the end of the 6-week double-blind period (while still taking *G biloba* and within 3 days of the end of the study), participants underwent neuropsychological evaluation including tests of learning, memory, attention and concentration, and expressive language.

In some cases the vernacular name is not the genus or species and should be provided as well to ensure that the reader understands which plant is intended.

> *Hypericum perforatum* (St John's wort) is a popular herbal product used to treat depression, but it has been implicated in drug interactions.

When referring to a specific product or formulation, as in a study, the specific proprietary name and manufacturer should be listed, because formulations vary by manufacturing technique.

> Participants were randomly assigned to 1 of 2 conditions: *Ginkgo biloba* (Ginkoba; Boehringer Ingelheim Pharmaceuticals, Ingelheim, Germany) or placebo control (1:1 ratio).
>
> A marketed enteric-coated preparation (Tegra; Hermes Arzneimittel GmbH, Grosshesselohe, Germany) containing 5 mg of steam-distilled garlic (*Allium sativum*) oil bound to a matrix of beta cyclodextrin and matching placebos, whose coating tasted like garlic, were used.
>
> Guggulipid, which is an extract from the plant *Commiphora mukul* (guggul), contains numerous other substances besides the small amounts of guggulsterones purported to be the active ingredients.

REFERENCES

1. *USP Dictionary of USAN and International Drug Names.* 41st ed. Rockville, MD: US Pharmacopoeia; 2005.
2. Guidance on INN. World Health Organization. http://www.who.int/medicines/services/inn/innquidance/en/index.html. Accessed June 14, 2006.
3. International Nonproprietary Names. World Health Organization. http://www.who.int/medicines/services/inn/en/. Accessed June 14, 2006.
4. Nies AS. Principles of therapeutics. In: Hardman JG, Limbird LE, eds. *Goodman & Gilman's The Pharmacological Basis of Therapeutics.* 10th ed. New York, NY: McGraw-Hill Book Co; 2001.
5. *Physicians' Desk Reference.* 59th ed. Montvale, NJ: Medical Economics; 2005.
6. Safety, efficacy and utilization of medicines. World Health Organization. http://www.who.int/medicines/areas/quality_safety/safety_efficacy/en/. Accessed June 14, 2006.
7. Van Laan S. Approved stems. USAN. http://www.ama-assn.org/ama/pub/category/4782.html. Updated July 20, 2006. Accessed September 22, 2006.
8. Orphan Drug Act, Pub L No. 97-414. http://www.fda.gov/orphan/oda.htm. Accessed June 14, 2006.

9. Toyer D, Holquist C. Bextra: valdecoxib or bucindolol? [FDA Safety Page]. *Drug Topics.* January 6, 2003:54.
10. Dietary Supplement: Health and Education Act of 1994. US Food and Drug Administration, Center for Food Safety and Applied Nutrition. http://vm.cfsan.fda.gov/~dms/dietsupp.html. December 1, 1995. Accessed September 22, 2006.
11. Overview of dietary supplements. US Food and Drug Administration. http://www.cfsan.fda.gov/~dms/ds-oview.html. January 3, 2001. Accessed September 22, 2006.
12. *Physicians' Desk Reference for Nonprescription Drugs and Dietary Supplements.* 25th ed. Montvale, NJ: Medical Economics; 2004.
13. *Physicians' Desk Reference for Herbal Medicines.* Montvale, NJ: Medical Economics; 1998.
14. American Botanical Council; Blumenthal M, Busse WR, Klein S, et al, eds. *The Complete German Commission E Monographs: Therapeutic Guide to Herbal Medicines.* Philadelphia, PA: Lippincott Williams & Wilkins; 1998.
15. Regulatory situation of herbal medicines: a worldwide review. World Health Organization. http://whqlibdoc.who.int/hq/1998/WHO_TRM_98.1.pdf. Accessed June 14, 2006.
16. General policy issues. *WHO Drug Inf.* 1998;12(3)129-135. http://www.who.int/druginformation/vol12/12-3.pdf. Accessed June 14, 2006.

ADDITIONAL READINGS AND GENERAL REFERENCES

Billups NF, Billups SM, eds. *American Drug Index.* 40th ed. St Louis, MO: Facts and Comparisons; 2004.

Drug Facts and Comparisons [looseleaf with monthly updates]. St Louis, MO: Wolters Kluwer Health Inc. Available for purchase at http://www.factsandcomparisons.com/Products/index.aspx?id=1042. Accessed June 14, 2006.

Food and Nutrition Board, Institute of Medicine. *Dietary Reference Intakes for Vitamin C, Vitamin E, Selenium, and Carotenoids.* Washington, DC: National Academy Press; 2000.

Food and Nutrition Board, Institute of Medicine. *Dietary Reference Intakes (DRI) for Vitamin A, Vitamin K, Arsenic, Boron, Chromium, Copper, Iodine, Iron, Maganese, Molybdenum, Nickel, Silicon, Vandadium, and Zinc.* Washington, DC: National Academy Press; 2000.

WHO Drug Information [published quarterly]. http://www.who.int/druginformation. Accessed June 14, 2006.

15.5 Equipment, Devices, and Reagents. As with drugs and isotopes, nonproprietary names or descriptive phrasing is preferred to proprietary names for devices, equipment, and reagents, particularly in the context of general statements and interchangeable items (eg, urinary catheters, intravenous catheters, pumps). However, if several brands of the same product are being compared or if the use of proprietary names is necessary for clarity or to replicate the study, proprietary names should be given at first mention along with the nonproprietary name. In such cases information regarding the manufacturer or supplier and location also is important, and authors should include this information in parentheses after the name or description. Authors should provide this information for any reagents, antibodies, enzymes, or probes used in investigations.

The following are examples where specific information is required:

> The positron emission tomography (PET) unit (4096 Plus; General Electric Systems, Milwaukee, Wisconsin) comprised 8 detector rings positioned in a cylindrical array. Image processing and reconstruction were performed with a VAX 4000-300 computer system and a VAX 3100 workstation (Digital Equipment, Marlboro, Massachusetts).
>
> All magnetic resonance angiography examinations were performed with a 1.5-T whole-body imager (General Electric Medical Systems, Milwaukee, Wisconsin).

The following are examples of general references:

> Some hearing loss may result from use of a portable radio or cassette player equipped with headphones (Walkman-style) played at high decibel levels.
>
> Currently, treatment by Nd:YAG laser is the accepted method to surgically open the opacified posterior capsule.

As with drugs and isotopes, proprietary names should be capitalized; the registered trademark symbol is not used.

If a device is described as "modified," the modification should be explained or an explanatory reference cited. If equipment or apparatus is provided free of charge by the manufacturer, this fact should be included in the acknowledgment (see 2.10.8, Manuscript Preparation, Acknowledgment Section, Funding/Support; 5.2.1, Ethical and Legal Considerations, Acknowledgments, Acknowledging Support, Assistance, and Contributions of Those Who Are Not Authors; and 5.5.2, Ethical and Legal Considerations, Conflicts of Interest, Reporting Funding and Other Support).

> *When new nomenclature is presented, it often looks odd to practising biochemists and is not always appreciated. Even systems such as the one-letter codes for amino acids, which have been universally adopted, met with some skepticism at first.*
>
> R. Cammack[1]

> *Every cell division involves the copying of 6 billion base pairs (bp) of DNA.*
>
> F. S. Collins and J. M. Trent[2]

15.6 Genetics

15.6.1 Nucleic Acids and Amino Acids. Standards for molecular nomenclature are set jointly by the International Union of Biochemistry and Molecular Biology (IUBMB) and the International Union of Pure and Applied Chemistry (IUPAC).[1] The recommendations in this section are based on conventions put forth by the IUBMB-IUPAC Joint Commission on Biochemical Nomenclature and the Nomenclature Committee of the IUBMB.[3,4]

DNA. The nucleic acids DNA and RNA are nucleotide polymers. Deoxyribonucleic acid, or DNA, is the embodiment of the genetic code and is contained in the chromosomes of higher organisms. It is made up of (1) molecules called *bases,* (2) the sugar 2-deoxyribose, and (3) phosphate groups. The bases fall into 2 classes: *pyrimidine* and *purine*.

Structurally, DNA is a helical polymer of deoxyribose linked by phosphate groups; 1 of 4 bases projects from each sugar molecule of the sugar-phosphate chain. A base-sugar unit is a *nucleoside*. A base-sugar-phosphate unit is a *nucleotide* (Figure 2). The carbons in the sugar moiety are numbered with prime symbols (not apostrophes), eg, 3′-carbon, 5′-carbon. The carbons and nitrogens of the bases are numbered 1 through 6 (pyrimidines) or 1 through 9 (purines), and the carbons of deoxyribose are designated by numbers with prime symbols, 1′ through 5′.

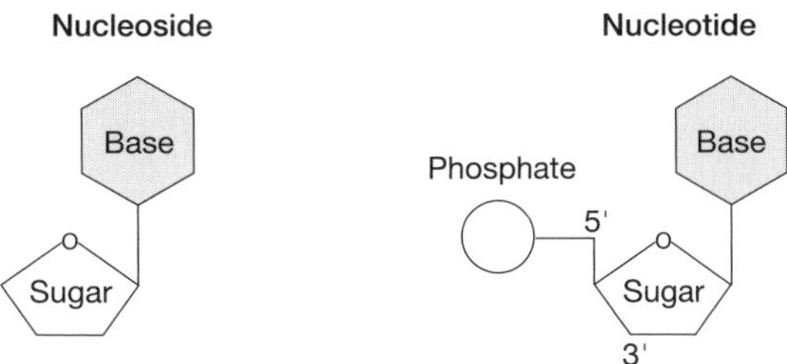

Figure 2. Nucleosides and nucleotides: general structure.

This section presents nomenclature for nucleotides of DNA, especially nomenclature used for DNA sequences, ie, nucleotide polymers. For nomenclature of nucleotides as DNA precursors and energy molecules, see the "Nucleotides as Precursors and Energy Molecules" section.

A 1-letter designation represents each base, nucleoside, or nucleotide. The letters are commonly used without expansion:

Abbreviation	*Base*	*Nucleoside; Nucleotide Residue in DNA*	*Molecular Class*
A	adenine	deoxyadenosine	purine
C	cytosine	deoxycytidine	pyrimidine
G	guanine	deoxyguanosine	purine
T	thymine	deoxythymidine	pyrimidine

The chemical structure of bases is illustrated in Figure 3. When a base (or nucleoside or nucleotide) is described that cannot be firmly identified as A, C, G, or T, other single-letter designators reflecting biochemical properties are used. Because these designations are not as well known as A, C, G, and T, it is best to define them, as shown below (table adapted by permission from Moss,[3] http://www.chem.qmw.ac.uk/iubmb/misc/naseq.html, Nomenclature for Incompletely Specified Bases in Nucleic Acid Sequences, 5. Discussion, copyright IUBMB):

Symbol	*Stands for*	*Derivation*
R	G or A	pu*r*ine
Y	T or C	p*y*rimidine

Symbol	*Stands for*	*Derivation*
M	A or C	a*m*ino
K	G or T	*k*eto
S	G or C	*s*trong interaction (3 hydrogen bonds)
W	A or T	*w*eak interaction (2 hydrogen bonds)
H	A or C or T	not G (H follows G in the alphabet)
B	G or T or C	not A (B follows A)
V	G or C or A	not T (V follows T; U is not used because it stands for uracil in RNA [see "RNA" section])
D	G or A or T	not C (D follows C)
N	G or A or T or C	a*n*y base

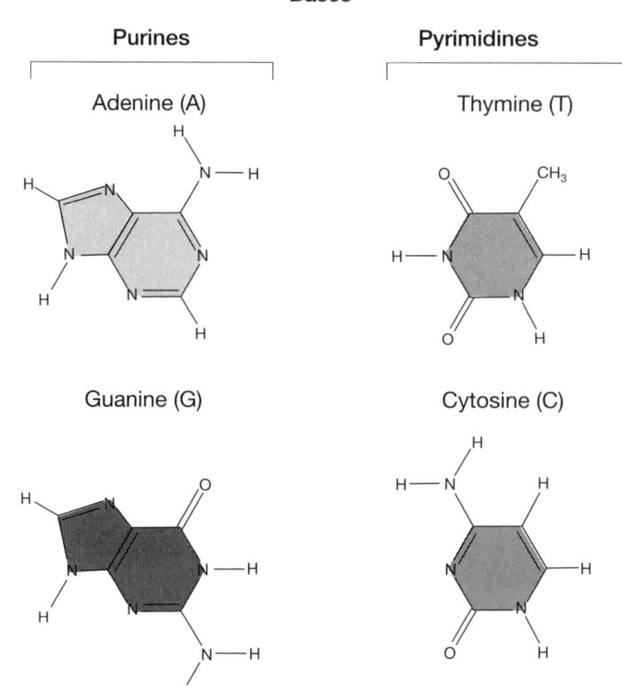

Figure 3. DNA bases: chemical structure.

Various forms of DNA are commonly abbreviated as follows; expand at first use:

bDNA	branched DNA
cDNA	complementary DNA, coding DNA
dsDNA	double-stranded DNA
gDNA	genomic DNA
hn-cDNA	heteronuclear cDNA (heterogeneous nuclear cDNA)

mtDNA	mitochondrial DNA
nDNA	nuclear DNA
rDNA	ribosomal DNA
scDNA	single-copy DNA
ssDNA	single-stranded DNA

There are several classes of DNA helixes, which differ in the direction of rotation and the tightness of the spiral (number of base pairs per turn):

A-DNA

B-DNA

C-DNA

D-DNA

Z-DNA (zigzag)

In eukaryotic cells, DNA is bound with special proteins associated with chromosomes (see 15.6.4, Human Chromosomes). This DNA-protein complex is known as *chromatin*. DNA in chromatin is organized into structures called *nucleosomes* by proteins known as *histones*. The 5 classes of histones are as follows:

H1

H2A

H2B

H3

H4

Almost all native DNA exists in the form of a double helix, in which 2 DNA polymers are paired, linked by hydrogen bonds between individual bases on each chain. Because of the biochemical structure of the nucleotides, A always pairs with T and C with G (Figure 4). Such pairs may be indicated as follows:

A · T, A = T

C · G, C ≡ G

Mispairings (which may occur as a consequence of a mutation or sequence variation) may be shown in the same way:

C · T

Unpaired DNA sequences are quantified by means of the terms base, kb (kilobase), and Mb (megabase). Paired DNA sequences use the terms bp (base pairs), kb (kilobase pairs), and Mb (megabase pairs). (Do not use "kbp" or "Mbp.") For example:

a 20-base fragment

a 235-bp repeat sequence

a 27-bp region

a 47-kb vector genome

1 Mb of DNA

The size of the human haploid genome is approximately 3×10^9 bp.

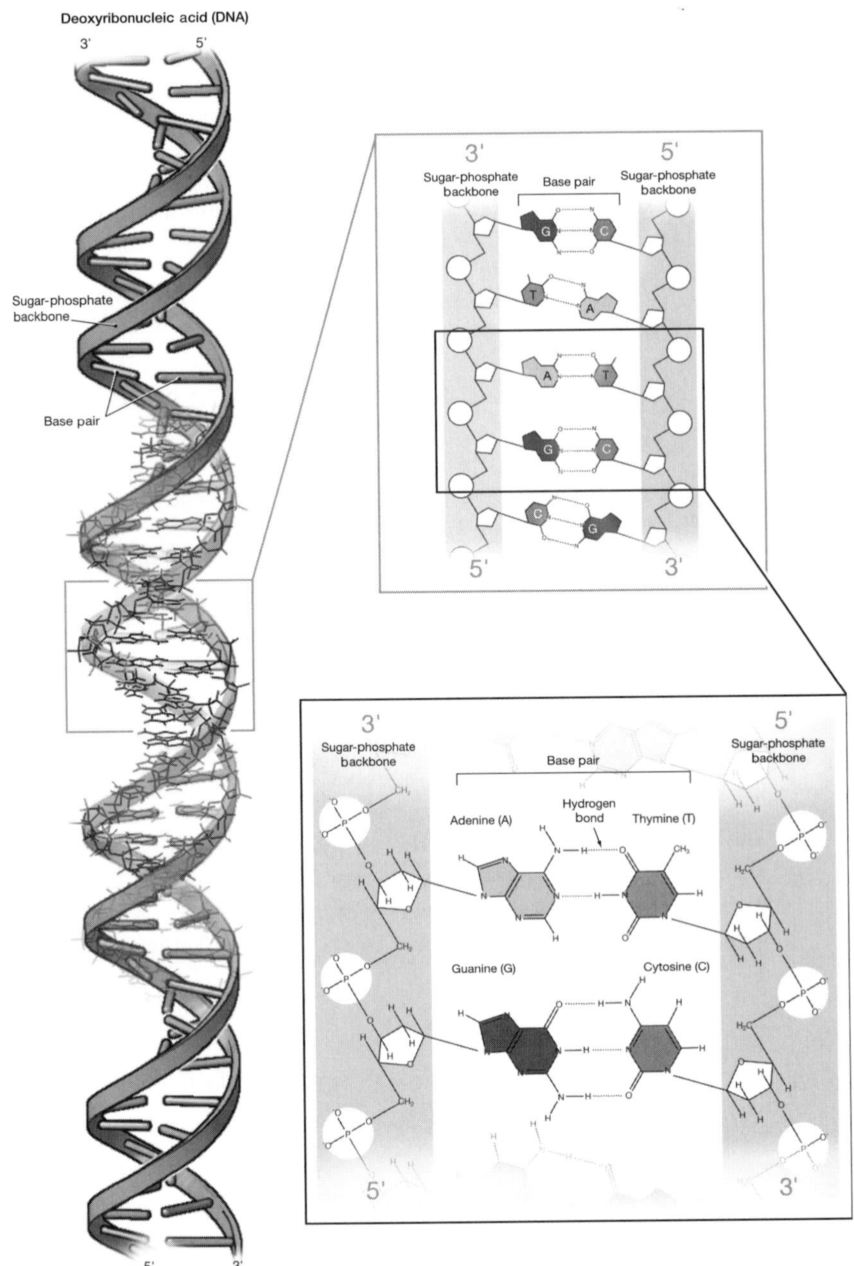

Figure 4. DNA double helix.

Sometimes the number of nucleotides in a DNA molecule is indicated using the suffix "mer":

> 20mer (20 nucleotides)
>
> 24mer (24 nucleotides)

(This formation is based on the terms *dimer, trimer, tetramer,* etc.)

A DNA sequence might be depicted as follows:

> GTCGACTG

Unknown bases may be depicted by using N (see previous table of symbols):

> GNCGANNGX

Instead of N, a lowercase n or a hyphen may be used for visual clarity:

> GnCGAnnG
>
> *or*
>
> G-CGA--G

A double-stranded sequence consisting of a strand of DNA and its complement would be as follows:

> GTCGACTG
CAGCTGAC

To show correct pairing between the bases in the 2 strands, sequences need to be aligned properly. In the sequence above, the first base pair is G · C, the next is T · A, etc. Note how the first G is directly above the first C, the first T above the first A, etc.

A codon is a sequence of 3 nucleotides in a DNA molecule that (ultimately) codes for an amino acid (see below), biosynthetic message, or signal (eg, start transcription, stop transcription). Codons are also referred to as codon triplets. Examples are as follows:

> CAT ATC ATT

The genetic code—the complete list of each codon and its specific product—is widely reproduced, eg, in medical dictionaries and textbooks and on the Internet.

Promoters are DNA sequences that promote transcription of DNA into RNA. They include the following:

> CAT box (CCAAT)
>
> CG island, CpG island (CG-rich sequence)
>
> GC box (GGGCGGG consensus sequence)
>
> 5′ UTR (5′ untranslated region) (5′ is defined below)
>
> TATA box

Sequences of repeating single nucleotides are named as follows:

> polyA
>
> polyC

polyG

polyT

Example: polyA tail

or, optionally, with lowercase d for deoxyribose:

poly(dT)

Repeating single-nucleotide pairs (in double-stranded DNA) are similarly named:

poly(dA-dT)

poly(dG-dC)

The phosphate groups linking the nucleotides are sometimes indicated with a lowercase p:

pGpApApTpTpC

CpG island

Methylated bases may be shown with a superscript lowercase m, which refers to the nucleotide residue to the right:

GAT^{m}CC

Sequences of repeating nucleotides, also known as tandem repeats, are indicated as follows (n stands for number of repeats):

$(TTAGGG)_n$

$(GT)_n$

$(CGG)_n$

Within a long sequence, the first repeat may be designated n, the next p, the next q, and so on:

$(TAGA)_n ATGGATAGATTA(GATG)_p AA(TAGA)_q$

The number of repeats may be specified:

$(GATG)_2$

$(TAGA)_{12}$

The phosphates that join the DNA nucleotides link the 3′-carbon of one deoxyribose to the 5′ carbon of the next deoxyribose. The end of the DNA strand with an unattached 5′ carbon is known as the 5′ end (or terminal), and the end with an unattached 3′ carbon as the 3′ end (or terminal) (Figure 4).

Sometimes chemical moieties are specified in connection with the 3′ and 5′ ends of DNA:

3′-hydroxyl end (3′-OH end)

5′-phosphate (5′-P) end

5′-OH end

(See also 14.13, Abbreviations, Elements and Chemicals.)

By convention in printed sequences, for single strands, the 5′ end is at the left and the 3′ end at the right; thus, a sequence such as the following:

CCCATCTCACTTAGCTCCAATG

would be assumed to have this directionality:

5′-CCCATCTCACTTAGCTCCAATG-3′

The complementary strands of dsDNA have opposite directionality; by convention, the top strand reads from the 5′ end to the 3′ end, while its complementary strand appears below it with the 3′ end on the left. The 5′-strand is the *sense strand* or *coding strand* or *positive strand*. The 3′-strand is the *antisense strand* or *template strand* or *negative strand*. In the example:

CCCATCTCACTTAGCTCCAATG
GGGTAGAGTGAATCGAGGTTAC

this directionality is implied:

5′-CCCATCTCACTTAGCTCCAATG-3′ (sense strand, coding strand)
3′-GGGTAGAGTGAATCGAGGTTAC-5′ (antisense strand, template strand)

Text should specify which strand, sense or antisense, is displayed. The sense strand "is the strand generally reported in the scientific literature or in databases."[5(p25)]

Long sequences pose special typesetting problems. Such sequences should be depicted as separate figures, rather than within text or tables, whenever possible.

For DNA, it must be made clear whether the sequence is single-stranded or double-stranded. A double-stranded sequence such as that of the following example:

CCCATCTCACTTAGCTCCAATG
GGGTAGAGTGAATCGAGGTTAC

might be mistaken for a single-stranded sequence and set as such:

CCCATCTCACTTAGCTCCAATGGGGTAGAGTGAATCGAGGTTAC

Conversely, mistaking a single-stranded sequence for a double-stranded sequence and typesetting accordingly should also be avoided.

Always maintain alignment in 2-stranded sequences—take care not to have this

CCCATCTCACTTAGCTCCAATG
GGGTAGAGTGAATCGAGGTTAC

become this:

CCCATCTCACTTAGCTCCAATG
GGGTAGAGTGAATCGAGGTTAC

Numbering and spacing may be used as visual aids in presenting sequences. A space every 3 bases indicates the codon triplets:

. . . GCA GAG GAC CTG CAG GTG GGG . . .

DNA sequences in most eukaryotic cells contain both exons (coding sequences of triplets) and introns (intervening noncoding sequences). An intron occurs within the sequence (examples from Cooper[6(p273)]):

intron: GTGAG . . . GGCAG

sequence in preceding example with intron included:

. . . GCA GAG GAC CTG CAG G GTGAG . . . GGCAG TG GGG . . .

Another way to display introns amid exons is to use lowercase letters for introns and uppercase letters for exons. There is a space on either side of the intron, and the next exon continues in the same frame or phase as before, to resume the correct codon sequence:

. . . GCA GAG GAC CTG CAG G gtgag . . . ggcag TG GGG . . .

In longer DNA sequences, spaces every 5 or 10 bases are customary visual aids:

GAATT CCTGA CCTCA GGTGA TCTGC CCGCC TCGGC CTCCC AAAGT GCTGG

GAATTCCTGA CCTCAGGTGA TCTGCCCGCC TCGGCCTCCC AAAGTGCTGG

Several types of numbering are further aids. In the following example (from Cooper[6(p133)]; "lowercase letters indicate uncertainty in the base call"), numbers on the left specify the number of the first base on that line:

```
  1   5′-GAATTCCTGA  CCTCAGGTGA  TCTGCCCGCC  TCGGCCTCCC  AAAGTGCTGG
 51      GATTTACAGG  CATGAGGCAC  CACACCTGGC  CAGTTGCTTA  GCTCTCTAAG
101      TCTTATTTGC  TTTACTTACA  AAATGGAGAT  ACAACCTTAT  AGAACATTCG
151      ACATATACTA  GGTTTCCATG  AACAGCAGCC  AGATCTCAAC  TATATAGGGA
201      CCAGTGAGAA  ACCAATCTCA  GGTAGCTGAT  GATGGGCAAa  GGgATGGGgA
251      CTGATATGCC  cNNNNNGACG  ATTCGAGTGA  CAAGCTACTA  TGTACCTCAG
301      CTTTtCATCT  tGATCTTCAC  CACCCATGGg  TAGGTGTCAC  TGAAaTT-3′
```

Alternatively, numbers may appear above bases of special interest:

```
     6                                 39
GAATTCCTGA CCTCAGGTGA TCTGCCCGCC TCGGCCTCCC AAAGTGCTGG
```

When the base number is large, the right-most digit should be directly over the base being designated:

```
                                21 857
21 831 ACATATACTA GGTTTCCATG AACAGCAGCC AGATCTCAAC TATATAGGGA
```

When a long sequence is run within text, use a hyphen at the right-hand end of the line to indicate the bond linking successive nucleotides:

GATTTACAGGCATGAGGCACCACACCTGGCCAGTTGCTTAGCTCTCTAAGTC-
TTATTGCTTTACTTACAAAATGGAGATACAACCTTATAGACATTCG

A hyphen is not necessary if spacing is used, as long as the break between groups occurs at the end of the line:

. . . 5′-CCT GGG

CAA AGC AAG GTA GG-3′

Recognition sequences are sections of a sequence recognized by proteins such as restriction enzymes that cleave DNA in specific locations (see the "Nucleic Acid Technology" section). To indicate sites of cleavage, virgules or carets may be used:

single-stranded:
GT/MKAC

GG/CGCGCC

C^TCGTG

double-stranded[7]*:*
CGWCG^
^GCWGC

G RGCY/C
C/YCGR G

Other conventions should be defined, in parentheses for text or in legends for tables and figures, eg[7]:

CACNN↓NNGTG (↓ indicates cleavage at identical position in both strands)

Sequence Variations, Nucleotides. Recommendations for mutation nomenclature have been one of the major activities of the HUGO Mutation Database Initiative, now the Human Genome Variation Society (HGVS).[8] Members devised the nomenclature after extensive community discussion.[9-14] Authors should consult the Recommendations page of the HGVS Web site (at www.hgvs.org [use the Recommendations Including Nomenclature Guidelines link] or www.hgvs.org/mutnomen) for the latest recommendations.[8] Basic style points are as follows (see also the "Sequence Variations, Amino Acids" section):

- For sequence variations described at the nucleotide level, the nucleotide number precedes the capital-letter nucleotide abbreviation.
- Numbers at the *end* of the term, if any, do not stand for the nucleotide number but rather indicate numbers of nucleotides involved in the change or, in the case of repeated sequences, numbers of repeats.
- The symbol > is used for substitutions. The following abbreviations are used: "ins," insertion; "del," deletion; "delins," deletion and insertion; "dup," duplication; "inv," inversion; "con," conversion; and "t," translocation.
- One set of brackets is used for 2 variations in a single allele, and 2 sets with a plus sign are used for 2 variations in paired alleles. An underscore character separates a range of affected nucleotide residues.
- The nucleotide number may be preceded by g plus dot (g.) for gDNA (genomic) or c plus dot (c.) for cDNA (complementary or coding).
- Nucleotide numbers may be positive or negative.

- The HGVS recommendations note a preference for the terms *sequence variant, sequence variation, alteration,* or *allelic variant* over the terms *mutation* and *polymorphism*.

Note the following examples. In general medical publications, textual explanations should accompany the shorthand terms at first mention.

Term	*Explanation*
1691G>A	G-to-A substitution at nucleotide 1691
253Y>N	pyrimidine at position 253 replaced by another base
[76A>C; 83G>C]	2 substitutions in single allele
[76A>C]+[87delG]	substitution and deletion in paired alleles
[76A>C (+) 83G>C]	2 sequence changes in 1 individual, alleles unknown
977insA	A inserted at nucleotide 977
186_187insC	C inserted between nucleotides 186 and 187
926ins11	insertion of 11 bases at position 926
185delAG	deletion of A and G at positions 185 and 186
617delT	deletion of T at position 617
188del11	11-bp deletion at nucleotide 188
1294del40	40-bp deletion at nucleotide 1294
c.5delA	A deleted at position 5 (cDNA)
c.5_7delAGG	AGG deleted at positions 5 through 7 (cDNA)
g.5_123del	nucleotides deleted from positions 5 through 123 (gDNA)
2316dupCCTGGA-TGAGACGGTC	duplicated sequence beginning at 2316
1007fs	frameshift mutation at codon 1007
112_117delinsTG 112_117delAGGTCAinsTG 112_117>TG	These are all acceptable ways of indicating a deletion from nucleotide 112 through 117 and insertion of TG.
203_506inv 203_506inv304	304 nucleotides inverted from positions 203 through 506
167(GT)6–22	6 to 22 GT repeats starting at position 167
g.167(GT)8	8 GT repeats starting at position 167 (gDNA)

Term	*Explanation*
[1263del55; 1326insT] [c.1226A>G; c.1448T>C]	variations in same allele indicated by brackets
[76A>C]+[76A>C] *or* 76A>C/A>C	changes in both alleles of same gene (heteroallelic)
76A>C; 137C>G	intra-allelic
c.827_XYZ:233del	examples[8] with hypothetical gene symbol *XYZ* incorporated (but not italicized) (see 15.6.2, Human Gene Nomenclature)
c.827_oXYZ:233del	o: opposite (antisense) strand

When a gene symbol is used with a sequence variation term, only the gene symbol is italicized (see 15.6.2, Human Gene Nomenclature).

ADRB1 1165C>G (not: *ADRB1 1165C>G*)

Note: Polymorphic variants are often indicated by using virgules, but this is not recommended.[14]

Avoid:	1721G/A
Preferred:	1721G, 1721A
Avoid:	2417A/G
Preferred:	2417A>G

In practice, means other than the symbol > are commonly used to indicate substitutions:

1691G-A

1691G→A

1691GtoA

1691G-to-A

Any symbol for substitution is better than no symbol; otherwise the expression may be misinterpreted as indicating a dinucleotide at the site. For instance, 1691GA would imply a change involving the dinucleotide GA (1691G and 1692A).

When genotype is being expressed in terms of nucleotides (eg, a polymorphic variant), italics and other punctuation for the nucleotides are not needed (see also 15.6.2, Human Gene Nomenclature):

MTHFR 677 CC and TT genotypes

For nucleotide numbering of a cDNA reference sequence, nucleotide +1 is the A of the ATG initiator codon. The 5′ nucleotide of the ATG initiator codon is −1. The nucleotide 3′ of the translation stop codon is *1. For introns, the first number is the position of the last nucleotide of the preceding exon or the first nucleotide of the following exon. For example:

c.77+2T cDNA, nucleotide 77 of preceding exon, position 2 in intron, T residue

c.78−1G cDNA, nucleotide 78 of next exon, position 1 in intron, G residue

Nucleotide numbering of a gDNA reference sequence is arbitrary (ie, there is no defined starting point as in cDNA). Therefore, authors should describe their numbering scheme. No plus signs or minus signs are used with gDNA reference sequences.

The recommendation to describe nucleotide variations with "IVS" (intervening sequence, referring to an intron and its number)[10] has been withdrawn[8]:

Preferred: c.88+2T>G

Replaces: c.IVS2+2T>G

Promoter variants (promoter polymorphisms) have been commonly expressed with terms such as:

−765G>A

which implies nucleotide numbering in terms of a cDNA reference sequence. However, authors are advised to instead (or additionally) describe the variant in relation to a gDNA reference sequence (see "Unique Identifiers" section) (J. den Dunnen, written communication, May 18, 2004):

L01531.1:g.1561C>T

Terms with a capital delta have been used to indicate exonic deletions, eg:

Δ ex 1a-15

Δ ex 1a-12

Δ ex 3

However, HGVS strongly recommends an alternative form of expression to facilitate inclusion in sequence variation databases, eg:

c.32-?_960+?del

See http://www.hgvs.org/mutnomen/disc.html#del? (from which the above example was taken) for further explanation.

Unique Identifiers. Official recommendations include mentioning a sequence variant's unique identifier, for instance, a number assigned by a locus-specific curator or the OMIM number.[15] (See also 15.6.2, Human Gene Nomenclature.) For a list of locus-specific database curators, see the Human Genome Variation Society Web site under Variation Databases and Related Sites (http://www.hgvs.org). For example:

1311C>T (OMIM 305900.0018)

880C>T (OMIM 600681.0002)

Database Identifiers for Genomic Sequences. Several databases record genomic sequence information:

Nucleotides:
GenBank (http://www.ncbi.nlm.nih.gov/Genbank/index.html)

RefSeq (http://www.ncbi.nlm.nih.gov/RefSeq/)

EMBL (European Molecular Biology Laboratory) (http://www.embl-heidelberg.de/)

DDBJ (DNA Data Bank of Japan) (http://www.ddbj.nig.ac.jp)

International HapMap Project (http://www.hapmap.org)

Proteins:
Swiss-Prot (http://www.expasy.ch/sprot/sprot-top.html)

PIR-PSD (Protein Information Resource: Protein Sequence Database) (http://pir.georgetown.edu)

For a review of databases in molecular biology, including several of the foregoing, see the 2005 Database Issue of the journal *Nucleic Acids Research*.[16]

Accession numbers are assigned when researchers submit unique sequences to any one of the databases. In published articles, accession numbers are useful in indicating specific sequences:

> Founder effects were investigated using 2 previously undescribed, highly polymorphic microsatellite markers that flank presenilin 1. The first is a GT repeat at position 33117 (GenBank accession No. AF109907). The second is a CA repeat at position 23,000 of this same sequence.[17]

Accession numbers should include the version (eg, .1, .2) if possible[8]:

NM_000130.1

NM_000130.2

L01538.1

The following example shows variation expressed with the accession number[8]:

NM_004006.1:c.3G>T

Common formatting for nucleotide data was determined in 1988 by representatives of GenBank, EMBL, and DDBJ, forming the International Nucleotide Sequence Database Collaboration (http://www.ncbi.nlm.nih.gov/projects/collab/).[18]

RNA. Functionally associated with DNA is ribonucleic acid (RNA). It contains the 3 bases adenine (A), cytosine (C), and guanine (G) but differs from DNA in having the base uracil (U) instead of thymine (T) and the sugar ribose rather than deoxyribose. The corresponding nucleosides are adenosine, cytidine, guanosine, and uridine.

An example of an RNA sequence is as follows:

5′-UUAGCACGUGCUAA-3′

Examples of RNA codons are as follows:

CAU UUG AUU

Expand these common abbreviations at first use:

cRNA	complementary RNA
dsRNA	double-stranded RNA
gRNA	genomic RNA
hnRNA	heteronuclear RNA (heterogeneous RNA)
mRNA	messenger RNA
miRNA	microRNA
mtRNA	mitochondrial RNA
nRNA	nuclear RNA
RNAi	RNA interference
rRNA	ribosomal RNA
siRNA	short interfering RNA
snRNA	small nuclear RNA
tRNA	transfer RNA

Types of tRNA may be further specified; follow typographic style closely (these need not be expanded):

$\mathrm{tRNA}^{\mathrm{Met}}$	tRNA specific for methionine
$\mathrm{Met\text{-}tRNA}^{\mathrm{Met}}$	methionyl-tRNA
$\mathrm{tRNA}^{\mathrm{fMet}}$	tRNA specific for formylmethionine
$\mathrm{fMet\text{-}tRNA}^{\mathrm{fMet}}$ *or* $\mathrm{fMet\text{-}tRNA}_{\mathrm{f}}$	*N*-formylmethionyl-tRNA
$\mathrm{tRNA}^{\mathrm{Ala}}$	tRNA specific for alanine
$\mathrm{tRNA}^{\mathrm{Val}}$	tRNA specific for valine

The 3-dimensional structure of tRNA has several different arms, which allow it to recognize a codon on mRNA and deliver the appropriate amino acid during protein synthesis:

AA (amino acid) arm

DHU (dihydrouridine) arm

anticodon arm

TψC arm (ψ for the unusual base pseudouridine)

RNA Sequence Variations. Style for abbreviated sequence variation terms described at the RNA level is essentially the same as for DNA (see the "Sequence Variations, Nucleotides" section). The main exception is that the RNA nucleotide abbreviations are lowercase. The prefix r. is used to signify RNA[14] but is not required.

78a>u

r.76a>c

RNA sequences are quantified by use of the same units as for DNA, ie, base, bp, kb, and Mb:

240-bp dsRNA

10-25 RNA bases

a 7.5-kb RNA probe

Nucleotides as Precursors and Energy Molecules. The nucleotides of DNA and RNA are also important individually as the precursors of DNA and RNA and as energy molecules. They may bind 1, 2, or 3 phosphate molecules, giving rise to compounds with the following abbreviations (see also 14.11, Abbreviations, Clinical, Technical, and Other Common Terms) or .lternative shorthand:

Ribonucleotides

Terms	*Abbreviation*	*Alternative Shorthand*
adenosine monophosphate, adenylic acid	AMP	pA
adenosine diphosphate	ADP	ppA
adenosine triphosphate	ATP	pppA
cytidine monophosphate, cytidylic acid	CMP	pC
cytidine diphosphate	CDP	ppC
cytidine triphosphate	CTP	pppC
guanosine monophosphate, guanylic acid	GMP	pG
guanosine diphosphate	GDP	ppG
guanosine triphosphate	GTP	pppG
uridine monophosphate, uridylic acid	UMP	pU
uridine diphosphate	UDP	ppU
uridine triphosphate	UTP	pppU

Deoxyribonucleotides

Term	*Abbreviation*	*Alternative Shorthand**
deoxyadenosine monophosphate, deoxyadenylic acid	dAMP	pdA
deoxyadenosine diphosphate	dADP	
deoxyadenosine triphosphate	dATP	
deoxycytidine monophosphate, deoxycytidylic acid	dCMP	pdC
deoxycytidine diphosphate	dCDP	
deoxycytidine triphosphate	dCTP	
deoxyguanosine monophosphate, deoxyguanylic acid	dGMP	pdG

Term	*Abbreviation*	*Alternative Shorthand**
deoxyguanosine diphosphate	dGDP	
deoxyguanosine triphosphate	dGTP	
deoxythymosine monophosphate, deoxythymidylic acid	dTMP	pdT
deoxythymosine diphosphate	dTDP	
deoxythymosine triphosphate	dTTP	

*Terms such as ppdA and pppdA are, by analogy with ribonucleotide shorthand, feasible but not commonly found.

In the foregoing examples, monophosphates are assumed to be phosphorylated at the 5′ position, and the more specific term may be used:

5′-AMP

The additional phosphate groups of diphosphates and triphosphates are linked sequentially to the first phosphate group. Other phosphate positions and variations may be specified as follows:

2′-UMP	
3′-UMP	Up
3′,5′-ADP	pAp
3′,5′-AMP	cAMP (cyclic AMP)

Note that the p follows the capital letter when 3′-phosphate is indicated.

Nucleic Acid Technology. Laboratory methods of analyzing DNA make use of special DNA sequences, which include the following:

RFLPs	restriction fragment length polymorphisms
SNPs	single-nucleotide polymorphisms
STRs	short tandem repeats
STRPs	STR polymorphisms
STSs	sequence tagged sites
VNTRs	variable number of tandem repeats

Note: Satellite DNA repeats, microsatellite repeats (or markers), and minisatellite repeats (or markers) are distinct types of tandem repeat sequences.

An SNP sequence may be preceded by rs (for reference SNP ID) or ss (for submitted SNP ID), used for accession numbers assigned by the National Center for Biotechnology Information:

rs1002138(-)

Methods of analysis include the following:

ASO	allele-specific oligonucleotide probes
DGGE	denaturing gradient gel electrophoresis

EMSA	electrophoretic mobility shift assay
FISH	fluorescence in situ hybridization
OSH	oligonucleotide-specific hybridization
PCR	polymerase chain reaction
PTT	protein truncation test
RT-PCR	reverse-transcriptase PCR
SKY	spectral karyotyping, a type of FISH
SSCP	single-stranded conformational polymorphism

Blotting. The first blotting technique, used for identifying specific DNA sequences in genomic DNA isolated in vitro by means of nucleic acid probes, was named Southern blotting for its originator, E. M. Southern. Similar techniques have since been named (with droll intent) for compass directions and include Northern blotting (RNA identified; nucleic acid probe), Western blotting (protein identified; antibody probe), Southwestern blotting (protein identified; DNA probe), and Far Western blotting (protein identified; protein probe).[5]

Recombinant DNA is DNA created by combining isolated DNA sequences of interest. Among the tools used in this process are cloning vectors, such as plasmids, phages (see 15.14.3, Organisms and Pathogens, Virus Nomenclature), and hybrids of these, cosmids and phagemids. Additional tools are bacterial artificial chromosomes, or BACs, and yeast artificial chromosomes, or YACs.

Basic explanations of these entities are available in medical dictionaries and textbooks. A few that present special nomenclatural problems are described here.

Cloning Vectors. Plasmids are typically named with a lowercase p followed by a letter or alphanumeric designation; spacing may vary:

pBR322

pJS97

pUC

pUC18

pSPORT

pSPORT 2

Phage cloning vectors are named for the phages, for example:

phage λ: λgt10, λgt11, λgt22A

M13 phage: M13KO7, M13mp

Restriction Enzymes. Restriction enzymes (or restriction endonucleases) are special enzymes that cleave DNA at specific sites. They are named for the organism from which they are isolated, usually a bacterial species or strain. An authoritative source of information is REBASE.[7] As originally proposed,[19] their names consist of a 3-letter term, italicized and beginning with a capital letter, taken from the organism of origin, eg:

Hpa for *Haemophilus parainfluenzae*

followed by a roman numeral, which is a series number, eg:

*Hpa*I

*Hpa*II

In some cases, the series number is preceded by a capital or lowercase letter (roman, not italic), an arabic numeral, or a number and letter combination, which refers to the strain of bacterium; there are no spaces between any of these elements of the term:

*Eco*RI

*Hin*fI

*Sau*96I

*Sau*3AI

Many variations in the form of the names of these enzymes have appeared, eg, *Hin* d III, *Hin* dIII, *Hin*d III, *Hind* III. It is currently recommended that italics and spacing be given as noted in the preceding paragraph, to differentiate the species name, strain designation, and enzyme series number. The following list gives examples:

Enzyme Name	*Organism of Origin*
*Acc*I	*Acinetobacter calcoaceticus*
*Alu*I	*Arthrobacter luteus*
*Alw*NI	*Acinetobacter lwoffi* N
*Bam*HI	*Bacillus amyloliquefaciens* H
*Bcl*I	*Bacillus caldolyticus*
*Bst*EII	*Bacillus stearothermophilus* ET
*Bst*XI	*Bacillus stearothermophilus* X
I-*Ceu*I	*Chlamydomonas eugametos*
*Dpn*I	*Streptococcus* (diplococcus) *pneumoniae* M
*Eco*RI	*Escherichia coli* RY13
*Eco*RII	*Escherichia coli* R245
*Hae*II	*Haemophilus aegyptius*
*Hinc*II	*Haemophilus influenzae* Rc
*Hin*dIII	*Haemophilus influenzae* Rd
*Hin*fI	*Haemophilus influenzae* Rf
*Mse*I	*Micrococcus* species
*Msp*I	*Moraxella* species
*Ple*I	*Pseudomonas lemoignei*
*Pml*I	*Pseudomonas maltophilia*
*Pst*I	*Providencia stuartii*
*Sau*3AI	*Staphylococcus aureus* 3A
*Sau*96I	*Staphylococcus aureus* PS96
*Sma*I	*Serratia marcescens*

Enzyme Name	*Organism of Origin*
*Sst*I	*Streptomyces stanford*
*Taq*I	*Thermus aquaticus* YT-1
*Xba*I	*Xanthomonas badrii*
*Xho*I	*Xanthomonas holicola*

Prefixes may further specify type of enzyme action, eg:

I-*Ceu*I	I: intron-coded endonuclease	*Chlamydomonas eugametos*
M.*Mly*I	M: methylase	*Micrococcus lylae*
N.*Mly*I	N: nicking enzyme	

Restriction enzyme names are often seen as modifiers, eg:

a *Bam*HI fragment

an *Eco*RI site

For information on recognition sequences, see the "DNA" section.

Modifying Enzymes. Enzymes exist that synthesize DNA and RNA (polymerases), cleave DNA (nucleases), join nucleic acid fragments (ligases), methylate nucleotides (methylases), and synthesize DNA from RNA (reverse transcriptases) (see also 15.10.3, Molecular Medicine, Enzyme Nomenclature). Those in laboratory use come from living systems, often from the same organisms that furnish restriction enzymes. Because the names may be similar, it is essential to specify the type of enzyme so that there is no confusion, eg:

*Alu*I methylase

Pfu DNA polymerase *(Pyrococcus furiosus)*

*Taq*I methylase

Taq DNA ligase

Modifying enzyme names are often seen as qualifiers, eg:

a *Taq*I RFLP

In the following enzyme terms, T plus numeral refers to the related phage (see 15.14.3, Organisms and Pathogens, Virus Nomenclature):

T7 DNA polymerase

T4 DNA polymerase

T4 polynucleotide kinase

T4 RNA ligase

DNA Families. Families of nongene DNA include the following:

Collective Term	*Example*
SINEs (short interspersed nuclear elements)	*Alu* family (named for *Alu*I; see "Restriction Enzymes" section)

Collective Term	*Example*
LINEs (long interspersed nuclear elements)	L1 family (from LINE 1 family)

Amino Acids. Twenty amino acids are ultimate products of the genetic code (see the "DNA" section) and constituents of proteins. Each has 1 or more distinct codons in DNA, eg, GCU, GCC, GCA, and GCG code for alanine.

The following tablulation gives the amino acids of proteins and their preferred 3- and single-letter symbols. Although these amino acids have systematic names (eg, alanine is 2-aminopropanoic acid), the trivial names are the most widely recognized and used. The single-letter symbols are usually used for longer sequences; otherwise, the 3-letter symbols are preferred. Do not mix single-letter and 3-letter amino acid symbols. In general publications, it may be helpful to define the single-letter symbols, eg, in a key, and to expand the 3-letter symbols at first mention as well.

Amino Acid	*3-Letter Symbol*	*Single-Letter Symbol*
alanine	Ala	A
arginine	Arg	R
asparagine	Asn	N
aspartic acid	Asp	D
asparagine or aspartic acid	Asx	B
cysteine	Cys	C
glutamine	Gln	Q
glutamic acid	Glu	E
glutamic acid or glutamine	Glx	Z
glycine	Gly	G
histidine	His	H
isoleucine	Ile	I
leucine	Leu	L
lysine	Lys	K
methionine	Met	M
phenylalanine	Phe	F
proline	Pro	P
serine	Ser	S
threonine	Thr	T
tryptophan	Trp	W
tyrosine	Tyr	Y
valine	Val	V
unspecified amino acid	Xaa	X

The symbols Asp and Glu apply equally to the anions aspartate and glutamate, respectively, the forms that exist under most physiological conditions.

The PE and PPE bacterial gene and protein families are named for Pro-Glu and Pro-Pro-Glu, sequence motifs in the proteins. The terms need not be expanded.

Other amino acids are also well known by their trivial names and have 3-letter codes. These, however, should always be expanded, as the example of cystine, whose 3-letter code is the same as that of cysteine, bears out:

citrulline	Cit
cystine	Cys
homocysteine	Hcy
homoserine	Hse
hydroxyproline	Hyp
ornithine	Orn
thyroxine	Thx

The side chains of amino acids are known as R groups, and the letter R is used in molecular formulas when indicating a nonspecified side chain, as in this general formula for an amino acid:

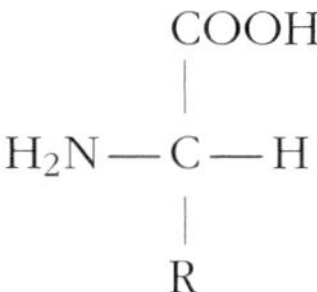

Do not confuse the R with the single-letter abbreviation for arginine (see tabluation above).

The carboxyl (COOH) group is referred to as the α-carboxyl group, which contains the C-1 carbon. The amino (NH_2) group (shown as H_2N above to indicate that C is linked with N) is referred to as the α-amino group, which contains the N-2 nitrogen. (The true structure is not neutral, as above, but rather contains NH_3^+ and COO^-. However, the structure above is often used, as it is herein, for purposes of discussion.)

Peptide bonds are bonds between the α-carboxyl group of one amino acid and the α-amino group of the next. Long peptide sequences are the backbones of proteins. A peptide sequence might be indicated as follows, with hyphens representing peptide bonds:

Gly-Ile-Val-Glu-Gln-Cys-Cys-Ala-Ser-Val-Cys-Ser-Leu-Tyr

By convention in such a sequence, the amino end of the peptide (the end whose amino acid has a free amino group, also known as the N terminal) is on the left and the carboxyl end (the end whose amino acid has a free carboxyl group, also known as the C terminal) is on the right. The symbols NH_2 and COOH may be included in the representation of the peptide sequence, as follows:

NH_2-Gly-Ile-Val-Glu-Gln-Cys-Cys-Ala-Ser-Val-Cys-Ser-Leu-Tyr-COOH

The same left-to-right convention applies to sequences using single letters. The above sequence using single letters would be

GIVEQCCASVCSLY

When the NH_2 group appears on the right of a sequence, it has a meaning other than amino end. For instance, in the following sequence, Val-NH_2 indicates the amide derivative of valine:

His-Phe-Arg-Lys-Pro-Val-NH_2

To indicate bonds other than the peptide bonds described above, lines, rather than hyphens, are used:

Glu ⌐ Cys-Gly or Glu └── Cys-Gly (glutathione)

Cys-Tyr-Ile-Gln-Asn-Cys-Pro-Leu-Gly-NH_2 (oxytocin)

(Adapted by permission from Moss[3] http://www.chem.qmw.ac.uk/iupac/AminoAcid/A1819.html, Nomenclature and Symbolism for Amino Acids and Peptides, 3AA-19.1. Peptide Chains; copyright IUPAC and IUBMB.)

For a multiline peptide sequence in running text, use a hyphen at the right end of one line to indicate a break and at the start of the next line to indicate the peptide bond:

Ala-Ser-Tyr-Phe-Ser-

-Gly-Pro-Gly-Trp-Arg

or, in figures, use a line:

Ala-Ser-Tyr-Phe-Ser ─┐
└─ Gly-Pro-Gly-Trp-Arg

(Adapted by permission from Moss,[3] http://www.chem.qmw.ac.uk/iupac/AminoAcid/A1819.html; 3AA-19.1. Peptide Chains, copyright IUPAC and IUBMB.)

In special cases, such as cyclic compounds, the bond from C-2 to N-2 can be shown with arrows, as follows:

→ Val → Orn → Leu → DPhe → Pro ─┐
└─ Pro ← DPhe ← Leu ← Orn ← Val ← (gramicidin S)

(Adapted by permission from Moss,[3] http://www.chem.qmw.ac.uk/iupac/AminoAcid/A1819.html; 3AA-19.5.1. Homodetic Cyclic Peptides, copyright IUPAC and IUBMB.)

As with nucleic acid sequences, alignment is important in protein sequences. In the following examples, the amino acid residues must remain aligned with the nucleic acid triplets:

```
   M et Se r I leGlnHis            Me t -S e r-I l e-Gl n-Hi s
AGTATGAGTATTCAACAT    or    AGT ATG AGT ATT CAA CAT
TCATACTCATAAGTTGTA          TCA TAC TCA TAA GTT GTA
```

(Adapted from Moss,[3] http://www.chem.qmw.ac.uk/iupac/AminoAcid/A1819.html#AA198, 3AA-19.8. Alignment of Peptide and Nucleic-Acid Sequences.)

An amino acid term plus number refers to the amino acid by codon number (when known) or by protein residue, eg:

Arg506

Sequence Variations, Amino Acids. Recently, HGVS has expressed a preference for the 3-letter amino-acid abbreviation to be used in shorthand descriptions of sequence variations in proteins, unless the change is very simple. Because this preference is recent, the 1-letter style still has currency. For sequence variations described at the protein level, recommended style for abbreviated terms is similar to that for nucleotides. (See also the "Sequence Variations, Nucleotides" section and Phenotype Terminology in 15.6.2, Human Gene Nomenclature). Note that the amino acid abbreviation begins the term, preceding the position number (in contrast to nucleotide sequence variant terms, in which the residue number precedes the residue abbreviation). Explanation of such terms at first mention is recommended. Use of the prefix p. (protein) is another recent recommendation.

3-Letter Style	*Single-Letter Style*	*Explanation*
Arg506Gln	R506Q	arginine at residue 506 replaced by glutamine (This amino acid substitution is the result of the G1691A subsitution.[15])
Leu10ins	L10ins	leucine inserted at position 10
Leu141del	L141del	leucine deleted at position 141
Gln318X *or* Gln318ter	Q318X	glutamine at 318 changed to stop codon (X or ter)
p.Trp26Cys	p.W26C	tryptophan at residue 26 replaced by cysteine

X is officially recommended as the symbol for the stop codon, but it can also be the single-letter abbreviation for unspecified or unknown amino acid. Therefore, when an amino acid sequence expressed with single letters that includes X is used, the X should be explained in the text.

When an amino acid sequence variation is used with a gene symbol, italicize only the gene symbol:

ADRB1 Arg389Gly (not: *ADRB1 Arg389Gly*)

(See also 15.6.2, Human Gene Nomenclature.)

Note: Residue numbering begins at the translation initiator methionine, +1.

For further details on expressing sequence variations in proteins, consult the HGVS recommendations.[8]

REFERENCES

1. Cammack R. The biochemical nomenclature committees. *IUBMB Life*. 2000;50(3): 159-161.
2. Collins FS, Trent JM. Cancer genetics. In: Braunwald E, Fauci AS, Isselbacher KJ, et al, eds. *Harrison's Online*. http://www.harrisonsonline.com. Accessed August 10, 2004.

3. Moss GP. International Union of Biochemistry and Molecular Biology recommendations on biochemical & organic nomenclature, symbols & terminology etc. http://www.chem.qmw.ac.uk/iubmb. Updated March 20, 2006. Accessed April 22, 2006.
4. Liébecq C. *Biochemical Nomenclature and Related Documents: A Compendium*. London, England: International Union of Biochemistry and Molecular Biology/Portland Press Ltd; 1992.
5. Nussbaum RL, McInnes RR, Willard HF. *Thompson and Thompson Genetics in Medicine*. 6th rev reprint ed. Philadelphia, PA: Saunders; 2004.
6. Cooper NG. *The Human Genome Project: Deciphering the Blueprint of Heredity*. Mill Valley, CA: University Science Books; 1994.
7. Roberts RJ, Macelis D. REBASE: the Restriction Enzyme Database. http://rebase.neb.com/rebase/rebase.html. Accessed August 23, 2005.
8. Human Genome Variation Society Web site. http://www.hgvs.org. Updated January 16, 2006. Accessed April 22, 2006.
9. den Dunnen JT, Antonarakis SE. Mutation nomenclature extensions and suggestions to describe complex mutations: a discussion. *Hum Mutat*. 2000;15(1):7-12.
10. Antonarakis SE; Nomenclature Working Group. Recommendations for a nomenclature system for human gene mutations. *Hum Mutat*. 1998;11(1):1-3.
11. Beutler E, McKusick VA, Motulsky AG, Scriver CR, Hutchinson F. Mutation nomenclature: nicknames, systematic names, and unique identifiers. *Hum Mutat*. 1996;8(3):203-206.
12. Ad Hoc Committee on Mutation Nomenclature. Update on nomenclature for human gene mutations. *Hum Mutat*. 1996;8(3):197-202.
13. Beaudet AL, Tsui L-C. A suggested nomenclature for designing mutations. *Hum Mutat*. 1993;2(4):245-248.
14. den Dunnen JT, Antonarakis E. Nomenclature for the description of human sequence variations. *Hum Genet*. 2001;109(1):121-124.
15. Online Mendelian Inheritance in Man (OMIM). National Center for Biotechnology Information Web site. http://www.ncbi.nlm.nih.gov/entrez/query.fcgi?db=OMIM. Accessed April 22, 2006.
16. 2005 Database Issue. *Nucleic Acids Res*. http://nar.oxfordjournals.org/content/vol33/suppl_1/. Accessed April 22, 2006.
17. Athan ES, Williamson J, Ciappa A, et al. A founder mutation in presenilin 1 causing early-onset Alzheimer disease in unrelated Caribbean Hispanic families. *JAMA*. 2001;286(18):2257-2263.
18. Rangel P, Giovannetti J. *Genfomes and Databases on the Internet: A Practical Guide to Functions and Applications*. Norfolk, England: Horizon Scientific Press; 2002.
19. Smith HO, Nathans D. A suggested nomenclature for bacterial host modification and restriction systems and their enzymes. *J Mol Biol*. 1973;81(3):419-423.

15.6.2 Human Gene Nomenclature. The International System for Human Gene Nomenclature (ISGN) was inaugurated in 1979[1,2] and has been continually updated. The Human Gene Mapping Nomenclature Committee, which developed the ISGN, put forth a "one human genome–one gene language" principle:

> Certainly there exists a genetic and molecular basis for a single human gene language without dialects. All human nuclear genes as we know them follow the same genetic, molecular, and evolutionary principles. . . . Thus it is

reasonable and logical to develop a standard and consolidated gene nomenclature system rather than have a human gene language based on different gene systems.[3(p12)]

The committee, known as the HUGO Gene Nomenclature Committee (HGNC), is 1 of 7 committees of the Human Genome Organisation (HUGO) and is "responsible for gene name validation."[4(p115)] Gene names and symbols are assigned by the HGNC.[5] The human genome is estimated to have approximately 30 000 genes, more than 20 000 of which are represented by active symbols,[6] with the remainder to be named in a consistent fashion as genes are discovered.

- *Gene Symbols:* A gene symbol is a short term, typically 3 to 7 characters long, that conveys in abbreviated form the name or other attribute of a gene. Human gene symbols usually consist of uppercase letters and may also contain (but never begin with) numerals. Approved gene symbols do not contain Greek letters, roman numerals, superscripts, or subscripts and usually contain no punctuation. In *JAMA* and the *Archives* Journals, gene symbols are italicized, per official recommendations.[7] Italicizing is a useful way to make clear that a gene, and not a similarly named entity such as a condition or product of the gene, is being discussed. Italics are not necessary in published catalogs of gene symbols.[7] For style rules for gene symbols, see Table 3.

Approved symbols may represent other entities, such as chromosomal regions, certain syndromes, genes whose existence is inferred (supported by linkage analysis or association with known markers), cloned DNA segments, pseudogenes, and DNA fragments.

Table 3. Style Rules for Gene Symbols (Examples)

Gene Description	Approved Gene Symbol	Rule Illustrated
α-fetoprotein	*AFP*	Greek letter changed to Latin letter (but not moved to end of symbol: exception to recommendation)
β_2-microglobulin	*B2M*	Greek letter changed to Latin letter; no subscripts or punctuation
α-galactosidase	*GLA*	Greek letter changed to Latin letter and moved to end of symbol
coagulation factor VIII	*F8*	roman numeral changed to arabic numeral
β_1-galactosidase	*GLB1*	Greek letter changed to Latin letter and moved with numeral to end of term; no subscripts or punctuation
heterogeneous nuclear ribonucleoprotein A2/B1	*HNRPA2B1*	no punctuation marks or spaces
MCF.2 cell line–derived transforming sequence	*MCF2*	no punctuation marks
5′-nucleotidase, cytosolic	*NT5C*	number moved from the start of symbol; no punctuation
5S RNA, cluster 1	*RN5S1@*	first character is letter, not number
thromboxane A_2 receptor	*TBXA2R*	no superscripts or subscripts

Within larger terms, only the gene symbol is italicized:

ADRB2 46G>A (*not: ADRB2 46G>A*)

ADRB2 Gly16Arg (*not: ADRB2 Gly16Arg*)

(For an explanation of 46G>A and Gly16Arg, see "Sequence Variations, Nucleotides," and "Sequence Variations, Amino Acids," in 15.6.1, Nucleic Acids and Amino Acids.)

Authors are encouraged to use the most up-to-date gene symbol, which may be verified at the HGNC Web site in the Human Gene Nomenclature Database (Searchgenes feature),[6,8,9] or Entrez Gene.[10] The records available in Searchgenes contain "23 fields, with 14 links to other resources," such as Online Mendelian Inheritance in Man (OMIM, see later in this section), LocusLink, and Swiss-Prot (see 15.6.1, Nucleic Acids and Amino Acids).[9] Consistent use of the approved gene symbol provides advantages when searching for information in multiple databases.[11]

- *Gene Names:* Genes are usually named for the molecular product of the gene, the function of the gene, or the condition associated with the gene if known. Gene names are not italicized. As shown directly below, the *approved* gene names, available in the above mentioned databases, expand Greek letters and do not use subscripts, etc (so that, for instance, in using Searchgenes to find a gene name with α, one would type in "alpha"). Descriptions based on the approved gene names but styled according to the journal in question (eg, using Greek letters and subscripts) or omitting some terms from the full name are permissible in general medical journals.

approved gene name: the alpha-fetoprotein gene

description: the α-fetoprotein gene

approved gene name: the gene for beta-2-microglobulin

description: the gene for β_2-microglobulin

A number of conventions are followed when gene symbols and names are officially designated. Related genes are often assigned symbols by sequentially numbering a stem, the root symbol for the gene family:

ABC: root symbol

genes: *ABCA1, ABCG4,* etc

TNF: root symbol

genes: *TNF, TNFAIP1, TNFAIP2, TNFAIP3,* etc

Other conventions involve stereotypic abbreviations, eg, *CR* will often signify a "chromosome region." (However, a given letter or letter combination does not always signify a conventional usage. For instance, *L* at or near the end of a symbol often, but not always, indicates "like.") In Table 4, the conventions in column 3 reflect HGNC recommendations.[7] (*Note:* DNA sequences are available from the Genome Database, http://gdbwww.gdb.org/gdb/.[7])

Table 4. Conventions for Gene Names and Gene Symbols (Examples)

Gene Description	Gene Symbol	Convention Illustrated
Angelman syndrome chromosome region	*ANCR*	*CR*: chromosome region
BRCA1-associated protein	*BRAP*	*AP:* associated protein
bromodomain containing 1	*BRD1*	*D:* domain-containing
chromosome 11 open reading frame 10	*C11orf10*	*orf:* lowercase exception for "open reading frame"
calcium modulating ligand	*CAMLG*	*LG*: ligand
caspase 1, 2, 3, etc, apoptosis-related cysteine protease	*CASP1, CASP2, CASP3,* etc	stem (*CASP*), sequentially numbered
cyclin-dependent kinase inhibitor 1 B	*CDKN1B*	*N:* inhibitor
Cornelia de Lange syndrome 1	*CDL1*	named for condition; *L* at end in this case does not signify "like"
carpal tunnel syndrome 1	*CTS1*	named for syndrome
cystic fibrosis transmembrane conductance regulator	*CFTR*	formerly *CF;* name modified after discovery of gene product
collagen (type VI, α_1), overlapping transcript 1	*COLOT1*	*OT:* overlapping transcript
DNA segment sequence	*D19S1177E*	*D*: DNA; *19*: chromosome 19; *S*: (unique DNA) segment; *E* expressed
Down syndrome chromosome region	*DCR*	*CR*: chromosome region
deafness, autosomal dominant 4	*DFNA4*	named for condition
DNA segment sequence	*DXS522E*	as above; *X*: X chromosome
DNA segment sequence	*DXYS155E*	as above; *XY*: sequence present at homologous sites on chromosomes X and Y
family with sequence similarity 7, member A1	*FAM7A1*	*FAM:* family with sequence similarity
fragile site, aphidicolin type, common, fra(10)(q11.2) (see also 15.6.4, Human Chromosomes)	*FRA10G*	*FRA:* fragile site; *10*: chromosome 10; *G:* series letter
fragile site, folic acid type, rare, fra(X)(q28)	*FRAXF*	*X*: X chromosome; final *F:* series letter
glucose 6-phosphatase, catalytic (glycogen storage disease type I, von Gierke disease)	*G6PC*	*C:* catalytic
glucose-6-phosphate dehydrogenase	*G6PD*	named for gene product
glucose-6-phosphate dehydrogenase–like	*G6PDL*	*L:* "like" sequence

Table 4. Conventions for Gene Names and Gene Symbols (Examples) *(cont)*

Gene Description	Gene Symbol	Convention Illustrated
hemoglobin, α_1	*HBA1*	named for gene product
hemoglobin, α_1 pseudogene	*HBAP1*	*P:* "pseudogene" (compare term directly above)
hair color 1 (brown)	*HCL1*	named for characteristic
human immunodeficiency virus 1 enhancer binding protein 2	*HIVEP2*	*P:* does not always signify "pseudogene"
major histocompatibility complex, class I, A	*HLA-A*	punctuation exception for HLA genes
homeobox A7	*HOXA7*	*HOX* signifies "homeobox" gene family
insulinlike growth factor 2, antisense	*IGF2AS*	*AS:* antisense
insulin-dependent diabetes mellitus 10	*IDDM10*	a type 1 diabetes susceptibility locus, number 10
interleukin 18 binding protein	*IL18BP*	*BP:* binding protein
insulin	*INS*	named for gene product
insulin receptor	*INSR*	*R:* receptor
insulin receptor–like	*INSRL*	*R:* receptor *L*: like
loss of heterozygosity 3, chromosomal region 2, gene A	*LOH3CR2A*	*LOH:* loss of heterozygosity
melanoma antigen, family A, 2	*MAGEA2*	named for condition and gene product
mitochondrial ribosomal protein 63	*MRP63*	*M:* mitochondrial *RP:* ribosomal protein
7S mitochondrial DNA	*MT7SDNA*	*MT:* mitochondrial
mitochondrially encoded 12S RNA	*MT-RNR1*	*MT:* mitochondrial, used with hyphen (punctuation exception)
programmed cell death 1	*PDCD1*	named for function
pepsinogen A gene cluster	*PGA@*	@: gene family or cluster
renin	*REN*	named for gene product
renin binding protein	*RENBP*	named for gene product; *BP:* binding protein
5S RNA, cluster 1	*RN5S1@*	@: gene family or cluster; *RN*: RNA
schwannomin interacting protein 1	*SCHIP1*	*IP:* interacting protein
T-cell, immune regulator 1	*TCIRG1*	*RG:* regulator
α_2-tubulin	*TUBA2*	named for gene product
zinc finger protein 160	*ZNF160*	initial *ZNF* indicates zinc finger protein

When a gene name or symbol has been changed, both the new and former names (previous symbols) are available in gene databases.[6,10] Authors should use the most up-to-date term. The previous symbol may be included parenthetically at first mention:

CYP2A6 (formerly *CYP2A3*)

SOD1 (formerly *ALS* and *ALS1*)

Writing About Genes and Italicizing Gene Symbols. Observing the rule of italicizing gene symbols makes clear whether the writer is referring to a gene or to another entity that might be confused with a gene.

In any discussion of a gene, it is recommended that the approved gene symbol be mentioned at some point, preferably in the title and abstract if relevant. However, the gene symbol need not be mentioned every time the writer refers to the gene. Authors may refer to genes (or gene loci) by their official gene names or other descriptive expression. Any of these is acceptable, depending on context and syntax. Of names, descriptions, and symbols, only the gene symbol is italicized. Examples are shown below:

Acceptable Expression	*Gene Description*	*Gene Symbol*
the breast and ovarian cancer susceptibility gene	breast cancer 1, early-onset gene	*BRCA1*
the cystic fibrosis locus	cystic fibrosis transmembrane conductance regulator gene	*CFTR*
the factor VIII locus	coagulation factor VIII, procoagulant component (hemophilia A) gene	*F8*
the hemophilia A locus	coagulation factor VIII, procoagulant component (hemophilia A) gene	*F8*
the gene for synapsin I	synapsin I gene	*SYN1*
the p53 gene	tumor protein p53 (Li-Fraumeni syndrome) gene	*TP53*

In the foregoing examples, the gene names and descriptions are readily distinguishable from the gene symbols. Sometimes, however, the gene symbol may be easily confused with the abbreviation for the product or condition associated with the gene unless the gene symbol is italicized; for instance:

Gene	*Potentially Confusing Nongene Term*
ABO	ABO blood group system (see also 15.1, Blood Groups, Platelet Antigens, and Granulocyte Antigens)
APOE	apoE (apolipoprotein E)
EPO	erythropoietin (Epo)
GRIFIN	GRIFIN protein (galectin-related interfiber protein)

Gene	*Potentially Confusing Nongene Term*
HLA-A, HLA-B, etc	HLA-A, HLA-B, etc (see also 15.8.5, Immunology, HLA/Major Histocompatibility Complex)
MS	multiple sclerosis (MS)
many hormone genes, eg, *CRH, GHRH, GNRHR, PTH, TRH*	hormone name abbreviations, eg, CRH, GHRH, GNRH receptor, PTH, TRH

In some expressions, italics may be moot, for instance, if a gene is named for an enzyme it produces:

Term	*Meaning*
TH gene	gene for tyrosine hydroxylase
TH gene	gene for tyrosine hydroxylase

In other expressions, italics distinguish different meanings:

Term	*Meaning*
HD	gene for huntingtin (protein), Huntington disease gene
HD	Huntington disease
person with *HD*	person with the *HD* gene, whether the disease-causing or normal form
person with HD	person with Huntington disease
prevalence of *HD*	prevalence of the *HD* gene
prevalence of HD	prevalence of Huntington disease; not necessarily equal to prevalence of the *HD* gene
TH deficiency	impaired functioning of the *TH* gene
TH deficiency	deficiency of the enzyme TH

Therefore, it is best to make clear by italicizing gene symbols and through context whether the gene or another entity is being discussed.

Gene symbols do not immediately follow the term in the gene name that they might seem to abbreviate, but rather, should relate to the word *gene*, usually following it:

> the guanylate cyclase 2D gene, *GUCY2D*
> *Not:* the guanylate cyclase 2D (*GUCY2D*) gene
>
> the Huntington disease gene, *HD*
>
> the tyrosine hydroxylase gene, *TH*
>
> The cystic fibrosis transmembrane conductance regulator gene, *CFTR,* is implicated in cystic fibrosis.

In the following examples, both gene aliases and approved symbols are used (see also 14.11, Abbreviations, Clinical, Technical, and Other Common Terms):

the retinal guanylate cyclase 2D (GUCY2D) gene, *GUCY2D*

the retinal guanylate cyclase 2D (RetGC1) gene, *GUCY2D*

Not: the guanylate cyclase 2D (*GUCY2D*) gene

the Huntington disease (HD) gene, *HD*

the tyrosine hydroxylase (TH) gene, *TH*

The cystic fibrosis (CF) transmembrane conductance regulator gene, *CFTR*, is implicated in CF.

In discussions of mutations, the gene symbol remains italicized; specific mutations, however, are *not* italicized (see "Sequence Variations, Nucleotides," and "Sequence Variations, Amino Acids" in 15.6.1, Nucleic Acids and Amino Acids):

ADRB2 46G>A

mutation of the *GUCY2D* gene

mutation of *GUCY2D*

GUCY2D mutation

mutated *GUCY2D* gene

Objective: To describe the phenotype in 4 families with dominantly inherited cone-rod dystrophy, 1 with an R838C mutation and 1 with an R838H mutation in the guanylate cyclase 2D gene (*GUCY2D*) encoding retinal guanylate cyclase-1.

$LRP5_{V171}$: valine substitution at codon 171 of the *LRP5* gene

In gene mapping, when the order of genes along the chromosome is known, the genes are listed from short-arm end (pter) to the centromere (cen) or long-arm end (qter) (see 15.6.4, Human Chromosomes):

pter-*ENO1-PGM1-AMY1*-cen

When the order of genes along the chromosome is not known, the genes are listed alphabetically and parentheses are used:

pter-*PGD-AK2-(ACTA,APOA2,REN)*-qter

Table 5 presents gene names and symbols from fields covered elsewhere in this chapter.

Table 5. Gene Names and Symbols From Fields Covered Elsewhere in This Chapter

Gene Symbol	Gene Description
	15.1, Blood Groups, Platelet Antigens, and Granulocyte Antigens
A4GALT	α-1,4-galactosyltransferase (P blood group)
ABO	ABO blood group (transferase A, α-1-3-*N*-acetylgalactosaminyltransferase; transferase B, α-1-3-galactosyltransferase)
ACHE	acetylcholinesterase (Yt blood group)

Table 5. Gene Names and Symbols From Fields Covered Elsewhere in This Chapter *(cont)*

Gene Symbol	Gene Description
	15.1, Blood Groups, Platelet Antigens, and Granulocyte Antigens
AQP1 (was *CO*)	aquaporin 1
ART4 (was *DO*)	ADP ribosyltransferase 4 (Dombrock blood group)
BCAM (was *LU*)	basic cell adhesion molecule (Lutheran blood group)
BSG	basigin (OK blood group)
C4A	complement component 4A
C4B	complement component 4B
CD44	CD44 antigen (homing function and Indian blood group system)
CD151 (was *MER2*)	antigen identified by monoclonal antibodies 1D12, 2F7
CR1	complement component (3b/4b) receptor 1, including Knops blood group system
CD55 (was *DAF*)	CD55, decay accelerating factor (DAF) for complement (Cromer blood group system)
DARC (was *FY*)	chemokine receptor (Duffy blood group)
ERMAP (was *SC*)	erythroblast membrane–associated protein (Scianna blood group)
FUT1	fucosyltransferase 1
FUT3	fucosyltransferase 3
GYPA	glycophorin A (includes MN blood group)
GYPB	glycophorin B (includes Ss blood group)
GYPC	glycophorin C (Gerbich blood group)
GYPE	glycophorin E
ICAM4	intercellular adhesion molecule 4, Landsteiner-Wiener blood group
KEL	Kell blood group
P1	P blood group (P1 antigen)
RHCE	Rh blood group, CcEe antigens
RHD	Rh blood group, D antigen
SLC4A1	solute carrier family 4, anion exchanger, member 1 (erythrocyte membrane protein band 3, Diego blood group)
SLC14A1	solute carrier family 14 (urea transporter), member 1 (Kidd blood group)
XG	Xg blood group (pseudoautosomal boundary-divided on the X chromosome)
XK	Kell blood group precursor (McLeod phenotype)
	15.2, Cancer (See Also 15.6.3, Oncogenes and Tumor Suppressor Genes)
ACTN1	α_1-actinin
ACTN2	α_1-actinin
BCL2	B-cell/CLL lymphoma 2

Table 5. Gene Names and Symbols From Fields Covered Elsewhere in This Chapter *(cont)*

15.2, Cancer (See Also 15.6.3, Oncogenes and Tumor Suppressor Genes)	
BCL7A	B-cell/CLL lymphoma 7A
CCND1 (formerly *BCL1*)	cyclin D1
CDC2	cell division cycle 2, G_1 to S and G_2 to M
CDK2	cyclin-dependent kinase 2
CDKN1A	cyclin-dependent kinase inhibitor 1A (p21, Cip1)
CTNNB1	β_1-catenin
MEN1	multiple endocrine neoplasia 1
RB1	retinoblastoma 1 (including osteosarcoma)
RET (formerly *MEN2A, MEN2B*)	ret proto-oncogene (multiple endocrine neoplasia and medullary thyroid carcinoma 1, Hirschsprung disease)
TGFA	transforming growth factor α
TGFB1	transforming growth factor β_1 (Camurati-Engelmann disease)
TNF	tumor necrosis factor (TNF superfamily, member 2)
TNFRSF1A	TNF receptor superfamily, member 1A
TP53	tumor protein p53 (Li-Fraumeni syndrome)
15.3, Cardiology	
ANK2 (formerly *LQT4*)	ankyrin 2 (neuronal; formerly long QT syndrome 4)
APOA1	apolipoprotein AI
APOB	apoliprotein B
APOC2	apoliprotein CII
APOD	apoliprotein D
APOE	apolipoprotein E
GPR1	G protein–coupled receptor 1
HDLBP	high-density lipoprotein-binding protein (vigilin)
KCNH2 (formerly *LQT2*)	potassium voltage-gated channel, subfamily H (eag-related), member 2
KCNQ1 (formerly *LQT1*)	potassium voltage-gated channel, KQT-like subfamily, member 1
LDLR	low-density lipoprotein receptor (familial hypercholesterolemia)
LPL	lipoprotein lipase
NOS1	nitric oxide synthase 1 (neuronal)
NOS2A	nitric oxide synthase 2A (inducible, hepatocytes)
NOS2B	nitric oxide synthase 2B
NOS2C	nitric oxide synthase 2C
NOS3	nitric oxide synthase 3 (endothelial cell)
PLAT	tissue plasminogen activator

Table 5. Gene Names and Symbols From Fields Covered Elsewhere in This Chapter *(cont)*

	15.3, Cardiology
SCN5A (formerly *LQT3*)	sodium channel, voltage-gated, type V, alpha polypeptide (long QT syndrome 3)
TNNC1	troponin C, slow
TNNC2	troponin C2, fast
TNNI1	troponin I, skeletal, slow
TNNI2	troponin I, skeletal, fast
TNNI3	troponin I, cardiac
TNNT1	troponin T1, skeletal, slow
TNNT2	troponin T2, cardiac
TNNT3	troponin T3, skeletal, fast
VLDLR	very-low-density lipoprotein receptor
	15.7, Hemostasis
A2M	α_2-macroglobulin
CALM1	calmodulin 1 (phosphorylase kinase, δ subunit)
CCL5	chemokine (C-C motif), ligand 5
CLEC3B (was *TNA*)	C-type lectin domain family 3, member B
F2	coagulation factor II (thrombin)
F2R	coagulation factor II (thrombin) receptor
F2RL1	coagulation factor II (thrombin) receptorlike 1
F3	coagulation factor III (tissue factor, thromboplastin)
F5	coagulation factor V
F7	coagulation factor VII
F7R	coagulation factor VII regulator
F8	coagulation factor VIII, procoagulant component (hemophilia A)
F8A1	coagulation factor VIII associated (intronic transcript) 1
F9	coagulation factor IX
F10	coagulation factor X
F11	coagulation factor XI
F12	coagulation factor XII
F13A1	coagulation factor XIII, A1 polypeptide
F13A2	coagulation factor XIII, A2 polypeptide
F13B	coagulation factor XIII, B polypeptide
FGA	fibrinogen A, α polypeptide
FGB	fibrinogen B, β polypeptide
FGG	fibrinogen, γ polypeptide

Table 5. Gene Names and Symbols From Fields Covered Elsewhere in This Chapter *(cont)*

	15.7, Hemostasis
FGL1	fibrinogenlike 1
FGL2	fibrinogenlike 2
GP5	glycoprotein V (platelet)
GP6	glycoprotein VI (platelet)
GP9	glycoprotein IX (platelet)
GP1BA	glycoprotein Ib, (platelet), α-polypeptide
ICAM1	intercellular adhesion molecule 1 (CD54)
ICAM2	intercellular adhesion molecule 2
ITGA1	α_1-integrin
ITGA2	α_2-integrin
ITGA2B	α_{2b}-integrin (platelet glycoprotein [Gp] IIb of IIb/IIIa complex, antigen CD41B)
ITGA3	α_3-integrin
ITGA6	α_6-integrin
ITGAV	α_v-integrin (vitronectin receptor, α polypeptide, antigen CD51)
ITGB1	β_1-integrin (fibronectin receptor, β polypeptide, antigen CD29)
ITGB3	integrin (platelet GpIIIa, antigen CD61)
ITPKA	inositol 1,4,5-triphosphate (IP_3) A
KLKB1	kallikrein B, plasma
KNG1	kininogen 1
NOS3	nitric oxide synthase 3 (endothelial cell)
PDGFA	platelet-derived growth factor α-polypeptide
PDGFC	platelet-derived growth factor C
PDGFRA	platelet-derived growth factor receptor, α-polypeptide
PDGFRL	platelet-derived growth factor receptor–like
PECAM1	platelet/endothelial cell adhesion molecule (CD31 antigen)
PLAT	plasminogen activator, tissue (tPA)
PLAU	plasminogen activator, urokinase (uPA)
PLAUR	uPA receptor
PLG	plasminogen
PLGLA1	plasminogenlike A1
PLGLB1	plasminogenlike B1
PPBP	proplatelet basic proteins (includes β-thromboglobulin)
PROC	protein C
PROS1	protein S
PROSP	protein S pseudogene
PROZ	protein Z, vitamin K–dependent plasma glycoprotein

Table 5. Gene Names and Symbols From Fields Covered Elsewhere in This Chapter *(cont)*

	15.7, Hemostasis
PTGDR	prostaglandin D_2 receptor
PTGDS	prostaglandin D_2 synthase
PTGFR	prostaglandin F receptor
PTGFRN	prostaglandin F2 receptor negative regulator
PTGIR	prostaglandin I2 (prostacyclin) receptor
PTGIS	prostaglandin I2 (prostacyclin) synthase
PTGS1	prostaglandin-endoperoxide synthase 1 (prostaglandin G/H synthase and cyclo-oxygenase)
SELE	E-selectin (endothelial adhesion molecule 1)
SELP	P-selectin
SERPINA1	serine (or cysteine) proteinase inhibitor, clade A (α_1-antiproteinase, antitrypsin), member 1
SERPINC1	serine (or cysteine) proteinase inhibitor, clade C (antithrombin), member 1
SERPINE1	serine (or cysteine) proteinase inhibitor, clade E (nexin, plasminogen activator inhibitor type 1), member 1
SERPINF2	serine (or cysteine) proteinase inhibitor, clade F (α_2-antiplasmin, pigment epithelium derived factor), member 2
TBXA2R	thromboxane A_2 receptor
TBXAS1	thromboxane A synthase 1
TFPI	tissue factor pathway inhibitor
TFPI2	tissue factor pathway inhibitor 2
THBD	thrombomodulin
VCAM1	vascular cell adhesion molecule 1
VWF	von Willebrand factor
VWFP	von Willebrand factor pseudogene
	15.8, Immunology
15.8.1, Chemokines	
CCL1	CCL1
CX3CL1	CX3CL1
CXCL1	CXCL1
PF4	platelet factor 4 (CXCL4)
XCL1	XCL1
15.8.2, CD Cell Markers	
CD14	CD14 antigen
CD19	CD19 antigen
CD1A	CD1a
CD3D	CD3δ

Table 5. Gene Names and Symbols From Fields Covered Elsewhere in This Chapter *(cont)*

	15.8, Immunology
CD46 (was *MCP*)	complement regulatory protein, CD46
CD55 (was *DAF*)	CD 55, DAF for complement (Cromer blood group system)
CD6	CD6
CD79A	CD79A, Igα
CD97	CD97
CR1	complement receptor type 1, CD35
FCGR3A	FcγRIIIa, CD16
ICAM3	intracellular adhesion molecule 3, CD50
MME	membrane metalloendopeptidase, CD10, CALLA
15.8.3, Complement	
C1QA	C1qα
C1QB	C1qβ
C1QBP	C1qbp
C1QR1	C1qR1
C1R	C1r
C1S	C1s
C2	C2
C3	C3
C4A	C4a
C4B	C4b
C4BPA	C4bp-α
C5	C5
C5AR1	C5aR1
C6	C6
C7	C7
C8A	C8α
C8B	C8β
C9	C9
CD55 (was *DAF*)	CD 55, DAF for complement (Cromer blood group system)
CFH	complement factor H
CFP	complement factor properdin
15.8.4, Cytokines	
CRLF1	cytokine receptorlike factor 1
CRLF2	cytokine receptorlike factor 2
CSF1	M-CSF

Table 5. Gene Names and Symbols From Fields Covered Elsewhere in This Chapter *(cont)*

	15.8, Immunology
CSF2	GM-CSF
CSF3	G-CSF
CSF3R	G-CSF receptor
EPO	erythropoietin (Epo)
EPOR	Epo receptor
GH1	growth hormone (GH) 1
GH2	GH 2
GHR	GH receptor
IFNA1	IFN-α1
IFNA2	IFN-α2
IFNB1	IFN-β1
IFNG	IFN-γ
IFNW1	IFN-ω
IL1A	IL-1α
IL1B	IL-1β
IL1R1	IL-1RI
IL1R2	IL-1RII
IL1RAP	IL-1R accessory protein
IL1RN	IL-1 receptor antagonist (IL-1ra)
IL2	IL-2
LEP	leptin
LEPR	leptin receptor
PRL	prolactin
SOCS1	suppressor of cytokine signaling 1
TGFA	transforming growth factor α (TGF-α)
TGFB1	TGF-β1 (Camurati-Engelmann disease)
THPO	thrombopoietin
TNF	tumor necrosis factor (TNF superfamily member 2)
15.8.5, HLA/Major Histocompatibility Complex	
HLA-A	HLA-A
HLA-B	HLA-B
HLA-C	HLA-C
HLA-DMA	HLA-DM α
HLA-DMB	HLA-DM β
HLA-DOA	HLA-DO α

Table 5. Gene Names and Symbols From Fields Covered Elsewhere in This Chapter *(cont)*

	15.8, Immunology
HLA-DOB	HLA-DO β
HLA-DPA1	HLA-DP α1
HLA-DQA1	HLA-DQ α1
HLA-DQB1	HLA-DQ β1
HLA-DRA	HLA-DR α
HLA-DRB1	HLA-DR β1
HLA-E	HLA-E
HLA-F	HLA-F
HLA-G	HLA-G
HLA-H	HLA-H (pseudogene)
HLA-J	HLA-J (pseudogene)
15.8.6, Immunoglobulins	
IGHA1	$C_{\alpha}1$
IGHA2	$C_{\alpha}2$
IGHD	C_{δ}
IGHD1-1	D_H1 subgroup member 1
IGHE	C_{ε}
IGHG1	$C_{\gamma}1$
IGHG2	$C_{\gamma}2$
IGHG3	$C_{\gamma}3$
IGHG4	$C_{\gamma}4$
IGHJ1	J_H1
IGHM	IgM μ C_H
IGHV@	V_H
IGHV1-2	V_H1 subgroup member 2
IGHV1-18	V_H1 subgroup member 18
IGKC	C_{κ}
IGKJ@	J_{κ}
IGKJ2	$J_{\kappa}2$
IGKV@	V_{κ}
IGKV1-5	$V_{\kappa}1$ subgroup member 5
IGLC@	C_{λ}
IGLC1	$C_{\lambda}1$
IGLJ@	J_{λ}
IGLJ1	$J_{\lambda}1$
IGLV@	V_{λ}

Table 5. Gene Names and Symbols From Fields Covered Elsewhere in This Chapter *(cont)*

	15.8, Immunology
IGLV10-54	V_λ10 subgroup member 54
15.8.7, Lymphocytes	
TRAC	T-cell receptor α chain (TCRα)
TRBC1	TCRβ1
TRBC2	TCRβ2
TRBV10-3	TCRβ variable 10 subgroup member 3
TRGC1	TCRγ C1
TRGJ1	TCRγ J1
TRGJ2	TCRγ J2
TRDC	TCRδ C
	15.10, Molecular Medicine
APBA1	amyloid-β peptide precursor
ADIPOQ	adiponectin (Acrp30), C1Q and collagen domain containing
ADIPOR1	adiponectin receptor 1
ADIPOR2	adiopnectin receptor 2
ACSL1	acyl-CoA synthetase long-chain family member 1
ADAMTS1	ADAM metallopeptidase with thrombospondin type 1 motif, 1
AHCY	*S*-adenosylhomocysteine (adoHcy)
AMD1	adenosylmethionine decarboxylase 1
AKT1	v-akt murine thymoma viral oncogene homolog 1
ATP1A1	ATPase, Na^+/K^+ transporting, alpha 1 polypeptide
BPGM	2,3-bisphosphoglycerate mutase
CALM1	calmodulin 1
CCAR1	cell division cycle and apoptosis regulator 1
CCPG1	cell cycle progression 1
CCRK	cell cycle–related kinase
CDC2	cell division cycle 2, G_1 to S and G_2 to M
CDCA1	cell division cycle–associated 1
CDK2	cyclin-dependent kinase (DCK) 2
CDK7	CDK-activating enzyme (CAK) cyclinH/CDK7
CDKN1A	CDK inhibitor 1A (p21)
CDKN1C	CDK inhibitor 1C (p57)
CDKN2A	cyclin-dependent kinase inhibitor 2A (melanoma, p16, inhibits CDK4 [$p16^{Ink4a}$])
COASY	coenzyme A (CoA) synthetase
COX4I1	cytochrome c oxidase subunit IV isoform 1

Table 5. Gene Names and Symbols From Fields Covered Elsewhere in This Chapter *(cont)*

	15.10, Molecular Medicine
COX5B	cytochrome c oxidase subunit Vb
CRP	C-reactive protein, pentraxin-related
CYP1A2	cytochrome P450 1A2 isozyme (CYP1A2)
DHFR	dihydrofolate reductase
DKK1	Dickkopf homolog 1
ERBB2	v-erb-b2 erythroblastic leukemia viral oncogene homolog 2, neuroblastoma-/glioblastoma-derived oncogene homolog (avian) (formerly *HER2/neu*)
FBP1	fructose 1,6-bisphosphatase 1
FDX1	ferredoxin (Fd) 1
FDX2	Fd 2
FHIT	fragile histidine triad (Fhit) gene
GNA12	G protein $G_{\alpha 12}$
GNG2	$G_{\gamma 2}$
GALNT1	GalNAc transferase 1
G6PD	glucose-6-phosphate dehydrogenase
B3GALT1	UDP-Gal:β-GlcNAc β-1,3-galactosyltransferase, polypeptide 1
CDKN2A	CDK4 inhibitor 2A
GFI1	growth factor independent 1
GRB2	growth factor receptor-bound protein 2
GRIN1	glutamate receptor, inotropic, *N*-methyl-D-aspartate (NMDA) 1
HBA1	hemoglobin (Hb) α_1
HBB	Hb β
HMGCS1	3-hydroxy-3-methylglutaryl CoA synthase 1
IGF1	insulinlike growth factor 1 (IGF-1)
IGF1R	IGF-1 receptor (IGF-R1)
IKBKB	IκB kinase β (IKKβ)
ITPKA	inositol 1,4,5-triphosphate (IP_3) A
MNAT1	menage a trois 1 (CAK assembly factor)
MB	myoglobin (Mb)
MCM2	Mcm 2 minichromosome maintenance deficient 2, mitotin (*Saccharomyces cerevisiae*)
NMNAT1	nicotinamide nucleotide adenyltransferase 1
NPY	neuropeptide
NPPA	natriuretic peptide precursor A
OGDH	oxoglutarate (α-ketoglutarate) dehydrogenase (lipoamide)
PIB5PA	phosphatidylinositol 4,5-biphosphate (PIP_2) 5-phosphatase A

Table 5. Gene Names and Symbols From Fields Covered Elsewhere in This Chapter *(cont)*

	15.10, Molecular Medicine
PYY	peptide YY
RBBP4	retinoblastoma binding protein 4
RNASE1	ribonuclease, RNase A family 1 (pancreatic)
SFPQ	splicing factor proline/glutamine-rich
SNCA	α-synuclein
TAF1	TAF1 RNA polymerase II, TATA box binding protein (TBP)–associated factor
TBP	TATA box binding protein
THPO	thrombopoietin
TNFSF11 (alias: *RANKL*)	TNF (ligand) superfamily member 11
TP53	tumor protein p53
UCP1	uncoupling protein 1 (UCP-1)
WNT1	wingless-type mouse mammary tumor virus (MMTV) integration site family, member 1
	15.11, Neurology
ACCN1	amiloride-sensitive cation channel 1, neuronal
ACHE	acetylcholinesterase (Yt blood group)
ADORA1	adenosine A1 receptor
ADRA1A	α_{1A}-adrenergic receptor
ADRB1	β_1-adrenergic receptor
BDNF	brain-derived neurotrophic factor
CACNA1A	Ca^{2+}, voltage-dependent, P/Q type, α1A subunit
CHRM1	cholinergic receptor, muscarinic 1
CHRNA1	cholinergic receptor, nicotinic, α-polypeptide 1 (muscle)
CNTF	ciliary neurotrophic factor
COMT	catechol-*O*-methyltransferase
DRD1	dopamine receptor D1
EGF	epidermal growth factor
GABBR1	γ-aminobutyric acid (GABA) B receptor 1
GDNF	glial cell line–derived neurotrophic factor
GRIA1	glutamate receptor, inotropic, α-amino-3-hydroxy-5-methyl-4-isoxazole propionic acid (AMPA) 1
GRIN1	glutamate receptor, NMDA 1
HRH1	histamine receptor 1
HTR1A	serotonin (5-hydroxytryptamine) receptor 1A
ITPKA	inositol 1,4,5-triphosphate (IP_3) A

Table 5. Gene Names and Symbols From Fields Covered Elsewhere in This Chapter *(cont)*

	15.11, Neurology
KCNJ3 (formerly *GIRK1*)	potassium inwardly rectifying channel, subfamily J, member 3
MAOA	monoamine oxidase A
NGFB	nerve growth factor β-polypeptide
NGFR	nerve growth factor receptor
NMB	neuromedin B
NOS1	nitric oxide synthase 1 (neuronal)
NPY	neuropeptide Y
NPY1R	neuropeptide Y receptor Y1
NRTN	neurturin
NTF3	neurotrophin 3
NTS	neurotensin
NTSR1	neurotensin receptor 1
OPRD1	opioid δ receptor
OPRK1	opioid κ receptor
OPRM1	opioid μ receptor
OPRS1	opioid receptor σ1
PCP2	Purkinje cell protein 2
SLC1A1(formerly *EAAT3*)	solute carrier family 1
SLC18A1	solute carrier family 18 (vesicular monoamine), member 1
SNAP25	synaptosomal-associated protein, 25 kDa
SNCA	α-synuclein
TAC1	tachykinin, precursor 1 (substance K, substance P, neurokinin 1, neurokinin 2, neuromedin L, neurokinin α, neuropeptide K, neuropeptide γ)
TAC3	tachykinin 3 (neuromedin K, neurokinin β)
TRPA1	transient receptor potential cation channel, subfamily A, member 1
TSNARE1	t-SNARE domain containing 1 [see 15.11, Neurology, for expansion]
VAMP1	vesicle-associated membrane protein 1 (synaptobrevin 1)
	15.14.3 and 15.4.4, Virus and Prion Nomenclature
AAVS1	adeno-associated virus integration site 2
BNIP1	BLC2/adenovirus E1B 19kDa interacting protein 1
CR2	complement component (3d/Epstein-Barr virus receptor 2)
CXADR	coxsackievirus and adenovirus receptor
CXB3S	coxsackievirus B3 sensitivity
E11S	echovirus (serotypes 4, 6, 11, 19) sensitivity
EBI2	Epstein-Barr virus–induced gene 2

Table 5. Gene Names and Symbols From Fields Covered Elsewhere in This Chapter *(cont)*

15.14.3 and 15.4.4, Virus and Prion Nomenclature	
EBVM1	Epstein-Barr virus modification site 1
EBVS1	Epstein-Barr virus insertion site 1
HAVCR1	hepatitis A virus cellular receptor 1
HBXAP	hepatitis B virus X-associated protein
HBXIP	hepatitis B virus X-interacting protein
HCVS	human coronavirus sensitivity
HIVE1	human immunodeficiency virus 1 (HIV-1) expression (elevated) 1
HPV6AI1	human papillomavirus type 6a integration site 1
HTLF	human T-cell leukemia virus enhancer factor
HV1S	herpes simplex virus type 1 sensitivity
ICAM1	intercellular adhesion molecule 1 (CD54), human rhinovirus receptor
MX1	myxovirus (influenza virus) resistance 1
PVR	poliovirus receptor
PRND	prion protein 2 (dublet)
PRNP	PrP27–30 (Creutzfeld-Jakob disease, Gerstmann-Strausler-Scheinker syndrome, fatal familial insomnia)
PRNPIP	prion protein interacting protein
PRNT	prion protein testis specific

Alleles. Alleles denote alternative forms of a gene. Alleles are often characterized by particular variant sequences (mutations). For variant sequence nomenclature see "Sequence Variations, Nucleotides, and Sequence Variations, Amino Acids," in 15.6.1, Nucleic Acids and Amino Acids.

Because alleles are alternative forms of a particular gene, they are expressed by means of both the gene name or symbol and an appendage that indicates the specific allele.

Classically, allele symbols consist of the gene symbol plus an asterisk plus the italicized allele designation,[7] eg:

*HBB*S* *S* allele of the *HBB* gene

As with gene terms, Greek letters are changed to Latin letters in allele terms:

*APOE*E4* allele producing the ε4 type of apolipoprotein E

If clear in context, the allele symbol may be used in a shorthand form that omits the gene symbol and includes only the asterisk and the allele designation that follows, eg:

**S*

**E4*

In the case of alleles of the major histocompatibility locus, which are not italicized (see 15.8.5, Immunology, HLA/Major Histocompatibility Complex), a portion of the gene name is usually included in the shortened form:

Full Name	_Shortened Form_
HLA-DRB1*0301	DRB1*0301

In practice, common or trivial names for alleles, which take various forms, are used. The same allele is often expressed in different ways that diverge from the recommended nomenclature. For example:

_s:_ short allele of serotonin transporter gene (_SLC6A4_)

_l:_ long allele of _SLC6A4_

As another example of common allele names, the following expressions are all used for _APOE*E4;_ follow author preference:

ε4 allele

epsilon 4 allele

E4 allele

APOE*4

apo e4

APOEE4

A system of nomenclature that takes evolutionary divergence into account has been proposed for alleles.[12] Stylistically, it is consistent with the above system of nomenclature, ie, asterisk followed by italicized alphanumeric allele designator. Examples (from Nebert[12]):

NAT2*4

_*1A1_

_*3A3_

_*7A28T17L47B88_

Genotype and Phenotype Terminology. The genotype comprises the set of alleles in an individual. Because individuals almost always have 2 of each autosome (nonsex chromosome) (see 15.6.4, Human Chromosomes), individuals have 2 alleles (which may be the same alleles or 2 different alleles) for each autosomal gene.

The simplest genotype term for an individual would describe 1 gene and consist of the names of 2 alleles. Larger genotypes would contain 2 or more allele symbol pairs.

As originally formulated in ISGN, allele groupings may be indicated by placement above and below a horizontal line or on the line. As seen in the following examples (from Shows et al[2,3]), such placement, as well as order, spacing, and punctuation marks (virgules [/], semicolons, spaces, and commas), has specific meanings.

Alleles of the same gene are indicated by placement above and below a horizontal line or with a virgule:

$$\frac{ADA*1}{ADA*2} \quad \text{or} \quad ADA*1/ADA*2$$

In theoretical discussions when a single letter is substituted for the allele symbol, the line or virgule may be dispensed with:

AA

Aa

aa

ss

ll

sl

Semicolons separate pairs of alleles at unlinked loci:

$$\frac{ADA^{*}1}{ADA^{*}2};\quad \frac{ADH1^{*}1}{ADH1^{*}1};\quad \frac{AMY1^{*}A}{AMY1^{*}B}$$

or

*ADA*1/ADA*2; ADH1*1/ADH1*1; AMY1*A/AMY1*B*

or

*ADA*1/*2; ADH*1/*1; AMY1*A/*B*

A single *space* separates alleles together on the same chromosome from alleles together on another chromosome (phase known):

$$\frac{AMY1^{*}A\ PGM1^{*}2}{AMY1^{*}B\ PGM1^{*}1}$$

or

*AMY1*A PGM1*2/AMY1*B PGM1*1*

Commas indicate that alleles above and below the line (or on either side of the virgule) are on the same chromosome pair, but not on which chromosome of the pair specifically (phase unknown):

$$\frac{PGM1^{*}1}{PGM1^{*}2},\ \frac{AMY1^{*}A}{AMY1^{*}B}$$

or

*PGM1*1/PGM1*2, AMY1*A/AMY1*B*

A special form for hemizygous males is

*G6PD*A/Y*

When genotype is being expressed in terms of nucleotides (eg, a polymorphism), italics and other punctuation are not needed (see also 15.6.1, Nucleic Acids and Amino Acids):

MTHFR 677 TT genotype

CC genotype

the "long/short" (5HTTLPR) polymorphism in *SLC6A4*

(LPR: length polymorphism region)

When the subject is being described in terms of the 2 possible amino acids at 1 position in the protein owing to a single nucleotide polymorphism (nonsynonymous mutation), the corresponding amino acids are separated by a virgule (see also 15.6.1, Nucleic Acids and Amino Acids):

Val/Val	(homozygous)
Met/Val	(heterozygous)
Met/Met	(homozygous)

Such terms should be explained at first mention with the amino acid terms expanded:

the common methionine/valine (Met/Val) polymorphism at codon 129

The virgule is not needed in expressions such as the following:

α_1-antitrypsin MZ heterozygotes

individuals with the ZZ phenotype

The phenotype is the collection of traits in an individual resulting from his or her genotype. When phenotypes are expressed in terms of the specific alleles, the phenotype term derives from the genotype term, but no italics are used, and, instead of asterisks, spaces are used. Genotypes usually contain pairs of symbols, while phenotypes contain single symbols. The following examples are from Shows et al[3]:

Genotype	*Phenotype*
*ADA*1/ADA*1*	ADA 1
*ADA*1/ADA*2*	ADA 1-2
*C2*C/C2*QO*	C2 C,QO
*HBB*A/HBB*6V*	HBB A,S [traditional, Hb A/S]
*ABO*A1/ABO*O*	ABO A1
*CFTR*N/CFTR*R*	CFTR N
*G6PD*A/Y*	G6PD A
*NAT2*4/*4*	rapid acetylator
*CYP2D6*4A/*5*	poor metabolizer

OMIM. Online Mendelian Inheritance in Man (OMIM) is a database of genetic syndromes.[13] The site is located at http://www.ncbi.nlm.nih.gov/entrez/query.fcgi?db=OMIM.

When a specific syndrome is mentioned, it is helpful to include the OMIM number:

bronchomalacia (Online Mendelian Inheritance in Man [OMIM] 211450)

DiGeorge syndrome (OMIM #188400)

Explanation of symbols that precede many OMIM numbers (eg, #, *, or %) is found in the OMIM frequently answered questions (FAQs) site, http://www.ncbi.nlm.nih.gov/Omim/omimfaq.html#numbering_system, and in Hamosh et al.[13]

REFERENCES

1. Klinger HP. Progress in nomenclature and symbols for cytogenetics and somatic-cell genetics. *Ann Intern Med.* 1979;91(3):487-488.
2. Shows TB, Alper CA, Bootsma D, et al. International system for human gene nomenclature (1979). *Cytogenet Cell Genet.* 1979;25(1-4):96-116.
3. Shows TB, McAlpine PJ, Boucheix C, et al. Guidelines for human gene nomenclature: an international system for human gene nomenclature (ISGN, HGM9). *Cytogenet Cell Genet.* 1987;46(1-4):11-28.
4. Rangel P, Giovannetti J. *Genomes and Databases on the Internet: A Practical Guide to Functions and Applications.* Norfolk, England: Horizon Scientific Press; 2002.
5. HUGO Gene Nomenclature Committee Web site. http://www.gene.ucl.ac.uk/nomenclature/. Updated March 29, 2006. Accessed April 21, 2006.
6. Searchgenes. Human Gene Nomenclature Database Search Engine. http://www.gene.ucl.ac.uk/cgi-bin/nomenclature/searchgenes.pl. Updated April 21, 2006. Accessed April 21, 2006.
7. Wain HM, Bruford EA, Lovering RC, Lush MJ, Wright MW, Povey S. Guidelines for human gene nomenclature. *Genomics.* 2002;79(4):464-470. Also available at http://www.gene.ucl.ac.uk/nomenclature/guidelines.html. Updated April 20, 2006. Accessed April 21, 2006.
8. Wain HM, Lush M, Ducluzeau F, Povey S. Genew: the Human Gene Nomenclature Database. *Nucleic Acids Res.* 2002;30(1):169-171.
9. Wain HM, Lush MJ, Ducluzeau F, Khodiyar VK, Povey S. Genew: the Human Gene Nomenclature Database, 2004 updates. *Nucleic Acids Res.* 2004;32(database issue): D255-D257. doi:10.1093/nar/gkh072.
10. Entrez Gene. http://www.ncbi.nlm.nih.gov/entrez/query.fcgi?db=gene. Accessed April 21, 2006.
11. HGNC FAQs. http://www.gene.ucl.ac.uk/nomenclature/information/FAQs.html. Updated April 20, 2006. Accessed April 24, 2006.
12. Nebert DW. Proposal for an allele nomenclature system based on the evolutionary divergence of haplotypes. *Hum Mutat.* 2002;20(6):463-472.
13. Hamosh A, Scott AF, Amberger JS, Bocchini CA, McKusick VA. Online Mendelian Inheritance in Man (OMIM), a knowledgebase of human genes and genetic disorders. *Nucl Acids Res.* 2005;33(database issue):D514-D517. doi:10.1093/nar/gki033.

Cancer is caused by an accumulation of genetic alterations that confer a survival advantage to the neoplastic cell.

J. L. Jameson[1(p73)]

15.6.3 Oncogenes and Tumor Suppressor Genes

Oncogenes: Oncogenes are "[g]enes that normally play a role in growth but, when overexpressed or mutated, can foster the growth of cancer."[2] Oncogenes were discovered and characterized in viruses and animal experimental systems. These genes exist widely outside the systems in which they were discovered, and their normal cellular homologues are important in cell division and differentiation.

Human oncogenes should be expressed according to style for human gene symbols (see 15.6.2, Human Gene Nomenclature). Mouse oncogenes (and other nonhuman oncogenes) should be expressed according to style for mouse gene symbols (see 15.6.5, Nonhuman Genetic Terms). Retroviral oncogenes are expressed in a style typical of microbial genes (see 15.6.5, Nonhuman Genetic Terms), namely, 3 letters, italicized, lowercase. The protein products of the oncogenes (oncoproteins) typically use the same term as the oncogene but in roman type. In humans, the protein is all capitals; in mice, the protein has an initial capital.

Retroviral Oncogenes	*Human Gene Homologue(s); Mouse Gene Homologue(s)*	*Human Protein Product(s); Mouse Protein Product(s); Retroviral Oncoprotein*	*Origin*
abl	*ABL1, ABL2* *Abl1, Abl2*	ABL1, ABL2 Abl1, Abl2 abl	Abelson murine leukemia virus
bcl-2	*BCL2* *Bcl2*	BCL2 Bcl2 bcl	B-cell CLL/lymphoma 2
erb	*ERBB2, ERBB3, ERBB4* *Erbb2, Erbb3, Erbb4*	ERBB2, ERBB3, ERBB4 Erbb2, Erbb3, Erbb4 erb	avian erythroblastic leukemia
ets	*ETS1, ETS2* *Ets1, Ets2*	ETS1, ETS2 Ets1, Ets2 ets	avian erythroblastosis
fes	*FES* *Fes*	FES Fes fes	feline sarcoma
fms	*CSF1R* (formerly *FMS*) *Csf1r* (formerly *Fms*)	colony stimulating factor 1 receptor (CSF1R)	McDonough feline sarcoma
fos	*FOS, FOSB* *Fos, Fosb*	FOS, FOSB Fos, Fosb fos	murine osteosarcoma
jun	*JUN, JUNB, JUND* *Jun, Junb, Jund*	JUN, JUNB, JUND Jun, Junb, Jund jun	avian sarcoma
kit	*KIT* *Kit*	KIT Kit kit	feline sarcoma

Retroviral Oncogenes	*Human Gene Homologue(s); Mouse Gene Homologue(s)*	*Human Protein Product(s); Mouse Protein Product(s); Retroviral Oncoprotein*	*Origin*
mos	*MOS* *Mos*	MOS Mos mos	Moloney sarcoma virus
myb	*MYB* *Myb*	MYB Myb myb	avian myeloblastosis
myc	*MYC* *Myc*	MYC Myc myc	avian myelocytomatosis
raf	*RAF1, ARAF, BRAF* *Raf1, Araf, Braf*	RAF1, ARAF1, BRAF Raf1, Araf, Braf raf	murine leukemia
ras	family with many human homologues, eg, *HRAS, NRAS, RAB9A, RRAS, RRAS2* *Hras1, Nras, Rab9, Rras, Rras2*	HRAS1, NRAS, RAB9A, RRAS, RRAS2 Rab9a, Rras, Rras2, Hras, Nras, Rab9 ras	retrovirus-associated DNA sequence
sis	*PDGFB* *Pdgfb*	PDGFB (platelet-derived growth factor, B chain) Pdgfb sis	simian sarcoma virus
src	*SRC* *Src*	SRC Src src	Rous sarcoma virus

Examples of use are as follows:

> ras activation and inactivation
>
> The *ras* protein, ras, functions as a signaling molecule.

HER2/neu. The symbol for the oncogene known as *HER2/neu* is actually *ERBB2*. *HER2* (from human epidermal growth factor receptor 2) and *NEU* have been shown to be the same as *ERBB2*[3,4] and are current aliases for *ERBB2*.[5] Because the term

HER2/neu is widely used and recognized, it may be included in parentheses after the first mention of *ERBB2*:

ERBB2 (formerly *HER2* or *HER2/neu*)

Commonly, the oncogene term contains a prefix that indicates the source or location of the gene: v- for virus or c- for the oncogene's cellular or chromosomal counterpart. The c- form is also known as a proto-oncogene and in standard gene nomenclature (see 15.6.2, Human Gene Nomenclature) is given in all capitals, as in the human gene homologues column of the tabulation above and the following examples:

c-*abl* (*ABL1*) c-*mos* (*MOS*)

v-*abl* v-*mos*

Editors should not substitute one type of term for another.

The protein product may be similarly prefixed:

c-abl c-mos

v-abl v-mos

Additional prefixes may further identify oncogenes. Expansions of some prefixes are given below, but it should not be inferred that the gene in question is associated only with the tumor it is named for:

Oncogene	*Prefix Expansion*
B-*lym*	B-cell lymphoma
L-*myc*	small cell lung carcinoma
N-*myc*	neuroblastoma
H-*ras*	Harvey rat sarcoma
c-H-*ras*	
v-H-*ras*	
K-*ras*	Kirsten rat sarcoma
c-K-*ras*	
v-K-*ras*	
N-*ras*	neuroblastoma

For example:

Hypothesis: The K-*ras* mutation assay is more sensitive than the conventional histologic diagnosis in detecting minute cancer invasion around the superior mesenteric artery.

Numbers or letters designate genes in a series, eg:

K-*ras*-2

H-*ras*-1

erb-b2

Fusion Oncogenes and Oncoproteins. The result of fusion of an oncogene and another gene is known as a *fusion oncogene*. The product of a fusion oncogene is a fusion oncoprotein. Terms for fusion oncogenes and their products may use traditional oncogene format or standard human gene format, as in the following examples:

Fusion Oncogene	*Fusion Oncoprotein*	*Explanation*
bcr-abl	bcr-abl	bcr: breakpoint cluster region
c-fos/c-jun	c-fos/c-jun	
gag-onc	gag-onc	general term for fusion proteins of viral *gag* (group-specific antigen) gene and oncogene
gag-jun	gag-jun	
PML-RARA	PML-RARα	promyelocytic leukemia-retinoic acid α

Tumor Suppressor Genes. Tumor suppressor genes are "[g]enes that normally restrain cell growth but, when missing or inactivated by mutation, allow cells to grow uncontrolled."[6] Examples are in the tabulation below:

Gene	*Gene Product*	*Explanation*
CDKN1A	p21	cyclin-dependent kinase (CDK) inhibitor 1A
CDKN1B	p27	CDK inhibitor 1B
CDKN1C	p57	CDK inhibitor 1C
DCC	a transmembrane receptor protein	deleted in colorectal carcinoma
GLTSCR1		glioma tumor suppressor candidate region gene 1
NF1	neurofibromin 1	
RB1	Rb protein	retinoblastoma 1
TP53	p53	a 53-kd protein
WT1	a zinc finger protein	Wilms tumor 1

REFERENCES

1. Jameson JL. Oncogenes and tumor suppressor genes. In: Jameson JL, Collins FS. *Principles of Molecular Medicine.* Totowa, NJ: Humana Press; 1998:73-82.
2. Terms and definitions (O). National Institutes of Health Office of Rare Diseases. http://ord.aspensys.com/asp/resources/glossary_n-r.asp#O. Accessed April 21, 2006.
3. V-ERB-B2 avian erythroblastic leukemia viral oncogene homolog 2; ERBB2. OMIM. http://www.ncbi.nlm.nih.gov/entrez/dispomim.cgi?id=164870. Updated January 30, 2006. Accessed April 21, 2006.
4. Di Fiore PP, Pierce JH, Kraus MH, Segatto O, King CR, Aaronson SA. *erb*B-2 is a potent oncogene when overexpressed in NIH/3T3 cells. *Science.* 1987;237(4811):178-182.
5. Searchgenes. Human Gene Nomenclature Database Search Engine. http://www.gene.ucl.ac.uk/cgi-bin/nomenclature/searchgenes.pl. Updated April 21, 2006. Accessed April 21, 2006.

6. Terms and definitions (T). National Institutes of Health Office of Rare Diseases. http://ord.aspensys.com/asp/resources/glossary_s-z.asp#T. Accessed April 21, 2006.

15.6.4 **Human Chromosomes.** Chromosomes are dark-staining, threadlike structures in the cell nucleus composed of DNA and chromatin that carry genetic information (definition after Nussbaum et al[1] and Mueller and Young[2]).

Formalized standard nomenclature for human chromosomes dates from 1960 and, since 1978, has been known as the International System for Human Cytogenetic Nomenclature (ISCN).

Material in this section is based on recommendations in *ISCN 2005*.[3] Earlier reports[4-6] have also been consulted.

Human chromosomes are numbered from largest to smallest[1] from 1 to 22. There are 2 additional chromosomes, X and Y. The numbered chromosomes are known as autosomes, X and Y as the sex chromosomes. Chromosomes stained using techniques that do not produce bands are grouped based on similar size and centromere position, as follows:

Group	*Chromosomes*
A	1-3
B	4, 5
C	6-12, X
D	13-15
E	16-18
F	19, 20
G	21, 22, Y

A chromosome may be referred to by number or by group:

chromosome 14

a D group chromosome

Chromosome Bands. Chromosome bands are elicited by special staining methods; terms in the left-hand column need not be expanded:

Banding Pattern	*Technique*
Q-banding, Q bands	quinacrine
G-banding, G bands	Giemsa
R-banding, R bands	reverse Giemsa
C-banding, C bands	constitutive heterochromatin
T-banding, T bands	telomeric
NOR	nucleolar organizing regions

Banding technique codes of several letters provide more information about the banding method. These abbreviations must be expanded, but the letters in the list above (Q, G, R, C, T, NOR) within those terms need not be expanded:

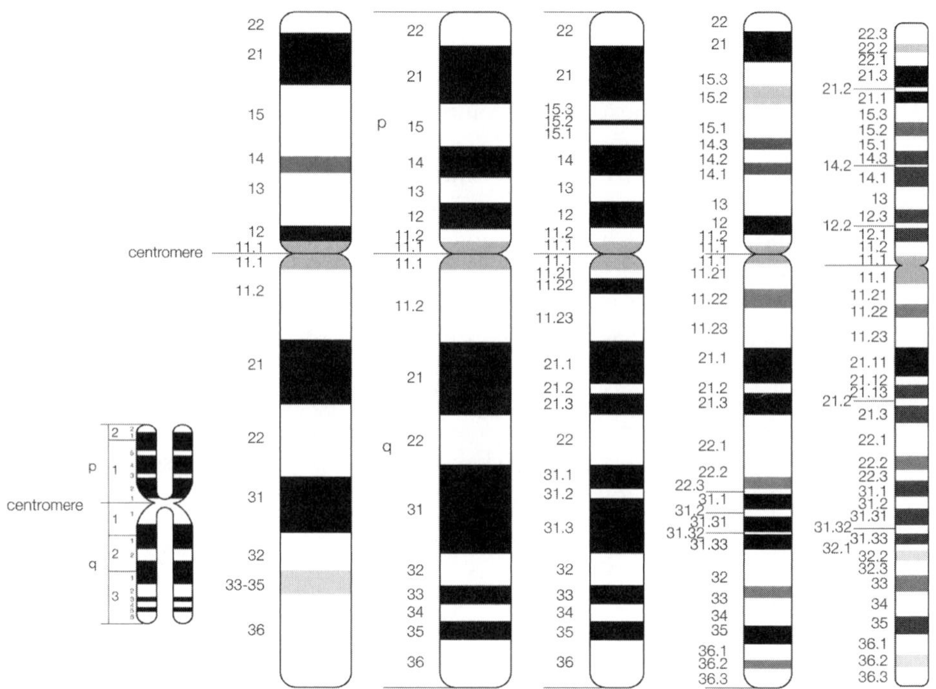

Figure 5. Diagram of chromosome 7 at different levels of resolution showing bands and subbands (reprinted from *ISBN 2005*[3] by permission of S Karger AG, Basel, Switzerland).

Abbreviation	*Expansion*
QF	Q bands by fluorescence
QFQ	Q bands by fluorescence using quinacrine
CBG	C bands by barium hydroxide using Giemsa stain
Ag-NOR	NOR staining, silver nitrate technique

Chromosomes contain short and long arms, which are joined at the centromere (Figure 5).

The short arm is designated by p, for *petit,* and the long arm by the next letter of the alphabet, q.[7] Arm designations follow the chromosome number:

17p	short arm of chromosome 17
3q	long arm of chromosome 3
Xq	long arm of the X chromosome

Expressions such as those on the left need not be expanded. It is incorrect to refer to chromosome arms as chromosomes:

Acceptable: chromosome arm 17p
short arm of 17
17p

Not: chromosome 17p

Regions are determined by major chromosome band landmarks. Chromosome arms contain 1 to 4 regions, numbered outward from the centromere. The region number follows the p or the q:

4q3	region 3 of long arm of chromosome 4

The regions are divided into bands, also numbered outward from the centromere. Bands have subdivisions or subbands. The band number follows the region number, and the subband number follows a period after the band number. When a subband is further subdivided, the sub-subband number follows the subband number without a period or other intervening punctuation:

11q23	chromosome 11, long arm, band 23 (region 2, band 3)
11q23.3	band in above subdivided, resulting in subband 23.3
20p11.23	chromosome 20, short arm, sub-subband 11.23 (region 1, band 1, subband 2, sub-subband 3)

It is correct usage to refer to the above expressions as "band 11q23," "band 11q23.3," and "band 20p11.23."

The centromere is designated band 10, as in the following:

p10 (portion of centromere facing short arm)

q10 (portion of centromere facing long arm)

Visualization of genomic information by chromosome region in humans and other organisms is available at the National Center for Biotechnology Information Map Viewer.[8]

Karyotype. *Karyotype* is the chromosome complement of an individual, tissue, or cell line. Karyotype is expressed as the number of chromosomes in a cell including the sex chromosomes, a description of the sex chromosome composition, and, whenever applicable, any chromosome abnormality.

The *karyogram* and the *idiogram* are graphic representations of karyotype. The karyogram is "a systemized array of the chromosomes" that has been prepared using methods such as photomicrography. An idiogram is "diagrammatic representation of the karyotype."[3(p6)]

In karyotype expressions, the sex chromosomes, which should always be specified, are separated from the number of chromosomes by a comma, as in the following examples:

46,XX	46 chromosomes (2 each of chromosomes 1-22 and 2 X chromosomes in human female karyotype)
46,XY	46 chromosomes (2 each of chromosomes 1-22, 1 X and 1 Y in human male karyotype)
45,X	45 chromosomes, 1 X chromosome (Turner syndrome)
47,XXY	47 chromosomes, 2 X chromosomes, 1 Y (Klinefelter syndrome)
47,XYY	47 chromosomes, 1 X, 2 Y chromosomes
69,XXX	3 each of chromosomes 1-22 and X

A virgule is used to indicate more than 1 karyotype in an individual, tumor, cell line, and so on:

45,X/46,XX

Descriptions of autosomal chromosome abnormalities are presented after the sex chromosomes and listed in numerical order irrespective of aberration type, separated from the sex chromosomes by a comma. For instance, the karyotype of a person with trisomy 21 (Down syndrome) with an extra chromosome 21 is specified as

47,XX,+21 (female)

47,XY,+21 (male)

A karyotype description may contain both constitutional and acquired elements. For instance, the karyotype of a tumor cell from a person with trisomy 21 could show both the constitutional anomaly and an acquired neoplastic anomaly, eg, an acquired extra chromosome 8, and would be expressed as

48,XX,+8,+21c

The lowercase c specifies that the trisomy 21 is constitutional, as distinguished from the acquired trisomy 8.

An individual with more than 1 karyotypic clone may have a *mosaic* (single-cell origin) karyotype or a *chimera* (multicell origin) karyotype, which should be specified with a 3-letter abbreviation at first mention of the karyotype, eg:

mos 45,X/46,XY

chi 46,XX/46,XY

Brackets indicate the number of cells observed in a clone:

chi 46,XX[25]/46,XY[10]X

A double slant (virgule), used in chimeras resulting from bone marrow transplants, separates recipient and donor cell lines. Recipient karyotype precedes the double slant, donor karyotype follows the double slant, and either or both may be specified, eg:

46,XY[3]//

//46,XX[17]

46,XY[3]//46,XX[17]

For details on order in such expressions, consult *ISCN 2005*.

Meiotic karyotypes may begin with a term such as MI and contain a haploid or near-haploid number of chromosomes, and may or may not have a comma between X and Y:

MI,23,XY

MI,24,X,Y

Chromosome Rearrangements. The abbreviations and symbols in Table 6 are used in descriptions of chromosomes, including chromosome rearrangements. The table is adapted from *ISCN 2005*.[3] Former designations based on *ISCN 1995* and *ISCN 1985* appear in parentheses. (A short online version of the information in Table 6 is available through the Cancer Genome Anatomy Project.[9])

Table 6. Chromosome Rearrangement Abbreviations and Symbols[a]

Abbreviation/Symbol	Explanation
AI	first meiotic anaphase
AII	second meiotic anaphase
ace	acentric fragment
add	additional material of unknown origin
arr	array
b	break
c	constitutional anomaly
cen	centromere
cgh	comparative genomic hybridization
chi	chimera
chr (cs [1985])	chromosome
cht (ct [1985])	chromatid
cp	composite karyotype
cx	complex chromatid interchanges
del	deletion
der	derivative
dia	diakinesis
dic	dicentric
dim	diminished
dip	diplotene
dir	direct
dis	distal
dit	dictyotene
dmin	double minute
dn (de novo [1995])	chromosome abnormality not inherited
dup	duplication
e	exchange
end	endoreduplication
enh	enhanced
fem	female
fis	fission
fra	fragile site
g	gap
h	heterochromatin
hsr	homogeneously staining region
i	isochromosome

Table 6. Chromosome Rearrangement Abbreviations and Symbols[a] *(cont)*

Abbreviation/Symbol	Explanation
idem	stemline karyotype in subclones
ider	isoderivative
idic	isodicentric
inc	incomplete karyotype
ins	insertion
inv	inversion or inverted
ish	in situ hybridization
lep	leptotene
MI	first meiotic metaphase
MII	second meiotic metaphase
mal	male
mar	marker chromosome
mat	maternal origin
med	medial
min	minute acentric fragment
ml	mainline
mn	modal number
mos	mosaic
neo	neocentromere
nuc	nuclear
oom	oogonial metaphase
or	alternative interpretation
p	short arm
PI	first meiotic prophase
pac	pachytene
pat	paternal origin
pcc	premature chromosome condensation
pcd	premature centromere division
prx	proximal
ps	satellited short arm
psu	pseudo-
pvz	pulverization
q	long arm
qdp	quadruplication
qr	quadriradial

Table 6. Chromosome Rearrangement Abbreviations and Symbols[a] *(cont)*

Abbreviation/Symbol	Explanation
qs	satellited long arm
r	ring chromosome
rcp	reciprocal
rea	rearrangement
rec	recombinant chromosome
rev	reverse
rob	robertsonian translocation
roman numerals	
I	univalent
II	bivalent
III	trivalent
IV	quadrivalent
s	satellite
sce	sister chromatid exchange
sct	secondary constriction
sdl	sideline
sl	stemline
spm	spermatogonial metaphase
stk	satellite stalk
subtel	subtelomeric region
t	translocation
tan	tandem
tas	telomeric association
ter	terminal end of chromosome or telomere (tel [1995])
tr	triradial
trc (tri [1985])	tricentric
trp	triplication
upd	uniparental disomy
var (v [1995], var [1985])	variant or variable region
xma	chiasma(ta)
zyg	zygotene
:	break
::	break and reunion
;	separates chromosomes and chromosome bands in structural rearrangements involving 2 or more chromosomes

Table 6. Chromosome Rearrangement Abbreviations and Symbols[a] *(cont)*

Abbreviation/Symbol	Explanation
→	from-to
+	gain
–	loss
~	intervals and boundaries in a chromosome segment
<>	angle brackets for ploidy
[ ]	square brackets for number of cells
=	number of chiasmata
×	multiple copies
?	questionable identification
/	separates clones
//	separates chimeric clones

[a] Adapted by permission of S Karger AG, Basel, Switzerland.

Single-letter abbreviations combined with other abbreviations are set closed up, eg:

chte chromatid exchange

Three-letter symbols combined are set with a space:

cht del chromatid deletion

psu dic pseudodicentric

The symbols in the list of chromosomes from *ISCN 2005* are part of an efficient shorthand that describes the exact changes in a karyotype containing rearranged chromosomes. In publications that range beyond the field of cytogenetics, the symbols should always be defined.

Chromosome rearrangement terms can be written using a "short system" or short form. Complex abnormalities are designated by the more specific "detailed system" or long form. The detailed form uses symbols such as arrows to describe individual derivative chromosomes resulting from complex rearrangements (even the short system can result in a complex expression), eg:

short:

46,XY,t(2;5)(q21;q31)

long:

46,XY,t(2;5)(2pter→2q21::5q31→5qter;5pter→5q31::2q21→2qter)

The complete nomenclature, formulated for consistency in the description of chromosomal rearrangements, is detailed in *ISCN 2005*.[3] The following sections contain terms that illustrate some of the basic principles of the ISCN. Terms such as these may stand alone or may be part of longer expressions such as those above.

Order. For aberrations involving more than 1 chromosome, the sex chromosome appears first, then other chromosomes in numerical order (or, less commonly, in group order if only group is specified).

t(X;13)(q27;q12) translocation involving bands Xq27 and 13q12

For 2 breaks in the same chromosome, the short arm precedes the long arm, and there is no internal punctuation, eg:

inv(2)(p21q31) inversion in chromosome 2

Exceptions to numerical order convey special conditions; for example, when a piece of one chromosome is inserted into another (3-break rearrangement), the recipient chromosome precedes the donor:

ins(5;2)(p14;q21q31) insertion of portion of long arm of chromosome 2 into short arm of chromosome 5

Plus and Minus Signs. A plus sign *preceding* a chromosome indicates addition of the entire chromosome:

+14 entire chromosome 14 gained

A plus sign *following* p or q and the chromosome number indicates an addition to that chromosome:

14p+ addition to 14p

Such a term is ambiguous; it might refer to one of many possible specific additions to 14p of an individual karyotype, to an unknown addition to 14p, or to additions to 14p in general. A term like 14p+ may be used after context has been provided. In the case of karyotype descriptions, this means using more specific terms incorporating symbols such as add, der, and ins:

Shorter Term	*Karyotype Term*
14p+	add(14)(p13)
14q+	add(14)(q32)

For example:

the 14q+ cytogenetic abnormality was found to be add(14)(q32).

A minus sign *preceding* a chromosome signifies loss of the *entire* chromosome:

−5 all of chromosome 5 missing

A minus sign *following* a chromosome arm signifies loss *from* that arm, but this should be reserved for text, while more specific notation is used in karyotype descriptions, eg:

Text	*Karyotype*
5q−	del(5)(q13q31)

A deletion of the entire long arm of a chromosome should not be expressed in text with a minus sign.

del(5q) (*not* 5q−)

(Use more specific terms in karyotypes.)

Punctuation

- *Parentheses:* the number of the affected chromosome follows the rearrangement symbol in parentheses:

  inv(2) inversion in chromosome 2

Details of the aberration follow in a second set of parentheses:

  inv(2)(p13p24) inversion in chromosome 2 involving bands 13 and 24 of the short arm

- *Semicolon:* In rearrangements involving 2 or more chromosomes, a semicolon is used:

  t(2;5)(q21;q31) translocation involving breaks at 2q21 and 5q31

- *Comma:* Commas separate the number of chromosomes, sex chromosomes, and each term describing an abnormality:

  46,XX,r(18)(p11q22) female karyotype with ring chromosome 18 with ends joined at bands p11 and q22

Underlining. In different clones within the same karyotype, an underline (underbar) distinguishes homologous aberrations of the same chromosome:

46,XX,der(1)t(1;3)(p34;q21)/46,XX,der(1̲)t(1̲;3)(p34;q21)

In manuscripts, authors should indicate that the underline is intended, so that it will not be set as italics, per typographic convention, in the published version.

Or. This word indicates "alternative interpretations of an aberration"[3(p50)] or alternative results (for instance, breaks appearing in consecutive bands using different techniques):

add(19)(p13 or q13)

add(10)(q22 or q23)

Spacing. As seen in previous examples, there is no spacing between the elements of a karyotype description (except following mos and chi, between 2 or more 3-letter abbreviations [eg, cht del, rev ish enh], and before and after "or").

Long Karyotypes. Multiline karyotypes carry over from 1 line of text to the next with no punctuation other than that of the original expression (eg, no hyphen at the end of the first line), as in the following tumor karyotype:

46,XX,t(8;21)(q22;q22)[12]/45,idem,−X[19]/46,idem,
−X,+8[5]/47,idem, X,+8,+9[8]

In Situ Hybridization. Style for terms describing karyotypes identified by means of this technique alone or along with cytogenetic analysis (traditional karyotyping techniques) is similar to that described above (see also 15.6.1, Nucleic Acids and

Table 7. In Situ Hybridization Abbreviations and Symbols[a]

Abbreviation/Symbol	Explanation
amp	amplified signal
arr	array
cgh	comparative genomic hybridization
con	connected signals
dim	diminished signal intensity
enh	enhanced signal intensity
fib ish	extended chromatin/DNA fiber in situ hybridization
FISH	fluorescence in situ hybridization
ish	in situ hybridization
nuc ish	nuclear or interphase in situ hybridization
pcp	partial chromosome paint
rev ish	reverse in situ hybridization
sep	separated signals
subtel	subtelomeric
wcp	whole chromosome paint
;	separates probes on different derivative chromosomes
.	[period] separates cytogenetic observations from results of in situ hybridization or array-based cgh
+	present on a specific chromosome
++	duplication on a specific chromosome
−	absent on a specific chromosome
×	precedes number of signals seen

[a] Adapted by permission of S Karger AG, Basel, Switzerland.

Amino Acids). Some symbol meanings may differ. Table 7 is adapted from *ISCN 2005*.[3]

Examples are as follows:

46,XY.ish del(22)(q11.2q11.2)(D22S75−)

47,XY,+mar.ish der(8)(D8Z1+)

(D22S75 refers to the probe for the DNA segment sequence *D22S75;* see 15.6.2, Human Gene Nomenclature.)

Marker Chromosomes, Derivative Chromosomes, and the Philadelphia Chromosome. A *marker chromosome* "is a structurally abnormal chromosome in which no part can be identified"[3(p73)] and might be included in a karyotype as in

47,XX,+mar

A structurally abnormal chromosome in which any part can be recognized is considered a *derivative chromosome*, defined as "a structurally rearranged chromosome generated by a rearrangement involving two or more chromosomes or by multiple aberrations within a single chromosome."[3(p62)]

A derivative chromosome is specified in parentheses, followed by the aberrations involved in the generation of the derivative chromosome. The aberrations are not separated by a comma. For instance:

der(1)t(1;3)(p32;q21)t(1;11)(q25;q13)

signifies a derivative chromosome 1 generated by 2 translocations, one involving the short arm with a breakpoint in 1p32 and the other involving the long arm with a breakpoint in 1q25.

Philadelphia chromosome is the name given to a particular derivative chromosome found in chronic myelogenous leukemia and some types of acute leukemia. The Philadelphia chromosome can be abbreviated as "Ph chromosome" or, if clear in context, "Ph." Appendages, as in Ph^1, Ph1, Ph_1, or Ph′, are not necessary, and Ph is the preferred form. The Ph chromosome is the derivative chromosome 22 resulting from the translocation t(9;22)(q34;q11) and may be described as follows:

der(22)t(9;22)(q34;q11.2)

The Ph chromosome is the result of a rearrangement that juxtaposes the oncogene *ABL* with the breakpoint cluster region gene *BCR* (see 15.6.2, Human Gene Nomenclature, and 15.6.3, Oncogenes and Tumor Suppressor Genes).

REFERENCES

1. Nussbaum RL, McInnes RR, Willard HF. *Thompson & Thompson Genetics in Medicine.* 6th rev reprint ed. Philadelphia, PA: Saunders; 2004.
2. Mueller RF, Young ID. *Emery's Medical Genetics.* New York, NY: Churchill Livingstone; 2001.
3. Shaffer LG, Tommerup N, eds. *ISCN 2005: An International System for Human Cytogenetic Nomenclature (2005).* Basel, Switzerland: S Karger AG; 2005.
4. Mitelman F, ed. *ISCN 1995: An International System for Human Cytogenetic Nomenclature 1995.* Basel, Switzerland: S Karger AG; 1995.
5. Mitelman F, ed. *ISCN (1991): Guidelines for Cancer Cytogenetics: Supplement to an International System for Human Cytogenetic Nomenclature.* Basel, Switzerland: S Karger AG; 1991.
6. Harnden DG, Klinger HP, eds. *ISCN (1985): An International System for Human Cytogenetic Nomenclature.* Basel, Switzerland: S Karger AG; 1985.
7. Qumsiyeh MB, Yilmaz Y. Molecular biology of cancer: cytogenetics. In: DeVita VT Jr, Hellman S, Rosenberg SA, eds. *Cancer: Principles and Practice of Oncology.* 7th ed. Philadelphia, PA: Lippincott Williams & Wilkins; 2005:34-43.
8. NCBI Map Viewer. http://www.ncbi.nlm.nih.gov/mapview/. Accessed April 21, 2006.
9. ISCN abbreviated terms and symbols. The Cancer Genome Anatomy Project. http://cgap.nci.nih.gov/Chromosomes/ISCNSymbols. Accessed April 21, 2006.

[T]he word mouse . . . comes originally from the Sanskrit mush derived from a verb meaning to steal. . . . Mice and rats, through their voracious activities in grain larders and as carriers of disease, inflicted considerable losses in food and lives upon ancient civilizations.

H. C. Morse III[1(p6)]

A very obvious gap in our understanding of human genome evolution lies in the complete absence of any mapping data from the eutherian orders most distantly related to man, particularly the edentates. We would urge anyone with an interest in the genetics of the aardvark and the armadillo to consider a unique mapping project which will be at the forefront (alphabetically, at least) of the comparative mapping effort.

J. A. Marshall Graves et al[2(p964)]

15.6.5 Nonhuman Genetic Terms. Comparative genome analysis has shown that eukaryote species share genes to a great extent.[3] Therefore, similar or identical names designate the same gene across species whenever possible. Italicization of gene symbols is uniformly observed.

Vertebrates. Animal gene symbols resemble human gene symbols (see 15.6.2, Human Gene Nomenclature, and below).[4,5] However, unlike human gene symbols, animal gene symbols typically use or include lowercase letters and punctuation marks. Editors of medical publications may follow author style for animal gene symbols.

Gene terminology for the laboratory mouse *(Mus musculus domesticus)* and laboratory rat *(Rattus norvegicus)*, often seen in medical publications because of the common use of those species in investigating diseases affecting humans, is prototypic of such style.

Mouse and Rat Gene Nomenclature. Mouse and rat gene nomenclature guidelines were unified in 2003 by the International Committee on Standardized Genetic Nomenclature for Mice and the Rat Genome and Nomenclature Committee.[6]

Mouse and rat gene symbols resemble human symbols in several respects.[6,7] They are descriptive, short (preferably 3 to 5 characters), and italicized. Symbols begin with letters, not numbers. They contain roman letters in place of Greek letters and arabic numerals in place of roman numerals.

Mouse and rat gene symbols differ from human symbols in using lowercase letters. Symbols usually contain an initial capital. Capital letters within a mouse gene symbol may indicate the laboratory code or code for another species/vector (see below). A symbol with all lowercase letters (ie, no initial capital) indicates a recessive trait. Mouse and rat gene symbols may contain hyphens and other punctuation.

Table 8. Style Rules for Mouse Gene Symbols and Comparison With Human Gene Symbols (Examples)

Mouse Gene Symbol	Mouse Gene Description	Rule Illustrated	Human Gene Symbol (When Known)
a	nonagouti	lowercase initial capital because named for mutant recessive trait	*ASIP*
Afp	α-fetoprotein	initial capital, otherwise lowercase, Greek letter changed to roman	*AFP*
B2m	β_2-microglobulin	no subscript	*B2M*
Gla	α-galactosidase	Greek letter changed to roman and moved to end of symbol	*GLA*
Gt(ROSA)26Sor	gene trap, ROSA 26, Philippe Soriano	parentheses may be used	
Rn4.5s	4.5S RNA	period permissible	
Rn5s	5S RNA	symbol does not begin with number	*RN5S1@* (@ signifies gene family; see 15.6.2, Human Gene Nomenclature)

The central source for mouse gene terms is the Mouse Genome Database (http://www.informatics.jax.org),[8] and for rats, RatMap (http://ratmap.gen.gu.se) and the Rat Genome Database (http://rgd.mcw.edu).[9] Gene names and symbols may be verified by means of the search features at those sites.

Style rules and conventions for mouse and rat gene symbols are shown in Tables 8 through 10. (*Note:* The gene descriptions in the tables that follow are based on but not identical to the approved gene names available in the Mouse Genome Informatics database, which are more complete and do not use Greek letters and other typographic variants. For instance, in searching for a term with α, one would type in "alpha.") The Mammalian Orthology Query Form (http://www.informatics.jax.org/searches/homology_form.shtml) allows comparative searches of 20 vertebrate species. Note that a given letter or letter combination often but not always signifies a conventional usage. For instance, *l* at or near the end of a symbol often, but not always, indicates "like."

Mouse Alleles. A mouse allele symbol consists of a mouse gene symbol often with a superscript. As with mouse gene symbols, mouse allele symbols are italicized.

Allele symbols can be verified within the records of a mouse gene:

- Search for the gene symbol at http://www.informatics.jax.org/javawi2/servlet/WIFetch?page=markerQF
- Click on link for the gene symbol that has been located
- Under Phenotypes, click on the numeric link after "all phenotypic alleles"

Allele searches are also available at http://www.informatics.jax.org/searches/allele_form.shtml.

Table 9. Conventions for Mouse Gene Symbols and Comparison With Human Gene Symbols (Examples)

Mouse Gene Symbol	Mouse Gene Description	Convention Illustrated	Human Gene Symbol (When Available)
Brca1	breast cancer 1	same as human symbol except for case	*BRCA1*
Cafq1	caffeine metabolism QTL 1	*q:* quantitative locus	
C4bp-ps1	complement component 4 binding protein, pseudogene 1	*-ps:* pseudogene	*C4BPB*
D10Mit1	DNA segment, Chr 10, Massachusetts Institute of Technology 1	symbol for DNA segment identified only in the mouse; includes laboratory code (see "Laboratory Codes")	
D17H21S56	DNA segment, Chr 17, human *D21S56*	*H21* indicates DNA segment resides on human chromosome 21	*D21S56*
G6pdx	glucose-6-phosphate dehydrogenase X-linked	similar but not identical to human gene symbol	*G6PD*
Gna-rs1	guanine binding protein, related sequence 1	*-rs:* related sequence	*GNL1*
Gtl10	gene trap locus 10	*Gt:* gene trap	
Gt(ROSA)26Sor	gene trap ROSA 26, Philippe Soriano	vector in parentheses; laboratory code indicated (see "Laboratory Codes" section)	
H2-Aa	histocompatibility 2, class II antigen A, α		*HLA-DQA1*
Hbb	hemoglobin β-chain complex	same as human symbol except for case	*HBB*
Hc9	heterochromatin, Chr 9	*Hc:* heterochromatin	
Hras1	Harvey rat sarcoma virus oncogene 1	see also 15.6.3, Oncogenes and Tumor Suppressor Genes	*HRAS*
Ighmbp2 (formerly *nmd*)	immunoglobulin heavy chain μ binding protein 2 (formerly neuromuscular degeneration)	name change with new information about gene	*IGHMBP2*
l17Wis9	lethal, Chr 17, University of Wisconsin 9	initial *l:* lethal	
Lamb1-1	β_1 laminin, subunit 1	hyphen separates 2 adjacent numbers	*LAMB1*
Lzp-s	P lysozyme structural	*s:* structural	
mt-Rnr1	12S RNA, mitochondrial	*mt:* mitochondrial	*MT-RNR1*
Mcptl	mast cell protease-like	*l:* like	

Table 9. Conventions for Mouse Gene Symbols and Comparison With Human Gene Symbols (Examples) *(cont)*

Mouse Gene Symbol	Mouse Gene Description	Convention Illustrated	Human Gene Symbol (When Available)
Nidd1, Nidd2, Nidd3, Nidd4	non-insulin-dependent diabetes mellitus 1, 2, 3, 4	same stem (root) for gene families	
Nup160	nucleoporin 160	name change (formerly *Gtl1-13*)	*NUP160*
Rnr13	rRNA, chromosome 13 cluster		
Tcrb	T-cell receptor β-chain		*TRB@* (formerly *TCRB;* @ signifies gene family; see 15.6.2 Human Gene Nomenclature)
Tel10p	telomeric sequence, Chr 10, centromere end	*Tel:* telomere; 10: Chr 10; p: short arm	
Tg(APOE)1Vln	transgene insertion 1, Fred Van Leuven	*Tg:* transgene; parenthetic material: inserted gene, in this case the human gene *APOE; Vln:* founder or "laboratory of" designation	

Table 10. Conventions for Mouse Gene Symbols Identified in Collaborative Sequencing Efforts (Examples)[a]

Mouse Gene Symbol	Mouse Gene Description	Convention Illustrated	Human Gene Symbol (When Available)
0610005C13Rik	RIKEN cDNA 0610005C13 gene	RIKEN symbol assigned to sequence that does not match known genes in other species; *Rik:* RIKEN Institute, Japan	
Cdc42ep3	CDC42 effector protein (Rho GTPase binding) 3; formerly *3200001F04Rik*	RIKEN symbol changed when gene identified in another organism	*CDC42EP3*
BC023055	cDNA sequence BC023055	*BC* indicates sequence from Mammalian Gene Collection of the National Institutes of Health	*C10orf83*
Aldob	aldolase 2, B isoform, formerly *BC016435*	Mammalian Gene Collection symbol changed when gene identified in another organism	*ALDOB*
AF179933	cDNA sequence AF179933	Genbank symbol for genes with no other information available in other organisms or sequencing efforts	

Table 10. Conventions for Mouse Gene Symbols Identified in Collaborative Sequencing Efforts (Examples)[a] *(cont)*

Mouse Gene Symbol	Mouse Gene Description	Convention Illustrated	Human Gene Symbol (When Available)
Ppt2	palmitoyl-protein thioesterase 2, formerly *AA672937* and *0610007M19Rik*	Genbank sequence ID withdrawn when gene identified in other organism	*PPT2*

[a] See also Database Identifiers for Genomic Sequences in 15.6.1, Nucleic Acids and Amino Acids.

Conventions and rules for mouse allele symbols are shown in Table 11. In a phenotype expression, a superscript plus sign indicates wild-type, eg:

$Nf1^{tm1Fcr}/Nf1^{+}$

which indicates a phenotype with a mutant neurofibromatosis allele (targeted mutation 1, Fredrick Cancer Research and Development Center) and the wild-type neurofibromatosis allele.

Table 11. Rules and Conventions for Mouse Allele Terms (Examples)

Allele Symbol	Allele Name	Convention or Rule Illustrated
abn	abnormal	recessive trait, thus begins with lowercase; because there is no superscript indicating an allelic term, use context to clarify
Dbf	doublefoot	dominant trait, thus begins with capital; because there is no superscript indicating an allelic term, use context to clarify
$Dnahc11^{iv}$	situs inversus viscerum allele of dynein, axon, heavy chain 11 gene	allele superscript designation is lowercase (recessive)
$Ins2^{Akita}$	Akita allele of insulin 2 gene	allele superscript designation has initial capital (dominant)
$Lama2^{dy\text{-}2J}$	dystrophia muscularis allele, Jackson 2, of α_2-laminin gene (second allele discovered at the Jackson Laboratory)	laboratory code included in superscript (see "Laboratory Codes" section); hyphens used
$Matp^{Uw\text{-}dbr}$	underwhite dominant brown alleles of membrane-associated transporter protein gene	multiple alleles separated by hyphen in superscript

Mouse Chromosomes. Chromosome nomenclature is similar for mice and humans (see 15.6.4, Human Chromosomes). However, in mice, rearrangement terms are capitalized. The following listing and subsequent examples are from the International Committee on Standardized Genetic Nomenclature for Mice[10]:

Cen	centromere
Del	deletion

Df	deficiency
Dp	duplication
Hc	pericentric heterochromatin
Hsr	homogeneous staining region
In	inversion
Is	insertion
MatDf	maternal deficiency
MatDi	maternal disomy
MatDp	maternal duplication
Ms	monosomy
Ns	nullisomy
PatDf	paternal deficiency
PatDi	paternal disomy
PatDp	paternal duplication
Rb	robertsonian translocation
T	translocation
Tc	transchromosomal
Tel	telomere
Tet	tetrasomy
Tg	transgenic insertion
Tp	transposition
Ts	trisomy
UpDf	uniparental deficiency
UpDi	uniparental disomy
UpDp	uniparental duplication

As with human chromosomes, lowercase p represents the short arm and lowercase q the long arm. When specific mouse chromosomes are referred to, the word Chromosome is capitalized (and abbreviated Chr after first mention), eg:

> Human chromosome 1 shows extensive homology to several mouse chromosomes, especially Chromosome (Chr) 4 and Chr 1.

Chromosome anomaly symbols usually include a unique laboratory code (see the "Laboratory Codes" section) and a series number, eg:

In5Rk	fifth inversion found by Roderick
T37H	37th translocation found at Harwell

Chromosome number appears in parentheses:

In(2)5Rk	inversion in Chr 2

Semicolons separate numbers of chromosomes involved in translocations:

T(4;X)37H	translocation involving Chr 4 and Chr X

Periods indicate the centromere in robertsonian translocations:

Rb(9.19)163H robertsonian translocation involving Chr 9 and Chr 19

In insertions, the donor chromosome number comes first:

Is(7;1)40H insertion from Chr 7 to Chr 1

For further rules and conventions for chromosomes, see the chromosome nomenclature section of the Mouse Genome Informatics Web site.[10]

Laboratory Codes. Laboratory registration codes appear as 1- to 4-letter symbols in animal genetic terminology, including chromosomal, DNA locus, and mouse strain nomenclature (see below). Such codes help identify specific colonies, useful in genetic studies that can extend over many generations. Laboratory codes are registered with the Institute of Laboratory Animal Resources at the National Academy of Sciences in Washington, DC, and may be located at http://dels.nas.edu/ilar_n/ilarhome.[11] These codes uniquely identify an investigator, laboratory, or institution that breeds rodents or rabbits. Laboratory codes have initial capitals and appear without expansion. Examples are as follows:

Arb: Arthritis and Rheumatism Branch, National Institute of Arthritis and Musculoskeletal and Skin Diseases

Ddd: University of Durham, Drug Dependence Group

J: The Jackson Laboratory

N: National Institutes of Health

Ty: Benjamin A. Taylor, The Jackson Laboratory

Wil: Jean Wilson, University of Texas

Mouse Strains. Mouse strain names[12] are registered at the Mouse Genome Informatics Web site (http://www.informatics.jax.org/mgihome/submissions/submissions_menu.shtml). Mouse strain names are available at http://www.informatics.jax.org/external/festing/search_form.cgi. (Rat strain names are registered at the Rat Genome Database.[9])

Mouse strain names consist of capital letters or combinations of capital letters and numbers:

A

BXH

CBA

C57BL

FVB

HDA32

A few earlier strains have names that are entirely numeric, eg:

129

A substrain is indicated by a term following the strain name after a virgule, usually the laboratory registration codes (see above), eg:

129/J

A/J

atherosclerosis in CBA/J mice

FVB/N mice used as controls

A serial number may precede the laboratory code, eg, the 10 before the J in this example:

C57BL/10J

Exceptions to the initial capital after the virgule exist in the case of 2 well-known strains (not substrains) of mouse:

BALB/c

C57BR/cd

Many standard laboratory mouse strains are derived from crosses dating back to the early 20th century or even older lines, and the names reflect abbreviations for characteristics:

A	albino
BALB	Bagg, albino
DBA	dilute, brown, nonagouti

However, mouse strain names are not expanded.

Strain names may be abbreviated using approved abbreviations, eg:

B	C57BL
C	BALB/c

Note that some abbreviations are the same as some names of different strains (eg, the strain C and the abbreviation C), so context must clarify. Additional abbreviations are available at http://www.informatics.jax.org/mgihome/nomen/strains.shtml.

Abbreviations and the letter X are used to indicate recombinant inbred strains (female parental strain first), eg:

CXB BALB/c x C57BL

Capital F followed by a number in parentheses may appear after a strain designation to indicate the number of inbred generations:

F(20) 20 inbred generations

For further guidelines on mouse strain nomenclature, see the Mouse Genome Informatics Web site at http://www.informatics.jax.org/mgihome/nomen/strains.shtml.[12]

Invertebrates

Drosophila melanogaster. Gene symbols for the fruitfly *Drosophila melanogaster* are generally capital and lowercase or all lowercase for recessive phenotypes. This convention is also observed for gene names. Gene symbols may include punctuation.[13,14] A source for background on *Drosophila* gene names is FlyNome.[15] Nomenclature rules and symbol search are available at FlyBase.[13]

Gene Symbol	*Name*
Ppi	Preproinsulinlike
SerT	Serotonin transporter
su(Hw)	suppressor of Hairy wing
tRNA:S7:23Ea	transfer RNA:ser7:23Ea (ser7: seventh isoform of serine; 23E: map position)

As with mouse alleles, *Drosophila* alleles are indicated with superscripts:

Hn^{r}, Hn^{r2} (Henna gene, eye color-defective alleles)

Caenorhabditis elegans. The gene symbols for this nematode (roundworm) consist of 3 lowercase letters, hyphen, arabic numeral (sometimes a decimal), and, sometimes, a roman numeral after a space[14,16]:

dpy-1

dpy-5 I

let-37 X

sir-2.1

Parentheses indicate mutation in the gene:

let-37(mn138)

Mutation symbols consist of 1- or 2-letter terms plus a number:

mn138

A characteristic of a mutation may be indicated by a 2-letter ending set in roman type:

*hc17*ts (ts: temperature sensitive)

OMIA. Online Mendelian Inheritance in Animals is the counterpart to Online Mendelian Inheritance in Man (OMIM; see 15.6.2, Human Gene Nomenclature).[17,18]

Microorganism Gene Nomenclature

Yeasts. Gene symbols for the fungus *Saccharomyces cerevisiae* consist of 3 capital letters plus a number (or, occasionally, a number-letter) ending[19]:

Gene Symbol	*Name*
ACT1	actin
CDC25	adenylate cyclase regulatory protein
COX5A	cytochrome c oxidase chain Va

This represents a change from earlier style in which all-lowercase symbols were used for loci named for recessive mutations (the preponderance of symbols) and all-capital symbols for loci named for dominant mutations. Allele symbols still follow the case convention (ie, capital for dominant, lowercase for recessive).

Bacterial Gene Nomenclature. Gene terms typically consist of an italicized lowercase 3-letter abbreviation often with an uppercase locus designator. The phenotype or encoded entity (eg, enzyme) is in all roman letters with an initial capital.[14,20,21]

Gene Symbol	*Phenotype (Explanation)*
araA	AraA (L-arabinose isomerase)
asr	Asr (acid shock protein)
imp (formerly *ostA*)	OstA (organic solvent intolerance; imp: increased membrane permeability)
katE	KatE (catalase)
sodA	SodA (superoxide dismutase, manganese)
sodB	SodB (superoxide dismutase, iron)

A number of bacterial genome databases are available on the Internet. The National Center for Biotechnology Information sponsors Entrez Genome (http://www.ncbi.nlm.nih.gov/entrez: under Search, select Gene, then search for the gene in question).

Alleles are designated with a number after the uppercase letter or following a hyphen, when not assigned to a locus. Wild-type alleles are designated with a superscript plus sign:

ara^{+}

araA1

ara-23

sodA1

Retroviral Gene Nomenclature. Human immunodeficiency virus and other retroviruses contain 3 main structural genes and a number of regulatory genes[22] (see also 15.6.3, Oncogenes and Tumor Suppressor Genes):

Structural:

env	envelope gene
gag	group-specific core antigen gene
pol	polymerase gene

Regulatory:

nef	negative factor
rev	regulator of viral protein expression
tat	transactivator of viral transcription
vif	viral infectivity
vpr	viral protein R
vpu	viral protein U
vpx	viral protein X

Compare typographic style of gene names and their products (p stands for protein, gp for glycoprotein):

Gene	*Gene Product (Protein or Polypeptide)*	*Protein Products (Examples)*
env	Env	gp41, gp120
gag	Gag	p6, p7, p17, p24
pol	Pol	p12, p32, p66/51
nef	Nef	p27
rev	Rev	p19
tat	Tat	p14
vif	Vif	p24
vpr	Vpr	p15
vpu	Vpu	p16
vpx	Vpx	p14

REFERENCES

1. Morse HC III. The laboratory mouse—a historical perspective. In: Foster HL, Fox F, eds. *The Mouse in Biomedical Research*. Vol 1. Orlando, FL: Academic Press Inc; 1981:6-10.
2. Marshall Graves JA, Wakefield MJ, Peters J, Searle AG, Womack JE, O'Brien SJ. Report of the Committee on Comparative Gene Mapping. In: Cuticchia AJ, ed. *Human Gene Mapping 1994: A Compendium*. Baltimore, MD: Johns Hopkins University Press; 1995:962-1016.
3. Gene Ontology Consortium. Gene ontology: tool for the unification of biology. *Nat Genet*. 2000; 25(1):25-29. Also available at http://www.geneontology.org/GO_nature_genetics_2000.pdf. Accessed April 21, 2006.
4. ARKdb. http://www.thearkdb.org. Accessed April 21, 2006.
5. RatMapGroup. RATMAP: the Rat Genome Database. http://ratmap.gen.gu.se/. Accessed April 21, 2006.
6. International Committee on Standardized Genetic Nomenclature for Mice and Rat Genome and Nomenclature Committee. Rules for nomenclature of genes, genetic markers, alleles, and mutations in mouse and rat. http://www.informatics.jax.org/mgihome/nomen/gene.shtml#genenom. Updated January 2005. Accessed April 21, 2006.
7. Maltais LJ, Blake JA, Chu T, Lutz CM, Eppig JT, Jackson I. Rules and guidelines for mouse gene, allele, and mutation nomenclature: a condensed version. *Genomics*. 2002;79(4):471-474. Also available at http://www.informatics.jax.org/mgihome/nomen/short_gene.shtml. Accessed April 21, 2006.
8. Jackson Laboratory. MGI: Mouse Genome Informatics. http://www.informatics.jax.org. Updated April 20, 2006. Accessed April 21, 2006.
9. RGD: Rat Genome Database. http://rgd.mcw.edu. Updated April 17, 2006. Accessed April 21, 2006.
10. International Committee on Standardized Genetic Nomenclature for Mice. Rules for nomenclature of chromosome aberrations. http://www.informatics.jax.org/mgihome/nomen/anomalies.shtml. Accessed April 21, 2006.

11. ILAR: Institute for Laboratory Animal Research. Laboratory Code Registry. http://dels.nas.edu/ilar_n/ilarhome. Accessed April 21, 2006.
12. International Committee on Standardized Genetic Nomenclature for Mice and Rat Genome and Nomenclature Committee. Rules for nomenclature of mouse and rat strains. http://www.informatics.jax.org/mgihome/nomen/strains.shtml. Updated January 2005. Accessed April 21, 2006.
13. FlyBase: a database of the *Drosophila* genome. http://flybase.net. Accessed April 21, 2006.
14. Stewart A, ed. *TIG Genetic Nomenclature Guide*. Tarrytown, NY: Elsevier Trends Journals; 1995.
15. FlyNome: a database of *Drosophila* nomenclature. http://www.flynome.com. Accessed April 21, 2006.
16. Hodgkin J. Recommended genetic nomenclature for *Caenorhabditis elegans*. http://elegans.swmed.edu/Genome/nomen.html.01_10_25. Accessed April 21, 2006.
17. Nicholas FW. Online Mendelian Inheritance in Animals (OMIA). http://www.angis.org.au/omia. Updated October 16, 2003. Accessed April 21, 2006.
18. Rangel P, Giovannetti J. *Genomes and Databases on the Internet: A Practical Guide to Functions and Applications*. Norfolk, England: Horizon Scientific Press; 2002.
19. SGD gene naming guidelines. http://www.yeastgenome.org/gene_guidelines.shtml. Accessed April 21, 2006.
20. Demerec M, Adelberg EA, Clark AJ, Hartman PE. A proposal for a uniform nomenclature in bacterial genetics. *Genetics*. 1966;54(1):61-76.
21. *Journal of Bacteriology* 2006 instructions to authors. http://jb.asm.org/misc/itoa.pdf. Accessed April 21, 2006.
22. Guatelli JC, Siliciano RF, Kuritzkes DR, Richman DD. Human immunodeficiency virus. In: Richman DD, Whitley RJ, Hayden FD, eds. *Clinical Virology*. 2nd ed. Washington, DC: ASM Press; 2002:685-729.

15.6.6 **Pedigrees.** Pedigree format recommendations are put forth by the Pedigree Standardization Task Force of the National Society of Genetic Counselors.[1] (See also 5.8.3, Legal and Ethical Considerations, Protecting Research Participants' and Patients' Rights in Scientific Publication, Rights in Published Reports of Genetic Studies.)

A square represents a male individual; a circle, a female individual; and a diamond, an individual whose sex is unknown:

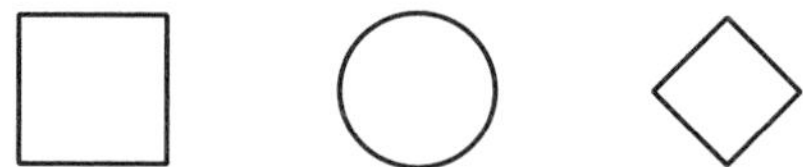

Shading indicates an affected individual. Partitions with different shading should be used for individuals with more than one condition. Define all shading in a legend or key.

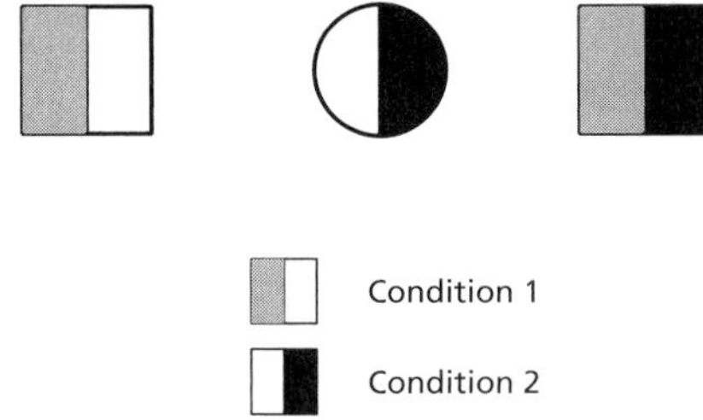

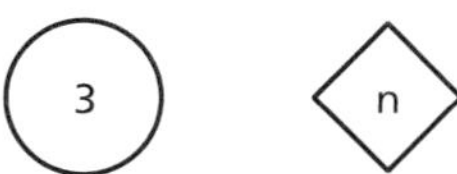

Multiple individuals are indicated by a number inside the shape. For unknown number, a roman n is preferred to a question mark:

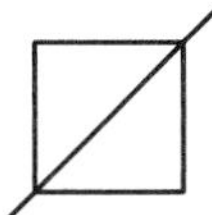

A slash mark indicates a deceased individual:

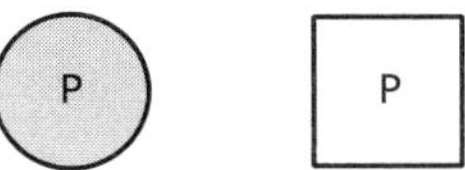

An individual in gestation is indicated with a capital P inside the shape:

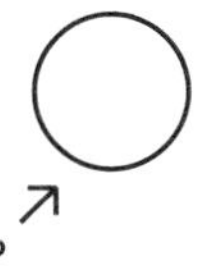

The proband ("first affected family member coming to medical attention"[1(p746)]) is indicated by a capital P with arrow:

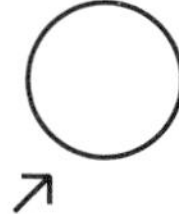

The consultand (person seeking medical attention) is indicated with an arrow:

Textual information appears below the individual symbol. Preferred order is age information, evaluation, and pedigree number:

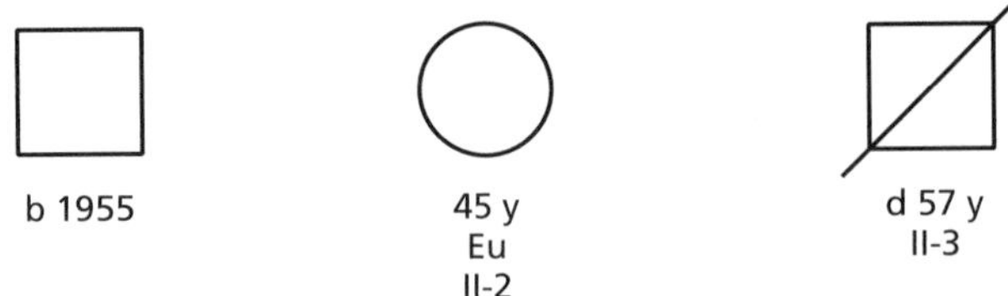

Eu: uninformative evaluation.

An obligate carrier (ie, unaffected individual inferred by pedigree analysis to carry a trait) is indicated with a central dot:

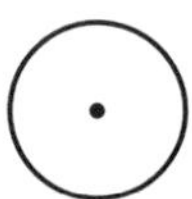

A small triangle indicates an individual in a pregnancy not carried to term. Sex, if known, is indicated with text. Shading is used as described above for affected individuals. "ECT" indicates ectopic pregnancy. A slash indicates termination of pregnancy.

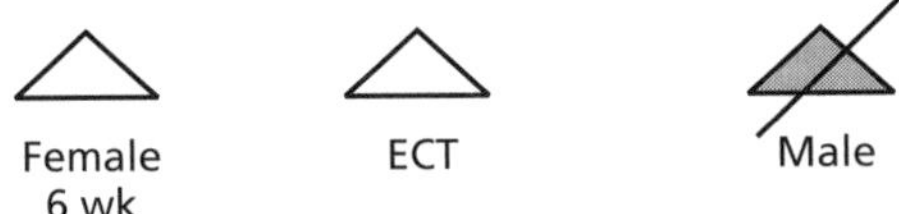

Stillborn individuals are represented by full-sized shapes with "SB" in the caption:

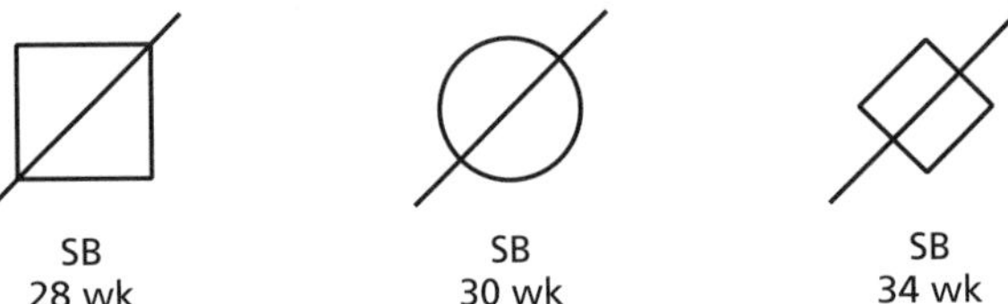

Partner relationships are indicated by a straight, horizontal line. It is preferred that the male partner be shown on the left.

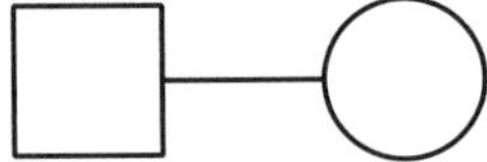

Siblings should appear in order of birth (oldest to the left), connected by lines as follows:

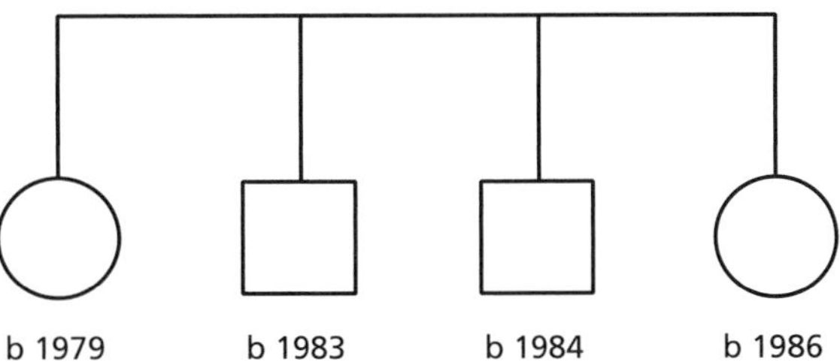

Offspring are indicated by vertical lines; a shorter line indicates a pregnancy not carried to term:

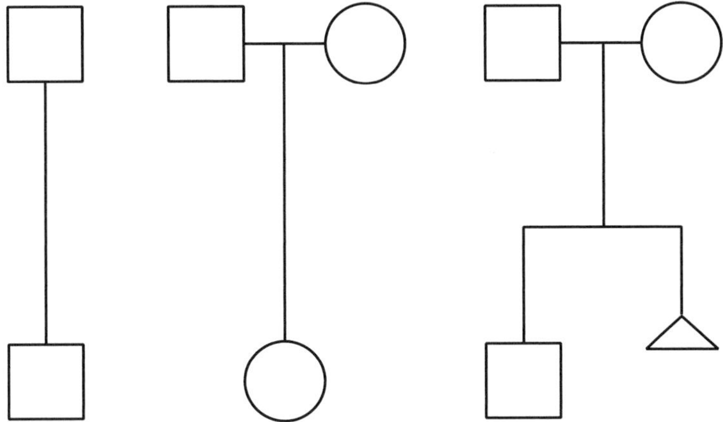

An ended relationship is indicated by a double slash:

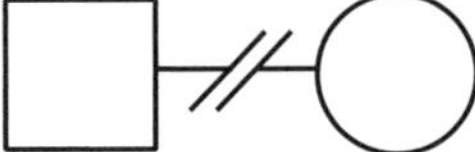

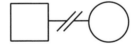

Consanguinity ("kinship because of common ancestry"[2(p401)]) is indicated by a double line:

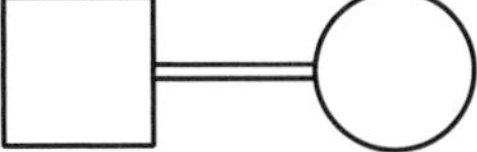

Diagonal lines indicate twins. A horizontal bar specifies monozygotic; no horizontal bar, dizygotic; and a question mark, unknown:

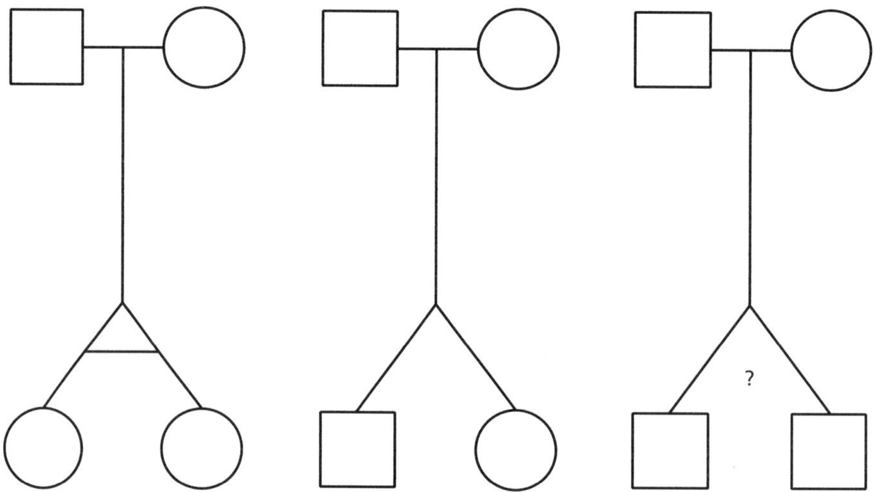

No issue is indicated by perpendicular lines; infertility, by perpendicular lines with a double horizontal line.

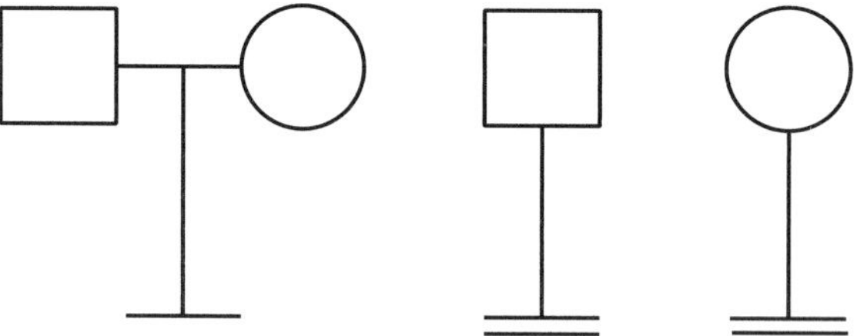

Brackets indicate an adopted individual and dashed lines social parentage, eg, step-parent (example from Bennett et al[1(p748)]):

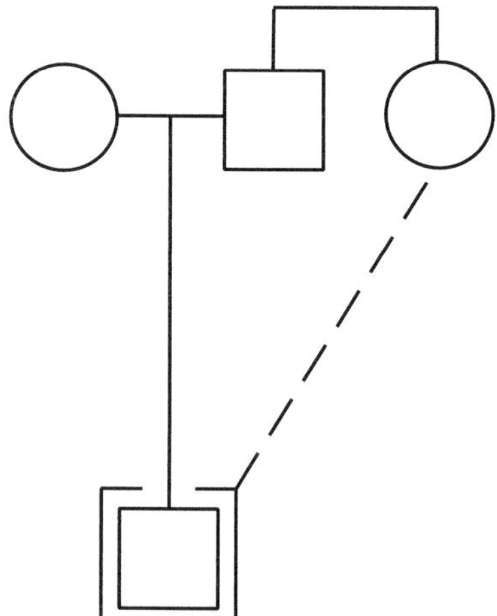

In pedigrees that show relationships defined by assisted reproductive technologies, D indicates donor (sperm or ovum) and S, surrogate carrier of the pregnancy.

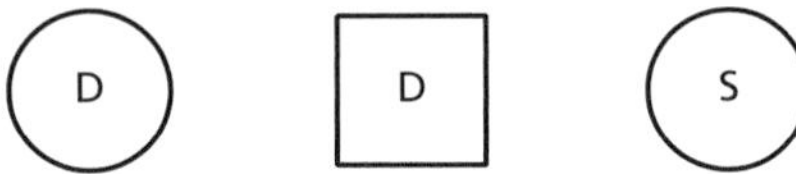

Diagonal lines indicate other parental relationships:

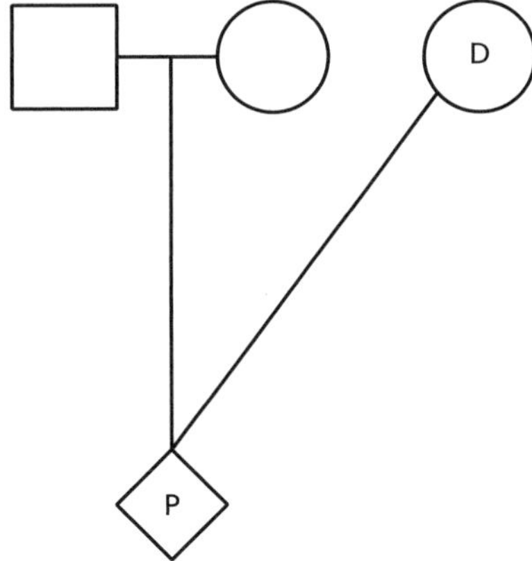

Haplotypes may be indicated with shaded rectangles below the individual. Meaning should be clarified by means of a key.

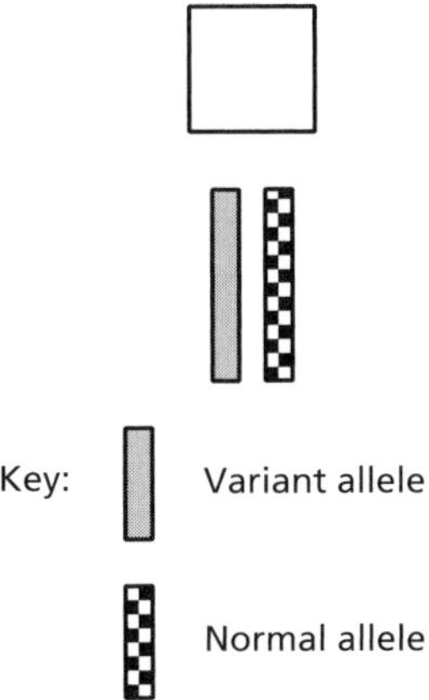

A sample complete pedigree follows (Figure 6):

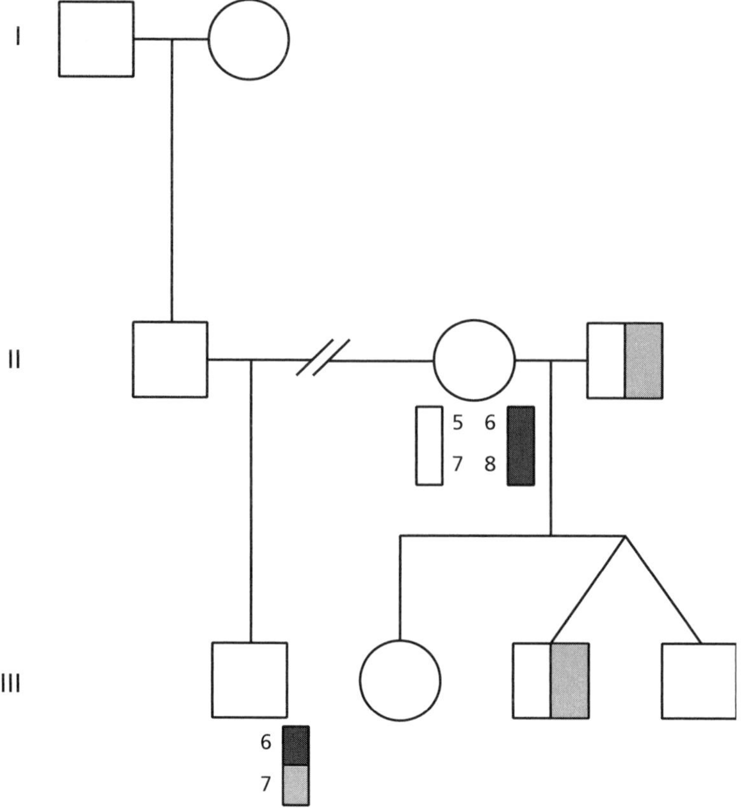

Figure 6. Pedigree showing 3 generations includes terminated relationship (double diagonal lines), condition common to father and 1 dizygotic twin son (half-shaded boxes), and haplotypes of mother and another son (rectangles with numbers). Roman numerals indicate generations.

REFERENCES

1. Bennett RL, Steinhaus KA, Uhrich SB, et al. Recommendations for standardized human pedigree nomenclature. *Am J Hum Genet*. 1995;56(3):745-752. Also published in *J Genet Counseling*. 1995;4(4):267-279.
2. *Stedman's Medical Dictionary*. 27th ed. Philadelphia, PA: Lippincott Williams & Wilkins; 2000.

Thrombosis may be regarded as an accident of nature that has not had time to adapt through the lengthy process of evolution to the advances of modern medicine, which allow patients to survive the hemostatic challenge of major surgery and trauma but leave them vulnerable to venous thrombosis.

R. W. Colman et al[1(p3)]

> *...each milliliter of blood contains enough clotting material to clot all the fibrinogen in the body in 10 to 15 s.*
>
> R. I. Handin[2(p340)]

15.7 Hemostasis. Hemostasis consists of platelet plug formation (primary hemostasis) and blood coagulation (secondary hemostasis, coagulation, clotting). Hemostasis and its control involve complex interactions of more than 50 procoagulants and anticoagulants. Description of hemostatic processes depends on consistent use of terms.

15.7.1 Primary Hemostasis. Note the typography of the following terms, which are found in descriptions of platelet hemostasis (use parenthetical abbreviated terms in accordance with 14.11, Abbreviations, Clinical, Technical, and Other Common Terms):

Term	*Abbreviation*
6-keto prostaglandin $F_{1\alpha}$	6-keto $PGF_{1\alpha}$
α-granules	
arachidonic acid	AA
ATP P2X1 receptor	P2X1
β-thromboglobulin	βTG *or* BTG
calcium calmodulin complex	Ca-CaM *or* Ca-CM
cyclooxygenase	CO *or* COX
diacylglycerol	DAG
G proteins (proteins that hydrolyze guanosine triphosphate; expansion not necessary)	
glycoprotein Ia/IIa complex	GpIa-IIa
glycoprotein Ib/IX complex	GpIb-IX
glycoprotein Ib/IX/V complex	GpIb-IX-V
glycoprotein IIb/IIIa complex	GpIIb-IIIa
glycoprotein IV (CD36; see also 15.8.7, Immunology, Lymphocytes)	GpIV
glycoprotein VI	GpVI
inositol triphosphate	IP_3
myosin light chain	MLC
myosin light chain kinase	MLCK
myosin light chain, phosphorylated	$MLC\text{-}PO_4$
phosphatidylinositol 4,5-biphosphate	PIP_2
phosphodiesterase 3A	PDE3A
phospholipase A_2	PLA_2
phospholipase C	PLC
platelet activating factor	PAF

Term	*Abbreviation*
platelet-derived growth factor	PDGF
platelet factor 3	PF3
platelet factor 4	PF4
platelet ADP P2T adenylate cyclase receptor	$P2T_{AC}$
platelet ADP P2X1 receptor	P2X1
platelet ADP P2Y1 receptor	P2Y1
prostacyclin, prostaglandin I_2	PGI_2
prostaglandin D_2	PGD_2
6-keto prostaglandin $F_{1\alpha}$	6-keto $PGF_{1\alpha}$
prostaglandin G_2	PGG_2
prostaglandin H_2	PGH_2
protein p47	p47
protein p47, phosphorylated	p47-PO_4
protein kinase C	PKC
thromboxane A_2	TXA_2
thromboxane B_2	TXB_2
β-thromboglobulin	βTG *or* BTG
von Willebrand factor (see also below)	vWF

See also 15.1.2, Blood Groups, Platelet Antigens, and Granulocyte Antigens, Platelet-Specific Antigens.

15.7.2 Endothelial Factors. Structures and products of endothelial cells—the cells lining blood vessels—maintain blood fluidity by preventing excessive clotting and prevent bleeding by promoting clotting. The following endothelium-associated terms are presented as a guide to style.

Class	*Term*	*Abbreviation*
cellular (or cell) adhesion molecules		CAMs
	intercellular adhesion molecule 1	ICAM-1
	intercellular adhesion molecule 2	ICAM-2
	platelet-endothelial CAM	PECAM
	vascular CAM 1	VCAM-1
cytokines (see also 15.8.4, Immunology, Cytokines)		
	gro (growth-stimulating factor)	

Class	*Term*	*Abbreviation*
	RANTES (regulated on activation, normal T-expressed, and presumably secreted[3])	
integrins		
	$\alpha_1\beta_1$ integrin	
	$\alpha_2\beta_3$ integrin	
	$\alpha_3\beta_1$ integrin	
	$\alpha_6\beta_1$ integrin	
	$\alpha_v\beta_1$ integrin	
	$\alpha_v\beta_3$ integrin	
miscellaneous		
	nitric oxide	NO
	endothelial (or epithelial) NO synthase	eNOS (also NOS3)
	endothelial-cell associated ADPase (CD39; see also 15.8.7, Immunology, Lymphocytes)	
	prostacyclin, prostaglandin I_2	PGI_2
	E-selectin	
	L-selectin	
	P-selectin	
	tissue plasminogen activator (see 15.7.4, Inhibition of Coagulation and Fibrinolysis)	tPA
	urokinase or urinary plasminogen activator (see 15.7.4, Inhibition of Coagulation and Fibrinolysis)	uPA

Three glycoprotein complexes are synonymous with 3 integrins and take part in hemostasis:

GpIa-IIa	$\alpha_2\beta_1$
GpIc-IIa	$\alpha_6\beta_1$
GpIIb-IIIa	$\alpha_{IIB}\beta_3$

15.7.3 **Secondary Hemostasis.** Blood coagulation is the phase of clot formation dependent on plasma coagulation factors (also known as clotting factors).

Pathways. The laboratory evaluation of plasma factor-dependent coagulation has been divided into 2 pathways (systems, phases). The following terms and synonyms are used:

Term	Synonym
intrinsic pathway	contact system-initiated pathway
extrinsic pathway	tissue factor-mediated or tissue factor-dependent pathway

Clotting Factors. An international system of nomenclature, formulated from 1954 through 1963,[4,5] clarified clotting factor terminology and, as Biggs[6] observed, scientific findings in coagulation, when factors identified and named independently by different groups were shown to be the same.[5] A major update to the standard nomenclature was published by Blomback et al[7,8] in the early 1990s.

A number of clotting factors were named for the patients whose disorders led to their discovery. Biggs considered this practice valuable in avoiding "'hypothetical implication.'"[5(p705)]

Roman numerals are used to designate most of the major plasma coagulation factors. These designations when formulated were seen as having advantages over eponyms and functional names for comprehension by readers of non-Western languages.[5] "The sequence of numbers in current terminology is . . . based on the historical order in which the coagulation factors were discovered."[5(p710)]

The following tabulation gives roman numeral designations, descriptive names, and synonyms for the plasma coagulation factors. Asterisks indicate preferred terms. Terms that are rarely used are enclosed in parentheses. If a term other than the preferred term is used, the preferred term should be given in parentheses at the first mention of a factor. Common abbreviations appear here, but their use should conform to guidelines in 14.11, Abbreviations, Clinical, Technical, and Other Common Terms. (The term "factor VI," originally designating activated factor V, is not used.)

Factor No.	Descriptive Name	Synonym(s)
(factor I)	fibrinogen*	
factor II	prothrombin*	prethrombin
(factor III)	tissue factor	thromboplastin tissue thromboplastin tissue extract
(factor IV)	calcium*	calcium ion Ca^{2+}
factor V*	proaccelerin	(labile factor) (accelerator globulin [AcG]) (Ac globulin) (thrombogen)
factor VII*	proconvertin	(stable factor) (serum prothrombin conversion accelerator [SPCA]) (autoprothrombin I)
factor VIII*	antihemophilic factor (AHF)	antihemophilic globulin (AHG) antihemophilic factor A (platelet cofactor 1) (thromboplastinogen)

Factor No.	*Descriptive Name*	*Synonym(s)*
factor IX*	plasma thrombo-plastin component (PTC)	Christmas factor antihemophilic factor B (autoprothrombin III) (platelet cofactor 2)
factor X*	Stuart factor	Prower factor Stuart-Prower factor (autoprothrombin III) (thrombokinase)
factor XI*	plasma thrombo-plastin antecedent (PTA)	(antihemophilic factor C)
factor XII*	Hageman factor	contact factor (glass factor)
factor XIII	fibrin stabilizing factor (FSF)	plasma transglutaminase fibrinoligase (Laki-Lorand factor [LLF]) (fibrinase)
. . .	prekallikrein*	Fletcher factor prokallikrein
. . .	high-molecular-weight kininogen (HMW kininogen, HMWK, HK)*	Fitzgerald factor Williams factor Flaujeac factor (contact activation factor) (Reid factor) (Washington factor)

A lowercase a designates the activated form of a factor, eg, IXa.

In diagrams of coagulation pathways, activation is indicated with a solid arrow:

X ——▸ Xa

and action on another factor, with a dashed arrow:

XIIa ----▸ XI

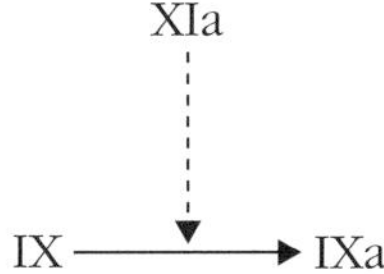

Additional terms related to secondary hemostasis are as follows:

Term	*Abbreviation*
γ-glutamyl carboxylic acid residues	Gla residues
tissue factor/VIIa complex	TF-VIIa complex
or	
VIIa/tissue factor complex	VIIa-TF complex
active factor XII fragment	XIIf

Clotting Factor Variants. Specific variants or abnormal forms may be named for locations, as follows:

factor V Cambridge

factor V Leiden

factor X San Antonio

fibrinogen Paris

protein C Vermont

prothrombin Barcelona

prothrombin Himi I

prothrombin Himi II

Clotting factor variants that have been characterized molecularly are specified by means of terms that indicate the molecular change, ie, nucleotide or amino acid alteration.[9] The abbreviations ins (insertion), del (deletion), In (intron), Ex (exon), and ter (termination codon) are used within such terms.[9] See Sequence Variations, Nucleotides, and Sequence Variations, Amino Acids, in 15.6.1, Genetics, Nucleic Acids and Amino Acids, for a more detailed description of such notation. Examples:

factor VIII Arg1689Cys *or* VIII R1689C

factor VIII Glu1987ter *or* VIII G1987ter

factor VIII Ex24-25del

A shorthand expression is permissible after the term is first defined:

> The factor II resulting from the 20210G→A variant (mutation) in the prothrombin gene (factor II A^{20210}) . . .

Thrombin. The protein thrombin is the end result of the coagulation factor cascade. Related terms include the following:

α-thrombin

β-thrombin

γ-thrombin

thrombin A loop, B loop, C loop, E loop, γ loop

β-thromboglobulin

Hemophilias and Thrombophilias. Hemophilias are bleeding disorders. Hemophilia A is associated with factor VIII deficiency, hemophilia B with factor IX deficiency, hemophilia C with factor XI deficiency, and von Willebrand disease with von Willebrand factor deficiency. (Factor IX was the originally named Christmas factor, after a patient's surname. That patient went on to become an influential advocate for safe blood supply.[5] Hemophilia B, known as Christmas disease, was reported in the Christmas 1952 issue of the *British Medical Journal*.[4,5]) Examples of subtypes include hemophilia A, CRM(+) variant (CRM: cross-reacting material), hemophilia B Leyden [*sic*], and hemophilia Bm.

Thrombophilias are excessive clot-forming disorders. One variety occurs with factor V Leiden.

See "Clotting Factor Variants" above for molecularly based nomenclature.

Von Willebrand Factor. Because factor VIII, involved in coagulation, and von Willebrand factor (vWF), involved in platelet adhesion, form a noncovalent bimolecular complex, they were originally difficult to distinguish biochemically and immunologically. Original nomenclature reflected this difficulty; for instance, what was first referred to as factor VIII-related antigen (abbreviated VIIIR:Ag) was found to be the factor that is deficient in von Willebrand disease.

Factor VIII and vWF, although functionally associated, are physiologically, genetically, and clinically distinct. In 1985 the International Committee on Coagulation and Thrombosis put forth preferred terminology that was meant (1) to distinguish VIII from vWF and (2) to clarify exactly which entity was being specified (Table 12). The committee noted that it is acceptable to use the term VIII-vWF for the biomolecular complex but not for either single component.[10,11]

The terms in column 1 of Table 12 are not only preferred but also familiar exactly as shown to those conversant with the field. However, for most audiences, authors should clarify the preferred term by including the synonym or an explanation (eg, column 4, "Meaning") at first mention.

Von Willebrand Disease. Variants of von Willebrand disease include the following:

Type	*Sample Molecular Variants*[12]
type I	vWF Arg854Gln, vWF Cys1149Arg
type IIA	vWF Ile865Thr, vWF Arg834Trp
type IIB	vWF Trp550Cys, vWF Arg545Cys
type III	vWF Arg1659ter, vWF Arg2635ter
Normandy 1	vWF Thr28Met

Table 12. Factor VII and von Willebrand Factor Terminology

Preferred	Synonym	Old (Avoid)	Meaning
factor VIII	antihemophilic factor (AHF)	VIII:C	factor VIII protein
VIII:Ag	factor VIII antigen	VIII:CAg	factor VIII antigen
VIII:c			factor VIII coagulant activity
vWF	von Willebrand factor	VIIIR:Ag VIII/vWF AHF-like protein	von Willebrand factor protein
vWF:Ag		VIIIR:Ag	von Willebrand factor antigen
ristocetin cofactor (RCoF)		VIIIR:RCoF VIII:R:RCo VIIIR:vWF	von Willebrand factor function, ie, platelet adhesion-promoting property of vWF in the presence of the drug ristocetin

Nomenclature for sequence variants (mutations and polymorphisms) of the *VWF* gene is indicated according to Sequence Variations, Nucleotides, and Sequence Variations, Amino Acids, in 15.6.1, Nucleic Acids and Amino Acids, as above or as in the following examples[13]:

1234G>A	adenine substituted for guanine at position 1234 in *VWF* cDNA sequence
g1234G>A	as above, in complete *VWF* sequence
1234insN	nucleotide insertion after nucleotide 1234 in *VWF* cDNA sequence
R123G	glycine substitute for arginine at position 123 in pre-pro VWF sequence
R123del	arginine deletion at position 123 in pre-pro VWF sequence
1234A/G	adenine/guanine polymorphism at position 1234 in *VWF* cDNA

15.7.4 Inhibition of Coagulation and Fibrinolysis

Inhibition of Coagulation. The following sample terms are included for reference. Expand at first mention in accordance with 14.11, Abbreviations, Clinical, Technical, and Other Common Terms.

Term	*Abbreviation*
α_1-antitrypsin	AAT
α_2-macroglobulin	AMG
antithrombin III	ATIII
α-ATIII isoform	α-ATIII
β-ATIII isoform	β-ATIII
ATIII/heparin complex	. . .
C1 inhibitor	C1 INH (see also 15.8.3, Immunology, Complement)
heparin cofactor II	. . .
lupus coagulation inhibitor (also called lupus anticoagulant)	LCI
protein C	. . .
activated protein C	APC
protein S	. . .
protein Z	. . .
serpin (serine protease inhibitor)	. . .
tissue factor pathway inhibitor	TFPI

Note: Protein C was named for an investigator's chromatographic fraction C in which it was discovered. The S in protein S refers to Seattle, where it was discovered. Protein S is not the same as S protein; see also 15.8.3, Complement.

Fibrinolysis (Fibrin Degradation, Clot Degradation, Thrombolysis). The following sample terms represent entities that take part in fibrinolysis or its inhibition. Expand at first mention in accordance with 14.11, Abbreviations, Clinical, Technical, and Other Common Terms:

Term	*Abbreviation*
α_2-plasmin inhibitor, α_2-antiplasmin	α_2PI
aminocaproic acid (amicar)	ACA
ε-ACA	EACA
dimerized plasmin fragment D	D-dimer
fibrin degradation products or fibrin split products	FDP or FSP
Glu-plasminogen (see also "Amino Acids" in 15.6.1, Genetics, Nucleic Acids and Amino Acids)	. . .
Lys-plasminogen (see also "Amino Acids" in 15.6.1, Genetics, Nucleic Acids and Amino Acids)	. . .
a plasminogen activator inhibitor	PAI-1
protein C inhibitor	PAI-3
thrombin-activated fibrinolytic inhibitor	TAFI
tissue plasminogen activator (when a specific therapeutic formulation of tPA is intended, use the USAN term; see 15.4, Drugs)	tPA
tPA receptor	tPAR
urokinase or urinary plasminogen activator	uPA
uPA receptor	uPAR

Tests of Coagulation. Two among several tests of coagulation are the prothrombin time (PT) and the partial thromboplastin time (PTT). When the more common activated partial thromboplastin time (aPTT) is used instead of the PTT, this should be specified.

Traditionally, the prothrombin ratio (PTR) had been reported as a ratio of the patient's PT to the mean laboratory control PT. Reporting the PTR has been refined by use of a modified PTR, the international normalized ratio (INR).[14-16] In accordance with a 1985 policy statement of the International Committee for Thrombosis and Hemostasis and the International Committee for Standardization in Hematology,[14] authors are encouraged to report the INR if at all possible. Unlike conversions between conventional and SI units (see 18.1, Units of Measure, SI Units), there is no simple conversion factor from the PTR to the INR since the international sensitivity index (ISI) of the thromboplastin used in the actual assay performed must be known. The INR is calculated as shown:

$$INR = PTR^{ISI}$$

Authors should specify the exact method by which their results were initially reported by the laboratory performing the assay and the method of conversion, if any, used on the original results.

REFERENCES

1. Colman RW, Marder VJ, Clowes AW, George JN, Goldhaber SZ. Overview of hemostasis. In: Colman RW, Hirsh J, Marder VJ, Clowes AW, George JN, eds. *Hemostasis and Thrombosis: Basic Principles and Clinical Practice.* 5th ed. Philadelphia, PA: Lippincott Williams & Wilkins; 2006:3-16.
2. Handin RI. Bleeding and thrombosis. In: Kasper DL, Braunwald E, Fauci AS, Hauser SL, Longo DL, Jameson JL, eds. *Harrison's Principles of Internal Medicine.* 16th ed. New York, NY: McGraw-Hill; 2005:337-343.
3. *Stedman's Medical Dictionary.* 27th ed. Baltimore, MD: Lippincott Williams & Wilkins; 2000.
4. Owen CA Jr. *A History of Blood Coagulation.* Rochester, MN: Mayo Foundation for Education and Research; 2001.
5. Giangrande PL. Six characters in search of an author: the history of the nomenclature of coagulation factors. *Br J Haematol.* 2003;121(5):703-712.
6. Biggs R. *Human Blood Coagulation, Haemostasis, and Thrombosis.* 2nd ed. Oxford, England: Blackwell Scientific Publications; 1976:15-16.
7. Blomback M, Abildgaard U, van den Besselaar AM, et al. Nomenclature of quantities and units in thrombosis and haemostasis (recommendation 1993): a collaborative project of the Scientific and Standardization Committee of the International Society on Thrombosis and Haemostasis (ISTH/SSC) and the Commission/Committee on Quantities and Units (in Clinical Chemistry) of the International Union of Pure and Applied Chemistry-International Federation of Clinical Chemistry (IUPAC-IFCC/CQU[CC]). *Thromb Haemost.* 1994;71(3):375-394.
8. ISTH: The International Society on Thrombosis and Haemostasis Web site. Working Group/Liaison Reports. http://www.med.unc.edu/isth/welcome. Accessed March 16, 2006.
9. Peake I, Tuddenham E. A standard nomenclature for factor VIII and factor IX gene mutations and associated amino acid alterations: on behalf of the ISTH SSC Subcommittee on Factor VIII and Factor IX. *Thromb Haemost.* 1994;72(3):475-476.
10. Marder VJ, Mannucci PM, Firkin BG, Hoyer LW, Meyer D. Standard nomenclature for factor VIII and von Willebrand factor: a recommendation by the International Committee on Thrombosis and Haemostasis. *Thromb Haemost.* 1985;54(4):871-872.
11. Marder VJ, Roberts HR. Proposed symbols for factor VIII and von Willebrand factor [letter]. *Ann Intern Med.* 1986;105(4):627.
12. OMIM: Online Mendelian Inheritance in Man. http://www.ncbi.nlm.nih.gov/entrez/query.fcgi?db=OMIM. Updated December 21, 2005. Accessed March 16, 2006.
13. Goodeve AC, Eikenboom JCJ, Ginsburg D, et al. A standard nomenclature for von Willebrand factor gene mutations and polymorphisms: on behalf of von Willebrand Factor Subcommittee of the Scientific and Standardization Committe [*sic*] of the International Society on Thrombosis and Haemostasis. http://www.med.unc

.edu/isth/SSC/communications/von_willebrand/vwfnomen.pdf. Posted October 30, 2000. Accessed March 16, 2006.

14. Loeliger EA. ICSH/ICTH recommendations for reporting prothrombin time in oral anticoagulant control. *Thromb Haemost*. 1985;53:155-156.
15. Hirsh J, Dalen JE, Deykin D, Poller L. Oral anticoagulants: mechanism of action, clinical effectiveness, and optimal therapeutic range. *Chest*. 1992;102:312S-326S.
16. Hirsh J, Poller L. The international normalized ratio: a guide to understanding and correcting its problems. *Arch Intern Med*. 1994;154(3):282-288.

15.8 Immunology

15.8.1 Chemokines.

Chemokines. Chemokines comprise a family of about 40 low-molecular-weight cytokines (see 15.8.4, Cytokines) with important roles in the immune system, as well as functions beyond it.[1-5] The name *chemokine,* a contraction of "chemotactic cytokine," reflects the common property, by which chemokines were originally identified, of promoting leukocyte chemotaxis.

Chemokines are classified into 4 subfamilies, based on their cysteine (C) residues and other amino-acid (X) residues (see 15.6.1, Genetics, Nucleic Acids and Amino Acids):

CXC	1 amino-acid residue between the 2 *N*-terminal cysteines
CC	*N*-terminal cysteines adjacent
XC	cysteines 1 and 3 not present
CX3C	3 amino acids between the cysteine residues

Examples of specific chemokines, by subfamily, are shown below:

Subfamily Name	*Synonym*	*Examples*[5]		*Receptors*
		Systematic Name	*Common Names and Abbreviation*	
CXC	α class	CXCL1	growth-related oncogene α (GRO-α), melanoma growth stimulatory activity protein (MGSA)	CXCR2
		CXCL4	platelet factor 4 (see 15.7, Hemostasis)	
		CXCL5	epithelial cell-derived neutrophil attractant 78 (ENA-78)	CXCR2
		CXCL6	granulocyte chemoattractant protein 2 (GCP-2)	CXCR1, CXCR2
		CXCL8	interleukin 8 (IL-8) (see 15.8.4, Cytokines)	CXCR1, CXCR2

Subfamily Name	*Synonym*	*Examples*[5]		*Receptors*
		Systematic Name	*Common Names and Abbreviation*	
		CXCL14	chemokine isolated from breast and kidney tissue (BRAK), bolekine	
CC	β class	CCL1	inducible 309 (I-309)	CCR8
		CCL3	macrophage inflammatory protein 1a or 1α (MIP-1α)	CCR1, CCR5
		CCL5	regulated on activation of normal T cells expressed and secreted (RANTES)	CCR1, CCR3, CCR5 (also called CD195; see 15.8.2, CD Cell Markers)
		CCL7	monocyte chemoattractant (or chemotactic) protein 3 (MCP-3)	CCR1, CCR2, CCR3
		CCL21	secondary lymphoid tissue chemokine (SLC), chemokine β-9 (CKβ-9), exodus 2, 6Ckine	CCR7 (also called CDw107; see 15.8.2, CD Cell Markers)
XC	γ class	XCL1	lymphotactin, activation-induced, T-cell-derived, and chemokine-related (ATAC), single cysteine motif 1α (SCM-1α)	XCR1
		XCL2	SCM-1β	XCR1
CX3C	δ class	CX3CL1	fractalkine	CX3CR1

Expanded common names of the chemokines are often unwieldy and uninformative and so are rarely used, though use of the abbreviations persists. Terms such as those in the tabulation above for chemokine, chemokine subfamily, and chemokine receptor do not need to be expanded, but context should provided at first mention, eg:

the CXC chemokine family

the chemokine CXCL1

chemokine receptor CXCR2

A useful reference on chemokines is the Cytokine Family Database (dbCFC): http://cytokine.medic.kumamoto-u.ac.jp.[6]

15.8.2 CD Cell Markers.

CD Cell Markers. Clusters of differentiation (CDs) are a system for identifying cellular surface markers, a number of which define lymphocyte subsets (see 15.8.7, Lymphocytes).[7-12] The system and its nomenclature were formalized in a 1982 international workshop. Originally CD terms specified the monoclonal antibodies (mAbs) that clustered statistically in their reactivities to target cells. More recently, the CD terms apply to the cellular molecules themselves. The CDs, which now number more than 200 (and may eventually number in the thousands[12]), are defined at the Human Cell Differentiation Molecules workshops (formerly Human Leukocyte Differentiation Antigen Workshops). Workshops involve "multiple laboratories examining coded panels of antibodies [with] multilaboratory blind analysis and statistical evaluation of the results."[11(p226)] Although reactivity and cellular expression originally were key in identifying CDs, gene-based molecular relatedness has become an important determinant.[11,12]

See the Human Cell Differentiation Molecules Web site (http://www.hlda8.org) for updates on the most recent workshop and conference, including confirmed, validated antibodies and newly assigned CDs.[13]

Some CDs are known most commonly by their CD designation. Other molecules have been assigned CD numbers retroactively; although they will be referred to by their common names, it is useful for authors to include the CD designations.[11] Terms related to CDs do not need to be expanded. See the following examples.

CD Terms	*Other Name(s)*[13]
CD1a	
CD3d	CD3 complex
CD4	(see also 15.8.7, Lymphocytes)
CD6	
CD8α	(see also 15.8.7, Lymphocytes)
CD10	CALLA (common acute lymphoblastic leukemia antigen), neprilysin; enkephalinase; membrane metalloendopeptidase
CD16a	FcγRIIIa (an Fc receptor; see also 15.8.6, Immunoglobulins)
CD35	C3b/C4b receptor; complement receptor type 1 (CR1; see also 15.8.3, Complement)
CD41	glycoprotein IIb (see also 15.1.2, Platelet-Specific Antigens)
CD44R	CD44 variant; CD44v1-10
CD46	membrane cofactor protein (MCP; see also the "Complement Regulators" section in 15.8.3, Complement)
CD50	intracellular adhesion molecule 3 (ICAM-3)
CD55	delay accelerating factor (DAF; see also 15.8.3, Complement)
CD62P	P-selectin; granule membrane protein-140 (GMP-140)
CD79a	Igα (see also 15.8.6, Immunoglobulins); MB-1

CD Terms	*Other Name(s)*[13]
CD97	BL-KDD/F12
CD107a	lysosomal-associated membrane protein 1 (LAMP-1)
CD120a	tumor necrosis factor receptor (TNFR) type 1; TNFR p55
CD139	
CD195	CCR5 (see 15.8.1, Chemokines)
CD213a2	IL-13Rα2 (see also the "Interleukins" section in 15.8.4, Cytokines)
CD220	insulin receptor
CD235a	glycophorin a
CD240CE	Rh blood group, CcEe antigens (see also 15.1.1, Blood Groups)

A lowercase w (for "workshop") signifies a provisional cluster (which is likely to become final, and have the w dropped, in an upcoming workshop[11]):

CDw186

The new designation of CDw128A is CD181.

Complexes of more than 1 CD molecule are indicated with a forward slash or virgule:

CD11a/CD18 (leukocyte functional antigen 1 [LFA-1])

CD11b/CD18 (CR3 or C3bi receptor; see 15.8.3, Complement)

CD49c/CD29

The CD nomenclature displaced previous terms, eg, CD8 for T8 or OKT8, CD4 for T4 or OKT4, CD5 for Leu-1, Lyt-1, CD5 for T1.

For therapeutic monoclonal antibody nomenclature, see 15.4, Drugs.

It is estimated that one C3b deposited on an organism can become four million in about 4 min.
M. K. Liszewski and J. P. Atkinson[14(p922)]

15.8.3 **Complement.**

The term *complement* refers to a group of serum proteins activated sequentially and rapidly in a cascade that produces molecules providing resistance to pathogens.[14-16] The system was named in 1899 for its complementarity with antibodies in destroying microbes.[15]

Current nomenclature derives largely from the 1968 World Health Organization Bulletin "Nomenclature of Complement,"[17] with subsequent modifications as mechanisms of action were further elucidated.

Three complement activation pathways are recognized: the classical pathway (activation by antibody), the alternative pathway (despite the name, the more phylogenetically ancient), and the lectin pathway. They culminate in a common terminal pathway. Components of the classical and terminal pathways are designated with a C and a number, reflective of the order of discovery of the component rather than the reaction sequence. (The prime, as in C′, has been discontinued.) Letters and abbreviations other than C typify the components of the other pathways. Complement component terms need not be expanded:

Pathway	*Components*
classical	C1, C4, C2
alternative	factors D, B, P (P for properdin ["destruction-bringing"[14]])
Lectin or MBLectin	mannose-binding lectin (MBL), MBL-associated serine protease 1 (MASP-1), MASP-2, MASP-3
terminal	C5, C6, C7, C8, C9
	C3 (common to all pathways)

Fragments. Appended lowercase letters indicate complement fragments. Usually, a lowercase b indicates the larger, active (membrane-binding) fragment and a lowercase a, the smaller, release fragment (released on cleavage of the parent molecule). However, C2 is inconsistent: C2a is the larger active fragment and C2b the smaller release fragment. Other letters represent fragments of b fragments.

C3a	C3b	C3c	C3d	Cdg	C3f
C4a	C4b	C4c	C4d		
C5a	C5b				
	Bb				

Subunits. The subunits of C1 are as follows:

C1q C1r C1s

Various notations combining the C1 subunits convey the stoichiometry (relative quantities of subunits) of the complex; all such styles are acceptable:

$(C1r)_2$

$C1r_2C1s_2$

$C1qC1r_2C1s_2$

$C1qr_2s_2$

C1s-C1r-C1r-C1s

Isotypes of C4 have capital letters appended:

C4A C4B

Protein chains have Greek letters appended:

C8α

C8β

C8γ

C3α is the α chain of C3.

Cleavage of C3α produces C3a and C3b.

An i signifies inactive forms:

iC3 *or* C3i

iC3b

Complement components that form a complex are written in a series without spaces:

C4b2a3b

C4bC2

Sometimes a hyphen is used to indicate a series:

C5b67 or C5b-7

C5-9

An asterisk shows nascent or metastable state:

C4b*

C3b*

C5b*

C5b-7*

Convertase complexes are linked complement fragments that activate other complement components. For example, the convertase that activates C3 is known as C3 convertase. As in the following examples, the convertases have different compositions, depending on which complement pathway generated them:

	Classical Pathway	*Alternative Pathway*
C3 convertase	C4b2a	C3bBb
		C3bBbP
		C3(H_2O)Bb(Mg^{2+})
C5 convertase	C4b2a3b	C3bBbC3b
		(C3b)2Bb

(*Note:* Occasionally, authors have changed the designation of the activated moiety of C2 from C2a to C2b, to be consistent with other complement components.[18,19(p8)] A tipoff to the change is the designation of classical pathway C3 convertase as C4b2b.)

A bar over the suffix was proposed in 1968 to designate activated complement, eg:

$C\overline{4}$ $C\overline{423}$ $C\overline{4b2a}$

but this convention has fallen from use.

Complement Regulators. Complement regulators include the following:

Name	*Other Terms*
C1 inhibitor (C1-INH)	C1 esterase inhibitor, C1 esterase INH
C3 membrane proteinases	

Name	*Other Terms*
C4 binding protein (C4bp)	
carboxypeptidases	
CD59	membrane inhibitor of reactive lysis (MIRL), membrane attack complex-inhibitory factor (MACIF), homologous restriction factor 20 (HRF20), P18, protectin
decorin	
delay accelerating factor (DAF)	CD55
factor H	formerly β_1H
factor I [letter I, not roman numeral "one"]	
factor H-like protein (FHL-1)	
membrane cofactor protein (MCP)	CD46
S protein*	vitronectin
SP-40,40	clusterin

(*Not the same as protein S; see 15.7.4, Hemostasis, Inhibition of Coagulation and Fibrinolysis.)

Complement Receptors. Complement receptors include the following:

Name	*Other Terms*
complement receptor type 1 (CR1)	C3b receptor, CD35
CR2	C3d receptor, CD21, CD21S (short isoform), CD21L (long isoform)
CR3	Mac-1, CD11b/CD18
CR4	p150/95, CD11c/CD18
C3Ar	
C4Ar	
C5Ar	CD88
cC1Qr	collectin receptor; c prefix: collagen region of C1q
gC1Qr	g prefix: globular head portion of C1q
$C1qR_p$	
factor H receptor (fH-R)	

. . . some viruses subvert the immune response by producing homologs of mammalian cytokines or their receptors.

J. J. Oppenheim and M. Feldmann[20(p7)]

15.8.4 **Cytokines.** Cytokines are proteins or glycoproteins produced after stimulation (such as activation of immune cells) that act at short distances in very low concentrations to produce various effects, such as immune and inflammatory reactions, repair processes, and cell growth and differentiation.[6,20-25] Each cytokine has multiple effects and overlaps with other cytokines, including structurally dissimilar ones, in those effects. The multiple effects (pleiotropy) are explained by the presence of cytokine receptors on a wide variety of cells, and the overlap (redundancy) by structural similarities of the intracellular portions of cytokine receptors.[26]

Cytokines were originally named by function. Because of their multiple and overlapping functions,[20] the interleukin nomenclature[27,28] was proposed to simplify terminology of this major class of cytokines and, it was hoped, subsequent regulatory immune system proteins. The more recent grouping of cytokines by receptor families and signaling pathways, however, does not necessarily correspond to previous groupings; eg, the interleukins fall into more than one family.

Cytokine Families and Subfamilies. Molecular similarity of cytokine receptors has resulted in their grouping into families and subfamilies[26]:

chemokine families (see 15.8.1, Chemokines)
interleukin 1/toll-like receptors (IL-1/TLR)
platelet-derived growth factor family (PDGF)
receptor tyrosine kinases
transforming growth factor β (TGF-β) receptor serine kinase family
tumor necrosis factor (TNF)
type 1 (hematopoietins)
  β_c-utilizing (common cytokine receptor β chain)
  γ_c-utilizing (common cytokine receptor γ chain)
  gp130-utilizing
  heterodimeric
  homodimeric
type 2 (interferons; IL-10 family receptors)
  heterodimeric

Cytokine signaling pathways are associated with the families and subfamilies.

Cytokine Signaling Pathways	*Expansion or Origin of Term*	*Associated Cytokine Family*
caspases		TNF
FADD	Fas-associated death domain	TNF
FAST-1	forkhead activin signal transducer	TGF-β receptor serine kinase family
IRAK	IL-1 receptor-associated kinase	IL-1/TLR
Jak1	Janus kinase 1	type 1
Jak2	Janus kinase 2	type 1
Jak3	Janus kinase 3	type 1

Cytokine Signaling Pathways	*Expansion or Origin of Term*	*Associated Cytokine Family*
MyD88	myeloid differentiation marker	IL-1/TLR
NF-κB	nuclear factor κB	IL-1/TLR
Ras/Raf/MAPK	ras protein, raf protein (see also 15.6.3, Oncogenes and Tumor Suppressor Genes), mitogen-activated protein kinases	type 1, receptor tyrosine kinases
SARA	SMAD anchor for receptor activation	TGF-β receptor serine kinase family
SMADs	mothers against decapentaplegic (dpp) signaling (MAD) in *Drosophila* and *Sma* genes from *Caenorhabditis elegans*[29]	TGF-β receptor serine kinase family
STAT1	signal transducer and activator of transcription 1	type 1
STAT2		type 1
STAT3		type 1
STAT4		type 1
STAT5		type 1
STAT5a		type 1
STAT5b		type 1
STAT6		type 1
TAK1	TGF-β-associated kinase	TGF-β receptor serine kinase family
TRADD	TNF receptor-associated death domain	TNF
TRAFs	TNF-α receptor-associated factors	TNF
TRAF6		IL-1/TLR
Tyk2	tyrosine kinase 2	type 1

The pathway terms need not be expanded, but context should be clear at first mention, eg:

the Jak1 signaling pathway

Chemokines. See 15.8.1, Chemokines.

Colony-Stimulating Factors. Colony-stimulating factors (CSFs) stimulate growth and differentiation of 1 or more blood cell types (neutrophils, eosinophils, monocytes/macrophages). Terms often include the letters SF, but not always (eg, interleukins 3, 4, and 5—IL-3, IL-4, IL-5—which are also CSFs). Expand CSF terms at first mention:

granulocyte-macrophage colony-stimulating factor	GM-CSF
granulocyte colony-stimulating factor	G-CSF
macrophage colony-stimulating factor	M-CSF

Hormones. These hormones are also considered cytokines:

erythropoietin	Epo
growth hormone	GH
leptin	
prolactin	PrL
thrombopoietin	Tpo

Interleukins. A subset of cytokines were designated as interleukins in 1978 for "their ability to act as communication signals between different populations of leukocytes."[27(p2929)] The interleukins have other biological effects as well. Their nomenclature was formalized in 1991.[28] They are designated by number in order of discovery, eg, interleukin 1, interleukin 18, interleukin 29, but in general have no structural or functional relationship to one another. Although most have now been recognized as members of larger cytokine families, they retain their original designations. Specific interleukins are mentioned most commonly in their abbreviated form (note hyphen):

IL-1
IL-18
IL-29

The IL-1 family includes 2 forms of IL-1:

IL-1α
IL-1β

and the IL-1 receptor antagonist:

IL-1ra

Receptors for interleukins are designated, at minimum, with the interleukin name plus a capital R, eg:

IL-2R
IL-4R

Receptor names designating subtypes may be even more specific:

IL-1RI
IL-1RII

Greek letters are used for subunits (chains) of the same receptor:

IL-2Rα	IL-2Rβ
IL-6Rα	IL-6Rβ
IL-12Rβ1	IL-12Rβ2

Terms for interleukins from different species should be expanded at first mention:

human IL-2	hIL-2
mouse IL-4	mIL-4
viral IL-10	vIL-10

For terminology for therapeutic interleukins, see 15.4.13, Drugs, Nomenclature for Biological Products.

Interferons. Interferons (IFNs) are another group of cytokines, originally discovered (and named) because of their interference with viral replication.

The type I IFNs, also known as *antiviral interferons,* are as follows:

IFN-α
IFN-β
IFN-λ1 (IL-29)
IFN-λ2 (IL-28A)
IFN-λ (IL-28B)
IFN-κ
IFN-ω
IFN-τ

Type II IFN, also known as *immune interferon,* is

IFN-γ

For terminology for therapeutic interferons, see 15.4.13, Drugs, Nomenclature for Biological Products.

Other Cytokines. Other cytokines include the following:

Term	*Abbreviation*
cardiotrophin 1	CT-1
ciliary neurotrophic factor	CNTF
endothelial growth factor	EGF
FLT-3/FLT-2 ligand	FL
high mobility group box chromosomal protein 1	HMGB-1
leukemia inhibitory factor	LIF
lymphotoxin α	LTα
oncostatin M	OSM
receptor activated nuclear factor-κB ligand	RANKL
stem cell factor	SCF, c-kit ligand
transforming growth factor β	TGFβ, TGFβ1, TGFβ2, TGFβ3
tumor necrosis factor α	TNF-α
tumor necrosis factor β	TNF-β

*[I]n transplantation, **H**istocompatibility **L**eads to **A**cceptance; in anthropology, **H**uman populations are **L**ocated by **A**llelic variation; in disease, **HLA** alleles in **L**inkage disequilibrium **A**ccount for disease. . . .*

Julia G. Bodmer[30(p7)]

15.8.5 **HLA/Major Histocompatibility Complex.** Antigens of what is known as the HLA system appear on virtually all nucleated cells of human tissues and on platelets. Just as red blood cell antigens determine blood type (see 15.1, Blood Groups, Platelet Antigens, and Granulocyte Antigens), HLA antigens determine tissue type.

HLA antigens were discovered to be determinants of the success of tissue transplantation (histocompatibility, *histo-* meaning "relating to tissue"). They were subsequently found to be critical for activating many immune responses, and certain HLA antigens are associated with particular diseases. Because of the great variation among individuals in these antigens (polymorphism), they have been used in forensic identification.

The molecules of the HLA system are encoded by at least 47 genes (among more than 200 genes, some related to immunity, some not) in a region of the short arm of chromosome 6 known as the *major histocompatibility complex* (MHC). Genes of the HLA system have multiple alleles, ie, are polymorphic; nearly 2000 had been officially named by 2005.[31] The magnitude of this polymorphism distinguishes the HLA system from other gene families and has resulted in a detailed system for naming alleles and antigens.

Originally identified by serologic and cellular assays, HLA alleles came to be defined by DNA sequencing techniques. Accordingly, in 1987, new nomenclature for these alleles consistent with the International System for Human Gene Nomenclature (see 15.6.2, Genetics, Human Gene Nomenclature) was built onto the original nomenclature.[32,33] A prime goal was for the nomenclature to reflect the relationship between serologically defined antigen specificities and those defined by DNA technology.[30] With increased emphasis on DNA technology, new alleles do not always have known serologic counterparts.[34]

Nomenclature. Nomenclature of the HLA system, first formalized in 1967,[35] is determined by the World Health Organization Nomenclature Committee for Factors of the HLA System. Full reports on HLA nomenclature, which present officially recognized antigens and alleles, appear annually, with monthly updates, in the journals *Human Immunology, European Journal of Immunogenetics,* and *Tissue Antigens* and are available on the Internet[36] on the Web site of the Anthony Nolan Research Institute[37] and at the IMGT/HLA Sequence Database at http://www.ebi.ac.uk/imgt/hla.[38] These reports are based on international workshops that take place every few years, with the participation of more than 400 laboratories.[36]

HLA. This abbreviation has come to signify *human leukocyte antigen(s),* but "HLA antigens" is a common and acceptable expression. (The original term was HL-A, the A being a simple letter designation, not an abbreviation for "antigen."[33]) The term

HLA applies both to the antigens on cells and to the loci (MHC) on the human genome responsible for those antigens. The term Mhc is used in nonhuman animals (see the "Animals" section below).

HLA Class I Antigens (Class I MHC Antigens). The class I antigens are as follows:

classical:	HLA-A	HLA-B	HLA-C
nonclassical (or class Ib):	HLA-E	HLA-F	HLA-G

The components of a class I MHC molecule include the following:

α chain or heavy chain (coded in the MHC) domains: α_1, α_2, α_3

β_2 chain (β_2 microglobulin; coded on chromosome 15, not on the MHC)

HLA Class II Antigens (Class II MHC Antigens). The class II antigens are as follows:

classical:	HLA-DR	HLA-DQ	HLA-DP
nonclassical:	HLA-DO	HLA-DM	

(DR originally signified "D-related"; the others were named alphabetically.)

The components of a class II MHC molecule include the following:

α chain domains: α_1, α_2

β chain domains: β_1, β_2

(*Note:* The α and β chains of class I and class II molecules are not identical, despite the similar naming convention, but rather are distinct proteins.)

Serologically Defined HLA Antigens. Antigen specificities of the major HLA loci are indicated with numbers following the major locus letter(s), eg:

HLA-A1 HLA-B27 HLA-DR1

A w (for "workshop") is used for 2 specificity groups:

HLA-C (to distinguish the C antigens from complement), eg, HLA-Cw1

HLA-Bw4 and Bw6

Parenthetical numbers indicate subtypes or "splits" of a given serologically defined antigen:

HLA-A23(9)	(A23 is a split of A9)
HLA-A24(9)	(A24 is a split of A9)
HLA-B49(21)	(B49 is a split of B21)
HLA-Cw9(w3)	(Cw9 is a split of Cw3)
HLA-DR14(6)	(DR14 is a split of DR6)
HLA-DQ7(3)	(DQ7 is a split of DQ3)

The term *cross-reactive group* (CREG) refers to serologically related groups of antigens. The abbreviation should be expanded at first mention. Note the following sample terms:

the HLA-A1 cross-reactive group (CREG)

the HLA-A2 CREG

the B5 cross-reactive group HLA-B51, B52, and B53

B7 CREG

Phrases such as the following may be used:

HLA-A, HLA-B, and HLA-C associations

possible associations with HLA-B18 and HLA-A2, and HLA-DQB1

testing for HLA-A (A2, A26) and HLA-B (B35, B44)

high prevalence of HLA-A1 (63%) and HLA-B8 (42%)

frequencies of HLA-A2 and A29

HLA Haplotypes. The HLA haplotype is the set of HLA alleles on 1 chromosome. Each person possesses 2 such haplotypes, 1 from each parent, and thus has 2 HLA antigens determined by each major locus, ie, 2 HLA-A antigens, 2 HLA-B antigens, etc. When HLA typing is performed serologically, antigen specificities of the individual's phenotype are presented as follows:

Phenotype	*Notes*
A3, A23, B51, B7, Cw2, Cw5, DR7, DR11	all antigens listed collectively
A23, B7, Cw5, DR7/A3, B51, Cw2, DR11	virgule separates antigens of one chromosome from those of other chromosome
A3, A23, B51, B7, Cw2, Cw5, DR11,-	hyphen indicates undetermined antigen
A1, B8, Cw4, DR17(3)/A2, B27, Cw5,-	DR for this haplotype not typed or untypable
A1, B8, Cw4, DR17(3)/A2, B27, Cw5, DR17(3)	2 identical DR specificities

Shorter haplotype expressions are shown below:

HLA-Cw6-bearing haplotype

the A1-B8-DR3 haplotypes

DRB1, DQA1, and DQB1 haplotypes

A25 B18 BFS DR11 haplotype

Other Histocompatibility Loci. HLA antigens represent only some of the products of the MHC. Others, also important in immunity, are as follows:

Class I loci

MIC (MHC class I-related chain)
specificities: MICA, MICB, MICC, MICD, MICE

Class II loci

TAP (transporter associated with antigen processing)
specificities: TAP1, TAP2

PSMB (proteosome-related sequence)
specificities: PSMB8 (formerly LMP7), PSMB9 (formerly LMP2)

Class III loci (loci for 4 components of complement; see also 15.8.3, Complement):

C2

C4

Bf (B factor, properdin)

A haplotype of complement types is called a *complotype,* eg:

BfS, C2C, C4AQO, C4B1

(QO designates a deficiency.)

Genetic and Allele Nomenclature. Use italics to distinguish HLA genes or gene loci from protein products, eg, *HLA-A, HLA-DRB1* (see also 15.6.2, Genetics, Human Gene Nomenclature). HLA alleles are distinguished from HLA antigens by their names, eg, the HLA-A1 antigen is coded by the HLA-A*0101 allele. The hyphen is retained in HLA gene expressions, an exception permitted in official gene nomenclature. Terms with asterisks indicate that HLA typing has been performed by molecular techniques. Terms with 2 digits (eg, A*02) indicate antigen typing with known serologic equivalent. Terms with 4 digits (eg, A*0201) represent alleles. In contrast to other alleles, HLA alleles are usually not italicized. Authors should make clear from context whether the gene or its product is being discussed.

The following tabulation, adapted from Marsh,[37] summarizes nomenclature for HLA designations:

Term	*Indicates*	*Change From Previous Nomenclature (If Any)*	*Former Term (If Any)*
HLA	HLA region, prefix for *HLA* gene		
HLA-DRB1 or *DRB1*	a particular HLA locus, ie, DRB1 (B refers to the β-chain locus; see directly below tabulation)		

Term	*Indicates*	*Change From Previous Nomenclature (If Any)*	*Former Term (If Any)*
HLA-DRB1*13	a group of alleles at the DRB1 locus that encode the DR13 antigen (antigen conferring DR13 specificity)		
HLA-DRB1*1301	a specific HLA allele, ie, DRB1*1301		
HLA-DRB1*1301N	a null (N) allele		
HLA-DRB1*130102	5th and 6th digits (02) indicate synonymous mutation	5th digit only (2) for synonymous mutation	HLA-DRB1*13012
HLA-DRB1*13010102	allele with mutation outside coding region		
HLA-DRB1*13010102N	null allele with mutation outside the coding region		
HLA-A*24020102L	low expression (L)		
HLA-B*44020102S	secreted (S)	new as of 2002 report	
	cytoplasm (C)	new as of 2002 report	
	aberrant (A) expression	new as of 2002 report	
HLA-A*3211Q	unconfirmed, ie, questionable (Q) effect of allele with mutation		
sHLA-G*0101	soluble (s) form		
mHLA-G*0101	membrane-bound (m) form		

For the HLA-D region, the gene name includes a letter for the chain that the gene codes for (A for α, B for β), often followed by a number for the chain gene (*not* the domain number, as described in the previous section on class I and class II molecules). For instance,

DRB1 gene for first DR β chain

DQA1 gene for first DQ α chain

The HLA prefix (including the hyphen) may be dropped from allele designations in series after first mention, eg:

comparative frequencies of HLA-DRB1*14, DQA1*03, DQA1*05, DQA1*01, DQB1*06

(*not:* HLA-DRB1*14, -DQA1*03, -DQA1*05, -DQA1*01, -DQB1*06)

The conjunction *and* may be used to separate haplotypes but is not used before the final element in any single haplotype:

HLA-B38, DRB1*0402, DRB4*0101, DQB1*0201, DQB1*0302 [*not* and DQB1*0302]

HLA-B38, DRB1*0402, DRB4*0101, DQB1*0201, DQB1*0302 and HLA-B*0702, DRB1*1601, DRB5*02, DQB1*0502 haplotypes

The portion of the term before the asterisk may be dropped in a series, provided it would be the same in each term:

DRB4*01010101, *01030102N, *010302, *010303, *0105

Commas signify *and*, and virgules (forward slashes) signify *or*.[39] Thus, commas indicate corresponding alleles from chromosome pairs (see the "Haplotypes" section above), eg:

Donor: A*01, 02; B*08, 44; DRB1*01, 03; DRB3.

Recipient: A*02, 11; B*40, 15; DRB1*09, 11; DRB3, DRB4

Virgules (forward slashes) indicate an ambiguous result in HLA typing, eg:

Term	*Meaning*
A*0201/0203/0205 (*also* A*0201/03/05)	A*0201 or A*0203 or A*0205 is present

Serologically defined antigens and the corresponding alleles may or may not be structurally similar and therefore may or may not be numerically similar.[37] Also, alleles not defined serologically may have no known associated antigenic specificity:

Specificity	*Allele Name*
A203	A*0203
B78	B*7801, B*780201, B*780202
B65(14)	B*1402
B50(21)	B*5001
DR53	DRB4 (various, eg, DRB4*0102, *010303)
none	the E alleles (E*0101, 0102, etc)
none	the F allele F*0101
none	the G alleles (G*010101, 010102, etc)

HLA pseudogenes (see also 15.6.2, Genetics, Human Gene Nomenclature) resemble and are located near the HLA loci but are not transcribed to produce functional products. The class I pseudogenes end in letters after *G*, and the class II pseudogenes end in numbers after *1*:

HLA-H	*HLA-J*	*HLA-K*	*HLA-L*	*HLA-N*
HLA-S	*HLA-X*	*HLA-Z*		

HLA-DRB2	*HLA-DRB6*	*HLA-DRB6*	*HLA-DRB8*	*HLA-DRB9*
HLA-DQA2	*HLA-DQB2*	*HLA-DQB3*	*HLA-DPA2*	*HLA-DPB2*

Animals. In animals, major histocompatibility locus is abbreviated Mhc, using uppercase and lowercase.

The names for the Mhc in other animals[40] usually correspond to the expression HLA for humans (but not always, eg, the prototypical mouse locus, H-2). In this convention, the name is based on a common name or species name combined with LA (leukocyte antigen):

cat	FLA
dog	DLA
domestic cattle	BoLA
domestic fowl	B
guinea pig	GPLA
horse	EqLA
mole rat	Smh
mouse	H-2
pig	SLA
rabbit	RLA
rat	RT1

Primate researchers use an alternative style based on the genus and species name (see 15.14, Organisms and Pathogens), which substitutes Mhc for LA.[40] Note the following examples:

Common Animal Name	*Species Designation*	*Mhc Term*	*Former LA Term*
chimpanzee	*Pan troglodytes*	MhcPatr	ChLA
gorilla	*Gorilla gorilla*	MhcGogo	GoLA
orangutan	*Pongo pygmaeus*	MhcPopy	OrLA
rhesus macaque	*Macaca mulatta*	MhcMamu	RhLA

. . . the antibody in serum is a mixture of perhaps 100 million slightly different types of molecule . . .
J. H. L. Playfair and B. M. Chain[41(p38)]

Plasma cells can release up to 2000 antibody molecules per second . . .
J. H. L. Playfair and B. M. Chain[41(p43)]

You are the antibody.
Smash Mouth

15.8.6 Immunoglobulins. Immunoglobulins are the glycoproteins that constitute antibodies. They were first recognized by serum electrophoresis and, because they were localized to the electrophoretic gamma zone, were originally referred to as γ-globulins.[42-47]

The term *immunoglobulin* and terminology for immunoglobulin classes were put forth in the 1960s.[48-53] The use of the abbreviation Ig (pronounced [eye-gee][54]) in preference to γ was suggested to avoid confusion with the IgG heavy chain, γ[55] (see the "Heavy Chains" section below). The class of immunoglobulin molecules most abundant in serum was named IgG, the G deriving from the electrophoretic gamma mobility. The M in IgM originates in an earlier designation as a macroglobulin.

The 5 classes of immunoglobulins, from most to least abundant, are as follows:

Class	*Origin of Name*[48,54]
IgG	gamma electrophoretic mobility
IgA	from β_{2A}-globulin, later α-immunoglobulin
IgM	macroglobulin
IgD	"process of elimination"[54(p66)]: B reserved for mice, C had no Greek equivalent
IgE	E-reactive antibody associated with erythema of allergy

Each can be found either on a cell surface (where it serves as an antigen receptor) or in tissue fluids such as blood (where it serves as a protective antibody).

Figure 7 shows schematically the basic structural unit of all immunoglobulin molecules, including many components defined herein. An immunoglobulin can be composed of 1 such unit (monomer) or more.

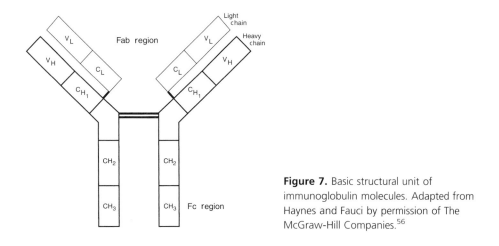

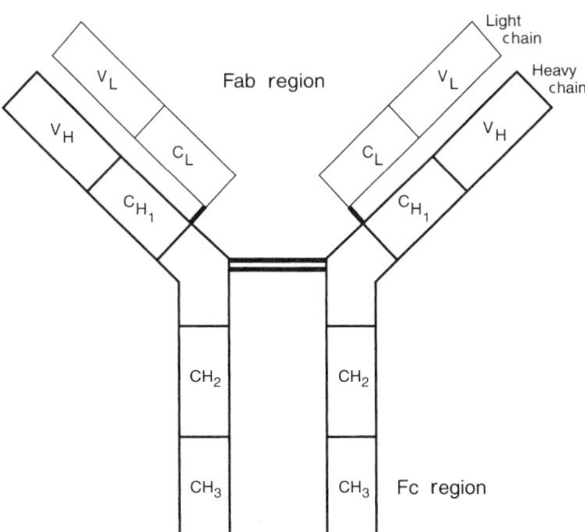

Figure 7. Basic structural unit of immunoglobulin molecules. Adapted from Haynes and Fauci by permission of The McGraw-Hill Companies.[56]

Enzyme cleavage and antibody engineering result in fragments of the immunoglobulin molecule with specific names. Expansion of these terms is not necessary:

Fab	antigen-binding fragment
Fab′	Fab with part of hinge
$F(ab')_2$	2 linked Fab′ fragments

Fabc	
Fb	
Fc	crystallizable fragment
F′c	
pFc′	
Fd	
Fv	variable part of Fab
scFv	single-chain Fv

Each immunoglobulin monomer contains 2 heavy chains and 2 light chains, abbreviated as follows:

H L

Each H chain and L chain in turn contains both constant and variable regions, abbreviated as follows:

C V

Regions of the Ig molecule may be indicated as follows:

V_H	variable region of heavy chain
V_L	variable region of light chain
C_H	constant region of heavy chain
C_L	constant region of light chain

Immunoglobulins have 3 or 4 C_H domains, depending on isotype, abbreviated as follows:

C_H1 C_H2 C_H3 C_H4

Heavy Chains. The type of heavy chain identifies the class (isotype) of immunoglobulin. Heavy chains are named with the Greek letter that corresponds to the class of immunoglobulin:

Heavy-Chain Name	*Immunoglobulin Class*
γ	IgG
α	IgA
μ	IgM
δ	IgD
ε	IgE

IgG and IgA subclasses and corresponding heavy chains are as follows:

Heavy-Chain Name	*Immunoglobulin Subclass*
γ1	IgG1
γ2	IgG2

Heavy-Chain Name	*Immunoglobulin Subclass*
$\gamma3$	IgG3
$\gamma4$	IgG4
$\alpha1$	IgA1
$\alpha2$	IgA2

C_H domains may be specified according to isotype:

$C_\varepsilon 2$ $C_\mu 4$ $C_\alpha 3$ $C_\gamma 3$

Light Chains. There are 2 types of light chain (named for initials of the discoverers' surnames[55]):

κ λ

Both types of light chain are associated with all 5 immunoglobulin classes; that is, an immunoglobulin molecule of any type might have κ or λ light chains (but not both types in the same molecule). In humans, there are 6 classes (isotypes) of λ chain:

λ1 λ2 λ3 λ4 λ5 λ6

C_L and V_L regions may be specified by light chain type, as follows:

C_κ C_λ

V_κ V_λ

The 3 specific hypervariable regions within the variable regions of an immunoglobulin H or L chain are known as complementarity-determining regions (CDRs) and are named as follows:

CDR1 CDR2 CDR3

Heavy- and light-chain CDRs are termed HCDR1, etc, and LCDR1, etc, respectively.

The 4 framework regions (relatively invariable regions between hypervariable regions) are designated as follows:

FR1 FR2 FR3 FR4

Ig Prefixes. The following are examples of terms combining Ig and a single-letter prefix. It is best to expand these terms at first mention (especially those with the letters m or s, each of which has more than 1 meaning):

mIgM	monomeric IgM
mIgM	membrane-bound IgM
pIg	polymeric immunoglobulin
pIgA	polymerized IgA
pIgR	receptor for polymeric immunoglobulin
sIg	surface immunoglobulin
sIgM	surface IgM
sIgA	secretory IgA

Other Immunoglobulin Components. The secretory forms of IgM and IgA contain an additional polypeptide, the J chain (not to be confused with the joining or J segments of the immunoglobulin gene loci; see the "Immunoglobulin Genetics" section below).

Secreted IgA also contains a secretory component, SC.

Molecular Formulas. These indicate the number of polypeptide chains that constitute an immunoglobulin molecule:

γ_2L_2	IgG monomer with 2 γ chains and 2 light chains
α_2L_2	IgA monomer with 2 α chains and 2 light chains
$(\alpha_2L_2)_2SCJ$	IgA dimer with 4 α chains, 4 light chains, an SC, and a J chain
$(\mu_2L_2)_5$	IgM pentamer with 10 μ chains and 10 light chains
$(\mu_2L_2)_5J$	IgM pentamer with 10 μ chains, 10 light chains, and a J chain
$\delta_2\kappa_2$	IgD monomer with 2 δ chains and 2 κ light chains
$\varepsilon_2\lambda_2$	IgE monomer with 2 ε chains and 2 λ light chains

Fc Fragments and Fc Receptors. Fc fragments may be specified by the heavy-chain class from which they arise[57]:

Fcγ1 Fcγ2 Fcγ3 Fcγ4

Fcα1 Fcα2

Fcμ

Fcδ

Fcε

Receptors for the Fc portion of immunoglobulin molecules are named as follows (cell surface marker identities, if applicable, are shown in parentheses; see 15.8.2, CD Cell Markers):

IgG receptors:

FcγRI	(CD64)
FcγRII	(CD32)
FcγRIIIA *or* FcγRIIIa	(CD16a)
FcγRIIIB *or* FcγRIIIb	(CD16b)

IgA receptor:

FcαR (CD89)

IgM receptor:

FcμR

IgE receptors:

FcεRI

FcεRII (CD23)

The 2 transmembrane accessory proteins associated with surface immunoglobulins on some immune cells should not be confused with terms for immunoglobulin classes or heavy chains:

Igα	(immunoglobulin-associated α; CD79a; this is not IgA or the α heavy chain)
Igβ	(immunoglobulin-associated β; CD79b)

Serologic markers associated with some heavy and light chains are indicated with roman letters and a lowercase m:

Marker	*Associated Chain*
G1m	γ1
G2m	γ2
G3m	γ3
A2m, A2m(1), A2m(2)[58]	α2
Em	ε
Km	κ

Immunoglobulin Genetics. Each immunoglobulin light chain gene is made up of a variable (V), joining (J), and constant (C) gene segment. Each immunoglobulin heavy chain is made up of V, J, C, and D (diversity) gene segments. These segments can be referred to as follows:

V_H V_L J_H J_L C_H C_L D_H

or, more specifically, as in the following (subscript numbers refer to the class of Ig):

V_κ V_λ J_κ $C_{\lambda 2}$ C_μ $C_{\alpha 2}$

Subgroups (various nonallelic forms) of V, D, J, and C gene segments are specified numerically (subscript numbers refer to the class of Ig, numbers set on the line refer to the subgroup), as in:

$V_\kappa 1$ $V_\lambda 3$ $D_H 1$ $D_H 3$ $C_{\alpha 2} 5$ $C_{\lambda 1} 1$ $C_\lambda 2$ $J_\kappa 2$ $J_H 1$

A superscript plus sign may be used to indicate expression of a specific segment, eg, by a particular B lymphocyte (see 15.8.7, Lymphocytes):

$V_\kappa 3^+$

The V, D, and J gene segments are brought together by DNA rearrangement. Descriptive terms for this process include the following:

V/J exon, segment, region, gene, recombination	in L-chain genes
V/D/J exon, segment, region, gene, recombination	in H-chain genes
V/(D)/J	L- and/or H-chain genes

VDJ, V/D/J, V-D-J, variable-diversity-joining	alternative terms

A leader segment (L), which codes for a leader (L) peptide, precedes each V segment. Note the following potential sources of confusion:

V, D, and J segments code for the variable (V) region of an immunoglobulin protein.

J segment does not refer to the J chain of the secretory forms of IgA and IgM (see the "Other Immunoglobulin Components" section above).

L (leader) gene segment and L (light) immunoglobulin chain are different entities. (Subscript L's, as in various terms in this section, typically refer to the light chain.)

Official Gene Terminology. Official gene symbols for specific genes of the types discussed above are presented in the following table (see 15.6.2, Genetics, Human Gene Nomenclature). Follow author usage.

Official Gene Symbol	*Immunogenetic Term*
IGHA1	$C_\alpha 1$
IGHD	C_δ
IGHD1-1	member of D_H1 subgroup
IGHE	C_ε
IGHG1	$C_\gamma 1$
IGHJ1	J_H1
IGHV@	V_H
IGHV1-2	member of V_H1 subgroup
IGKC	C_κ
IGKJ@	J_κ
IGKJ2	$J_\kappa 2$
IGKV@	V_κ
IGKV1-5	member of $V_\kappa 1$ subgroup
IGLC@	C_λ
IGLC1	$C_\lambda 1$
IGLJ@	J_λ
IGLJ1	$J_\lambda 1$
IGLV@	V_λ
IGLV1-36	member of $V_\lambda 1$ subgroup

Alleles. Alleles are indicated with an asterisk and number following the gene name:

IGHA1*01

IGHD*02

IGHD1-7*01

IGHE*03

IGHG3*04

IGHM*03

IGLJ1*01

IGLV2-11*01

For more detailed molecular information about immunoglobulin genetics, consult the International ImMunoGeneTics database (http://imgt.cines.fr).[59]

The normal adult human body contains on the order of a trillion (10^{12}) lymphocytes. . . . Together, the thymus and marrow produce approximately 10^9 mature lymphocytes each day, which are then released into the circulation.

Tristram G. Parslow[60(pp40-41)]

15.8.7 Lymphocytes

Lymphocytes. Lymphocytes are the cells that carry out antigen-specific immune responses.[60-62] The 2 main types are the T lymphocyte and the B lymphocyte, also called the T cell and the B cell. A hyphen does not appear in these terms, unless they are used adjectivally.

T lymphocyte	T cell	T-cell lymphoma
B lymphocyte	B cell	B-cell signaling

Historically, the letters T and B reflected the anatomic sites of maturation of the 2 groups of cells, the thymus and the bursa of Fabricius, respectively. (The bursa of Fabricius is an organ of birds.) Because in human adults B cells mature in the bone marrow, the letter B is sometimes taken as signifying *bone marrow.*

A third group of lymphocytes is known as natural killer cells, abbreviated NK cells.

B Lymphocytes. In the context of B-lymphocyte development, the prefixes pre- and pro- are encountered; note hyphenation:

pro-B cell

pre-B cell

B-cell subsets are named in various ways, eg:

$CD5^+$ B cells

B1 B cells

B-cell antigen receptors (BCRs) are membrane complexes of membrane immunoglobulins and the molecules Igα and Igβ (see 15.8.6, Immunoglobulins).

T Lymphocytes. The main types of T lymphocyte are as follows (expand at first mention):

helper T cells: T_H cells

cytotoxic T cells: T_C cells, also called cytotoxic lymphocytes (CTL)

Most helper T cells express the cell marker CD4, and most cytotoxic T cells express the cell marker CD8 (see 15.8.2, CD Cell Markers), giving rise to the following terms:

CD4 cells   CD8 cells

When presence or absence of a marker on a T cell is emphasized, superscript plus or minus signs are used. Presence and absence of the CD4 and CD8 markers are often indicated by the terms *positive* and *negative* (eg, "double-positive lymphocyte"), as below:

$CD4^+$		
$CD4^-$		
$CD4^+CD8^-$	single positive	a CD4 cell
$CD4^-$ $CD8^+$	single positive	a CD8 cell
$CD4^-$ $CD8^-$	double negative	
$CD2^+CD4^-$ $CD8^-$	double negative	
$CD4^+CD8^+$	double positive	
$CD2^+CD4^+CD8^-$	single positive	a CD4 cell
$CD2^+CD4^-$ $CD8^+$	single positive	a CD8 cell
$CD3^+CD4^+CD8^-$	single positive	a CD4 cell
$CD3^+CD4^-CD8^+$	single positive	a CD8 cell

Because other cells, eg, monocytes, may express CD4, authors should use terms more specific than "CD4 cells," unless context has made clear which cells are referred to, eg:

CD4 lymphocyte count (*not* CD4 cell count)

Subtypes of helper T cells are as follows:

T_H0 T_H1 T_H2 T_H3

The theoretical helper T precursor to these subtypes is abbreviated:

T_Hp

T-Cell Receptors. T-cell receptors (TCRs) are protein complexes on the surface of T cells.[63] The T-cell receptor-CD3 complex (abbreviated TCR-CD3) is a structure that recognizes antigen. Its subunits, or chains, are designated by Greek letters:

α chain

β chain

γ chain

δ chain

ε chain

ζ chain

η chain

(Do not confuse these chains with the components of MHC or Ig molecules, although there is some homology among them; see 15.8.5, HLA/Major Histocompatibility Complex, and 15.8.6, Immunoglobulins.)

The α and β chains are also referred to as follows:

TCRα and TCRβ

Linked α and β chains and linked γ and δ chains result in these terms:

αβ dimer	γδ dimer
αβ heterodimer	γδ heterodimer
αβ receptor	γδ receptor
αβ cell	γδ cell
αβ T cell	γδ T cell
T αβ	T γδ
CD8αβ	

The γ, δ, ε, ζ, and η chains constitute the CD3 complex. The CD3 chains are also referred to individually and as dimers:

CD3γ CD3δ CD3ε CD3ζ CD3η

CD3γε CD3δε CD3ζζ CD3ζη

There are 2 subtypes of the γ chain:

γ1 γ2

The TCR protein has variable (V) and constant (C) regions or domains. The gene for TCRα is made up of variable (V), joining (J), and constant (C) segments, as is the β chain, which also has a diversity (D) segment. (These are analogous to the segments of the immunoglobulin genes; see 15.8.6, Immunoglobulins.) These segments may also be referred to as follows:

V_α V_β J_α J_β D_β C_α C_β

Subgroups (various nonallelic forms) of the V, D, or J segments are specified numerically, eg:

$V_\alpha 2$ $J_\beta 7$

T-cell expression of a particular segment may be indicated by using a superscript plus sign:

$V_\beta 2^+$

T-Cell Receptor Gene Terminology. Because the V, D, and J gene segments together encode the variable (V) region of the protein, it is unusual to refer to D or J regions of the protein.[63]

The V, D, and J gene segments are brought together by DNA rearrangement. Descriptive terms include the following:

V/J exon, segment, region, gene, recombination	for α or γ chain genes

V/D/J exon, segment, region, gene, recombination	for β or δ chains
V/(D)/J	of α and γ or β and δ chains
VDJ, V/D/J,V-D-J, variable-diversity-joining	alternative terms

Official Gene Terminology. Official gene symbols for specific genes of the types discussed above are presented in 15.6.2, Genetics, Human Gene Nomenclature. The TCR genes begin with *TR* and use roman letters that correspond to the Greek letters of the TCR component chains, and they contain V, C, D, and J corresponding to the above terms. Like other immune genes, they may contain hyphens:

TRAC *TRBC* *TRBV10-3* *TRGC1* *TRGJ* *TRDC*

Alleles. Alleles are indicated with an asterisk and number following the gene name:

TRBV7-1*01

REFERENCES

1. IUIS/WHO Subcommittee on Chemokine Nomenclature. Chemokine/chemokine receptor nomenclature. *J Interferon Cytokine Res.* 2002;22(10):1067-1068.
2. Zlotnik A, Yoshie O. Chemokines: a new classification system and their role in immunity. *Immunity.* 2000;12(2):121-127.
3. Murphy PM. Chemokines. In: Paul WE, ed. *Fundamental Immunology.* 5th ed. Philadelphia, PA: Lippincott Williams & Wilkins; 2003:801-840.
4. Rich RR, Fleisher T, Shearer WT, Kotzin BL, Schroeder HW Jr, eds. *Clinical Immunology: Principles and Practice.* St Louis, MO: Mosby; 2001.
5. Thomson AW, Lotze MT. *The Cytokine Handbook.* 4th ed. San Francisco, CA: Academic Press; 2003.
6. Cytokine Family Database (dbCFC). http://cytokine.medic.kumamoto-u.ac.jp. Updated February 27, 2006. Accessed April 3, 2006.
7. Bernard A, Boumsell L. The clusters of differentiation (CD) defined by the First International Workshop on Human Leukocyte Differentiation Antigens. *Hum Immunol.* 1984;11(1):1-10.
8. Bernard A, Bernstein I, Boumsell L, et al. Differentiation human leukocyte antigens: a proposed nomenclature. *Immunol Today.* 1984;5(6):158-159.
9. IUIS/WHO Subcommittee on CD Nomenclature. Nomenclature for clusters of differentiation (CD) of antigens defined on human leukocyte populations. *Bull World Health Organ.* 1984;62(5):809-811.
10. Singer NG, Todd RF, Fox DA. Structures on the cell surface: update from the Fifth International Workshop on Human Leukocyte Differentiation Antigens. *Arthritis Rheum.* 1994;37(8):1245-1248.
11. Zola H. The CD nomenclature: a brief historical summary of the CD nomenclature, why it exists and how CDs are defined. *J Biol Regul Homeost Agents.* 1999;13(4): 226-228.
12. Zola H, Swart B. The human leucocyte differentiation antigens (HLDA) workshops: the evolving role of antibodies in research, diagnosis and therapy. *Cell Res.* 2005;15(9):691-694.

13. HCDM: Human Cell Differentiation Molecules. http://www.hlda8.org/. Accessed May 27, 2006.
14. Liszewski MK, Atkinson JP. The complement system. In: Paul WE, ed. *Fundamental Immunology*. 3rd ed. New York, NY: Raven Press; 1993:917-939.
15. Prodinger WM, Würzner R, Erdei A, Dierich MP. Complement. In: Paul WE, ed. *Fundamental Immunology*. 4th ed. Philadelphia, PA: Lippincott-Raven; 1999: 967-996.
16. Prodinger WM, Würzner R, Stoiber H, Dierich MP. Complement. In: Paul WE, ed. *Fundamental Immunology*. 5th ed. Philadelphia, PA: Lippincott Williams & Wilkins; 2003:1077-1103.
17. World Health Organization. Nomenclature of complement. *Bull World Health Organ*. 1968;39(6):935-938.
18. Letendre P. Complement: to be or not to be? *Transfusion*. 1990;30(5):478-479.
19. Playfair JHL, Lydyard PM. *Medical Immunology Made Memorable*. 2nd ed. New York, NY: Churchill Livingstone; 2000.
20. Oppenheim JJ, Feldmann M. Introduction to the role of cytokines in innate host defense and adaptive immunity. In: Durum SK, Hirano T, Vilcek J, Nicola NA, eds. *Cytokine Reference: A Compendium of Cytokines and Other Mediators of Host Defense*. San Diego, CA: Academic Press; 2001:3-20.
21. Leonard WJ. Type I cytokines and interferons and their receptors. In: Paul WE, ed. *Fundamental Immunology*. 4th ed. Philadelphia, PA: Lippincott-Raven; 1999: 741-774.
22. Krakauer T, Vilcek J, Oppenheim JJ. Proinflammatory cytokines: TNF and IL-1 families, chemokines, TGF-β, and others. In: Paul WE, ed. *Fundamental Immunology*. 4th ed. Philadelphia, PA: Lippincott-Raven; 1999:775-812.
23. O'Shea JJ, Frucht DM, Duckett CS. Cytokines and cytokine receptors. In: Rich RR, Fleisher TA, Shearer WT, Kotzin BL, Schroeder HW Jr, eds. *Clinical Immunology: Principles and Practice*. 2nd ed. St Louis, MO: Mosby; 2001:12.1-12.22.
24. Rich RR, Fleisher TA, Shearer WT, Kotzin BL, Schroeder HW Jr, eds. *Clinical Immunology: Principles and Practice*. 2nd ed. St Louis, MO: Mosby; 2001:A12-A14.
25. Leonard WJ. Type I cytokines and interferons and their receptors. In: Paul WE. *Fundamental Immunology*. 5th ed. Philadelphia, PA: Lippincott Williams & Wilkins; 2003:701-474.
26. Fitzgerald KA, O'Neill LAJ, Gearing AJH, Callard RE. *The Cytokine FactsBook*. 2nd ed. San Diego, CA: Academic Press; 2001.
27. Aarden LA, Brunner TK, Cerottini J-C, et al. Revised nomenclature for antigen-nonspecific T cell proliferation and helper factors [letter]. *J Immunol*. 1979;123(6): 2928-2929.
28. Paul WE, Kishimoto T, Melchers F, et al. Nomenclature for secreted regulatory proteins of the immune system (interleukins). *Clin Exp Immunol*. 1992;88(2):367.
29. Lagna G, Hata A, Hemmati-Brivanlou A, Massague J. Partnership between DPC4 and SMAD proteins in TGF-beta signalling pathways. *Nature*. 1996;383(6603): 832-836.
30. Bodmer WF. HLA 1991. In: Tsuji K, Aizawa M, Sasazuki S, eds. *HLA 1991: Proceedings of the Eleventh International Histocompatibility Workshop and Conference Held in Yokohama, Japan, 6-13 November, 1991*. New York, NY: Oxford University Press; 1992:7-16.

31. Marsh SGE, Albert ED, Bodmer WF, et al. Nomenclature for factors of the HLA system, 2004. *Tissue Antigens.* 2005;65(4):30-369. doi:10.1111/j.1399-0039.2005.00379.x.
32. Bodmer WF, Albert E, Bodmer JG, et al. Nomenclature for factors of the HLA system, 1987. *Hum Immunol.* 1989;26(1):3-14.
33. International Histocompatibility Working Group. A brief history of the international histocompatibility workshops. http://www.ihwg.org/history/history.htm. Accessed April 6, 2006.
34. Marsh SGE, Albert ED, Bodmer WF, et al. Nomenclature for factors of the HLA system, 2002. *Tissue Antigens.* 2002;60(5):407-464. doi:10.1034/j.1399-0039.2002.600509.x.
35. Bodmer JG. Nomenclature 1991 foreword. *Hum Immunol.* 1992;34(1):2-3.
36. Marsh SGE, Parham P, Barber LD. *The HLA FactsBook.* San Diego, CA: Academic Press; 2000.
37. Marsh SGE. Nomenclature for factors of the HLA System. http://www.anthonynolan.com/HIG/lists/nomenc.html. Updated January 1, 2006. Accessed April 6, 2006.
38. Robinson J, Waller MJ, Parham P, et al. IMGT/HLA and IMGT/MHC: sequence databases for the study of the major histocompatibility complex. *Nucleic Acids Res.* 2003;31(1):311-314. Also available at http://nar.oupjournals.org/cgi/content/full/31/1/311?ijkey=W/BIuukIQ8mf2&keytype=ref&siteid=nar. Accessed April 6, 2006.
39. Tiercy J-M, Marsh SGE, Schreuder GMT, Albert E, Fischer G, Wassmuth R. Guidelines for nomenclature usage in HLA reports: ambiguities and conversion to serotypes. *Eur J Immunogenet.* 2002;29(3):273-274.
40. Klein J, Bontrop RE, Dawkins RL, et al. Nomenclature for the major histocompatibility complexes of different species: a proposal. *Immunogenetics.* 1990;31(4):217-219.
41. Playfair JHL, Chain BM. *Immunology at a Glance.* 7th ed. Malden, MA: Blackwell Science; 2001.
42. Haynes BF, Fauci AS. Introduction to the immune system. In: Kasper DL, Braunwald E, Fauci AS, Hauser SL, Longo DL, Jameson JL, eds. *Harrison's Principles of Internal Medicine.* 16th ed. New York, NY: McGraw-Hill; 2005:1907-1930.
43. Frazer JK, Capra JD. Immunoglobulins: structure and function. In: Paul WE, ed. *Fundamental Immunology.* 4th ed. Philadelphia, PA: Lippincott-Raven; 1999:37-74.
44. Nairn R, Helbert M. *Immunology for Medical Students.* St Louis, MO: Mosby; 2002.
45. Lefranc M-P, Lefranc G. *The Immunoglobulin FactsBook.* San Diego, CA: Academic Press; 2001.
46. Parslow TG. Immunoglobulins and immunoglobulin genes. In: Parslow TG, Stites DP, Terr AI, Imboden JB, eds. *Medical Immunology.* 10th ed. New York, NY: Lange Medical Books/McGraw-Hill; 2001:95-114.
47. Kolar GR, Capra JD. Immunoglobulins: structure and function. In: Paul WE, ed. *Fundamental Immunology.* 5th ed. Philadelphia, PA: Lippincott Williams & Wilkins; 2003:47-68.
48. Kao NL. How immunoglobulins were named. *Ann Intern Med.* 1992;117(5):445.
49. Ceppellini R, Dray S, Edelman G, et al. Nomenclature for human immunoglobulins. *Bull World Health Organ.* 1964;30:447-449.
50. Ishizaka K, Ishizaka T, Hornbrook MM. Physico-chemical properties of human reaginic antibody, IV: presence of a unique immunoglobulin as a carrier of reaginic activity. *J Immunol.* 1966;97(1):75-85.

51. Rowe DS, Fahey JL. A new class of human immunoglobulins, I: a unique myeloma protein. *J Exp Med.* 1965;121:171-184.
52. Rowe DS, Fahey JL. A new class of human immunoglobulins, II: normal serum IgD. *J Exp Med.* 1965;121:185-199.
53. Kunkel HG, Fahey JL, Franklin EC, Osserman EF, Terry WD. Notation for human immunoglobulin subclasses [letter]. *Int Arch Allergy Appl Immunol.* 1967;32(2): 247-248.
54. Black CA. A brief history of the discovery of the immunoglobulins and the origin of the modern immunoglobulin nomenclature. *Immunol Cell Biol.* 1997;75(1):65-68.
55. Recommendations for the nomenclature of human immunoglobulins. *Biochemistry.* 1972;11(18):3311-3312.
56. Haynes BF, Fauci AS. Introduction to the immune system. In: *Harrison's Online.* http://harrisons.accessmedicine.com. Accessed September 20, 2004.
57. IUIS Subcommittee on Nomenclature. Nomenclature of the Fc receptors. *Bull World Health Organ.* 1989;67(4):449-450.
58. IUIS/WHO Subcommittee on IgA Nomenclature. Nomenclature of immunoglobulin A and other proteins of the mucosal immune system. *J Immunol Methods.* 1999;223(2):263-264. Also published in *Eur J Immunol.* 1999;29(3):1057-1058.
59. LeFranc M-P. International ImMunoGeneTics Information System. http://imgt.cines.fr. Accessed April 6, 2006.
60. Parslow TG. Lymphocytes and lymphoid tissues. In: Parslow TG, Stites DP, Terr AI, Imboden JB, eds. *Medical Immunology.* 10th ed. New York, NY: Lange Medical Books/McGraw-Hill; 2001:40-60.
61. DeFranco AL. B-cell development and the humoral immune response. In: Parslow TG, Stites DP, Terr AI, Imboden JB, eds. *Medical Immunology.* 10th ed. New York, NY: Lange Medical Books/McGraw-Hill; 2001:115-130.
62. Imboden JB, Seaman WE. T lymphocytes and natural killer cells. In: Parslow TG, Stites DP, Terr AI, Imboden JB, eds. *Medical Immunology.* 10th ed. New York, NY: Lange Medical Books/McGraw-Hill; 2001:131-147.
63. LeFranc M-P, LeFranc G. *The T Cell Receptor FactsBook.* San Diego, CA: Academic Press; 2001.

15.9 **Isotopes.**

Isotopes may be referred to in the medical literature alone or as a component of a radiopharmaceutical administered for therapeutic or diagnostic purposes. The nomenclature for the isotopes incorporated in radiopharmaceuticals follows the international nonproprietary name (INN) drug nomenclature and therefore differs from that of isotopes that occur as elements alone.

15.9.1 **Elements.**

An isotope referred to as an element rather than as part of the name of a chemical compound may be described at first mention by providing the name of the element spelled out followed by the isotope number in the same typeface and type size (no hyphen, subscript, or superscript is used). The element abbreviation may be listed in parentheses at first mention and used thereafter in the article, with the isotope number preceding the element symbol as a superscript.

> Of the 13 known isotopes of iodine, only iodine 128 (^{128}I) is not radioactive. The investigators used ^{128}I to avoid the difficulty and expense of disposing of radioactive waste.

The symbol representing a single element should not be used as an abbreviation for a compound (eg, do not abbreviate the compound sodium arsenate As 74 as ^{74}As).

15.9.2 **Radiopharmaceuticals.** The INN designations for radioactive pharmaceuticals consist of "the name of the compound serving as the carrier for the radioactivity, the symbol for the radioactive isotope, and the atomic weight."[1(p11)] Since the nonproprietary name comprises all these components, the complete name should be provided at first mention unless the radiopharmaceuticals being referred to are a general category. Subsequently, a shorter term may be used, such as *iodinated albumin* or *gallium scan*.

Although the nonproprietary name for the radiopharmaceutical may appear to contain redundant information, maintaining consistent terminology is important for clarity. For example, technetium Tc 99m is contained in more than 40 nonproprietary radiopharmaceuticals, from technetium Tc 99m albumin to technetium Tc 99m teboroxime.[1(pp844-846)] The isotope number appears in the same type (not superscript) as the rest of the drug name, and it is not preceded by a hyphen. A few commonly used drugs appear below. For drugs not listed here, consult the most recent edition of the *USP Dictionary*.[1]

> cyanocobalamin Co 60
>
> fibrinogen I 125
>
> fludeoxyglucose F 18
>
> gallium citrate Ga 67
>
> indium In 111 altumomab pentetate
>
> indium In 111 satumomab pentedine
>
> iodohippurate sodium I 131
>
> potassium bromide Br 82
>
> sodium iodide I 125
>
> Strontium chloride 89 can be used to treat pain from skeletal metastases.
>
> In an earlier study, 50 patients underwent lung imaging with technetium Tc 99m sulfur colloid.
>
> The patient underwent an exercise stress test with injection of thallous chloride Tl 201 (thallium stress test).

In a discussion that does not refer to administration of a specific drug, the more general term may be used.

> For a patient recuperating from a myocardial infarction who wishes to begin an exercise program, a treadmill test with or without thallium imaging may be useful to determine whether the patient is at high risk for recurrent ischemia.

At the beginning of a sentence, the name rather than the element symbol should be used.

> The patient was treated with sodium iodide I 131 after she was found to have hyperthyroidism. Iodine 131 levels were then monitored by measuring the amount of radioactivity in the patient's urine.

15.9.3 Radiopharmaceutical Compounds Without Approved Names. Compounds may be combined with radioisotopes for research purposes. Such compounds would not receive an INN if no commercial use is intended. In lieu of an INN, standard chemical nomenclature should be followed (see 15.9.1, Elements, or consult the *CRC Handbook of Chemistry and Physics*[2] for more information).

After first mention, the name of the substance can be abbreviated. Use the superscript form of the isotope number to the left of the element symbol. Enclose the isotope symbol in brackets and close up with the compound name if the nonradioactive isotope of the element is normally part of the compound.

glucose labeled with radioactive carbon (^{14}C) [or glucose tagged with carbon 14]

[^{14}C]glucose (not glucose C 14)

Use no brackets and separate the element and compound name with a hyphen if the compound does not normally contain the isotope element.

amikacin labeled with iodine 125

^{125}I-amikacin

If uncertain as to whether the isotope element is normally part of a compound, consult the *USP Dictionary*[1] for drugs and *The Merck Index*[3] for other compounds.

15.9.4 Radiopharmaceutical Proprietary Names. In proprietary names of radiopharmaceuticals, isotope numbers may appear in the same position as in the approved nonproprietary names, but they are usually joined to the rest of the name by a hyphen and are not necessarily preceded by the element symbol. Follow the *USP Dictionary*[1] or the usage of individual manufacturers.

Proprietary	*Nonproprietary (Preferred)*
Iodotope I-131	sodium iodide I 131
Glofil-125	iothalamate sodium I 125

15.9.5 Uniform Labeling. The abbreviation ul (for uniformly labeled) may be used without expansion in parentheses:

[^{14}C]glucose (ul)

Similarly, terms such as *carrier-free*, *no carrier added*, and *carrier added* may be used. In general medical publications, these terms should be explained at first mention, since not all readers will be familiar with them.

15.9.6 Hydrogen Isotopes. Two isotopes of hydrogen have their own specific names, deuterium and tritium, which should be used instead of "hydrogen 2" and "hydrogen 3." In text, the specific names are also preferred to the symbols ^2H or D (for deuterium, which is stable) and ^3H (for tritium, which is radioactive). The 2 forms of heavy water, D_2O and ^3H_2O, should be referred to by the approved nonproprietary names deuterium oxide and tritiated water, respectively.

15.9.7 Metastable Isotopes. The abbreviation m, as in krypton Kr 81m or technetium Tc 99m, stands for *metastable*. The abbreviation should never be deleted, since the term without the *m* designates a different radionuclide isomer.

REFERENCES

1. *USP Dictionary of USAN and International Drug Names.* 41st ed. Rockville, MD: US Pharmacopoeia; 2005.
2. Lide DR, ed. *CRC Handbook of Chemistry and Physics.* 85th ed. Boca Raton, FL: CRC Press; 2004.
3. O'Neil MJ, Smith A, Heckelman PE, Budavari S, eds. *The Merck Index: An Encyclopedia of Chemicals, Drugs, & Biologicals.* 13th ed. Whitehouse Station, NJ: Merck & Co Inc; 2001.

Naming things is essential for people to understand one another, no matter what language or field of interest is involved. This is as true for enzymes, genes and chemicals as it is for birds, food, flowers, etc.
Keith Tipton and Sinéad Boyce[1(p34)]

15.10 Molecular Medicine. Molecules and their interactions underlie every area of medicine. Many classes of molecules are described according to rules or conventions, some of which are covered in other sections of this chapter. The Joint Commission on Biochemical Nomenclature (JCBN) formulates nomenclature policy for classes of biochemicals; see http://www.chem.qmul.ac.uk/iupac/jcbn/index.html#1. (JCBN enzyme nomenclature is described in 15.10.3, Enzyme Nomenclature.) The National Center for Biotechnology Information (http://www.ncbi.nlm.nih.gov/) is a searchable information resource on molecular biology with links to databases.

This section provides information on various molecular terms, including expansions, derivations, typography, and usage information (but not rules for naming molecules). It is meant to assist the editor or reader encountering an unfamiliar term and to guide the author in employing such terms. For terms not described herein, helpful sources include the MeSH database of the National Library of Medicine (http://www.ncbi.nlm.nih.gov/entrez/query.fcgi?db=mesh), medical texts and dictionaries, and Internet searches. For a review of molecular biology databases, see the 2005 Database Issue of *Nucleic Acids Research*.[2]

15.10.1 Molecular Terminology: Other Sections of Chapter 15. The following sections of chapter 15 have subsections on molecular terms: 15.2, Cancer; 15.3, Cardiology; and 15.11, Neurology. The following sections of chapter 15 substantially deal with molecular terminology: 15.1, Blood Groups, Platelet Antigens, and Granulocyte Antigens; 15.6, Genetics; 15.7, Hemostasis; and 15.8, Immunology.

The following tabulation gives molecular terms associated with subjects covered elsewhere in this chapter:

Entity	*Section*
amino acids	15.6.1, Genetics, Nucleic Acids and Amino Acids

Entity	*Section*
antitrypsins, antithrombins	15.7.4, Hemostasis, Inhibition of Coagulation and Fibrinolysis
apolipoproteins	15.3.12, Cardiology, Cellular and Molecular Cardiology
bacterial strains and proteins	15.14.2, Organisms and Pathogens, Bacteria: Additional Terminology
blood gas terminology (eg, Pao_2)	15.16, Pulmonary, Respiratory, and Blood Gas Terminology
cancer molecules	15.2.5, Cancer, Molecular Cancer Terminology 15.6.3, Genetics, Oncogenes and Tumor Suppressor Genes
cellular adhesion molecules	15.7.2, Hemostasis, Endothelial Factors 15.8, Immunology
chemokines	15.8, Immunology
chromosomes	15.6.4, Genetics, Human Chromosomes
cloning vectors	15.6.1, Genetics, Nucleic Acids and Amino Acids
clotting factors	15.7.3, Hemostasis, Secondary Hemostasis
clusters of differentiation (CDs)	15.8, Immunology 15.1.2, Blood Groups, Platelet Antigens, and Granulocyte Antigens, Platelet-Specific Antigens
codons	15.6.1, Genetics, Nucleic Acids and Amino Acids
colony-stimulating factors	15.8, Immunology
complement	15.8, Immunology
creatine kinases	15.3.12, Cardiology, Cellular and Molecular Cardiology
cytokines	15.8, Immunology
D-dimer	15.7.4, Hemostasis, Inhibition of Coagulation and Fibrinolysis
DNA	15.6.1, Genetics, Nucleic Acids and Amino Acids
genes	15.6.2, Genetics, Human Gene Nomenclature 15.6.3, Genetics, Oncogenes and Tumor Suppressor Genes 15.6.5, Genetics, Nonhuman Genetic Terms
glycoproteins	15.1.2, Blood Groups, Platelet Antigens, and Granulocyte Antigens, Platelet-Specific Antigens

Entity	*Section*
	15.7.1, Hemostasis, Primary Hemostasis 15.7.2, Hemostasis, Endothelial Factors
guanine nucleotides	15.3.12, Cardiology, Cellular and Molecular Cardiology 15.6.1, Genetics, Nucleic Acids and Amino Acids
hemostatic molecules	15.7.1, Hemostasis, Primary Hemostasis
hepatitis antigens and antibodies	15.14.3, Virus Nomenclature
histones	15.6.1, Genetics, Nucleic Acids and Amino Acids
HLA antigens	15.8, Immunology
immunoglobulins	15.8, Immunology
influenza types and strains	15.14.3, Organisms and Pathogens, Virus and Prion Nomenclature
integrins	15.7.2, Hemostasis, Endothelial Factors
interferon	15.8, Immunology
interleukins	15.8, Immunology
ion channels	15.11.5, Neurology, Molecular Neuroscience
lipoproteins	15.3.12, Cardiology, Cellular and Molecular Cardiology
muscle cell components	15.3.12, Cardiology, Cellular and Molecular Cardiology
mutations	15.6.1, Genetics, Nucleic Acids and Amino Acids
myosin chains	15.7.1, Hemostasis, Primary Hemostasis
neurotransmitters and receptors	15.11.5, Neurology, Molecular Neuroscience
nitric oxide synthase	15.3.12, Cardiology, Cellular and Molecular Cardiology 15.7.2, Hemostasis, Endothelial Factors
nodal cells	15.3.12, Cardiology, Cellular and Molecular Cardiology
nucleic acid technology (eg, polymerase chain reaction [PCR], single nucleotide repeats [SNPs], short tandem repeats [STRs])	15.6.1, Genetics, Nucleic Acids and Amino Acids
nucleosides, nucleotides	15.6.1, Genetics, Nucleic Acids and Amino Acids

Entity	*Section*
phages	15.14.3, Organisms and Pathogens, Virus Nomenclature
phospholipase	15.7.1, Hemostasis, Primary Hemostasis
plasminogen activators	15.3.12, Cardiology, Cellular and Molecular Cardiology 15.7.2, Hemostasis, Endothelial Factors
platelet-activating factors	15.7.1, Hemostasis, Primary Hemostasis
prions	15.14.4, Organisms and Pathogens, Prions
prostaglandins	15.7.1, Hemostasis, Primary Hemostasis
restriction enzymes	15.6.1, Genetics, Nucleic Acids and Amino Acids
retrovirus gene terms	15.6.3, Genetics, Oncogenes and Tumor Suppressor Genes 15.6.5, Genetics, Nonhuman Genetic Terms
RNA	15.6.1, Genetics, Nucleic Acids and Amino Acids
serotonin	15.11.5, Neurology, Molecular Neuroscience
thromboxanes	15.7.1, Hemostasis, Primary Hemostasis
troponins	15.3.12, Cardiology, Cellular and Molecular Cardiology
von Willebrand factor	15.7.3, Hemostasis, Secondary Hemostasis

15.10.2 Molecular Terms: Considerations and Examples. Molecular terms often are more familiar in unexpanded form; their expansions may be obscure. Molecular terms often mix numbers, letters, and cases. They may be abbreviations or abbreviations within abbreviations (for instance, see TAF and subsequent entries in Table 13). Molecular terms differ from standard abbreviations, which typically are uppercase initialisms (eg, premature ventricular contraction, PVC). In contrast, many molecular terms are (or incorporate) contractions of single words, using all lowercase letters or mixing capital and lowercase letters (eg, apo, apolipoprotein; Hb, hemoglobin).

Letter prefixes (including Greek letters) and numeric prefixes are linked to the main term by hyphens.

α_1-antitrypsin

β-catenin

γ-tubulin

glucose 6-phosphate

However, these terms are not hyphenated:

α helix

β sheet

Hyphens are added in adjectival usages, eg:

β-pleated sheet

glucose-6-phosphate dehydrogenase

Hyphens are used as follows in numbers that interrupt a word:

propan-1,2-diol (propanol)

flavan-3-ol

For letter or number suffixes, hyphens typically are not used with expanded terms but are handled in various ways with abbreviated terms (see examples in sections cited in Table 13):

interleukin 1 (IL-1)

phosphodiesterase 3A (PDE3A)

6-keto prostaglandin $F_{1\alpha}$ (6-keto $PGF_{1\alpha}$)

The chemical prefixes L (levo) and D (dextro) are small capitals:

L-folinic acid

D-glyceraldehyde

Element symbols in chemical names, such as *S* (sulfur) and *N* (nitrogen), are italicized. Other capital letters are not italicized.

N-acetyl-D-glucosamine

cytochrome P450

N-terminal, C-terminal

A subscript letter indicates a modifier of the main term.

P_i (inorganic phosphate)

Plus signs and minus signs indicating charges are set superscript. Numerals indicating quantities of an element within a molecule are set subscript. Numerals indicating a charge are superscript.

HCO_3^-

Fe^{3+}

Proteins are often expressed as p plus a numeral signifying the atomic weight in kilodaltons, eg, p53, a 53-kDa protein. Affixes, such as superscripts, further specify the protein (important because different proteins may have the same weight). See the examples in Table 13. Although the gene symbols for such proteins are often given as the same term italicized, eg, the tumor suppressor gene *p53*, the correct gene symbols should be used, eg, in humans *TP53*; in mice, *Tp53*. Use the search feature at the HUGO Gene Nomenclature Committee Web site (http://www.gene.ucl.ac.uk/nomenclature/; see also 15.6, Genetics).

The term *stem cell* has the general meaning of a precursor, pluripotent, or progenitor cell. Research articles should specify the type(s) of stem cell referred to, eg, *adult, embryonic, germline, hematopoietic, mesenchymal, neural, peripheral blood, somatic, umbilical cord–derived, unrestricted somatic*, and so forth. (The preceding terms are not all mutually exclusive.)

Terms in Table 13 are included as a reference. Some context or explanation of such terms is desirable at first mention, but, in contrast to abbreviations (see 14.0, Abbreviations), first mention need not be a literal expansion and the term may be stated as an appositive, rather than in parentheses, eg:

the cyclin-dependent kinase CDK2

When an abbreviation is used in the Suggested Usage at First Mention column, it is assumed that in the article the abbreviated term has already been introduced and defined or expanded; eg, if INK4 is defined as "inhibitors of CDK4" at first mention, it is assumed that CDK4 was previously defined or expanded. Providing more information is often helpful. For instance, at first mention, p21 may be referred to as "the protein p21" or "the CDKI protein p21" or given additional context.

Table 13. Molecular Terms

Term	Explanation	Suggested Usage at First Mention
Aβ peptide, $Aβ_{42}$	amyloid-β peptide	amyloid-β peptide (Aβ), $Aβ_{42}$ peptide, *or* 42-residue form of Aβ
Aβ*56	56-kDa Aβ fragment	56-kDa Aβ fragment
Ach	acetylcholine	acetylcholine
Acrp30 (*or* adiponectin)	adipocyte-complement related 30 kDa-protein	the protein Acrp30 *or* adiponectin
acyl-CoA	acyl derivatives of coenzyme A	acyl coenzyme A
acyl-*S*-CoA	sulfonated acyl-CoA	sulfonated acyl-CoA
ADAMTS [see Apte[3]]	a disintegrinlike and metalloprotease domain (reprolysin-type) with thrombospondin type 1 motifs	ADAMTS protease
specific ADAMTS, eg, ADAMTS-13	ADAMTS-13; trivial name von Willebrand factor (vWF) protease (*see also* 15.7, Hemostasis)	ADAMTS-13 *and/or* vWF protease
adoHcy	*S*-adenosylhomocysteine	S-adenosylhomocysteine
adoMet (also SAM)	*S*-adenosylmethionine	S-adenosylmethionine
Akt kinase	a serine-threonine kinase, also known as protein kinase B, related to *akt* oncogene (origin: AKT retrovirus isolated from AKR mouse thymoma)	Akt protein kinase
allo-SCT	allogenic stem cell transplantation	allogenic stem cell transplantation
ATCase	aspartate transcarbamoylase	aspartate transcarbamoylase
ATPase	adenosine triphosphatase	adenosine triphosphatase
BNP	brain (*or* b-type) natriuretic peptide	brain (*or* b-type) natriuretic peptide

Table 13. Molecular Terms *(cont)*

Term	Explanation	Suggested Usage at First Mention
1,3-BPG	1,3-bisphosphoglycerate	1,3-bisphosphoglycerate
CAK (=cyclinH/CDK7)	CDK-activating enzyme	the CDK-activating enzyme (CAK) cyclinH/CDK7
CaM	calmodulin	calmodulin
CDK2, CDK3, CDK7, etc	cyclin-dependent kinases	the cyclin-dependent kinase CDK2, etc
CDKI	CDK inhibitors (*see also* INK4 below)	CDK inhibitors
CoA	coenzyme A	coenzyme A
COX-1, COX-2	cyclooxygenases 1 and 2	cyclooxygenase 1, cyclooxygenase 2
C-reactive protein	protein reactive to pneumococcal cell wall C polysaccharide	C-reactive protein (CRP)
cyclin D/CDK4/CDK6, cyclin E/CDK2	cyclin-CDK complexes	the cyclin D/CDK4/CDK6 complex; the cyclin E/CDK2 complex
CYP1A2, CYP2C9, CYP2C19, CYP2D6, CYP3A4	isoforms of cytochrome P450 enzymes (*also* cytochrome P450 isozymes) [P: pigment; 450: 450-nm absorbance]	various, eg, cytochrome P450 1A2 isozyme (CYP1A2); cytochrome P450 3A4 isozyme (CYP3A4 *or* P450 3A4 *or* 3A4)
Dkk-1	Dickkopf-1	the inhibitor protein Dkk-1
F_0 (subscript is zero, not capital O)	portion of mitochondrial ATP synthase (F: energy-coupling factor)	context, eg, F_0 portion of mitochondrial ATP synthase, proton channel portion of ATP synthase, etc
F_0F_1	complex portion of mitochondrial ATP synthase	context, eg, F_0F_1 mitochondrial ATP synthase, F_0F_1 complex, etc
F_1	portion of mitochondrial ATP synthase	context, eg, F_1 portion of mitochondrial ATP synthase, catalytic portion of ATP synthase, etc
F1P, F6P	fructose 1-phosphate, fructose 6-phosphate	fructose 1-phosphate, fructose 6-phosphate
FAD	flavin adenine dinucleotide	flavin adenine dinucleotide
$FADH_2$	reduced (hydrogenated) FAD	$FADH_2$ *or* reduced (*or* hydrogenated) FAD
FBPase-1, FBPase-2	fructose 1,6-bisphosphatase, fructose 2, 6-bisphosphatase	fructose 1,6-bisphosphatase, fructose 2,6-bisphosphatase
Fd	ferredoxin	ferredoxin
Fhit	fragile histidine triad protein	fragile histidine triad protein
FMN	flavin mononucleotide	flavin mononucleotide
$FMNH_2$	reduced (hydrogenated) FMN	$FMNH_2$ *or* reduced (*or* hydrogenated) FMN

Table 13. Molecular Terms *(cont)*

Term	Explanation	Suggested Usage at First Mention
Fp	flavoprotein	flavoprotein (Fp)
G_0	quiescent state of cell cycle	G_0 phase
G_1	growth *or* gap 1 phase of cell cycle	G_1 phase
G_2	growth *or* gap 2 phase of cell cycle	G_2 phase
G protein	guanine triphosphate (GTP)-binding protein	G protein
G_α, G_β, G_γ	G protein families	G_α, G_β, G_γ protein *or* family
$G_{\alpha 12}$, $G_{\alpha 13}$	members of G_α	$G_{\alpha 12}$, $G_{\alpha 13}$ protein
$G_{\beta\gamma}$, $\beta\gamma$	G_β subunit or complex	$G_{\beta\gamma}$, $\beta\gamma$ subunit *or* complex
G1P, G6P	glucose 1-phosphate, glucose 6-phosphate	glucose 1-phosphate, glucose 6-phosphate
GalN	D-galactosamine	D-galactosamine
GalNAc	*N*-acetyl-D-galactosamine	*N*-acetyl-D-galactosamine
G_i	inhibitory G protein	inhibitory G protein
Glc *or* D-Glc	D-glucose	glucose *or* D-glucose
G_q, $G_{q/11}$	classes of G protein	G_q, $G_{q/11}$ protein
G_s	stimulatory G protein	stimulatory G protein
GlcA	D-gluconic acid	gluconic acid or *D*-gluconic acid
GlcNAc (also NAG)	*N*-acetyl-D-glucosamine	*N*-acetyl-D-glucosamine GlcNAc
GlcUA	D-glucuronic acid	D-glucuronic acid
Grb2	growth factor receptor-bound protein 2	the protein Grb2
H_2F (also DHF)	dihydrofolate *or* 7,8-dihydrofolate	dihydrofolate (H_2F *or* DHF) *or* 7,8-dihydrofolate (H_2F *or* DHF)
H_4F (also THF)	tetrahydrofolate *or* 5,6,7,8-tetrahydrofolate	tetrahydrofolate *or* 5,6,7,8-tetrahydrofolate
Hb	hemoglobin	hemoglobin
HbA_{1a}, HbA_{1b}, HbA_{1c}	glycated (*not* glycosylated[4-7]) hemoglobin fractions	preferred: glycated hemoglobin A_{1c}, etc (also: glycohemoglobin A_{1c})
HbCO	carbon monoxyhemoglobin, carboxyhemoglobin	carbon monoxyhemoglobin
HbO_2	oxyhemoglobin	oxyhemoglobin
HER2/neu	from human epidermal growth factor receptor 2; preferred term is now ERBB2; *see also* 15.6.3, Genetics, Oncogenes and Tumor Suppressor Genes	ERBB2 (formerly HER2 *or* HER2/neu)

Table 13. Molecular Terms *(cont)*

Term	Explanation	Suggested Usage at First Mention
HMG-CoA	β-hydroxy-β-methylglutaryl-CoA	β-hydroxy-β-methylglutaryl-CoA
IKKβ	IκB kinase β (I: inhibitor)	IκB kinase β
INK4	inhibitors of CDK4 (*see also* CDKI above and $p16^{Ink4}$, etc, below)	inhibitors of CDK4
IGF-1, IGF-2	insulinlike growth factor, type 1 and type 2	insulinlike growth factor 1, insulinlike growth factor 2
IGF-R1, IGF-R2	IGF-1 receptor, IGF-2 receptor	IGF-1 receptor, IGF-2 receptor
IP_3	inositol 1,4,5-triphosphate	inositol 1,4,5-triphosphate
α-KG	α-ketoglutarate	α-ketoglutarate
lac	lactose	lactose
M	mitosis (phase of cell cycle)	M phase
Man	D-mannose	D-mannose
Mb	myoglobin (don't confuse with Mb, megabase, or MB, megabyte)	myoglobin
MbO_2	oxymyoglobin	oxymyoglobin
M-CDK	M-cyclin-CDK complex	M-phase CDK
Mcm proteins	minichromosome maintenance proteins	Mcm proteins
M-cyclin	M-kinase-cyclin complex	M-cyclin
M-kinase	mitosis-phase kinase	M-kinase
Mur	muramic acid	muramic acid
Mur2Ac (also NAM)	*N*-acetylmuramic acid	*N*-acetylmuramic acid
NAD	nicotinamide adenine dinucleotide	nicotinamide adenine dinucleotide *or* the nicotinamide coenzyme NAD
NAD^+	oxidized NAD	NAD^+
NADH	reduced (hydrogenated) NAD	reduced (*or* hydrogenated) NAD *or* NADH
NADH hydrogenase		NADH hydrogenase
NADP	NAD phosphate	NAD phosphate *or* NADP
NADPH	reduced (hydrogenated) NADP	reduced (*or* hydrogenated) NADP *or* NADPH
NAG	(*see* GlcNAc above)	
Neu5Ac	*N*-acetylneuraminic acid (sialic acid)	*N*-acetylneuraminic acid
NFκB	nuclear factor-κB	nuclear factor-κB

Table 13. Molecular Terms *(cont)*

Term	Explanation	Suggested Usage at First Mention
NMDA	*N*-methyl-D-aspartate	*N*-methyl-D-aspartate
NMN	nicotinamide mononucleotide	nicotinamide mononucleotide
NMN^+	oxidized NMN	NMN^+
NMNH	reduced (hydrogenated) NMN	reduced *or* hydrogenated NMN
NMP	nucleoside monophosphate	nucleoside monophosphate
NOx	nitrogen oxides, such as nitrate, nitrite, and nitrosothiols; nitric oxide (NO) metabolites	nitrogen oxides
NPY	neuropeptide Y	neuropeptide Y
NT-proBNP	N-terminal fragment of the prohormone brain natriuretic peptide (*see* 15.6.1, Genetics, Nucleic Acids and Amino Acids under "Amino Acids")	N-terminal fragment of the prohormone brain natriuretic peptide
$p16^{Ink4}$, $p15^{Ink4B}$, $p18^{Ink4C}$, $p19^{Ink4D}$	INK4s	the INK4 $p16^{Ink4}$, etc
p21	21-kDa protein	the protein p21
$p21^{WAFI/CIP1}$, $p27^{KIP1}$, $p57^{KIP2}$	other CDKI; WAFI: wild type p53-activated protein 1; CIP1: CDK-interacting protein 1; KIP: kinase inhibitor protein	the CDKI $p21^{WAFI/CIP1}$, etc
p53	53-kDa protein	the protein p53 (or simply p53 if a similarly named protein has already been introduced)
p57	57-kDa protein	the protein p57 (*or* p57)
PE, PPE	protein or gene family named for amino acid sequence motif (PE: Pro-Glu, PPE: Pro-Pro-Glu); see 15.6.1, Genetics, Nucleic Acids and Amino Acids	PE and PPE protein families, PE/PPE gene families, etc
P-gp	P-glycoprotein	P-glycoprotein
P_i	inorganic phosphate	inorganic phosphate
PI	phosphatidylinositol	phosphatidylinositol
PIP_2	phosphatidylinositol 4,5-bisphosphate	phosphatidylinositol 4,5-bisphosphate
Pol	polymerase (eg, DNA, RNA)	polymerase
PP_i	inorganic pyrophosphate	inorganic pyrophosphate
pRb	retinoblastoma protein	retinoblastoma protein
$PYY_{3\text{-}36}$	NPY receptor agonist (P: peptide; Y: NPY; Y: Y2 receptor; 3-36: 34 amino acid residue numbers)	peptide $YY_{3\text{-}36}$, the gut hormone $PYY_{3\text{-}36}$

Table 13. Molecular Terms *(cont)*

Term	Explanation	Suggested Usage at First Mention
RANKL	receptor-activated nuclear factor-κB ligand	receptor-activated nuclear factor-κB ligand
RecA protein, RecA	recombinase A	recombinase A
RNAi	RNA interference	RNA interference
R point	restriction point (of cell cycle)	R point
RNase	ribonuclease	ribonuclease
rTpo	recombinant thrombopoietin	recombinant thrombopoietin
S	DNA synthesis phase of cell cycle	S phase or DNA synthesis phase
S-cyclin	S-kinase-cyclin complex	S-cyclin
sFlt-1	soluble fms-like tyrosine kinase 1 (fms: McDonough feline sarcoma [oncogene])	soluble fms-like tyrosine kinase 1
S-kinase	synthesis-phase kinase	S-kinase
αSp22	22-kDa glycosylated form of α-synuclein	22-kDa glycosylated α-synuclein
αSyn	α-synuclein	α-synuclein
TAF	TBP-associated factor	TATA-binding protein (TBP)–associated factor
TAF_{II}	a class of TAFs	a class of factors associated with TBP
TATA box	a DNA sequence rich in adenine (A) and thymidine (T)	TATA box
TBP	TATA-binding protein	TATA-binding protein
$TF_{II}D$	complex of TBP and several $TAF_{II}s$	TBP-TAF_{II} complex
UCP-1, UCP-2, UCP-3	uncoupling proteins	uncoupling protein 1, etc
UDP-Gal	uridine diphosphate galactose	UDP-galactose
UDP-Glc	UDP-glucose	UDP-glucose
uE_3	unconjugated estriol	unconjugated E_3
Wnt	named for *Drosophila melanogaster* wingless mutant integration site	the developmental protein Wnt, the Wnt signaling pathway, etc

15.10.3 **Enzyme Nomenclature.**[8] Enzyme nomenclature was formalized in the 1950s.[1] It is formulated by the International Union of Biochemistry (IUB) and the International Union of Pure and Applied Chemistry (IUPAC), more specifically, the Nomenclature Committee of the International Union of Biochemistry and Molecular Biology (NC-IUBMB) and the IUPAC-IUB Joint Commission on Biochemical Nomenclature.

There are around 3500 listed enzymes. Officially assigned names and numbers for enzymes are available at the Enzyme Nomenclature Database: http://www.chem.qmul.ac.uk/iubmb/enzyme/. Rules for enzyme nomenclature are available at http://www.chem.qmul.ac.uk/iubmb/enzyme/rules.html.

There are 3 types of enzyme name: recommended name (common, working, or trivial name), systematic name, and Enzyme Commission (EC) number. The recommended name is the name by which the enzyme is commonly known. The systematic name incorporates the reaction the enzyme catalyzes. The EC number is a unique identifier assigned to each enzyme.

Because systematic names can be unwieldy and recommended names are well known, recommended names are used in general medical publications. For unambiguous identification, the EC number, the systematic name, or both may be included at first mention.

The parts of the EC number are as follows:

class

subclass

sub-subclass

serial number within sub-subclass

The enzyme classes are as follows:

EC1:	oxidoreductases
EC2:	transferases
EC3:	hydrolases
EC4:	lyases
EC5:	isomerases
EC6:	ligases

Examples are shown below:

EC No.	*Recommended Name*	*Systematic Name*
EC 1.11.1.7	peroxidase	donor:hydrogen-peroxide oxidoreductase
EC 2.3.3.10 (was EC 4.1.3.5)	hydroxymethylglutaryl-CoA synthase	acetyl-CoA:acetoacetyl-CoA *C*-acetyltransferase
EC 2.7.1.1	hexokinase	ATP:D-hexose 6-phosphotransferase
EC 3.1.1.7	acetylcholinesterase	acetylcholine acetylhydrolase
EC 3.5.2.6	β-lactamase	β-lactam hydrolase
EC 5.4.2.2	phosphoglucomutase	α-D-glucose 1,6-phosphomutase

EC No.	*Recommended Name*	*Systematic Name*
EC 6.5.1.1	DNA ligase (ATP)	poly(deoxyribonucleotide): poly(deoxyribonucleotide) ligase (AMP-forming)

REFERENCES

1. Tipton K, Boyce S. History of the enzyme nomenclature system. *Bioinformatics.* 2000:16(1):34-40.
2. 2005 Database Issue. *Nucl Acids Res.* http://nar.oxfordjournals.org/content/vol33/suppl_1/. Accessed April 20, 2006.
3. Apte SS. ADAMTS Nomenclature. http://www.lerner.ccf.org/bme/apte/adamts/nomenclature.php. Published September 30, 2004. Accessed April 20, 2006.
4. Fuentes-Arderiu X. "Glycohemoglobin," not "glycated hemoglobin" or "glycosylated hemoglobin." *Clin Chem.* 1990;36(6):1254.
5. Roth M. "Glycated hemoglobin," not "glycosylated" or "glucosylated." *Clin Chem.* 1983;29(11):1991.
6. Sharon N. Nomenclature of glycoproteins, glycopeptides and peptidoglycans. *Pure Appl Chem.* 1988;60(9):1389-1394.
7. Glycated proteins. JCBN/NC-IUB Newsletter 1984. http://www.chem.qmul.ac.uk/iubmb/newsletter/misc/glypro.html. Accessed June 6, 2006.
8. Moss GP; Nomenclature Committee of the International Union of Biochemistry and Molecular Biology (NC-IUBMB) in consultation with the IUPAC-IUBMB Joint Commission on Biochemical Nomenclature (JCBN). Enzyme nomenclature: recommendations of the Nomenclature Committee of the International Union of Biochemistry and Molecular Biology on the Nomenclature and Classification of Enzyme-Catalysed Reactions. http://www.chem.qmul.ac.uk/iubmb/enzyme/. Updated March 13, 2006. Accessed April 20, 2006.

15.11 Neurology

15.11.1 Nerves. Most nerves have names (eg, ulnar nerve or nervus ulnaris). English names are preferred to Latin. For terminology, consult a medical dictionary, anatomy text, or *Terminologia Anatomica.*[1]

Cranial Nerves. The cranial nerves are as follows:

Nerve	*English Name*	*Latin Name*
I	olfactory	olfactorius
II	optic	opticus
III	oculomotor	oculomotorius
IV	trochlear	trochlearis
V	trigeminal	trigeminus
VI	abducens	abducens
VII	facial	facialis
VIII	vestibulocochlear	vestibulocochlearis (acoustic)
IX	glossopharyngeal	glossopharyngeus
X	vagus	vagus

Nerve	*English Name*	*Latin Name*
XI	accessory	accessorius
XII	hypoglossal	hypoglossus

Use roman numerals or English names when designating cranial nerves:

> Cranial nerves III, IV, and VI are responsible for ocular movement.
>
> The oculomotor, trochlear, and abducens nerves are responsible for ocular movement.

Use ordinals when the numeric adjectival form is used:

> The third, fourth, and sixth cranial nerves are responsible for ocular movement.

Vertebrae, Spinal Nerves, Spinal Levels, Dermatomes, and Somites. These entities share a common nomenclature, deriving from spinal anatomic regions: cervical (neck), thoracic (trunk), lumbar (lower back), sacral (pelvis), and coccygeal (coccyx or tailbone).

Spinal nerves C1 through C7 are named for the vertebrae above which they emerge, while T1 through S5 are named for the vertebrae below which they emerge. Spinal nerve C8 emerges below vertebra C7; there is no C8 vertebra.

Vertebrae and spinal nerves are as follows.

Region	*Vertebrae*	*Spinal Nerves*
cervical	C1 through C7	C1 through C8
thoracic	T1 through T12	T1 through T12
lumbar	L1 through L5	L1 through L5
sacrum	S1 through S5	S1 through S5
coccyx	4 fused, not individually designated	coccygeal nerve

The alphanumeric terms need not be expanded and, when clear in context, "vertebra" and "nerve" need not be repeated:

> The first cervical vertebra is also known as the atlas, C2 as the axis, and C7 as the vertebra prominens.

Portions of a vertebra may be referred to as follows, ie, without the term *vertebra*:

> C5 spinous process
>
> L3 lamina
>
> T12 transverse process

Hyphens are used for intervertebral spaces (including neural foramina) and intervertebral disks, as follows:

Space	*Disk*
C2-3 (space between C2 and C3)	C2-3 disk
T2-3 (space between T2 and T3)	T2-3 disk
L2-3 (space between L2 and L3)	L2-3 disk

Space	*Disk*
C7-T1 (space between C7 and T1)	C7-T1 disk
L5-S1 (space between L5 and S1)	L5-S1 disk

L4-5 diskectomy

(*Note: Terminologia Anatomica* uses *disc*, not *disk*. See also 11.0, Correct and Preferred Usage.)

The sacrum, because its vertebrae are fused, does not contain intervertebral spaces. Its 4 paired foramina are commonly referred to as the first sacral foramen (or S1 foramen), second sacral foramen (or S2 foramen), etc.

Ranges of vertebrae are expressed as in the following examples; use letters for both the first and last vertebra in the indicated range:

C3 through C7	third through seventh cervical vertebrae (not C3 through 7)
T6 through S1	sixth thoracic through first sacral vertebrae

Ranges of vertebrae *when used as modifiers* have one or more hyphens, eg:

C1-C3 arthrodesis

C2-T1 spinous processes

C4-T3 fusion

L1-L2-L3 motion segments

L1-L4 bone mass density

L2-S1 canal stenosis

L3-L4-L5 fusion

L4-L5 laminectomy

erosion of T9-T12 vertebrae

The same abbreviations are used for spinal segments or levels, spinal dermatomes, and somites. Text should indicate which is being referred to, eg, vertebra, spinal nerve (or root, radiculopathy, or distribution), spinal level, dermatome, or somite. Within a clear context, as noted above, the words *vertebra*, *nerve*, etc, need not be repeated.

> Serious injury of the cervical cord at the level of the C2-C5 vertebrae causes respiratory paralysis due to injury of spinal nerves C3 through C5.
>
> The first patient had herpes zoster in the T9 dermatomal distribution, the second patient in the C5 distribution.
>
> L1-S2 radiculopathy
>
> L3-L4-L5 periradicular infiltration

15.11.2 Electroencephalographic Terms.[2,3(pp12-34),4,5] Guidelines for electroencephalography (EEG) are available through the American Clinical Neurophysiology Society (formerly the American Electroencephalographic Society; http://www.acns.org)[6] and at the International Federation of Clinical Neurophysiology Web site (IFCN; http://www.ifcn.info; formerly the International Federation of Societies for Electroencephalography and Clinical Neurophysiology).[7]

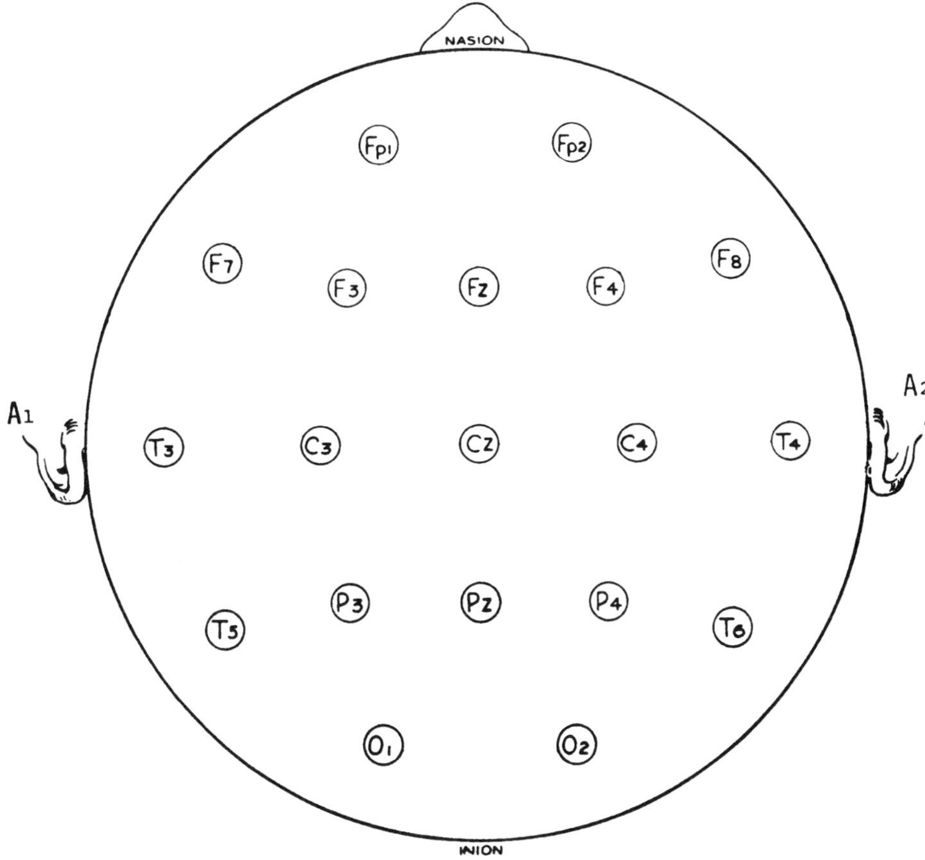

Figure 8. Electroencephalographic lead positions, from *EEG in Clinical Practice,* 2nd ed, by J. R. Hughes, Boston, MA, Butterworth-Heinemann; 1994:2. Reprinted by permission of Elsevier.

The International 10-20 System specifies placement of electrodes used in electroencephalography. The 10-20 System, which originated in the 1950s,[8,9] is so named because electrodes are spaced 10% or 20% apart along the head (Figure 8).

The terms used in the 10-20 System are widely used and recognized. They are systematically derived, as follows:

- Letters refer to anatomic areas (primarily of the skull, which do not necessarily coincide with the brain areas from which the electrodes register electrical activity).
- Odd numbers are for electrodes placed on the left side, even numbers are for electrodes placed on the right side, and the letter z ("zero") is for midline electrodes.

Electrode Designation	*Location*
A1, A2	earlobe
Cz, C3, C4	central
F7, F8	lateral frontal (anterior temporal)

Electrode Designation	*Location*
Fp1, Fp2	frontal pole or prefrontal
Fz, F3, F4	superior frontal
O1, O2	occipital
Pz, P3, P4	parietal
T3, T4	midtemporal
T5, T6	posterior temporal

Additional electrodes and other placement systems may be used, for instance, the "modified combinatorial nomenclature" also known as the extended 10-20 electrode system or the 10% system, which adds electrodes at intermediate 10% positions.[7,10-12] The same electrode may have a different name in the 10-20 and the 10% systems.[4] The added electrodes result in additional numeric designations for existing regional electrodes (eg, C5, F10) and in new letters or letter-number combinations, as in the following examples:

Electrode Designation	*Location*
AFz, AF3, AF4, AF7, AF8	anterior frontal
C1, C2, C5, C6,	centrotemporal
CPz, CP1-CP6	centroparietal
FCz, FC1-FC10	frontocentral
Fpz	midprefrontal
FT7, FT8, FT9, FT10	frontotemporal
Iz	inion
Nz	nasion
Oz	midoccipital
P1, P2, P5-P10	parietal-posterior temporal
POz, PO3, PO4, PO7, PO8	parieto-occipital
Sp1, Sp2	sphenoidal
T1, T2	true anterior temporal
T7-T10	centrotemporal
TP7-TP10	temporal-posterior

Neonatal electrodes may be placed differently (eg, the 12.5% to 25% system of the Children's Hospital of British Columbia) and may (or may not) have different designations,[4] eg:

LaF	left anterior frontal
LaT	left anterior temporal
LFC	left frontocentral
LO	left occipital
LP	left parietal
LST	left superior temporal

RaF	right anterior frontal
RaT	right anterior temporal
RFC	right frontocentral
RO	right occipital
RP	right parietal
RST	right superior temporal

In figures showing EEGs, electrode symbols usually will be paired. Usually, the symbols will be beside and to the left of each channel of the tracing but may be above and below each channel with connecting lines. Authors should include with tracings a time marker and an indicator of voltage, as in the top tracing (Figure 9).

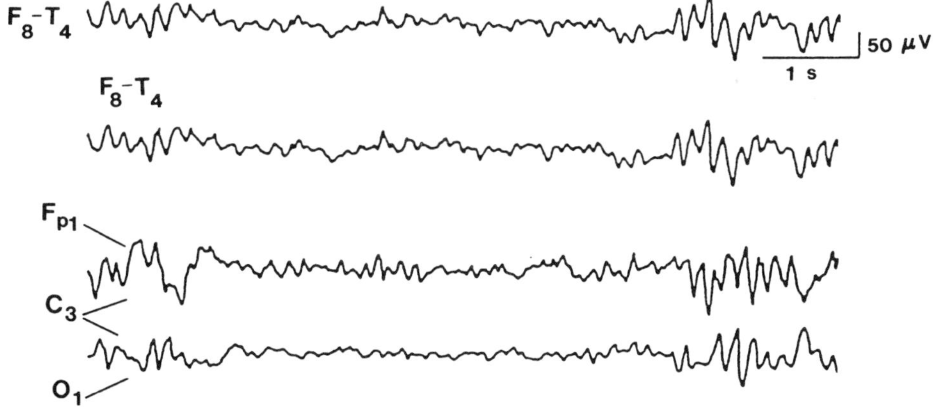

Figure 9. Sample electroencephalographic tracings (schematic).

Descriptions of EEG potentials include many qualitative terms for waveforms and frequencies. The following are a few of numerous descriptive terms (note that Greek letters are spelled out):

> alpha rhythm, beta activity, polymorphic delta activity, sleep spindles, spike-wave complexes, paroxysms, spikes, sharp waves, delta brush, frontal sharp transient, mu rhythm, lambda waves

A comprehensive glossary of EEG terms has been provided by the IFCN.[13]

Frequency is given per second (/s). For cycles (c) per second, hertz (Hz) is preferred to c/s (see 18.1, Units of Measure, SI Units):

> 10-Hz alpha activity
>
> a theta frequency of 5 to 7.5 Hz
>
> 15-Hz spindles
>
> 60-Hz artifact
>
> background rhythm of 8 to 10 Hz

15.11.3 Evoked Potentials.[2(pp34-41),3,14-17] Several types of evoked potentials (stimulated electrical signals) may be recorded: brainstem auditory evoked potentials (BAEPs), somatosensory evoked potentials (SSEPs, including various types such as the following, which are not mutually exclusive: short-latency, upper extremity, lower extremity, median nerve, posterior tibial nerve), and visual evoked potentials (VEPs, including pattern [PVEP] and flash [FVEP]). As in EEG, evoked potential testing uses recording electrodes and produces tracings.

Electrode terminology resembles that of EEGs (see above), with additional or modified electrodes such as the following,[3] which may be used without expansion:

BAEP electrodes:

Ac	contralateral earlobe
Ai	ipsilateral earlobe
EAM	external auditory meatus
EAMc	contralateral EAM
EAMi	ipsilateral EAM
M1 M2	mastoid process
Mc	contralateral M
Mi	ipsilateral M

SSEP electrodes:

AC	anterior cervical
C1′, C2′, C3′, C4′	near EEG C1, C2, C3, C4
C2S, C5S	C2, C5 spinous processes
Cc	contralateral C3′ or C4′
Ci	ipsilateral C3′ or C4′
CP	midway between C3 or C4 and P3 or P4
CPc	contralateral CP
CPi	ipsilateral CP
Cz′	near 10-20 Cz
EP	Erb point
EP1, EP2	left and right EP
EPi	ipsilateral EP
Fpz′	near EEG Fpz
IC	iliac crest
L2S, L3S	L2, L3 spinous processes
LN	lateral neck
LNi	ipsilateral LN
PFd, PFp	popliteal fossa (distal, proximal)
REF	reference
T6S, T10S, T12S	T6, T10, T12 spinous processes

VEP electrodes:

I	inion
LO	left occipital
LT	left posterior temporal
MF	midfrontal
MO	midoccipital
MP	midparietal
RO	right occipital
RT	right posterior temporal
V	vertex

Waveforms recorded in evoked potential testing are identified with P for positive or N for negative plus a number indicating milliseconds between stimulus and response in normal adults:

VEP: N75, N100, N155, P75, P100, P135

SSEP: N9, N11, N13, N15, N18, N20, N34, N35, P9, P11, P13, P15, P27, P37

SSEPs were . . . recorded from the brachial plexus (Erb potential), cervical spine at C2 (N13), and the contralateral parietal area (N19) with a frontal (Fz) reference.

SSEPs showed normal Erb point and cervical potentials and significant delay of scalp components (N20 latency >>3 SDs, N13-N20 central conduction time >3 SDs, bilaterally).

Persistent delay of the P100 wave of the pattern-reversal VEP after an episode of optic neuritis is considered to be compatible with residual demyelination within the optic nerve.

An additional SSEP wave is the LP (lumbar potential).

Other waves, eg, in BAEP, are designated with roman numerals:

I through VII	vertex-positive waves
I′ through VI′	vertex-negative waves

BAEPs of the proband showed normal wave I, increased latency of waves II and III (>3 SDs), and absent IV and V components despite normal hearing acuity.

I-III interpeak interval

V/I amplitude ratio

15.11.4 Polysomnography and Sleep Stages.[3,18] Polysomnography is the monitoring of various physiologic parameters simultaneously during sleep, including the following:

- EEG: standard electrodes are used (see 15.11.2, Electroencephalographic Terms)
- Electro-oculogram (EOG): tracings are obtained from the left eye and right eye
- Electromyogram (EMG): submental (chin) EMG, leg muscle EMG, eg, left anterior tibialis, right anterior tibialis
- Respiratory function, eg, oxygen saturation ($Sa{O_2}$), expired CO_2, and tidal volume (V_T) (see 15.16, Pulmonary, Respiratory, and Blood Gas Terminology)
- Electrocardiogram (ECG): see 15.3.1, Cardiology, Electrocardiographic Terms

Sleep stages are as follows[19]:

rapid-eye movement sleep (REM sleep)

non-rapid eye movement (non-REM) sleep (NREM sleep)
sleep stage 1
sleep stage 2
sleep stage 3
sleep stage 4

15.11.5 Molecular Neuroscience. The following terms are provided for reference (a major source is Nestler et al[20]) (see also 15.10, Molecular Medicine). Terms with asterisks need not be expanded; others should be expanded at first mention.

Term	*Expansion or Explanation*
α-adrenergic receptor, α receptor* (subtypes: α_{1A}, α_{1B}, α_{1D}, α_{2A}, α_{2B}, α_{2C})	
α-synuclein	
A_1, A_2*	neuropeptide adenosine receptors (also known as purine receptors P_1, P_2; see also 15.6.1, Genetics, Nucleic Acids and Amino Acids)
ACh	acetylcholine
AChE	acetylcholinesterase
AMPA	α-amino-3-hydroxy-5-methyl-4-isoxazole propionic acid class of glutamate receptor
β-adrenergic receptor, β receptor* (subtypes: β_1, β_2, β_3)	
BDNF	brain-derived neurotrophic factor
CCR3, CCR5, CXCR4	chemokine receptors (see 15.8.1, Immunology, Chemokines)
Ch1 through Ch8	cholinergic nuclei
CNTF	ciliary neurotrophic factor
COMT	catechol-*O*-methyltransferase
cytokines	(see 15.8.4, Immunology, Cytokines)

Term	*Expansion or Explanation*
δ-receptor	opioid δ receptor
D_1 through D_5	dopamine receptors
DAT	dopamine transporters
EAAT1 EAAT2 EAAT3 EAAT4 EAAT5	excitatory amino acid reuptake transporters
EGF	epidermal growth factor
GABA	γ-aminobutyric acid
$GABA_A$, $GABA_B$	GABA receptor classes
GABAergic	GABA-mediated
GABA-T	GABA transaminase
GAT-1, GAT-2, GAT-3, GAT-4	GABA family transporters
GDNF	glial cell line-derived neurotrophic factor
GFR	GDNF-neurturin receptor
GIRKs	G protein-coupled Kir3 channels
H_1, H_2, H_3	histamine receptors
5-HT	5-hydroxytryptamine, serotonin (preferred expansion)
5-HT_{1A}, 5-HT_{1B}, 5-HT_{2A}, 5-HT_{5B}, 5-HT_7	5-HT receptors
5-HTT	serotonin transporter
5HTTLPR	a polymorphism of the serotonin transporter gene (LPR: length polymorphism region) (see also 15.6.2, Genetics, Human Gene Nomenclature)
interleukins	(see 15.8.4, Immunology, Cytokines)
IP_3	inositol triphosphate
κ-receptor	opioid κ receptor
K(ATP) channel	potassium channel
K(Ca)	Ca^{2+}-gated K^+ channel
Kir1, Kir2, Kir3, Kir4, Kir5*	inwardly rectifying K^+ channels
L channels, L-type channels*	large-current or long-open-time Ca^{2+} channels
μ-receptor	opioid μ receptor
M_1 through M_5*	muscarinic receptors
MAO	monoamine oxidase
MAO_A, MAO_B	major forms of MAO
N channels*	neuronal Ca^{2+} channels
nAChRs	nicotinic acetylcholine receptors

Term	*Expansion or Explanation*
NET	norepinephrine GABA family transporter
neuromedin B*	
neuromedin K*	
neuropeptide Y*	
NGF	nerve growth factor
NK_1 NK_2 NK_3	neuromedin K tachykinin receptors
NMDA	*N*-methyl-D-aspartate class of glutamate receptor
nNOS (*also* NOS1)	neuronal nitric oxide synthetase
NSF	*N*-ethylmaleamide sensitive factor
NT-3, NT-4	neurotrophin 3 and neurotrophin 4
NTS_1, NTS_2	neurotensin receptors
P channels*	Purkinje Ca^{2+} channels
P_1, P_2*	neuropeptide purine receptors (also known as adenosine receptors A_1, A_2; see also 15.6.1, Genetics, Nucleic Acids and Amino Acids)
R-PTK	receptor-associated protein tyrosine kinase
σ-receptor	opioid σ receptor
SERT	serotonin GABA family transporter
SNAP-25	synaptosomal associated protein of 25 kDa
SNAPs	soluble NSF attachment proteins (note different expansion of SNAP than for SNAP-25)
SNARE proteins	SNAP receptors
SNAREpins	hairpin forms of SNARE proteins
substance P*	
T channels*	transient Ca^{2+} channels
t-SNARES	t: target membranes
VAChT	vesicular transporters of ACh
VAMP	vesicle-associated membrane protein, synaptobrevin
VGAT	vesicular transporter for GABA
VGlutT1	vesicular transporter for glutamate
VMAT1	vesicular transporter for monoamines
v-SNARE	v: vesicle
Y_1, Y_2, Y_4, Y_5, Y_6	neuropeptide Y receptors

Gene symbols for many of the above terms are found in the list of genes in 15.6.2, Genetics, Human Gene Nomenclature. For reference, gene symbols are given below for terms in the preceding list whose abbreviations do not closely resemble the gene symbol:

Term	*Gene Symbol*
A_1	*ADORA1*
AMPA	*GRIA1*
δ receptor	*OPRD1*
D1	*DRD1*
H1	*HRH1*
5-HT_{1A}	*HTR1A*
κ receptor	*OPRK1*
μ receptor	*OPRM1*
M1	*CHRM1*
nAChR	*CHRNA1*
neuromedin K	*TAC3*
NMDA	*GRIN1*
σ receptor	*OPRS1*
substance P	*TAC1*
transporters (various)	*SLC* genes (various, eg, *SLC6A1*)
Y1	*NPY1R*

REFERENCES

1. Federative Committee on Anatomical Terminology. *Terminologia Anatomica.* Stuttgart, Germany: Georg Thieme Verlag; 1998.
2. Victor M, Ropper AH. *Adams and Victor's Principles of Neurology.* 7th ed. New York, NY: McGraw-Hill; 2001:27-41.
3. Gilmore RL, ed. American Electroencephalographic Society Guidelines in Electroencephalography, Evoked Potentials, and Polysomnography. *J Clin Neurophysiol.* 1994;11(1):1-158.
4. Connolly MB, Sharbrough FW, Wong KH. Electrical fields and recording techniques. In: Ebersole JS, Pedley TA, eds. *Current Practice of Clinical Electroencephalography.* 3rd ed. Philadelphia, PA: Lippincott Williams & Wilkins; 2003:72-99.
5. Reilly EL. EEG recording and operation of the apparatus. In: Niedermeyer E, Lopes da Silva F, eds. *Electroencephalography: Basic Principles, Clinical Applications, and Related Fields.* 5th ed. Philadelphia, PA: Lippincott Williams & Wilkins; 2005:139-159.
6. American Clinical Neurophysiology Society Web site. http://www.acns.org. Accessed April 20, 2006.
7. Nuwer MR, Comi G, Emerson R, et al. IFCN standards for digital recording of clinical EEG. *Electroencephalogr Clin Neurophysiol.* 1998;106(3):259-261. Also available at http://www.ifcn.info. (See IFCN Publications, then IFCN Standards under Useful Links.) Accessed April 20, 2006.
8. Jasper HH. Report of the Committee on Methods of Clinical Examination in Electroencephalography: 1957. *Electroencephalogr Clin Neurophysiol.* 1958;10:370-375.
9. Rowan AJ, Tolunsky E. *Primer of EEG: With a Mini-Atlas.* Philadelphia, PA: Butterworth-Heinemann; 2003.
10. Sharbrough F, Chatrian G-E, Lesser RP, Lüders H, Nuwer M, Picton TW; Electrode Position Nomenclature Committee. American Electroencephalographic Society guidelines for standard electrode position nomenclature. *J Clin Neurophysiol.* 1991;8(2):200-202.

11. Chatrian G-E, Lettich E, Nelson PL. Modified nomenclature for the "10%" electrode system. *J Clin Neurophysiol.* 1988;5(2):183-186.
12. Nuwer MR. Recording electrode site nomenclature. *J Clin Neurophysiol.* 1987; 4(2):121-133.
13. Noachtar S, Binnie C, Ebersole J, Mauguière F, Sakamoto A, Westmoreland B. A glossary of terms most commonly used by clinical electroencephalographers and proposal for the report form for the EEG findings. *Electroencephalogr Clin Neurophysiol Suppl.* 1999;52:21-41.
14. American Association of Electrodiagnostic Medicine. Guidelines in electrodiagnostic medicine, 6: guidelines in somatosensory evoked potentials. *Muscle Nerve.* 1999;22: S123-S138.
15. Celesia GG, Bodis-Wollner I, Chatrian GE, Harding GFA, Sokol S, Spekreijse H. Recommended standards for electroretinograms and visual evoked potentials: report of an IFCN committee. *Electroencephalogr Clin Neurophysiol.* 1993;87(6):421-436. Also available at: http://www.ifcn.info. (See IFCN Publications, then IFCN Standards under Useful Links.) Accessed April 20, 2006.
16. Nuwer MR, Aminoff M, Goodin D, et al. IFCN recommended standards for brain-stem auditory evoked potentials: report of an IFCN committee. *Electroencephalogr Clin Neurophysiol.* 1994;91(1):12-17. Also available at http://www.ifcn.info. (See IFCN Publications, then IFCN Standards under Useful Links.) Accessed April 20, 2006.
17. Deutschl G, Eisen A, eds. Recommendations for the practice of clinical neurophysiology: guidelines of the International Federation of Neurophysiology. *Electroencephalogr Clin Neurophysiol.* 1999;S52:1-304.
18. Radtke RA. Sleep disorders: laboratory evaluation. In: Ebersole JS, Pedley TA, eds. *Current Practice of Clinical Electroencephalography.* 3rd ed. Philadelphia, PA: Lippincott Williams & Wilkins; 2003:803-832.
19. American Academy of Sleep Medicine. *The International Classification of Sleep Disorders, Revised: Diagnostic and Coding Manual.* Chicago, IL: American Academy of Sleep Medicine; 2001. Also available at http://www.absm.org/PDF/ICSD.pdf. Accessed April 20, 2006.
20. Nestler EJ, Hyman SE, Malenka RC. *Molecular Neuropharmacology: A Foundation for Clinical Neuroscience.* New York, NY: McGraw-Hill; 2001.

15.12 Obstetric Terms.

15.12 Obstetric Terms. Two colloquial shorthand expressions quantify an individual's obstetric history: GPA and TPAL. The GPA and TPAL expressions are familiar and widely used clinically. However, they are also recognized as imprecise and lacking in standardization.[1-3]

15.12.1 GPA.

15.12.1 GPA.[4(pp225-226)] The letters G, P, and A (or Ab) accompanied by numbers indicate number of pregnancies, births of viable offspring, and number of spontaneous or induced abortions, respectively. Definitions of viability vary and in articles should be specified. In the expansions below, the clinical meaning associated with the GPA shorthand appears; the Latin terms refer to the individual (see any medical dictionary):

Letter	*Expansion of Letter*	*Clinical Meaning*
G	gravida	pregnancies
P	para	births of viable offspring
A or Ab	aborta	abortions

For example, G3, P2, A1 would indicate 3 pregnancies, 2 births of viable offspring, and 1 abortion. In published articles, however, it is preferable to write out the expression, eg:

gravida 3, para 2, aborta 1

Although some sources, including medical dictionaries, feature roman numerals with these expressions, use arabic numerals.

Quantifying prefixes combine with the terms *gravida* and *para* (see list below). Noun forms are *gravidity* and *parity* (with prefixes, *nulligravidity, multiparity,* etc). Adjective forms are *gravid* and *parous* (with prefixes, *multigravid, nulliparous, primiparous,* etc).

Term	*Meaning*
nulligravida	gravida 0
primigravida	gravida 1
secundigravida	gravida 2
multigravida	gravida >1
nullipara	para 0
primipara	para 1
multipara	para >1
grand multipara	para ≥5

Even these Latin-derived terms are somewhat imprecise.[5] Therefore, in addition to use of expansions, further specification (eg, single or multiple births, ectopic pregnancy) is required in scientific articles.

15.12.2 TPAL.[4(pp225-226)]

The letters in this expression indicate obstetric history as follows:

Letter	*Expansion*
T	term deliveries
P	premature deliveries
A	abortions
L	living children

Often, 4 numbers separated by hyphens are recorded, eg:

TPAL: 3-1-1-4 *or* 3-1-1-4

which would indicate 3 term deliveries, 1 premature delivery, 1 abortion, and 4 living children. However, the text of a manuscript should define the numerical expressions and not give the numbers alone.

15.12.3 Apgar Score.[4(p387-389),6-8]

This score is an assessment of a newborn's physical well-being based on the 5 parameters of heart rate, breathing, muscle tone, reflex irritability, and color, each of which is rated 0, 1, or 2; the 5 ratings are then summed. The Apgar score is often reported as 2 numbers, from 0 to 10, separated by a virgule or forward slash, reflecting assessment at 1 minute and 5 minutes after birth. In general medical journals, however, it is best to specify the time intervals, especially as the Apgar score may be assessed at other intervals, eg, 10, 15, or 20 minutes.

Ambiguous: Apgar of 9/10

Preferred: Apgar score of 9/10 at 1 and 5 minutes

or

Apgar score of 9 at 1 minute and 10 at 5 minutes

The score is named after the late anesthesiologist Virginia Apgar, MD; thus, "Apgar" is *not* printed in all capital letters as though for an acronym (although versions of such an acronym have been created as a mnemonic device).

REFERENCES

1. Ely JW. Summarizing the obstetric history [question]. *JAMA*. 1991;266(23):3344.
2. Pun TC, Ng JC. "Madame is a 30-year-old housewife, gravida X, para Y. . . ." *Obstet Gynecol*. 1989;73(2):276-277.
3. Woolley RJ. Parity clarity: proposal for a new obstetric shorthand. *J Fam Pract*. 1993;36(3):265-266.
4. Cunningham FG, Gant NF, Leveno KJ, Gilstrap LC III, Hauth JC, Wenstrom KD. *Williams Obstetrics*. 21st ed. New York, NY: McGraw-Hill; 2001.
5. Dirckx JH. Summarizing the obstetric history [answer]. *JAMA*. 1991;266(23):3344.
6. Committee on Fetus and Newborn, American Academy of Pediatrics, and Committee on Obstetric Practice, American College of Obstetricians and Gynecologists. Use and abuse of the Apgar score. *Pediatrics*. 1996;98(1):141-142.
7. Apgar V. A proposal for a new method of evaluation of the newborn infant. *Curr Res Anesth Analg*. 1953;32(4):260-267. http://www.neonatology.org/classics/apgar.html. Modified April 27, 2002. Accessed April 20, 2006.
8. Apgar V, Holaday DA, James LS, Weisbrot IM, Berrien C. Evaluation of the newborn infant: second report. *JAMA*. 1958;168(15):1985-1988.

15.13 Ophthalmology Terms. Some of the terms described in this section are specific to ophthalmology, and others have special usage requirements in ophthalmology. See also 11.0, Correct and Preferred Usage.

adnexa oculi—Although often used as a synonym for eyelids, the term *adnexa oculi* (which is plural) properly includes the eyelids, lacrimal apparatus, and other appendages of the eye and should be used with its inclusive meaning.

diopter—The diopter is a measure of the power of an optical lens and is the reciprocal of the focal length in meters. Diopter is abbreviated D when used with a number.

diopter sphere

diopter cylinder

conversion from diopters to millimeters

correction of 10.5 D

The prism diopter is a measure of the power of a prism and represents a 1-cm deflection of an image at a distance of 1 m. Its symbol, Δ, may be used with numbers after first mention.

The left eye showed an improvement, with only 25-prism diopter hypotropia.

distance exotropia = 35 prism diopters (Δ); near exotropia = 5Δ

disc; cup-disc ratio—For the optic disc, spell as *disc* (not *disk*). The cup-disc ratio refers to the ratio of the diameter of the optic cup (a central area of the optic disc) to the diameter of the optic disc:

> cup-disc ratio of 0.6

It can be useful to specify whether the ratio is vertical, horizontal, or other, eg:

> The mean horizontal cup-disc ratio by contour estimated from stereophotography was 0.36 ± 0.18 (mean ± SD).

disc diameters and disc areas—Disc diameters (DD) may be used to indicate location or dimension of findings on the ocular fundus with relative distances expressed as diameters of the optic disc, eg:

> 2 DD inferior to the fovea
>
> Lesions varied from 0.5 to 4.5 disc diameters (DD; median, 2.0 DD) for the first group, 0.75 to 7.5 DD (median, 2.5 DD) for the second group, and 1.0 to 9.0 DD (median, 4.0 DD) for the last group.

Disc areas (DA) are also used to indicate relative sizes of findings on the ocular fundus, as well as in considerations of the size of the disc, eg:

> The scar measured 3 DA.
>
> Significant ischemia was defined as greater than 10 disc areas of retinal capillary nonperfusion.
>
> reduced disc areas (DA) . . . mean (SD) DA of 2.57 (0.71) mm^2

electroretinogram—Waves of the electroretinogram (ERG) are as follows:

> a_1 a_2 b

An ERG may be described as normal, subnormal, or negative. Do not substitute one of these terms for another. (For visual evoked potentials, see 15.11.3, Neurology, Evoked Potentials.) Waves of the pattern electroretinogram (PERG)[1] are as follows:

> a_{pt} b_{pt} c_{pt}

Two main components of the PERG are the P50 wave, a positive-deflection waveform, and the N95 wave, a negative-deflection waveform. The terms P50 and N95 may be used without expansion.

fovea and macula—The central retinal fovea is a central portion of the retinal macula. The terms *fovea* and *macula* should be used specifically and not interchangeably.

Goldmann perimetry—This is a method of assessing the visual field. The test stimuli are described by means of a 3-part term: spot size is designated with roman numerals I through V, and luminance is designated with arabic numerals 1 through 4 and letters a through e. For example:

> I-4-e isopter area
>
> I-2-e test object
>
> V-4-e light

greatest linear dimension—This is the greatest dimension between 2 points on the boundary of a lesion.

> Lesion size was less than or equal to 9 disc areas, and greatest linear dimension was less than or equal to 5400 μm.

injection—When used to indicate excess blood, engorgement, or dilation of a vessel, should be changed to *hyperemia* or *vasodilation,* eg, *conjunctival hyperemia* or *conjunctival vasodilation* (not *conjunctival injection*).

intraocular pressure—Measurements of intraocular pressure should include the method used, eg, Goldmann applanation tonometry and, if determined, the corneal thickness measurement.

lasers—Lasers used in ophthalmology include the following:

argon laser
erbium:YAG laser
eximer laser
holmium:YAG laser
krypton laser
Nd:YAG laser
photodynamic therapy laser
Q-switched Nd:YAG laser
transpupillary thermal therapy

The term Nd:YAG (neodymium:yttrium-aluminum-garnet) may be used without expansion.

lids—*Lids* should be changed to *eyelids*.

masked—*Masked*, rather than *blinded*, should be used in the ophthalmologic literature, when referring to randomization, if there could be confusion.

OD, OS, OU—These abbreviations may be used without expansion only with numbers, eg, 20/25 OU, or descriptive assessments of acuity (eg, counting fingers OS; see ***visual acuity, vision***, below):

Abbreviation	*Derivation*	*Expansion*
OD	oculus dexter	right eye
OS	oculus sinister	left eye
OU	oculus uterque	each eye

Note that OU does not mean both eyes, although it is often used incorrectly to imply a vision measurement (eg, visual acuity or visual field) with both eyes at the same time.

See also ***visual acuity, vision***, below.

orbit—*Orbit* refers to the bony cavity that contains the eyeball and its adnexa (muscles, vessels, nerves). It should be clear to readers whether authors are referring to the orbit, the specific bones that compose it, the structures that fill the orbit, or a combination of these.

visual acuity, vision—Distinguish between *vision,* a general term, and *visual acuity,* measurable clearness of vision. If a measurement is given, eg, 20/20 (see below), use "visual acuity." Change "unaided vision" to "acuity without correction." (See also 11.0, Correct and Preferred Usage.)

distance acuity—The Snellen eye chart is a well-known method of assessing distance visual acuity, resulting in the Snellen fraction, an expression such as 20/20, 20/15, or 20/60. The first number represents the testing distance from chart to patient; the second number represents the smallest row of letters that the patient can read. For example, acuity of 20/40 indicates that at 20 ft the smallest line read is readable by a normal eye at 40 ft.

The units for distance acuity are feet (eg, 20 ft) or meters (eg, 6 m). By convention, acuity is expressed without these units specified, eg, 20/20. *JAMA* and the *Archives* Journals follow the author's preference in expressing distance acuity equivalents as metric, eg, 6/6, or English, eg, 20/20, and do not convert English fractions to metric or vice versa. Only one type, English or metric, should be used throughout a manuscript.

Visual acuity is assessed separately for each eye. Other means are also used to assess visual acuity, eg, counting fingers (CF), hand motions (HM), and light perception (LP), which is indicated as LP with projection, LP without projection, or no LP (NLP). Express visual acuity, including numerical measures and other means, by using OD or RE (right eye) and OS or LE (left eye). (See also ***OD, OS, OU***, above).

> The visual acuity was 20/40 OD and counting fingers OS.
>
> (*Not:* . . . 20/40 OD and counting fingers in the left eye.)

Another method of assessing visual acuity makes use of the Bailey-Lovie acuity chart and designates acuity using the base 10 logarithm of the minimum angle of resolution, or logMAR. A logMAR of 0.0 is equivalent to 20/20 Snellen. LogMAR visual acuities always should be expressed in logMAR.

near visual acuity—Near visual acuity (reading vision) may be reported by means of Snellen equivalents or the Jaeger system (J values), eg, J7. J1 is equivalent to Snellen 20/23.[2]

visual field—The extent of the visual field is described by means of degrees from a central point from 0° through 90°:

> 85° temporally
>
> 65° nasally
>
> 56° up and nasally

REFERENCES

1. Celesia GG, Bodis-Wollner I, Chatrian GE, Harding GFA, Sokol S, Spekreijse H. Recommended standards for electroretinograms and visual evoked potentials: report of an IFCN committee. *Electroencephalogr Clin Neurophysiol.* 1993;87(6): 421-436. Also available at http://www.ifcn.info. (See IFCN Publications, then IFCN Standards under Useful Links.) Accessed April 20, 2006.
2. Millodot M, Laby DM. *Dictionary of Ophthalmology.* Woburn, MA: Butterworth-Heinemann; 2002.

Intemperate language should not be used in any discussion or writing which involves zoological nomenclature, and all debates should be conducted in a courteous and friendly manner.

Code of Ethics, *International Code of Zoological Nomenclature*[1(p124)]

I know the scientific names of beings animalculous.

W. S. Gilbert

15.14 Organisms and Pathogens

15.14.1 Biological Nomenclature

Scientific and Vernacular Names. Scientific names are labels used in place of lengthy descriptions. A scientific name corresponds to a set of formally defined attributes. The meanings of scientific names are internationally understood.[2]

Vernacular names or common names are also labels. Vernacular names seen in medical publications include fungi, prokaryotes, meningococcus, and St John's wort. Vernacular names cannot be assumed to correspond to formally defined sets of attributes and vary by region and language.

In scientific writing, scientific names should be used when the labeled entity verifiably corresponds to the set of attributes associated with the scientific name, at least at first mention. Subsequently vernacular names (including collective genus terms, described later in this section) may be used.

Parenthetic mention of the vernacular name when the scientific name is used, and vice versa, is helpful. For instance:

	First Mention	*Subsequent Mention*
Vernacular name	St John's wort (*Hypericum perforatum*)	St John's wort; eg, "participants who reported taking St John's wort tablets"
Scientific name	*Hypericum perforatum* (St John's wort)	*H perforatum,* or St John's wort, depending on context; eg, "participants given tablets prepared from a pure extract of *H perforatum*"

Biological Nomenclature. Biological nomenclature is the scientific naming of organisms and is the source of scientific names. Taxonomy comprises the principles and practices of classifying organisms[2] to reflect their relatedness. Nomenclature "is the assignment of names to the taxonomic groups according to international rules."[3(p27)]

Biological nomenclature—the nomenclature of living things—derives from the paradigm of the 18th-century taxonomist Linnaeus, who used 2-word labels to replace the long descriptive Latin phrases appended to the genus name.[4,5] Since

Linnaeus' time, international bodies have continued to formalize biological nomenclature, resulting in the current principal codes:

Code	*Content*
International Code of Zoological Nomenclature[1]	animals, including protozoa and parasites
International Code of Botanical Nomenclature[6]	fungi and noncultivated plants, including algae
International Code of Nomenclature of Bacteria[7]	bacteria
International Code of Nomenclature for Cultivated Plants[8]	cultivated plants
International Code of Virus Classification and Nomenclature	viruses (see 15.14.3, Organisms and Pathogens, Virus Nomenclature)

The codes contain principles, rules, and recommendations for name derivations, priority, validity, and spelling. For a name to have international standing, the codes stipulate valid publication according to specific requirements.

An effort has been made to unify biological nomenclature for all organisms with a single code, the BioCode, under the auspices of the International Committee on Bionomenclature (a joint committee of the International Union of Microbiological Societies and the International Union of Biological Sciences).[5,9-11] Another proposed unifying code is the PhyloCode, which is meant to reflect phylogeny and to be used concurrently with the extant codes, at least initially.[12,13]

"The essence of the Linnaean revolution was the recognition that the function of the specific 'name' was merely to label a concept rather than to describe an entity."[5(p5)] Scientific names change when taxonomy changes, but not when new knowledge indicates that the original name is no longer an apt descriptor. (For instance, it was learned several decades after its discovery that the bacterium *Haemophilus influenzae* did not cause influenza,[14] but the name was not changed.[7]) The stability of names is crucial, and name changes may cause harm[5(p75),6(preamble)] (see "perilous name" in the bacteriologic code[7]).

Resources. A useful source of names of organisms available on the Web, particularly plant and animal names, is the Index to Organism Names.[15] Other resources are available at the National Center for Biotechnology Information Entrez Taxonomy Homepage (http://www.ncbi.nlm.nih.gov/entrez/query.fcgi?db=taxonomy).[16]

Style for Scientific Names. This section presents style that applies to scientific names. The nomenclature codes differ in some style recommendations, but most publications, when possible, will apply style consistently for all scientific names, eg, will use abbreviations in the same way for animals, plants, and bacteria. Therefore, style applied to animals, plants, and bacteria is presented together in this section. (See also 15.14.2, Bacteria: Additional Terminology, and 15.14.3, Virus Nomenclature.)

Organisms are classified in taxonomic groups, also called taxa (singular: taxon), within different ranks, eg:

Rank	*Taxon*
genus	*Homo*
species	*Homo sapiens*

Major ranks, from most inclusive to most specific, are kingdom, domain (bacteria), phylum (animals, fungi, and bacteria) or division (plants and bacteria), class, order, family, genus, and species.

Stylistic hallmarks of biological nomenclature differentiate scientific names from vernacular names.[2,4] These hallmarks are latinization, italics, and a 2-word term for species: the binomial, also called binary or binominal, eg, *Homo sapiens*. (Within a code, the names of ranks above species usually must be unique; the same species designator, however, can be used with multiple genera, eg, *Klebsiella pneumoniae, Streptococcus pneumoniae*. Across codes, names may be the same at any rank, eg, the bacterial genus *Bacillus,* the stick and leaf insect genus *Bacillus*.)

According to the international codes, initial capitals are used for all taxa, except for the second portion of the binomial. (That portion is called the *specific name* in the zoological code and the *specific epithet* in the botanical and bacteriological codes.) Italics are always used for the genus and species components of the binomial. Diacritical marks (accents) and ligatures (eg, æ) are not used. Hyphens occasionally may be used in the specific epithet, eg, the butterfly *Polygonia c-album,* which has a c-shaped wing mark.[2]

All codes capitalize scientific names of taxa but differ on italicizing higher taxa. The bacterial code recommends italicizing all scientific names but recognizes that journals may wish to style all organism names similarly. In *JAMA* and the *Archives* Journals, taxa above genus are not italicized. The following examples of taxonomic classification according to the 3 codes illustrate style in *JAMA* and the *Archives* Journals for capitalization and italicization (see also 10.3.6, Capitalization, Proper Nouns, Organisms). The suffixes are typical and specified in each code (eg, family: -idae [animals], -aceae [plants and bacteria]), although exceptions are found:

Animal		*Fungi*		*Bacteria*	
Rank	*Taxon*	*Rank*	*Taxon*	*Rank*	*Taxon*
kingdom	Animalia	kingdom	Fungi (Mycota)	kingdom	Procaryotae
phylum	Chordata	phylum	Ascomycota	division	Firmicutes
class	Mammalia	class	Ascomycetes	class	Firmibacteria
order	Primates	order	Onygenales	order	(not applicable in example; ending: *-ales*)
family	Hominidae	family	Onygenaceae	family	Bacillaceae
genus	*Homo*	genus	*Ajellomyces*	genus	*Staphylococcus*
species	*Homo sapiens*	species	*Ajellomyces capsulatus*	species	*Staphylococcus aureus*

(Another scheme for bacterial taxonomic rank uses domain and phylum, rather than kingdom and division.[4])

Subranks and superranks follow the same style, eg:

Animal		*Fungi*	
Rank	*Taxon*	*Rank*	*Taxon*
subphylum	Vertebrata		
		subclass	Peronosporomycetidae
suborder	Anthropoidea		
superfamily	Hominoidea		

(See also the sections "Subgenus" and "Subspecific Ranks, Ternary Names," below.)

Abbreviation of Genus and Other Abbreviations. As described in 14.11, Abbreviations, Clinical, Technical, and Other Common Terms, treat each manuscript portion (title, abstract, text, etc) separately. After first mention of the binomial species name, abbreviate the genus portion of the name. (*JAMA* and the *Archives* Journals do not use a period.) Do not abbreviate the specific name. Do not begin a sentence with an abbreviated genus name; either expand or reword.

> *Staphylococcus aureus* is a common cause of hospital-acquired infection. Nosocomial *S aureus* infection is also a source of community-acquired infection.

When the genus name is repeated but used with a new specific name, do not abbreviate the genus name until subsequent mention.

> *Staphylococcus aureus* and *Staphylococcus epidermidis* may be components of normal flora or pathogens in clinically significant infections, although *S aureus* is the more serious pathogen of the two.

Do not abbreviate the specific name, and do not abbreviate the genus name when used alone.

> *Not:* . . . *S au* is the more serious pathogen . . .
>
> *Not:* . . . the more serious pathogen in the genus *S* . . .

When organisms with genus names that begin with the same letter are mentioned in the same article, in *JAMA* and the *Archives* Journals, genus is abbreviated after first mention, for instance:

> hospital infections caused by *Staphylococcus aureus* and *Streptococcus faecalis* and bacteriuria with *S aureus* and *S faecalis*

Style variations in such instances are permissible (eg, if the editor thinks there is any possibility of confusing genera), and author requests to expand the genus names should be honored. *JAMA* and the *Archives* Journals do not use multiletter abbreviations for genus name, eg:

> *S aureus* and *S faecalis* (not *Sta aureus* or *Str faecalis*)

Do not use 2-letter abbreviations for the binomial, eg, do not use SA for *Staphylococcus aureus* or SE for *S epidermidis*. However, longer expressions that include the scientific name may be abbreviated:

CoNS	coagulase-negative *Staphylococcus* species
EHEC	enterohemorrhagic *Escherichia coli*
MRSA	methicillin-resistant *Staphylococcus aureus*

Abbreviations such as sp nov (*species nova,* new species) and gen nov (*genus novum,* new genus) are used in published proposals of new genus and species designations, eg:

Corynebacterium nigricans sp nov

Roseomonas mucosa sp nov and *Roseomonas gilardii* subsp *rosea* subsp nov[17]

Wigglesworthia glossinidia sp nov[18]

Wigglesworthia gen nov[18]

New proposals for higher taxa are indicated as in the following examples[19-22]:

Cycliophora, new phylum

Eucycliophora, new class

Symbiida, new order

Symbiidae, new family

Symbion gen nov

Symbion pandora sp nov

Pfiesteria piscicida gen et sp nov (Pfiesteriaceae fam nov)

Parachlamydiaceae fam nov and Simkaniaceae fam nov

The "nov" abbreviations should be mentioned prominently in the article, eg, in the title, but need not be included with every mention of the organism name.

Synonyms are expressed as follows:

Fugomyces cyanescens (syn *Sporothrix cyanescens, Cerinosterus cyanescens*)

Mesocestoides vogae (syn *M corti*)

Subgenus. Subgenus is capitalized, italicized, and placed in parentheses, sometimes with the abbreviation "subgen," eg:

Mus (Mus) musculus

Moraxella (subgen *Branhamella) catarrhalis*

Parentheses. For other uses of parentheses within species names, such as name changes, use quotation marks or a qualifier such as "formerly," eg:

Bartonella (formerly *Rochalimaea) henselae*

Helicobacter (formerly *Campylobacter*) *pylori*

Issatchenkia orientalis (anamorph *Candida krusei*)

Indicate a change in species name with the entire binomial in parentheses as follows:

Bacteroides ureolyticus (formerly *Bacteroides corrodens*)

Authorship of the scientific name may be indicated by personal names, which are not italicized, following the species name. Sometimes parentheses are used. Within and among codes, conventions for such references vary. Editors should not restyle such terms but rather should verify with authors that the proper form has been used. "L." alone is the common abbreviation for "Linneaus," eg, *Culex pipiens* L., but "Linnaeus" should be written in full in publications whose readers are unlikely to know of this convention. Examples:

Aedes aegypti (Linnaeus)

Culex pipiens Linnaeus

Escherichia coli (Migula) Castellani and Chalmers

Serratia marcescens Bizio

The parentheses indicate that the organism, after initial description, was transferred into another genus by others, in the case of *E coli* by Castellani and Chalmers.

Year of published discovery may be included, eg:

Escherichia coli (Migula 1895) Castellani and Chalmers 1919

Serratia marcescens Bizio 1823

Subspecific Ranks, Ternary Names. Subspecific ranks receive ternary or trinomial names. Subspecific designations are handled differently for animals, plants, and bacteria, as in the following examples. (The term *var* as a synonym for subspecies was removed from the bacterial nomenclature code in 1990.)

Type of Organism	*Subspecific Rank (Designator)*	*Example*
Animal		
Higher animal	subspecies (no designator)	*Mus musculus domesticus*
Protozoon		*Trypanosoma brucei gambiense*
Fungus	variety (var)	*Histoplasma capsulatum* var *duboisii*
Bacteria		
Bacterium	subspecies (subsp)	*Campylobacter fetus* subsp *fetus* *Mycobacterium avium* subsp *paratuberculosis*

Plant names may use *var*, as above, *subsp*, *f* (form), and other subspecific epithets, which are not interchangeable, in ternary names, eg:

Satureja parnassica subsp *parnassica*

Not all 3-word combinations are ternary names:

Ixodes scapularis larvae

Legionella pneumophila pneumonia

Schistosoma mansoni miracidium

Trypanosoma brucei procyclin

Infrasubspecific Subdivisions. Subdivisions below the subspecies level (infrasubspecific subdivisions) include the serovar (serologically differentiated) and the biovar (biochemically or physiologically differentiated). The suffix -type is most often used in the clinical literature, eg, biotype, serotype. But to avoid confusion with nomenclatural type ("the element of the taxon with which the name is permanently associated"[7(p17)]), the suffix -var is often preferred in microbiological literature.

Infrasubspecific subdivisions are designated with various numbers, letters, or terms; follow author usage:

Brucella suis biovar 4

Cryptococcus neoformans serovar A

Fusarium oxysporum f sp *radicis lycopersici* [f sp: *forma specialis*]

Haemophilus influenzae biotype I

H influenzae biotype VII

Pseudomonas fluorescens biovar I

Staphylococcus aureus subsp *aureus* biotype A

S simulans biovar *staphylolyticus*

Ureaplasma urealyticum parvo biovar

U urealyticum T960 biovar

Yersinia enterocolitica serovar O:8

Anglicized and Vernacular (Trivial, Common) Terms. In medical publications, uncapitalized anglicized forms are often used for taxa in ranks above genus (see also 9.4, Plurals, Microorganisms)[23]:

Anglicized Term	*Formal Term*
vertebrates	Vertebrata
primates	Primates
hominids	Hominidae
fungi	Fungi
moniliaceous molds	Moniliaceae
prokaryotes	Procaryotae
mycobacteria	Mycobacteriaceae
chlamydiae	Chlamydiales

Collective Genus Terms. Many organisms possess traditional generic plural designations, which are verifiable in the dictionary. Some also have special adjectival forms. It is also acceptable to add the word *organisms* or *species* to the italicized genus name. See the examples below.

Genus	*Plural Noun Form*	*Adjectival Form*
Cryptococcus	*Cryptococcus* species	cryptococcal
Escherichia	*Escherichia* organisms	
Legionella	legionellae	
Macaca	macaques	
Mycobacterium	mycobacteria	mycobacterial
Pseudomonas	pseudomonads	pseudomonal
Salmonella	salmonellae	
Staphylococcus	staphylococci	staphylococcal
Streptococcus	streptococci	streptococcal
Treponema	treponemes	treponemal
Trypanosoma	trypanosomes	trypanosomal

a novel *Yersinia* species

Loxosceles species (brown recluse) spider venom

group A streptococcal infection

viridans streptococcal endocarditis

Genus names often qualify other terms, eg:

Candida endocarditis

Lactobacillus serogroups

Legionella pneumonia

Unspecified Species. The name of a genus used alone implies the genus as a whole:

Toxocara infections are frequently acquired from household pets.

The term *species* is used in cases in which the genus is certain but the species cannot be determined. For instance, if an author knew that a skin test reaction indicated presence of *Toxocara* organisms but was unsure whether the reaction resulted from *Toxocara canis* infection or *Toxocara cati* infection, the author might write:

The source of the patient's infection was *Toxocara* species.

In the latter example, *Toxocara* organisms would also be acceptable, but *Toxocara* alone would be incorrect.[24,25]

Name Changes. Two recent new names have been adopted more readily by microbiologists than clinicians: *Chlamydophila* (see 15.14.2, Bacteria: Additional Terminology) and *Pneumocystis jiroveci*.[26-29]

The fungal genus *Pneumocystis* now includes 2 authentic species. The name of the species infective of rats is *P carinii*. The human pathogen was transitionally named *P carinii* f sp *hominis* and is now known as *P jiroveci*.[26,27] The familiar abbreviation PCP may be retained for *Pneumocystis* pneumonia in human and nonhuman hosts.[26]

When a name is very new or in dispute, authors are advised to include both versions at first mention:

> *Chlamydophila* (formerly *Chlamydia) pneumoniae*
>
> *Chlamydia pneumoniae* (proposed new name *Chlamydophila pneumoniae)*

Usage. In text dealing with infectious conditions, it is important to distinguish between the infectious agent and the condition. Infectious agents, infections, and diseases are not equivalent.

Incorrect:	*Legionella pneumophila* may be serious or subclinical.
Preferred:	Infection with *Legionella pneumophila* may be serious or subclinical.
Incorrect:	*Legionella pneumophila* may be severe.
Preferred:	*Legionella pneumophila* pneumonia may be severe.

There is no "official" classification of bacteria. . . . [B]acterial classifications are devised for microbiologists, not for the entities being classified. Bacteria show little interest in the matter of their classification.

D. J. Brenner, J. T. Staley, and N. R. Krieg[3(p31)]

. . . the majority of bacteria in nature have not been grown or characterized.

R. G. E. Murray and John G. Holt[30(p2)]

15.14.2 Bacteria: Additional Terminology

General. For general guidelines on biological nomenclature that apply to bacteria, see 15.14.1, Biological Nomenclature. Rules for bacterial nomenclature are found in the *International Code of Nomenclature of Bacteria.*[7] Sources of bacterial names available on the Web are the List of Prokaryotic Names With Standing in Nomenclature[31] and the German Collection of Microorganisms and Cell Cultures bacterial nomenclature search page.[32] General references consulted in preparation of this section are Murray et al[33] and Brooks et al.[34]

Bacterial Genes. Bacterial gene nomenclature is covered in 15.6.5, Genetics, Nonhuman Genetic Terms.

Chlamydia *and* Chlamydophila. A proposed change in taxonomy has resulted in a number of changes, including name changes of 2 medically important organisms.[22,35] *Chlamydia pneumoniae* has become *Chlamydophila pneumoniae* and *Chlamydia psittaci* has become *Chlamydophila psittaci. Chlamydia trachomatis* remains so named. The proposal has been questioned,[36] and as of this writing the older terminology persists in medical journals and textbooks. The new terminology is used by the Centers for Disease Control and Prevention and major compendia of bacterial names.[31-33,37]

The TWAR biovar of *Chlamydophila pneumoniae* was named "after the laboratory designation of the first 2 isolates—TW-183 and AR-39."[38(p161)-40]

Escherichia coli. The O:K:H serotype profile of *Escherichia coli* is based on the somatic O antigen, capsular K antigen, and flagellar H antigen. The O is a capital letter O, not a zero. The abbreviations O, K, and H within the terms need not be expanded. Expansion of other components is not necessary but can be helpful (NM, nonmotile; NT, not typeable; Orough, O antigen, rough). Note the following examples:

Escherichia coli O6:K13:H1

E coli O157:H7

O157:NM

ONT:NM

Orough:H9

non-O157

O111:NM (or H-)

Prominent serogroups include O26, O103, O111, and O128.

Diarrheogenic *E coli* strains are abbreviated as follows (expand at first mention in accordance with 14.11, Abbreviations, Clinical, Technical, and Other Common Terms):

EAggEC	enteroaggregative *E coli*
EIEC	enteroinvasive *E coli*
EPEC	enteropathogenic *E coli*
ETEC	enterotoxigenic *E coli*
STEC	Shiga toxin-producing *E coli* (also called enterohemorrhagic *E coli* [EHEC])
VTEC	verotoxin-producing *E coli*

Serotype and strain are often mentioned together in various combinations:

O157:H7 STEC

strains of STEC serotypes other than O157:H7

STEC O103

Note the following terms representing Shiga toxins:

stx1

stx2

Gram-Positive, Gram-Negative. Bacteria are often grouped according to reaction to the Gram stain. Note capitalization style in the following (see also 10.3, Capitalization, Proper Nouns):

gram-negative bacilli

gram-positive cocci

Gram stain

Haemophilus. *Haemophilus influenzae* strains are defined by capsular antigens, designated types a through f, for instance:

Haemophilus influenzae type b (Hib)

The name of the vaccine should be expanded at first mention:

Haemophilus influenzae type b (Hib) vaccine . . . Hib vaccine

H influenzae type b (Hib) vaccination

Haemophilus aegyptius has been shown to be *H influenzae* biogroup *aegyptius*; *aegypticus* is a misspelling.

Laboratory Media. Microorganism names applied to laboratory media are given lowercase and roman:

bacteroides bile esculin agar

brucella agar

Capitalization indicates a product name:

Haemophilus ID Quad agar

Lactobacillus *GG.* *Lactobacillus* GG refers to a strain of *Lactobacillus rhamnosus* named for the authors who isolated it.[41]

L Forms. L phase variants, or L forms, are forms of various bacteria with deficient or defective cell walls. Examples of usage are as follows:

Helicobacter pylori L-form infection

L-form *Bacillus subtilis*

L-form bioluminescence

the L form of *Mycobacterium tuberculosis*

Macrolide Resistance. Macrolide-resistance phenotypes are expressed as follows:

M phenotype (M: macrolide)

MLSB (L: lincosamide; SB: streptogramin B)

cMLSB (c: constitutive, includes resistance to clindamycin)

iMLSB (i: inducible by macrolides but not by clindamycin)

Mycobacterium avium-intracellulare. This term indicates that in a particular context, the 2 species *Mycobacterium avium* and *M intracellulare* are indistinguishable.

Neisseria meningitidis. Clinically important serogroups of this organism include the following:

serogroups A, B, C, Y, and W-135

The vernacular name of this organism is meningococcus.

Salmonella. Nomenclature of salmonellae is complex and evolving.[42-45] What had been considered separate species were shown to be strains. The main stylistic change is that the traditional binomial species designation is no longer applied to serotypes, eg:

Salmonella Typhi, *not Salmonella typhi*

Editors should query authors if the latter term and its like are used (except, for instance, in discussions of nomenclature) but otherwise should follow author preference and apply style as in the following examples:

Species: *Salmonella enterica, S bongori* (formerly subspecies V)

Subspecies, *S enterica:*

S enterica subsp *enterica*	subspecies I
S enterica subsp *salamae*	subspecies II
S enterica subsp *arizonae*	subspecies IIIa
S enterica subsp *diarizonae*	subspecies IIIb
S enterica subsp *houtenae*	subspecies IV
S enterica subsp *indica*	subspecies VI

Serotypes (serovars) of subspecies I use italics, roman, and capitals as follows:

Salmonella ser Typhi (equivalent to *S enterica* subsp *enterica* ser Typhi)

After first mention, ser may be omitted:

Salmonella Enteritidis

Salmonella Typhi

Salmonella Typhimurium

When the genus name is repeated, it may be abbreviated:

S Typhi

Serovars of *Salmonella* are defined by the O (somatic), Vi (capsular), and H (flagellar) antigens. In contrast to *E coli* strains, when *Salmonella* serotype is expressed with those antigens, the letters O, H, and Vi are not included in the serotype designation. Colons separate the O, Vi, and H designations, which take a variety of forms (letter, numeric, etc):

Salmonella enterica subsp *salamae* ser 50:z:e,n,x

Salmonella serotype II 50:z:e,n,x

Salmonella serotype IV 45:g,z_{51}:-

Salmonella serotype IIIa 41:z_4z_{23}:-

Salmonella subsp *arizonae* serovar 50:z_4z_{24}:-

Salmonella Typhimurium 1,4,5,12:1:1,2

Alternatively, geographic or other designations are used:

Salmonella ser Brookfield

Salmonella Typhimurium MR-DT104

Salmonella Typhimurium DT204b

O antigen groups (O groups) are A, B, C_1, C_2, D, E, and F, eg:

Salmonella group E

a group D *Salmonella* outbreak

Strain and Group Designations. Strains and groups are designated in various ways, sometimes alone, sometimes following the binomial species name. These additional designations are not italicized. Strains are sometimes designated by the abbreviation of a culture collection repository and number. Such abbreviations need not be expanded when used in strain names only, but should be otherwise.[24]

ATCC 27853 strain of *Pseudomonas aeruginosa*

CDC EO-2 [EO: eugonic oxidizer]

CDC group WO-2 [WO: weak oxidizer]

Escherichia coli ATCC 25922

Staphylococcus aureus NCTC 83

the control strain, NCTC 8325

Geobacillus stearothermophilus (DSMZ 22; equivalent to ATCC 12980) cultures obtained from the American Type Culture Collection, Manassas, Virginia

Streptococci. Clinically important groups of streptococci are designated in various ways. Capital letters refer to Lancefield serologic groups, eg:

α-hemolytic streptococci

group A β-hemolytic streptococci

group A *Streptococcus pyogenes*

group B β-hemolytic streptococci (*S agalactiae*)

group C streptococci

viridans streptococci

Proteins of *Streptococcus pyogenes* include the following:

M protein

class I M protein

class II M protein

P substance

R protein

T substance

The cell wall C polysaccharide of *S pneumoniae* is the basis of the term "C-reactive protein" (an acute-phase inflammatory protein that reacts with the C polysaccharide).

Do not confuse the M protein with the M phenotype of various streptococci and other bacteria (see the "Macrolide Resistance" section above) or C polysaccharide with group C streptococci.

The vernacular name of *Streptococcus pneumoniae* is pneumococcus.

Vibrio. *Vibrio cholerae* serogroups are expressed as in these examples:

Vibrio cholerae O1

V cholerae O139

REFERENCES

1. International Commission on Zoological Nomenclature. *International Code of Zoological Nomenclature.* 4th ed. London, England: International Trust for Zoological Nomenclature; 1999. Also available at http://www.iczn.org/iczn/. Accessed April 20, 2006.
2. Jeffrey C. *Biological Nomenclature.* 3rd ed. London, England: Edward Arnold; 1989.
3. Brenner DJ, Staley JT, Krieg NR. Classification of procaryotic organisms and the concept of bacterial speciation. In: Boone DR, Castenholz RW, eds. *Bergey's Manual of Systematic Bacteriology.* 2nd ed. *Vol 1: The* Archaea *and the Deeply Branching and Phototrophic Bacteria.* New York, NY: Springer-Verlag; 2001:27-31.
4. Sneath PHA. Bacterial nomenclature. In: Boone DR, Castenholz RW, eds. *Bergey's Manual of Systematic Bacteriology.* 2nd ed. *Vol 1: The* Archaea *and the Deeply Branching and Phototrophic Bacteria.* New York, NY: Springer-Verlag; 2001:83-88.
5. Melville RV. *Towards Stability in the Names of Animals: A History of the International Commission on Zoological Nomenclature 1895-1995.* London, England: International Trust for Zoological Nomenclature; 1995.
6. Greuter W, McNeill J, Barrie FR, et al, eds. *International Code of Botanical Nomenclature (St Louis Code).* Vienna, Austria: International Association for Plant Taxonomy; Königstein, Germany: Koeltz Scientific Books; 1999. Also available at http://www.bgbm.org/IAPT/Nomenclature/Code/SaintLouis/0001ICSLContents.htm. Updated February 12, 2001. Accessed April 20, 2006.
7. Lapage SP, Sneath PHA, Lessel EF, Skerman VBD, Seeliger HPR, Clark WA. *International Code of Nomenclature of Bacteria and Statutes of the International Committee on Systematic Bacteriology and Statutes of the Bacteriology and Applied Microbiology Section of the International Union of Microbiological Societies.* Washington, DC: International Union of Microbiological Societies, American Society for Microbiology; 1992.
8. Trehane P, Brickell CD, Baum BR, et al, eds. *International Code of Nomenclature for Cultivated Plants.* Wimborne, England: Quarterjack Publishing; 1995.
9. International Committee on Bionomenclature (ICB). http://www.rom.on.ca/biodiversity/biocode/bioicb1997.html. Accessed September 13, 2005.
10. Ride WDL. Introduction. In: International Commission on Zoological Nomenclature. *International Code of Zoological Nomenclature.* 4th ed. London, England: International Trust for Zoological Nomenclature; 1999:xix-xxix

11. International Union of Biological Sciences Web site. http://www.iubs.org. Accessed April 20, 2006.
12. Robinson P, Kommedahl T. Phylocode: a new system of nomenclature. *Sci Editor.* 2002;25(2):52.
13. Phylocode. http://www.ohiou.edu/phylocode. Modified April 20, 2006. Accessed April 21, 2006.
14. Kolata G. *Flu: The Story of the Great Influenza Pandemic of 1918 and the Search for the Virus That Caused It.* New York, NY: Touchstone; 1999.
15. Biosis. Index to organism names. http://www.organismnames.com. Accessed April 21, 2006.
16. NCBI Entrez Taxonomy Homepage. http://www.ncbi.nlm.nih.gov/entrez/query.fcgi?db=taxonomy. Accessed April 21, 2006.
17. Han XY, Pham AS, Tarrand JJ, Rolston KV, Helsel LO, Levett PN. Bacteriologic characterization of 36 strains of *Roseomonas* species and proposal of *Roseomonas mucosa* sp nov and *Roseomonas gilardii* subsp *rosea* subsp nov. *Am J Clin Pathol.* 2003;120(2):256-264.
18. Aksoy S. *Wigglesworthia* gen. nov. and *Wigglesworthia glossinidia* sp. nov., taxa consisting of the mycetocyte-associated, primary endosymbionts of tsetse flies. *Int J Syst Bacteriol.* 1995;45(4):848-851.
19. Funch P, Kristensen RM. Cycliophora is a new phylum with affinities to Entoprocta and Ectoprocta. *Nature.* 1995;378(6558):711-714.
20. Morris SC. A new phylum from the lobster's lips. *Nature.* 1995;378(6558):661-662.
21. Steidinger KA, Burkholder JM, Glasgow HB, et al. *Pfiesteria piscicida* gen. et sp. nov. (Pfiesteriaceae fam. nov.), a new toxic dinoflagellate with a complex life cycle and behavior. *J Phycol.* 1996;32(1):157-164.
22. Everett KD, Bush RM, Andersen AA. Emended description of the order Chlamydiales, proposal of Parachlamydiaceae fam. nov. and Simkaniaceae fam. nov., each containing one monotypic genus, revised taxonomy of the family Chlamydiaceae, including a new genus and five new species, and standards for the identification of organisms. *Int J Syst Bacteriol.* April 1999;49:415-440.
23. Ursing JB. Bacteriologic nomenclature. In: Maisonneuve H, Enckell PH, Polderman AKS, Thapa R, Vekony M, eds. *Science Editors' Handbook.* West Clandon, England: European Association of Science Editors; 2003;3-4.1:1-4.
24. *ASM Style Manual for Journals and Books.* Washington, DC: American Society for Microbiology: 1991.
25. Style notes: taxonomic names in microbiology and their adjectival derivatives [editorial]. *Ann Intern Med.* 1989;110(6):419-420.
26. Stringer JR, Beard CB, Miller RF, Wakefield AE. A new name (*Pneumocystis jiroveci*) for *Pneumocystis* from humans. *Emerg Infect Dis.* 2002;8(9):891-896.
27. Cushion MT. *Pneumocystis.* In: Murray PR, Baron EJ, Jorgensen JH, Pfaller MA, Yolken RH, eds. *Manual of Clinical Microbiology.* 8th ed. Washington, DC: ASM Press; 2003:1712-1725.
28. Hughes WT. *Pneumocystis carinii* vs. *Pneumocystis jiroveci:* another misnomer (response to Stringer et al). *Emerg Infect Dis.* 2003;9(2):276-277.
29. Stringer JR, Beard CB, Miller RF, Cushion MT. A new name (*Pneumocystis jiroveci*) for *Pneumocystis* from humans (response to Hughes). *Emerg Infect Dis.* 2003;9(2):277-279.
30. Murray RGE, Holt JG. The history of *Bergey's Manual.* In: Boone DR, Castenholz RW, eds. *Bergey's Manual of Systematic Bacteriology.* 2nd ed. *Vol 1: The* Archaea *and the*

Deeply Branching and Phototrophic Bacteria. New York, NY: Springer-Verlag; 2001:1-13.

31. Euzéby JP. List of prokaryotic names with standing in nomenclature. http://www.bacterio.cict.fr/ or http://www.bacterio.net. Updated April 19, 2006. Accessed April 21, 2006.
32. DSMZ. Bacterial nomenclature search page. http://www.dsmz.de/bactnom/bactname. Accessed April 24, 2006.
33. Murray PR, Baron EJ, Jorgensen JH, Pfaller MA, Yolken RH, eds. *Manual of Clinical Microbiology*. 8th ed. Washington, DC: ASM Press; 2003:991-1004.
34. Brooks GF, Butel JS, Morse SA. *Jawetz, Melnick, and Adelberg's Medical Microbiology*. 22nd ed. New York, NY: Lange Medical Books/McGraw-Hill; 2001.
35. Mahony JB, Coombes BK, Chernesky MA. *Chlamydia* and *Chlamydophila*. In: Murray PR, Baron EJ, Jorgensen JH, Pfaller MA, Yolken RH, eds. *Manual of Clinical Microbiology*. 8th ed. Washington, DC: ASM Press; 2003:991-1004.
36. Schachter J, Stephens RS, Timms P, et al. Radical changes to chlamydial taxonomy are not necessary just yet. *Int J Syst Evol Microbiol*. 2001;51(pt 1):249.
37. Boone DR, Castenholz RW, eds. *Bergey's Manual of Systematic Bacteriology*. 2nd ed. *Vol 1: The* Archaea *and the Deeply Branching and Phototropoic Bacteria*. New York, NY: Springer-Verlag; 2001.
38. Grayston JT, Kuo C-C, Wang S-P, Altman J. A new *Chlamydia psittaci* strain, TWAR, isolated in acute respiratory tract infections. *N Engl J Med*. 1986;315(3):161-168.
39. Grayston JT, Kuo C-C, Campbell LA, Wang SP. *Chlamydia pneumoniae* sp. nov. for *Chlamydia* sp: strain TWAR. *Int J Syst Bacteriol*. 1989;39(1):88-90.
40. Saikku P, Wang SP, Kleemola M, Brander E, Rusanan E, Grayston JT. An epidemic of mild pneumonia due to an unusual strain of *Chlamydia psittaci*. *J Infect Dis*. 1985;151(5):832-839.
41. Gorbach SL, Chang TW, Goldin B: Successful treatment of relapsing *Clostridium difficile* colitis with *Lactobacillus* GG. *Lancet*. 1987;2(8574):1519.
42. Euzéby JP. *Salmonella* nomenclature. http://www.bacterio.cict.fr/salmonellanom.html. Updated March 19, 2005. Accessed September 13, 2005.
43. Farmer JJ III. Enterobacteriaceae: introduction and identification. In: Murray PR, Baron EJ, Jorgensen JH, Pfaller MA, Yolken RH, eds. *Manual of Clinical Microbiology*. 8th ed. Washington, DC: ASM Press; 2003:636-653.
44. Bopp CA, Brenner FW, Fields PI, Wells JG, Strockbine NA. *Escherichia, Shigella,* and *Salmonella*. In: Murray PR, Baron EJ, Jorgensen JH, Pfaller MA, Yolken RH, eds. *Manual of Clinical Microbiology*. 8th ed. Washington, DC: ASM Press; 2003:654-671.
45. Brenner FW, Villar RG, Angulo FJ, Tauxe R, Swaminathan B. Guest commentary: *Salmonella* nomenclature. *J Clin Microbiol*. 2000;38(7):2465-2467.

Viruses evolve rapidly. . . . [A]denovirus, for example, may produce 250 000 DNA molecules in an infected cell. . . .

Leslie Collier and John Oxford[1(p12)]

Taxonomy lies at the uneasy interface between biology and logic.

L. Andrew Ball[2(p3)]

If you wanted to call one of your children home for dinner would you go into the street and shout "Homo sapiens"*?*

Michael A. Drebot, Eric Henchal, Brian Hjelle, et al[3(p2468)]

15.14.3 Virus Nomenclature. Most medical articles describe concrete viral entities and, therefore, use the common (vernacular, informal) names of viruses (eg, cytomegalovirus, Hantaan virus, orthopoxviruses). To indicate taxonomic groups, formal virus names are used (eg, *Human herpesvirus 5, Hantaan virus,* the genus *Orthopoxvirus*).

Style Rules of Thumb. A virus term that ends in -virales, -viridae, or -virinae should be capitalized, eg, change paramyxovirinae to Paramyxovirinae. Terms that end in *-virus* may or may not be formal terms (and may be genuses, species, or subspecific entities); editors should follow author usage. Authors should distinguish formal and common terms and style them accordingly. It is useful to give the formal, taxonomic identity of a virus at first mention in an article; afterward the informal name is typically used (unless the article is discussing taxonomy per se). Formal names are used for species and above, so subspecific viral entities (strains, serotypes, isolates etc) are not capitalized or italicized. Abbreviations may be used for common names.

Reference sources for viral terms include the latest nomenclature reports[2] and online databases[4,5] (more below). See Table 14 (at the end of the section on viruses) for formal names, common names, and abbreviations of human (and related) viruses.

Background and further style specifics follow.

The Viral Code. International virus taxonomy dates from 1966 and the first published report from 1971. Viral taxonomy and nomenclature are put forth by the International Committee on Taxonomy of Viruses (ICTV) in the International Code of Virus Classification and Nomenclature of ICTV.[2,6] (The ICTV is a committee of the Virology Division, International Union of Microbiology Societies.) The code is the work of more than 500 virologists worldwide, including 82 study groups.[7] The eighth report was issued in 2005.[2]

Official virus names for species and higher taxa are available in book form[2] with updates published in *Archives of Virology.* Online, official names and updates are to be available at the ICTV Web site, http://www.danforthcenter.org/iltab/ictvnet/asp/_MainPage.asp,[4] and at ICTVdb, http://phene.cpmc.columbia.edu (US mirror site: http://www.ncbi.nlm.nih.gov/ICTVdb/).[5] The ICTVdb site also provides information about isolates (eg, serotypes, strains) with links to genome sequence databases. (It is hoped that this linkage will bring needed consistency between official viral nomenclature and viral entries in gene sequence databases.[7])

As with bacterial, animal, and plant nomenclature, viral nomenclature aims for stability and clarity. (See also 15.14.1, Biological Nomenclature.) Names of viral taxa have standing when approved by the members of the full ICTV.[8] Proposals for new names or changes should be submitted to the ICTV Web site.[4]

The viral code applies to the ranks of order, family, subfamily, genus, and species (but not lower ranks). A virus may not yet be classified at each rank, eg, a viral species may belong to a family but not a genus, and a viral genus may not be assigned to a family. The rank of species was added to the code in 1991[6,9] and is reflected in the approximately 1950 viral species names found in the eighth report.[2] (There are around 5500 viruses recognized in the latest report.[2]) International specialty groups are responsible for viral nomenclature below the rank of species, eg, types, strains. The code does not govern artificially created and laboratory hybrid viruses.

Formal vs Vernacular Virus Names. Formal virus names are used for taxonomic groups (order, family, subfamily, genus, and species) in the abstract state.[2,10-12] Use of the formal name indicates that the group has official standing according to the ICTV code. Vernacular (common, informal) virus species names are used for actual entities, eg, laboratory material or outbreak specimens: "concrete viral objects that cause diseases. . . ."[12(p2247)]

Style of Virus Names. For examples of the typographic conventions described in this section, see Table 14, Viruses of Humans, at the end of the section.[2,9,13,14]

Typical endings for order, family, subfamily, genus, and species are as follows:

	Viruses		*Bacteria Ending*
	Example	*Ending*	
Order	Mononegavirales	-virales	-ales
Family	Paramyxoviridae	-viridae	-aceae
Subfamily	Paramyxovirinae	-virinae	-oideae
Genus	*Respirovirus*	*-virus*	(varies)
Species	*Human parainfluenzavirus 1*	*-virus*	(varies)

Latin and English Forms. Formal names of viral genus and above are latinized. Formal names of species "are English names derived from vernacular common names."[9(p3)] English, the scientific lingua franca during the era of viral discovery, is used for formal virus species names no matter what the language of publication.

Initial Capitals. Formal virus names at each rank have initial capital letters. Other capitals are used when a proper noun is part of the name, eg:

St Louis encephalitis virus

West Nile virus

Vernacular names do not use initial capitals unless a proper noun is part of the name, eg:

La Crosse virus

Italics. Although the viral nomenclature code recommends italicizing all scientific virus names (ie, species through order), codes for other organisms differ on using italics for names of higher taxa. For reasons of internal consistency, *JAMA* and the *Archives* Journals do not italicize names of viral taxa above genus. *JAMA* and the *Archives* Journals do italicize formal viral genus and species names. (Italicization of species is a change from previous ICTV nomenclature reports that was introduced in 1998, to indicate formal approval.[15] It is consistent with style in other areas of biological nomenclature.) Vernacular names are never italicized.

How to Style a Virus Term. An editor encountering a term ending in -virales, -viridae, or -virinae would capitalize the term; for instance, an editor would change parvoviridae to Parvoviridae. An editor encountering a term ending in -virus can use context to determine whether it is a formal or vernacular name (more below) and revise as necessary, querying the author. For instance, an editor might leave the term poliovirus as is or might change it to the formal species term *Poliovirus*. Terms for strains, types, serogroups, isolates, etc, are never italicized or capitalized (see the section on those entities below). In legends to figures depicting actual viral entities, eg, electron micrographs, italics and capitals would not be used for the actual entity depicted.[15] Legends to schematic depictions of viruses, however, probably refer to classes of virus, and formal style should be used.

Formal and Vernacular Names in Articles. Formal names are used for abstract entities, vernacular names for physical entities:

> *West Nile virus* is a member of the genus *Flavivirus*. The presence of West Nile virus was confirmed in mosquitoes and dead crows. . . .
>
> "We used polymerase chain reaction assays to detect RNA of West Nile virus (family *Flaviviridae,* genus *Flavivirus,* species *West Nile virus*) . . ."[16(p505)]

It is useful, for purposes of identification, to include the formal name initially in an article discussing actual viral entities (with the vernacular name used thereafter)[2,3,10,11,13]:

> *Hepatitis C virus* . . . hepatitis C virus
>
> *Human herpesvirus 4* . . . Epstein-Barr virus
>
> *Human herpesvirus 3* . . . varicella-zoster virus
>
> *Human immunodeficiency virus 1* . . . HIV-1

In such articles, the virus and its higher taxonomic classification may be usefully included early on, eg:

> "Sin Nombre virus (family *Bunyaviridae,* genus *Hantavirus*, species *Sin Nombre virus*) is an etiologic agent of hantavirus pulmonary syndrome, a potentially fatal illness of humans."[3(p2469)]

The formal name remains in English, the vernacular name in the language of publication, eg:

> *Measles virus* . . . virus de la rougeole . . . [12,13]
>
> *Hepatitis B virus* . . . el virus de la hepatitis B

Abbreviations. Formal viral species names should not be abbreviated. Common names of viral species names may be abbreviated. Recommended abbreviations are given in the international code (see Table 14, Viruses of Humans, at the end of this section).[2] Note that related gene symbols and virus abbreviations may differ (see 15.6.2, Genetics, Human Gene Nomenclature):

Gene symbol:	Gene description with virus abbreviation:
HVBS4	hepatitis B virus (HBV) integration site 4

The viral code recommends that rank always be specified with formal names and that it precede the virus name:

the family Paramyxoviridae

the genus *Respirovirus* (formerly the genus *Paramyxovirus*)

the species *Human parainfluenzavirus 1*

Virus names used as adjectives are not italicized,[15] eg:

human immunodeficiency virus infection

murine leukemia virus polymerase

vaccinia immune globulin

West Nile virus surveillance

Official style calls for temporary names (recognized taxa whose names are not yet formally approved) to be presented in roman type within quotation marks:

Sapovirus (formerly "Sapporo-like virus")

"T4-like viruses"

Formal style is unambiguous. Vernacular style can be ambiguous, because the ending *-virus* occurs in common names at all taxonomic ranks and in other informal designations (eg, arboviruses, which includes several families). It is therefore helpful for authors to specify rank with vernacular terms as well:

the family of retroviruses

Hantaan virus, a species of the genus *Hantavirus*

the paramyxovirus family

the paramyxovirus subfamily

Plant Virus Alternative. Many plant virologists favor a different style for formal species names, which uses a binomial term that includes species and genus.[6,11,17,18] (Despite the designation "binomial," it may contain more than 2 words.) Plant virus names in this style consist of an English species name followed by the genus name:

plant alternative:	Tobacco mosaic *tobamovirus*
ICTV style:	*Tobacco mosaic virus* (genus *Tobamovirus*)

Binomial Proposal. Formal virus species names do not currently follow the binomial style typical of other organisms (see 15.14.1, Biological Nomenclature), which includes the genus name and a specific epithet. Confusion exists between terms for abstract virus species and actual virus entities, which often are distinguished only typographically. Virologists have indicated a preference for a binomial style for official virus species names.[10,12] Such a style would resemble the plant style described above, giving species and then genus. (For instance, *Measles virus* would become *Measles morbillivirus*. The vernacular term measles virus would remain in use for actual measles-virus entities.) That proposal is under study.[10,11,12,17]

Derivations. For derivations of virus names, consult the reports of the ICTV.[2]

Some virus names are combinations of words; such names are known as *sigla*. Examples include *echovirus* (*e*nteric *c*ytopathic *h*uman *o*rphan *virus*) and picornavirus (*pico-*, *RNA virus*). Variant capitalization—eg, ECHOvirus, picoRNAvirus—is not used.

Strains, Types, and Isolates. In clinical and laboratory articles dealing with actual entities, most terms will refer to strains, serotypes, serogroups, or viral isolates, ie, ranks below species. Such terms are not capitalized (unless they include proper nouns) or italicized. Such terms often contain numbers, letters, or names, eg:

coxsackievirus A1, coxsackievirus A24

Desert Shield virus (a strain of *Norwalk virus)*

human adenovirus 2 (a strain of *Human adenovirus C)*

human astrovirus 3, Berlin isolate

Hantaan virus 76-118 (a serotype of *Hantaan virus)*

hepatitis C virus (HCV) genotype 1

HCV subtype (or genotype) 3a

hepatitis D virus genotype 1

human poliovirus 1, poliovirus 1, or poliovirus type 1

human poliovirus 2, poliovirus 2, or poliovirus type 2

human poliovirus 3, poliovirus 3, or poliovirus type 3

human respiratory syncytial virus A2

La Crosse virus (a serotype of *California encephalitis virus*)

Norwalk virus (a strain of *Norwalk virus)*

rotavirus B strain IDIR

tick-borne encephalitis virus European subtype

Formal species names may also include numbers or letters (eg, *Human herpesvirus 1, hepatitis B virus*; see Table 14, Viruses of Humans, at the end of this section).

Hepatitis Terms. Antigens of hepatitis B virus and antibodies to hepatitis B virus are expressed as follows:

Antigen	*Abbreviation*	*Antibody*
hepatitis B surface antigen	HBsAg	anti-HBs
hepatitis B core antigen	HBcAg	anti-HBc
hepatitis B e antigen	HBeAg	anti-HBe
hepatitis B X antigen	HBxAg	anti-HBx

Do not confuse hepatitis e antigen with hepatitis E virus or anti-HBe with anti-hepatitis E virus (anti-HEV).

Influenza Types and Strains. Strains of influenza A virus are identified by antigenic subtypes, defined by the surface proteins hemagglutinin (H) and neuraminidase (N), eg:

influenza A(H3N2)

The H,N suffix is used only for influenza A, but the 3 species of influenza virus may also contain suffixes with terms for the host of origin (if nonhuman), geographic origin (or a proper name in older strains), laboratory strain number, and year of isolation, separated by virgules (forward slashes) and, in the case of influenza A, followed by the H and N designations in parentheses:

influenza A/New York/55/2004(H3N2)

influenza A/chicken/Hong Kong/317.5/01(H5N1)

influenza B/Jiangsu/10/2003

influenza C/California/78

Phages. Phages are viruses that infect bacteria. The term *phage* is shortened from "bacteriophage." Although the current ICTV nomenclature code prohibits Greek letters in new virus names, older names with Greek letters have not been changed. Spelled-out Greek letters are also found, and letters may be uppercase or lowercase; follow author style. Vernacular terms often include the word *phage*, eg:

phage T4 *or* T4 phage

Phage groups or genera are sometimes referred to with general terms such as the following: T-even phages, actinophages, coliphages, T7 phage group.

Examples of formal phage names include the following:

Species	*Abbreviation*	*Genus*
Acholeplasma phage L51	L51	*Plectrovirus*
Enterobacteria phage λ	λ	"λ-like viruses"
Enterobacteria phage PRD1	PRD1	*Tectivirus*
Enterobacteria phage Qβ	Qβ	*Allolevivirus*
Enterobacteria phage T1	T1	"T1-like viruses"
Enterobacteria phage T4	T4	"T4-like viruses"
Enterobacteria phage Mu	Mu	"Mu-like viruses"
Halobacterium phage øH	øH	"øH-like viruses"
Lactococcus phage c2	c2	"c2-like viruses"
Pseudomonas phage ø6	ø6	*Cystovirus*

All of the above phage viruses have identically named strains, and many more strains belong to species of similar names. Follow author usage.

Enterobacteria phages Qβ and M11 are strains of *Enterobacteria phage Qβ*.

(For phage cloning vectors, see 15.6.1, Genetics, Nucleic Acids and Amino Acids, "Cloning Vectors.")

Genes. For genes related to human viruses, see 15.6.2, Genetics, Human Gene Nomenclature. For retrovirus gene terms, see 15.6.3, Genetics, Oncogenes and Tumor Suppressor Genes, and 15.6.5, Nonhuman Genetic Terms.

Table 14. Viruses of Humans

Common and Infraspecific Names[a]	Formal Species Names	Basic Abbreviation[b]	Genus	Family
adeno-associated virus	*Adeno-associated virus 1, Adeno-associated virus 2, Adeno-associated virus 3, etc*	AAV	*Dependovirus*	Parvoviridae (subfamily: Parvovirinae)
Alfuy virus	*Murray Valley encephalitis virus*	ALFV	*Flavivirus*	Flaviviridae
astrovirus	*Human astrovirus*	HAstV	*Mamastrovirus*	Astroviridae
Babanki virus	*Sindbis virus*		*Alphavirus*	Togaviridae
BK virus	*BK polyomavirus*	BKPyV	*Polyomavirus*	Polyomaviridae
Bunyamwera virus	*Bunyamwera virus*	BUNV	*Orthobunyavirus*	Bunyaviridae
California encephalitis virus	*California encephalitis virus*	CEV	*Orthobunyavirus*	Bunyaviridae
Colorado tick fever virus	*Colorado tick fever virus*	CTFV	*Coltivirus*	Reoviridae
coronavirus: *see* human coronavirus				
coxsackieviruses, eg, coxsackievirus A10, coxsackievirus B6, coxsackievirus A24	*Human enterovirus A, Human enterovirus B, Human enterovirus C*	CV	*Enterovirus*	Picornaviridae
Crimean-Congo hemorrhagic fever virus	*Crimean-Congo hemorrhagic fever virus*	CCHFV	*Nairovirus*	Bunyaviridae
cytomegalovirus	*Human herpesvirus 5*	HHV-5	*Cytomegalovirus*	Herpesviridae (subfamily: Betaherpesvirinae)
dengue virus	*Dengue virus*	DENV	*Flavivirus*	Flaviviridae
Desert Shield virus	*Norwalk virus*	Hu/NV/DSV	*Norovirus*	Calciviridae
Eastern equine encephalitis virus	*Eastern equine encephalitis virus*	EEEV	*Alphavirus*	Togaviridae
Ebola viruses, eg, Cote D'Ivoire ebolavirus, Reston ebolavirus Texas, Sudan Ebola virus Maleo, Zaire Ebola virus Gabon	*Cote d'Ivoire ebolavirus, Reston ebolavirus, Sudan ebolavirus, Zaire ebolavirus*	CIEBOV REBOV SEBOV, ZEBOV	*Ebolavirus*	Filoviridae

echoviruses, eg, echovirus 1, echovirus 2	*Human enterovirus B*	E	*Enterovirus*	Picornaviridae
enterovirus 68 enterovirus 70	*Human enterovirus D*	EV	*Enterovirus*	Picornaviridae
Epstein-Barr virus	*Human herpesvirus 4*	HHV-4	*Lymphocryptovirus*	Herpesviridae (subfamily: Gammaherpesvirinae)
Eyach virus	*Eyach virus*	EYAV	*Coltivirus*	Reoviridae
GB virus A GB virus C	*GB virus A, GB virus C*	GBV-A, GBV-C	unassigned	Flaviviridae
GB virus B	*GB virus B*	GBV-B	*Hepacivirus* (tentative)	Flaviviridae
Hantaan virus	*Hantaan virus*	HTNV	*Hantavirus*	Bunyaviridae
Hendra virus	*Hendravirus*	HeV	*Henipavirus*	Paramyxoviridae (subfamily: Paramyxovirinae)
hepatitis A virus	*Human hepatitis A virus*	HHAV	*Hepatovirus*	Picornaviridae
hepatitis B virus hepatitis B virus-A hepatitis B virus-B, etc	*Hepatitis B virus*	HBV	*Orthohepadnavirus*	Hepadnaviridae
hepatitis C virus HCV clade 1 HCV genotype 1a, etc	*Hepatitis C virus*	HCV	*Hepacivirus*	Flaviviridae
hepatitis D virus	*Hepatitis delta virus*	HDV	*Deltavirus*	unassigned
hepatitis E virus	*Hepatitis E virus*	HEV	*Hepevirus*	Hepeviridae
hepatitis G virus	*GB virus C*	HGV	unassigned	Flaviviridae
herpes simplex virus type 1, herpes simplex virus type 2	*Human herpesvirus 1,* *Human herpesvirus 2*	HHV-1, HHV-2	*Simplexvirus*	Herpesviridae (subfamily: Alphaherpesvirinae)
herpesvirus simiae (also simian herpes B virus)	*Cercopithecine herpesvirus 1*	CeHV-1	*Simplexvirus*	Herpesviridae (subfamily: Alphaherpesvirinae)
human adenoviruses, eg human adenovirus 2	*Human adenovirus A* through *F*, eg, *Human adenovirus C*	HAdV HAdV-2	*Mastadenovirus*	Adenoviridae

Table 14. Viruses of Humans *(cont)*

Common and Infraspecific Names[a]	Formal Species Names	Basic Abbreviation[b]	Genus	Family
human coronavirus 229E human coronavirus OC43	*Human coronavirus 229E,* *Human coronavirus OC43*	HCoV-229E, HCoV-OC43	*Coronavirus*	*Coronaviridae*
human herpesvirus 6, herpesvirus 7	*Human herpesvirus 6,* *Human herpesvirus 7*	HHV-6, HHV-7	*Roseolovirus*	Herpesviridae (subfamily: Betaherpesvirinae)
human immunodeficiency virus	*Human immunodeficiency virus 1,* *Human immunodeficiency virus 2*	HIV-1, HIV-2	*Lentivirus*	Retroviridae (subfamily: Orthoretrovirinae)
human papillomavirus	*Human papillomavirus 5, etc*	HPV-5, etc	*Betapapillomavirus*	Papillomaviridae
human papillomavirus	*Human papillomavirus 4, etc*	HPV-4, etc	*Gammapapillomavirus*	Papillomaviridae
human papillomavirus	*Human papillomavirus 1,* *Human papillomavirus 63*	HPV-1, HPV-63	*Mupapillomavirus*	Papillomaviridae
human papillomavirus	*Human papillomavirus 32, etc*	HPV-32	*Alphapapillomavirus*	Papillomaviridae
human papillomavirus	*Human papillomavirus 41*	HPV-41	*Nupapillomavirus*	Papillomaviridae
human T-lymphotropic virus 1 human T-lymphotropic virus 2	*Primate T-lymphotropic virus 1* *Primate T-lymphotropic virus 2*	HTLV-1 HTLV-2	*Deltaretrovirus*	Retroviridae (subfamily: Orthoretrovirinae)
influenza A virus influenza A/PR8/34 (H1N1)	*Influenza A virus*	FLUAV	*Influenzavirus A*	Orthomyxoviridae
influenza B virus influenza B/Lee/40	*Influenza B virus*	FLUBV	*Influenzavirus B*	Orthomyxoviridae
influenza C virus influenza C/California/78	*Influenza C virus*	FLUCV	*Influenzavirus C*	Orthomyxoviridae
Japanese encephalitis virus	*Japanese encephalitis virus*	JEV	*Flavivirus*	Flaviviridae
JC virus	*JC polyomavirus*	JCPyV	*Polyomavirus*	Polyomaviridae
Kaposi sarcoma-associated herpesvirus	*Human herpesvirus 8*	HHV-8	*Rhadinovirus*	Herpesviridae (subfamily: Gammaherpesvirinae)
Kunjin virus	*West Nile virus*	KUNV	*Flavivirus*	Flaviviridae
Kyasanur Forest disease virus	*Kyasanur Forest disease virus*	KFDV	*Flavivirus*	Flaviviridae

La Crosse virus	*California encephalitis virus*	LACV	*Orthobunyavirus*	Bunyaviridae
Lassa virus	*Lassa virus*	LASV	*Arenavirus*	Arenaviridae
Lebombo virus	*Lebombo virus*	LEBV	*Orbivirus*	Reoviridae
lymphocytic choriomeningitis virus	*Lymphocytic choriomeningitis virus*	LCMV	*Arenavirus*	Arenaviridae
Marburg virus	*Lake Victoria marburgvirus*	MARV	*Marburgvirus*	Filoviridae
measles virus	*Measles virus*	MeV	*Morbillivirus*	Paramyxoviridae (subfamily: Paramyxovirinae)
metapneumovirus	*Human metapneumovirus*	HMPV	*Metapneumovirus*	Paramyxoviridae (subfamily: Pneumovirinae)
molluscum contagiosum virus	*Molluscum contagiosum virus*	MOCV	*Molluscipoxvirus*	Poxviridae (subfamily: Chordopoxvirinae)
monkeypox virus monkeypox virus Zaire-96-I-16	*Monkeypox virus*	MPXV	*Orthopoxvirus*	Poxviridae (subfamily: Chordopoxvirinae)
mumps virus	*Mumps virus*	MuV	*Rubulavirus*	Paramyxoviridae (subfamily: Paramyxovirinae)
Murray Valley encephalitis virus	*Murray Valley encephalitis virus*	MVEV	*Flavivirus*	Flaviviridae
Nipah virus	*Nipah virus*	NiV	*Henipavirus*	Paramyxoviridae (subfamily: Paramyxovirinae)
Norwalk virus	*Norwalk virus*	NV	*Norovirus*	Calciviridae
O'nyong-nyong virus	*O'nyong-nyong virus*	ONNV	*Alphavirus*	Togaviridae
Omsk hemorrhagic fever virus	*Omsk hemorrhagic fever virus*	OHFV	*Flavivirus*	Flaviviridae
orf virus	*Orf virus*	ORFV	*Parapoxvirus*	Poxviridae (subfamily: Chordopoxvirinae)
Orungo virus	*Orungo virus*	ORUV	*Orbivirus*	Reoviridae
papillomavirus: see human papillomavirus				
parainfluenza virus 1, parainfluenzavirus 3	*Human parainfluenzavirus 1, Human parainfluenzavirus 3*	HPIV-1, HPIV-3	*Respirovirus*	Paramyxoviridae (subfamily: Paramyxovirinae)

Table 14. Viruses of Humans *(cont)*

Common and Infraspecific Names[a]	Formal Species Names	Basic Abbreviation[b]	Genus	Family
parainfluenzavirus 2, parainfluenzavirus 4	*Human parainfluenzavirus 2, Human parainfluenzavirus 4*	HPIV-2, HPIV-4	*Rubulavirus*	Paramyxoviridae (subfamily: Paramyxovirinae)
parvovirus B19-A6 parvovirus B19-Au	*Human parvovirus B19*	B19V	*Erythrovirus*	Parvoviridae (subfamily: Parvovirinae)
poliovirus 1 poliovirus 2 poliovirus 3	*Poliovirus*	PV	*Enterovirus*	Picornaviridae
rabies virus	*Rabies virus*	RABV	*Lyssavirus*	Rhabdoviridae
respiratory syncytial virus human respiratory syncytial virus A2	*Human respiratory syncytial virus*	HRSV	*Pneumovirus*	Paramyxoviridae (subfamily: Pneumovirinae)
rhinoviruses, eg, rhinovirus A, human rhinovirus 37, rhinovirus B, human rhinovirus 100	*Human rhinovirus A, Human rhinovirus B*	HRV	*Rhinovirus*	Picornaviridae
Rift Valley fever virus	*Rift Valley fever virus*	RVFV	*Phlebovirus*	Bunyaviridae
Ross River virus	*Ross River virus*	RRV	*Alphavirus*	Togaviridae
rotavirus	*Rotavirus B, Rotavirus C*	RV-B, HRV-C	*Rotavirus*	Reoviridae
rubella virus	*Rubella virus*	RUBV	*Rubivirus*	Togaviridae
Sagiyama virus	*Ross River virus*		*Alphavirus*	Togaviridae
Sapporo virus	*Sapporo virus*	Hu/SV	*Sapovirus* (formerly "Sapporo-like viruses")	Calciviridae
SARS virus or SARS-associated coronavirus	*Severe acute respiratory syndrome coronavirus*	SARS-CoV	*Coronavirus*	Coronaviridae
simian hepatitis A virus	*Human hepatitis A virus*	SHAV	*Hepatovirus*	Picornaviridae
simian herpes B virus (also herpesvirus simiae)	*Cercopithecine herpesvirus 1*	CeHV-1	*Simplexvirus*	Herpesviridae (subfamily: Alphaherpesvirinae)

simian T-lymphotropic virus	*Primate T-lymphotropic virus 1*	STLV-1	*Deltaretrovirus*	Retroviridae (subfamily: Orthoretrovirinae)
Sin Nombre virus	*Sin Nombre virus*	SNV	*Hantavirus*	Bunyaviridae
Sindbis virus	*Sindbis virus*	SINV	*Alphavirus*	Togaviridae
St Louis encephalitis virus	*St Louis encephalitis virus*	SLEV	*Flavivirus*	Flaviridae
tanapox virus	*Tanapox virus*	TANV	*Yatapoxvirus*	Poxviridae (subfamily: Chordopoxvirinae)
tick-borne encephalitis virus	*Tick-borne encephalitis virus*	TBEV	*Flavivirus*	Flaviviridae
vaccinia virus vaccinia virus Ankara vaccinia virus Copenhagen	*Vaccinia virus*	VACV	*Orthopoxvirus*	Poxviridae (subfamily: Chordopoxvirinae)
varicella-zoster virus	*Human herpesvirus 3*	HHV-3	*Varicellovirus*	Herpesviridae (subfamily: Alphaherpesvirinae)
variola virus	*Variola virus*	VARV	*Orthopoxvirus*	Poxviridae (subfamily: Chordopoxvirinae)
Venezuelan equine encephalitis virus	*Venezuelan equine encephalitis virus*	VEEV	*Alphavirus*	Togaviridae
vesicular stomatitis virus	*Vesicular stomatitis Alagoas virus, Vesicular stomatitis Indiana virus, Vesicular stomatitis New Jersey virus*	VSAV, VSIV, VSNJV	*Vesiculovirus*	Rhabdoviridae
West Nile virus	*West Nile virus*	WNV	*Flavivirus*	Flaviviridae
Western equine encephalitis virus	*Western equine encephalitis virus*	WEEV	*Alphavirus*	Togaviridae
yellow fever virus	*Yellow fever virus*	YFV	*Flavivirus*	Flaviviridae

[a] Entries in this column are not complete listings of all members of the corresponding species. Entries may include species names, strains, serogroups, etc.

[b] Use abbreviations in accordance with recommendations in 14.0, Abbreviations.

15.14.4 **Prions.** The following are disease names and abbreviations of transmissible spongiform encephalopathies[2,19-21]:

Disease	*Abbreviation*
bovine spongiform encephalopathy ("mad cow disease")	BSE
Creutzfeldt-Jakob disease	CJD
familial CJD	fCJD
iatrogenic CJD	iCJD
sporadic CJD	sCJD
variant CJD (formerly new variant CJD [nvCJD])	vCJD
chronic wasting disease of mule deer and elk	CWD
exotic ungulate encephalopathy (nyala, greater kudu, oryx)	EUE
fatal familial insomnia	FFI
feline spongiform encephalopathy	FSE
Gerstmann-Sträussler-Scheinker syndrome	GSS
kuru	
scrapie	
transmissible mink encephalopathy	TME
transmissible spongiform encephalopathy	TSE

(Do not confuse "kudu" and "kuru.")

The infectious agents of TSEs are known as *TSE agents* or *prions*. The term *prion* (from "proteinaceous infectious particle") reflects the agents' proposed association or identity with spongiform encephalopathy-related pathologic proteins. Follow author preference for the terms *TSE agent* and *prion*.

Proteins related to spongiform encephalopathies in humans are designated as follows:

PrP	prion protein
PrP27-30	PrP of 27-30 kD
$\mathrm{PrP^{C}}$	cellular PrP
$\mathrm{PrP^{Sc}}$	scrapie-type PrP
PrP-res	protease-resistant PrP
PrP-sen	protease-sensitive PrP
rPrP	recombinant PrP
$\mathrm{BovPrP^{Sc}}$	(bovine)
$\mathrm{FePrP^{Sc}}$	(feline)
$\mathrm{HuPrP^{CJD}}$	(human)
$\mathrm{HuPrP^{Sc}}$	(human)
$\mathrm{MDePrP^{Sc}}$	(mule deer and elk)

$MkPrP^{Sc}$	(mink)
MoPrP	(mouse)
$NyaPrP^{Sc}$	(nyala and greater kudu)
$OvPrP^{Sc}$	(ovine [scrapie])
Tg(HuPrP)	(transgenic)
Tg(MoPrP-P101L)	

The last term refers to a transgenic mouse line with a proline to leucine mutation at residue 101 (see also 15.6.1, Genetics, Nucleic Acids and Amino Acids).

For prion-related genes, see 15.6.2, Genetics, Human Gene Nomenclature.

REFERENCES

1. Collier L, Oxford J. *Human Virology: A Text for Students of Medicine, Dentistry, and Microbiology*. New York, NY: Oxford University Press; 1993.
2. Fauquet CM, Mayo MA, Maniloff J, Desselberger U, Ball LA. *Virus Taxonomy: Classification and Nomenclature of Viruses: Eighth Report of the International Committee on Taxonomy of Viruses*. San Diego, CA: Elsevier Academic Press; 2005.
3. Drebot MA, Henchal E, Hjelle B, et al. Improved clarity of meaning from the use of both formal species names and common (vernacular) virus names in virological literature. *Arch Virol*. 2002;147(12):2465-2471.
4. Donald Danforth Plant Science Center. ICTVNet. http://www.danforthcenter.org/iltab/ictvnet/asp/_MainPage.asp. Accessed April 21, 2006.
5. Büchen-Osmond C. ICTVdb: The Universal Virus Database of the International Committee on Taxonomy of Viruses. http://phene.cpmc.columbia.edu and http://www.ncbi.nlm.nih.gov/ICTVdb/. Updated February 18, 2005. Accessed April 21, 2006.
6. Van Regenmortel MHV, Fauquet CM, Bishop DHL, et al, eds. *Virus Taxonomy: Classification and Nomenclature of Viruses: Seventh Report of the International Committee on Taxonomy of Viruses*. San Diego, CA: Academic Press; 2000.
7. Fauquet CM, Fargette D. International Committee on Taxonomy of Viruses and the 3,142 unassigned species. *Virol J*. 2005;2:64. doi:10.1186/1743-422X-2-64.
8. Mayo MA, Fauquet CM, Maniloff J. Taxonomic proposals on the Web: new ICTV consultative procedures. *Arch Virol*. 2003;148(3):609-611.
9. Van Regenmortel MHV. Virus nomenclature. In: Maisonneuve H, Enckell PH, Polderman AKS, Thapa R, Vekony M, eds. *Science Editors' Handbook*. West Clandon, England: European Association of Science Editors; 2003;§3-4.2:1-4.
10. Van Regenmortel MHV, Mahy BWJ. Emerging issues in virus taxonomy. *Emerg Infect Dis*. 2004;10(1):8-13.
11. Van Regenmortel MHV. Viruses are real, virus species are man-made, taxonomic constructions. *Arch Virol*. 2003;148(12):2481-2488.
12. Van Regenmortel MHV, Fauquet CM. Only italicised species names of viruses have a taxonomic meaning. *Arch Virol*. 2002;147(11):2247-2250.
13. Van Regenmortel MHV. On the relative merits of italics, Latin and binomial nomenclature in virus taxonomy. *Arch Virol*. 2000;145(2):433-441.
14. Van Regenmortel MHV, Mayo MA, Fauquet CM, Maniloff J. Virus nomenclature: consensus versus chaos. *Arch Virol*. 2000;145(10):2227-2232.
15. Van Regenmortel MHV. How to write the names of virus species. *Arch Virol*. 1999;144(5):1041-1042.

16. Calisher CH, Mahy BWJ. Taxonomy: get it right or leave it alone. *Am J Trop Med Hyg.* 2003;68(5):505-506.
17. Van Regenmortel MHV. Perspectives on binomial names of virus species. *Arch Virol.* 2001;146(8):1637-1640.
18. Brunt A, Crabtree K, Dallwitz M, Gibbs A, Watson L, Zurcher E, eds. Plant Viruses Online: Descriptions and Lists From the VIDE Database. http://image.fs.uidaho.edu/vide/refs.htm#names. Accessed December 4, 2006.
19. Asher DM. Transmissible spongiform encephalopathies. In: Murray PR, Baron EJ, Jorgensen JH, Pfaller MA, Yolken RH, eds. *Manual of Clinical Microbiology.* 8th ed. Washington, DC: ASM Press; 2003:1592-1604.
20. Prusiner SB. Novel proteinaceous infectious particles cause scrapie. *Science.* 1982;216(4542):136-144.
21. Prusiner SB. Prion diseases and the BSE crisis. *Science.* 1997;278(5336):245-251.

15.15 Psychiatric Terminology

15.15.1 *Diagnostic and Statistical Manual of Mental Disorders (DSM).*

The American Psychiatric Association has published 5 editions of a manual for the classification of mental disorders. Each edition has been titled *Diagnostic and Statistical Manual of Mental Disorders* and has used the abbreviation *DSM*:

DSM-I (1952)

DSM-II (1968)

DSM-III (1980)

DSM-III-R (1987)

DSM-IV (1994)

Using *DSM-IV* as an example, these books should be cited as follows:

> American Psychiatric Association. *Diagnostic and Statistical Manual of Mental Disorders.* 4th ed. Washington, DC: American Psychiatric Association; 1994.

A text revision of *DSM-IV* was published in 2000 as *Diagnostic and Statistical Manual of Mental Disorders, Fourth Edition, Text Revision*, abbreviated *DSM-IV-TR*. This book is a revision of the text describing the diagnostic and associated features, prevalence, course, and differential diagnosis of the disorders included in the *DSM-IV* diagnostic categories. However, the diagnostic classification and criteria in *DSM-IV-TR* are unchanged from those in the 1994 *DSM-IV* diagnostic manual. If *DSM-IV-TR* is cited for diagnostic criteria, it gives the misleading impression that the criteria used differ from those of *DSM-IV* and date from 2000 rather than 1994. Thus, a citation for the *DSM-IV* diagnostic criteria should be to *DSM-IV* (1994). There are no *DSM-IV-TR* diagnostic criteria per se. If a reference citation pertains to the updated descriptive material in *DSM-IV-TR*, that should be cited. If a citation pertains to both the *DSM-IV* criteria and the updated descriptive material in *DSM-IV-TR*, it would be best to clarify that in the text.

Beginning with *DSM-III*, the diagnostic system involves an assessment on several axes as follows:

Axis I	Clinical Disorders
	Other Conditions That May Be a Focus of Clinical Attention

Axis II	Personality Disorders
	Mental Retardation
Axis III	General Medical Conditions
Axis IV	Psychosocial and Environmental Problems
Axis V	Global Assessment of Functioning

For proper expressions of editions of *DSM,* see 14.11, Abbreviations, Clinical, Technical, and Other Common Terms. For proper capitalization of designators of axes in *DSM,* eg, Axis I, see 10.4, Capitalization, Designators.

15.15.2 Other Psychiatric Terminology. For appropriate use of terms such as *manic* and *schizophrenic*, see 11.1, Correct and Preferred Usage, Correct and Preferred Usage of Common Words and Phrases.

For molecular terms, see 15.11.5, Neurology, Molecular Neuroscience.

15.16 Pulmonary, Respiratory, and Blood Gas Terminology.

Standardization of symbols in respiratory physiology dates from at least 1950.[1]

Despite the familiarity of abbreviations in pulmonary and respiratory medicine, authors and editors are encouraged to expand all terms at first mention, except as noted.

Symbols and abbreviations are both used. Symbols consist of separate elements in various combinations whose letters may differ from the initial letters of the expansion, eg, $\dot{Q}$ (perfusion). Abbreviations are usually initialisms.

15.16.1 Symbols.

Symbols and their subgrouping into main symbols and modifiers are consistent with approved nomenclature formulated circa 1980 by the Commission of Respiratory Physiology (International Union of Physiological Sciences) and the Publications Committee of the American Physiological Society.[2,3] The following groupings of pulmonary-respiratory symbols are adapted from Fishman.[2]

Main symbols are typically capital letters set on the line and are the first elements of an expression. The same letter may stand for one entity in respiratory mechanics and another in gas exchange (eg, P stands for pressure in respiratory mechanics and partial pressure in gas exchange). The following are examples (note dots above some letters to indicate flow):

C	compliance, concentration
D	diffusing capacity
F	fractional concentration in a dry gas
P	pressure, partial pressure
Q	volume of blood
$\dot{Q}$	perfusion (volume of blood per unit time or blood flow)
R	resistance, gas (respiratory) exchange ratio
S	saturation
sG	specific conductance
V	volume of gas
$\dot{V}$	ventilation (volume per unit time)

Modifiers are set as small capitals (not subscript):

A	alveolar
B	barometric
DS	dead space
E	expired, expiratory
ET	end-tidal
I	inspired, inspiratory
L	lung
T	tidal

Lowercase-letter modifiers (which are not subscript) follow small-capital modifiers, if both appear; note bar in last term:

a	arterial
aw	airway
b	blood
c	capillary
c′	pulmonary end-capillary
i	ideal
max	maximum
p	pulse oximetry
v	venous
$\bar{v}$	mixed venous

Gas abbreviations are usually the last element of the symbol, given as small capitals:

CO	carbon monoxide
CO_2	carbon dioxide
N_2	nitrogen
O_2	oxygen

(*Note:* At other times, when gas abbreviations are used on their own, large capitals are used, eg, carbon monoxide [CO].)

The main symbols and modifiers are combined in various ways to derive terms; common examples are the following:

Term	*Expansion*	*Typical Units of Measure*[2,4-8]
Pco_2	partial pressure of carbon dioxide	mm Hg *or* kPa
$Paco_2$	partial pressure of carbon dioxide, arterial	mm Hg *or* kPa
Po_2	partial pressure of oxygen	mm Hg *or* kPa
Pao_2	partial pressure of oxygen, arterial	mm Hg *or* kPa

(*Note:* The above 4 terms may be given without expansion at first mention; see also 14.11, Abbreviations, Clinical, Technical, and Other Common Terms, and 18.0, Units of Measure.)

Term	*Expansion*	*Typical Units of Measure*[2,4-8]
P_{AO_2}	partial pressure of oxygen, alveolar	mm Hg *or* kPa
$P_{\bar{v}O_2}$	partial pressure of oxygen, mixed venous	mm Hg *or* kPa
P_B	barometric pressure	mm Hg *or* kPa
P_{AO_2} - Pa_{O_2}	alveolar-arterial difference (or gradient) in partial pressure of oxygen (preferred to AaD_{O_2})	mm Hg *or* kPa
Ca_{O_2}	oxygen concentration (or content), arterial	mL/dL *or* mmol/L
Cc'_{O_2}	oxygen concentration (or content), pulmonary end-capillary	mL/dL
C_L	lung compliance	L/cm H_2O *or* L/mm Hg *or* L/kPa
D_{LCO}	diffusing capacity of lung for carbon monoxide	$mL \cdot min^{-1} \cdot mm\ Hg^{-1}$
F_{EN_2}	fractional concentration of nitrogen in expired gas	fraction
F_{IO_2}	fraction of inspired oxygen	fraction
P_{Emax}	maximum expiratory pressure	cm H_2O *or* mm Hg
P_{Imax}	maximum inspiratory pressure	cm H_2O *or* mm Hg
Raw	airway resistance	$cm\ H_2O \cdot L^{-1} \cdot s^{-1}$ *or* $kPa \cdot L^{-1} \cdot s^{-1}$
Sa_{O_2}	arterial oxygen saturation	%
sGaw	specific airway conductance	$L \cdot s^{-1} \cdot cm\ H_2O^{-1}$ *or* $L \cdot s^{-1} \cdot kPa^{-1}$
Sp_{O_2}	oxygen saturation as measured by pulse oximetry	%
V_{DS}	volume of dead space	mL *or* L
$\dot{V}_E$	expired volume per unit time	L/min
$\dot{V}_{O_2}$	oxygen consumption	mL/min *or* L/min *or* mmol/min
$\dot{V}_{O_2}max$	maximum oxygen consumption	mL/min *or* L/min *or* mmol/min
$\dot{V}/\dot{Q}$	ventilation perfusion ratio (also $\dot{V}_A/\dot{Q}$)	ratio
V_T	tidal volume	mL *or* L

**Note:* Sometimes quantities are given per unit body weight, eg, V_T in liters per kilogram.

15.16.2 Abbreviations. The following are some common abbreviations from pulmonary function testing; they should always be expanded at first mention:

Term	*Expansion*	*Typical Unit of Measure*
CC	closing capacity	L
CV	closing volume	L
ERV	expiratory reserve volume	L
FEF	forced expiratory flow	L/min
$FEF_{25\%-75\%}$	FEF, midexpiratory phase	L/min *or* L/s
$FEF_{200-1200}$	FEF between 200 and 1200 mL of forced vital capacity (FVC)	L/min *or* L/s
FEV	forced expiratory volume	L
FEV_1	FEV in the first second of expiration	L
FIVC	forced inspiratory vital capacity	L
FRC	functional residual capacity	mL *or* L
FVC	forced vital capacity	L
IRV	inspiratory reserve volume	L
IVC	inspiratory vital capacity	L
MVV	maximum voluntary ventilation	L/min
PEF, PEFR	peak expiratory flow rate	L/min
RV	residual volume	L
TLC	total lung capacity	L
VC	vital capacity	L

15.16.3 Mechanical Ventilation. The following should be expanded at first mention:

APRV	airway pressure release ventilation
BiPAP	bilevel positive airway pressure (cm H_2O)
CPAP	continuous positive airway pressure (cm H_2O)
ECMO	extracorporeal membrane oxygenation
ET tube	endotracheal tube
HFV	high-frequency ventilation
NIPPV	noninvasive positive pressure ventilation
NIV	noninvasive ventilation
PAV	proportional assist ventilation
PEEP	positive end-expiratory pressure (cm H_2O)

REFERENCES

1. Pappenheimer JR, Comroe JH, Cournand A, et al. Standardization of definitions and symbols in respiratory physiology. *Fed Proc.* 1950;9:602-605.
2. Fishman AP, ed. *Handbook of Physiology: A Critical, Comprehensive Presentation of Physiological Knowledge and Concepts.* Vol 2, section 3, pt 1. Bethesda, MD: American Physiological Society; 1986:endpapers.

3. Macklem PT. Symbols and abbreviations. In: Fishman AP, ed. *Handbook of Physiology: A Critical Comprehensive Presentation of Physiological Knowledge and Concepts.* Vol 2, section 3, pt 1. Bethesda, MD: American Physiological Society; 1986:ix.
4. West JB. *Pulmonary Pathophysiology: The Essentials.* 6th ed. Philadelphia, PA: Lippincott Williams & Wilkins; 2003.
5. West JB. *Respiratory Physiology: The Essentials.* 7th ed. Philadelphia, PA: Lippincott Williams & Wilkins; 2005.
6. Kasper DL, Braunwald E, Fauci AS, Hauser SL, Longo DL, Jameson JL, eds. *Harrison's Principles of Internal Medicine.* 16th ed. New York, NY: McGraw-Hill; 2005:A-14.
7. Albert RK, Spiro SG, Jett JR. *Clinical Respiratory Medicine.* 2nd ed. Philadelphia, PA: Mosby; 2004.
8. McMillan JA, DeAngelis CD, Feigin R, Warshaw JB. *Oski's Pediatrics.* 3rd ed. Philadelphia, PA: Lippincott Williams & Wilkins; 1999.

15.17 Radiology Terms

15.17.1 Resources. Available radiologic glossaries include the following[1]:

- Thoracic radiology: "Glossary of Terms for Thoracic Radiology"[2]
- Computed tomography of the lung: "Glossary of Terms for CT of the Lungs"[3]
- Breast imaging: BI-RADS Atlas[4]
- Magnetic resonance: *ACR Glossary of MRI Terms,*[5] Glossary of Magnetic Resonance Terms[6]
- Ultrasonography: *Recommended Ultrasound Terminology*[7]
- General, for laypersons and nonspecialists: RadiologyInfo[8]

In addition to the terminology explained in this section, see 11.0, Correct and Preferred Usage, for terms such as *radiography*, *roentgen*, and *x-ray;* 14.14, Abbreviations, Radioactive Isotopes, and 15.9, Isotopes; and 18.0, Units of Measure, for units such as H (Hounsfield) and keV (kiloelectron volt).

15.17.2 Terms. The following terms are commonly used in radiology.[9]

b value—The *b factor* or *b value* is associated with diffusion-weighted magnetic resonance imaging (diffusion-weighted MRI or DWI). It measures "strength (intensity and timing) of the diffusion gradient"[9]; units are seconds per square millimeter.

> maximum b value of 1221 s/mm^2
>
> Four gradient strengths were applied, resulting in b values of 0 and 1000 s/mm^2 applied sequentially in the X, Y, and Z gradient directions.

Doppler—See 15.3.6, Cardiology, Echocardiography.

echo train—A sequence of echoes. "*Echo train* is not a unit of measure"[9] but is expressed as in these examples:

> echo train length 5
>
> echo train length 18

echo train length 16

echo train length 20

a long echo-train-length 3-dimensional fast-spin echo sequence

k-space—This term refers to mathematical space with frequency and phase as coordinates, rather than spatial coordinates.[6]

Our pulse sequences collected data spirally in k-space.

k-space filtering

k-space sampling

number of excitations/signals—Change "number of excitations" to "number of signals acquired" (applies to MRI).

T1, T1ρ, T2, T2*—These are types of relaxation time in magnetic resonance imaging.[5,6] They need not be expanded.

T1	spin-lattice or longitudinal relaxation time
T1ρ	spin-lattice relaxation time in the rotating frame
T2	spin-spin or transverse relaxation time
T2*	time constant for loss of phase coherence among spins

TE, TR—Expand echo time (TE) and repetition time (TR) as in this example:

cardiac-gated repetition time (TR) greater than 2400 milliseconds; echo times (TEs), 20 and 80 milliseconds

REFERENCES

1. Skryd PJ. Radiologic nomenclature and abbreviations. *Radiology*. 2001;218(1):10-11. Also available at http://radiology.rsnajnls.org/cgi/content/full/218/1/10. Accessed September 22, 2005.
2. Tuddenham WJ. Glossary of terms for thoracic radiology: recommendations of the Nomenclature Committee of the Fleischner Society. *AJR Am J Roentgenol*. 1984;143(3):509-517.
3. Austin JHM, Müller NL, Friedman PJ, et al. Glossary of terms for CT of the lungs: recommendations of the Nomenclature Committee of the Fleischner Society. *Radiology*. 1996;200(2):327-331.
4. American College of Radiology. BI-RADS Atlas. http://www.acr.org/s_acr/sec.asp?CID=97&DID=142. Accessed September 22, 2005.
5. Hendrick RE, Bradley WG Jr, Harms SE, et al. ACR Revised Glossary 2005 (*ACR Glossary of MRI Terms*. 5th ed.) Chicago, IL: American College of Radiology; 2005. http://www.acr.org/s_acr/sec.asp?CID=3614&DID=22815. Accessed April 21, 2006.
6. European Magnetic Resonance Forum. Glossary of magnetic resonance terms. http://www.emrf.org/Education%20and%20Training/Glossary%20Page%20E.html. Accessed April 21, 2006.
7. *Recommended Ultrasound Terminology*. 2nd ed. Laurel, MD: American Institute of Ultrasound in Medicine; 1997.
8. RadiologyInfo. http://www.radiologyinfo.com/glossary/glossary1.cfm. Accessed April 21, 2006.
9. Lang D. Usage and nomenclature. In: *Radiological Society of North America (RSNA) In-House Style Manual*. Oak Brook Terrace, IL: RSNA; 2001.

16 Eponyms

Eponyms are names or phrases derived from or including the name of a person or place. These terms are used in a descriptive or adjectival sense[1] in medical and scientific writing to describe entities such as diseases, syndromes, signs, tests, methods, and procedures. These eponymous terms should be distinguished from true possessives (eg, Homer's *Iliad*). Medical eponyms are numerous (a Web site[2] devoted to medical eponyms lists more than 7000), are frequently used in medical publications, and are treated in dictionaries of eponyms covering general medicine[3] and some specialties, eg, neurology.[4]

Eponyms historically have indicated the name of the describer or presumptive discoverer of the disease (eg, Alzheimer disease) or sign (eg, Murphy sign), the name of a person or kindred found to have the disease described (eg, Christmas disease), or, when based on the name of a place (technically, *toponyms*), the geographic location in which the disease was found to occur (eg, Lyme disease). Traditionally, eponyms named after the describer or discoverer took the possessive form (-*'s*) and those named for other persons or for places took the nonpossessive form. As the use of the possessive form for all eponyms has become progressively less common (see 16.2, Nonpossessive Form), this formal distinction has faded.

Correct use of eponyms should be considered with a view toward clarity and consistency, the awareness that meanings can change over time and across cultures, and a desire to minimize misunderstanding in an increasingly global medical community.

16.1 **Eponymous vs Noneponymous Terms.** Use of eponyms in the biomedical literature should be considered with regard to their usefulness in transmitting medical information. Although some eponyms are evanescent, many are permanently integrated into the body of medical knowledge. Eponyms have a degree of historical and cultural value and sometimes become well known. In the converse of historical value, it has been argued that certain eponyms should not be used because the named individual was involved in war crimes.[5] In any case, many eponyms can be replaced with a noneponymous term consisting of a descriptive word or phrase that applies to the same disease, condition, or procedure. For example:

> osteitis deformans, instead of Paget disease of bone
> hemolytic uremic syndrome, instead of Gasser syndrome

The use of the noneponymous term may provide information about location or function and may serve the goal of clarity in international biomedical communication. The noneponymous term may be preferred in such contexts. This will also avoid confusing distinctly different disease entities with similar eponymous names (eg, Paget disease of bone, Paget disease of the nipple).

In some cases readers may be more familiar with the eponymous term. To insist on the use of either the noneponymous or the eponymous term would be contrary to a major purpose of scientific writing, which is to disseminate information that can be quickly understood by all. Placing the descriptive term(s) in parentheses after first mention of the eponymous term is another option that may be helpful, for example:

Stein-Leventhal (polycystic ovary) syndrome
Stevens-Johnson syndrome (bullous erythema multiforme)

The eponym, but not the noun or article that accompanies it, should be capitalized:

Babinski sign
Osler nodes
the Fisher exact test

Derivative adjectival forms of proper names are not capitalized, eg:

parkinsonian gait (from Parkinson disease)

16.2 **Nonpossessive Form.** There is some continuing debate over the use of the possessive form for eponyms, but a transition toward the nonpossessive form has taken place. A major step toward preference for the nonpossessive form occurred when the National Down Syndrome Society advocated the use of *Down syndrome*, rather than *Down's syndrome*, arguing that the syndrome does not actually belong to anyone.[6] The previous (ninth) edition of this manual,[7] the seventh edition of the Council of Science Editors style manual,[8] the *Dictionary of Medical Eponyms,*[3] and the 27th edition of *Stedman's Medical Dictionary*[9] recommend and use the nonpossessive form for eponymous terms. However, the 30th edition of *Dorland's Illustrated Medical Dictionary* takes an intermediate position, stating, "The use of the possessive form ending in *'s* for eponyms is becoming progressively less common, and the entries for eponymic terms in this Dictionary reflect this ongoing change in usage. The Dictionary therefore presents an inconsistent mixture of forms."[10]

One reason for preferring the nonpossessive form is that, although eponyms are possessive nouns using proper names, they are structurally adjectival and should not convey a true possessive sense.[1] For example, the name *Addison*, as used in describing "Addison's disease," is used as a noun modifier, with the sense of the modifier being clearly nonpossessive. Some possessive eponyms have evolved into the form of derived adjectives, as exemplified in the term *addisonian crisis*. Even when eponyms are used in an attributive sense, they have commonly lost possessive endings over time (eg, Nobel Prize, Petri dish). Thus, the transition of eponyms to the nonpossessive form is consistent with a linguistic perspective and also with trends in English usage.[1]

Use of the nonpossessive form of eponyms has become standard in medical genetics, and such usage, recommended by McKusick in *Mendelian Inheritance in Man: A Catalog of Human Genes and Genetic Disorders*,[11] is appropriate in other areas of medicine. McKusick's reasons for avoiding the possessive form of eponyms included the comment that "the eponym is merely a 'handle'; often the person whose name is used was not the first to describe the condition . . . or did not describe the full syndrome as it has subsequently become known."[11] Hence, even the initial description may not belong to the named individual, providing an additional reason to avoid the possessive form.

The following examples illustrate the advantages of the nonpossessive form in particular categories of eponymous terms with regard to spelling and pronunciation.

- When the word following begins with a sibilant *c*, *s*, or *z* (eg, *syndrome*, *sign*, *zone*)[11]:

Bitot spots	Looser zones
Cullen sign	Reye syndrome
Korsakoff psychosis	Schwann cell

- When an eponym ends in *ce*, *s*, or *z*[11]:

Betz cell	Homans sign
Colles fracture	Meigs syndrome
Fordyce disease	Posadas mycosis
Graves disease	Wilms tumor
Grawitz tumor	Yates correction

- When a hyphenated name is involved:

Brown-Séquard syndrome

- When 2 or more names are involved:

Charcot-Marie-Tooth disease
Dejerine-Sottas dystrophy

- When an article (*a*, *an*, *the*) precedes the term:

an Opie paradox
a Schatzki ring

Occasionally, the nonpossessive eponymous term may appear awkward. This can often be addressed by using *the* before the term:

the Avogadro number	the Starling law
the Pascal principle	the Tukey test

Alternative stylings for eponymous terms may include the use of *of*:

angle of Virchow
circle of Willis

The possessive form is used when it is part of an established nonmedical eponymous name:

Russell's viper
St John's wort

The possessive form is retained if it is part of the name of an organization or was used in the original of a quotation or citation:

The Alzheimer's Association

The possessive form is also retained for noneponymous terms describing disorders characteristic of certain occupations or activities:

coal workers' pneumoconiosis
woolsorter's disease
gamekeeper's thumb

In view of the adjectival and descriptive, rather than possessive, sense of eponyms, the advantages of the nonpossessive form in particular instances, the recommendations of authorities, and in keeping with the desire to promote clarity and consistency in scientific writing, we recommend (with the exceptions noted above) that the nonpossessive form be used for eponymous terms.

ACKNOWLEDGMENTS

Principal author: Richard M. Glass, MD

This chapter is a revision of the chapter on eponyms in the previous edition of this manual. Jeanette M. Smith, MD, *JAMA,* was the principal author of that chapter.

REFERENCES

1. Anderson JB. The language of eponyms. *J R Coll Physicians Lond*. 1996;30(2):174-177.
2. Who named it? http://www.whonamedit.com. Accessed December 8, 2006.
3. Firkin BG, Whitworth JA. *Dictionary of Medical Eponyms*. 2nd ed. Pearl River, NY: Parthenon Publishing Group Inc; 1996.
4. Koehler PJ, Bruyn GW, Pearce JMS, eds. *Neurological Eponyms*. New York, NY: Oxford University Press; 2000.
5. Jeffcoate WJ. Should eponyms be actively detached from diseases? *Lancet*. 2006;367(9519):1296-1297.
6. Thumbs-up on Down syndrome? *Copy Editor*. April/May 1994:1, 7.
7. Iverson C, Flanagin A, Fontanarosa PB, et al. *American Medical Association Manual of Style: A Guide for Authors and Editors*. 9th ed. Baltimore, MD: Williams & Wilkins; 1998.
8. Style Manual Committee, Council of Science Editors. *Scientific Style and Format: The CSE Manual for Authors, Editors, and Publishers*. 7th ed. New York, NY: Rockefeller University Press, in cooperation with the Council of Science Editors, Reston, VA; 2006:83.
9. *Stedman's Medical Dictionary*. 27th ed. Baltimore, MD: Lippincott Williams & Wilkins; 2000:xxxii.
10. *Dorland's Illustrated Medical Dictionary*. 30th ed. Philadelphia, PA: Saunders; 2003:xx.
11. McKusick VA. *Mendelian Inheritance in Man: A Catalog of Human Genes and Genetic Disorders*. 11th ed. Baltimore, MD: Johns Hopkins University Press; 1994:xl, xlii.

17 Greek Letters

Greek letters are frequently used in statistical formulas and notations, in mathematical composition, in certain chemical names for drugs, and in clinical and technical terms (see 14.11, Abbreviations, Clinical, Technical, and Other Common Terms; 14.12, Abbreviations, Units of Measure; 15.0, Nomenclature; 20.0, Study Design and Statistics; and 21.0, Mathematical Composition).

β-adrenergic
κ light chain
IFN-λ
^{123}I-β-CIT
nuclear factor κβ

17.1 Greek Letter vs Word. The editors of *JAMA* and the *Archives* Journals prefer the use of Greek letters rather than spelled-out words, unless usage dictates otherwise. Consult *Dorland's* and *Stedman's* medical dictionaries for general terms. These sources may differ in the representation of terms, ie, α-fetoprotein (symbol) (*Stedman's*) and alpha fetoprotein (*Dorland's*). If the Greek letter, rather than the word, is found in either of these sources for the item in question, use the letter in preference to the word.

- For chemical terms, the use of Greek letters is almost always preferred.

  β-pinene

- For electroencephalographic terms, use the word (see 15.11.2, Nomenclature, Neurology, Electroencephalographic Terms).

  lambda waves

- For drug names that contain Greek letters, consult the sources listed in 15.4, Nomenclature, Drugs, for preferred usage. In some cases, when the Greek letter is part of the word, as in *betamethasone*, the Greek letter is spelled out and set closed up. For some names, the approved nonproprietary name takes the word and not the letter, as in *beta carotene*, with an intervening space. (However, the chemical name for beta carotene is β-carotene.)

17.2 Capitalization After a Greek Letter. In titles, subtitles (except in references), headings, table column heads, line art, and at the beginning of sentences, the first non-Greek letter after a lowercase Greek letter should be capitalized.

β-Blocker use during pregnancy increases the risk that an infant will be small for gestational age.

Do not capitalize the Greek letter itself, unless the word itself normally includes a Greek capital letter. In this case, the first non-Greek letter after the capital letter should be lowercased.

β-Hemolytic streptococci were identified.

Δ^1-3,4-*trans*-tetrahydrocannabinol is 1 of 2 psychoactive isometric principles in cannabis.

For hyphenation in words that contain Greek letters, consult Special Combinations in 8.3.1, Punctuation, Hyphens and Dashes, Hyphen.

17.3 Greek Alphabet. Capital and lowercase Greek letters are listed below.

Name of Letter	*Greek Lowercase*	*Greek Capital*
Alpha	α	A
Beta	β	B
Gamma	γ	Γ
Delta	δ	Δ
Epsilon	ε	E
Zeta	ζ	Z
Eta	η	H
Theta	θ	Θ
Iota	ι	I
Kappa	κ	K
Lambda	λ	Λ
Mu	μ	M
Nu	ν	N
Xi	ξ	Ξ
Omicron	ο	O
Pi	π	Π
Rho	ρ	P
Sigma	σ	Σ
Tau	τ	T
Upsilon	υ	Y
Phi	φ	Φ
Chi	χ	X
Psi	ψ	š
Omega	α	Ω

17.4 Page Composition and Electronic Formats. If Greek letters need to be marked or modified on page proofs, this can be done by writing the letters "Gk" in the margin, followed by a description of the character (eg, "Gk lowercase mu").

Greek letters can pose problems for some Internet browsers. The best solution for editors is to make sure their text outputs Greek letters in a universal, platform-independent, nonproprietary standard for character encoding, such as Unicode. Most word processing and typesetting programs can generate Greek letters that already are Unicode encoded. Greek letters in running text should never be saved as graphics; these files are much larger than text and take much longer to download. Also, Web graphics are not scalable and tend not to print well.

ACKNOWLEDGMENT

Principal author: Brenda Gregoline, ELS

Section

4 Measurement and Quantitation

18 Units of Measure

The presentation of quantitative scientific information is an integral component of biomedical publication. Accurate communication of scientific knowledge and presentation of numerical data require a scientifically informative system for reporting units of measure.

18.1 SI Units.

SI Units. The International System of Units (Le Système International d'Unités or SI) represents a modified version of the metric system that has been established by international agreement and currently is the official measurement system of most nations of the world.[1] The SI promotes uniformity of quantities and units, minimizes the number of units and multiples used in other measurement systems, and can express virtually any measurement in science, medicine, industry, and commerce.

In 1977, the World Health Organization recommended the adoption of the SI by the international scientific community. Since then, many biomedical publications throughout the world have adopted SI units as their preferred and primary method for reporting scientific measurements. However, in the United States, most physicians and other health care professionals use conventional units for many common clinical measurements (eg, blood pressure), and many clinical laboratories report most laboratory values by means of conventional units. Accordingly, some biomedical publications, including *JAMA* and the *Archives* Journals, have adopted an approach for reporting units of measure that includes a combination of SI units and conventional units. (See 18.5, Conventional Units and SI Units in *JAMA* and the *Archives* Journals.) Authors, scientists, clinicians, editors, and others involved in preparing and processing manuscripts for biomedical publication should be familiar with appropriate use of units of measure and should ensure that the presentation and reporting of scientific information is clear and accurate, including any necessary conversion from conventional units to SI units, or vice versa.

18.1.1 **Base Units.** The SI is based on 7 fundamental units (base units) that refer to 7 basic quantities of measurement (see the tabulation below). These units form the structure from which other measurement quantities are composed.

Quantity	*Base Unit Name*	*SI Unit Symbol*
Length	meter	m
Mass	kilogram	kg
Time	second	s
Electric current	ampere	A
Thermodynamic temperature	kelvin	K
Luminous intensity	candela	cd
Amount of substance	mole	mol

Although not included among the 7 base units, the liter is widely used in the SI as a fundamental measure of capacity or volume. The liter is the recommended unit for measurement of volume for liquids and gases, whereas the cubic meter is the SI unit of volume for solids. Although the kelvin is the SI unit for thermodynamic temperature, the degree Celsius is used with the SI for temperature measurement in biomedical settings.

18.1.2 **Derived Units.** Other SI measurement quantities are referred to as *derived units* and are expressed as products or quotients of the 7 base units. Certain derived SI units have special names and symbols and may be used in algebraic relationships to express other derived units. See the following tabulation.

Quantity	*Name*	*SI Symbol*	*Derivation From Base Unit*
Area	square meter	m^2	m^2
Volume	cubic meter	m^3	m^3
Speed, velocity	meter per second	m/s	m/s
Density, mass density	kilogram per cubic meter	kg/m^3	kg/m^3
Specific volume	cubic meter per kilogram	m^3/kg	m^3/kg
Concentration	mole per cubic meter	mol/m^3	mol/m^3
Frequency	hertz	Hz	s^{-1}
Force	newton	N	$kg \cdot m \cdot s^{-2}$
Pressure, stress	pascal	Pa	$kg \cdot m^{-1} \cdot s^{-2}$ (N/m^2)
Work, energy	joule	J	$kg \cdot m^2 \cdot s^{-2}$ ($N \cdot m$)

Quantity	*Name*	*SI Symbol*	*Derivation From Base Unit*
Luminous flux	lumen	lm	$m^2 \cdot m^{-2} \cdot cd = cd$
Power, radiant flux	watt	W	$m^2 \cdot kg \cdot s^{-3}$ (J/s)
Electric potential	volt	V	$m^2 \cdot kg \cdot s^{-3} \cdot A^{-1}$
Electric charge	coulomb	C	$A \cdot s$
Electric resistance	ohm	Ω	$m^2 \cdot kg \cdot s^{-3} \cdot A^{-2}$ (V/A)
Capacitance	farad	F	$m^{-2} \cdot kg^{-1} \cdot s^4 \cdot A^2$ (C/V)
Magnetic flux	weber	Wb	$m^2 \cdot kg \cdot s^{-2} \cdot A^{-1}$ (V · s)
Magnetic flux density	tesla	T	$kg \cdot s^{-2} \cdot A^{-1}$ (Wb/m^2)
Inductance	henry	H	$m^2 \cdot kg \cdot s^{-2} \cdot A^{-2}$

18.1.3 **Prefixes.** Prefixes are combined with base units and derived units to form multiples of SI units. The factors designated by prefixes are powers of 10, and most prefixes involve exponents that are simple multiples of 3, thereby facilitating conversion procedures using successive multiplications by 10^3 or 10^{-3}.

Factor	*Prefix*	*Symbol*
10^{24}	yotta	Y
10^{21}	zetta	Z
10^{18}	exa	E
10^{15}	peta	P
10^{12}	tera	T
10^{9}	giga	G
10^{6}	mega	M
10^{3}	kilo	k
10^{2}	hecto	h
10^{1}	deka (deca)	da
10^{-1}	deci	d
10^{-2}	centi	c
10^{-3}	milli	m
10^{-6}	micro	μ
10^{-9}	nano	n
10^{-12}	pico	p
10^{-15}	femto	f
10^{-18}	atto	a
10^{-21}	zepto	z
10^{-24}	yocto	y

Compound prefixes formed by the combination of 2 or more SI prefixes generally are not used. It is preferable to use an expression with a single prefix.

Preferred: nm (nanometer)

Avoid: mμm (millimicrometer)

The kilogram is the only SI base unit with a prefix as part of its name and symbol (kg). However, because compound prefixes are not recommended, prefixes relating to mass are combined with gram (g) rather than kilogram (kg).

Preferred: mg (milligram)

Avoid: μkg (microkilogram)

18.2 Expressing Unit Names and Symbols. The SI includes conventions for expressing unit names and abbreviations (often referred to as symbols) and for displaying them in text.

18.2.1 Capitalization. The SI unit names are written lowercase (eg, kilogram) when spelled out, except for Celsius (as in "degrees Celsius"), which is capitalized. Abbreviations or symbols for SI units also are written lowercase, with the following exceptions:

- Abbreviations derived from a proper name should be capitalized (eg, N for newton, K for kelvin, A for ampere), although nonabbreviated SI unit names derived from a proper name are not capitalized (eg, newtons, amperes).
- An uppercase letter L is used as the abbreviation for liter to avoid confusion with the lowercase letter l and the number 1.
- Certain SI prefixes are capitalized to distinguish them from similar lowercase abbreviations:
  - M denotes the prefix *mega* (10^6), whereas m denotes the prefix *milli* (10^{-3})
  - mg denotes *milligram* (10^{-3} g), whereas MHz denotes *megahertz* (10^6 Hz)
  - P denotes the prefix *peta* (10^{15}), whereas p denotes the prefix *pico* (10^{-12})

18.2.2 Products and Quotients of Unit Symbols. The product of 2 or more SI units should be indicated by a space between them or by a raised multiplication dot. The multiplication dot must be positioned properly to distinguish it from a decimal point, which is set on the baseline. (See 21.6, Mathematical Composition, Expressing Multiplication and Division.) When the unit of measure is the product of 2 or more units, either abbreviations (symbols) or nonabbreviated units should be used. Abbreviated and nonabbreviated forms should not be combined in products.

Preferred: newton meter is expressed as newton meter or N m or N · m

Avoid: newton · m or N · meter

When numerals are used to denote a quantity of measurement, it is preferable to use the abbreviated form of the SI unit.

Preferred: 50 N · m

Avoid: 50 newton meter

The quotient of SI unit symbols may be expressed by the forward slash or virgule (/) or by the use of negative exponents. If the derived unit is formed by 2 abbreviated units of measure (eg, μg/L), the quotient also may be expressed by means of the forward slash or negative exponents.

Preferred: μg/L or μg L^{-1} or μg · L^{-1}

Avoid: μg per L

When the unit names are spelled out in a quotient or in text, the word *per* should be used.

Preferred: The power output was measured in joules per second.

Avoid: The power output was measured in joules/second [or J/s].

Expressions with 2 or more units of measure may require use of the forward slash, dot products, negative exponents, or parentheses. (See 21.6, Mathematical Composition, Expressing Multiplication and Division.)

$mL \cdot kg^{-1} \cdot min^{-1}$ or mL/kg/min

$m^2 \cdot kg \cdot s^{-2} \cdot A^{-2}$ or $(m^2 \cdot kg)/(s^2 \cdot A^2)$

18.3 **Format, Style, and Punctuation.** The format, style, and punctuation guidelines generally apply for SI reporting but also are used for reporting most values in conventional units.

18.3.1 **Exponents.** SI reporting style uses exponents rather than certain abbreviations, such as *cu* and *sq*.

Preferred: m^2

Avoid: sq m

Preferred: m^3

Avoid: cu m

18.3.2 **Plurals.** The same symbol is used for single and multiple quantities. Unit symbols are not expressed in the plural form.

Preferred:	1 L	70 L
Avoid:	1 Ls	70 Ls
Preferred:	1 g	1500 g
Avoid:	1 gs	1500 gs

18.3.3 **Subject-Verb Agreement.** Units of measure are treated as collective singular (not plural) nouns and require a singular verb.

To control the patient's fever, 500 mg of acetaminophen was [not *were*] administered at the time of admission and 1000 mg was required 4 hours later.

18.3.4 **Beginning of Sentence, Title, Subtitle.** A unit of measure that follows a number at the beginning of a sentence, title, or subtitle should not be abbreviated, even though the same unit of measure is abbreviated if it appears elsewhere in the same sentence.

(See 19.2.1, Numbers and Percentages, Spelling Out Numbers, Beginning a Sentence, Title, Subtitle, or Heading; and 19.2.2, Numbers and Percentages, Spelling Out Numbers, Common Fractions.)

18.3.5 **Abbreviations.** Most units of measure are abbreviated when used with numerals or in a virgule construction. Certain units of measure should be spelled out at first mention, with the abbreviated form in parentheses. Thereafter, the abbreviated form should be used in text. (See 14.12, Abbreviations, Units of Measure.)

18.3.6 **Punctuation.** Symbols or abbreviations of units of measure are not followed by a period, unless the symbol occurs at the end of a sentence.

The patient's weight was 80 kg [*not* 80 kg.] and had increased by 10%.

18.3.7 **Hyphens.** A hyphen is used to join 2 spelled-out units of measure.

pascal-second

A hyphen is used to join a unit of measure and the number associated with it when the combination is used as an adjective. (See Temporary Compounds in 8.3.1, Punctuation, Hyphens and Dashes, Hyphen.)

an 8-L container a 10-mm strip

18.3.8 **Spacing.** With the exception of the percent sign, the degree sign (for temperature and angles), and normal and molar solutions (see 18.5.7, Conventional Units and SI Units in *JAMA* and the *Archives* Journals, Solutions and Concentration), a full space should appear between the arabic numeral indicating the quantity and the unit of measure.

140 nmol/L (not 140nmol/L)

135-150 nmol/L

120 mm Hg

40% adherence rate

40%-50%

45° angle

temperature of 37.5°C (not 37.5° C or 37.5 °C)

18.4 Use of Numerals With Units

18.4.1 **Expressing Quantities.** Arabic numerals are used for quantities with units of measure (see 19.1, Numbers and Percentages, Use of Numerals). By SI convention, it is preferable to use only numbers between 0.1 and 1000 and to use the appropriate prefix for expressing quantities. For example, 0.003 mL is expressed as 3 μL; 15 000 g is expressed as 15 kg.

Some clinical measurements are expressed in quantities and units that may have numbers outside this preferred range. For such values, the use of scientific notation is acceptable.

20 000 000 A may be expressed as 20 million amperes or as 2×10^7 A

Reported SI values should follow recommendations for preserving the proper number of significant digits. (See 20.8.2, Study Design and Statistics, Significant Digits and Rounding Numbers, Rounding.) The use of these increments is intended to eliminate reporting results beyond the appropriate level of precision.

18.4.2 **Decimal Format.** The decimal format is recommended for numbers used with units of measure. Numerical values less than 1 require placement of 0 before the decimal marker.

Preferred: 0.123

Avoid: .123

However, certain statistical values, such as α levels and P values, should be reported without the use of 0 before the decimal marker. (See 19.7.1, Numbers and Percentages, Forms of Numbers, Decimals; and 20.9, Study Design and Statistics, Glossary of Statistical Terms.)

The sample size was based on detecting a 10% difference in the primary outcome measure, using a 2-sided α level of .05.

Statistical significance was defined as $P < .01$.

Fractions should not be used with SI units.

Preferred: 2.5 kg

Avoid: 2½ kg

Mixed fractions occasionally are used in text to indicate less precise measurements and most commonly involve units of measure representing time.

After more than 7½ years of investigation, the effort to develop a new vaccine was abandoned.

The decimal format also could be used:

After more than 7.5 years of investigation, the effort to develop a new vaccine was abandoned.

18.4.3 **Number Spacing.** By SI convention, the decimal point is the only punctuation mark permitted in numerals, and it is used to separate the integer and decimal parts of the number. The SI does not use commas in numbers, in particular because the comma is used in some countries as the decimal sign. Integers (whole numbers) with more than 4 digits are separated into groups of 3 (using a thin space) with respect to the decimal point. Four-digit integers are closed up (without a space). Decimal digits also are grouped in sets of 3 digits beginning at the decimal sign, with the same closed-up spacing for 4-digit groups. (See also 19.1.1, Numbers and Percentages, Use of Numerals, Numbers of 4 or More Digits to Either Side of the Decimal Point).

Preferred	*Avoid*
1234	1,234
123 456	123,456
12 345.678 901	12,345.678901
1234.567 89	1,234.56789
1 234 567.8901	1,234,567.8901

However, certain types of numerals that have more than 4 digits are expressed without spacing, such as street addresses, postal codes, page numbers, and numerals combined with letters, including trial registration identifiers.

Chicago, IL 60610

This study was supported by grant MCH-110624.

Trial Registration: clinicaltrials.gov Identifier: NCT00381954

18.4.4 Multiplication of Numbers. Multiplication of numbers should be indicated by the multiplication sign (×) and may be used to express area (eg, a $15 \times 35\text{-cm}^2$ burn), volume (eg, a $5.2 \times 3.7 \times 6.9\text{-m}^3$ cube), matrixes (eg, 2 × 2 table), magnification (×30 000), or scientific notation (eg, $3.6 \times 10^9/\text{L}$).

18.4.5 Indexes. An index generally refers to a quantity derived from a ratio of 2 (or more) measurable quantities and often is used to compare individuals with each other or with normal values. Except for products or quotients representing specific derived SI units of measure (see also 18.2.2, Expressing Unit Names and Symbols, Products and Quotients of Unit Symbols), the ratio of SI units used to create indexes does not represent an SI convention.

At first mention in the text, the formula used to calculate the index should be described; thereafter, the numerical value for the index may be given without units attached to it. For figures or tables, the formula should be included in legends or in footnotes, respectively. However, the formula used to calculate an index need not be included in the abstract of an article.

body mass index (BMI), calculated as the weight in kilograms divided by height in meters squared

cardiac index, calculated as cardiac output in liters per minute divided by body surface area in square meters (L/min/m^2)

18.5 Conventional Units and SI Units in *JAMA* and the *Archives* Journals.

In the United States, most physicians and other health care professionals use conventional units for most commonly encountered clinical measurements (eg, blood pressure), and most clinical laboratories report many laboratory values by means of conventional units. To serve these readers, but also to serve the needs of readers in countries where SI units are used, *JAMA* and the *Archives* Journals have adopted an approach for reporting units of measure that includes a combination of SI units and conventional units.

18.5.1 Length, Area, Volume, Mass. Measurements of length, area, volume, and mass are reported by means of metric units rather than English units (Table 1). In less formal, nonscientific texts such as essays, use of nonmetric units, such as miles or inches, and the use of idioms, such as "An ounce of prevention is worth a pound of cure," are acceptable. In addition, if the nonmetric unit was used as part of a survey or questionnaire, the original measure should be retained.

The patients were asked, "Do you have difficulty walking 15 feet?"

Table 1. Conversions to Metric Measures

Symbol	Known Quantity	Multiply by	To Find	Metric Symbol
		Length		
in	inches	2.54	centimeters	cm
ft	feet	30	centimeters	cm
ft	feet	0.3	meters	m
yd	yards	0.9	meters	m
	miles	1.6	kilometers	km
		Area		
sq in	square inches	6.5	square centimeters	cm^2
sq ft	square feet	0.09	square meters	m^2
sq yd	square yards	0.8	square meters	m^2
	square miles	2.6	square kilometers	km^2
		Mass		
oz	ounces	28	grams	g
lb	pounds	0.45	kilograms	kg
		Volume		
tsp	teaspoons	5	milliliters	mL
tbsp	tablespoons	15	milliliters	mL
fl oz	fluid ounces	30	milliliters	mL
c	cups	0.24	liters	L
pt	US pints	0.47	liters	L
qt	US quarts	0.95	liters	L
gal	US gallons	3.8	liters	L
cu ft	cubic feet	0.03	cubic meters	m^3
cu yd	cubic yards	0.76	cubic meters	m^3

18.5.2 **Temperature.** The Celsius scale (°C) is used for temperature measurement rather than the base SI unit for temperature, the kelvin (K), which has little application in medicine. Although both kelvin and Celsius scales have the same interval value for temperature differences, they differ in their absolute values. For example, a temperature of 273.15°K is equal to 0°C. Temperature values generally are reported in degrees Celsius, and values given in degrees Fahrenheit (°F) are converted to degrees Celsius (°C).

$$(°F - 32)(0.556) = °C$$

18.5.3 **Time.** The SI unit for time is the second, although minute, hour, and day also are used. Other units of time, such as week, month, and year, are not part of the SI but also are used. The abbreviations for minute, hour, and day are min, h, and d, respectively, and the abbreviations for week, month, and year are wk, mo, and y, respectively. These abbreviations are used in tables, figures, virgule constructions, and within parentheses. (See 14.12, Abbreviations, Units of Measure.)

18.5.4 **Visual Acuity.** Visual acuity should be reported on the basis of how the measurement was determined. For example, using the Snellen fraction with English units, 20/20 or 20/100 indicates that the person being evaluated can see at 20 ft what a person with "normal visual acuity" can see at 20 ft or at 100 ft, respectively. The equivalent metric measurements for visual acuity are 6/6 and 6/30, respectively. (See 15.13, Nomenclature, Ophthalmology Terms.)

18.5.5 **Pressure.** Blood pressure and intraocular pressure are reported in millimeters of mercury (mm Hg); cerebrospinal fluid pressure is reported as centimeters of water (cm H_2O). The pascal (newton per square meter [N/m^2]) is the recommended SI unit for pressure but generally is not used for reporting these common physiologic pressure measurements. Partial pressure of gases (eg, of oxygen and carbon dioxide) may be reported as millimeters of mercury (mm Hg) or as kilopascals (kPa). (See also 15.16, Nomenclature, Pulmonary, Respiratory, and Blood Gas Terminology.)

18.5.6 **pH.** Although SI nomenclature could be used to express values of hydrogen ion concentration (nmol/L), the pH scale (1-14) is used.

18.5.7 **Solutions and Concentration.** A *molar* solution contains 1 mol (1 g molecular weight) of solute in 1 L of solution. The SI style for reporting molar solutions is mol/L; for solutions with millimolar concentrations, mmol/L is used; and for solutions with micromolar concentrations, µmol/L is used. The concentration is given as 4-mmol/L potassium chloride, *not* 4 mmol/L *of* potassium chloride.

> The gel was incubated at 40°C after applying 10 mL of a solution of 4-mmol/L potassium chloride and 5 mL of a solution of 1-mol/L sodium chloride.

Molar concentrations of solutions and reagents also may be expressed by using M to designate molar and SI prefixes to denote concentration (eg, mM for millimolar; µM for micromolar). Note that the molar concentration unit is set closed up to the number.

> The gel was incubated at 40°C after applying 10 mL of a solution of 4mM potassium chloride and 5 mL of a solution of 1M sodium chloride.

A *normal* solution contains a concentration of 1 gram-equivalent of solute per liter. To show the concentration of a solution in relation to normality (N), the abbreviation N is used, with no space between the numerical value and the N.

normal	N
half normal	0.5N or N/2

18.5.8 **Energy.** The calorie is the unit of measure often used in chemistry and biochemistry for reporting heat energy. A value of 1 calorie is the amount of energy (heat) required to raise the temperature of 1 g of pure water by 1°C. The joule is the preferred SI unit for energy, and calories and kilocalories may be converted to joules (J) and kilojoules (kJ) by using the following formulas:

1 calorie = 4.186 J

1 kilocalorie = 4.186 kJ

JAMA and the *Archives* Journals prefer to report heat energy in calories or kilocalories.

Formerly a distinction was made between this "small calorie" (with a lowercase c) and the "large calorie," designated as Calorie (with a capital C and abbreviated Cal)[2] and equivalent to 1000 calories or 1 kilocalorie (kcal). In metabolic studies, the Calorie is the amount of heat energy required to raise or lower 1 kg of pure liquid water by 1°C.[2] The Calorie also is used in nutrition to express the energy content of food.[3] By convention, the use of capitalized C in dietary Calories indicates kilocalories (ie, 1 Cal is equivalent to 1 kcal or 1000 cal). For example, if the label on a food package indicates that a serving contains 300 Cal, that serving would yield 300 kcal (not 300 cal) of heat energy when subjected to complete combustion. *JAMA* and the *Archives* Journals prefer Calories or kilocalories for expresssing the energy content of food.

Energy expenditure also is reported as Calories (or kilocalories) to reflect the amount of energy required for the work done. The values for Calorie expenditure are based on the metabolic cost, expressed as METs, or metabolic equivalents. One MET represents the metabolic rate for an adult at rest (ie, set at 3.5 mL of oxygen consumed per kilogram of body mass per minute) or approximately 1 kcal/kg/h.[3] Activities with MET values near 1 are sedentary activities (eg, sitting quietly), whereas activities with higher MET values involve higher levels of energy expenditure (eg, brisk walking has a MET value of 3, or 3 times the resting metabolic rate).

18.5.9 **Drug Doses.** Drug doses are expressed in conventional metric mass units (eg, milligrams or milligrams per kilogram), rather than in molar SI units. Moreover, certain drugs (such as insulin or heparin) may be prepared as mixtures and have no specific molecular weight, thereby precluding their expression in mass units. Although other drug dose units such as drops (for ophthalmologic preparations), grains (for aspirin), and various apothecary system measurements (eg, teaspoonfuls, ounces, and drams) may be encountered clinically, these units generally are not used. Also, the units for drug doses are often different from the units used to measure drug concentrations, such as in therapeutic drug levels.

18.5.10 **Laboratory Values.** In *JAMA* and the *Archives* Journals, laboratory values for clinical chemistry analyses, hematologic tests, immunologic assays, metabolic and endocrine tests, therapeutic drug monitoring, toxicology determinations, and urinalysis are reported by means of conventional laboratory units. Table 2 provides examples of conventional units and SI units for clinical laboratory measurement and is intended to facilitate conversion from conventional units to SI units (and vice versa). However, laboratory reference values and units may vary substantially among individual laboratories and are highly dependent on the analytic methods used. Several resources[4-8] contain detailed information about these topics as well as tables with laboratory reference values and SI conversion factors.

Table 2. Selected Laboratory Tests, With Reference Ranges and Conversion Factors[a]

Analyte	Specimen	Reference Range, Conventional Unit	Conventional Unit	Conversion Factor (Multiply by)	Reference Range, SI Unit	SI Unit
Acetaminophen	Serum, plasma	10-30	μg/mL	6.614	66-200	μmol/L
Acetoacetate	Serum, plasma	< 1	mg/dL	97.95	< 100	μmol/L
Acetone	Serum, plasma	< 1.0	mg/dL	0.172	< 0.17	mmol/L
Acid phosphatase	Serum	< 5.5	U/L	16.667	< 90	nkat/L
Activated partial thromboplastin time (APTT)	Whole blood	25-40	s	1.0	25-40	s
Adenosine deaminase	Serum	11.5-25.0	U/L	16.667	190-420	nkat/L
Adrenocorticotropic hormone (ACTH)	Plasma	< 120	pg/mL	0.22	< 26	pmol/L
Alanine	Plasma	1.87-5.89	mg/dL	112.2	210-661	μmol/L
Alanine aminotransferase (ALT)	Serum	10-40	U/L	0.0167	0.17-0.68	μkat/L
Albumin	Serum	3.5-5.0	g/dL	10	35-50	g/L
Alcohol dehydrogenase	Serum	< 2.8	U/L	16.667	< 47	nkat/L
Aldolase	Serum	1.0-7.5	U/L	0.0167	0.02-0.13	μkat/L
Aldosterone	Serum, plasma	2-9	ng/dL	27.74	55-250	pmol/L
Alkaline phosphatase	Serum	30-120	U/L	0.0167	0.5-2.0	μkat/L
Alprazolam	Serum, plasma	10-50	ng/mL	3.24	32-162	nmol/L
Amikacin	Serum, plasma	20-30	μg/mL	1.708	34-52	μmol/L
α-Aminobutyric acid	Plasma	0.08-0.36	mg/dL	96.97	8-35	μmol/L
δ-Aminolevulinic acid	Serum	15-23	μg/dL	0.0763	1.1-8.0	μmol/L
Amiodarone	Serum, plasma	0.5-2.5	μg/mL	1.55	0.8-3.9	μmol/L
Amitriptyline	Plasma	120-250	ng/mL	3.605	433-903	nmol/L
Ammonia (as nitrogen)	Serum, plasma	15-45	μg/dL	0.714	11-32	μmol/L
Amobarbital	Serum	1-5	μg/mL	4.42	4-22	μmol/L

Amphetamine	Serum, plasma	20-30	ng/mL	7.4	148-222	nmol/L
Amylase	Serum	27-131	U/L	0.01667	0.46-2.23	μkat/L
Androstenedione	Serum	75-205	ng/dL	0.0349	2.6-7.2	nmol/L
Angiotensin I	Plasma	< 25	pg/mL	0.772	< 15	pmol/L
Angiotensin II	Plasma	10-60	pg/mL	0.957	0.96-58	pmol/L
Angiotensin-converting enzyme	Serum	< 40	U/L	16.667	< 670	nkat/L
Anion gap $Na^+ - (Cl^- + HCO_3^-)$	Serum, plasma	8-16	mEq/L	1.0	8-16	mmol/L
Antidiuretic hormone (ADH)	Plasma	1-5	pg/mL	0.923	0.9-4.6	pmol/L
Antithrombin III	Plasma	21-30	mg/dL	10	210-300	mg/L
α_1-Antitrypsin	Serum	78-200	mg/dL	0.184	14.5-36.5	μmol/L
Apolipoprotein A-I	Serum	80-151	mg/dL	0.01	0.8-1.5	g/L
Apolipoprotein B	Serum, plasma	50-123	mg/dL	0.01	0.5-1.2	g/L
Arginine	Serum	0.37-2.40	mg/dL	57.05	21-138	μmol/L
Arsenic	Whole blood	< 2-23	μg/L	0.0133	0.03-0.31	μmol/L
Ascorbic acid (see Vitamin C)						
Asparagine	Plasma	0.40-0.91	mg/dL	75.689	30-69	μmol/L
Aspartate aminotransferase (AST)	Serum	10-30	U/L	0.01667	0.17-0.51	μkat/L
Aspartic acid	Plasma	< 0.3	mg/dL	75.13	< 25	μmol/L
Atrial natriuretic hormone	Plasma	20-77	pg/mL	0.325	6.5-2.5	pmol/L
Bands (see White blood cell count)						
Basophils (see White blood cell count)						
Base excess	Whole blood	−2 to 3	mEg/L	1.0	− 2 to 3	mmol/L
Bicarbonate	Serum	21-28	mEq/L	1.0	21-28	mmol/L
Bile acids (total)	Serum	0.3-2.3	μg/mL	2.448	0.73-5.63	μmol/L
Bilirubin, total	Serum	0.3-1.2	mg/dL	17.104	5.0-21.0	μmol/L
Bilirubin, direct (conjugated)	Serum	0.1-0.3	mg/dL	17.104	1.7-5.1	μmol/L

Table 2. Selected Laboratory Tests, With Reference Ranges and Conversion Factors[a] *(cont)*

Analyte	Specimen	Reference Range, Conventional Unit	Conventional Unit	Conversion Factor (Multiply by)	Reference Range, SI Unit	SI Unit
Biotin	Serum	200-500	pg/mL	0.00409	0.82-2.05	nmol/L
Bismuth	Whole blood	1-12	μg/L	4.785	4.8-57.4	nmol/L
Blood gases						
Carbon dioxide, Pco_2	Arterial blood	35-45	mm Hg	0.133	4.7-5.9	kPa
pH	Arterial blood	7.35-7.45		1.0	7.35-7.45	
Oxygen, Po_2	Arterial blood	80-100	mm Hg	0.133	11-13	kPa
Brain-type natriuretic peptide (BNP)	Plasma	< 167	pg/mL	1.0	< 167	ng/L
Bromide (toxic)	Serum	> 1250	μg/mL	0.0125	> 15.6	mmol/L
C1 esterase inhibitor	Serum	12-30	mg/dL	10	120-300	mg/L
C3 complement	Serum	1200-1500	μg/mL	0.001	1.2-1.5	g/L
C4 complement	Serum	350-600	μg/mL	0.001	0.35-0.60	g/L
Cadmium	Whole blood	0.3-1.2	μg/L	8.896	2.7-10.7	nmol/L
Caffeine	Serum, plasma	3-15	μg/L	0.515	2.5-7.5	μmol/L
Calcitonin	Plasma	3-26	pg/mL	0.292	0.8-7.6	pmol/L
Calcium, ionized	Serum	4.60-5.08	mg/dL	0.25	1.15-1.27	mmol/L
Calcium, total	Serum	8.2-10.2	mg/dL	0.25	2.05-2.55	mmol/L
Cancer antigen (CA) 125	Serum	< 35	U/mL	1.0	< 35	kU/L
Carbamazepine	Serum, plasma	8-12	μg/mL	4.233	34-51	μmol/L
Carbon dioxide (total)	Serum, plasma	22-28	mEq/L	1.0	22-28	mmol/L
Carboxyhemoglobin, toxic	Whole blood	> 20	%	0.01	> 0.2	Proportion of 1.0
Carcinoembryonic antigen (CEA)	Serum	< 3.0	ng/mL	1.0	< 3.0	μg/L
β-Carotene	Serum	10-85	μg/dL	0.01863	0.2-1.6	μmol/L
Carotenoids	Serum	50-300	μg/dL	0.01863	0.9-5.6	μmol/L

Ceruloplasmin	Serum	20-40	mg/dL	10	200-400	mg/L
Chloramphenicol	Serum	10-25	μg/mL	3.095	31-77	μmol/L
Chlordiazepoxide	Serum, plasma	0.4-3.0	μg/mL	3.336	1.3-10.0	μmol/L
Chloride	Serum, plasma	96-106	mEq/L	1.0	96-106	mmol/L
Chlorpromazine	Plasma	50-300	ng/mL	3.126	157-942	nmol/L
Chlorpropamide	Plasma	75-250	mg/L	3.61	270-900	μmol/L
Cholecalciferol (see Vitamin D)						
Cholesterol (total)						
Desirable	Serum, plasma	< 200	mg/dL	0.0259	< 5.18	mmol/L
Borderline high	Serum, plasma	200-239	mg/dL	0.0259	5.18-6.18	mmol/L
High	Serum, plasma	≥240	mg/dL	0.0259	≥ 6.21	mmol/L
Cholesterol, high-density (HDL) (low level)	Serum, plasma	< 40	mg/dL	0.0259	< 1.03	mmol/L
Cholesterol, low-density (LDL) (high level)	Serum, plasma	> 160	mg/dL	0.0259	4.144	mmol/L
Cholinesterase	Serum	5-12	mg/L	2.793	14-39	nmol/L
Chorionic gonadotropin (β-hCG) (nonpregnant)	Serum	5.0	mIU/mL	1.0	5.0	IU/L
Chromium	Whole blood	0.7-28.0	μg/L	19.232	13.4-538.6	nmol/L
Citrate	Serum	1.2-3.0	mg/dL	52.05	60-160	μmol/L
Citrulline	Plasma	0.2-1.0	mg/dL	57.081	12-55	μmol/L
Clonazepam	Serum	10-50	ng/mL	0.317	0.4-15.8	nmol/L
Clonidine	Serum, plasma	1.0-2.0	ng/mL	4.35	4.4-8.7	nmol/L
Clozapine	Serum	200-350	ng/mL	0.003	0.6-1.0	μmol/L
Coagulation factor I	Plasma	0.15-0.35	g/dL	29.41	4.4-10.3	μmol/L
(Fibrinogen)	Plasma	150-350	mg/dL	0.01	1.5-3.5	g/L
Coagulation factor II (prothrombin)	Plasma	70-130	%	0.01	0.70-1.30	Proportion of 1.0

Table 2. Selected Laboratory Tests, With Reference Ranges and Conversion Factors[a] *(cont)*

Analyte	Specimen	Reference Range, Conventional Unit	Conventional Unit	Conversion Factor (Multiply by)	Reference Range, SI Unit	SI Unit
Coagulation factor V	Plasma	70-130	%	0.01	0.70-1.30	Proportion of 1.0
Coagulation factor VII	Plasma	60-140	%	0.01	0.60-1.40	Proportion of 1.0
Coagulation factor VIII	Plasma	50-200	%	0.01	0.50-2.00	Proportion of 1.0
Coagulation factor IX	Plasma	70-130	%	0.01	0.70-1.30	Proportion of 1.0
Coagulation factor X	Plasma	70-130	%	0.01	0.70-1.30	Proportion of 1.0
Coagulation factor XI	Plasma	70-130	%	0.01	0.70-1.30	Proportion of 1.0
Coagulation factor XII	Plasma	70-130	%	0.01	0.70-1.30	Proportion of 1.0
Cobalt	Serum	4.0-10.0	μg/L	16.968	67.9-169.7	nmol/L
Cocaine (toxic)	Serum	> 1000	ng/mL	3.297	> 3300	nmol/L
Codeine	Serum	10-100	ng/mL	3.34	33-334	nmol/L
Coenzyme Q10 (ubiquinone)	Plasma	0.5-1.5	μg/mL	1.0	0.5-1.5	mg/L
Copper	Serum	70-140	μg/dL	0.157	11-22	μmol/L
Coproporphyrin	Urine	< 200	μg/24 h	1.527	< 300	μmol/d
Corticotropin	Plasma	< 120	pg/mL	0.22	< 26	pmol/L
Cortisol	Serum, plasma	5-25	μg/dL	27.588	140-690	nmol/L
Cotinine	Plasma	0-8	μg/L	5.675	0-45	nmol/L
C-peptide	Serum	0.5-2.5	ng/mL	0.331	0.17-0.83	nmol/L
C-reactive protein	Serum	0.08-3.1	mg/L	9.524	0.76-28.5	nmol/L
Creatine	Serum	0.1-0.4	mg/dL	76.25	8-31	μmol/L
Creatine kinase (CK)	Serum	40-150	U/L	0.0167	0.67-2.5	μkat/L
Creatine kinase-MB fraction	Serum	0-7	ng/mL	1.0	0-7	μg/L
Creatinine	Serum, plasma	0.6-1.2	mg/dL	88.4	53-106	μmol/L

Creatinine clearance	Serum, plasma	75-125	mL/min/1.73 m^2	0.0167	1.24-2.08	mL/s/m^2
Cyanide (toxic)	Whole blood	> 1.0	μg/mL	23.24	> 23	μmol/L
Cyclic adenosine monophosphate (cAMP)	Plasma	4.6-8.6	ng/mL	3.04	14-26	nmol/L
Cyclosporine	Serum	100-400	ng/mL	0.832	83-333	nmol/L
Cystine	Plasma	0.40-1.40	mg/dL	41.615	16-60	μmol/L
D-dimer	Plasma	< 0.5	μg/mL	5.476	< 3.0	nmol/L
Dehydroepiandrosterone (DHEA)	Serum	1.8-12.5	ng/mL	3.47	6.2-43.3	nmol/L
Dehydroepiandrosterone sulfate (DHEA-S)	Serum	50-450	μg/dL	0.027	1.6-12.2	μmol/L
Deoxycorticosterone	Serum	2-19	ng/dL	30.5	61-576	nmol/L
Desipramine	Serum, plasma	50-200	ng/mL	3.754	170-700	nmol/L
Diazepam	Serum, plasma	100-1000	ng/mL	0.0035	0.35-3.51	μmol/L
Digoxin	Plasma	0.5-2.0	ng/mL	1.281	0.6-2.6	nmol/L
Diltiazem	Serum	< 200	mg/L	2.412	< 480	μmol/L
Disopyramide	Serum, plasma	2.8-7.0	μg/mL	2.946	8.3-22.0	μmol/L
Dopamine	Plasma	< 87	pg/mL	6.528	< 475	pmol/L
Doxepin	Serum, plasma	30-150	ng/mL	3.579	108-538	nmol/L
Electrophoresis (protein)						
Proportion of total protein						
Albumin	Serum	52-65	%	0.01	0.52-0.65	Proportion of 1.0
α_1-Globulin	Serum	2.5-5.0	%	0.01	0.025-0.05	Proportion of 1.0
α_2-Globulin	Serum	7.0-13.0	%	0.01	0.07-0.13	Proportion of 1.0
β-Globulin	Serum	8.0-14.0	%	0.01	0.08-0.14	Proportion of 1.0
γ-Globulin	Serum	12.0-22.0	%	0.01	0.12-0.22	Proportion of 1.0

Table 2. Selected Laboratory Tests, With Reference Ranges and Conversion Factors[a] *(cont)*

Analyte	Specimen	Reference Range, Conventional Unit	Conventional Unit	Conversion Factor (Multiply by)	Reference Range, SI Unit	SI Unit
Concentration						
Albumin	Serum	3.2-5.6	g/dL	10.0	32-56	g/L
α_1-Globulin	Serum	0.1-0.4	g/dL	10.0	1-10	g/L
α_2-Globulin	Serum	0.4-1.2	g/dL	10.0	4-12	g/L
β-Globulin	Serum	0.5-1.1	g/dL	10.0	5-11	g/L
γ-Globulin	Serum	0.5-1.6	g/dL	10.0	5-16	g/L
Eosinophils (see White blood cell count)						
Ephedrine (toxic)	Serum	> 2	μg/mL	6.052	> 12.1	μmol/L
Epinephrine	Plasma	< 60	pg/mL	5.459	< 330	pmol/L
Erythrocyte count (see Red blood cell count)						
Erythrocyte sedimentation rate	Whole blood	0-20	mm/h	1.0	0-20	mm/h
Erythropoietin	Serum	5-36	IU/L	1.0	5-36	IU/L
Estradiol (E_2)	Serum	30-400	pg/mL	3.671	110-1470	pmol/L
Estriol (E_3)	Serum	5-40	ng/mL	3.467	17.4-138.8	nmol/L
Estrogens (total)	Serum	60-400	pg/mL	1.0	60-400	ng/L
Estrone (E_1)	Serum, plasma	1.5-25.0	pg/mL	3.698	5.5-92.5	pmol/L
Ethanol (ethyl alcohol)	Serum, whole blood	< 20	mg/dL	0.2171	< 4.3	mmol/L
Ethchlorvynol (toxic)	Serum, plasma	> 20	μg/mL	6.915	> 138	μmol/L
Ethosuximide	Serum	40-100	mg/L	7.084	280-700	μmol/L
Ethylene glycol (toxic)	Serum, plasma	> 30	mg/dL	0.1611	> 5	mmol/L
Fatty acids (nonesterified)	Serum, plasma	8-25	mg/dL	0.0355	0.28-0.89	mmol/L
Fecal fat (as stearic acid)	Stool	2.0-6.0	g/d	1.0	2-6	g/24 h

Fenfluramine	Serum	0.04-0.30	μg/mL	4.324	0.18-1.30	μmol/L
Fentanyl	Serum	0.01-0.10	μg/mL	2.972	0.02-0.30	μmol/L
Ferritin	Serum	15-200	ng/mL	2.247	33-450	pmol/L
α_1-Fetoprotein	Serum	< 10	ng/mL	1.0	< 10	μg/L
Fibrin degradation products	Plasma	< 10	μg/mL	1.0	< 10	mg/L
Fibrinogen	Plasma	200-400	mg/dL	0.0294	5.8-11.8	μmol/L
Flecanide	Serum, plasma	0.2-1.0	μg/mL	2.413	0.5-2.4	μmol/L
Fluoride	Whole blood	< 0.05	mg/dL	0.5263	< 0.027	mmol/L
Fluoxetine	Serum	200-1100	ng/mL	0.00323	0.65-3.56	μmol/L
Flurazepam (toxic)	Serum, plasma	> 0.2	μg/mL	2.5	> 0.5	μmol/L
Folate (folic acid)	Serum	3-16	ng/mL	2.266	7-36	nmol/L
Follicle-stimulating hormone (FSH)	Serum, plasma	1-100	mIU/mL	1.0	1-100	IU/L
Fructosamine	Serum	36-50	mg/L	5.581	200-280	mmol/L
Fructose	Serum	1-6	mg/dL	55.506	55-335	μmol/L
Galactose	Serum, plasma	< 20	mg/dL	0.0555	< 1.10	mmol/L
Gastrin	Serum	25-90	pg/mL	0.481	12-45	pmol/L
Gentamicin	Serum	6-10	μg/mL	2.090	12-21	μmol/L
Glucagon	Plasma	20-100	pg/mL	1.0	20-100	ng/L
Glucose	Serum	70-110	mg/dL	0.0555	3.9-6.1	mmol/L
Glucose-6-phosphate dehydrogenase	Whole blood	10-14	U/g hemoglobin	0.0167	0.17-0.24	nkat/g hemoglobin
Glutamic acid	Plasma	0.2-2.8	mg/dL	67.967	15-190	μmol/L
Glutamine	Plasma	6.1-10.2	mg/dL	68.423	420-700	μmol/L
γ-Glutamyltransferase (GGT)	Serum	2-30	U/L	0.01667	0.03-0.51	μkat/L
Glutethimide	Serum	2-6	μg/mL	4.603	9-28	μmol/L
Glycerol (free)	Serum	0.3-1.72	mg/dL	0.1086	0.32-0.187	mmol/L

Table 2. Selected Laboratory Tests, With Reference Ranges and Conversion Factors[a] *(cont)*

Analyte	Specimen	Reference Range, Conventional Unit	Conventional Unit	Conversion Factor (Multiply by)	Reference Range, SI Unit	SI Unit
Glycine	Plasma	0.9-4.2	mg/dL	133.2	120-560	μmol/L
Gold	Serum	< 10	μg/dL	50.770	< 500	nmol/L
Growth hormone (GH)	Serum	0-18	ng/mL	1.0	0-18	μg/L
Haloperidol	Serum, plasma	6-24	ng/mL	2.66	16-65	nmol/L
Haptoglobin	Serum	26-185	mg/dL	10	260-1850	mg/L
Hematocrit	Whole blood	41-50	%	0.01	0.41-0.50	Proportion of 1.0
Hemoglobin	Whole blood	14.0-17.5	g/dL	10.0	140-175	g/L
Mean corpuscular hemoglobin (MCH)	Whole blood	26-34	pg/cell	1.0	26-34	pg/cell
Mean corpuscular hemoglobin concentration (MCHC)	Whole blood	33-37	g/dL	10	330-370	g/L
Mean corpuscular volume (MCV)	Whole blood	80-100	μm^3	1.0	80-100	fL
Hemoglobin A_{1c} (glycated hemoglobin)	Whole blood	4-7	% of total hemoglobin	0.01	0.04-0.07	Proportion of total hemoglobin
Hemoglobin A_2	Whole blood	2.0-3.0	%	0.01	0.02-0.03	Proportion of 1.0
Histamine	Plasma	0.5-1.0	μg/L	8.997	4.5-9.0	nmol/L
Histidine	Plasma	0.5-1.7	mg/dL	64.45	32-110	μmol/L
Homocysteine	Plasma	0.68-2.02	mg/L	7.397	5-15	μmol/L
Homovanillic acid	Urine	1.4-8.8	mg/24 h	5.489	8-48	μmol/d
Hydrocodone	Serum	< 0.02	μg/mL	3.34	< 0.06	μmol/L
Hydromorphone	Serum	0.008-0.032	μg/mL	3504	28-112	nmol/L
β-Hydroxybutyric acid	Plasma	< 3.0	mg/dL	96.06	< 300	μmol/L
5-Hydroxyindoleacetic acid (5-HIAA)	Urine	2-6	mg/24 h	5.23	10.4-31.2	μmol/d
Hydroxyproline	Plasma	< 0.55	mg/dL	76.266	< 42	μmol/L

Ibuprofen	Serum	10-50	μg/mL	4.848	50-243	μmol/L
Imipramine	Plasma	150-250	ng/mL	3.566	536-893	nmol/L
Immunoglobulin A (IgA)	Serum	40-350	mg/dL	10	400-3500	mg/L
Immunoglobulin D (IgD)	Serum	0-8	mg/dL	10	0-80	mg/L
Immunoglobulin E (IgE)	Serum	0-1500	μg/L	0.001	0-1.5	mg/L
Immunoglobulin G (IgG)	Serum	650-1600	mg/dL	0.01	6.5-16.0	g/L
Immunoglobulin M (IgM)	Serum	54-300	mg/dL	10	550-3000	mg/L
Insulin	Serum	2.0-20	μIU/mL	6.945	14-140	pmol/L
Insulinlike growth factor	Serum	130-450	ng/mL	0.131	18-60	nmol/L
Iodine	Serum	58-77	μg/L	7.880	450-580	nmol/L
Iron	Serum	60-150	μg/dL	0.179	10.7-26.9	μmol/L
Iron-binding capacity	Serum	250-450	μg/dL	0.179	44.8-80.6	μmol/L
Isoleucine	Plasma	0.5-1.3	mg/dL	76.236	40-100	μmol/L
Isoniazid	Plasma	1-7	μg/mL	7.291	7-51	μmol/L
Isopropanol (toxic)	Serum, plasma	>400	mg/L	0.0166	>6.64	mmol/L
Kanamycin	Serum, plasma	25-35	μg/mL	2.08	52-72	μmol/L
Ketamine	Serum	0.2-6.3	μg/mL	4.206	0.8-26	μmol/L
17-Ketosteroids	Urine	3-12	mg/24 h	3.33	10-42	μmol/d
Lactate	Plasma	5.0-15	mg/dL	0.111	0.6-1.7	mmol/L
Lactate dehydrogenase (LDH)	Serum	100-200	U/L	0.0167	1.7-3.4	μkat/L
LDH isoenzymes						
LD_1	Serum	17-27	%	0.01	0.17-0.27	Proportion of 1.0
LD_2	Serum	27-37	%	0.01	0.27-0.37	Proportion of 1.0
LD_3	Serum	18-25	%	0.01	0.18-0.25	Proportion of 1.0
LD_4	Serum	3-8	%	0.01	0.03-0.08	Proportion of 1.0

Table 2. Selected Laboratory Tests, With Reference Ranges and Conversion Factors[a] *(cont)*

Analyte	Specimen	Reference Range, Conventional Unit	Conventional Unit	Conversion Factor (Multiply by)	Reference Range, SI Unit	SI Unit
LD_5	Serum	0-5	%	0.01	0-0.05	Proportion of 1.0
Lead	Serum	< 10-20	μg/dL	0.0483	< 0.5-1.0	μmol/L
Leucine	Plasma	1.0-2.3	mg/dL	76.237	75-175	μmol/L
Leukocytes (see White blood cell count)						
Lidocaine	Serum, plasma	1.5-6.0	μg/mL	4.267	6.4-25.6	μmol/L
Lipase	Serum	31-186	U/L	0.01667	0.5-3.2	μkat/L
Lipoprotein(a) [Lp(a)]	Serum	10-30	mg/dL	0.0357	0.35-1.0	μmol/L
Lithium	Serum	0.6-1.2	mEq/L	1.0	0.6-1.2	mmol/L
Lorazepam	Serum	50-240	ng/mL	3.114	156-746	nmol/L
Luteinizing hormone (LH)	Serum, plasma	1-104	mIU/mL	1.0	1-104	IU/L
Lycopene	Serum	0.15-0.25	mg/L	1.863	0.28-0.46	μmol/L
Lymphocytes (see White blood cell count)						
Lysergic acid diethylamide	Serum	< 0.004	μg/mL	3726	< 15	nmol/L
Lysine	Plasma	1.2-3.5	mg/dL	68.404	80-240	μmol/L
Lysozyme	Serum, plasma	0.4-1.3	mg/dL	10	4-13	mg/L
Magnesium	Serum	1.3-2.1	mEq/L	0.50	0.65-1.05	mmol/L
Manganese	Whole blood	10-12	μg/L	18.202	182-218	nmol/L
Maprotiline	Plasma	200-600	ng/mL	1.0	200-600	μg/L
Melatonin	Serum	10-15	ng/L	4.305	45-66	pmol/L
Meperidine	Serum, plasma	400-700	ng/mL	4.043	1620-2830	nmol/L
Mercury	Serum	< 5	μg/L	4.985	< 25	nmol/L
Metanephrine (total)	Urine	< 1.0	mg/24 h	5.07	< 5	μmol/d
Metformin	Serum	1-4	μg/mL	7.742	8-30	μmol/L

Methadone	Serum, plasma	100-400	ng/mL	0.00323	0.32-1.29	μmol/L
Methamphetamine	Serum	0.01-0.05	μg/mL	6.7	0.07-0.34	μmol/L
Methanol	Plasma	< 200	μg/mL	0.0312	< 6.2	mmol/L
Methaqualone	Serum, plasma	2-3	μg/mL	4.0	8-12	μmol/L
Methemoglobin	Whole blood	< 0.24	g/dL	155	< 37.2	μmol/L
Methemoglobin	Whole blood	< 1.0	% of total hemoglobin	0.01	< 0.01	Proportion of total hemoglobin
Methicillin	Serum	8-25	mg/L	2.636	22-66	μmol/L
Methionine	Plasma	0.1-0.6	mg/dL	67.02	6-40	μmol/L
Methotrexate	Serum, plasma	0.04-0.36	mg/L	2200	90-790	nmol/L
Methyldopa	Plasma	1-5	μg/mL	4.735	5.0-25	μmol/L
Metoprolol	Serum, plasma	75-200	ng/mL	3.74	281-748	nmol/L
β_2-Microglobulin	Serum	1.2-2.8	mg/L	1.0	1.2-2.8	mg/L
Morphine	Serum, plasma	10-80	ng/mL	3.504	35-280	nmol/L
Myoglobin	Serum	19-92	μg/L	0.0571	1.0-5.3	nmol/L
Naproxen	Serum	26-70	μg/mL	4.343	115-300	μmol/L
Niacin (nicotinic acid)	Urine	2.4-6.4	mg/24 h	7.30	17.5-46.7	μmol/d
Nickel	Whole blood	1.0-28.0	μg/L	17.033	17-476	nmol/L
Nicotine	Plasma	0.01-0.05	mg/L	6.164	0.062-0.308	μmol/L
Nitrogen (nonprotein)	Serum	20-35	mg/dL	0.714	14.3-25.0	mmol/L
Nitroprusside (as thiocyanate)		6-29	μg/mL	17.2	103-500	μmol/L
Norepinephrine	Plasma	110-410	pg/mL	5.911	650-2423	pmol/L
Nortriptyline	Serum, plasma	50-150	ng/mL	3.797	190-570	nmol/L
Ornithine	Plasma	0.4-1.4	mg/dL	75.666	30-106	μmol/L
Osmolality	Serum	275-295	mOsm/kg	1.0	275-295	mmol/kg
Osteocalcin	Serum	3.0-13.0	ng/mL	1.0	3.0-13.0	μg/L

Table 2. Selected Laboratory Tests, With Reference Ranges and Conversion Factors[a] *(cont)*

Analyte	Specimen	Reference Range, Conventional Unit	Conventional Unit	Conversion Factor (Multiply by)	Reference Range, SI Unit	SI Unit
Oxalate	Serum	1.0-2.4	mg/mL	11.107	11-27	μmol/L
Oxazepam	Serum, plasma	0.2-1.4	μg/mL	3.487	0.7-4.9	μmol/L
Oxycodone	Serum	10-100	ng/mL	3.171	32-317	nmol/L
Oxygen, partial pressure (Po_2)	Arterial blood	80-100	mm Hg	0.133	11-13	kPa
Paraquat	Whole blood	0.1-1.6	μg/mL	5.369	0.5-8.5	μmol/L
Parathyroid hormone	Serum	10-65	pg/mL	0.1053	10-65	ng/L
Pentobarbital	Serum, plasma	1-5	μg/mL	4.439	4.0-22	μmol/L
Pepsinogen	Serum	28-100	ng/mL	1.0	28-100	μg/L
pH (see Blood gases)						
Phencyclidine (toxic)	Serum, plasma	90-800	ng/mL	4.109	370-3288	nmol/L
Phenobarbital	Serum, plasma	15-40	μg/mL	4.31	65-172	μmol/L
Phenylalanine	Plasma	0.6-1.5	mg/dL	60.544	35-90	μmol/L
Phenylpropanolamine	Serum	0.05-0.10	μg/mL	6613	330-660	nmol/L
Phenytoin	Serum, plasma	10-20	mg/L	3.968	40-79	μmol/L
Phosphorus (inorganic)	Serum	2.3-4.7	mg/dL	0.323	0.74-1.52	mmol/L
Placental lactogen	Serum	0.5-1.1	μg/mL	46.296	23-509	nmol/L
Plasminogen (antigenic)	Plasma	10-20	mg/dL	0.113	1.1-2.2	μmol/L
Plasminogen activator inhibitor	Plasma	4-40	ng/mL	19.231	75-750	pmol/L
Platelet count (thrombocytes)	Whole blood	150-350	$\times 10^3/\mu L$	1.0	150-350	$\times 10^9/L$
Porphyrins (total)	Urine	20-120	μg/L	1.203	25-144	nmol/L
Potassium	Serum	3.5-5.0	mEq/L	1.0	3.5-5.0	mmol/L
Prealbumin	Serum	19.5-35.8	mg/dL	10	195-358	mg/L
Pregnanediol	Urine	< 2.6	mg/24 h	3.12	< 8	μmol/d

Pregnanetriol	Urine	< 2.5	mg/24 h	2.972	< 7.5	µmol/d
Primidone	Serum, plasma	5-12	µg/mL	4.582	23-55	µmol/L
Procainamide	Serum, plasma	4-10	µg/mL	4.25	17-42	µmol/L
Progesterone	Serum	0.15-25	ng/mL	3.18	0.5-79.5	nmol/L
Prolactin	Serum	3.8-23.2	µg/L	43.478	90-140	pmol/L
Proline	Plasma	1.2-3.9	mg/dL	86.858	104-340	µmol/L
Propoxyphene	Plasma	0.1-0.4	µg/mL	2.946	0.3-1.2	µmol/L
Propranolol	Serum	50-100	ng/mL	3.856	193-386	nmol/L
Prostate-specific antigen	Serum	< 4.0	ng/mL	1.0	< 4.0	µg/L
Protein (total)	Serum	6.0-8.0	g/dL	10.0	60-80	g/L
Prothrombin time (PT)	Plasma	10-13	s	1.0	10-13	s
Protoporphyrin	Red blood cells	15-50	µg/dL	0.0178	0.27-0.89	µmol/L
Protriptyline	Serum, plasma	70-250	µg/dL	3.787	266-950	nmol/L
Pyridoxine (see Vitamin B_6)						
Pyruvate	Plasma	0.5-1.5	mg/dL	113.56	60-170	µmol/L
Quinidine	Serum	2.0-5.0	µg/mL	3.082	6.2-15.4	µmol/L
Red blood cell count	Whole blood	3.9-5.5	$\times 10^6/\mu L$	1.0	3.9-5.5	$\times 10^{12}/L$
Renin	Plasma	30-40	pg/mL	0.0237	0.7-1.0	pmol/L
Reticulocyte count	Whole blood	25-75	$\times 10^3/\mu L$	1.0	25-75	$\times 10^9/L$
Reticulocyte count	Whole blood	0.5-1.5	% of red blood cells	0.01	0.005-0.015	Proportion of red blood cells
Retinol (see Vitamin A)						
Riboflavin (see Vitamin B_2)						
Rifampin	Serum	4-40	mg/L	1.215	5-49	µmol/L
Salicylates	Serum, plasma	150-300	µg/mL	0.0724	1086-2172	µmol/L
Selenium	Serum, plasma	58-234	µg/L	0.0127	0.74-2.97	µmol/L

Table 2. Selected Laboratory Tests, With Reference Ranges and Conversion Factors[a] *(cont)*

Analyte	Specimen	Reference Range, Conventional Unit	Conventional Unit	Conversion Factor (Multiply by)	Reference Range, SI Unit	SI Unit
Serine	Plasma	0.7-2.0	mg/dL	95.156	65-193	µmol/L
Serotonin (5-hydroxytryptamine)	Whole blood	50-200	ng/mL	0.00568	0.28-1.14	µmol/L
Sex hormone–binding globulin	Serum	1.5-2.0	µg/mL	8.896	13-17	nmol/L
Sodium	Serum	136-142	mEq/L	1.0	136-142	mmol/L
Somatomedin C (Insulinlike growth factor)	Serum	130-450	ng/mL	0.131	18-60	nmol/L
Somatostatin	Plasma	< 25	pg/mL	0.6110	< 15	pmol/L
Streptomycin	Serum	7-50	mg/L	1.719	12-86	µmol/L
Strychnine	Whole blood	< 0.5	mg/L	2.99	< 1.5	µmol/L
Substance P	Plasma	< 240	pg/mL	0.742	< 180	pmol/L
Sulfate	Serum	10-32	mg/L	31.188	310-990	µmol/L
Sulfmethemoglobin	Whole blood	< 1.0	% of total hemoglobin	0.01	< 0.010	Proportion of total hemoglobin
Taurine	Plasma	0.3-2.1	mg/dL	79.91	24-168	µmol/L
Testosterone	Serum	300-1200	ng/dL	0.0347	10.4-41.6	nmol/L
Tetrahydrocannabinol	Serum	< 0.20	µg/mL	3.180	< 0.60	µmol/L
Theophylline	Serum, plasma	10-20	µg/mL	5.55	56-111	µmol/L
Thiamine (see Vitamin B_1)						
Thiopental	Serum, plasma	1-5	µg/mL	4.144	4.1-20.7	µmol/L
Thioridazine	Serum, plasma	1.0-1.5	µg/mL	2.699	2.7-4.1	µmol/L
Threonine	Plasma	0.9-2.5	mg/dL	84	75-210	µmol/L
Thrombin time	Plasma	16-24	s	1.0	16.24	s
Thrombocytes (see Platelet count)						

Thyroglobulin	Serum	3-42	ng/mL	1.0	3-42	μg/L
Thyroid-stimulating hormone (TSH)	Serum	0.4-4.2	mIU/L	1.0	0.4-4.2	mIU/L
Thyroxine, free (FT_4)	Serum	0.9-2.3	ng/dL	12.871	12-30	pmol/L
Thyroxine, total (T_4)	Serum	5.5-12.5	μg/dL	12.871	71-160	nmol/L
Thyroxine-binding globulin	Serum	16.0-24.0	μg/mL	17.094	206-309	nmol/L
Tissue plasminogen activator	Plasma	< 0.04	IU/mL	1000	< 40	IU/L
Tobramycin	Serum, plasma	5-10	μg/mL	2.139	10-21	μmol/L
Tocainide	Serum	4-10	μg/mL	5.201	21-52	μmol/L
α-Tocopherol (see Vitamin E)						
Tolbutamide	Serum	80-240	μg/mL	3.70	296-888	μmol/L
Transferrin	Serum	200-400	mg/dL	0.0123	2.5-5.0	μmol/L
Triglycerides	Serum	< 160	mg/dL	0.0113	1.8	mmol/L
Triiodothyronine, free (FT_3)	Serum	1.4-4.4	pg/mL	0.0154	0.22-6.78	pmol/L
Triiodothyronine, total (T_3)	Serum	60-180	ng/dL	0.0154	0.92-2.76	nmol/L
Troponin I	Serum	0-0.4	ng/mL	1.0	0-0.4	μg/L
Troponin T	Serum	0-0.1	ng/mL	1.0	0-0.1	μg/L
Tryptophan	Plasma	0.5-1.5	mg/dL	48.967	25-73	μmol/L
Tyrosine	Plasma	0.4-1.6	mg/dL	55.19	20-90	μmol/L
Urea nitrogen	Serum	8-23	mg/dL	0.357	2.9-8.2	mmol/L
Uric acid	Serum	4.0-8.0	mg/dL	59.485	240-480	μmol/L
Urobilinogen	Urine	1-3.5	mg/24 h	1.7	1.7-5.9	μmol/d
Valine	Plasma	1.7-3.7	mg/dL	85.361	145-315	μmol/L
Valproic acid	Serum, plasma	50-100	μg/mL	6.934	346-693	μmol/L
Vancomycin	Serum, plasma	20-40	μg/mL	0.690	14-28	μmol/L
Vanillylmandelic acid (VMA)	Urine	2.1-7.6	mg/24 h	5.046	11-38	μmol/d
Vasoactive intestinal polypeptide	Plasma	< 50	pg/mL	0.2960	< 15	pmol/L

Table 2. Selected Laboratory Tests, With Reference Ranges and Conversion Factors[a] *(cont)*

Analyte	Specimen	Reference Range, Conventional Unit	Conventional Unit	Conversion Factor (Multiply by)	Reference Range, SI Unit	SI Unit
Vasopressin	Plasma	1.5-2.0	pg/mL	0.923	1.0-2.0	pmol/L
Verapamil	Serum, plasma	100-500	ng/mL	2.20	220-1100	nmol/L
Vitamin A (retinol)	Serum	30-80	μg/dL	0.0349	1.05-2.80	μmol/L
Vitamin B_1 (thiamine)	Serum	0-2	μg/dL	29.6	0-75	nmol/L
Vitamin B_2 (riboflavin)	Serum	4-24	μg/dL	26.6	106-638	nmol/L
Vitamin B_3	Whole blood	0.2-1.8	μg/mL	4.56	0.9-8.2	μmol/L
Vitamin B_6 (pyridoxine)	Plasma	5-30	ng/mL	4.046	20-121	nmol/L
Vitamin B_{12}	Serum	160-950	pg/mL	0.7378	118-701	pmol/L
Vitamin C (ascorbic acid)	Serum	0.4-1.5	mg/dL	56.78	23-85	μmol/L
Vitamin D (1,25 dihydroxyvitamin D)	Serum	25-45	pg/mL	2.6	60-108	pmol/L
Vitamin D (25-hydroxyvitamin D)	Plasma	14-60	ng/mL	2.496	35-150	nmol/L
Vitamin E (α-tocopherol)	Serum	5-18	μg/mL	23.22	12-42	μmol/L
Vitamin K	Serum	0.13-1.19	ng/mL	2.22	0.29-2.64	nmol/L
Warfarin	Serum, plasma	1.0-10	μg/mL	3.247	3.2-32.4	μmol/L
White blood cell count	Whole blood	4500-11 000	/μL	0.001	4.5-11.0	$\times 10^9$/L
Differential count						
Neutrophils-segmented	Whole blood	1800-7800	/μL	0.001	1.8-7.8	$\times 10^9$/L
Neutrophils-bands	Whole blood	0-700	/μL	0.001	0-0.70	$\times 10^9$/L

Lymphocytes	Whole blood	1000-4800	/μL	0.001	1.0-4.8	$\times 10^9$/L
Monocytes	Whole blood	0-800	/μL	0.001	0-0.80	$\times 10^9$/L
Eosinophils	Whole blood	0-450	/μL	0.001	0-0.45	$\times 10^9$/L
Basophils	Whole blood	0-200	/μL	0.001	0-0.20	$\times 10^9$/L
Differential count (number fraction)						
Neutrophils-segmented	Whole blood	56	%	0.01	0.56	Proportion of 1.0
Neutrophils-bands	Whole blood	3	%	0.01	0.03	Proportion of 1.0
Lymphocytes	Whole blood	34	%	0.01	0.34	Proportion of 1.0
Monocytes	Whole blood	4	%	0.01	0.04	Proportion of 1.0
Eosinophils	Whole blood	2.7	%	0.01	0.027	Proportion of 1.0
Basophils	Whole blood	0.3	%	0.01	0.003	Proportion of 1.0
Zidovudine	Serum, plasma	0.15-0.27	μg/mL	3.7	0.56-1.01	μmol/L
Zinc	Serum	75-120	μg/dL	0.153	11.5-18.5	μmol/L

[a] The laboratory values and reference ranges are provided for illustration only and are not intended to be comprehensive or definitive. Each laboratory determines its own values, and reference ranges are highly method dependent. Reference values given are for adults. For some entries for which specific molecular masses are not known (eg, proteins), reference values in SI are given as mass amounts per liter.

The information in this table is adapted from and based on the following sources: (1) Kratz A, Ferraro M, Sluss PM, Lewandrowski KB. Laboratory reference values. *N Engl J Med.* 2004;351(15):1548-1563; (2) Young DS, Huth EJ. *SI Units for Clinical Measurement*. Philadelphia, PA: American College of Physicians; 1998; (3) Henry JB, ed. *Clinical Diagnosis and Management by Laboratory Methods*. 20th ed. Philadelphia, PA: WB Saunders; 2001; (4) Kasper DL, Braunwald E, Fauci AS, et al, eds. *Harrison's Principles of Internal Medicine*, 16th ed. New York, NY: McGraw Hill; 2004; and (5) Goldman L, Ausiello D. *Cecil Textbook of Medicine*. 22nd ed. Philadelphia, PA: WB Saunders; 2004.

For laboratory values reported in *JAMA* and in the *Archives* Journals, factors for converting conventional units to SI units should be provided in the article. In text, the conversion factor should be given once, at first mention of the laboratory value, in parentheses following the conventional unit.

> The blood glucose concentration of 126 mg/dL (to convert to millimoles per liter, multiply by 0.055) was used as a criterion for diagnosing diabetes.

For articles in which several laboratory values are reported in text, the conversion factors may be listed in a paragraph at the end of the "Methods" section. For figures or tables, the conversion factors should be included in legends or in footnotes, respectively, but not in the abstract of the article. (See Footnotes in 4.1.3, Visual Presentation of Data, Tables, Table Components.)

> Hematologic values should be reported by means of conventional units.
>
> The complete blood cell count showed a hemoglobin level of 13.4 g/dL, hematocrit of 41%, platelet count of 180 000/μL, and white blood cell count of 6500/μL.

For enzymatic activity, the international unit (IU) is used; 1 IU equals the amount of enzyme generating 1 μmol of product per minute.

> The peak follicle-stimulating hormone level was 48 mIU/mL.

18.5.11 **Radiation.** Measurements of ionizing radiation and radioactivity should be reported by means of SI units. The SI units for radiation are established by international agreement.[1] The unit for activity of a radionuclide is the becquerel; the absorbed dose of radiation (absorbed per unit weight of tissue) is the gray (Gy); and the dose equivalent used to indicate the detrimental effects of an absorbed radiation dose on biological tissue is the sievert (Sv).

A 1-Gy dose is equivalent to 1 joule (J) of radiation energy absorbed per kilogram of organ or tissue weight. Rad is the older, non-SI term and is still in use as a unit of absorbed dose (100 rad = 1 Gy). However, equal doses of all types of ionizing radiation are not equally harmful. Alpha particles produce greater harm than beta particles, γ rays, and x-rays for a given absorbed dose. To account for this difference, radiation dose is expressed as equivalent dose in sieverts (Sv).[9]

SI units for radiation and factors to convert values from SI units to conventional units are shown below.

Quantity	*SI Unit (Symbol)*	*Conversion Factors*	*Non-SI Unit*
Radioactivity	becquerel (Bq)	1 Bq = 2.7×10^{-11} Ci (approx)	curie
		1 Ci = 3.7×10^{10} Bq	
		1 Bq = 27 picocurie (pCi)	
Absorbed dose	gray (Gy)	1 Gy = 100 rad	rad
		1 rad = 0.01 Gy[a]	

Quantity	*SI Unit (Symbol)*	*Conversion Factors*	*Non-SI Unit*
"Dose" equivalent	sievert (Sv)	1 Sv = 100 rem	rem
		1 rem = 0.01 Sv	

[a] Although 1 rad = 1 cGy, the *centi-* prefix is generally not preferred in SI. Therefore, despite the appeal of one-to-one conversion, rad should be converted to gray, not centigray.

Although SI units are preferred, authors of some articles, such as those reporting studies involving nuclear medicine or radiation oncology, may prefer to report results in both SI units and non-SI units. As with units for laboratory results, conversion factors to convert radiation units from SI units to conventional units should be provided in the article, either in the text, in footnotes to tables or figures, or in the "Methods" section.

18.5.12 **Currency.** Amounts of money in US, Canadian, and British currency are expressed as a decimal number or whole number preceded by the symbol for the unit of measure for the currency.

> The cost-effectiveness analysis suggested a $7000 difference between the 2 treatment strategies.

Table 3. Selected International Currencies and Symbols

Country	Currency	Symbol or Abbreviation
Argentina	Argentine peso	$
Australia	Australian dollar	A$
Austria	Austrian shillings	ATS
Bahamas	Bahamian dollar	B$
Belgium	Euro (replaces Belgian franc)	€
Bermuda	Bermuda dollar	Bd$
Bolivia	boliviano	$
Brazil	Brazilian real	R$
Canada	Canadian dollar	Can$
Chile	Chilean peso	Ch$
China	yuan renminbi	¥
Colombia	Colombian peso	Col$
Cuba	Cuban peso	$
Czech Republic	Czech koruna	Kč
Denmark	Danish krone	kr
Dominican Republic	Dominican peso	RD$
Egypt	Egyptian pound	£
European Union	Euro	€
Finland	Euro (replaces markka)	€
France	Euro (replaces franc)	€

Table 3. Selected International Currencies and Symbols *(cont)*

Country	Currency	Symbol or Abbreviation
Germany	Euro (replaces deutsche mark)	€
Greece	drachma	$\mathcal{D}_{\rho}$*
Hong Kong	Hong Kong dollar	HK$
Hungary	forint	ft
India	rupee	Rs
Iran	rial	IRR
Iraq	new Iraqi dinar	IQD
Ireland	Euro (replaces pound)	€
Israel	Israeli new sheqel	₪
Italy	Euro (replaces lira)	€
Japan	yen	¥
Jordan	Jordanian dinars	JD
Korea	won	₩
Lebanon	Lebanese pound	LBP
Luxembourg	Euro (replaces franc)	€
Mexico	Mexican peso	Mex$
The Netherlands	Euro (replaces guilder)	€
New Zealand	New Zealand dollar	NZ$
Norway	Norwegian krone	kr
Pakistan	rupee	Rs
Peru	neuvos soles	S/
Poland	zloty	Zl
Portugal	Euro (replaces escudo)	€
Russia	ruble	R
Saudi Arabia	Saudi riyal	SR
Singapore	Singapore dollar	SGD
South Africa	rand	R
Spain	Euro (replaces pesata)	€
Sweden	Swedish krona	Sk
Switzerland	Swiss franc	Sw₣
Taiwan	Taiwanese new dollar	NT$
Thailand	baht	฿
Turkey	Turkish new lira	T£
United Kingdom	pound sterling	£
United States of America	US dollar	$
Vietnam	dong	₫

In *JAMA* and the *Archives* Journals, for amounts reported in non-US currency, the current exchange rate should be used to calculate the amount in US dollars, and that amount should be shown in parentheses. A list of some international currencies and their symbols is provided in Table 3. Online currency converter programs also are available.[10,11]

> The baseline amount for the cost-benefit analysis was estimated from the procedure cost of CaD $3000 (US $2800).
>
> The projected cost of the new research laboratory was €25 million (US $47.7 million).

ACKNOWLEDGMENTS

Principal authors: Phil B. Fontanarosa, MD, MBA, and Stacy Christiansen, MA

I thank Lupe Morales, *JAMA*, for her assistance with preparation of the tables in this chapter.

REFERENCES

1. Bureau International des Poids et Mesures. *The International System of Units (SI)*. 8th ed. http://www1.bipm.org/utils/common/pdf/si_brochure_8.pdf. Accessed August 7, 2006.
2. *Dorland's Illustrated Medical Dictionary*. 30th ed. Philadelphia, PA: WB Saunders Co; 2000.
3. Kriska AM, Caspersen CJ. Introduction to a collection of physical activity questionnaires. *Med Sci Sports Exerc*. 1997;29(6):S5-S9.
4. Kratz A, Ferraro M, Sluss PM, Lewandrowski KB. Laboratory reference values. *N Engl J Med*. 2004;351(15):1548-1563.
5. Young DS, Huth EJ. *SI Units for Clinical Measurement*. Philadelphia, PA: American College of Physicians; 1998.
6. Henry JB, ed. *Clinical Diagnosis and Management by Laboratory Methods*. 20th ed. Philadelphia, PA: WB Saunders Co; 2001.
7. Goldman L, Ausiello D. *Cecil Textbook of Medicine*. 22nd ed. Philadelphia, PA: WB Saunders Co; 2004.
8. Kasper DL, Braunwald E, Fauci AS, et al, eds. *Harrison's Principles of Internal Medicine*. 16th ed. New York, NY: McGraw-Hill; 2004.
9. Canadian Centre for Occupational Health and Safety. What is ionizing radiation? www.ccohs.ca/oshanswers/phys_agents/ionizing.html. Accessed August 7, 2006.
10. Codes for representation of currencies and funds. Geneva, Switzerland: International Organization for Standardization; 2004. http://www.xe.com/iso4217.htm. Accessed August 7, 2006.
11. Oanda.com Quick Converter. www.oanda.com/converter/classic. Accessed August 7, 2006.

19 Numbers and Percentages

Any policy on the use of numbers in text must take into account the reader's impression that numbers written as numerals (symbols) appear to emphasize quantity more strongly than numbers spelled out as words. Because numerals convey quantity more efficiently than spelled-out numbers, they are generally preferable in technical writing. In literary writing, by contrast, spelled-out numbers may be more compatible with style. Despite these general principles, usage may appear inconsistent when a publication chooses to use numerals in some instances and words in others. The guidelines outlined in this section attempt to reduce these inconsistencies and avoid use of numerals that may be jarring to the reader. In situations that are not governed by these guidelines, common sense and editorial judgment should prevail.

19.1

Use of Numerals. In scientific writing, numerals are used to express numbers in most circumstances. Exceptions are the following:

- Numbers that begin a sentence, title, subtitle, or heading
- Common fractions
- Accepted usage such as idiomatic expressions and numbers used as pronouns
- Other uses of "one" in running text
- Ordinals *first* through *ninth*
- Numbers spelled out in quotes or published titles. (See 19.2, Spelling Out Numbers.)

Note the following examples of numerals in text:

The relative risk of exposed individuals was nearly 3 times that of the controls.

In the second phase of the study, 3 of the investigators administered the 5 tests to the 7 remaining subjects. The test scores showed a 2- to 2.4-fold improvement over those of the first phase.

In 2 of the 17 patients in whom both ears were tested, we were unable to obtain responses from either ear. While testing patient 3, we experienced technical problems consisting of unmanageable electrical artifacts.

Groups 1 and 2 were similar in terms of demographic and clinical characteristics (Table 1). Table 2 lists the 4 tests that were performed.

A 3-member committee from the Food and Drug Administration visited the researchers.

19.1.1 **Numbers of 4 or More Digits to Either Side of the Decimal Point.** Commas are not used in large numbers. In 4-digit numbers, the digits are set closed up. For numbers of 10 000 or greater, a half-space or thin space is used to separate every 3 digits starting from the right-most integer (or, in numbers with decimals, from the left of the decimal point). For numbers with 5 or more digits to the right of the decimal point, a half-space is used between every 3 digits starting from the right of the decimal point (see also 18.4, Units of Measure, Use of Numerals With Units).

The exact weight of the salt was 8.453 98 g, but its reported value was rounded to 8.4540 g.

Our analytical sample included all 2455 community-dwelling individuals 65 years or older, representing 32 294 810 elderly persons in the United States.

19.1.2 **Mixed Fractions.** For less precise measurements, mixed fractions may be used instead of decimals. These expressions usually involve time. Common fractions are typically spelled out (see 19.2.2, Spelling Out Numbers, Common Fractions).

The surgery lasted 3¼ hours.

The patient was hospitalized for 5½ days.

Of the patients returning for a second visit, half received the intervention.

19.1.3 **Measures of Time.** Measures of time usually are expressed as numerals (see also 14.3, Abbreviations, Days of the Week, Months, Eras). When dates are provided, numerals should be used for day and year; the month should be spelled out unless listed in a table. Conventional form for time and dates (11:30 PM on February 25, 1961) is preferred to European or military form (2330 on 25 February 1961). However, use of military time may clarify the time course in figures that depict a 24-hour experiment, times of drug dosing, and the like. For time, if the hour of the day is given, AM or PM is used and set in small capitals (see also 22.0, Typography). When referring to time on the hour, the minutes may be omitted (eg, 3 PM). With 12 o'clock, simply use noon or midnight, whichever is intended.

At 5:45 AM, October 15, 1994, the researchers completed the final experiment.

The 21st century officially began just after midnight on January 1, 2001.

When referring to a position as it would appear on a clock face, express the position by means of numerals followed by "o'clock."

The needle was inserted at the 9-o'clock position.

But: The procedure was scheduled to begin at 9 AM.

See 8.2.3 (Punctuation, Comma, Semicolon, Colon, Colon) for punctuation in expressions of time.

19.1.4 **Measures of Temperature.** Use the degree symbol with Celsius or Fahrenheit measures of temperature. The degree symbol should be closed up (see 18.3.8, Units of Measure, Format, Style, and Punctuation, Spacing).

The plates were cultured at 17°C, 3°C lower than usual.

19.1.5 **Measures of Currency.** For sums of money, use the appropriate symbol to indicate the type of currency (eg, $, €, £; see also 18.5.12, Units of Measure, Conventional Units and SI Units in *JAMA* and the *Archives* Journals, Currency).

His charge for the medication was $55.60 plus $0.95 for shipping.

The equivalent sum in euros was €30.

19.2 **Spelling Out Numbers.** Use words to express numbers that occur at the beginning of a sentence, title, subtitle, or heading; for common fractions; for accepted usage and numbers used as pronouns; for ordinals *first* through *ninth*; and when part of a published quote or title in which the number is spelled out. When spelling out numerals, hyphenate *twenty-one* through *ninety-nine* when these numbers occur alone or as part of a larger number. When numbers greater than 100 are spelled out, do not use commas or *and* (eg, one hundred thirty-two).

19.2.1 **Beginning a Sentence, Title, Subtitle, or Heading.** Use words for any number that begins a sentence, title, subtitle, or heading. However, it may be better to reword the sentence so that it does not begin with a number.

Three hundred twenty-eight men and 126 women were included in the study.
Better: The study population comprised 328 men and 126 women.

Participants: Seventy-two thousand three hundred thirty-seven postmenopausal women aged 34 to 77 years.
Better: **Participants:** A total of 72 337 postmenopausal women aged 34 to 77 years.

Three patients were identified; 2 had hypertension and 1 had diabetes.

Numerals may be used in sentences that begin with a specific year, but avoid beginning sentences with years if possible.

1995 marked the 50th anniversary of the bombing of Hiroshima.
Better: The year 1995 marked the 50th anniversary of the bombing of Hiroshima.

2005 was the medical school's centennial year.
Better: The medical school's centennial year was 2005.

When a unit of measure follows a number that begins a sentence, it too must be written out, even if the same unit is abbreviated elsewhere in the same sentence. Because this construction can be cumbersome, rewording the sentence may be preferable (see 18.3, Units of Measure, Format, Style, and Punctuation).

Two milligrams of haloperidol was administered at 9 PM, followed by 1 mg at 3:30 AM.
Better: At 9 PM, 2 mg of haloperidol was administered, followed at 3:30 AM by 1 mg.

19.2.2 Common Fractions. Common fractions are expressed with hyphenated words, whether the fraction is used as an adjective or a noun. Mixed fractions are typically expressed in numerals (see 19.1.2, Use of Numerals, Mixed Fractions).

Of those attending, nearly three-fourths were members of the association.

There was a half-second delay before the concert hall was illuminated.

We require a two-thirds majority for consensus.

In some cases, fractions can be expressed with an indefinite article preceding the denominator. Such constructions do not use the hyphen.

The test concluded after half an hour.

A quarter may be used in place of *one-fourth*.

A quarter of the consensus panel dissented.

19.2.3 *One* Used as a Pronoun. The word *one* should be spelled out when used as a pronoun or noun.

The investigators compared a new laboratory method with the standard one.

These differences may be concealed if one looks only at the total group.

William James uses the idea of the one and the many as the great challenge of the philosophical mind.

19.2.4 Accepted Usage. Spell out numbers for generally accepted usage, such as idiomatic expressions. *One* frequently appears in running text without referring to a quantity per se and may appear awkward if expressed as a numeral. When *one* may be replaced by *a* or *a single* without changing the meaning, the word *one* rather than the numeral is usually appropriate. Other numbers, most often *zero, two,* and large rounded numbers, also may be written as words in circumstances in which use of the numeral would place an unintended emphasis on a precise quantity or would be confusing.

Any one of the 12 individuals might have been holding the winning ticket. [In this example, *one* may be superfluous. Depending on the intent, the following may be an equivalent sentence: Any of the 12 individuals might have been holding the winning ticket.]

The study was plagued by one problem after another.

In the article, one researcher estimated that firearms are used for protective purposes in the United States several hundred thousand times annually.

Models were developed to allow for the inclusion of one-time variables.

We appear to be moving from one extreme to another.

On the one hand, the blood glucose concentrations were substantially improved; on the other hand, the patient felt worse.

Medical futility has become one of the dominant topics in medical ethics in recent years.

In one recent case, the bonus amounted to $1 billion.

We ought to bring together in one place all that we have learned on a given subject.

The outcome was a zero-sum gain.

A zero should not be placed to the left of the decimal point of a *P* value, both because it could be confused with the letter O, and because a *P* value is always less than 1.0.

Conventional wisdom has it that there are at least two sides to every issue.

Please include an example or two of the following scales.

I would like to ask the patient a question or two about her perception of her illness.

He quoted the Ten Commandments. [See also 10.0, Capitalization.]

Many of the mass-vaccination campaigns have been large, with tens of thousands of persons immunized, and expensive, costing as much as a half-million dollars.

During one of the laboratory runs, it was observed that samples from cases 1, 3, and 9 had faint electrophoretic bands due to suboptimal DNA quality. *But:* During 1 of the 17 laboratory runs, it was observed. . . . [See 19.3.2, Combining Numerals and Words, Consecutive Numerical Expressions.]

19.2.5 Ordinals. Ordinal numbers generally express order or rank, rather than a precise quantity. Because they usually address nontechnical aspects of the objects they modify, ordinals are often found in literary writing. The numerical expression of commonly used ordinals (1st, 2nd, 3rd, 4th, etc) may appear jarring and interrupt the flow of the text. For this reason the ordinals *first* through *ninth* are spelled out.

The third patient was not available for reevaluation.

It has become second nature.

The numeric form of ordinals greater than *ninth* is well established in literary texts (10th, 11th, and so on) except at the beginning of a sentence, title, subtitle, or heading. Use the following suffixes: *-st*, *-nd*, *-rd*, *-th*. These suffixes should not be superscripted.

> Eleventh-hour negotiations settled the strike.
>
> The pandemic will continue well into the 21st century.
>
> He celebrated his 80th birthday.
>
> *But:* Some forms are spelled out by convention, eg, Twenty-fifth Amendment.

If a sentence contains 2 or more ordinals, at least 1 of which is greater than *ninth*, all should be expressed in numeric form.

> Children in the 5th and 10th grades were included in the survey.
>
> The first and third patients treated experienced complete remissions.

19.3 Combining Numerals and Words. Use a combination of numerals and words to express rounded large numbers and consecutive numerical expressions.

19.3.1 Rounded Large Numbers. Rounded large numbers, such as those starting with *million,* should be expressed with numerals and words.

> The disease affects 5 million to 6 million people. [Note that the word *million* is repeated to avoid ambiguity.]

The word *million* signifies the quantity 10^6, while *billion* signifies the quantity 10^9. Although *billion* has traditionally signified 10^{12} (1 million million) in Britain, many British medical journals[1] now use *billion* to indicate the quantity 10^9. A number may be expressed in *million* rather than *billion* if the latter term could create ambiguity. In that case, the decimal should be moved 3 places to the right. *Trillion* should be used to denote the quantity 10^{12}.

> The projected budget is £2.5 billion.
> *Or:* The projected budget is £2500 million.
>
> The budget deficit is expected to expand to $1 trillion by 2020.

19.3.2 Consecutive Numerical Expressions. When 2 numbers appear consecutively in a sentence, either reword the sentence or spell out 1 of the numbers for clarity.

> Study participants were provided twenty 5-mL syringes.
>
> *Avoid:* In the cohort of 1500, 690 were men.
> *Better:* In the cohort of fifteen hundred, 690 were men.
> *Or:* In the cohort, 690 of the 1500 individuals were men.
>
> The envelope contained 3 copies of the manuscript and one 3.5-in diskette.

However, numerals may be listed consecutively if they refer to items in an array. As always, clarity and common sense should guide usage.

The life expectancy of groups 1, 2, and 3 was 69, 83, and 75 years, respectively.

Abbreviations or symbols may follow numbers. In this case, if there is potential for misunderstanding, it is preferable to reword the sentence.

There are 2 D_2 dopamine receptor isoforms.
Better: The D_2 dopamine receptor has 2 isoforms.

The investigators were able to identify 3 γ-aminobutyric acid-mediated sites.
Better: The investigators were able to identify 3 sites mediated by γ-aminobutyric acid.

Superscripts that indicate references may be mistaken for exponents if they immediately follow a numeral.

Increased morbidity has been associated with a BMI less than 18[2] and greater than 27[3]. [This can be reworded: Smith and Jones[2] found that a BMI of less than 18 was associated with increased morbidity. They also found that patients with a BMI greater than 27 had increased morbidity.[3]]

19.4 **Use of Digit Spans and Hyphens.** Digits should not be omitted when indicating a span of years or page numbers in the text. Hyphens may be used in text when a year span is used as the identifying characteristic of a study (eg, the 1982-1984 NHANES survey), but only when the actual dates of the study have been defined previously in the text; if the dates are not defined in the text, the hyphen is ambiguous and may or may not mean that the dates indicated are inclusive. In certain circumstances, such as fiscal year or academic year, the actual span may be understood and no definition is required; in these cases the hyphen is acceptable at first mention and throughout the text.

The students participated in the study during the 1994-1995 academic year.

Substantial profits were anticipated for fiscal years 1996-1998.

Sir William Osler (1849-1919)

Use of *to* also may introduce ambiguity. *To* should be used rather than *through* only when the final digit is not included in the span and *through* instead of *to* when the final digit is included in the span. However, in some circumstances, such as life span, historical periods, fiscal or academic year, page numbers in text, or age ranges, the meaning is clear without making a distinction between *to* and *through,* and *to* may be used.

The participants ranged in age from 23 to 56 years.

The second enrollment period spanned January 30, 1991, to September 1, 1993. [In this example, the enrollment period ended on August 31.]
Or: The second enrollment period spanned January 31, 1991, through August 31, 1993.

We looked at the following 3 periods: 1964 through 1967, 1968 through 1978, and 1979 through 1992.

Time spans may be referred to by means of hyphens between years once the meaning has been made clear at the first mention.

> The mortality rate ratio of 2.01 (95% CI, 1.80-2.24) indicates that the mortality rate during 1968-1978 was about twice that during 1979-1992.

A hyphen may be used within parentheses or in tables to indicate spans, including confidence intervals, without further definition, provided the meaning is clear. However, if one of the values in the span includes a minus sign (most commonly found in confidence intervals), the word *to* should be used to avoid ambiguity. The word *to* should then be used in place of the hyphen throughout the table and text for consistency. (See also 8.3, Punctuation, Hyphens and Dashes, and 20.8, Study Design and Statistics, Significant Digits and Rounding Numbers.)

> The mean number of years of life gained was 1.7 (95% confidence interval, 1.3-2.1).

> The mean number of years of disease-free life gained was 0.4 (95% confidence interval, −0.1 to 0.9).

> After the drug was injected, the seizures continued for a brief period (20-30 seconds), then ceased.

> The fourth edition contains a discussion of recommended preventive measures (pp 1243-1296).

> The median age of the individuals in the sample was 56 years (range, 31-92 years).

If the unit of measure for the quantity is set closed up with the number, the unit should be repeated for each number.

> The temperature remained normal throughout the day (96.5°C-97.3°C).

> The differences between groups were relatively small (5%-8%).

> *But:* The pressure gradient varied widely (10-60 mm Hg) throughout the day.

If the unit of measure changes within the parentheses, *to* is used.

> Because of the wide range of measurements (2 mg to 3.7×10^4 kg), we displayed our results on a logarithmic scale.

19.5 **Enumerations.**

Indicate a short series of enumerated items by numerals run in and enclosed within parentheses in the text (see also 8.5, Punctuation, Parentheses and Brackets).

> The testing format focused on 6 aspects: (1) alertness and concentration, (2) language, (3) naming, (4) calculations, (5) construction, and (6) memory.

For long or complex enumerations, indented numbers followed by a period, without parentheses, may be used.

> In response to other issues:
>
> 1. The study was conducted under 2 protocols that prespecified that the data would be pooled for the analyses.
> 2. A particular regression procedure (model selection stepdown) was applied individually for clinical outcomes.

3. The relative risk of all serious adverse events was comparable to the relative risk at 6 months.

If enumerated items contain further enumerations of their own, it is best to provide this information in a box or table.

Bullets without enumeration may be used for emphasis and clarity when the specific order of the items is not important. If the items are complete sentences, begin each item with a capital letter and end it with a period.

The current labeling provides the following instructions:

- Use should be limited to physicians experienced in emergency treatment of anaphylaxis.
- Initial dosage should be based on skin testing.
- The patient should be observed for at least 20 minutes after injection.
- Immunotherapy should be withheld when a β-blocker is used.

If the bulleted items are not complete sentences, no end punctuation is needed and the use of a capital or lowercase letter on the first word of each item is a matter of judgment, often determined by length (capital letters on initial letter of longer items, lowercase on initial letters of shorter items), with consistency within a single list.

Anorexia nervosa includes the following:

- Low body weight with refusal to maintain a healthy weight
- Fear of being overweight despite having an extremely low body weight
- Disturbed body image or denial of the degree of underweight
- Absence of a menstrual period

Signs and symptoms of cardiogenic shock may include

- hypotension
- cold, clammy skin
- low urine output
- confusion

19.6 Abbreviating *Number*. The word *number* may be abbreviated *No.* in the body of tables and line art or in the text when used as a specific designator. Do not use the number sign (#) in place of the abbreviation. The word *number* should always be spelled out when it is used as a proper noun (eg, "Social Security number").

	Drug	*Placebo*
No. of participants	49	48

A No. 10 catheter was placed in the femoral artery.

When referring to numbers of individuals in a study—in tables, figures, and within parentheses—the abbreviation N is used when referring to the entire sample; n refers to a subsample. (See also 20.9, Study Design and Statistics, Glossary of Statistical Terms.)

Patients were enrolled at each study site (N = 2758) and randomized to intervention (n = 1378) or placebo (n = 1380).

19.7 Forms of Numbers

19.7.1 Decimals. The decimal form should be used when a fraction is given with an abbreviated unit of measure (eg, 0.5 g, 2.7 mm) to reflect the precision of the measurement (eg, 38.0 kg should not be rounded to 38 kg if the scale was accurate to tenths of a kilogram). (See also 18.4.2, Units of Measure, Use of Numerals With Units, Decimal Format.)

The patient was receiving gentamicin sulfate, 3.5 mg/kg, every 8 hours. Her serum gentamicin level reached a peak of 5.8 μg/mL and a trough of 0.7 μg/mL after the third dose.

Place a zero before the decimal point in numbers less than 1, except when expressing the 3 values related to probability: P, α, and β. These values cannot equal 1, except when rounding (see 20.9, Study Design and Statistics, Glossary of Statistical Terms). Because they appear frequently, eliminating the zero can save substantial space in tables and text. (Although other statistical values also may never equal 1, their use is less frequent, and to simplify usage, the zero before the decimal point is included.)

$P = .16$

$1 - \beta = .80$

Our predetermined α level was .05.

But: $\kappa = 0.87$

Note, however, that α and β may sometimes be used to indicate other statistics, and in some of these cases their values may be 1 or greater.

Cronbach $\alpha = 0.78$

standardized β coefficient $= 2.34$

By convention, a zero is not used in front of the decimal point of the measure of the bore of a firearm.

.22-caliber rifle

19.7.2 Percentages. The term *percent* derives from the Latin *per centum*, meaning by the hundred, or in, to, or for every hundred. The term *percent* and the symbol % should be used with specific numbers. *Percentage* is a more general term for any number or amount that can be stated as a percent. *Percentile* is defined as the value on a scale of 100 that indicates the percentage of the distribution that is equal to or below it.

Ten percent of the work remained to be done.

Heart disease was present in a small percentage of the participants. (*But:* Five percent of the participants had heart disease.)

Her body mass index placed her in the 95th percentile of the study group.

Unless otherwise indicated, data in the table are expressed as number (percentage).

Use arabic numerals and the symbol % for specific percentages. The symbol is set closed up to the numeral and is repeated with each number in a series or range of percentages. Include the symbol % with a percentage of zero.

A 5% incidence (95% confidence interval, 1%-9%) was reported.

The prevalence in the populations studied varied from 0% to 20%.

At the beginning of a sentence, spell out both the number and the word *percent*, even if the percentage is part of a series or range. Often it is preferable to reword the sentence so that a comparison between percentages is more readily apparent.

Twenty percent to 30% of patients reported gastrointestinal symptoms.

Better: The percentage of patients who reported gastrointestinal symptoms ranged from 20% to 30%.

Or: Between 20% and 30% of the patients reported gastrointestinal symptoms.

When referring to a percentage derived from a study sample, include with the percentage the numbers from which the percentage is derived. This is particularly important when the sample size is less than 100 (see also 20.8, Study Design and Statistics, Significant Digits and Rounding Numbers). To give primacy to the original data, it is preferable to place the percentage in parentheses.

Of the 26 adverse events, 19 (73%) occurred in infants.

Any discrepancy in the sum of percentages in a tabulation (eg, due to rounding numbers, missing values, or multiple procedures) should be explained in the text, table footnote, or figure legend.

The terms *percent change, percent increase,* and *percent decrease* are often used in place of *percentage of change*. Although these less formal terms are acceptable, their usage must be precise. They generally are computed as the difference between an index value and either an earlier or later value, divided by the index value. Although a percent increase may exceed 100%, a percent decrease generally cannot. A percent decrease can also be expressed as a negative percent increase.

These terms must be differentiated from *percentage point change, increase,* or *decrease*, which are obtained by subtracting one percentage value from another. For example, a change in rate from 20% to 30% can be referred to either as an increase of 10 percentage points, as in "the intervention group improved 10 percentage points," or as a 50% increase (percent change), as in "The intervention group showed a 50% improvement" ([30%-20%]/20%). The 2 terms are *not* interchangeable. Since the percent change does not indicate the actual beginning or ending values or the magnitude of the change, the actual values should be provided whenever possible.

19.7.3 **Reporting Proportions and Percentages.** Whenever possible, proportions and percentages should be accompanied by the actual numerator (*n*) and denominator (*d*) from which they were derived. The numerator and denominator should be expressed as "*n* of *d*," not by the virgule construction "*n*/*d*," which could imply that the numbers were computed in an arithmetic operation.

Death occurred in 6 of 200 patients.

Not: Death occurred in 6/200 patients.

For clarity, when a numerator and denominator are accompanied by a resulting proportion or percentage, the proportion or percentage should not intervene between the numerator and denominator.

Death occurred in 6 of 200 patients (3%).

Death occurred in 3% (6 of 200) of patients.

Of the 200 patients, death occurred in 6 (3%).

Of the 200 patients, 6 (3%) died.

Not: Death occurred in 6 (3%) of 200 patients.

The denominator may be omitted if it is clear from the context.

Death occurred in 3 patients (1%).

In expressing a series of proportions or percentages drawn from the same sample, the denominator need be provided only once.

Of the 200 patients, 6 (3%) died, 18 (9%) experienced an adverse event, and 22 (11%) were lost to follow-up.

19.7.4 **Reporting Rates and Ratios.** Use the virgule construction for rates when placed in parentheses (eg, 1/2) but never in running text. A colon is used for ratios (eg, 1:2). Rates should use the decimal format when the denominator is understood to be 100; otherwise, the denominator should be specified.

Of all individuals exposed, children were affected at a rate of 0.05.

The infant mortality rate was 3 per 10 000 live births.
Not: The infant mortality rate was 3/10 000 live births.

19.7.5 **Roman Numerals.** Use roman numerals with proper names (eg, Henry Ford III). Note that no comma is used before the numeral. However, arabic numerals should be used as designators in all other cases (eg, round 2, Table 4, year 5; see also 10.4, Capitalization, Designators) unless roman numerals are part of formally established nomenclature (see 15.0, Nomenclature).

Step I diet

level I trauma center

schedule II drug

Axis I diagnosis

But: type 2 diabetes mellitus, phase 3 study

Use roman numerals for cancer stages and arabic numerals for cancer grades (see also 15.2, Nomenclature, Cancer). In pedigree charts, use roman numerals to indicate generations and arabic numerals to indicate families or individual family members (see also Pedigrees in 4.2.2, Visual Presentation of Data, Figures, Diagrams). Roman numerals also may be used in outline format (see 4.1, Visual Presentation of Data, Tables).

In bibliographic material (eg, references or book reviews), do not use roman numerals to indicate volume number, even though roman numerals may have been used in the original. However, if roman numerals were used in the original title or in an outline, refer to the title or outline as it was published, with roman numerals. Retain lowercase roman numerals that refer to pages in a foreword, preface, or introduction. Roman numerals may also be used to number supplements to journals, so that roman numerals appear adjacent to page numbers in references to the work. In this case, the roman numerals should be retained.

For the use of roman numerals in biblical and classical references, follow the most recent edition of the *Chicago Manual of Style* (see also 3.0, References).

The following list indicates the roman equivalents for arabic numerals. In general, roman numerals to the right of the greatest numeral are added to that numeral, and numerals to the left are subtracted. A horizontal bar over a roman numeral multiplies its value by 1000.

1	I	20	XX
2	II	30	XXX
3	III	40	XL
4	IV	50	L
5	V	60	LX
6	VI	70	LXX
7	VII	80	LXXX
8	VIII	90	XC
9	IX	100	C
10	X	200	CC
11	XI	300	CCC
12	XII	400	CD
13	XIII	500	D
14	XIV	600	DC
15	XV	700	DCC
16	XVI	800	DCCC
17	XVII	900	CM
18	XVIII	1000	M
19	XIX	5000	$\overline{\text{V}}$

ACKNOWLEDGMENT

Principal authors: Stephen J. Lurie, MD, PhD, and Margaret A. Winker, MD

REFERENCE

1. Billion bites the dust [opinion]. *Nature.* 1992;358(6381):2.

ADDITIONAL READINGS AND GENERAL REFERENCES

American Psychological Association. *Publication Manual of the American Psychological Association.* 5th ed. Washington, DC: American Psychological Association; 2001.

The Chicago Manual of Style. 15th ed. Chicago, IL: University of Chicago Press; 2003.

Style Manual Committee, Council of Science Editors. *Scientific Style and Format: The CSE Manual for Authors, Editors, and Publishers.* 7th ed. New York, NY: Rockefeller University Press, in cooperation with the Council of Science Editors, Reston, VA; 2006.

20 Study Design and Statistics

The essence of life is statistical improbability on a grand scale.

Richard Dawkins[1]

There are three kinds of lies: lies, damn lies, and statistics.

Attributed to Disraeli by Mark Twain[1]

Statistical concepts, such as the margin of error in a public opinion poll or the probability of rain or snow, appear in everyday conversation. But, just as one may understand how the heart functions and how blood circulates but not be able to perform a cardiac catheterization, an understanding of statistical concepts does not enable one to perform the work of a statistician. Although the concepts may be familiar, the tools of statistics may be misapplied and the results misinterpreted without a statistician's help.

In medical research, the quality of the statistical analysis and clarity of presentation of statistical results are critical to a study's validity. Decisions about statistical analysis are best made at the time that the study is designed and generally should not be deferred until after the data have been collected. Even the most sophisticated statistical analysis cannot salvage a fundamentally flawed study. Regardless of the statistician's role, authors (who may include statisticians) are responsible for the appropriate design, analysis, and presentation of the study's results.

Many excellent statistical texts are available, and a comprehensive approach is far beyond the scope of this chapter. However, authors, editors, and manuscript editors should have a general understanding of study designs, statistical terms and concepts, and the use of statistical tests and presentation. Although few rules exist to guide how statistics should be presented, presenting statistics briefly but completely and consistently should improve the reader's understanding of the analysis.

20.1 **The Manuscript: Presenting Study Design, Rationale, and Statistical Analysis.** Each portion of the manuscript should contribute to the reader's understanding of why and how the study was done and should help persuade the reader that (1) the hypothesis or study question is clearly stated, carefully considered, and important, (2) the methods are designed to answer the question and the analysis is appropriate, (3) the results are credible, and (4) the implications are placed in context and the limitations do not preclude interpretation of the results.

Words used herein that are defined in the glossary (see 20.9, Glossary of Statistical Terms) are given in a different font.

20.1.1 **Abstract and Introduction.** The structured abstract should enable the reader to assess the study hypothesis and methods quickly and easily.[2] The context for the study question and the hypothesis (objective) should be clearly stated (eg, "To determine whether enalapril reduces left ventricular mass . . ."), the study design and population and setting from which the sample was drawn described, and the main outcome measures explained. The results should include some explanation of effect size, if appropriate, with point estimates and confidence intervals used to describe the results. The conclusions should follow from the results without overinterpreting the data. Abstract format is too brief to permit detailed explanation of statistical analyses, but a basic description may be appropriate (eg, "The screening test was validated by means of a bootstrap procedure and performance tested with a receiver operating characteristic curve.").

The introduction should include a concise review of the relevant literature to provide a context for the study question and a rationale for the choice of a particular method. The study hypothesis or purpose should be clearly stated in the last sentence(s) before the "Methods" section. Results or conclusions do not belong in the introduction.

20.1.2 **Methods.** The "Methods" section should include enough information to enable a knowledgeable reader to replicate the study and, given the original data, verify the reported results. Components should include as many of the following as are applicable to the study design:

- Study design (see sections 20.2-20.7).
- Year(s) (and exact dates if appropriate) when the study was conducted.
- Disease or condition to be studied—how was it defined?
- Setting in which participants were studied (eg, community based, referral population, primary care clinic), as well as geographic location and, if applicable, name of institution.

- Individuals or other data studied—who or what was eligible; **inclusion** and **exclusion criteria**; if all participants were not included in each analysis, reason for exclusions; informed consent and approval by institutional review board or ethics committee when appropriate (see 5.8.1, Ethical and Legal Considerations, Protecting Research Participants' and Patients' Rights in Scientific Publication, Ethical Review of Studies and Informed Consent). If results for any of the participants have been previously described, provide citations for all reports or ensure that different reports of the same study can be easily identified (eg, by using a unique study name).

- Any remuneration or other compensation for participants.

- Intervention(s), including their length. In general, authors should provide sufficient detail to allow readers to replicate the interventions. This would also permit comparison with other studies. Treatment of any control or comparison groups should also be described in detail.

- Outcomes and how they were measured, including **reliability** of measures and whether investigators determining outcomes were **blinded** to which group received the intervention or underwent the exposure.

- Other variables and how they were measured—for example, demographic variables and risk factors for the disease. Such variables are often used to assess or adjust for **confounding** of the relationship between the **dependent** and **independent variables**.

- Preliminary analyses: if the study is a preliminary analysis of an ongoing study, the reason for publishing data before the end of the study should be clearly stated, along with information regarding whether and when the study is to be completed. Authors should indicate whether such analyses were preplanned at the time the study began.

- Source to obtain original or additional data if other than from the authors. For example, data tapes are often obtained from the US government; the source should be stated. The Web can be used to store or display data or information that could not be included in the manuscript. For information essential to the study, the information should be included in the manuscript, if at all possible. If this is not possible, the editors should request and consider retaining a copy, as Web sites and uniform resource locators (URLs) may change and become inaccessible. The source also may be listed in the acknowledgment.

- Statistical methods, including procedures used for each analysis, what α level was considered acceptable, **power** of the study (which should have been calculated before the study was conducted to determine sample size), assumptions made, any data transformations or **multiple comparisons procedures** performed, steps used for developing a model in **multivariate analysis**, and pertinent references for statistical tests and type of software used. Authors should provide evidence that the data meet the assumptions of the statistical tests used. Test statistics should include **degrees of freedom** whenever applicable. It is always preferable for results to be presented in terms of **point estimates** and **confidence intervals**, which convey more information than do ***P* values**.

- If the study has been registered in a central trial registry, the name of the registry and the trial number should be provided. (See 20.2, Randomized Controlled Trials.)

20.1.3 **Results.** The "Results" section should include the number of individuals or other data units initially eligible for study, the number at its inception, and the number who were excluded, dropped out, or were lost to follow-up at each point in the study. For example, *JAMA* requires a figure showing the flow of participants through controlled trials (see 20.2, Randomized Controlled Trials). Authors should provide descriptive statistics about the sample and, if appropriate, the individual subgroups. Primary outcome measures should be discussed after the study population is described, followed by secondary outcome measures. **Post hoc analyses** may be presented, but they should be identified as such. Results of post hoc analyses may be unreliable, and thus such analyses should be used for generating rather than testing hypotheses (see **type I error**). If one statistical test has been used throughout the manuscript, the test should be clearly stated in the "Methods" section. If more than one statistical test has been used, the statistical tests performed should be discussed in the methods and the specific test used reported along with the corresponding results. Tests of relative results (eg, **relative risk, odds ratio**) may overstate the real magnitude of differences between groups, particularly when such values are very small. Thus, when presenting relative results, authors should also report a measure of the actual **central tendency** of the groups (ie, mean or median).

20.1.4 **Discussion (Comment).** Whether the hypothesis was supported or refuted by the results should be addressed. The study result should be placed in context of published literature. The limitations of the study should be discussed, especially possible sources of **bias** and how these problems might affect conclusions and generalizability. Evidence to support or refute the problems introduced by the limitations should be provided. The implications for clinical practice, if any, and specific directions for future research may be offered. The conclusions should not go beyond the data and should be based on the study results and limited to the specific **population** represented by the study **sample**.

20.2 **Randomized Controlled Trials.** The randomized controlled trial (RCT) generally leads to the strongest inferences about the effect of medical treatments.[3] Randomized controlled trials assess efficacy of the treatment intervention in controlled, standardized, and highly monitored settings, and usually among highly selected samples of patients. Thus, their results might not reflect the effects of the treatment in real-world settings, or in other groups of individuals who were not enrolled in the trial. Information from RCTs may thus be supplemented by results of observational studies (see 20.3, Observational Studies) as well as other types of studies.

The methods of RCTs must be described in detail to allow the reader to judge the quality of the study, replicate the study intervention, and extract pertinent information for comparison with other studies. The CONSORT statement[4] provides a checklist (Table 1) to help ensure complete reporting of RCTs. *JAMA* and the *Archives* Journals require that authors complete the checklist, and the International Committee of Medical Journal Editors (ICMJE) (www.icmje.org) recommends following this reporting procedure. While completing the checklist does not guarantee that a study has been performed well, it can help ensure that the information critical to interpretation of the study is provided and accessible to editors, reviewers, and, if published, readers. Journal editors may nonetheless also ask authors to provide a more detailed description of the study protocol. Although such information may not necessarily appear in the published article, it may help reviewers and editors to more thoroughly evaluate the manuscript.

A flow diagram is also important to outline the flow of participants in the study, including when and why participants dropped out or were lost to follow-up and how many participants were evaluated for the study end points. Authors should include a flow diagram (Figure 1), and, if the manuscript is accepted for publication, the flow diagram generally should be published with the study. The number of groups after randomization shown in the diagram should correspond to the number of intervention and control groups in the study. CONSORT continues to be adapted to specific types of RCTs.[5] Current information is available from the CONSORT Web site (www.consort-statement.org).

The report should include a comparison of characteristics of the participants in the different groups in the trial, usually as a table. However, performing **significance** testing on the baseline differences between groups is controversial. (Even with perfect random assignment, an average of 1 in every 20 comparisons will be appear to be "significant" at the .05 level by chance alone; such random findings illustrate the dangers of **post hoc analyses**.) Furthermore, in small studies, large differences may nonetheless be statistically nonsignificant due to limited statistical **power**. Nonetheless, it is usually helpful for authors to report statistical comparisons between groups. Such information should be interpreted not as a test of a **null hypothesis** of baseline differences between groups, but rather as a general estimate of the magnitude of any baseline differences that may have been confounded with the intervention. These results should be reported either in a table or in running text. This information would help the reader decide whether the authors should have accounted for these baseline differences in their statistical analysis of the prespecified outcomes.

In analyzing the data from a randomized trial, it is usually best to report the results of an **intention-to-treat (ITT) analysis**. That is, the final results are based on analysis of data from all of the participants who were originally randomized, whether or not they actually completed the trial. Such participants may have varying degrees of missing data, however, and thus ITT analyses usually involve some method for **imputation** of these missing results. For noninferiority and equivalence trials, however, ITT analysis may overstate the equivalence of experimental conditions. In these trial designs, results should also be reported only for those participants who completed the trial (as-treated analysis, completers' analysis, etc). (See 20.2.3, Randomized Controlled Trials, Equivalence and Noninferiority Trials.)

There is ongoing debate about the circumstances in which it may be unethical to perform an RCT.[6,7] There is general agreement, however, that RCTs are unethical if the intervention is already known to be superior to the control in the population under investigation, or if participants could be unduly harmed by any condition in the experiment.

The decision to perform specific interim analyses is usually made before the study begins.[8(pp130,258)] (Data and safety monitoring boards, however, may monitor adverse events continually throughout the course of the study.) Investigators also usually define prospective **stopping rules** for such analyses; if the stopping rule is met, this generally means that collection of additional data would not change the interpretation of the study. If the criteria for the stopping rules have not been met, the

Table 1. Checklist of Items to Include When Reporting a Randomized Trial[a]

Section and Topic	Item No.	Descriptor	Reported on Page No.
Title and abstract	1	How participants were allocated to interventions (eg, "random allocation," "randomized," or "randomly assigned").	
Introduction Background	2	Scientific background and explanation of rationale.	
Methods Participants	3	Eligibility criteria for participants and the settings and locations where the data were collected.	
Interventions	4	Precise details of the interventions intended for each group and how and when they were actually administered.	
Objectives	5	Specific objectives and hypotheses.	
Outcomes	6	Clearly defined primary and secondary outcome measures and, when applicable, any methods used to enhance the quality of measurements (eg, multiple observations, training of assessors).	
Sample size	7	How sample size was determined and, when applicable, explanation of any interim analyses and stopping rules.	
Randomization Sequence generation	8	Method used to generate the random allocation sequence, including details of any restriction (eg, blocking, stratification).	
Allocation concealment	9	Method used to implement the random allocation sequence (eg, numbered containers or central telephone), clarifying whether the sequence was concealed until interventions were assigned.	
Implementation	10	Who generated the allocation sequence, who enrolled participants, and who assigned participants to their groups.	
Blinding (masking)	11	Whether or not participants, those administering the interventions, and those assessing the outcomes were blinded to group assignment. If done, how the success of blinding was evaluated.	
Statistical methods	12	Statistical methods used to compare groups for primary outcome(s); methods for additional analyses, such as subgroup analyses and adjusted analyses.	
Results Participant flow	13	Flow of participants through each stage (a diagram is strongly recommended). Specifically, for each group report the numbers of participants randomly assigned, receiving intended treatment, completing the study protocol, and analyzed for the primary outcome. Describe protocol deviations from study as planned, together with reasons.	
Recruitment	14	Dates defining the periods of recruitment and follow-up.	
Baseline data	15	Baseline demographic and clinical characteristics of each group.	
Numbers analyzed	16	Number of participants (denominator) in each group included in each analysis and whether the analysis was by "intention-to-treat." State the results in absolute numbers when feasible (eg, 10 of 20, not 50%).	

Table 1. Checklist of Items to Include When Reporting a Randomized Trial[a] (*cont*)

Section and Topic	Item No.	Descriptor	Reported on Page No.
Outcomes and estimation	17	For each primary and secondary outcome, a summary of results for each group, and the estimated effect size and its precision (eg, 95% confidence interval).	
Ancillary analyses	18	Address multiplicity by reporting any other analyses performed, including subgroup analyses and adjusted analyses, indicating those prespecified and those exploratory.	
Adverse events	19	All important adverse events or side effects in each intervention group.	
Comment Interpretation	20	Interpretation of the results, taking into account study hypotheses, sources of potential bias or imprecision, and the dangers associated with multiplicity of analyses and outcomes.	
Generalizability	21	Generalizability (external validity) of the trial findings.	
Overall evidence	22	General interpretation of the results in the context of current evidence.	

[a] From Moher et al.[4]

results of interim analyses should not be reported unless the treatment has important adverse effects and reporting is necessary for patient safety. If a report is an interim analysis, this should be clearly stated in the manuscript with the reason for reporting the interim results. The plans for interim analyses and reports contained in the original study protocol should be described and, if the interim analysis deviates from those plans, the reasons for the change should be justified. If a manuscript reports the final results of a study for which an interim analysis was previously published, the reason for publishing both reports should be stated and the interim analysis referenced.

Publication bias is the tendency of authors to submit and journals to preferentially publish studies with statistically significant results (see also 20.4, Meta-analysis). To address the problem of publication bias, the ICMJE now requires, as a condition of publication, that a clinical trial be registered in a public trials registry.[9] The ICMJE policy applies to any clinical trial starting enrollment after July 1, 2005. For trials that began enrollment prior to this date, the ICMJE member journals required registration by September 13, 2005. The policy defines a clinical trial as "any research project that prospectively assigns human subjects to intervention or comparison groups to study the cause-and-effect relationship between a medical intervention and a health outcome."

20.2.1 Parallel-Design Double-blind Trials. In this study design, participants are assigned to only 1 treatment group of the study. These trials are generally designed to assess whether 1 or more treatments are superior to the others. Participants and those administering the intervention should all be unaware of which intervention individual participants are receiving ("double-blinding"). Ideally, those rating the outcomes should also be blinded to treatment assignment ("triple-blinding"). Blinded

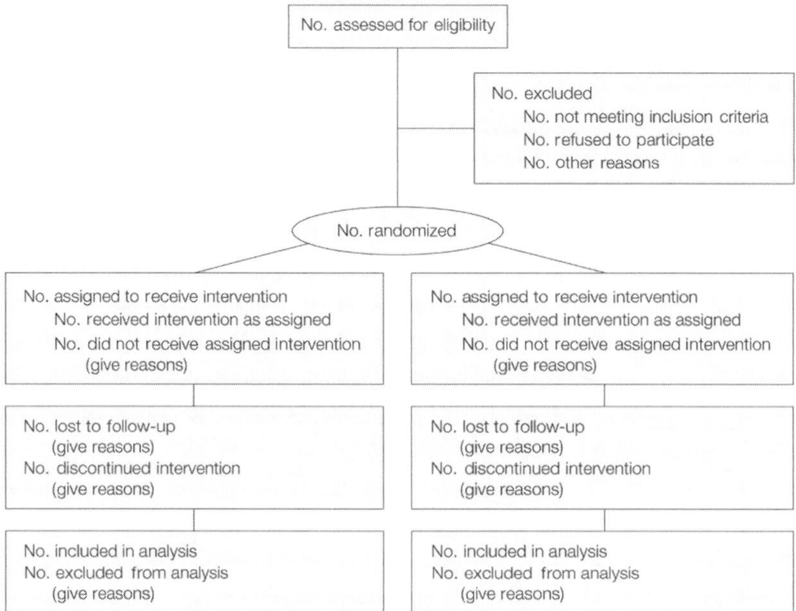

Figure 1. CONSORT flow diagram showing the progress of patients throughout the trial. From Instructions for Authors. *JAMA.* 2006;296(1):107-115.

parallel-design trials are often the optimal design to compare 2 or more types of drug or other therapy, since known and unknown potentially confounding factors should be randomly distributed between intervention and control groups. The CONSORT diagram should clearly indicate how many participants were assigned to each treatment group, how many were lost at various stages of the trial, and the reasons that individuals did not complete the trial. Methods of randomization, allocation concealment, and assessment of the success of blinding should be reported. If there is no significant difference between groups, authors cannot claim that the treatments are equivalent; such a conclusion would require an equivalence or noninferiority trial (see 20.2.3, Randomized Controlled Trials, Equivalence and Noninferiority Trials).

20.2.2 **Crossover Trials.** In a crossover trial, participants receive more than 1 of the treatments under investigation, usually in a randomly determined sequence, and with a prespecified amount of time (a **"washout period"**) between sequential treatments. The participants and the investigators are generally **blinded** to the treatment assignment (double-blinded). This experimental design is often used for evaluating drug treatments. Each participant serves as his or her own control, thereby eliminating variability when comparing treatment effects and reducing the sample size needed to detect a **significant** effect. Most considerations of parallel-design randomized trials apply. Rather than indicating which participants were assigned to which condition, the CONSORT flow diagram should indicate how many were assigned to each sequence of conditions. Other information important to this study design includes possible carryover effects (ie, effect of intervention persists after completion of the intervention) and length of **washout period** (intervention effects should have ended completely before crossover to the other treatment). If the actual period of crossover differs from the original study protocol, how and why decisions were made to cross over to the alternate treatment and when the crossover occurred should be stated. The treatment sequence should be randomized to ensure that investigators remain blinded and that no systematic differences arise because of treatment order. Otherwise, unblinding is likely, treatment order may confound the analysis, and carryover effects will be more difficult to assess. The amount of time between each intervention (the washout period) should also be prespecified. If carryover effects are significant, or if a washout period with no treatment is undesirable or unethical, a parallel-group design (possibly with a larger sample size) may be necessary.

20.2.3 **Equivalence and Noninferiority Trials.** It is sometimes desirable to compare a less expensive treatment or intervention against a treatment or intervention that is already known to be effective. In these cases, it would be unethical to expose participants to an inactive placebo. Thus, these trial designs assess whether the treatment or intervention under study (the "new intervention") is no worse than an existing alternative (the "active control").

In equivalence and noninferiority trials, authors must prespecify a margin of noninferiority (Δ), within which the new intervention can be assumed to be no worse than the active control. There are a number of methods for arriving at the value Δ. Because different methods of estimating Δ may be more defensible in some situations than others, authors should provide clear explanations of their method and rationale for arriving at their value for Δ. Noninferiority trials test the 1-sided hypothesis that the effect of the new intervention is no more than Δ units less than the active control. Equivalence trials, which are less common than noninferiority trials, test the 2-sided hypothesis that the effect of the new treatment lies within the range of Δ to $-\Delta$.

Although use of intention-to-treat (ITT) analysis is optimal in trials that test whether one treatment is superior to another, use of such analysis can bias the results of equivalence and noninferiority trials. Thus, in addition to ITT analysis, authors should report results for only participants who completed the trial.

Interpretation of the results depends on the confidence interval for the difference between the new intervention and the active placebo, and whether this confidence interval crosses Δ, $-\Delta$, and 0. See Table 2.

Authors should refer to specific CONSORT guidelines for reporting the design and results of equivalence and noninferiority trials.[10]

20.3 **Observational Studies.** In an observational study, the researcher identifies a condition or outcome of interest and then measures factors that may be related to that outcome. Although observational studies cannot lead to strong causal inferences, they may nonetheless suggest certain causal hypotheses. To infer causation in observational studies, investigators attempt to establish a sequence of events—if event A generally precedes event B in time, then it is possible that A may be responsible for causing B. Such studies may be either retrospective (the investigator tries to reconstruct what happened in the past) or prospective (the investigator identifies a group of individuals and then observes them for a specified period of time). Prospective studies generally yield more reliable conclusions than do retrospective studies.

Cross-sectional studies observe individuals at a single point in time. Such studies may be helpful for suggesting relationships among variables but cannot address whether one condition may precede or follow another. Thus, cross-sectional studies

Table 2. Checklist of Items for Reporting Noninferiority or Equivalence Trials (Additions or Modifications to the CONSORT Checklist Are Indicated in Footnotes)[a]

Paper Section and Topic	Item No.	Noninferiority or Equivalence Trials
Title and abstract	1[b]	How participants were allocated to interventions (eg, "random allocation," "randomized," or "randomly assigned"), specifying that the trial is a noninferiority or equivalence trial.
Introduction Background	2[b]	Scientific background and explanation of rationale, including the rationale for using a noninferiority or equivalence design.
Methods Participants	3[b]	Eligibility criteria for participants (details whether participants in the noninferiority or equivalence trial are similar to those in any trial(s) that established efficacy of the reference treatment) and the settings and locations where the data were collected.
Interventions	4[b]	Precise details of the intervention intended for each group, detailing whether the reference treatment in the noninferiority or equivalence trial are identical (or very similar) to that in any trial(s) that established efficacy, and how and when they were actually administered.
Objectives	5[b]	Specific objective and hypotheses, including the hypothesis concerning noninferiority or equivalence.
Outcomes	6[b]	Clearly defined primary and secondary outcome measures, detailing whether the outcomes in the noninferiority or equivalence trial are identical (or very similar) to those in any trial(s) that established efficacy of the reference treatment and, when applicable, any methods used to enhance the quality of measurements (eg, multiple observations, training of assessors).
Sample size	7[b]	How sample size was determined, detailing whether it was calculated using a noninferiority or equivalence criterion and specifying the margin of equivalence with the rationale for its choice. When applicable, explanation of any interim analysis and stopping rules (and whether related to a noninferiority or equivalence hypothesis).
Randomization Sequence generation	8	Method used to generate the random allocation sequence, including details of any restriction (eg, blocking, stratification).
Allocation concealment	9	Method used to implement the random allocation sequence (eg, numbered containers or central telephone), clarifying whether the sequence was concealed until interventions were assigned.
Implementation	10	Who generated the allocation sequence, who enrolled participants, and who assigned participants to their groups.
Blinding (masking)	11	Whether or not participants, those administering the interventions, and those assessing the outcomes were blinded to group assignment. When relevant, how the success of blinding was evaluated.
Statistical methods	12[b]	Statistical methods used to compare groups for primary outcome(s), specifying whether a 1- or 2-sided confidence interval approach was used. Methods for additional analyses, such as subgroup analyses and adjusted analyses.

Table 2. Checklist of Items for Reporting Noninferiority or Equivalence Trials (Additions or Modifications to the CONSORT Checklist Are Indicated in Footnotes)[a] (*cont*)

Paper Section and Topic	Item No.	Noninferiority or Equivalence Trials
Results Participant flow	13	Flow of participants through each stage (a diagram is strongly recommended). Specifically, for each group report the numbers of participants randomly assigned, receiving intended treatment, completing the trial protocol, and analyzed for the primary outcome. Describe protocol deviations from trial as planned, together with reasons.
Recruitment	14	Dates defining the periods of recruitment and follow-up.
Baseline data	15	Baseline demographic and clinical characteristics of each group.
Numbers analyzed	16[a]	Number of participants (denominator) in each group included in each analysis and whether "intention-to-treat" and/or alternative analyses were conducted. State the results in absolute numbers when feasible (eg, 10 of 20, not 50%).
Outcomes and estimation	17[a]	For each primary and secondary outcome, a summary of results for each group and the estimated effect size and its precision (eg, 95% confidence interval). For the outcome(s) for which noninferiority or equivalence is hypothesized, a figure showing confidence intervals and margins of equivalence may be useful.
Ancillary analyses	18	Address multiplicity by reporting any other analyses performed, including subgroup analyses and adjusted analyses, indicating those prespecified and those exploratory.
Adverse events	19	All important adverse events or side effects in each intervention group.
Comment Interpretation	20[a]	Interpretation of the results, taking into account the noninferiority or equivalence hypothesis and any other trial hypotheses, sources of potential bias or imprecision, and the dangers associated with multiplicity of analyses and outcomes.
Generalizability	21	Generalizability (external validity) of the trial findings.
Overall evidence	22	General interpretation of the results in the context of current evidence.

[a] From Piaggio et al.[10]
[b] Expansion of corresponding item on CONSORT checklist.[4,11]

cannot establish **causation**, but they may nonetheless be helpful for suggesting hypotheses to guide more rigorous studies.

Because individuals in observational studies are not randomly assigned to conditions, there are often large baseline differences between groups in such studies. For instance, individuals with better exercise habits often differ in a number of important ways (eg, education, income, diet, smoking) from those who do not exercise regularly. Because exercise is **confounded** with these variables, it is difficult to know whether exercise itself is responsible for any differences in health outcomes. Researchers may use several different statistical techniques to minimize the effects of confounding, including **matching**, **stratification**, **multivariate analysis**, and **propensity analysis**.

Even with the most extensive attempts to minimize confounding, it is always possible that results of observational studies may in fact be due to other variables that the authors did not measure. Because of this unavoidable possibility of **residual confounding** in observational studies, the results are generally not as reliable as those of RCTs. Sometimes the results of observational studies may differ significantly from those of RCTs.[12] On the other hand, because observational studies are more often based on the outcomes of a large range of people in realistic situations, they may add useful insights to disease processes as they occur beyond the limited conditions of RCTs. Furthermore, observational studies may be the only way to investigate certain problems (eg, automobile crashes, exposure to toxic chemicals) for which it would be unethical to perform RCTs.

There are currently no standardized guidelines for reporting the various types of observational studies. Although the CONSORT group is currently developing such guidelines for case-control and cohort studies, it is unclear at this time whether they will become as widely accepted as the CONSORT guidelines for RCTs. Current information can be found on the CONSORT Web site (www.consort-statement.org).

20.3.1 **Cohort Studies.** A prospective cohort study follows a group or **cohort** of individuals who are initially free of the outcome of interest. Individuals in a cohort generally share some underlying characteristic, such as age, sex, or exposure to a **risk factor**. Some studies may comprise several different cohorts. The study is usually conducted for a predetermined period, long enough for some members of the cohort to develop the outcome of interest. Individuals who developed the outcome are compared with those who did not. The report of the study should include a description of the cohort and the length of follow-up, what **independent variables** were measured and how, and what outcomes were measured and how. The number of individuals unavailable for follow-up and whether they differed from those with complete follow-up should also be included. All adverse events should be reported.

Any previous published reports of closely related studies from the same cohort should be cited in the text or should be clear from the study name (eg, the Framingham Study). All previous reports on the same or similar outcomes should be cited.

Retrospective cohort studies may be appropriate if investigators are blinded to study outcomes when formulating the **hypothesis** and determining the **dependent** and **independent variables**, but many of the strengths of prospective cohort studies are lost with retrospective studies, such as identifying the population to study and defining the variables and outcomes before the events occur.

20.3.2 **Case-Control Studies.** Case-control studies, which are always retrospective, compare those who have had an outcome or event (**cases**) with those who have not (**controls**). Cases and controls are then evaluated for exposure to various **risk factors** and thus should never be selected on the basis of their exposure to the risk factors under investigation. Cases and controls generally are matched according to specific characteristics (eg, age, sex, or duration of disease) to reduce **confounding** by these variables. However, if the matched variables are inextricably linked with the exposure of interest (not necessarily with the disease or outcome of interest), matching may confound the analysis (see also **overmatching**). The **independent variable** is exposure to an item of interest (eg, a drug or disease). Information about the source of both cases and controls must be included, and **inclusion** and **exclusion criteria** must be listed for each. Cases and controls should be drawn from the same or similar **populations** to avoid **selection bias**. Pairs (1:1 match) or groups (eg, 1:2 or 1:3 match) of cases and controls may be matched on 1 or more variables. The analysis generally is unpaired, however, because of the difficulty in matching every important characteristic. Nonetheless, paired analysis reduces the necessary sample size to detect a difference and may be justified if individuals are well matched. **Recall bias** is common in all retrospective studies and is especially a concern when participants believe that a factor related to the independent variable may be associated with the outcome. If recall bias may have occurred, the authors should discuss how they addressed this possibility.

In a nested case-control study, the cases and controls are drawn from some larger population or **cohort** that may have been convened for some other purpose. In these instances, authors should clearly indicate how the original sample was defined, the size of the original sample, and how the cases and controls were selected from it.

20.3.3 Case Series.

A case series describes characteristics of a group of patients with a particular disease or patients who have undergone a particular procedure. A case series may also involve observation of larger units such as groups of hospitals or municipalities, as well as smaller units such as laboratory samples. Case series may be used to formulate a case definition of a disease or describe the experience of an individual or institution in treating a disease or performing a type of procedure. Case series should comprise consecutive patients or observations seen by the individual or institution to minimize **selection bias**. A case series is not used to test a hypothesis because there is no comparison group. (Occasionally comparisons are made with historical controls or published studies, but these comparisons are informal and should not include formal statistical analysis.) A report of a case series should include the rationale for publishing the population description and inclusion and exclusion criteria. Case series are subject to several types of **biases**, and therefore authors should be particularly careful about the kinds of conclusions that can be drawn from them.

20.4 Meta-analysis.

Meta-analysis is a systematic pooling of the results of 2 or more studies to address a question of interest or hypothesis. According to Moher and Olkin,[13]

> [Meta-analyses] provide a systematic and explicit method for synthesizing evidence, a quantitative overall estimate (and confidence intervals) derived from the individual studies, and early evidence as to the effectiveness of treatments, thus reducing the need for continued study. They also can address questions in specific subgroups that individual studies may not have examined.

A meta-analysis quantitatively summarizes the evidence regarding a treatment, procedure, or association. It is a more statistically powerful test of the null hypothesis than is provided by the separate studies themselves because the sample size is substantially larger than those in the individual studies. However, a number of issues make meta-analysis a much-debated form of analysis.[14-19] To help standardize the presentation of meta-analysis, *JAMA* recommends use of the QUOROM flow diagram and checklist (http://www.consort-statement.org/QUOROM.pdf) for reporting meta-analyses of RCTs, and the MOOSE checklist (http://www.consort-statement.org/Initiatives/MOOSE/moose.pdf) for reporting meta-analyses of observational studies.

To ensure that the meta-analysis accurately reflects the available evidence, the methods of identifying possible studies for inclusion should be explicitly stated (eg, literature search, reference search, and contacting authors regarding other or unpublished work). Authors should state the dates that their search covered and the search terms used. A search strategy that includes several approaches to identify articles is preferable to a single database search.[20] Authors should make all attempts to include results of non-English-language articles.

Publication bias, or the tendency of authors and journals to publish articles with positive results, is a potential limitation of any systematic review of the literature.[21] Unpublished studies may be included in a meta-analyses if they meet predefined inclusion criteria. One approach to addressing whether publication bias might affect the result is to define the number of negative studies that would be needed to change the results of a meta-analysis from positive to negative. Authors may also provide **funnel plots**.

To address the problem of publication bias, the ICMJE now requires, as a condition of publication, that a clinical trial be registered in a public trials registry.[9] The ICMJE policy applies to any clinical trial starting enrollment after July 1, 2005. For trials that began enrollment prior to this date, the ICMJE member journals required registration by September 13, 2005. The policy defines a clinical trial as "any research project that prospectively assigns human subjects to intervention or comparison groups to study the cause-and-effect relationship between a medical intervention and a health outcome."

Other controversial issues include which study designs are acceptable for inclusion, whether and how studies should be rated for quality,[22] and whether and how to combine results from studies with disparate study characteristics. While few would disagree that meta-analysis of RCTs is most appropriate when possible, many topics include too few randomized trials to permit meta-analysis or cannot be studied in a trial.

Gerbarg and Horwitz[23] have suggested that criteria for combining studies should be similar to those for multicenter trials and should include similar prognostic factors, which would justify combining them. Whether studies can be appropriately combined can be determined statistically by analyzing the degree of **heterogeneity** (ie, the variability in outcomes across studies). Assessment of heterogeneity includes examining the **effect size**, the sample size in each group, and whether the effect sizes from different studies are homogeneous. If statistically significant heterogeneity is found, then combining the studies into a single analysis may not be valid.[24] Another concern is the influence a small number of large trials may have on the results; large trials in a small pool of studies can dominate the analysis, and the meta-analysis may reflect little more than the individual large trial. In such cases, it may be appropriate to perform **sensitivity analyses** comparing results with and without inclusion of the large trial(s).

Meta-analyses are often analyzed by means of both **fixed-effects** and **random-effects models** to determine how different assumptions affect the results. An example of how results of a meta-analysis may be depicted graphically is shown in 4.2.2, Visual Presentation of Data, Figures, Diagrams (Example F13). The more conservative random-effects model is generally preferred.

A meta-analysis is useful only as long as it reflects current literature. Thus, a concern of meta-analysts and clinicians is that the meta-analyses should be updated as new studies are published. One international effort, the Cochrane Collaboration, publishes and frequently updates a large number of systematic reviews and meta-analyses on a variety of topics.[25]

20.5 Cost-effectiveness Analysis, Cost-Benefit Analysis. Although a treatment or screening technique may be shown to be effective in an RCT, recommending it in general practice would not necessarily be rational. Such interventions may be prohibitively expensive, or they may benefit only a small number of people at the expense of a large number of people, or they may lead to significant "downstream" costs that would eventually negate any immediate savings or benefit. Thus, it is possible that interventions that appear less effective may actually lead to the greatest societal benefits over the long term.

Cost-effectiveness and cost-benefit analyses comprise a set of mathematical techniques to model these complex consequences of medical interventions. Cost-effectiveness analysis "compares the net monetary costs of a health care intervention with some measure of clinical outcome or effectiveness such as mortality rates or life-years saved."[26] Cost-benefit analysis is similar but converts clinical measures of outcomes into monetary units, allowing both costs and benefits to be expressed on a single scale. This use of a common metric thus enables comparisons between different treatment or screening strategies.

The results of a cost-effectiveness analysis are usually expressed in terms of a cost-effectiveness ratio, for example, the cost per year of life gained. The use of **quality-adjusted life-years (QALYs)** or **disability-adjusted life-years (DALYs)** permits direct comparison of different types of interventions using the same measure for outcomes. The use of such composite measures allows researchers to weigh the relative benefits of length and quality of life.

The complexity of these analyses and the many decisions required when selecting data and choosing assumptions may be of particular concern when the analysis is performed by an investigator or company with financial interest in the treatment being evaluated.[27] Such analyses may have biases that are difficult to detect even with the most rigorous peer review process.[28]

One approach frequently used by cost-effectiveness analysts is to define a base case that represents the choices to be considered, perform an analysis for the base case, and then perform **sensitivity analyses** to determine how varying the data used and assumptions made for the base case affects the results. Sometimes authors test their conclusions by performing **bootstrap** or **jackknife** analyses. This involves taking a very large number of repeated random samples from the data and then observing whether this procedure generally replicates the previous analytic conclusions. A number of journals have published guidelines and approaches to cost-effectiveness analysis, but consensus has yet to emerge on their reporting[29-32] or interpretation.[33] Nonetheless, authors should clearly indicate all sources of data for both treatment effects and costs. Graphical approaches may help readers better understand the basic conclusions of the analysis.[34] *JAMA* requires authors of cost-effectiveness analyses and decision analyses to submit a copy of the decision tree comprising their model. Although this need not necessarily be included in the body of the published article, such information is necessary for reviewers and editors to assess the details of the model and its analysis.

20.6 Studies of Diagnostic Tests. Correct treatment depends on accurate diagnosis. Diagnostic tests may include simple procedures such as physical signs or physical examination, as well as blood tests and radiologic imaging. Few diagnostic tests, however, can be relied on to yield accurate diagnoses 100% of the time. Thus, it is important to study the performance of diagnostic tests. Bossuyt et al[35] stated:

> Exaggerated and biased results from poorly designed and reported diagnostic studies can trigger their premature dissemination and lead physicians into making incorrect treatment decisions. A rigorous evaluation process of diagnostic tests before introduction into clinical practice could not only reduce the number of unwanted clinical consequences related to misleading estimates of test accuracy, but also limit health care costs by preventing unnecessary testing.

Studies to determine the diagnostic accuracy of a test are a vital part in this evaluation process. *JAMA* recommends that authors use the Standards for Reporting of Diagnostic Accuracy (STARD) checklist in reporting such analyses (www.consort-statement.org/Initiatives/newstand.htm).

Studies of diagnostic tests generally yield estimates of **likelihood ratios**, **sensitivity**, **specificity**, **positive predictive values**, and **negative predictive values**. Authors should report **confidence intervals** associated with these statistics. It is also common for these studies to report **receiver operating characteristic curves**.

20.7 Survey Studies. In a survey study, a representative sample of individuals are asked to describe their opinions, attitudes, or behaviors. For surveys of behavior (eg, diet, exercise, smoking), authors should provide evidence that the survey instrument correlates with the actual, observed behaviors of a similar sample of individuals. That is, the survey instrument should have been shown to have **validity**. If the survey instrument is different in any way from that given to the previous validation sample (eg, wording, order, or omission of questions), then it may no longer be a valid measure of those behaviors.

For surveys, as for other studies, it is critical to describe explicit inclusion and exclusion criteria, as well as how and when individuals left the study once they were initially identified. Flow diagrams can be a useful way of presenting this information. There is currently no standard reporting format for survey studies, however, and authors have usually reported no more than a single **response rate** for their survey. To address this situation, the American Association for Public Opinion Research (AAPOR) has published a set of expanded definitions.[36] The AAPOR document defines response rate as "the number of complete interviews with reporting units divided by the number of eligible reporting units in the sample." The document points out that this general definition allows for at least 6 different ways of actually computing this statistic, depending on how the numbers of "complete interviews" and the "number of eligible reporting units" are defined. The document goes on to define 4 possible equations for cooperation rates (the proportion of all cases interviewed of all eligible units ever contacted), 3 equations for refusal rates (the proportion of all cases in which a housing unit or respondent refuses to do an interview), and 3 equations for contact rates (the proportion of all cases in which some responsible member of the housing unit was reached by the survey). Thus, authors should be clear about how they assigned individuals to categories and which categories they used to compute these statistics.

The AAPOR document defines specific reporting procedures for the 3 most common survey designs: random-digit-dial telephone surveys, in-person surveys, and mail surveys. Future updates of the AAPOR document will discuss Internet-based surveys. As with observational studies, meta-analyses, and cost-benefit studies, there are currently no universally agreed-upon reporting criteria for survey studies.

Survey studies may be either longitudinal (the same respondents are surveyed at several time points) or cross-sectional. Causality may be cautiously inferred from longitudinal surveys, but never from cross-sectional surveys. Case-control studies (see 20.3.2) and cohort studies (see 20.3.1) may exclusively use survey methodology to obtain their **dependent variables**, and thus in practice the distinction between observational studies and survey studies may be nuanced.

20.8 **Significant Digits and Rounding Numbers.** When numbers are expressed in scientific and biomedical articles, they should reflect the degree of accuracy of the original measurement. Numbers obtained from mathematical calculations should be rounded to reflect the original degree of precision.

20.8.1 **Significant Digits.** The use of a numeral in a numbers column (eg, the ones column) implies that the method of measurement is accurate to that level of precision. For example, when a reporter attempts to estimate the size of a crowd, the estimate might be to the nearest tens of number of people, but would not be expressed as an exact number, such as 86, unless each individual was counted. Similarly, when an author provides a number with numerals to the right of the decimal point, the numerals imply that the measurement used to obtain the number is accurate to the last place a numeral is shown. Therefore, numbers should be rounded to reflect the precision of the instrument or measurement; for example, for a scale accurate to 0.1 kg, a weight should be expressed as 75.2 kg, not 75.23 kg. Similarly, the instrument used to measure a concentration is accurate only to a given fraction of the concentration, for example, 15.6 mg/L, not 15.638 mg/L (see Table 2 in 18.5.10, Units of Measure, Conventional Units and SI Units in *JAMA* and the *Archives* Journals, Laboratory Values, for the appropriate number of significant digits). Numbers that result from calculations, such as means and SDs, should be expressed to no more than 1 significant digit beyond the accuracy of the instrument. Thus, the mean (SD) of weights of individuals weighed on a scale accurate to 0.1 kg should be expressed as 62.45 (4.13) kg. Adult age is reported rounded to 1-year increments, so the mean could be expressed as, for example, 47.7 years.

20.8.2 **Rounding.** The digits to the right of the last significant digit are rounded up or down. If the digit to the right of the last significant digit is less than 5, the last significant digit is not changed. If the digit is greater than 5, the last significant digit is rounded up to the next higher digit. (For example, 47.746 years is rounded to 47.7 years and 47.763 years is rounded to 47.8 years.) If the digit immediately to the right of the last significant digit is 5, with either no digits or all zeros after the 5, the last significant digit is rounded up if it is odd and not changed if it is even. (For example, 47.7500 would become 47.8; 47.65 would become 47.6.) If the digit to the right of the last significant digit is 5 followed by any number other than 0, the last significant digit is rounded up (47.6501 would become 47.7).

P values and other statistical expressions raise particular issues about rounding. For more information about how and why to round *P* values and other statistical terms, see ***P* value** in 20.9, Glossary of Statistical Terms. Briefly, *P* values should be expressed to 2 digits to the right of the decimal point (regardless of whether the *P* value is significant), unless $P < .01$, in which case the *P* value should be expressed to

Table 3. Selection of Commonly Used Statistical Techniques[a]

	Scale of Measurement		
	Interval[b]	**Ordinal**	**Nominal**[c]
2 Treatment groups	Unpaired *t* test	Mann-Whitney rank sum test	χ^2 Analysis-of-contingency table; Fisher exact test if ≤6 in any cell
≥3 Treatment groups	Analysis of variance	Kruskal-Wallis statistic	χ^2 Analysis-of-contingency table; Fisher exact test if ≤6 in any cell
Before and after 1 treatment in same individual	Paired *t* test	Wilcoxon signed rank test	McNemar test
Multiple treatments in same individual	Repeated-measures analysis of variance	Friedman statistic	Cochran *Q*
Association between 2 variables	Linear regression and Pearson product moment correlation	Spearman rank correlation	Contingency coefficients

[a] Adapted with permission from Glantz, *Primer of Biostatistics.*[39] © The McGraw-Hill Companies, Inc.

[b] Assumes normally distributed data. If data are not normally distributed, then rank the observations and use the methods for data measured on an ordinal scale.

[c] For a nominal dependent variable that is time dependent (such as mortality over time), use life-table analysis for nominal independent variables and Cox regression for continuous and/or nominal independent variables.

3 digits to the right of the decimal point. (One exception to this rule is when rounding *P* from 3 digits to 2 digits would result in *P* appearing nonsignificant, such as $P = .046$. In this case, expressing the *P* value to 3 places may be preferred by the author. The same holds true for rounding confidence intervals that are significant before rounding but nonsignificant after rounding.) The smallest *P* value that should be expressed is $P < .001$, since additional zeros do not convey useful information.[37]

P values should never be rounded up to 1.0 or down to 0. While such a procedure might be justified arithmetically, the results are misleading. Statistical inference is based on the assumption that events occur in a probabilistic, rather than deterministic, universe. *P* values may approach infinitely close to these upper and lower bounds, but never close enough to establish that the associated observation was either absolutely predestined ($P = 1.0$) or absolutely impossible ($P = 0$) to occur. Thus, very large and very small *P* values should always be expressed as $P > .99$ and $P < .001$, respectively.

20.9 Glossary of Statistical Terms.

Glossary of Statistical Terms. In the glossary that follows, terms defined elsewhere in the glossary are printed in **this font**. An arrowhead (➔) indicates points to consider in addition to the definition. For detailed discussion of these terms, the referenced texts and the resource list at the end of the chapter are useful sources.

Eponymous names for statistical procedures often differ from one text to another (eg, the Newman-Keuls and Student-Newman-Keuls test). The names provided in this glossary follow the *Dictionary of Statistical Terms*[38] published for the International Statistical Institute. Although statistical texts use the possessive form for most eponyms, the possessive form for eponyms is not used in *JAMA* and the *Archives* Journals (see 16.0, Eponyms).

Most statistical tests are applicable only under specific circumstances, which are generally dictated by the scale properties of both the independent variable and the dependent variable. Table 3 presents a guide to selection of commonly used statistical techniques. This table is not meant to be exhaustive but rather to indicate the appropriate applications of commonly used statistical techniques.

abscissa: horizontal or **x-axis** of a graph.

absolute risk: probability of an event occurring during a specified period. The absolute risk equals the **relative risk** times the average probability of the event during the same time, if the **risk factor** is absent.[40(p327)] See **absolute risk reduction**.

absolute risk reduction: proportion in the control group experiencing an event minus the proportion in the intervention group experiencing an event. The inverse of the absolute risk reduction is the **number needed to treat**. See **absolute risk**.

accuracy: ability of a test to produce results that are close to the true measure of the phenomenon.[40(p327)] Generally, assessing accuracy of a test requires that there be a **criterion standard** with which to compare the test results. Accuracy encompasses a number of measures including **reliability, validity**, and lack of **bias**.

actuarial life-table method: see **life table, Cutler-Ederer method**.

adjustment: statistical techniques used after the collection of data to adjust for the effect of known or potential **confounding variables**.[40(p327)] A typical example is adjusting a result for the independent effect of age of the participants (age is the **independent variable**).

aggregate data: data accumulated from disparate sources.

agreement: statistical test performed to determine the equivalence of the results obtained by 2 tests when one test is compared with another (one of which is usually but not always a **criterion standard**).

➔ Agreement should not be confused with **correlation**. Correlation is used to test the degree to which changes in a variable are related to changes in another, whereas agreement tests whether 2 variables are equivalent. For example, an investigator compares results obtained by 2 methods of measuring hematocrit. Method A gives a result that is always exactly twice that of method B. The correlation between A and B is perfect since A is always twice B, but the agreement is very poor; method A is not equivalent to method B (written communication, George W. Brown, MD, September 1993). One appropriate way to assess agreement has been described by Bland and Altman.[41]

algorithm: systematic process carried out in an ordered, typically branching sequence of steps; each step depends on the outcome of the previous step.[42(p6)] An algorithm may be used clinically to guide treatment decisions for an individual patient on the basis of the patient's clinical outcome or result.

α (alpha), α level: size of the likelihood acceptable to the investigators that a relationship observed between 2 variables is due to chance (the probability of a **type I error**); usually $\alpha = .05$. If $\alpha = .05$, $P < .05$ will be considered significant.

analysis: process of mathematically summarizing and comparing data to confirm or refute a **hypothesis**. Analysis serves 3 functions: (1) to test hypotheses regarding differences in large **populations** based on samples of the populations, (2) to control for confounding variables, and (3) to measure the size of differences between groups or the strength of the relationship between variables in the study.[40(p25)]

analysis of covariance (ANCOVA): statistical test used to examine data that include both **continuous** and **nominal independent variables** and a continuous **dependent variable**. It is basically a hybrid of **multiple regression** (used for continuous independent variables) and **analysis of variance** (used for nominal independent variables).[40(p299)]

analysis of residuals: see **linear regression**.

analysis of variance (ANOVA): statistical method used to compare a **continuous dependent variable** and more than 1 **nominal independent variable**. The **null hypothesis** in ANOVA is tested by means of the **F test**.

In 1-way ANOVA there is a single **nominal independent variable** with 2 or more levels (eg, age categorized into strata of 20 to 39 years, 40 to 59 years, and 60 years and older).When there are only 2 mutually exclusive categories for the nominal independent variable (eg, male or female), the 1-way ANOVA is equivalent to the ***t* test**.

A 2-way ANOVA is used if there are 2 independent variables (eg, age strata and sex), a 3-way ANOVA if there are 3 independent variables, etc. If more than 1 nonexclusive independent variable is analyzed, the process is called *factorial ANOVA*, which assesses the **main effects** of the independent variables as well as their **interactions**. An analysis of main effects in the 2-way ANOVA above would assess the independent effects of age group or sex; an association between female sex and systolic blood pressure that exists in one age group but not another would mean that an interaction between age and sex exists. In a factorial 3-way ANOVA with independent variables A, B, and C, there is one 3-way interaction term ($A \times B \times C$), 3 different 2-way interaction terms ($A \times B$, $A \times C$, and $B \times C$), and 3 main effect terms (A, B, and C). A separate F test must be computed for each different main effect and interaction term.

If **repeated measures** are made on an individual (such as measuring blood pressure over time) so that a matched form of analysis is appropriate, but potentially confounding factors (such as age) are to be controlled for simultaneously, repeated-measures ANOVA is used. Randomized-block ANOVA is used if treatments are assigned by means of **block randomization**.[40(pp291-295)]

➔ An ANOVA can establish only whether a significant difference exists among groups, not which groups are significantly different from each other. To determine which groups differ significantly, a pairwise analysis of a continuous dependent variable and more than 1 nominal variable is performed by a procedure such as the **Newman-Keuls test** or **Tukey test**, as well as many others. These **multiple comparison procedures** avoid the potential of a **type I error** that might occur if the *t* test were applied at this stage. Such comparisons may also be computed through the use of orthogonal contrasts.

➔ The F ratio is the statistical result of ANOVA and is a number between 0 and infinity. The F ratio is compared with tables of the **F distribution**, taking into account the α **level** and **degrees of freedom (*df*)** for the numerator and denominator, to determine the *P* value.

> *Example:* The difference was found to be significant by 1-way ANOVA ($F_{2,63}$=61.07; $P < .001$).[43]

The *df*s are provided along with the F statistic. The first subscript (2) is the *df* for the numerator; the second subscript (63) is the *df* for the denominator. The *P* value can be obtained from an F statistic table that provides the *P* value that corresponds to a given F and *df*. In practice, however, the *P* value is generally calculated by a computerized **algorithm**. Because ANOVA does not determine which groups are significantly different from each other, this example would normally be accompanied by the results of the **multiple comparisons procedure.**[43] Other models such as **Latin square** may also be used.

ANCOVA: see **analysis of covariance.**

ANOVA: see **analysis of variance.**

Ansari-Bradley dispersion test: rank test to determine whether 2 distributions known to be of identical shape (but not necessarily of **normal distribution**) have equal **parameters** of scale.[35(p6)]

area under the curve (AUC): technique used to measure the performance of a test plotted on a **receiver operating characteristic (ROC) curve** or to measure drug clearance in pharmacokinetic studies.[42(p12)] When measuring test performance, the larger the AUC, the better the test performance. When measuring drug clearance, the AUC assesses the total exposure of the individual, as measured by levels of the drug in blood or urine, to a drug over time. The curve of drug clearance used to calculate the AUC is also used to calculate the drug half-life.

➔ The method used to determine the AUC should be specified (eg, the trapezoidal rule).

artifact: difference or change in measure of occurrence of a condition that results from the way the disease or condition is measured, sought, or defined.[40(p327)]

> *Example:* An artifactual increase in the incidence of AIDS was expected because the definition of AIDS was changed to include a larger number of AIDS-defining illnesses.

assessment: in the statistical sense, evaluating the outcome(s) of the **study** and **control groups.**

assignment: process of distributing individuals to study and control groups. See also **randomization.**

association: statistically significant relationship between 2 variables in which one does not necessarily cause the other. When 2 variables are measured simultaneously, association rather than **causation** generally is all that can be assessed.

Example: After confounding factors were controlled for by means of multivariate regression, a significant association remained between age and disease prevalence.

attributable risk: disease that can be attributed to a given risk factor; conversely, if the risk factor were eliminated entirely, the amount of the disease that could be eliminated.[40(pp327-328)] Attributable risk assumes a causal relationship (ie, the factor to be eliminated is a cause of the disease and not merely associated with the disease). See attributable risk percentage and attributable risk reduction.

attributable risk percentage: the percentage of risk associated with a given factor among those with the risk factor.[40(pp327-328)] For example, risk of stroke in an older person who smokes and has hypertension and no other risk factors can be divided among the risks attributable to smoking, hypertension, and age. Attributable risk percentage is often determined for a population and is the percentage of the disease related to the risk factor. See population attributable risk percentage.

attributable risk reduction: the number of events that can be prevented by eliminating a particular risk factor from the population. Attributable risk reduction is a function of 2 factors: the strength of the association between the risk factor and the disease (ie, how often the risk factor causes the disease) and the frequency of the risk factor in the population (ie, a common risk factor may have a lower attributable risk in an individual than a less common risk factor, but could have a higher attributable risk reduction because of the risk factor's high prevalence in the population). Attributable risk reduction is a useful concept for public health decisions. See also attributable risk.

average: the central tendency of a number of measurements. This is often used synonymously with mean, but can also imply the median, mode, or some other statistic. Thus, the word should generally be avoided in favor of a more precise term.

Bayesian analysis: theory of statistics involving the concept of prior probability, conditional probability or likelihood, and posterior probability.[38(p16)] For interpreting studies, the prior probability is based on previous studies and may be informative, or, if no studies exist or those that exist are not useful, one may assume a uniform prior. The study results are then incorporated with the prior probability to obtain a posterior probability. Bayesian analysis can be used to interpret how likely it is that a positive result indicates presence of a disease, by incorporating the prevalence of the disease in the population under study and the sensitivity and specificity of the test in the calculation.

➔ Bayesian analysis has been criticized because the weight that a particular study is given when prior probability is calculated can be a subjective decision. Nonetheless, the process most closely approximates how studies are considered when they are incorporated into clinical practice. When Bayesian analysis is used to assess posterior probability for an individual patient in a clinic population, the process may be less subjective than usual practice because the prior probability, equal to the prevalence of the disease in the clinic population, is more accurate than if the prevalence for the population at large were used.[32]

β (beta), β level: probability of showing no significant difference when a true difference exists; a false acceptance of the null hypothesis.[42(p57)] One minus β is the statistical power of the test to detect a true difference; the smaller the β, the greater the power. A value of .20 for β is equal to .80 or 80% power. A β of .1 or .2 is most frequently used in power calculations. The β error is synonymous with **type II error**.[43]

bias: a systematic situation or condition that causes a result to depart from the true value in a consistent direction. Bias refers to defects in study design (often **selection bias**) or measurement.[40(p328)] One method to reduce measurement bias is to ensure that the investigator measuring outcomes for a participant is unaware of the group to which the participant belongs (ie, **blinded assessment**).

bimodal distribution: nonnormal distribution with 2 peaks, or **modes**. The **mean** and **median** may be equivalent, but neither will describe the data accurately. A **population** composed entirely of schoolchildren and their grandparents might have a mean age of 35 years, although everyone in the population would in fact be either much younger or much older.

binary variable: variable that has 2 mutually exclusive subgroups, such as male/female or pregnant/not pregnant; synonym for **dichotomous variable**.[44(p75)]

binomial distribution: probability with 2 possible mutually exclusive outcomes; used for modeling cumulative **incidence** and **prevalence** rates[42(p17)] (for example, the probability of a person having a stroke in a given **population** over a given period; the outcome must be stroke or no stroke). In a binomial sample with a probability p of the event and n number of participants, the predicted mean is $p \times n$ and the predicted variance is $p(p-1)$.

biological plausibility: evidence that an **independent variable** can be expected to exert a biological effect on a **dependent variable** with which it is associated. For example, studies in animals were used to establish the biological plausibility of adverse effects of passive smoking.

bivariable analysis: see **bivariate analysis**.

bivariate analysis: used when 1 **dependent** and 1 **independent variable** are to be assessed.[40(p263)] Common examples include the **t test** for 1 **continuous variable** and 1 **binary variable** and the **χ^2 test** for 2 binary variables. Bivariate analyses can be used for hypothesis testing in which only 1 independent variable is taken into account, to compare baseline characteristics of 2 groups, or to develop a model for multivariate regression. See also **univariate** and **multivariate analysis**.

➔ Bivariate analysis is the simplest form of hypothesis testing but is often used incorrectly, either because it is used too frequently, resulting in an increased likelihood of a **type I error**, or because tests that assume a **normal distribution** (eg, the ***t* test**) are applied to nonnormally distributed data.

Bland-Altman plot: a method to assess **agreement** (eg, between 2 tests) developed by Bland and Altman.[41]

blinded (masked) assessment: evaluation or categorization of an outcome in which the person assessing the outcome is unaware of the treatment assignment. **Masked assessment** is the term preferred by some investigators and journals, particularly those in ophthalmology.

➔ Blinded assessment is important to prevent **bias** on the part of the investigator performing the assessment, who may be influenced by the study question and consciously or unconsciously expect a certain test result.

blinded (masked) assignment: assignment of individuals participating in a prospective study (usually random) to a study group and a **control group** without the investigator or the participants being aware of the group to which they are assigned. Studies may be single-blind, in which either the participant or the person administering the intervention does not know the treatment assignment, or double-blind, in which neither knows the treatment assignment. The term *triple-blinded* is sometimes used to indicate that the persons who analyze or interpret the data are similarly unaware of treatment assignment. Authors should indicate who exactly was blinded. The term **masked assignment** is preferred by some investigators and journals, particularly those in ophthalmology.

block randomization: type of **randomization** in which the unit of randomization is not the individual but a larger group, sometimes stratified on particular variables such as age or severity of illness to ensure even distribution of the variable between randomized groups.

Bonferroni adjustment: one of several statistical adjustments to the ***P* value** that may be applied when **multiple comparisons** are made. The **α level** (usually .05) is divided by the number of comparisons to determine the α level that will be considered statistically significant. Thus, if 10 comparisons are made, an α of .05 would become $\alpha = .005$ for the study. Alternatively, the *P* value may be multiplied by the number of comparisons, while retaining the α of .05.[44(pp31-32)] Alternatively, the *P* value may be multiplied by the number of comparisons, while retaining the α of .05. For example, a *P* value of .02 obtained for 1 of 10 comparisons would be multiplied by 10 to get the final result of $P = .20$, a nonsignificant result.

➔ The Bonferroni test is a conservative adjustment for large numbers of comparisons (ie, less likely than other methods to give a significant result) but is simple and used frequently.

bootstrap method: statistical method for validating a new diagnostic **parameter** in the same group from which the parameter was derived. Thus, the validation of the method is based on a simulated sample, rather than a new sample. The parameter is first derived from the entire group, then applied sequentially to subsegments of the group to see whether the parameter performs as well for the subgroups as it does for the entire group (derived from "pulling oneself up by one's own bootstraps").[42(p32)]

For example, a number of prognostic indicators are measured in a **cohort** of hospitalized patients to predict mortality. To determine whether the model using the indicators is equally predictive of mortality for subsegments of the group, the bootstrap method is applied to the subsegments and **confidence intervals** are calculated to determine the predictive ability of the model. The **jackknife dispersion** test also uses the same sample for both derivation and validation.

➔ Although the preferable means for validating a model is to apply the model to a new sample (eg, a new cohort of hospitalized patients in the previous example), the bootstrap method can be used to reduce the time, effort, and expense necessary to complete the study. However, the bootstrap method provides less assurance than validation in a new sample that the model is generalizable to another **population**.

Brown-Mood procedure: test used with a **regression** model that does not assume a **normal distribution** or common variance of the errors.[38(p26)] It is an extension of the **median test**.

C statistic: a measure of the area under a **receiver operating characteristic curve**.

case: in a study, an individual with the outcome or disease of interest.

case-control study: **retrospective study** in which individuals with the disease (**cases**) are compared with those who do not have the disease (**controls**). Cases and controls are identified without knowledge of exposure to the **risk factors** under study. Cases and controls are matched on certain important variables, such as age, sex, and year in which the individual was treated or identified. A case-control study on individuals already enrolled in a cohort study is referred to as a **nested case-control study**.[42(p111)] This type of case-control study may be an especially strong study design if characteristics of the cohort have been carefully ascertained. See also 20.3.2, Observational Studies, Case-Control Studies.

→ Cases and controls should be selected from the same **population** to minimize confounding by factors other than those under study. Matching cases and controls on too many characteristics may obscure the association of interest, because if cases and controls are too similar, their exposures may be too similar to detect a difference (see **overmatching**).

case-fatality rate: probability of death among people diagnosed as having a disease. The rate is calculated as the number of deaths during a specific period divided by the number of persons with the disease at the beginning of the period.[44(p38)]

case series: retrospective descriptive study in which clinical experience with a number of patients is described. See 20.3.3, Observational Studies, Case Series.

categorical data: counts of members of a category or class; for the analysis each member or item should fit into only 1 category or class[38(p29)] (eg, sex or race/ethnicity). The categories have no numerical significance. Categorical data are summarized by proportions, percentages, fractions, or simple counts. Categorical data is synonymous with **nominal data**.

cause, causation: something that brings about an effect or result; to be distinguished from **association**, especially in cohort studies. To establish something as a cause it must be known to precede the effect. The concept of causation includes the **contributory cause**, the **direct cause**, and the **indirect cause**.

censored data: censoring has 2 different statistical connotations: (1) data in which extreme values are reassigned to some predefined, more moderate value; (2) data in which values have been assigned to individuals for whom the actual value is not known, such as in **survival analyses** for individuals who have not experienced the outcome (usually death) at the time the data collection was terminated.

The term *left-censored data* means that data were censored from the low end or left of the distribution; *right-censored data* come from the high end or right of the distribution[42(p26)] (eg, in survival analyses). For example, if data for falls are categorized as individuals who have 0, 1, or 2 or more falls, falls exceeding 2 have been right-censored.

central limit theorem: theorem that states that the mean of a number of samples with **variances** that are not large relative to the entire sample will increasingly approximate a **normal distribution** as the sample size increases. This is the basis for the importance of the normal distribution in statistical testing.[38(p30)]

central tendency: property of the distribution of data, usually measured by **mean, median,** or **mode.**[42(p41)]

χ^2 test (chi-square test): a test of significance based on the χ^2 statistic, usually used for **categorical data**. The observed values are compared with the expected values under the assumption of no **association**. The χ^2 **goodness-of-fit test** compares the observed with expected frequencies. The χ^2 test can also compare an observed **variance** with hypothetical variance in normally distributed samples.[38(p33)] In the case of a continuous **independent variable** and a nominal **dependent variable**, the χ^2 test for trend can be used to determine whether a linear relationship exists (for example, the relationship between systolic blood pressure and stroke).[40(pp284-285)]

➔ The ***P* value** is determined from χ^2 tables with the use of the specified α level and the *df* calculated from the number of cells in the χ^2 table. The χ^2 statistic should be reported to no more than 1 decimal place; if the **Yates correction** was used, that should be specified. See also **contingency table**.

> *Example:* The exercise intervention group was least likely to have experienced a fall in the previous month ($\chi^2_3 = 17.7$, $P = .02$).

Note that the *df* for χ^2_3 is specified using a subscript 3; it is derived from the number of cells in the χ^2 table (for this example, 4 cells in a 2×2 table). The value 17.7 is the χ^2 value. The *P* value is determined from the χ^2 value and *df*.

Results of the χ^2 test may be biased if there are too few observations (generally 5 or fewer) per cell. In this case, the **Fisher exact test** is preferred.

choropleth map: map of a region or country that uses shading to display quantitative data.[42(p28)] See also 4.2.3, Visual Presentation of Data, Figures, Maps.

chunk sample: subset of a **population** selected for convenience without regard to whether the sample is random or representative of the population.[38(p32)] A synonym is **convenience sample**.

Cochran *Q* test: method used to compare percentage results in matched samples (see **matching**), often used to test whether the observations made by 2 observers vary in a systematic manner. The analysis results in a *Q* statistic, which, with the *df*, determines the ***P* value**; if significant, the variation between the 2 observers cannot be explained by chance alone.[38(p25)] See also **interobserver bias**.

coefficient of determination: square of the **correlation coefficient**, used in linear or multiple **regression analysis**. This statistic indicates the proportion of the variation of the **dependent variable** that can be predicted from the **independent variable**.[40(p328)] If the analysis is **bivariate**, the correlation coefficient is indicated as *r* and the coefficient of determination is r^2. If the correlation coefficient is derived from **multivariate analysis**, the correlation coefficient is indicated as *R* and the coefficient of determination is R^2. See also **correlation coefficient**.

Example: The sum of the R^2 values for age and body mass index was 0.23. [Twenty-three percent of the variance could be explained by those 2 variables.]

➔ When R^2 values of the same dependent variable total more than 1.0 or 100%, then the independent variables have an interactive effect on the dependent variable.

coefficient of variation: ratio of the **standard deviation** (SD) to the **mean**. The coefficient of variation is expressed as a percentage and is used to compare **dispersions** of different **samples**. The smaller the coefficient of variation, the greater the **precision**.[43] The coefficient of variation is also used when the SD is dependent on the mean (eg, the increase in height with age is accompanied by an increasing SD of height in the **population**).

cohort: a group of individuals who share a common exposure, experience, or characteristic, or a group of individuals followed up or traced over time in a **cohort study**.[38(p31)]

cohort effect: change in rates that can be explained by the common experience or characteristic of a group or **cohort** of individuals. A cohort effect implies that a current pattern of variables may not be generalizable to a different cohort.[38(p328)]

Example: The decline in socioeconomic status with age was a cohort effect explained by fewer years of education among the older individuals.

cohort study: study of a group of individuals, some of whom are exposed to a variable of interest (eg, a drug treatment or environmental exposure), in which participants are followed up over time to determine who develops the outcome of interest and whether the outcome is associated with the exposure. Cohort studies may be concurrent (prospective) or nonconcurrent (retrospective).[40(pp328-329)] See also 20.3.1, Observational Studies, Cohort Studies.

➔ Whenever possible, a participant's outcome should be assessed by individuals who do not know whether the participant was exposed (see **blinded assessment**).

concordant pair: pair in which both individuals have the same trait or outcome (as opposed to **discordant pair**). Used frequently in twin studies.[42(p35)]

conditional probability: **probability** that an event E will occur given the occurrence of F, called the conditional probability of E given F. The reciprocal is not necessarily true: the probability of E given F may not be equal to the probability of F given E.[44(p55)]

confidence interval (CI): range of numerical expressions within which one can be confident (usually 95% confident, to correspond to an α **level** of .05) that the **population** value the study is intended to estimate lies.[40(p329)] The CI is an indication of the **precision** of an estimated population value.

➔ Confidence intervals used to estimate a population value usually are symmetric or nearly symmetric around a value, but CIs used for **relative risks** and **odds ratios** may not be. Confidence intervals are preferable to ***P* values** because they convey information about **precision** as well as statistical **significance** of **point estimates**.

→ Confidence intervals are expressed with a hyphen separating the 2 values. To avoid confusion, the word *to* replaces hyphens if one of the values is a negative number. Units that are closed up with the numeral are repeated for each CI; those not closed up are repeated only with the last numeral. See also 20.8, Significant Digits and Rounding Numbers, and 19.4, Numbers and Percentages, Use of Digit Spans and Hyphens.

> *Example:* The odds ratio was 3.1 (95% CI, 2.2-4.8). The prevalence of disease in the **population** was 1.2% (95% CI, 0.8%-1.6%).

confidence limits (CLs): upper and lower boundaries of the **confidence interval**, expressed with a comma separating the 2 values.[42(p35)]

> *Example:* The mean (95% confidence limits) was 30% (28%, 32%).

confounding: (1) a situation in which the apparent effect of an exposure on risk is caused by an **association** with other factors that can influence the outcome; (2) a situation in which the effects of 2 or more causal factors as shown by a set of data cannot be separated to identify the unique effects of any of them; (3) a situation in which the measure of the effect of an exposure on risk is distorted because of the association of exposure with another factor(s) that influences the outcome under study.[42(p35)] See also **confounding variable**.

confounding variable: variable that can cause or prevent the outcome of interest, is not an intermediate variable, and is associated with the factor under investigation. Unless it is possible to adjust for confounding variables, their effects cannot be distinguished from those of the factors being studied. Bias can occur when adjustment is made for any factor that is caused in part by the exposure and also is correlated with the outcome.[25(p35)] **Multivariate analysis** is used to control the effects of confounding variables that have been measured.

contingency coefficient: the coefficient *C* (*Note:* not to be confused with the **C statistic**), used to measure the strength of **association** between 2 characteristics in a **contingency table**.[44(pp56-57)]

contingency table: table created when **categorical variables** are used to calculate expected frequencies in an analysis and to present data, especially for a **χ^2 test** (2-dimensional data) or **log-linear models** (data with at least 3 dimensions). A 2×3 contingency table has 2 rows and 3 columns. The *df* are calculated as (number of rows − 1)(number of columns −1). Thus, a 2 × 3 contingency table has 6 cells and 2 *df*.

continuous data: data with an unlimited number of equally spaced values.[40(p329)] There are 2 kinds of continuous data: ratio data and interval data. Ratio-level data have a true 0, and thus numbers can meaningfully be divided by one another (eg, weight, systolic blood pressure, cholesterol level). For instance, 75 kg is half as heavy as 150 kg. Interval data may be measured with a similar precision but lack a true 0 point. Thus, 32°C is not half as warm as 64°C, although temperature may be measured on a precise continuous scale. Continuous data include more information than **categorical**, **nominal**, or **dichotomous** data. Use of **parametric statistics** requires that continuous data have a normal distribution, or that the data can be transformed to a **normal distribution** (eg, by computing logarithms of the data).

contributory cause: independent variable (cause) that is thought to contribute to the occurrence of the dependent variable (effect). That a cause is contributory should not be assumed unless all of the following have been established: (1) an association exists between the putative cause and effect, (2) the cause precedes the effect in time, and (3) altering the cause alters the probability of occurrence of the effect.[40(p329)] Other factors that may contribute to establishing a contributory cause include the concept of biological plausibility, the existence of a dose-response relationship, and consistency of the relationship when evaluated in different settings.

control: in a case-control study, the designation for an individual without the disease or outcome of interest; in a cohort study, the individuals not exposed to the independent variable of interest; in a randomized controlled trial, the group receiving a placebo or standard treatment rather than the intervention under study.

controlled clinical trial: study in which a group receiving an experimental treatment is compared with a control group receiving a placebo or an active treatment. See also 20.2.1, Randomized Controlled Trials, Parallel-Design Double-blind Trials.

convenience sample: sample of participants selected because they were available for the researchers to study, not because they are necessarily representative of a particular population.

➔ Use of a convenience sample limits generalizability and can confound the analysis depending on the source of the sample. For instance, in a study comparing cardiac auscultation, echocardiography, and cardiac catheterization, the patients studied, simply by virtue of their having undergone cardiac catheterization and echocardiography, likely are not comparable to an unselected population.

correlation: description of the strength of an association among 2 or more variables, each of which has been sampled by means of a representative or naturalistic method from a population of interest.[40(p329)] The strength of the association is described by the correlation coefficient. See also agreement. There are many reasons why 2 variables may be correlated, and thus correlation alone does not prove causation.

➔ The Kendall τ rank correlation test is used when testing 2 ordinal variables, the Pearson product moment correlation is used when testing 2 normally distributed continuous variables, and the Spearman rank correlation is used when testing 2 nonnormally distributed continuous variables.[43]

➔ Correlation is often depicted graphically by means of a scatterplot of the data (see Example F4 in 4.2.1, Visual Presentation of Data, Figures, Statistical Graphs). The more circular a scatterplot, the smaller the correlation; the more linear a scatterplot, the greater the correlation.

correlation coefficient: measure of the association between 2 variables. The coefficient falls between −1 and 1; the sign indicates the direction of the relationship and the number the magnitude of the relationship. A positive sign indicates that the 2 variables increase or decrease together; a negative sign indicates that increases in one are associated with decreases in the other. A value of 1 or −1 indicates that the sample values fall in a straight line, while a value of 0 indicates no relationship. The correlation coefficient should be followed by a measure of the significance of the correlation, and the statistical test used to measure correlation should be specified.

Example: Body mass index increased with age (Pearson $r = 0.61$; $P < .001$); years of education decreased with age (Pearson $r = -0.48$; $P = .01$).

➔ When 2 variables are compared, the correlation coefficient is expressed by r; when more than 2 variables are compared by **multivariate analysis**, the correlation coefficient is expressed by R. The symbol r^2 or R^2 is termed the **coefficient of determination** and indicates the amount of variation in the **dependent variable** that can be explained by knowledge of the **independent variable**.

cost-benefit analysis: economic analysis that compares the costs accruing to an individual for some treatment, process, or procedure and the ensuing medical consequences, with the benefits of reduced loss of earnings resulting from prevention of death or premature disability. The cost-benefit ratio is the ratio of marginal benefit (financial benefit of preventing 1 case) to marginal cost (cost of preventing 1 case).[42(p38)] See also 20.5, Cost-effectiveness Analysis, Cost-Benefit Analysis.

cost-effectiveness analysis: comparison of strategies to determine which provides the most clinical value for the cost.[43] A preferred intervention is the one that will cost the least for a given result or be the most effective for a given cost.[30(pp38-39)] Outcomes are expressed by the cost-effectiveness ratio, such as cost per year of life saved. See also 20.5, Cost-effectiveness Analysis, Cost-Benefit Analysis.

cost-utility analysis: form of economic evaluation in which the outcomes of alternative procedures are expressed in terms of a single **utility**-based measurement, most often the **quality-adjusted life-year (QALY)**.[42(p39)]

covariates: variables that may mediate or confound the relationship between the **independent** and **dependent variables**. Because patterns of covariates may differ systematically between groups in a trial or observational study, their effect should be accounted for during the analysis. This can be accomplished in a number of ways, including **analysis of covariance**, **multiple regression**, **stratification**, or **propensity matching**.

Cox-Mantel test: method for comparing 2 survival curves that does not assume a particular distribution of data,[44(p63)] similar to the **log-rank test**.[45(p113)]

Cox proportional hazards regression model (Cox proportional hazards model): in **survival analysis**, a procedure used to determine relationships between survival time and treatment and prognostic **independent variables** such as age.[37(p290)] The **hazard function** is modeled on the set of independent variables and assumes that the hazard function is independent of time. Estimates depend only on the order in which events occur, not on the times they occur.[44(p64)] Thus, authors should generally indicate that they have tested the proportionality assumption of the Cox model, which assumes that the ratio of the hazards between groups is similar at all points in time. The proportionality assumption would not be met, for instance, if one group experienced an early surge in mortality while the other group did not. In this case, the ratio of the hazards would be different early vs late during the time of follow-up.

criterion standard: test considered to be the diagnostic standard for a particular disease or condition, used as a basis of comparison for other (usually noninvasive) tests. Ideally, the **sensitivity** and **specificity** of the criterion standard for the disease should be 100%. (A commonly used synonym, *gold standard*, is considered jargon by some.[42(p70)]) See also **diagnostic discrimination**.

Cronbach α: index of the internal consistency of a test,[44(p65)] which assesses the **correlation** between the total score across a series of items and the comparable score that would have been obtained had a different series of items been used.[42(p39)] The Cronbach α is often used for psychological tests.

cross-design synthesis: method for evaluating outcomes of medical interventions, developed by the US General Accounting Office, which pools results from databases of randomized controlled trials and other study designs. It is a form of meta-analysis (see 20.4, Meta-analysis).[42(p39)]

crossover design: method of comparing 2 or more treatments or interventions. Individuals initially are randomized to one treatment or the other; after completing the first treatment they are crossed over to 1 or more other **randomization** groups and undergo other courses of treatment being tested in the experiment. Advantages are that a smaller sample size is needed to detect a difference between treatments, since a paired analysis is used to compare the treatments in each individual, but the disadvantage is that an adequate washout period is needed after the initial course of treatment to avoid carryover effect from the first to the second treatment. Order of treatments should be randomized to avoid potential bias.[44(pp65-66)] See 20.2.2, Randomized Controlled Trials, Crossover Trials.

cross-sectional study: study that identifies participants with and without the condition or disease under study and the characteristic or exposure of interest at the same point in time.[40(p329)]

➔ Causality is difficult to establish in a cross-sectional study because the outcome of interest and associated factors are assessed simultaneously.

crude death rate: total deaths during a year divided by the midyear population. Deaths are usually expressed per 100 000 persons.[44(p66)]

cumulative incidence: number of people who experience onset of a disease or outcome of interest during a specified period; may also be expressed as a rate or ratio.[42(p40)]

Cutler-Ederer method: form of **life-table** analysis that uses actuarial techniques. The method assumes that the times at which follow-up ended (because of death or the outcome of interest) are uniformly distributed during the time period, as opposed to the **Kaplan-Meier method**, which assumes that termination of follow-up occurs at the end of the time block. Therefore, Cutler-Ederer estimates of risk tend to be slightly higher than Kaplan-Meier estimates.[40(p308)] Often an intervention and **control group** are depicted on 1 graph and the curves are compared by means of a **log-rank test**. This is also known as the **actuarial life-table method**.

cut point: in testing, the arbitrary level at which "normal" values are separated from "abnormal" values, often selected at the point 2 SDs from the mean. See also **receiver operating characteristic curve**.[42(p40)]

DALY: see **disability-adjusted life-years**.

data: collection of items of information.[42(p42)] (*Datum*, the singular form of this word, is rarely used.)

data dredging (aka "fishing expedition"): jargon meaning **post hoc analysis**, with no a priori **hypothesis**, of several variables collected in a study to identify that have a statistically significant association for purposes of publication.

➔ Although post hoc analyses occasionally can be useful to generate hypotheses, data dredging increases the likelihood of a **type I error** and should be avoided. If post hoc analyses are performed, they should be declared as such and the number of post hoc comparisons performed specified.

decision analysis: process of identifying all possible choices and outcomes for a particular set of decisions to be made regarding patient care. Decision analysis generally uses preexisting data to estimate the likelihood of occurrence of each outcome. The process is displayed as a decision tree, with each node depicting a branch point representing a decision in treatment or intervention to be made (usually represented by a square at the branch point), or possible outcomes or chance events (usually represented by a circle at the branch point). The relative worth of each outcome may be expressed as a utility, such as the **quality-adjusted life-year**.[42(p44)] See Figure 2.

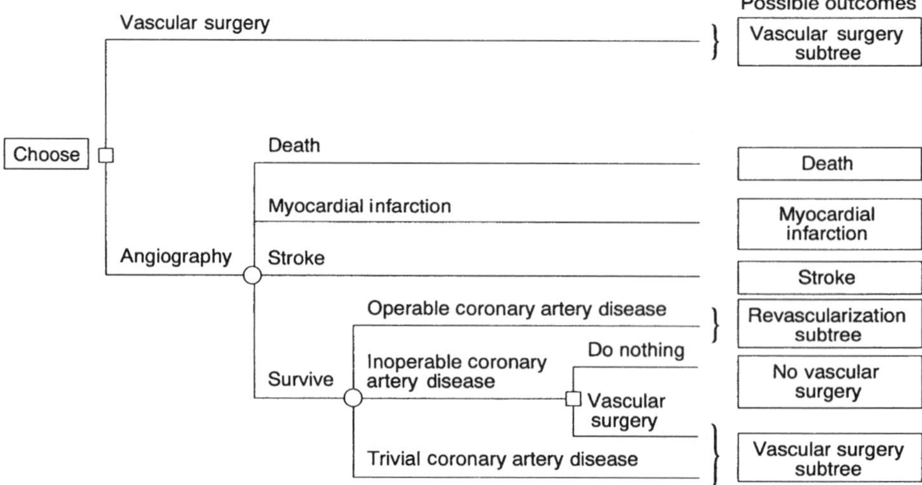

Figure 2. Decision tree showing decision nodes (squares) and chance outcomes (circles). End branches are labeled with outcome states. The subtrees to which the decision tree refers are depicted in a separate figure for simplicity. Adapted from Mason JJ, Owens DK, Harris RA, Cooke JP, Hlatky MA. The role of coronary angiography and coronary revascularization before noncardiac vascular surgery. *JAMA.* 1995;273(24):1919-1925.

degrees of freedom (*df*): see *df*.

dependent variable: outcome variable of interest in any study; the outcome that one intends to explain or estimate[40(p329)] (eg, death, myocardial infarction, or reduction in blood pressure). **Multivariate analysis** controls for **independent variables** or **covariates** that might modify the occurrence of the dependent variable (eg, age, sex, and other medical diseases or risk factors).

descriptive statistics: method used to summarize or describe data with the use of the **mean, median, SD, SE,** or **range,** or to convey in graphic form (eg, by using a **histogram,** shown in Example F5 in 4.2.1, Visual Presentation of Data, Figures, Statistical Graphs) for purposes of data presentation and analysis.[44(p73)]

***df* (degrees of freedom)** (*df* is not expanded at first mention): the number of arithmetically independent comparisons that can be made among members of a sample. In a **contingency table,** *df* is calculated as (number of rows − 1)(number of columns − 1).

➔ The *df* should be reported as a subscript after the related statistic, such as the ***t* test, analysis of variance,** and **χ^2 test** (eg, $\chi^2_3 = 17.7$, $P = .02$; in this example, the subscript 3 is the number of *df*).

diagnostic discrimination: statistical assessment of how the performance of a clinical diagnostic test compares with the **criterion standard.** To assess a test's ability to distinguish an individual with a particular condition from one without the condition, the researcher must (1) determine the variability of the test, (2) define a **population** free of the disease or condition and determine the normal range of values for that population for the test (usually the central 95% of values, but in tests that are quantitative rather than qualitative, a **receiver operating characteristic curve** may be created to determine the optimal cut point for defining normal and abnormal), and (3) determine the criterion standard for a disease (by definition, the criterion standard should have 100% sensitivity and specificity for the disease) with which to compare the test. Diagnostic discrimination is reported with the performance measures **sensitivity, specificity, positive predictive value,** and **negative predictive value; false-positive rate;** and the **likelihood ratio.**[40(pp151-163)] See Table 4.

➔ Because the values used to report diagnostic discrimination are ratios, they can be expressed either as the ratio, using the decimal form, or as the percentage, by multiplying the ratio by 100.

> *Example:* The test had a sensitivity of 0.80 and a specificity of 0.95; the false-positive rate was 0.05.
> *Or:* The test had a sensitivity of 80% and a specificity of 95%; the false-positive rate was 5%.

Table 4. Diagnostic Discrimination

Test Result	Disease by Criterion Standard	Disease Free by Criterion Standard
Positive	a (true positives)	b (false positives)
Negative	c (false negatives)	d (true negatives)
	a + c = total number of persons with disease	b + d = total number of persons without disease
	Sensitivity $= \frac{a}{a+c}$	Specificity $= \frac{d}{b+d}$
	Positive predictive value $= \frac{a}{a+b}$	Negative predictive value $= \frac{d}{c+d}$

➔ When the diagnostic discrimination of a test is defined, the individuals tested should represent the full spectrum of the disease and reflect the population on whom the test will be used. For example, if a test is proposed as a screening tool, it should be assessed in the general population.

dichotomous variable: a variable with only 2 possible categories (eg, male/female, alive/dead); synonym for **binary variable**.[44(p75)]

➔ A variable may have a **continuous** distribution during data collection but is made dichotomous for purposes of analysis (eg, age <65 years/age ≥ 65 years). This is done most often for nonnormally distributed data. Note that the use of a **cut point** generally converts a **continuous variable** to a dichotomous one (eg, normal vs abnormal).

direct cause: **contributory cause** that is believed to be the most immediate cause of a disease. The direct cause is dependent on the current state of knowledge and may change as more immediate mechanisms are discovered.[40(p330)]

> *Example:* Although several other causes were suggested when the disease was first described, the human immunodeficiency virus is the direct cause of AIDS.

disability-adjusted life-years (DALY): A quantitative indicator of burden of disease that reflects the years lost due to premature mortality and years lived with disability, adjusted for severity.[45]

discordant pair: pair in which the individuals have different **outcomes**. In twin studies, only the discordant pairs are informative about the **association** between exposure and disease.[42(pp47-48)] Antonym is **concordant pair**.

discrete variable: variable that is counted as an integer; no fractions are possible.[44(p77)] Examples are counts of pregnancies or surgical procedures, or responses to a **Likert scale**.

discriminant analysis: analytic technique used to classify participants according to their characteristics (eg, the **independent variables**, signs, symptoms, and diagnostic test results) to the appropriate **outcome** or **dependent variable**,[44(pp77-78)] also referred to as discriminatory analysis.[37(pp59-60)] This analysis tests the ability of the independent variable model to correctly classify an individual in terms of outcome. Conceptually, this may be thought of as the opposite of **analysis of variance**, in that the predictor variables are **continuous**, while the dependent variables are **categorical**.

dispersion: degree of scatter shown by observations; may be measured by **SD**, various **percentiles** (eg, tertiles, quantiles, quintiles), or **range**.[38(p60)]

distribution: group of ordered values; the frequencies or relative frequencies of all possible values of a characteristic.[40(p330)] Distributions may have a **normal distribution** (bell-shaped curve) or a **nonnormal distribution** (eg, **binomial** or **Poisson distribution**).

dose-response relationship: relationship in which changes in levels of exposure are associated with changes in the frequency of an **outcome** in a consistent direction. This supports the idea that the agent of exposure (most often a drug) is responsible for the effect seen.[40(p330)] May be tested statistically by using a χ^2 **test** for trend.

Duncan multiple range test: modified form of the Newman-Keuls test for multiple comparisons.[44(p82)]

Dunnett test: multiple comparisons procedure intended for comparing each of a number of treatments with a single control.[44(p82)]

Dunn test: multiple comparisons procedure based on the Bonferroni adjustment.[44(p84)]

Durbin-Watson test: test to determine whether the residuals from linear regression or multiple regression are independent or, alternatively, are serially correlated.[44(p84)]

ecological fallacy: error that occurs when the existence of a group association is used to imply, incorrectly, the existence of a relationship at the individual level.[40(p330)]

effectiveness: extent to which an intervention is beneficial when implemented under the usual conditions of clinical care for a group of patients,[40(p330)] as distinguished from efficacy (the degree of beneficial effect seen in a clinical trial) and efficiency (the intervention effect achieved relative to the effort expended in time, money, and resources).

effect of observation: bias that results when the process of observation alters the outcome of the study.[40(p330)] See also Hawthorne effect.

effect size: observed or expected change in outcome as a result of an intervention. Expected effect size is used during the process of estimating the sample size necessary to achieve a given power. Given a similar amount of variability between individuals, a large effect size will require a smaller sample size to detect a difference than will a smaller effect size.

efficacy: degree to which an intervention produces a beneficial result under the ideal conditions of an investigation,[40(p330)] usually in a randomized controlled trial; it is usually greater than the intervention's effectiveness.

efficiency: effects achieved in relation to the effort expended in money, time, and resources. Statistically, the precision with which a study design will estimate a parameter of interest.[42(pp52-53)]

effort-to-yield measures: amount of resources needed to produce a unit change in outcome, such as number needed to treat[43]; used in cost-effectiveness and cost-benefit analyses. See 20.5, Cost-effectiveness Analysis, Cost-Benefit Analysis.

error: difference between a measured or estimated value and the true value. Three types are seen in scientific research: a false or mistaken result obtained in a study; measurement error, a random form of error; and systematic error that skews results in a particular direction.[42(pp56-57)]

estimate: value or values calculated from sample observations that are used to approximate the corresponding value for the population.[40(p330)]

event: end point or outcome of a study; usually the dependent variable. The event should be defined before the study is conducted and assessed by an individual blinded to the intervention or exposure category of the study participant.

exclusion criteria: characteristics of potential study participants or other data that will exclude them from the study sample (such as being younger than 65 years, history of cardiovascular disease, expected to move within 6 months of the beginning of the study). Like **inclusion criteria**, exclusion criteria should be defined before any individuals are enrolled.

explanatory variable: synonymous with **independent variable**, but preferred by some because "independent" in this context does not refer to statistical independence.[38(p98)]

extrapolation: conclusions drawn about the meaning of a study for a **target population** that includes types of individuals or data not represented in the study sample.[40(p330)]

factor analysis: procedure used to group related variables to reduce the number of variables needed to represent the data. This analysis reduces complex correlations between a large number of variables to a smaller number of independent theoretical factors. The researcher must then interpret the factors by looking at the pattern of "loadings" of the various variables on each factor.[43] In theory, there can be as many factors as there are variables, and thus the authors should explain how they decided on the number of factors in their solution. The decision about the number of factors is a compromise between the need to simplify the data and the need to explain as much of the variability as possible. There is no single criterion on which to make this decision, and thus authors may consider a number of indexes of **goodness of fit**. There are a number of **algorithms** for rotation of the factors, which may make them more straightforward to interpret. Factor analysis is commonly used for developing scoring systems for rating scales and questionnaires.

false negative: negative test result in an individual who has the disease or condition as determined by the **criterion standard**.[40(p330)] See also **diagnostic discrimination**.

false-negative rate: proportion of test results found or expected to yield a false-negative result; equal to 1 − sensitivity.[40] See also **diagnostic discrimination**.

false positive: positive test result in an individual who does not have the disease or condition as determined by the **criterion standard**.[40(p330)] See also **diagnostic discrimination**.

false-positive rate: proportion of tests found to or expected to yield a false-positive result; equal to 1 − specificity.[40] See also **diagnostic discrimination**.

***F* distribution:** ratio of the distribution of 2 **normally distributed independent variables**; synonymous with **variance ratio distribution**.[42(p61)]

Fisher exact test: assesses the independence of 2 variables by means of a 2 × 2 **contingency table**, used when the frequency in at least 1 cell is small[44(p96)] (usually <6). This test is also known as the Fisher-Yates test and the Fisher-Irwin test.[38(p77)]

fixed-effects model: model used in meta-analysis that assumes that differences in treatment effect in each study all estimate the same true difference. This is not often the case, but the model assumes that it is close enough to the truth that the results will not be misleading.[46(p349)] Antonym is **random-effects model**.

Friedman test: a **nonparametric** test for a design with 2 factors that uses the ranks rather than the values of the observations.[38(p80)] Nonparametric analog to **analysis of variance**.

F test (score): alternative name for the **variance ratio** test (or F ratio),[42(p74)] which results in the F score. Often encountered in **analysis of variance**.[44(p101)]

Example: There were differences by academic status in perceptions of the quality of both primary care training ($F_{1,682} = 6.71$, $P = .01$) and specialty training ($F_{1,682} = 6.71$, $P = .01$). [The numbers set as subscripts for the F test are the ***df*** for the numerator and denominator, respectively.]

funnel plot: in meta-analysis, a graph of the sample size or **standard error** of each study plotted against its **effect size**. Estimates of effect size from small studies should have more variability than estimates from larger studies, thus producing a funnel-shaped plot. Departures from a funnel pattern suggest **publication bias**.

gaussian distribution: see **normal distribution**.

gold standard: see **criterion standard**.

goodness of fit: agreement between an observed set of values and a second set that is derived wholly or partly on a hypothetical basis.[38(p86)] The **Kolmogorov-Smirnov test** is one example.

group association: situation in which a characteristic and a disease both occur more frequently in one group of individuals than another. The association does not mean that all individuals with the characteristic necessarily have the disease.[40(p331)]

group matching: process of matching during assignment in a study to ensure that the groups have a nearly equal distribution of particular variables; also known as frequency matching.[40(p331)]

Hartley test: test for the equality of variances of a number of **populations** that are **normally distributed**, based on the ratio between the largest and smallest sample variations.[38(p90)]

Hawthorne effect: effect produced in a study because of the participants' awareness that they are participating in a study. The term usually refers to an effect on the **control group** that changes the group in the direction of the outcome, resulting in a smaller effect size.[44(p115)] A related concept is **effect of observation**. The Hawthorne effect is different than the **placebo effect**, which relates to participants' expectations that an intervention will have specific effects.

hazard rate, hazard function: theoretical measure of the likelihood that an individual will experience an event within a given period.[42(p73)] A number of hazard rates for specific intervals of time can be combined to create a hazard function.

hazard ratio: the ratio of the hazard rate in one group to the hazard rate in another. It is calculated from the **Cox proportional hazards model**. The interpretation of the hazard ratio is similar to that of the **relative risk**.

heterogeneity: inequality of a quantity of interest (such as variance) in a number of groups or populations. Antonym is **homogeneity**.

histogram: graphical representation of data in which the frequency (quantity) within each class or category is represented by the area of a rectangle centered on the class interval. The heights of the rectangles are proportional to the observed frequencies. See also Example F5 in 4.2.1, Visual Presentation of Data, Figures, Statistical Graphs.

Hoeffding independence test: **bivariate** test of **nonnormally distributed continuous data** to determine whether the elements of the 2 groups are independent of each other.[42(p93)]

Hollander parallelism test: determines whether 2 **regression lines** for 2 **independent variables** plotted against a **dependent variable** are parallel. The test does not require a **normal distribution**, but there must be an equal and even number of observations corresponding to each line. If the lines are parallel, then both independent variables predict the **dependent variable** equally well. The Hollander parallelism test is a special case of the **signed rank test**.[38(p94)]

homogeneity: equality of a quantity of interest (such as **variance**) specifically in a number of groups or **populations**.[38(p94)] Antonym is **heterogeneity**.

homoscedasticity: statistical determination that the variance of the different variables under study is equal.[42(p78)] See also **heterogeneity**.

Hosmer-Lemeshow goodness-of-fit test: a series of statistical steps used to assess **goodness of fit**; approximates the χ^2 statistic.[47]

Hotelling *T* statistic: generalization of the ***t* test** for use with **multivariate data**; results in a *T* statistic. Significance can be tested with the **variance ratio distribution**.[38(p94)]

hypothesis: supposition that leads to a prediction that can be tested to be either supported or refuted.[42(p80)] The **null hypothesis** is generally that there is no difference between groups or relationships among variables and that any such difference or relationship, if found, would occur strictly by chance. Hypothesis testing includes (1) generating the study hypothesis and defining the null hypothesis, (2) determining the level below which results are considered statistically significant, or **α level** (usually $\alpha = .05$), and (3) identifying and applying the appropriate statistical test to accept or reject the null hypothesis.

imputation: a group of techniques for replacing missing data with values that would have been likely to have been observed. Among the simplest methods of imputation is last-observation-carried-forward, in which missing values are replaced by the last observed value. This provides a conservative estimate in cases in which the condition is expected to improve on its own, but may be overly optimistic in conditions that are known to worsen over time. Missing values may also be imputed based on the patterns of other variables. In *multiple imputation*, repeated random samples are simulated, each of which produces a set of values to replace the missing values. This provides not only an estimate of the missing values but also an estimate of the uncertainty with which they can be predicted.

incidence: number of new cases of disease among persons at risk that occur over time,[42(p82)] as contrasted with **prevalence**, which is the total number of persons with the disease at any given time. Incidence is usually expressed as a percentage of individuals affected during an interval (eg, year) or as a rate calculated as the number of individuals who develop the disease during a period divided by the number of person-years at risk.

> *Example:* The incidence rate for the disease was 1.2 cases per 100 000 per year.

inclusion criteria: characteristics a study participant must possess to be included in the study population (such as age 65 years or older at the time of study enrollment and willing and able to provide informed consent). Like **exclusion criteria**, inclusion criteria should be defined before any participants are enrolled.

independence, assumption of: assumption that the occurrence of one event is in no way linked to another event. Many statistical tests depend on the assumption that each **outcome** is independent.[42(p83)] This may not be a valid assumption if repeated tests are performed on the same individuals (eg, blood pressure is measured sequentially over time), if more than 1 outcome is measured for a given individual (eg, myocardial infarction and death or all hospital admissions), or if more than 1 intervention is made on the same individual (eg, blood pressure is measured during 3 different drug treatments). Tests for **repeated measures** may be used in those circumstances.

independent variable: variable postulated to influence the **dependent variable** within the defined area of relationships under study.[42(p83)] The term does not refer to statistical independence, so some use the term **explanatory variable** instead.[38(p98)]

Example: Age, sex, systolic blood pressure, and cholesterol level were the independent variables entered into the multiple logistic regression.

indirect cause: contributory cause that acts through the biological mechanism that is the direct cause.[40(p331)]

Example: Overcrowding in the cities facilitated transmission of the tubercle bacillus and precipitated the tuberculosis epidemic. [Overcrowding is an indirect cause; the tubercle bacillus is the direct cause.]

inference: process of passing from observations to generalizations, usually with calculated degrees of uncertainty.[42(p85)]

Example: Intake of a high-fat diet was significantly associated with cardiovascular mortality; therefore, we infer that eating a high-fat diet increases the risk of cardiovascular death.

instrument error: error introduced in a study when the testing instrument is not appropriate for the conditions of the study or is not accurate enough to measure the study **outcome**[40(p331)] (may be due to deficiencies in such factors as calibration, **accuracy**, and **precision**).

intention-to-treat analysis, intent-to-treat analysis: analysis of outcomes for individuals based on the treatment group to which they were randomized, rather than on which treatment they actually received and whether they completed the study. The intention-to-treat analysis generally avoids biases associated with the reasons that participants may not complete the study and should be the main analysis of a randomized trial.[44(p125)] See 20.2, Randomized Controlled Trials.

➔ Although other analyses, such as evaluable patient analysis or per-protocol analyses, are often performed to evaluate outcomes based on treatment actually received, the intention-to-treat analysis should be presented regardless of other analyses because the intervention may influence whether treatment was changed and whether participants dropped out. Intention-to-treat analyses may bias the results of equivalence and noninferiority trials; for those trials, additional analyses should be presented. See 20.2.3, Randomized Controlled Trials, Equivalence and Noninferiority Trials.

interaction: see **interactive effect**.

interaction term: variable used in **analysis of variance** or **analysis of covariance** in which 2 independent variables interact with each other (eg, when assessing the effect of energy expenditure on cardiac output, the increase in cardiac output per unit increase in energy expenditure might differ between men and women; the interaction term would enable the analysis to take this difference into account).[40(p301)]

interactive effect: effect of 2 or more **independent variables** on a **dependent variable** in which the effect of an independent variable is influenced by the presence of another.[38(p101)] The interactive effect may be additive (ie, equal to the sum of the 2 effects present separately), synergistic (ie, the 2 effects together have a greater effect than the sum of the effects present separately), or antagonistic (ie, the 2 effects together have a smaller effect than the sum of the effects present separately).

interim analysis: data analysis carried out during a clinical trial to monitor treatment effects. Interim analysis should be determined as part of the study protocol prior to patient enrollment and specify the **stopping rules** if a particular treatment effect is reached.[7(p130)]

interobserver bias: likelihood that one observer is more likely to give a particular response than another observer because of factors unique to the observer or instrument. For example, one physician may be more likely than another to identify a particular set of signs and symptoms as indicative of religious preoccupation on the basis of his or her beliefs, or a physician may be less likely than another physician to diagnose alcoholism in a patient because of the physician's expectations.[44(p25)] The **Cochran *Q* test** is used to assess interobserver bias.[44(p25)]

interobserver reliability: test used to measure agreement among observers about a particular measure or **outcome**.

➔ Although the proportion of times that 2 observers agree can be reported, this does not take into account the number of times they would have agreed by chance alone. For example, if 2 observers must decide whether a factor is present or absent, they should agree 50% of the time according to chance. The **κ statistic** assesses agreement while taking chance into account and is described by the equation [(observed agreement) – (agreement expected by chance)]/(1 – agreement expected by chance). The value of κ may range from 0 (poor agreement) to 1 (perfect agreement) and may be classified by various descriptive terms, such as slight (0-0.20), fair (0.21-0.40), moderate (0.41-0.60), substantial (0.61-0.80), and near perfect (0.81-0.99).[48(pp27-29)]

➔ In cases in which disagreement may have especially grave consequences, such as one pathologist rating a slide "negative" and another rating a slide "invasive carcinoma," a weighted κ may be used to grade disagreement according to the severity of the consequences.[48(p29)] See also **Pearson product moment correlation**.

interobserver variation: see **interobserver reliability**.

interquartile range: the distance between the 25th and 75th percentiles, which is used to describe the dispersion of values. Like other quantiles (eg, tertiles, quintiles), such a range more accurately describes **nonnormally distributed** data than does the **SD**. The interquartile range describes the inner 50% of values; the interquintile range describes the inner 60% of values; the interdecile range describes the inner 80% of values.[38(pp102-103)]

interrater reliability: reproducibility among raters or observers; synonymous with interobserver reliability.

interval estimate: see confidence interval.[40(p331)]

intraobserver reliability (or variation): reliability (or, conversely, variation) in measurements by the same person at different times.[40(p331)] Similar to interobserver reliability, intraobserver reliability is the agreement between measurements by one individual beyond that expected by chance and can be measured by means of the κ statistic or the Pearson product moment correlation.

intrarater reliability: synonym for intraobserver reliability.

jackknife dispersion test: technique for estimating the variance and bias of an estimator, applied to a predictive model derived from a study sample to determine whether the model fits subsamples from the model equally well. The estimator or model is applied to subsamples of the whole, and the differences in the results obtained from the subsample compared with the whole are analyzed as a jackknife estimate of variance. This method uses a single data set to derive and validate the model.[48(p131)]

➔ Although validating a model in a new sample is preferable, investigators often use techniques such as jackknife dispersion or the bootstrap method to validate a model to save the time and expense of obtaining an entirely new sample for purposes of validation.

Kaplan-Meier method: nonparametric method of compiling life tables. Unlike the Cutler-Ederer method, the Kaplan-Meier method assumes that termination of follow-up occurs at the end of the time block. Therefore, Kaplan-Meier estimates of risk tend to be slightly lower than Cutler-Ederer estimates.[40(p308)] Often an intervention and control group are depicted on one graph and the groups are compared by a log-rank test. Because the method is nonparametric, there is no attempt to fit the data to a theoretical curve. Thus, Kaplan-Meier plots have a jagged appearance, with discrete drops at the end of each time interval in which an event occurs. This method is also known as the product-limit method.

κ (kappa) statistic: statistic used to measure nonrandom agreement between observers or measurements.[42(p94)] See interobserver and intraobserver reliability.

Kendall τ (tau) rank correlation: rank correlation coefficient for ordinal data.[48(p134)]

Kolmogorov-Smirnov test: comparison of 2 independent samples of continuous data without requiring that the data be normally distributed[44(p136)]; may be used to test goodness of fit.[43]

Kruskal-Wallis test: comparison of 3 or more groups of nonnormally distributed data to determine whether they differ significantly.[44(p137)] The Kruskal-Wallis test is a nonparametric analog of analysis of variance and generalizes the 2-sample Wilcoxon rank sum test to the multiple-sample case.[38(p111)]

kurtosis: the way in which a unimodal curve deviates from a normal distribution; may be more peaked (leptokurtic) or more flat (platykurtic) than a normal distribution.[44(p137)]

Latin square: form of complete treatment crossover design used for crossover drug trials that eliminates the effect of treatment order. Each patient receives each drug, but each drug is followed by another drug only once in the array. For example, in the following 4×4 array, letters A through D correspond to each of 4 drugs, each row corresponds to a patient, and each column corresponds to the order in which the drugs are given.[8(p142)]

	First Drug	*Second Drug*	*Third Drug*	*Fourth Drug*
Patient 1	C	D	A	B
Patient 2	A	C	B	D
Patient 3	D	B	C	A
Patient 4	B	A	D	C

See also 20.2.2, Randomized Controlled Trials, Crossover Trials.

lead-time bias: artifactual increase in survival time that results from earlier detection of a disease, usually cancer, during a time when the disease is asymptomatic. Lead-time bias produces longer survival from the time of diagnosis but not longer survival from the time of onset of the disease.[40(p331)] See also **length-time bias**.

➔ Lead-time bias may give the appearance of a survival benefit from screening, when in fact the increased survival is only artifactual. Lead-time bias is used more generally to indicate a systematic error arising when follow-up of groups does not begin at comparable stages in the natural course of the condition.

least significant difference test: test for comparing mean values arising in **analysis of variance**. An extension of the ***t* test**.[40(p115)]

least squares method: method of estimation, particularly in **regression analysis**, that minimizes the sum of the differences between the observed responses and the values predicted by the model.[44(p140)] The regression line is created so that the sum of the squares of the **residuals** is as small as possible.

left-censored data: see **censored data**.

length-time bias: bias that arises when a sampling scheme is based on patient visits, because patients with more frequent clinic visits are more likely to be selected than those with less frequent visits. In a screening study of cancer, for example, screening patients with frequent visits is more likely to detect slow-growing tumors than would sampling patients who visit a physician only when symptoms arise.[44(p140)] See also **lead-time bias**.

life table: method of organizing data that allows examination of the experience of 1 or more groups of individuals over time with varying periods of follow-up. For each increment of the follow-up period, the number entering, the number leaving, and the number dying of disease or developing disease can be calculated. An assumption of the life-table method is that an individual not completing follow-up is exposed for half the incremental follow-up period.[44(p143)] (The **Kaplan-Meier method** and the **Cutler-Ederer method** are also forms of life-table analysis but make different assumptions about the length of exposure.) See Figure 3.

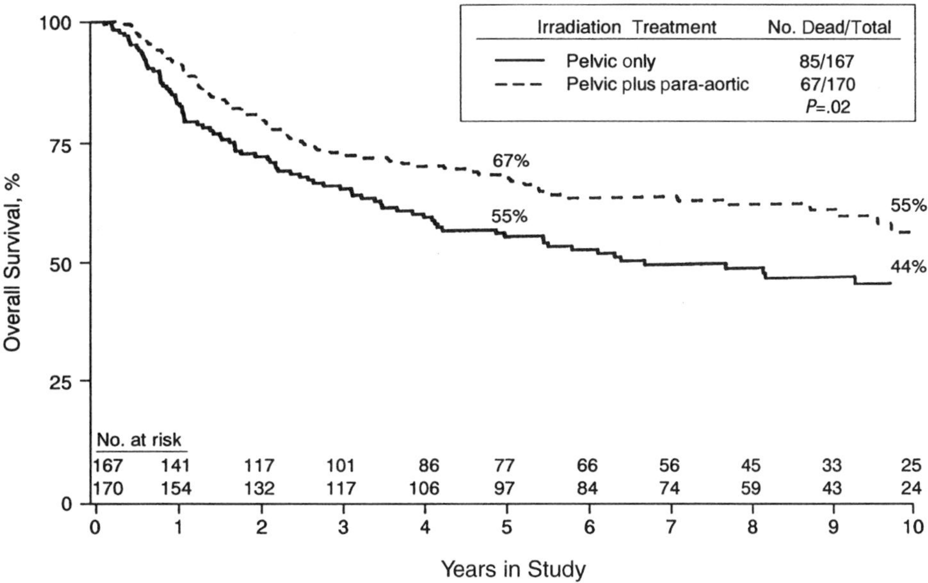

Figure 3. Survival curve showing outcomes for 2 treatments groups with number at risk at each time point. While numbers at risk are not essential to include in a survival analysis figure, this presentation conveys more information than the curve alone would. Adapted from Rotman M, Pajak TF, Choi K, et al. Prophylactic extended-field irradiation of para-aortic lymph nodes in stages IIB and bulky IB and IIA cervical carcinomas: ten-year treatment results of RTOG 79-20. *JAMA.* 1995;274(5):387-393.

➔ The clinical life table describes the outcomes of a cohort of individuals classified according to their exposure or treatment history. The cohort life table is used for a cohort of individuals born at approximately the same time and followed up until death. The current life table is a summary of mortality of the population over a brief (1- to 3-year) period, classified by age, often used to estimate life expectancy for the population at a given age.[42(p97)]

likelihood ratio: probability of getting a certain test result if the patient has the condition relative to the probability of getting the result if the patient does not have the condition. For **dichotomous variables**, this is calculated as **sensitivity**/(1 − **specificity**). The greater the likelihood ratio, the more likely that a positive test result will occur in a patient who has the disease. A ratio of 2 means a person with the disease is twice as likely to have a positive test result as a person without the disease.[43] The likelihood ratio test is based on the ratio of 2 likelihood functions.[38(p118)] See also **diagnostic discrimination**.

Likert scale: scale often used to assess opinion or attitude, ranked by attaching a number to each response such as 1, strongly agree; 2, agree; 3, undecided or neutral; 4, disagree; 5, strongly disagree. The score is a sum of the numerical responses to each question.[44(p144)]

Lilliefors test: test of normality (using the **Kolmogorov-Smirnov test** statistic) in which **mean** and **variance** are estimated from the data.[38(p118)]

linear regression: statistical method used to compare **continuous dependent** and **independent variables.** When the data are depicted on a graph as a **regression line**, the independent variable is plotted on the **x-axis** and the dependent variable on the **y-axis**. The **residual** is the vertical distance from the data point to the regression line[43(p110)]; analysis of residuals is a commonly used procedure for **linear regression**. (See Example F4 in 4.2.1, Visual Presentation of Data, Figures, Statistical Graphs.) This method is frequently performed using **least squares** regression.[37(pp202-203)]

➔ The description of a linear regression model should include the equation of the fitted line with the slope and 95% **confidence interval** if possible, the fraction of variation in y explained by the x variables (correlation), and the variances of the fitted coefficients a and b (and their **SDs**).[37(p227)]

> *Example:* The regression model identified a significant positive relationship between the dependent variable weight and height (slope = 0.25; 95% CI, 0.19-0.31; $y = 12.6 + 0.25x$; $t_{451} = 8.3$, $P < .001$; $r^2 = 0.67$).[43]

(In this example, the slope is positive, indicating that as one variable increases the other increases; the **t test** with 451 *df* is significant; the regression line is described by the equation and includes the slope 0.25 and the constant 12.6. The coefficient of determination r^2 demonstrates that 67% of the variance in weight is explained by height.)[43]

➔ Four important assumptions are made when linear regression is conducted: the dependent variable is sampled randomly from the population; the spread or dispersion of the dependent variable is the same regardless of the value of the independent variable (this equality is referred to as homogeneity of variances or **homoscedasticity**); the relationship between the 2 variables is linear; and the independent variable is measured with complete precision.[40(pp273-274)]

location: central tendency of a **normal distribution**, as distinguished from dispersion. The location of 2 curves may be identical (**means** are the same), but the **kurtosis** may vary (one may be peaked and the other flat, producing small and large **SDs**, respectively).[49(p28)]

logistic regression: type of **regression** model used to analyze the relationship between a **binary dependent variable** (expressed as a natural log after a logit transformation) and 1 or more **independent variables.** Often used to determine the independent effect of each of several explanatory variables by controlling for several factors simultaneously in a multiple logistic regression analysis. Results are usually expressed by **odds ratios** or **relative risks** and 95% **confidence intervals.**[40(pp311-312)] (The multiple logistic regression equation may also be provided but, because these involve exponents, they are substantially more complicated than linear regression equations. Therefore, in *JAMA* and the *Archives* Journals, the equation is generally not published but can be made available on request from authors. Alternatively, it may be placed on the Web.)

➔ To be valid, a multiple regression model must have an adequate sample size for the number of variables examined. A rough rule of thumb is to have at least 25 individuals in the study for each explanatory variable examined.

log-linear model: linear models used in the analysis of **categorical data.**[38(p122)]

log-rank test: method of using the relative death rates in subgroups to compare overall differences between survival curves for different treatments; same as the Mantel-Haenszel test.[38(pp122,124)]

main effect: estimate of the independent effect of an explanatory (independent) variable on a dependent variable in analysis of variance or analysis of covariance.[44(p153)]

Mann-Whitney test: nonparametric equivalent of the *t* test, used to compare ordinal dependent variables with either nominal independent variables or continuous independent variables converted to an ordinal scale.[42(p100)] Similar to the Wilcoxon rank sum test.

MANOVA: multivariate analysis of variance. This involves examining the overall significance of all dependent variables considered simultaneously and thus has less risk of type I error than would a series of univariate analysis of variance procedures on several dependent variables.

Mantel-Haenszel test: another name for the log-rank test.

Markov process: process of modeling possible events or conditions over time that assumes that the probability that a given state or condition will be present depends only on the state or condition immediately preceding it and that no additional information about previous states or conditions would create a more accurate estimate.[44(p155)]

masked assessment: synonymous with blinded assessment, preferred by some investigators and journals to the term *blinded*, especially in ophthalmology.

masked assignment: synonymous with blinded assignment, preferred by some investigators and journals to the term *blinded*, especially in ophthalmology.

matching: process of making study and control groups comparable with respect to factors other than the factors under study, generally as part of a case-control study. Matching can be done in several ways, including frequency matching (matching on frequency distributions of the matched variable[s]), category (matching in broad groups such as young and old), individual (matching on individual rather than group characteristics), and pair matching (matching each study individual with a control individual).[42(p101)]

McNemar test: form of the χ^2 test for binary responses in comparisons of matched pairs.[42(p103)] The ratio of discordant to concordant pairs is determined; the greater the number of discordant pairs with the better outcome being associated with the treatment intervention, the greater the effect of the intervention.[44(p158)]

mean: sum of values measured for a given variable divided by the number of values; a measure of central tendency appropriate for normally distributed data.[49(p29)]

➔ If the data are not normally distributed, the median is preferred. See also average.

measurement error: estimate of the variability of a measurement. Variability of a given parameter (eg, weight) is the sum of the true variability of what is measured (eg, day-to-day weight fluctuations) plus the variability of the instrument or observer measurement, or variability caused by measurement error (error variability, eg, the scale used for weighing). The intraclass correlation coefficient *R* measures the relationship of these 2 types of variability: as the error variability declines with respect to true variability, R increases, up to 1 when error variance is 0. If all variability is a result of error variability, then $R = 0$.[46(p30)]

median: midpoint of a distribution chosen so that half the values for a given variable appear above and half occur below.[40(p332)] For data that do not have a normal distribution, the median provides a better measure of central tendency than does the mean, since it is less influenced by outliers.[47(p29)]

median test: nonparametric rank-order test for 2 groups.[38(p128)]

meta-analysis: See 20.4, Meta-analysis.

missing data: incomplete information on individuals resulting from any of a number of causes, including loss to follow-up, refusal to participate, and inability to complete the study. Although the simplest approach would be to remove such participants from the analysis, this would violate the intention-to-treat principle. Furthermore, certain health conditions may be systematically associated with the risk of having missing data, and thus removal of these individuals could bias the analysis. It is generally better to attempt imputation of these missing values, which are then included in the analysis.

mode: in a series of values of a given variable, the number that occurs most frequently; used most often when a distribution has 2 peaks (bimodal distribution).[49(p29)] This is also appropriate as a measure of central tendency for categorical data.

Monte Carlo simulation: a family of techniques for modeling complex systems for which it would otherwise be difficult to obtain sufficient data. In general, Monte Carlo simulations use a computer algorithm to generate a large number of random "observations." The patterns of these numbers are then assessed for underlying regularities.

mortality rate: death rate described by the following equation: [(number of deaths during period) × (period of observation)]/(number of individuals observed). For values such as the crude mortality rate, the denominator is the number of individuals observed at the midpoint of observation. See also crude death rate.[44(p66)]

➔ Mortality rate is often expressed in terms of a standard ratio, such as deaths per 100 000 persons per year.

Moses ranklike dispersion test: rank test of the equality of scale of 2 identically shaped populations, applicable when the population medians are not known.[38(p134)]

multiple analyses problem: problem that occurs when several statistical tests are performed on one group of data because of the potential to introduce a type I error. The problem is particularly an issue when the analyses were not specified as primary outcome measures. Multiple analyses can be appropriately adjusted for by means of a Bonferroni adjustment or any of several multiple comparisons procedures.

multiple comparisons procedures: any of several tests used to determine which groups differ significantly after another more general test has identified that a significant difference exists but not between which groups. These tests are intended to avoid the problem of a type I error caused by sequentially applying tests, such as the *t* test, not intended for repeated use. Authors should specify whether these tests were planned a priori, or whether the decision to perform them was post hoc.

→ Some tests result in more conservative estimates (less likely to be significant) than others. More conservative tests include the **Tukey test** and the **Bonferroni adjustment**; the **Duncan multiple range test** is less conservative. Other tests include the **Scheffé test**, the **Newman-Keuls test**, and the Gabriel test,[38(p137)] as well as many others. There is ongoing debate among statisticians about when it is appropriate to use these tests.

multiple regression: general term for analysis procedures used to estimate values of the **dependent variable** for all measured **independent variables** that are found to be associated. The procedure used depends on whether the variables are **continuous** or **nominal**. When all variables are continuous variables, multiple **linear regression** is used and the mean of the dependent variable is expressed using the equation $Y = \alpha + \beta_1\chi_1 + \beta_2\chi_2 + \cdots + \beta_k\chi_k$, where Y is the dependent variable and k is the total number of independent variables. When independent variables may be either nominal or continuous and the dependent variable is continuous, **analysis of covariance** is used. (Analysis of covariance often requires an **interaction term** to account for differences in the relationship between the independent and dependent variables.) When all variables are nominal and the dependent variable is time-dependent, **life-table** methods are used. When the independent variables may be either continuous or nominal and the dependent variable is nominal and time-dependent (such as incidence of death), the **Cox proportional hazards model** may be used. Nominal dependent variables that are not time-dependent are analyzed by means of **logistic regression** or **discriminant analysis**.[37(pp296-312)]

multivariable analysis: another name for **multivariate analysis**.

multivariate analysis: any statistical test that deals with 1 **dependent variable** and at least 2 **independent variables**. It may include **nominal** or **continuous** variables, but **ordinal** data must be converted to a nominal scale for analysis. The multivariate approach has 3 advantages over bivariate analysis: (1) it allows for investigation of the relationship between the dependent and independent variables while controlling for the effects of other independent variables; (2) it allows several comparisons to be made statistically without increasing the likelihood of a **type I error**; and (3) it can be used to compare how well several independent variables individually can estimate values of the dependent variable.[40(pp289-291)] Examples include **analysis of variance**, **multiple** (**logistic** or **linear**) **regression**, **analysis of covariance**, **Kruskal-Wallis test**, **Friedman test**, **life table**, and **Cox proportional hazards model**.

N: total number of units (eg, patients, households) in the sample under study.

> *Example:* We assessed the diagnoses of admission all patients admitted from the emergency department during a 1-month period (N = 127).

n: number of units in a subgroup of the sample under study.

> *Example*: Of the patients admitted from the emergency department (N = 127), the most frequent admission diagnosis was unstable angina (n = 38).

natural experiment: investigation in which a change in a risk factor or exposure occurs in one group of individuals but not in another. The distribution of individuals into a particular group is nonrandom and, as opposed to controlled clinical trials, the change is not brought about by the investigator.[40(p332)] The natural experiment is often used to study effects that cannot be studied in a controlled trial, such as the incidence of medical illness immediately after an earthquake. This is also referred to as a "found" experiment.

naturalistic sample: set of observations obtained from a sample of the population in such a way that the distribution of independent variables in the sample is representative of the distribution in the population.[40(p332)]

necessary cause: characteristic whose presence is required to bring about or cause the disease or outcome under study.[50(p332)] A necessary cause may not be a sufficient cause.

negative predictive value: the probability that an individual does not have the disease (as determined by the criterion standard) if the test result is negative.[40(p334)] This measure takes into account the prevalence of the condition or the disease. A more general term is posttest probability. See diagnostic discrimination.

nested case-control study: case-control study in which cases and controls are drawn from a cohort study. The advantages of a nested case-control study over a case-control study are that the controls are selected from participants at risk at the time of occurrence of each case that arises in a cohort, thus avoiding the confounding effect of time in the analysis, and that cases and controls are by definition drawn from the same population.[40(p111)] See also 20.3.1, Observational Studies, Cohort Studies, and 20.3.2, Observational Studies, Case-Control Studies.

Newman-Keuls test: a type of multiple comparisons procedure, used to compare more than 2 groups. It first compares the 2 groups that have the highest and lowest means, then sequentially compares the next most extreme groups, and stops when a comparison is not significant.[39(p92)]

n-of-1 trial: randomized controlled trial that uses a single patient and an outcome measure agreed on by the patient and physician. The n-of-1 trial may be used by clinicians to assess which of 2 or more possible treatment options is better for the individual patient.[50]

nominal variable: also called categorical variable. There is no arithmetic relationship among the categories, and thus there is no intrinsic ranking or order between them (for example, sex, gene alleles, race, eye color). The nominal or discrete variable usually is assessed to determine its frequency within a population.[40(p332)] The variable can have either a binomial or Poisson distribution (if the nominal event is extremely rare, eg, a genetic mutation).

nomogram: a visual means of representing a mathematical equation.

nonconcurrent cohort study: cohort study in which an individual's group assignment is determined by information that exists at the time a study begins. The extreme of a nonconcurrent cohort study is one in which the outcome is determined retrospectively from existing records.[40(p332)]

nonnormal distribution: data that do not have a normal (bell-shaped curve) distribution; includes binomial, Poisson, and exponential distributions, as well as many others.

→ Nonnormally distributed continuous data must be either transformed to a normal distribution to use **parametric** methods or, more commonly, analyzed by **nonparametric** methods.

nonparametric statistics: statistical procedures that do not assume that the data conform to any theoretical distribution. Nonparametric tests are most often used for **ordinal** or **nominal** data, or for nonnormally distributed continuous data converted to an **ordinal** scale[40(p332)] (for example, weight classified by tertile).

normal distribution: **continuous data** distributed in a symmetrical, bell-shaped curve with the mean value corresponding to the highest point of the curve. This distribution of data is assumed in many statistical procedures.[40(p330)] This is also called a **gaussian distribution**.

→ Descriptive statistics such as **mean** and **SD** can be used to accurately describe data only if the values are normally distributed or can be transformed into a normal distribution.

normal range: measure of the range of values on a particular test among those without the disease. **Cut points** for abnormal tests are arbitrary and are often defined as the central 95% of values, or the **mean** of values ± 2 **SDs**.

null hypothesis: the assertion that no true association or difference in the study **outcome** or comparison of interest between comparison groups exists in the larger population from which the study samples are obtained.[40(p332)] In general, statistical tests cannot be used to prove the null hypothesis. Rather, the results of statistical testing can reject the null hypothesis at the stated α likelihood of a **type I error**.

number needed to harm: computed similarly to **number needed to treat**, but number of patients who, after being treated for a specific period of time, would be expected to experience 1 bad **outcome** or not experience 1 good outcome.

number needed to treat (NNT): number of patients who must be treated with an intervention for a specific period to prevent 1 bad **outcome** or result in 1 good outcome.[40(pp332-333)] The NNT is the reciprocal of the **absolute risk reduction**, the difference between event rates in the intervention and placebo groups in a clinical trial. See also **number needed to harm**.

→ The study patients from whom the NNT is calculated should be representative of the **population** to whom the numbers will be applied. The NNT does not take into account adverse effects of the intervention.

odds ratio (OR): ratio of 2 odds. Odds ratio may have different definitions depending on the study and therefore should be defined. For example, it may be the odds of having the disease if a particular risk factor is present to the odds of not having the disease if the risk factor is not present, or the odds of having a risk factor present if the person has the disease to the odds of the risk factor being absent if the person does not have the disease.

→ The odds ratio typically is used for a case-control or cohort study. For a study of incident cases with an infrequent disease (for example, <2% incidence), the odds ratio approximates the **relative risk**.[42(p118)] When the incidence is relatively frequent, the odds ratio may be arithmetically corrected to better approximate the **relative risk**.[51]

➔ The odds ratio is usually expressed by a point estimate and 95% **confidence interval** (CI). An odds ratio for which the CI includes 1 indicates no statistically significant effect on risk; if the point estimate and CI are both less than 1, there is a statistically significant reduction in risk; if the point estimate and CI are both greater than 1, there is a statistically significant increase in risk.

1-tailed test: test of statistical significance in which deviations from the **null hypothesis** in only 1 direction are considered.[40(p333)] Most commonly used for the ***t* test**.

➔ One-tailed tests are more likely to produce a statistically significant result than are **2-tailed tests**. Since the use of a 1-tailed test implies that the intervention could have only 1 direction of effect, ie, beneficial or harmful, the use of a 1-tailed test must be justified.

ordinal data: type of data with a limited number of categories with an inherent ordering of the category from lowest to highest, but without fixed or equal spacing between increments.[40(p333)] Examples are Apgar scores, heart murmur rating, and cancer stage and grade. Ordinal data can be summarized by means of the **median** and **quantiles** or **range**.

➔ Because increments between the numbers for ordinal data generally are not fixed (eg, the difference between a grade 1 and a grade 2 heart murmur is not quantitatively the same as the difference between a grade 3 and a grade 4 heart murmur), ordinal data should be analyzed by **nonparametric statistics**.

ordinate: vertical or **y-axis** of a graph.

outcome: dependent variable or end point of an investigation. In retrospective studies such as case-control studies, the outcomes have already occurred before the study is begun; in prospective studies such as cohort studies and controlled trials, the outcomes occur during the time of the study.[40(p333)]

outliers (outlying values): values at the extremes of a **distribution**. Because the **median** is far less sensitive to outliers than is the **mean**, it is preferable to use the median to describe the **central tendency** of data that have extreme outliers.

➔ If outliers are excluded from an analysis, the rationale for their exclusion should be explained in the text. A number of tests are available to determine whether an outlier is so extreme that it should be excluded from the analysis.

overmatching: the phenomenon of obscuring by the matching process of a case-control study a true causal relationship between the **independent** and **dependent variables** because the variable used for matching is strongly related to the mechanism by which the independent variable exerts its effect.[40(pp119-120)] For example, matching cases and controls on residence within a certain area could obscure an environmental cause of a disease. Overmatching may also be used to refer to matching on variables that have no effect on the dependent variable, and therefore are unnecessary, or the use of so many variables for matching that no suitable controls can be found.[42(p120)]

oversampling: in survey research, a technique that selectively increases the likelihood of including certain groups or units that would otherwise produce too few responses to provide reliable estimates.

paired samples: form of matching that can include self-pairing, where each participant serves as his or her own **control**, or artificial pairing, where 2 participants are matched on prognostic variables.[42(p186)] Twins may be studied as pairs to attempt to separate the effects of environment and genetics. Paired analyses provide greater power to detect a difference for a given sample size than do nonpaired analyses, since interindividual differences are minimized or eliminated. **Pairing** may also be used to match participants in **case-control** or **cohort studies**. See Table 3.

paired *t* test: ***t* test** for paired data.

parameter: measurable characteristic of a **population**. One purpose of statistical analysis is to estimate population parameters from sample observations.[40(p333)] The statistic is the numerical characteristic of the sample; the parameter is the numerical characteristic of the population. Parameter is also used to refer to aspects of a model (eg, a regression model).

parametric statistics: tests used for continuous data and that require the assumption that the data being tested are **normally distributed**, either as collected initially or after transformation to the ln or log of the value or other mathematical conversion.[40(p121)] The ***t* test** is a parametric statistic. See Table 3.

Pearson product moment correlation: test of **correlation** between 2 groups of **normally distributed** data. See **diagnostic discrimination**.

percentile: see **quantile**.

placebo: a biologically inactive substance administered to some participants in a clinical trial. A placebo should ideally appear similar in every other way to the experimental treatment under investigation. Assignment, allocation, and assessment should be **blinded**.

placebo effect: refers to specific expectations that participants may have of the intervention. These can make the intervention appear more effective than it actually is. Comparison of a group receiving **placebo** vs those receiving the active intervention allows researchers to identify effects of the intervention itself, as the placebo effect should affect both groups equally.

point estimate: single value calculated from sample observations that is used as the estimate of the **population** value, or **parameter**[40(p333)]; in most circumstances accompanied by an interval estimate (eg, 95% **confidence interval**).

Poisson distribution: distribution that occurs when a **nominal** event (often disease or death) occurs rarely.[42(p125)] The Poisson distribution is used instead of a **binomial distribution** when sample size is calculated for a study of events that occur rarely.

population: any finite or infinite collection of individuals from which a sample is drawn for a study to obtain estimates to approximate the values that would be obtained if the entire population were sampled.[44(p197)] A population may be defined narrowly (eg, all individuals exposed to a specific traumatic event) or widely (eg, all individuals at risk for coronary artery disease).

population attributable risk percentage: percentage of risk within a **population** that is associated with exposure to the **risk factor**. Population **attributable risk** takes into account the frequency with which a particular event occurs and the frequency with which a given risk factor occurs in the population. Population attributable risk does not necessarily imply a cause-and-effect relationship. It is also called attributable fraction, attributable proportion, and etiologic fraction.[40(p333)]

positive predictive value: proportion of those participants or individuals with a positive test result who have the condition or disease as measured by the **criterion standard**. This measure takes into account the **prevalence** of the condition or the disease. Clinically, it is the probability that an individual has the disease if the test result is positive.[40(p334)] See Table 4 and **diagnostic discrimination**.

posterior probability: in **Bayesian analysis**, the probability obtained after the **prior probability** is combined with the probability from the study of interest.[42(p128)] If one assumes a **uniform prior** (no useful information for estimating probability exists before the study), the posterior probability is the same as the probability from the study of interest alone.

post hoc analysis: analysis performed after completion of a study and not based on a hypothesis considered before the study. Such analyses should be performed without prior knowledge of the relationship between the **dependent** and **independent variables**. A potential hazard of post hoc analysis is the **type I error**.

➔ While post hoc analyses may be used to explore intriguing results and generate new hypotheses for future testing, they should not be used to test hypotheses, because the comparison is not hypothesis-driven. See also **data dredging**.

posttest probability: the probability that an individual has the disease if the test result is positive (**positive predictive value**) or that the individual does not have the disease if the test result is negative (**negative predictive value**).[40(p158)]

power: ability to detect a significant difference with the use of a given sample size and **variance**; determined by frequency of the condition under study, magnitude of the effect, study design, and sample size.[40(p128)] Power should be calculated before a study is begun. If the sample is too small to have a reasonable chance (usually 80% or 90%) of rejecting the **null hypothesis** if a true difference exists, then a negative result may indicate a **type II error** rather than a true failure to reject the null hypothesis.

➔ Power calculations should be performed as part of the study design. A statement providing the power of the study should be included in the "Methods" section of all randomized controlled trials (see Table 1) and is appropriate for many other types of studies. A power statement is especially important if the study results are negative, to demonstrate that a **type II error** was unlikely to have been the reason for the negative result. Performing a post hoc power analysis is controversial, especially if it is based on the study results. Nonetheless, if such calculations were performed, they should be described in the "Comment" section and their post hoc nature clearly stated.

> *Example:* We determined that a sample size of 800 patients would have 80% power to detect the clinically important difference of 10% at $\alpha = .05$.

precision: inverse of the variance in measurement (see measurement error)[42(p129)]; the degree of reproducibility that an instrument produces when measuring the same event. Note that precision and accuracy are independent concepts; if a blood pressure cuff is poorly calibrated against a standard, it may produce measurements that are precise but inaccurate.

pretest probability: see prevalence.

prevalence: proportion of persons with a particular disease at a given point in time. Prevalence can also be interpreted to mean the likelihood that a person selected at random from the population will have the disease (synonym: pretest probability).[40(p334)] See also incidence.

principal components analysis: procedure used to group related variables to help describe data. The variables are grouped so that the original set of correlated variables is transformed into a smaller set of uncorrelated variables called the principal components.[42(p131)] Variables are not grouped according to dependent and independent variables, unlike many forms of statistical analysis. Principal components analysis is similar to factor analysis.

prior probability: in Bayesian analysis, the probability of an event based on previous information before the study of interest is considered. The prior probability may be informative, based on previous studies or clinical information, or not, in which case the analysis uses a uniform prior (no information is known before the study of interest). A reference prior is one with minimal information, a clinical prior is based on expert opinion, and a skeptical prior is used when large treatment differences are not expected.[44(p201)] When Bayesian analysis is used to determine the posterior probability of a disease after a patient has undergone a diagnostic test, the prior probability may be estimated as the prevalence of the disease in the population from which the patient is drawn (usually the clinic or hospital population).

probability: in clinical studies, the number of times an event occurs in a study group divided by the number of individuals being studied.[40(p334)]

product-limit method: see Kaplan-Meier method.

propensity analysis: in observational studies, a way of minimizing bias by selecting controls who have similar statistical likelihoods of having the outcome or intervention under investigation. In general, this involves examining a potentially large number of variables for their multivariate relationship with the outcome. The resulting model is then used to predict cases' individual propensities to the outcome or intervention. Each case can then be matched to a control participant with a similar propensity. Propensity analysis is thus a way of correcting for underlying sources of bias when computing relative risk.

proportionate mortality ratio: number of individuals who die of a particular disease during a span of time, divided by the number of individuals who die of all diseases during the same period.[40(p334)] This ratio may also be expressed as a rate, ie, a ratio per unit of time (eg, cardiovascular deaths per total deaths per year).

prospective study: study in which participants with and without an exposure are identified and then followed up over time; the outcomes of interest have not occurred at the time the study commences.[44(p205)] Antonym is retrospective study.

pseudorandomization: assigning of individuals to groups in a nonrandom manner, eg, selecting every other individual for an intervention or assigning participants by Social Security number or birth date.

publication bias: tendency of articles reporting positive and/or "new" results to be submitted and published, and studies with negative or confirmatory results not to be submitted or published; especially important in meta-analysis, but also in other systematic reviews. Substantial publication bias has been demonstrated from the "file-drawer" problem.[52] See **funnel plot**.

purposive sample: set of observations obtained from a **population** in such a way that the sample distribution of independent variable values is determined by the researcher and is not necessarily representative of distribution of the values in the population.[40(p334)]

***P* value:** probability of obtaining the observed data (or data that are more extreme) if the **null hypothesis** were exactly true.[44(p206)]

➔ While **hypothesis** testing often results in the *P* value, *P* values themselves can only provide information about whether the null hypothesis is rejected. **Confidence intervals** (CIs) are much more informative since they provide a plausible range of values for an unknown **parameter**, as well as some indication of the **power** of the study as indicated by the width of the CI.[37(pp186-187)] (For example, an odds ratio of 0.5 with a 95% CI of 0.05 to 4.5 indicates to the reader the [im]precision of the estimate, whereas $P = .63$ does not provide such information.) Confidence intervals are preferred whenever possible. Including both the CI and the *P* value provides more information than either alone.[37(187)] This is especially true if the CI is used to provide an interval estimate and the *P* value to provide the results of hypothesis testing.

➔ When any *P* value is expressed, it should be clear to the reader what parameters and groups were compared, what statistical test was performed, and the **degrees of freedom (*df*)** and whether the test was **1-tailed** or **2-tailed** (if these distinctions are relevant for the statistical test).

➔ For expressing *P* values in manuscripts and articles, the actual value for *P* should be expressed to 2 digits for $P \geq .01$, whether or not *P* is **significant**. (When rounding a *P* value expressed to 3 digits would make the *P* value nonsignificant, such as $P = .049$ rounded to .05, the *P* value can be left as 3 digits.) If $P < .01$, it should be expressed to 3 digits. The actual *P* value should be expressed ($P = .04$), rather than expressing a statement of inequality ($P < .05$), unless $P < .001$. Expressing *P* to more than 3 significant digits does not add useful information to $P < .001$, since precise *P* values with extreme results are sensitive to biases or departures from the statistical model.[37(p198)]

P values should not be listed simply as *not significant* or *NS*, since for **meta-analysis** the actual values are important and not providing exact *P* values is a form of incomplete reporting.[37(p195)] Because the *P* value represents the result of a statistical test and not the strength of the association or the clinical importance of the result, *P* values should be referred to simply as statistically significant or not significant; terms such as *highly significant* and *very highly significant* should be avoided.

➔ *JAMA* and the *Archives* Journals do not use a zero to the left of the decimal point, since statistically it is not possible to prove or disprove the null hypothesis completely when only a sample of the population is tested (P cannot equal 0 or 1, except by rounding). If $P < .00001$, P should be expressed as $P < .001$ as discussed. If $P > .999$, P should be expressed as $P > .99$.

qualitative data: data that fit into discrete categories according to their attributes, such as **nominal** or **ordinal data**, as opposed to **quantitative data**.[42(p136)]

qualitative study: form of study based on observation and interview with individuals that uses inductive reasoning and a theoretical sampling model, with emphasis on **validity** rather than **reliability** of results. Qualitative research is used traditionally in sociology, psychology, and group theory but also occasionally in clinical medicine to explore beliefs and motivations of patients and physicians.[53]

quality-adjusted life-year (QALY): method used in economic analyses to reflect the existence of chronic conditions that cause impairment, disability, and loss of independence. Numerical weights representing severity of residual disability are based on assessments of disability by study participants, parents, physicians, or other researchers made as part of **utility** analysis.[42(p136)]

quantile: method used for grouping and describing dispersion of data. Commonly used quantiles are the tertile (3 equal divisions of data into lower, middle, and upper ranges), quartile (4 equal divisions of data), quintile (5 divisions), and decile (10 divisions). Quantiles are also referred to as **percentiles**.[38(p165)]

➔ Data may be expressed as median (quantile range), eg, length of stay was 7.5 days (interquartile range, 4.3-9.7 days). See also **interquartile** range.

quantitative data: data in numerical quantities such as **continuous** data or counts[42(p137)] (as opposed to **qualitative data**). **Nominal** and **ordinal data** may be treated either qualitatively or quantitatively.

quasi-experiment: experimental design in which variables are specified and participants assigned to groups, but interventions cannot be controlled by the experimenter. One type of quasi-experiment is the **natural experiment**.[42(p137)]

***r*:** **correlation coefficient** for **bivariate analysis**.

***R*:** **correlation coefficient** for **multivariate analysis**.

r^2: **coefficient of determination** for **bivariate analysis**. See also **correlation coefficient**.

R^2: **coefficient of determination** for **multivariate analysis**. See also **correlation coefficient**.

random-effects model: model used in meta-analysis that assumes that there is a universe of conditions and that the effects observed in the studies are only a sample, ideally a **random sample**, of the possible effects.[34(p349)] Antonym is **fixed-effects model**.

randomization: method of assignment in which all individuals have the same chances of being assigned to the conditions in a study. Individuals may be randomly assigned at a 2:1 or 3:1 frequency, in addition to the usual 1:1 frequency. Participants may or may not be representative of a larger **population**.[37(p334)] Simple methods of randomization include coin flip or use of a random numbers table. See also **block randomization**.

randomized controlled trial: see 20.2.1, Randomized Controlled Trials, Parallel-Design Double-blind Trials.

random sample: method of obtaining a sample that ensures that every individual in the population has a known (but not necessarily equal, for example, in weighted sampling techniques) chance of being selected for the sample.[40(p335)]

range: the highest and lowest values of a variable measured in a sample.

> *Example:* The mean age of the participants was 45.6 years (range, 20-64 years).

rank sum test: see **Mann-Whitney test** or **Wilcoxon rank sum test**.

rate: measure of the occurrence of a disease or outcome per unit of time, usually expressed as a decimal if the denominator is 100 (eg, the surgical mortality rate was 0.02). See also 19.7.3, Numbers and Percentages, Forms of Numbers, Reporting Proportions and Percentages.

ratio: fraction in which the numerator is not necessarily a subset of the denominator, unlike a proportion[40(p335)] (eg, the assignment ratio was 1:2:1 for each drug dose [twice as many individuals were assigned to the second group as to the first and third groups]).

recall bias: systematic error resulting from individuals in one group being more likely than individuals in the other group to remember past events.[42(p141)]

➔ Recall bias is especially common in **case-control studies** that assess risk factors for serious illness in which individuals are asked about past exposures or behaviors, such as environmental exposure in an individual who has cancer.[40(p335)]

receiver operating characteristic curve (ROC curve): graphic means of assessing the extent to which a test can be used to discriminate between persons with and without disease,[42(p142)] and to select an appropriate cut point for defining normal vs abnormal results. The ROC curve is created by plotting **sensitivity** vs (1 − **specificity**). The area under the curve provides some measure of how well the test performs; the larger the area, the better the test. See Figure 4. The **C statistic** is a measure of the area under the ROC curve.

➔ The appropriate cut point is a function of the test. A screening test would require high **sensitivity**, whereas a diagnostic or confirmatory test would require high **specificity**. See Table 2 and **diagnostic discrimination**.

reference group: group of presumably disease-free individuals from which a sample of individuals is drawn and tested to establish a range of normal values for a test.[40(p335)]

regression analysis: statistical techniques used to describe a **dependent variable** as a function of 1 or more **independent variables**; often used to control for confounding variables.[40(p335)] See also **linear regression, logistic regression**.

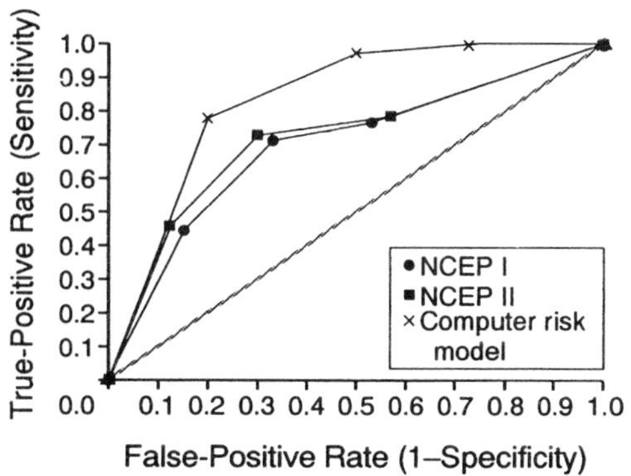

Figure 4. Receiver operating characteristic curve. The 45° line represents the point at which the test is no better than chance. The area under the curve measures the performance of the test; the larger the area under the curve, the better the test performance. Adapted from Grover SA, Coupal L, Hu X-P. Identifying adults at increased risk of coronary disease: how well do the current cholesterol guidelines work? *JAMA.* 1995;274(10):801-806.

regression line: diagrammatic presentation of a **linear regression** equation, with the **independent variable** plotted on the **x-axis** and the **dependent variable** plotted on the **y-axis**. As many as 3 variables may be depicted on the same graph.[42(p145)]

regression to the mean: the principle that extreme values are unlikely to recur. If a test that produced an extreme value is repeated, it is likely that the second result will be closer to the mean. Thus, after repeated observations results tend to "regress to the **mean**." A common example is blood pressure measurement; on repeated measurements, individuals who are initially hypertensive often will have a blood pressure reading closer to the **population** mean than the initial measurement was.[40(p335)]

relative risk (RR): probability of developing an **outcome** within a specified period if a **risk factor** is present, divided by the probability of developing the outcome in that same period if the risk factor is absent. The relative risk is applicable to randomized clinical trials and **cohort studies**[40(p335)]; for **case-control studies** the **odds ratio** can be used to approximate the relative risk if the outcome is infrequent.

> ➔ The relative risk should be accompanied by **confidence intervals**.
>
> *Example:* The individuals with untreated mild hypertension had a relative risk of 2.4 (95% confidence interval, 1.9-3.0) for stroke or transient ischemic attack. [In this example, individuals with untreated mild hypertension were 2.4 times more likely than were individuals in the comparison group to have a stroke or transient ischemic attack.]

relative risk reduction (RRR): proportion of the control group experiencing a given **outcome** minus the proportion of the treatment group experiencing the outcome, divided by the proportion of the control group experiencing the outcome.

reliability: ability of a test to replicate a result given the same measurement conditions, as distinguished from **validity**, which is the ability of a test to measure what it is intended to measure.[42(p145)]

repeated measures: analysis designed to take into account the lack of independence of events when measures are repeated in each participant over time (eg, blood pressure, weight, or test scores). This type of analysis emphasizes the change measured for a participant over time, rather than the differences between participants over time.

repeated-measures ANOVA: see analysis of variance.

reporting bias: a bias in assessment that can occur when individuals in one group are more likely than individuals in another group to report past events. Reporting bias is especially likely to occur when different groups have different reasons to report or not report information.[40(pp335-336)] For example, when examining behaviors, adolescent girls may be less likely than adolescent boys to report being sexually active. See also recall bias.

reproducibility: ability of a test to produce consistent results when repeated under the same conditions and interpreted without knowledge of the prior results obtained with the same test[40(p336)]; same as reliability.

residual: measure of the discrepancy between observed and predicted values. The residual SD is a measure of the goodness of fit of the regression line to the data and gives the uncertainty of estimating a point y from a point x.[38(p176)]

residual confounding: in observational studies, the possibility that differences in outcome may be caused by unmeasured or unmeasurable factors.

response rate: number of complete interviews with reporting units divided by the number of eligible units in the sample.[36] See 20.7, Survey Studies.

retrospective study: study performed after the outcomes of interest have already occurred[42(p147)]; most commonly a case-control study, but also may be a retrospective cohort study or case series. Antonym is prospective study.

right-censored data: see censored data.

risk: probability that an event will occur during a specified period. Risk is equal to the number of individuals who develop the disease during the period divided by the number of disease-free persons at the beginning of the period.[40(p336)]

risk factor: characteristic or factor that is associated with an increased probability of developing a condition or disease. Also called a risk marker, a risk factor does not necessarily imply a causal relationship. A modifiable risk factor is one that can be modified through an intervention[42(p148)] (eg, stopping smoking or treating an elevated cholesterol level, as opposed to a genetically linked characteristic for which there is no effective treatment).

risk ratio: the ratio of 2 risks. See also relative risk.

robustness: term used to indicate that a statistical procedure's assumptions (most commonly, normal distribution of data) can be violated without a substantial effect on its conclusions.[42(p149)]

root-mean-square: see standard deviation.

rule of 3: method used to estimate the number of observations required to have a 95% chance of observing at least 1 episode of a serious adverse effect. For example, to observe at least 1 case of penicillin anaphylaxis that occurs in about 1 in 10 000 cases treated, 30 000 treated cases must be observed. If an adverse event occurs 1 in 15 000 times, 45 000 cases need to be treated and observed.[40(p114)]

run-in period: a period at the start of a trial when no treatment is administered (although a placebo may be administered). This can help to ensure that patients are stable and will adhere to treatment. This period may also be used to allow patients to discontinue any previous treatments, and so is sometimes also called a washout period.

sample: subset of a larger population, selected for investigation to draw conclusions or make estimates about the larger population.[52(p336)]

sampling error: error introduced by chance differences between the estimate obtained from the sample and the true value in the population from which the sample was drawn. Sampling error is inherent in the use of sampling methods and is measured by the standard error.[40(p336)]

Scheffé test: see multiple comparisons procedures.

SD: see standard deviation.

SE: see standard error.

SEE: see standard error of the estimate.

selection bias: bias in assignment that occurs when the way the study and control groups are chosen causes them to differ from each other by at least 1 factor that affects the outcome of the study.[40(p336)]

➔ A common type of selection bias occurs when individuals from the study group are drawn from one population (eg, patients seen in an emergency department or admitted to a hospital) and the control participants are drawn from another (eg, clinic patients). Regardless of the disease under study, the clinic patients will be healthier overall than the patients seen in the emergency department or hospital and will not be comparable controls. A similar example is the "healthy worker effect": people who hold jobs are likely to have fewer health problems than those who do not, and thus comparisons between these groups may be biased.

SEM: see standard error of the mean.

sensitivity: proportion of individuals with the disease or condition as measured by the criterion standard who have a positive test result (true positives divided by all those with the disease).[40(p336)] See Table 4 and diagnostic discrimination.

sensitivity analysis: method to determine the robustness of an assessment by examining the extent to which results are changed by differences in methods, values of variables, or assumptions[40(p154)]; applied in decision analysis to test the robustness of the conclusion to changes in the assumptions.

signed rank test: see Wilcoxon signed rank test.

significance: statistically, the testing of the null hypothesis of no difference between groups. A significant result rejects the null hypothesis. Statistical significance is highly dependent on sample size and provides no information about the clinical significance of the result. Clinical significance, on the other hand, involves a judgment as to whether the **risk factor** or intervention studied would affect a patient's **outcome** enough to make a difference for the patient. The level of clinical significance considered important is sometimes defined prospectively (often by consensus of a group of physicians) as the minimal clinically important difference, but the cutoff is arbitrary.

sign test: a **nonparametric** test of significance that depends on the signs (positive or negative) of variables and not on their magnitude; used when combining the results of several studies, as in **meta-analysis**.[42(p156)] See also **Cox-Stuart trend test**.

skewness: the degree to which the data are asymmetric on either side of the **central tendency**. Data for a variable with a longer tail on the right of the **distribution** curve are referred to as positively skewed; data with a longer left tail are negatively skewed.[44(pp238-239)]

snowball sampling: a sampling method in which survey respondents are asked to recommend other respondents who might be eligible to participate in the survey. This may be used when the researcher is not entirely familiar with demographic or cultural patterns in the population under investigation.

Spearman rank correlation (ρ): statistical test used to determine the covariance between 2 **nominal** or **ordinal variables**.[44(p243)] The nonparametric equivalent to the **Pearson product moment correlation**, it can also be used to calculate the **coefficient of determination**.

specificity: proportion of those without the disease or condition as measured by the **criterion standard** who have negative results by the test being studied[40(p326)] (true negatives divided by all those without the disease). See Table 4 and **diagnostic discrimination**.

standard deviation (SD; does not need to be expanded at first mention): commonly used descriptive measure of the spread or **dispersion** of data; the positive square root of the **variance**.[40(p336)] The mean ± 2 SDs represents the middle 95% of values obtained.

➔ Describing data by means of SD implies that the data are **normally distributed**; if they are not, then the **interquartile range** or a similar measure involving **quantiles** is more appropriate to describe the data, particularly if the mean ± 2 SDs would be nonsensical (eg, mean [SD] length of stay = 9 [15] days, or mean [SD] age at evaluation = 4 [5.3] days). Note that the format mean (SD) should be used, rather than the ± construction.

standard error (SE; does not need to be expanded at first mention): positive square root of the **variance** of the sampling distribution of the statistic.[38(p195)] Thus, the SE provides an estimate of the precision with which a parameter can be estimated. There are several types of SE; the type intended should be clear.

In text and tables that provide descriptive statistics, SD rather than SE is usually appropriate; by contrast, **parameter** estimates (eg, regression coefficients) should be accompanied by SEs. In figures where error bars are used, the 95% **confidence interval** is preferred[54] (see Example F10 in 4.2.1, Visual Presentation of Data, Figures, Statistical Graphs).

standard error of the difference: measure of the dispersion of the differences between samples of 2 **populations**, usually the differences between the **means** of 2 **samples**; used in the ***t* test**.

standard error of the estimate: **SD** of the observed values about the **regression line**.[38(p195)]

standard error of the mean (SEM): An inferential statistic, which describes the certainty with which the **mean** computed from a random **sample** estimates the true mean of the **population** from which the sample was drawn.[39(p21)] If multiple samples of a population were taken, then 95% of the samples would have means would fall within ± 2 SEMs of the mean of all the sample means. Larger sample sizes will be accompanied by smaller SEMs, because larger samples provide a more precise estimate of the population mean than do smaller samples.

➔ The SEM is not interchangeable with SD. The SD generally describes the observed dispersion of data around the mean of a sample. By contrast, the SEM provides an estimate of the precision with which the true population mean can be inferred from the sample mean. The mean itself can thus be understood as either a descriptive or an inferential statistic; it is this intended interpretation that governs whether it should be accompanied by the SD or SEM. In the former case the mean simply describes the **average** value in the sample and should be accompanied by the SD, while in the latter it provides an estimate of the population mean and should be accompanied by the SEM. The interpretation of the mean is often clear from the text, but authors may need to be queried to discern their intent in presenting this statistic.

standard error of the proportion: **SD** of the **population** of all possible values of the proportion computed from **samples** of a given size.[39(p109)]

standardization (of a rate): adjustment of a rate to account for factors such as age or **sex**.[40(pp336-350)]

standardized mortality ratio: ratio in which the numerator contains the observed number of deaths and the denominator contains the number of deaths that would be expected in a comparison **population**. This ratio implies that confounding factors have been controlled for by means of indirect **standardization**. It is distinguished from **proportionate mortality ratio**, which is the mortality rate for a specific disease.[40(p337)]

standard normal distribution: a **normal distribution** in which the raw scores have been recomputed to have a mean of 0 and an SD of 1.[44(p245)] Such recomputed values are referred to as ***z* scores** or **standard scores**. The **mean**, **median**, and **mode** are all equal to zero.

standard score: see ***z* score**.[38(p196)]

statistic: value calculated from **sample** data that is used to estimate a value or **parameter** in the larger **population** from which the **sample** was obtained,[40(p337)] as distinguished from **data**, which refers to the actual values obtained via direct observation (eg, measurement, chart review, patient interview).

stochastic: type of measure that implies the presence of a random variable.[38(p197)]

stopping rule: rule, based on a test **statistic** or other function, specified as part of the design of the trial and established before patient enrollment, that specifies a limit for the observed treatment difference for the primary **outcome** measure, which, if exceeded, will lead to the termination of the trial or one of the study groups.[7(p258)] The stopping rules are designed to ensure that a study does not continue to enroll patients after a significant treatment difference has been demonstrated that would still exist regardless of the treatment results of subsequently enrolled patients.

stratification: division into groups. Stratification may be used to compare groups separated according to similar **confounding** characteristics. Stratified sampling may be used to increase the number of individuals sampled in rare categories of **independent variables**, or to obtain an adequate sample size to examine differences among individuals with certain characteristics of interest.[29(p337)]

Student-Newman-Keuls test: see **Newman-Keuls test**.

Student *t* test: see ***t* test**. W. S. Gossett, who originated the test, wrote under the name Student because his employment precluded individual publication.[42(p166)] Simply using the term *t* test is preferred.

study group: in a **controlled clinical trial**, the group of individuals who undergo an intervention; in a **cohort study**, the group of individuals with the exposure or characteristic of interest; and in a **case-control study**, the group of cases.[40(p337)]

sufficient cause: characteristic that will bring about or cause the disease.[40(p337)]

supportive criteria: substantiation of the existence of a contributory cause. Potential supportive criteria include the strength and consistency of the relationship, the presence of a **dose-response relationship**, and **biological plausibility**.[40(p337)]

surrogate end points: in a clinical trial, **outcomes** that are not of direct clinical importance but that are believed to be related to those that are. Such variables are often physiological measurements (eg, blood pressure) or biochemical (eg, cholesterol level). Such end points can usually be collected more quickly and economically than clinical end points, such as myocardial infarction or death, but their clinical relevance may be less certain.

survival analysis: statistical procedures for estimating the survival function and for making inferences about how it is affected by treatment and prognostic factors.[42(p163)] See **life table**.

target population: group of individuals to whom one wishes to apply or extrapolate the results of an investigation, not necessarily the **population** studied.[40(p337)] If the target population is different from the population studied, whether the study results can be extrapolated to the target population should be discussed.

τ (tau): see **Kendall τ rank correlation**.

trend, test for: see **χ^2 test**.

trial: controlled experiment with an uncertain **outcome**[38(p208)]; used most commonly to refer to a randomized study.

triangulation: in qualitative research, the simultaneous use of several different techniques to study the same phenomenon, thus revealing and avoiding **biases** that may occur if only a single method were used.

true negative: negative test result in an individual who does not have the disease or condition as determined by the **criterion standard**.[40(p338)] See also Table 4.

true-negative rate: number of individuals who have a negative test result and do not have the disease by the **criterion standard** divided by the total number of individuals who do not have the disease as determined by the criterion standard; usually expressed as a decimal (eg, the true-negative rate was 0.85). See also Table 4.

true positive: positive test result in an individual who has the disease or condition as determined by the **criterion standard**.[40(p338)] See also Table 4.

true-positive rate: number of individuals who have a positive test result and have the disease as determined by the **criterion standard** divided by the total number of individuals who have the disease as measured by the criterion standard; usually expressed as a decimal (eg, the true-positive rate was 0.92). See also Table 4.

***t* test:** statistical test used when the **independent variable** is **binary** and the **dependent variable** is **continuous**. Use of the *t* test assumes that the dependent variable has a **normal distribution**; if not, **nonparametric statistics** must be used.[40(p266)]

→ Usually the *t* test is **unpaired**, unless the data have been measured in the same individual over time. A paired *t* test is appropriate to assess the change of the **parameter** in the individual from baseline to final measurement; in this case, the dependent variable is the change from one measurement to the next. These changes are usually compared against 0, on the **null hypothesis** that there is no change from time 1 to time 2.

→ Presentation of the *t* statistic should include the **degrees of freedom** (***df***), whether the *t* test was paired or unpaired, and whether a **1-tailed** or **2-tailed test** was used. Since a 1-tailed test assumes that the study effect can have only 1 possible direction (ie, only beneficial or only harmful), justification for use of the 1-tailed test must be provided. (The 1-tailed test at $\alpha = .05$ is similar to testing at $\alpha = .10$ for a 2-tailed test and therefore is more likely to give a significant result.)

> *Example:* The difference was significant by a 2-tailed test for paired samples ($t_{15} = 2.78$, $P = .05$).

→ The *t* test can also be used to compare different **coefficients of variation**.

Tukey test: a type of **multiple comparisons procedure**.

2-tailed test: test of statistical **significance** in which deviations from the **null hypothesis** in either direction are considered.[40(p338)] For most **outcomes**, the 2-tailed test is appropriate unless there is a plausible reason why only 1 direction of effect is considered and a **1-tailed test** is appropriate. Commonly used for the ***t* test**, but can also be used in other statistical tests.

2-way analysis of variance: see **analysis of variance**.

type I error: a result in which the **sample** data lead to a rejection of the **null hypothesis** despite the fact that the null hypothesis is actually true in the **population**. The α level is the size of a type I error that will be permitted, usually .05.

➔ A frequent cause of a type I error is performing **multiple comparisons**, which increase the likelihood that a significant result will be found by chance. To avoid a type I error, one of several **multiple comparisons** procedures can be used.

type II error: the situation where the **sample** data lead to a failure to reject the **null hypothesis** despite the fact that the null hypothesis is actually false in the **population**.

➔ A frequent cause of a type II error is insufficient sample size. Therefore, a **power** calculation should be performed when a study is planned to determine the sample size needed to avoid a type II error.

uncensored data: **continuous data** reported as collected, without adjustment, as opposed to **censored data**.

uniform prior: assumption that no useful information regarding the **outcome** of interest is available prior to the study, and thus that all individuals have an equal **prior probability** of the outcome. See **Bayesian analysis**.

unity: synonymous with the number 1; a **relative risk** of 1 is a relative risk of unity, and a **regression line** with a slope of 1 is said to have a slope of unity.

univariable analysis: another name for **univariate analysis**.

univariate analysis: statistical tests involving only 1 **dependent variable**; uses measures of **central tendency** (**mean** or **median**) and **location** or **dispersion**. The term may also apply to an analysis in which there are no **independent variables**. In this case, the purpose of the analysis is to describe the sample, determine how the sample compares with the **population**, and determine whether chance has resulted in a skewed distribution of 1 or more of the variables in the study. If the characteristics of the sample do not reflect those of the population from which the sample was drawn, the results may not be generalizable to that population.[40(pp245-246)]

unpaired analysis: method that compares 2 treatment groups when the 2 treatments are not given to the same individual. Most **case-control studies** also use unpaired analysis.

unpaired *t* test: see ***t* test**.

***U* test:** see **Wilcoxon rank sum test**.

utility: in decision theory and clinical decision analysis, a scale used to judge the preference of achieving a particular **outcome** (used in studies to quantify the value of an outcome vs the discomfort of the intervention to a patient) or the discomfort experienced by the patient with a disease.[42(p170)] Commonly used methods are the time trade-off and the standard gamble. The result is expressed as a single number along a continuum from death (0) to full health or absence of disease (1.0). This quality number can then be multiplied by the number of years a patient is in the health state produced by a particular treatment to obtain the **quality-adjusted life-year**. See also 20.5, Cost-effectiveness Analysis, Cost-Benefit Analysis.

validity (of a measurement): degree to which a measurement is appropriate for the question being addressed or measures what it is intended to measure. For example, a test may be highly consistent and reproducible over time, but unless it is compared with a **criterion standard** or other validation method, the test cannot be considered valid (see also **diagnostic discrimination**). *Construct validity* refers to the extent to which the measurement corresponds to theoretical concepts. Because there are no criterion standards for constructs, construct validity is generally established by comparing the results of one method of measurement with those of other methods. *Content validity* is the extent to which the measurement samples the entire domain under study (eg, a measurement to assess delirium must evaluate cognition). *Criterion validity* is the extent to which the measurement is correlated with some quantifiable external criterion (eg, a test that predicts reaction time). Validity can be concurrent (assessed simultaneously) or predictive (eg, ability of a standardized test to predict school performance).[42(p171)]

➔ Validity of a test is sometimes mistakenly used as a synonym of **reliability**; the two are distinct statistical concepts and should not be used interchangeably. Validity is related to the idea of **accuracy**, while reliability is related to the idea of **precision**.

validity (of a study): *internal validity* means that the observed differences between the control and comparison groups may, apart from sampling error, be attributed to the effect under study; *external validity* or *generalizability* means that a study can produce unbiased inferences regarding the target **population**, beyond the participants in the study.[42(p171)]

Van der Waerden test: **nonparametric** test that is sensitive to differences in **location** for 2 samples from otherwise identical **populations**.[38(p216)]

variable: characteristic measured as part of a study. Variables may be **dependent** (usually the **outcome** of interest) or **independent** (characteristics of individuals that may affect the dependent variable).

variance: variation measured in a set of data for one **variable**, defined as the sum of the squared deviations of each data point from the mean of the variable, divided by the ***df*** (number of observations in the sample − 1).[44(p266)] The **SD** is the square root of the variance.

variance components analysis: process of isolating the sources of variability in the **outcome** variable for the purpose of analysis.

variance ratio distribution: synonym for ***F*** **distribution**.[42(p61)]

visual analog scale: scale used to quantify subjective factors such as pain, satisfaction, or values that individuals attach to possible outcomes. Participants are asked to indicate where their current feelings fall by marking a straight line with 1 extreme, such as "worst pain ever experienced," at one end of the scale and the other extreme, such as "pain-free," at the other end. The feeling (eg, degree of pain) is quantified by measuring the distance from the mark on the scale to the end of the scale.[42(p268)]

washout period: see 20.2.2, Randomized Controlled Trials, Crossover Trials.

Wilcoxon rank sum test: a **nonparametric** test that ranks and sums observations from combined samples and compares the result with the sum of ranks from 1 sample.[38(p220)] *U* is the statistic that results from the test. Alternative name for the **Mann-Whitney test**.

Wilcoxon signed rank test: **nonparametric** test in which 2 treatments that have been evaluated by means of matched samples are compared. Each observation is ranked according to size and given the sign of the treatment difference (ie, positive if the treatment effect was positive and vice versa) and the ranks are summed.[38(p220)]

Wilks Λ (lambda): a test used in **multivariate analysis of variance (MANOVA)** that tests the effect size for all the dependent variables considered simultaneously. It thus adjusts significance levels for **multiple comparisons**.

x-axis: horizontal axis of a graph. By convention, the **independent variable** is plotted on the x-axis. Synonym is **abscissa**.

Yates correction: continuity correction used to bring a distribution based on discontinuous frequencies closer to the continuous χ^2 distribution from which χ^2 tables are derived.[42(p176)]

y-axis: vertical axis of a graph. By convention, the **dependent variable** is plotted on the y-axis. Synonym is **ordinate**.

z-axis: third axis of a 3-dimensional graph, generally placed so that it appears to project out toward the reader. The z-axis and x-axis are both used to plot **independent variables** and are often used to demonstrate that the 2 independent variables each contribute independently to the **dependent variable**. See **x-axis** and **y-axis**.

***z* score:** score used to analyze **continuous variables** that represents the deviation of a value from the mean value, expressed as the number of **SDs** from the mean. The *z* score is frequently used to compare children's height and weight measurements, as well as behavioral scores.[42(p176)] It is sometimes referred to as the **standard score**.

20.10 Statistical Symbols and Abbreviations.

The following may be used without expansion except where noted by an asterisk. For a term expanded at first mention, the abbreviation may be placed in parentheses after the expanded term and the abbreviation used thereafter (see also 14.11, Abbreviations, Clinical, Technical, and Other Common Terms). Most terms other than mathematical symbols can also be found in 20.9, Glossary of Statistical Terms.

Symbol or Abbreviation	*Description*
|x|	absolute value
Σ	sum
>	greater than
≥	greater than or equal to
<	less than
≤	less than or equal to
^	hat, used above a parameter to denote an estimate
ANOVA	analysis of variance*
ANCOVA	analysis of covariance*

Symbol or Abbreviation	*Description*
α	alpha, probability of type I error
$1 - \alpha$	confidence coefficient
β	beta, probability of type II error; or population regression coefficient
$1 - \beta$	power of a statistical test
b	sample regression coefficient
CI	confidence interval*
CV	coefficient of variation $(s/\bar{x}) \times 100$*
D	difference
df	degrees of freedom (v is the international symbol[55] and also may be used if familiar to readers)
D^2	Mahalanobis distance, distance between the means of 2 groups
Δ	delta, change
δ	delta, true sampling error
ε	epsilon, true experimental error
e	exponential
$E(x)$	expected value of the variable x
f	frequency; or a function of, usually followed by an expression in parentheses, eg, $f(x)$
$F_{v1,v2}(1 - \alpha)$	F test, ratio of 2 variances, with $df = v_1,v_2$ for numerator and denominator, respectively, and $(1 - \alpha)$ = confidence coefficient
$G^2(df)$	likelihood ratio χ^2
H_0	null hypothesis
H_1	alternate hypothesis; specify whether 1- or 2-sided
κ	kappa statistic
λ_i	lambda, hazard function for interval i; eigenvalue; or estimate of parameter for log-linear models
Λ	Wilks lambda
ln	natural logarithm
log	logarithm to base 10
MANOVA	multivariate analysis of variance*
μ	population mean
n	size of a subsample
N	total sample size
$n!$	(n) factorial

Symbol or Abbreviation	*Description*
OR	odds ratio*
P	statistical probability
χ^2_3	χ^2 test or statistic, with 3 *df* shown as an example
r	bivariate correlation coefficient
R	multivariate correlation coefficient
r^2	bivariate coefficient of determination
R^2	multivariate coefficient of determination
RR	relative risk*
ρ	rho, population correlation coefficient
S_D	standard deviation of a difference D
s^2	sample variance
σ^2	sigma squared, population variance
σ	sigma, population SD
SD	standard deviation of a sample
SE	standard error
SEM	standard error of the mean
t	Student *t*; specify α level, *df*, 1-tailed vs 2-tailed
τ	Kendall tau
T^2	Hotelling T^2 statistic
U	Mann-Whitney *U* (Wilcoxon) statistic
$\bar{x}$	arithmetic mean
z	*z* score

ACKNOWLEDGMENTS

Principal authors: Margaret A. Winker, MD; updated by Stephen J. Lurie, MD, PhD

Dedicated to George W. Brown, MD, whose patient but persistent teaching led to this chapter.

Many thanks to John C. Bailar III, MD, PhD; Thomas B. Cole, MD, MPH; Theodore Colton, ScD; Peter Cummings, MD, PhD; Robert M. Golub, MD; and Naomi Vaisrub, PhD, for reviewing prior versions of this chapter.

REFERENCES

1. Partington A, ed. *The Oxford Dictionary of Quotations*. 4th ed. Oxford, England: Oxford University Press; 1992.
2. Haynes RB, Mulrow CD, Huth EJ, Altman DG, Gardner MJ. More informative abstracts revisited. *Ann Intern Med*. 1990;113(1):69-76.
3. Guyatt G, Rennie D, eds. *Users' Guides to the Medical Literature: A Manual for Evidence-Based Clinical Practice*. Chicago, IL: AMA Press; 2002:7.

4. Moher D, Schulz KF, Altman D; for the CONSORT Group. The CONSORT statement: revised recommendations for improving the quality of reports of parallel-group randomized trials. *JAMA*. 2001;285(15):1987-1991.
5. Campbell MJ. Extending CONSORT to include cluster trials. *BMJ*. 2004;328(7441):654-655.
6. Weijer C, Shapiro SH, Cranley Glass K. For and against: clinical equipoise and not the uncertainty principle is the moral underpinning of the randomised controlled trial. *BMJ*. 2000;321(72263):756-758.
7. Hellman D. Evidence, belief, and action: the failure of equipoise to resolve the ethical tension in the randomized clinical trial. *J Law Med Ethics*. 2002;30(3):375-380.
8. Meinert CL. *Clinical Trials Dictionary: Terminology and Usage Recommendations*. Baltimore, MD: Harbor Duvall Graphics; 1996.
9. DeAngelis CD, Drazen JM, Frizelle FA, et al. Clinical trial registration: a statement from the International Committee of Medical Journal Editors. *JAMA*. 2004;292(11):1363-1364.
10. Piaggio G, Elbourne DR, Altman DG, Pocock SJ, Evans SJW; for the CONSORT Group. Reporting of noninferiority and equivalence randomized trials: an extension of the CONSORT statement. *JAMA*. 2006;295(10):1152-1160.
11. D. Moher D, Schulz KF, Altman DG, for the CONSORT Group. The CONSORT statement: revised recommendations for improving the quality of reports of parallel-group randomized trials. *Ann Intern Med*. 2001;134(8):657-662.
12. Rossouw JE, Anderson GL, Prentice RL, et al; Writing Group for the Women's Health Initiative Investigators. Risks and benefits of estrogen plus progestin in healthy postmenopausal women: principal results from the Women's Health Initiative randomized controlled trial. *JAMA*. 2002;288(3):321-333.
13. Moher D, Olkin I. Meta-analysis of randomized controlled clinical trials: a concern for standards. *JAMA*. 1995;274(24):1962-1964.
14. Bailar JC III. The practice of meta-analysis. *J Clin Epidemiol*. 1995;48(1):149-157.
15. Shapiro S. Meta-analysis/shmeta-analysis. *Am J Epidemiol*. 1994;140(9):771-778.
16. Pettiti DB. Of babies and bathwater. *Am J Epidemiol*. 1994;140(9):779-782.
17. Greenland S. Can meta-analysis be salvaged? *Am J Epidemiol*. 1994;140(9):783-787.
18. Chalmers TC, Lau J. Meta-analytic stimulus for changes in clinical trials. *Stat Methods Med Res*. 1993;2(2):161-172.
19. Jadad AR, McQuay HJ. Meta-analyses to evaluate analgesic interventions: a systematic qualitative review of their methodology. *J Clin Epidemiol*. 1996;49(2):235-243.
20. Sampson M, Barrowman NJ, Moher D, et al. Should meta-analysts search EMBASE in addition to MEDLINE? *J Clin Epidemiol*. 2003;56(10):943-955.
21. Easterbrook PJ, Berlin J, Gopalan R, Matthews DR. Publication bias in clinical research. *Lancet*. 1991;337(8746):867-872.
22. Dickersin K, Scherer R, Lefebvre C. Identifying relevant studies for systematic reviews. *BMJ*. 1994;309(6964):1286-1291.
23. Gerbarg ZB, Horwitz RI. Resolving conflicting clinical trials: guidelines for meta-analysis. *J Clin Epidemiol*. 1988;41(5):502-509.
24. Thompson SG. Why sources of heterogeneity in meta-analysis should be investigated. *BMJ*. 1994;309(6965):1351-1355.
25. Bero L, Rennie D. The Cochrane Collaboration: preparing, maintaining, and disseminating systematic reviews of the effects of health care. *JAMA*. 1995;274(24):1935-1938.

26. Udvarhelyi IS, Colditz GA, Rai A, Epstein AM. Cost-effectiveness and cost-benefit analyses in the medical literature: are the methods being used correctly? *Ann Intern Med.* 1992;116(3):238-244.
27. Kassirer JP, Angell M. The Journal's policy on cost-effectiveness analyses. *N Engl J Med.* 1994;331(10):669-670.
28. Hill SR, Mitchell AS, Henry DA. Problems with the interpretation of pharmacoeconomic analyses: a review of submissions to the Australian Pharmaceutical Benefits Scheme. *JAMA.* 2000;283(16):2116-2121.
29. Russell LB, Gold MR, Siegel JE, Daniels N, Weinstein MC. The role of cost-effectiveness analysis in health and medicine. *JAMA.* 1996;276(14):1172-1177.
30. Siegel JE, Weinstein MC, Russell LB, Gold MR. Recommendations for reporting cost-effectiveness analyses: Panel on Cost-effectiveness in Health and Medicine. *JAMA.* 1996;276(16):1339-1341.
31. Drummond MF, Jefferson TO. Guidelines for authors and peer reviewers of economic submissions to the *BMJ. BMJ.* 1996;313(7052):275-283.
32. Drummond MF, Richardson WS, O'Brien BJ, Levine M, Heyland D; for the Evidence-Based Medicine Working Group. Users' guides to the medical literature: how to use an article on economic analyses of clinical practice, A: are the results of the study valid? *JAMA.* 1996;277(19):1552-1557.
33. Saha S, Hoerger TJ, Pignone MP, Teutsch SM, Helfand M, Mandelblatt JS; Cost Work Group, Third US Preventive Services Task Force. The art and science of incorporating cost effectiveness into evidence-based recommendations for clinical preventive services. *Am J Prev Med.* 2001;20(3)(suppl):36-43.
34. Mark DM. Visualizing cost-effectiveness analysis. *JAMA.* 2002;287(18):2428-2429.
35. Bossuyt PM, Reitsma JB, Bruns DE, et al; for the STARD group. Towards complete and accurate reporting of studies of diagnostic accuracy: the STARD Initiative. *Clin Radiol.* 2003;58(8):575-580.
36. American Association for Public Opinion Research. Standard definitions: final dispositions of case codes and outcome rates for surveys. http://www.aapor.org/pdfs/standarddefs_4.pdf. Accessed August 1, 2006.
37. Bailar JC, Mosteller F. *Medical Uses of Statistics.* 2nd ed. Boston, MA: NEJM Books; 1992.
38. Marriott FHC. *A Dictionary of Statistical Terms.* 5th ed. Essex, England: Longman Scientific & Technical; 1990.
39. Glantz SA. *Primer of Biostatistics.* 2nd ed. New York, NY: McGraw-Hill Book Co Inc; 1981.
40. Reigelman RK, Hirsch RP. *Studying a Study and Testing a Test.* 2nd ed. Boston, MA: Little Brown & Co Inc; 1989.
41. Bland JM, Altman DG. Statistical methods for assessing agreement between two methods of clinical measurement. *Lancet.* 1986;1(8476):307-310.
42. Last JM. *A Dictionary of Epidemiology.* 3rd ed. New York, NY: Oxford University Press; 1995.
43. Lang TA, Secic M. *Reporting Statistical Information in Medicine: Annotated Guide for Authors, Editors, and Reviewers.* Philadelphia, PA: American College of Physicians; 1997.
44. Everitt BS. *The Cambridge Dictionary of Statistics in the Medical Sciences.* Cambridge, England: Cambridge University Press; 1995.

45. Homedes N. The disability-adjusted life year (DALY) definition, measurement and potential use. http://www.worldbank.org/html/extdr/hnp/hddflash/workp/wp_00068.html. Accessed April 30, 2005.
46. Ingelfinger JA, Mosteller F, Thibodeau LA, Ware JH. *Biostatistics in Clinical Medicine.* 3rd ed. New York, NY: McGraw-Hill Book Co Inc; 1994.
47. Hosmer DW, Lemeshow S. *Applied Logistic Regression.* New York, NY: John Wiley & Sons Inc; 1989.
48. Everitt BS. *Statistical Methods for Medical Investigations.* 2nd ed. New York, NY: John Wiley & Sons Inc; 1994.
49. Colton T. *Statistics in Medicine.* Boston, MA: Little Brown & Co Inc; 1974.
50. Guyatt G, Sackett D, Taylor DW, et al. Determining optimal therapy: randomized trial in individual patients. *N Engl J Med.* 1986;314(14):889-892.
51. Zhang J, Yu KF. What's the relative risk? a method of correcting the odds ratio in cohort studies of common outcomes. *JAMA.* 1998;280(19):1690-1691.
52. Scherer RW, Dickersin K, Langenberg P. Full publication of results initially presented as abstracts: a meta-analysis. *JAMA.* 1994;272(2):158-162.
53. Pope C, Mays N. Reaching the parts other methods cannot reach: an introduction to qualitative methods in health and health services research. *BMJ.* 1995;311(6996):42-45.
54. Brown GW. Standard deviation, standard error: which "standard" should we use? *AJDC.* 1982;136(10):937-941.
55. Geng D. Conventions in statistical symbols and abbreviations. *CBE Views.* 1992; 15(5):95-96.

ADDITIONAL READINGS AND GENERAL REFERENCES

Friedman LM, Furberg CD, DeMets DL. *Fundamentals of Clinical Trials.* 3rd ed. St Louis, MO: Mosby-Year Book Inc; 1996.

Norman GR, Streiner DL. *PDQ Statistics.* 3rd ed. Philadelphia, PA: BC Decker Inc; 2003.

Sackett DL, Haynes RB, Guyatt GH, Tugwell P. *Clinical Epidemiology: A Basic Science for Clinical Medicine.* 2nd ed. Boston, MA: Little Brown & Co Inc; 1991.

Streiner DL, Norman GR. PDQ *Epidemiology.* 2nd ed. St Louis, MO: Mosby-Year Book Inc; 1996.

21 Mathematical Composition

Mathematical formulas and other expressions involving special symbols, character positions, and relationships may present difficulties in clarity in print and online publications. Careful markup (clarifying the symbols used and superior and inferior characters), avoidance of ambiguity through proper use of parentheses and brackets, and adherence to typographic conventions and capitalization rules in equations require special note (see also 8.5, Punctuation, Parentheses and Brackets, and 22.0, Typography).

21.1 Copy Marking.

Copy Marking. It is essential to mark carefully each character, letter, and symbol that may be mistaken for another form (eg, x, X, χ^2, $\times 2$, $2x$, x_2).

The following examples show correct markup for complex relations between elements of equations:

Superior	x2	x^2
Inferior	x2	x_2
Inferior to superior	xxi	x^{x_i}
Superior to superior	xx2	x^{x^2}
Inferior to inferior	xri	x_{r_i}
Superior to inferior	xr2	x_{r^2}
Inferior with superior and subinferior	x2xi (set subscript directly under superscript)	$x_2^{x_i}$

In expressions that involve both superscripts and subscripts, the subscript is usually aligned directly under the superscript. In online publication, this alignment can generally be created only by using an image.

21.2 Displayed vs Run-In. Simple formulas may remain within the text of the manuscript if they can be set on the line:

> The pulmonary vascular resistance index (PVRI) was calculated as follows: PVRI = (MPAP − PCWP)/CI, where MPAP indicates mean pulmonary artery pressure; PCWP, pulmonary capillary wedge pressure; and CI, cardiac index.

Long or complicated formulas should be centered on a separate line. In either case, symbols and signs should be marked in detail. Such formulas may be handled either as copy or as prepared art, depending on the availability of special characters and use of software for equation preparation. For online publications, formulas that require more than 1 line must either be shown as an image or depicted by means of specialized mathematical software.

Whether run into the text or centered, an equation is an element of the sentence that contains it. Punctuation and grammatical rules thus apply to it, just as they do to all other sentence elements. For example, if the equation is the last element in a sentence, it must be followed by a period. If there are 3 equations in a list, they must be separated by commas and the final equation must be preceded by "and."

If there are numerous equations in a manuscript, or if equations are related to each other or are referred to after initial presentation, they should be numbered consecutively. Numbered equations should each be set on a separate line, centered, with the parenthetical numbers set flush left.

(1) $$x = r\cos\theta$$

(2) $$y = r\sin\theta$$

(3) $$z = (x + y)$$

Standard abbreviations should be used in expressing units of measure (see 14.12, Abbreviations, Units of Measure). For short, simple equations, it may be preferable to express an equation as words in the running text, rather than to set it off as an actual formula:

> Attributable risk is calculated by subtracting the incidence among the nonexposed from the incidence among the exposed.

21.3 Stacked vs Unstacked. Stacking of fractions (ie, separating numerator and denominator by a horizontal line) should be avoided in favor of "unstacking" (ie, using a slash in place of the horizontal line) unless this sacrifices clarity (see 8.4.4, Punctuation, Forward Slash [Virgule, Solidus], In Equations).

$$y = (x_1 + x_2)/(x_1 - x_2) \text{ instead of } y = \frac{x_1 + x_2}{x_1 - x_2}$$

Whenever a fraction is unstacked, parentheses, brackets, and braces (collectively called "fences" in mathematical notation) should be used as appropriate to avoid ambiguity. For instance, the expression

$$a + \frac{b + c}{d} + e,$$

if written as $a + b + c/d + e$, is ambiguous and could have several interpretations, such as

$$\frac{a+b+c}{d+e}$$

or

$$a+b+\frac{c}{d}+e.$$

The expression's meaning is unambiguous if set off as follows:

$$a+[(b+c)/d]+e.$$

Parentheses should be used to set off simple expressions. If additional fences are needed for clarity, parenthetical expressions should be set off in brackets, and bracketed expressions should be set off with braces. Note that parentheses are thus always the *innermost* fences (see In Formulas in 8.5.2, Punctuation, Parentheses and Brackets, Brackets). All fences should be present in matched pairs.

$$\{[(a+b)/c]+[(d+e)/f]\}+g$$

21.4 Exponents

21.4.1 Fractional Exponents vs Radicals. Use of radicals may sometimes be avoided by substituting a fractional exponent:

$(a^2 - b^2)^{1/2}$ instead of $\sqrt{a^2 - b^2}$.

As with unstacking fractions, if clarity is sacrificed by making the equation fit within the text, it is preferable to set it off. For example, $E = 1.96\ \{[P\ (1 - P)]/m\}^{1/2}$ fits within the text, but the centered

$$E = 1.96\sqrt{\frac{P(1-P)}{m}}$$

might be more easily understood.

21.4.2 Negative Exponents. A negative exponent denotes the reciprocal of the expression, as illustrated in these examples:

$$x^{-n} = 1/x^n \qquad A^{-1} = 1/A \qquad B^{-2} = 1/B^2$$

A negative exponent may simplify some expressions within running text:

$\frac{A}{(x+y)^2}$ may also be written as $A(x+y)^{-2}$ or $A/(x+y)^2$.

21.4.3 Logarithmic Expressions. The term *log* is an abbreviation of *logarithm*. A system of logarithms may be based on any number, although logarithmic systems based on the numbers 10, 2, and the irrational number *e* are most common. The base should be subscripted and follow the word *log*. In the following examples, note that logarithms are always computed from exponents of the number that forms their basis.

$\log_{10} 1000 = 3$ (because $1000 = 10^3$)

$\log_2 8 = 3$ (because $8 = 2^3$)

Logarithms based on e (which is approximately 2.71) are called *natural logarithms* and are often represented as *ln*.

$$\ln 2.71 = 1$$

The terms "e^x" and "exp x" are identical in meaning and are interchangeable. The latter is preferable for constructions involving additional subscripts or superscripts. For instance, "exp ($x^3 - 1$)" is identical to "e^{x^3-1}," but the former is preferred because it is easier to set and to read.

21.5 Long Formulas. Long formulas may be given in 2 or more lines by breaking them at operation signs outside brackets or parentheses and keeping the indention the same whenever possible (some formulas may be too long to permit indention). If lines begin with an operation sign, they should be lined up with the first character to the right of the relation sign in the line above.

$$\begin{aligned} Y =& [(a_1 + b_1)/(a_2 - b_2)] \\ & +[(\sigma_1 + \sigma_2)/(\sigma_2 - \sigma_1)] \\ & +[(s_1 + s_2)/(t_1 + t_2)] \end{aligned}$$

However, if a formula loses comprehensibility by being unstacked and broken up, and/or if it fits the width of the column, it is preferable to leave it stacked.

$$\begin{aligned} \text{Percent Excess Weight Loss} =& \text{(Baseline Weight} - \text{Ideal Weight)} \\ & - \frac{\text{(Follow-up Weight} - \text{Ideal Weight)}}{\text{Baseline Weight} - \text{Ideal Weight}} \times 100 \end{aligned}$$

21.6 Expressing Multiplication and Division. The product of 2 or more terms, including units of measure, is conventionally indicated by a raised multiplication dot (·) (eg, 7 kg · m^2) or by 2 or more characters closed up (eg, $y = mx + b$). However, in scientific notation the times sign (×) is used (eg, 3×10^{-10} cm) (see 18.4.4, Units of Measure, Use of Numerals With Units, Multiplication of Numbers). An asterisk should not be used to represent multiplication, despite its use in this role in computer programs. *Note:* However, there may be occasions on which the asterisk may be used to provide the reader with the exact equation used in the analysis (eg, regression models).

A forward slash, a horizontal line, a negative exponent, or the word *per* may be used to express rates, which are generally obtained by dividing one unit by another. For example, velocity (meters per second) may be expressed as

$$\text{m/s} \quad \text{or} \quad \frac{\text{m}}{\text{s}} \quad \text{or} \quad \text{m·s}^{-1}$$

Complex rates involve division of a rate by another unit. Complex rates that are used frequently are conventionally indicated by 2 slashes in the same expression, eg:

The dose was 25 mg/kg/d.

Plasma renin activity was 1.3 ng/mL/h.

Acceleration at the surface of the earth is 9.8 m/s/s (or 9.8 m/s^2).

Most complex rates, however, are developed for particular applications. For clarity, these less commonly used rates should be expressed as "*a*/*b* per *c*." For instance,

The infusion was 2 mL/kg per minute.

Negative exponents may also be used to express such a rate when appropriate: 2 mL·kg^{-1}·min^{-1} (see 18.2.2, Units of Measure, Expressing Unit Names and Symbols, Products and Quotients of Unit Symbols). Common sense and clarity should guide this decision.

21.7 Commonly Used Symbols.

Some commonly used symbols are as follows:

Symbol	*Description*
$>$	greater than
$\geq$	greater than or equal to
$>>$	much greater than
$<$	less than
$\leq$	less than or equal to
$<<$	much less than
$\pm$	plus or minus (This symbol should *not* be used to indicate variability around a central tendency (eg, "The control group had a mean [SD] value of 12 [7]," *not* "The control group had a mean of 12 $\pm$ 7.")
$\int_a^b$	integral from value of a to value of b
$\sum_{a=1}^{30}$	summation from $a = 1$ to $a = 30$
$\prod_{a=1}^{30}$	product of $a = 1$ to $a = 30$
Δ	delta (change, difference between values)
f	function
$\neq$	not equal to
$\approx$	approximately equal to
$\sim$	similar to (reserve for use in geometry and calculus; use words in other cases where "approximately" is meant)
$\cong$	congruent to
$\equiv$	defined as
∞	infinity
!	factorial, eg, $n! = n(n - 1)(n - 2) \ldots 1$

The following symbols are usually reserved for specific values

π	pi (approximately 3.1416). Do not confuse with uppercase Π.
e	base of the system of natural logarithms (approximately 2.7183). See 21.4.3, Exponents, Logarithmic Expressions. In statistical equations, however, "e" may also represent the error term in a regression equation.
i	the square root of -1

For a list of additional symbols that are used in statistics, see 20.10, Study Design and Statistics, Statistical Symbols and Abbreviations.

The following are examples of these commonly used mathematical expressions:

$>10^5$ CFUs/mL	$\int_{10}^{13} 2x\, dx$
24.5 ± 0.5	$F \sim \frac{m_1 m_2}{r^2}$
$\mathrm{L} \approx 2 \times 10^{10}$ m	$r!\,(n - r)!$
$f(x) = x + \Delta x$	$(e^x + e^{-x})/2$
$y = dx/dt$	$Y = \beta_1 + \beta_2 + e$
$P < .001$	$\mathrm{kg} \cdot \mathrm{m} \cdot \mathrm{s}^{-2}$

$\sum_{i=0}^{n} a_i x_i$

$x + \frac{x^2}{2} + \frac{x^3}{3} + \frac{x^4}{4} + \cdots + \frac{x^n}{n}$ (note that in this case the operation sign is indicated on both sides of the ellipses)

Online journals should ensure that any symbols rendered in HTML are compatible across most commonly used browser platforms. An image should be used if incompatibility is possible. The World Wide Web consortium (http://www.w3.org) provides updated information about browser compatibility issues.

21.8 **Typography and Capitalization.** In general, variables, unknown quantities, and constants (eg, *x*, *y*, *z*, *A*, *B*, *C*) are set in italics, while units of measure (eg, kg, mL, s, m), symbols (including Greek characters [see 17.0, Greek Letters]), and numbers are set roman. Also, subscripts or superscripts used as modifiers are set roman:

C_{in} = clearance of inulin.

Arrays (A) and vectors (V) should be set boldface. Mathematical functions, such as sin, cos, ln, and log, are set roman.

$$\mathbf{V} = oai + bj + ck$$

$$\mathbf{A} = \begin{bmatrix} a_{11} & a_{12} & a_{13} \\ a_{21} & a_{22} & a_{23} \\ a_{31} & a_{32} & a_{33} \end{bmatrix}$$

For equations that are set off from the text, the words and letters should be set roman and the equation should be capitalized by the same rules that apply to titles (see 10.2, Capitalization, Titles and Headings):

$$U = \frac{\text{Efficacy}}{\text{Toxicity} - \text{Risk}} \times \frac{\text{Money Saved by Its Use}}{\text{Cost of Contrast Medium}}$$

$$\text{Age-Specific Attributable Risk} = (RR_i - 1)/RR_i$$

21.9 **Punctuation.** Punctuation after a set-off equation is helpful and often clarifies the meaning. Display equations are often preceded by punctuation.

In the linear quadratic equation model, the survival probability for cells receiving a *j* increment of radiation, D_j, is as follows:

$$\mathrm{S} = \exp(-\alpha D_j - \beta D_j),$$

where α and β are the parameters of the linear quadratic equation model.

Do not use periods after a set-off equation if the equation is preceded by a period.

21.10 **Spacing With Mathematical Symbols.** Thin spaces should be used before and after the following mathematical symbols: $\pm$, $=$, $<$, $>$, $\leq$, $\geq$, $+$, $-$, $\div$, $\times$, $\cdot$, $\approx$, $\sim$, $\cap$, $\int$, Π, $\sum$, and $|$.

$$a \pm b \quad a = b \quad a + b \quad a - b \quad a \div b \quad a \times b \quad a \cdot b \quad a > b \quad b < a$$

Symbols are set close to numbers, superscripts and subscripts, and parentheses, brackets, and braces.

$2a$	$(a + b)$
a^2	$[a - b]$
x_2	$\{a + b\}$

ACKNOWLEDGMENT

Principal author: Stephen J. Lurie, MD, PhD

ADDITIONAL READINGS AND GENERAL REFERENCES

Style Manual Committee, Council of Science Editors. *Scientific Style and Format: The CSE Manual for Authors, Editors, and Publishers*. 7th ed. New York, NY: Rockefeller University Press, in cooperation with the Council of Science Editors, Reston, VA; 2006.

Swanson E, O'Sean A, Schleyer A. *Mathematics Into Type*. Updated ed. Providence, RI: American Mathematical Society; 1999.

Section

5 Technical Information

22 Typography

Typography is the efficient means to an essentially, and only accidentally esthetic, end, for the enjoyment of patterns is rarely the reader's chief aim. . . . any disposition of printing material which, whatever the intention, has the effect of coming between author and reader is wrong.

Stanley Morison
(inventor of Times New Roman font)[1]

Good design is a blend of function and form, and the greater of these is function. This is as true of typography as it is of an opera house or space shuttle. Typography fails if it allows the reader's interest to decline. It fails absolutely if it contributes to the destruction of the reader's interest.

Colin Wheildon[1]

Typography is broadly defined as the composed arrangement and appearance of text and other elements on a surface that involves elements of design. The editor and graphic designer often cooperate in the process of creating the typography and design for a book, monograph, or journal (in print or online), with the goal of achieving a balance of form and readability.

According to typographer Edmund Arnold, good design and typography for English-language publications follow the linear flow of the Latin alphabet and support the act of reading.[1] The English language is read from left to right and from top to bottom. According to Arnold, when a reader of such language begins to read a printed page, the eyes first fall naturally to the top left corner and then move across and down the page, first from left to right and then in a right-to-left sweep to the next line, until reaching the bottom right corner. Any design or typographic element that forces the reader to work against this natural flow (reading gravity) interrupts the reading rhythm and should be avoided.[1] Wheildon conducted a controlled study in which half of the participants read an article with a design that followed Arnold's "reading gravity" principles and half read the same article but with a design that did not follow these principles. Rates of comprehension for those reading the article designed to comply with the principles of reading gravity were better (67% good, 19% fair, and 14% poor) than those reading the same article that disregarded the principles of reading gravity (32% good, 30% fair, and 38% poor).[1]

Typography for reading on a computer or other digital medium should follow the basic principles of reading as described above. There are a number of shared design considerations (eg, consistency and size of typeface; use of boldface for emphasis, subheadings, or calling out citations to tables or figures in text; concerns about overly long or wide tables or figures). However, online typography has additional attributes and concerns that are not seen in print and must reflect standards that address a different set of reading, browsing, and searching habits. For example, a Web page must work across different computer platforms, browsers, and screen sizes, and the publisher cannot control how the typographic elements (such as typeface, font, size, and color) appear on different users' screens; the Web is designed for interactivity and scrolling, so links and navigational buttons need to be clearly marked; and brightly lit screens may lead to eye strain so that online text must be presented in a different format than the same text designed for print. This chapter focuses primarily on typography for the printed page and for Latin character sets. Resources for design and typography for the Web are listed among the Additional Resources and General References at the end of the chapter. Many of the technical terms and concepts of design, typography, and composition mentioned in this chapter are listed in 24.0, Glossary of Publishing Terms.

22.1 **Basic Elements of Design.**

Good design arranges text and objects in a manner that invites and leads the reader through the composed page or material and enhances legibility and comprehension.[1,2] The basic elements of design that affect typography include the following:

- **Contrast**: This refers to the contrast between dark and light type and large and small units of information (such as title and byline, side heads and subheads, and text). In addition, the evenness of darkness or blackness of letters and characters affects legibility; this evenness depends on the specific typeface used as well as spacing between letters, words, and lines (see also 22.3, Spacing).[2]

- **Rhythm**: The rhythm of the design refers to repetition of similar units, in both opposition and juxtaposition, eg, spacing and proportion of type to the page and other design elements, and repetition of graphic contrasts or similarities.

- **Size**: The size of type and other elements affects legibility and the overall appearance of a composed page. The size relationships within the design refer to the optical images of the type and graphic elements and the relevant and proportional manners in which they appear on the page.

- **Color**: In this context, color has 2 meanings: (1) the darkness or density of the type (letters and characters) and the typeset page and (2) the use of contrasting nonblack colors, which attracts attention and creates associations. In scholarly publishing, however, the use of color for these purposes is limited.

- **Movement and Focal Points**: The elements of a page should guide the reader's eye along the lines of composition unconsciously, from large to small, from top to bottom, from left to right, from dark to light, and should follow the gravity of reading.

In scholarly publishing, a number of typographic and design elements, such as prescribed text format, titles and headings, bylines, abstracts, tables, figures, lists, equations, block quotations, and reference citations and lists, must be considered and incorporated. Consistent use of typographic style within a specific work (eg, journal, book) enhances readability and is recommended for scholarly publications. This often requires programmed style sheets based on standards for a specific publication.

The examples of journal pages shown in Figures 1 and 2 include some of these typographic elements of design as they are used in the print versions of *JAMA* and the *Archives* Journals.

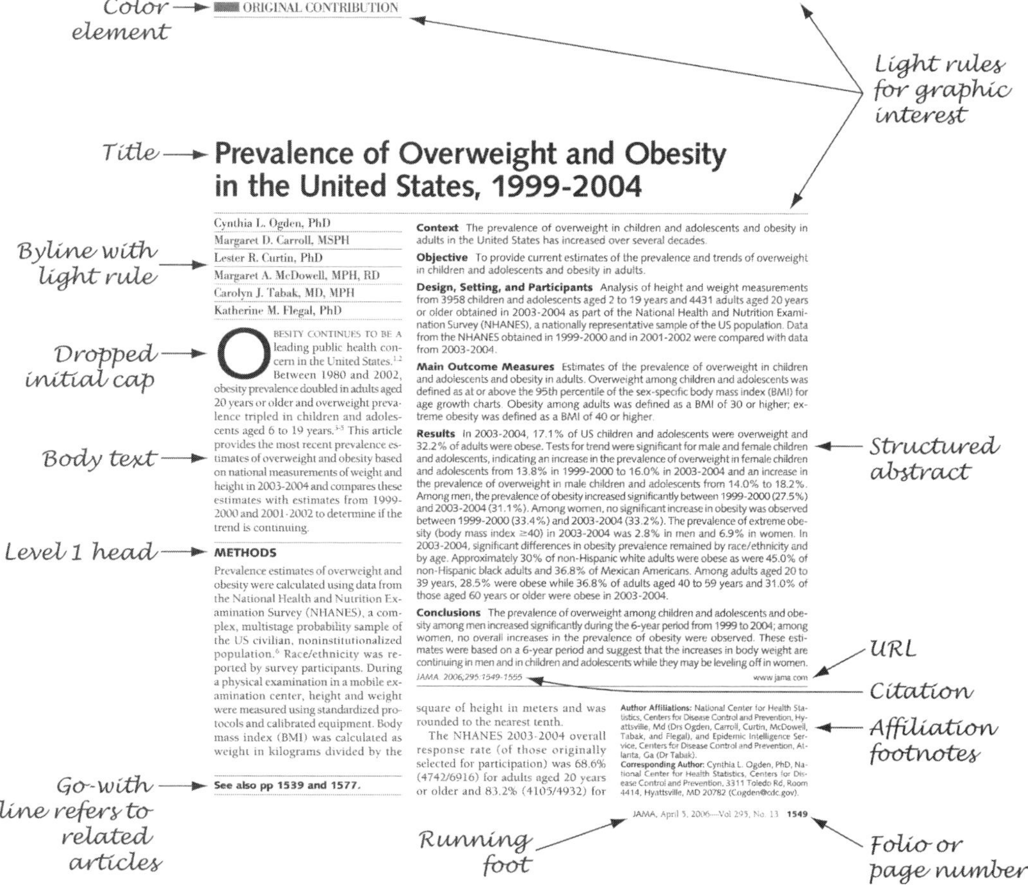

ORIGINAL CONTRIBUTION

Prevalence of Overweight and Obesity in the United States, 1999-2004

Cynthia L. Ogden, PhD
Margaret D. Carroll, MSPH
Lester R. Curtin, PhD
Margaret A. McDowell, MPH, RD
Carolyn J. Tabak, MD, MPH
Katherine M. Flegal, PhD

OBESITY CONTINUES TO BE A leading public health concern in the United States.[1,2] Between 1980 and 2002, obesity prevalence doubled in adults aged 20 years or older and overweight prevalence tripled in children and adolescents aged 6 to 19 years.[3-5] This article provides the most recent prevalence estimates of overweight and obesity based on national measurements of weight and height in 2003-2004 and compares these estimates with estimates from 1999-2000 and 2001-2002 to determine if the trend is continuing.

METHODS

Prevalence estimates of overweight and obesity were calculated using data from the National Health and Nutrition Examination Survey (NHANES), a complex, multistage probability sample of the US civilian, noninstitutionalized population.[6] Race/ethnicity was reported by survey participants. During a physical examination in a mobile examination center, height and weight were measured using standardized protocols and calibrated equipment. Body mass index (BMI) was calculated as weight in kilograms divided by the

See also pp 1539 and 1577.

Context The prevalence of overweight in children and adolescents and obesity in adults in the United States has increased over several decades.

Objective To provide current estimates of the prevalence and trends of overweight in children and adolescents and obesity in adults.

Design, Setting, and Participants Analysis of height and weight measurements from 3958 children and adolescents aged 2 to 19 years and 4431 adults aged 20 years or older obtained in 2003-2004 as part of the National Health and Nutrition Examination Survey (NHANES), a nationally representative sample of the US population. Data from the NHANES obtained in 1999-2000 and in 2001-2002 were compared with data from 2003-2004.

Main Outcome Measures Estimates of the prevalence of overweight in children and adolescents and obesity in adults. Overweight among children and adolescents was defined as at or above the 95th percentile of the sex-specific body mass index (BMI) for age growth charts. Obesity among adults was defined as a BMI of 30 or higher; extreme obesity was defined as a BMI of 40 or higher.

Results In 2003-2004, 17.1% of US children and adolescents were overweight and 32.2% of adults were obese. Tests for trend were significant for male and female children and adolescents, indicating an increase in the prevalence of overweight in female children and adolescents from 13.8% in 1999-2000 to 16.0% in 2003-2004 and an increase in the prevalence of overweight in male children and adolescents from 14.0% to 18.2%. Among men, the prevalence of obesity increased significantly between 1999-2000 (27.5%) and 2003-2004 (31.1%). Among women, no significant increase in obesity was observed between 1999-2000 (33.4%) and 2003-2004 (33.2%). The prevalence of extreme obesity (body mass index ≥40) in 2003-2004 was 2.8% in men and 6.9% in women. In 2003-2004, significant differences in obesity prevalence remained by race/ethnicity and by age. Approximately 30% of non-Hispanic white adults were obese as were 45.0% of non-Hispanic black adults and 36.8% of Mexican Americans. Among adults aged 20 to 39 years, 28.5% were obese while 36.8% of adults aged 40 to 59 years and 31.0% of those aged 60 years or older were obese in 2003-2004.

Conclusions The prevalence of overweight among children and adolescents and obesity among men increased significantly during the 6-year period from 1999 to 2004; among women, no overall increases in the prevalence of obesity were observed. These estimates were based on a 6-year period and suggest that the increases in body weight are continuing in men and in children and adolescents while they may be leveling off in women.

JAMA. 2006;295:1549-1555 www.jama.com

square of height in meters and was rounded to the nearest tenth.

The NHANES 2003-2004 overall response rate (of those originally selected for participation) was 68.6% (4742/6916) for adults aged 20 years or older and 83.2% (4105/4932) for

Author Affiliations: National Center for Health Statistics, Centers for Disease Control and Prevention, Hyattsville, Md (Drs Ogden, Carroll, Curtin, McDowell, Tabak, and Flegal), and Epidemic Intelligence Service, Centers for Disease Control and Prevention, Atlanta, Ga (Dr Tabak).
Corresponding Author: Cynthia L. Ogden, PhD, National Center for Health Statistics, Centers for Disease Control and Prevention, 3311 Toledo Rd, Room 4414, Hyattsville, MD 20782 (Cogden@cdc.gov).

JAMA, April 5, 2006—Vol 295, No. 13 **1549**

Figure 1. Layout of page 1 of a *JAMA* article.

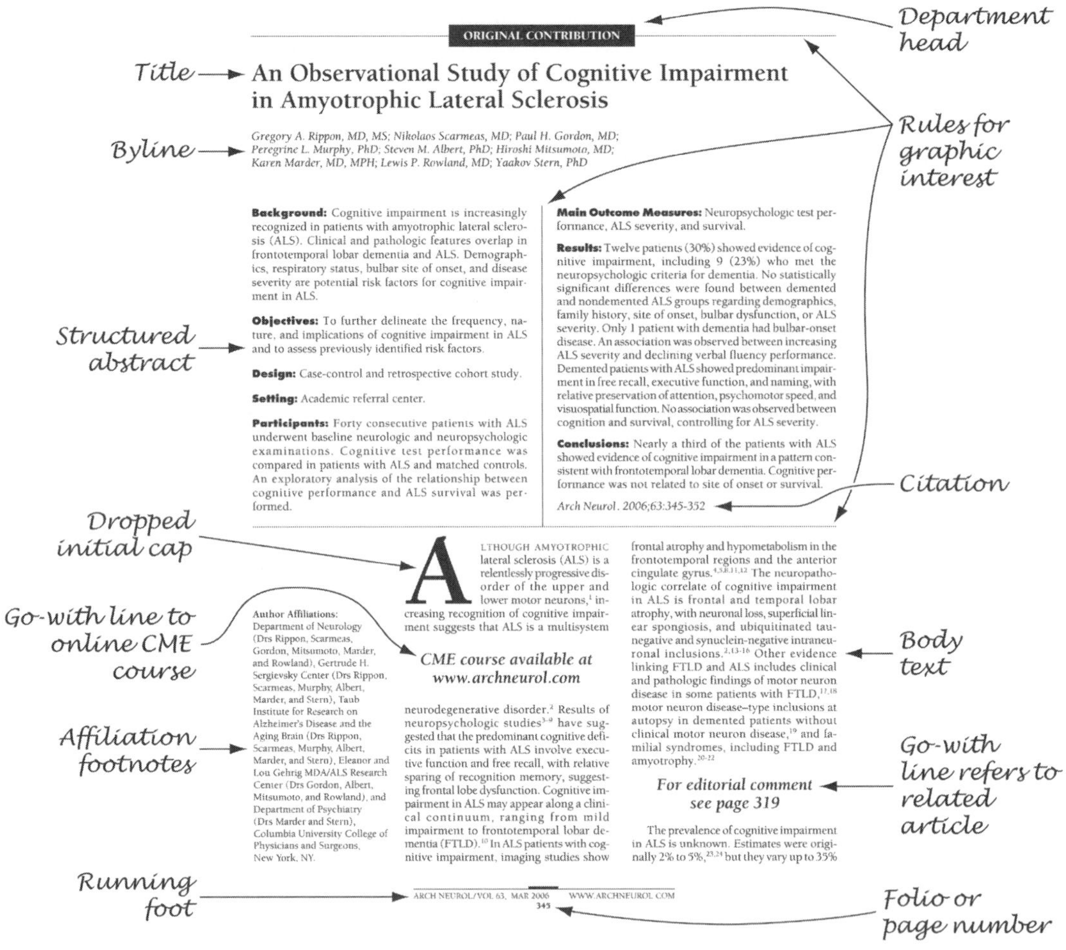

ORIGINAL CONTRIBUTION

An Observational Study of Cognitive Impairment in Amyotrophic Lateral Sclerosis

Gregory A. Rippon, MD, MS; Nikolaos Scarmeas, MD; Paul H. Gordon, MD; Peregrine L. Murphy, PhD; Steven M. Albert, PhD; Hiroshi Mitsumoto, MD; Karen Marder, MD, MPH; Lewis P. Rowland, MD; Yaakov Stern, PhD

Background: Cognitive impairment is increasingly recognized in patients with amyotrophic lateral sclerosis (ALS). Clinical and pathologic features overlap in frontotemporal lobar dementia and ALS. Demographics, respiratory status, bulbar site of onset, and disease severity are potential risk factors for cognitive impairment in ALS.

Objectives: To further delineate the frequency, nature, and implications of cognitive impairment in ALS and to assess previously identified risk factors.

Design: Case-control and retrospective cohort study.

Setting: Academic referral center.

Participants: Forty consecutive patients with ALS underwent baseline neurologic and neuropsychologic examinations. Cognitive test performance was compared in patients with ALS and matched controls. An exploratory analysis of the relationship between cognitive performance and ALS survival was performed.

Main Outcome Measures: Neuropsychologic test performance, ALS severity, and survival.

Results: Twelve patients (30%) showed evidence of cognitive impairment, including 9 (23%) who met the neuropsychologic criteria for dementia. No statistically significant differences were found between demented and nondemented ALS groups regarding demographics, family history, site of onset, bulbar dysfunction, or ALS severity. Only 1 patient with dementia had bulbar-onset disease. An association was observed between increasing ALS severity and declining verbal fluency performance. Demented patients with ALS showed predominant impairment in free recall, executive function, and naming, with relative preservation of attention, psychomotor speed, and visuospatial function. No association was observed between cognition and survival, controlling for ALS severity.

Conclusions: Nearly a third of the patients with ALS showed evidence of cognitive impairment in a pattern consistent with frontotemporal lobar dementia. Cognitive performance was not related to site of onset or survival.

Arch Neurol. 2006;63:345-352

Author Affiliations: Department of Neurology (Drs Rippon, Scarmeas, Gordon, Mitsumoto, Marder, and Rowland), Gertrude H. Sergievsky Center (Drs Rippon, Scarmeas, Murphy, Albert, Marder, and Stern), Taub Institute for Research on Alzheimer's Disease and the Aging Brain (Drs Rippon, Scarmeas, Murphy, Albert, Marder, and Stern), Eleanor and Lou Gehrig MDA/ALS Research Center (Drs Gordon, Albert, Mitsumoto, and Rowland), and Department of Psychiatry (Drs Marder and Stern), Columbia University College of Physicians and Surgeons, New York, NY.

ALTHOUGH AMYOTROPHIC lateral sclerosis (ALS) is a relentlessly progressive disorder of the upper and lower motor neurons,[1] increasing recognition of cognitive impairment suggests that ALS is a multisystem

CME course available at www.archneurol.com

neurodegenerative disorder.[2] Results of neuropsychologic studies[3-9] have suggested that the predominant cognitive deficits in patients with ALS involve executive function and free recall, with relative sparing of recognition memory, suggesting frontal lobe dysfunction. Cognitive impairment in ALS may appear along a clinical continuum, ranging from mild impairment to frontotemporal lobar dementia (FTLD).[10] In ALS patients with cognitive impairment, imaging studies show frontal atrophy and hypometabolism in the frontotemporal regions and the anterior cingulate gyrus.[4,5,8,11,12] The neuropathologic correlate of cognitive impairment in ALS is frontal and temporal lobar atrophy, with neuronal loss, superficial linear spongiosis, and ubiquitinated tau-negative and synuclein-negative intraneuronal inclusions.[2,13-16] Other evidence linking FTLD and ALS includes clinical and pathologic findings of motor neuron disease in some patients with FTLD,[17,18] motor neuron disease–type inclusions at autopsy in demented patients without clinical motor neuron disease,[19] and familial syndromes, including FTLD and amyotrophy.[20-22]

For editorial comment see page 319

The prevalence of cognitive impairment in ALS is unknown. Estimates were originally 2% to 5%,[23,24] but they vary up to 35%

ARCH NEUROL/VOL 63, MAR 2006 WWW.ARCHNEUROL.COM
345

Figure 2. Layout of page 1 of *Archives* Journal article.

22.2 Typefaces, Fonts, and Sizes.

A typeface is a design for a set of characters (eg, Times Roman, Arial). A font of type is the complete assortment of characters, qualities (eg, size, pitch, and spacing), and styles (eg, bold, italics) of a particular typeface (Figure 3). (Note: The term *font* is often used incorrectly as a synonym for *typeface*.)

Times New Roman
Times New Roman Italic
Times New Roman Bold
Times New Roman Bold Italic

Figure 3. A family of type.

The typeface for the body text of this book is ITC Garamond Light, and Frutiger is used for the chapter titles, heads, and subheads.

There are 2 common forms of typeface: serif and sans serif (Figure 4). Serif typefaces (eg, Times Roman) have a short, light line (serif) projecting from a letter's main strokes. Sans serif typefaces (eg, Arial) are unadorned letters without the short line projections. Serif type is generally believed to be more readable than sans serif type for large amounts of print text because serifs on the letters guide the eyes along a line of copy and the modulated thick and thin strokes of serif types help distinguish individual letters and words to be read.[1-3] Thus, for print publications, serif type is generally used for body text because of its readability; sans serif type is used for contrasting and complementary elements and to attract attention (eg, titles, heads).[1-3]

Aa Aa

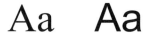

Figure 4. Serif and sans serif letters.

The font for a publication typically includes 7 styles: roman lowercase letters, roman capitals (uppercase letters), boldface capitals, boldface lowercase letters, italic capitals, italic lowercase letters, and small capitals. Each of these styles may also include different weights or heaviness of stroke (eg, light, regular, heavy, black, extra bold, condensed). Each font also includes numerals, punctuation marks, commonly used symbols and diacritical marks (eg, accents, tildes, umlauts), and ligatures and diphthongs (2 or more letters joined together); ligatures (eg, *æ* and *fi*) may be vowels and consonants, whereas diphthongs (eg, *œ*) are vowels only. It is important to note that not all serif and sans serif typefaces share similar characteristics and not all typefaces include all font characteristics. For more discussion on typeface characteristics, see Binghurst's *The Elements of Typographic Style*.[2]

The size of type is conventionally referred to as its point size. The height of characters in a specific font is measured in points; each point is approximately $\frac{1}{72}$ inch, 12 points equals 1 pica, and 6 picas equals 1 inch. The height of a letter in a specific font is measured by its x-height (so named because it is derived from the height of a lowercase *x*). The x-height is the distance between the baseline of a line of type and the top of the main part of the lowercase letter, not including ascenders and descenders. An ascender is the part of a letter that rises above the x-height of the font as seen in the letters *b, d, f, h, k,* and *t.* A descender refers to the part of the letter that dips below the baseline (eg, *p, q, y,* and *Q*) (see Figure 5). The width of a specific character is measured by pitch, which refers to how many characters can fit in an inch.

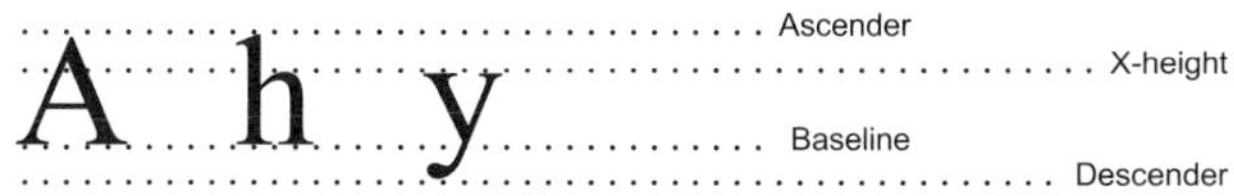

Figure 5. The x-height, ascenders, and descenders of letters.

Typefaces are commonly available and used in 6-point to 72-point sizes. Type sizes below 14 points are generally used for body text, and sizes of 14 points and above are generally used for display types (eg, titles and headlines). Optimal body-text type sizes range between 9 and 12 points.[4] The point size of the body text for this book is 9.75. In Figure 1, the point size of the body text is 10, and the size of the title is 26.

Points are also used to measure the space between lines of type (leading). The pica is used to measure the length of a line and the depth of the type area.

The horizontal spacing of type is measured in *ems*, which is a measure for each size of type whose value varies with size, specifically the size of a lowercase "m." For example, in 9-point type, the em is 9 points; for 12-point type, the em is 12 points.[2] Multiple conventions suggest an optimal number of characters per line for speed and comprehension of reading of journal articles and books and to avoid excessive hyphenation or a page spotted with erratic and distracting white spaces between words (eg, ladders, rivers).[2,4] The optimal number varies according the typeface, type size, column format (eg, 3-, 2-, or 1-column), and publication (journal vs book). One convention suggests that readability is best when 45 to 75 characters (including punctuation and spaces) fit on 1 line of the column.[2] Higher numbers of characters are best suited to single-column designs. For multiple-column formats such as those used in scholarly journals, conventions suggest that 40 to 50 characters per line is ideal or that the column width should accommodate 1½ alphabets (approximately 39 characters) of the typeface per line. In each case, a column width that is too narrow results in excessive hyphenation at line endings, while one that is too wide results in a line too long for the eye to easily complete.

22.3 **Spacing.** Readability of type depends on the spacing between letters, words, and lines; none of these is independent of the others.[2]

22.3.1 **Letterspacing.** Letterspacing refers to the space between letters and other characters. Ideally, the spaces between letters should be balanced. There are no absolute values for optimal letterspacing, but type size and column width are interdependent in design and may affect reading comprehension. Kerning (adjusting the space between characters) is often used to modify spacing between pairs of characters to bring letters closer together or further apart in an attempt to fit words into a defined space (ie, in text that uses justified columns rather than ragged right line ends). Kerning is typically done in units of 1, 2, or 3. The more kerning units used, the closer the letters become. Kerning should be used cautiously to avoid the merging of letters and reducing legibility.[1-3] See Figure 6 for examples of changes in the appearance of a line of type that occur by changing the letterspacing.

No letterspacing
Letterspacing. Note that the typesize

2-Point letterspacing
L e t t e r s p a c i n g . N o t e t h a t t h e t y p e s i z e

4-Point letterspacing
L e t t e r s p a c i n g .   N o t e   t h a t   t h e   t y p e s i z e

Figure 6. Letterspacing.

22.3.2 **Word Spacing.** Typefaces have predetermined spacing between words that is dictated by the point size and width of a typestyle, the darkness or density of the typeface, and the openness or tightness of the letterspacing. For text set ragged right (unjustified), word spacing may be fixed and unchanging. However, for text that is set flush left and flush right (justified), the spacing may need to be more flexible. For justified text, an average word space of a fourth of an em is ideal, with a minimum and maximum range of a fifth of an em to half an em.[2]

22.3.3 **Line Spacing.** Line spacing refers to the vertical distance between the base of 1 line of text and the base of the next line of text. Line spacing is traditionally known as *leading* for the strips of lead once used between lines of printer type. The space between lines of type is measured in points. Generally, leading is 20% larger than the copy size.[3] For example, 10-point copy would be set on 12 points of leading or line spacing (10/12), as is shown for the body copy in Figure 1. Optimal line spacing requires consideration of the type size, layout density, and line length. Generally, longer lines call for increased line spacing for optimal readability. See Figure 7 for different examples of changes in line spacing that change the appearance of the text. More open line spacing also calls for wider margins; tighter line spacing can be done within narrower margins.

No line spacing
Line spacing (or leading). Note that the type size and style are identical in each line; only the space between the lines changes.

1-Point line spacing
Line spacing (or leading). Note that the type size and style are identical in each line; only the space between the lines changes.

2-Point line spacing
Line spacing (or leading). Note that the type size and style are identical in each line; only the space between the lines changes.

Figure 7. Line spacing.

The conventions for letterspacing and word spacing vary depending on the amount of spacing between lines, column width and depth, and whether the text is justified (set as a squared-off block) or unjustified (set with a ragged right margin). For example, a smaller type size may be used on a wider column if the line spacing is adequate for readability. The nature of the composed material will suggest whether variations in typography may be effectively used.

22.4 **Layout.** Layout is the arrangement of all the elements of design and typography on the page for optimal readability, taking into account the context and aesthetic requirements of the text. To create emphasis, complementary typefaces and various fonts within a typeface may be used. However, only a few compatible typefaces should be used at once. Multiple typefaces on a single page can compete for attention, are distracting, and impede readability.[1,3] Two typefaces (a serif for body text and a sans serif for titles and subheads) with appropriate use of styles, such as bold and italics, will most often suffice for a scholarly publication.[3] The typesize and weight create emphasis or continuity, as needed. Headings and subheadings create the outline within the text to frame the article. In page layout for a scholarly journal, all of the elements of design and typography come together. See Figures 1 and 2 for examples. For more details on overall design elements, see resources at the end of this chapter.

Examples of some specific uses of lowercase and capital letters, italic and boldface fonts, and small capital letters are provided in 22.5, Specific Uses of Fonts, with cross-references to other chapters and sections.

22.5 Specific Uses of Fonts

22.5.1 **Lowercase.** Lowercase letters are smaller than capital (or uppercase) letters and are differently configured (eg, a, A). The term *lowercase* originates from the earlier use of manually set wooden or metal characters that were kept by compositors in 2 cases; the lower case contained the smaller letters and the upper case contained the larger capital letters.[1] Sentences are typically set with the initial letter of the first word of a sentence as a capital letter and all other letters lowercase. In titles, the initial letter of each major word is set as a capital letter and all other letters are lowercase. Some publications use sentence-style lowercase for titles, with only the initial letter of the first word being a capital. *JAMA* and the *Archives* Journals use a more traditional mix of initial uppercase and lowercase letters for titles (see also 10.2, Capitalization, Titles and Headings).

> Heterogeneity in Incidence Rates of Schizophrenia and Other Psychotic Syndromes
>
> Depressive Symptoms, Vascular Disease, and Mild Cognitive Impairment: Findings From the Cardiovascular Health Study

The format recommended herein for bibliographic references follows sentence-style lowercase for article titles and mixed capitals and lowercase for book titles (see also 3.9.1, References, Titles, English-Language Titles).

22.5.2 **Capital (Uppercase).** Capital letters are larger than lowercase letters and are used as initial letters in the first word of sentences and for proper names. They are also often used as the initial letter of major words in titles, heads, and subheads. (*Caput* is Latin for head.[1]) Use of all capital letters in large blocks of text should be avoided as legibility is decreased; other ways should be used to add emphasis if needed.[1,3] *JAMA* and the *Archives* Journals use all capital letters sparingly (eg, for level 1 heads).

A *dropped cap* (a form of *initial cap*) is an oversized capital letter of the first word that begins a paragraph and drops through several lines of text. It may be used in a complicated page to draw the reader's attention to the beginning of an article, chapter, or important section (see Figure 1 for an example). An initial cap may also be a raised cap when the capital letter is raised above the main line of text.

22.5.3 **Boldface.** A general scheme of heads and side heads may call for the use of boldface type for first- and second-level heads and for first-level side heads in the text, although heading styles and formats vary among journals (see also 2.8, Manuscript Preparation, Parts of a Manuscript, Headings, Subheadings, and Side Headings). For example:

> **METHODS** (level 1 head, flush left, bold caps)
>
> **Statistical Analysis** (level 2 head, bold caps and lowercase)
>
> **Clustering Data.**—(level 3 head or first-level side head, paragraph indent, run into the text, bold caps and lowercase).

Boldface may also be used in text to call out references to figures or tables.

> Demographic data for the participants in the study are shown in **Table 1**.

22.5.4 Italics. Italics is a form of roman type style that slants to the right. Italics have multiple uses. However, setting large blocks of body text in italics should be avoided because legibility is reduced. Use italics as follows:

- For level 4 heads (second-level side heads)
- When terms are described as terms, and letters as letters (see also 8.6.7, Punctuation, Quotation Marks, Coined Words, Slang, and 8.7.5, Punctuation, Apostrophe, Using Apostrophes to Form Plurals):

  > The page number is called the *folio.*
  > In his handwriting the *n*'s look like *u*'s.

- For titles of books and journals, proceedings, symposia, plays, paintings, long poems, musical compositions, space vehicles, planes, and ships (see also 10.2, Capitalization, Titles and Headings):

  > *Archives of General Psychiatry*
  > USS *Constitution*
  > Verdi's *Requiem*

- For epigraphs set at the beginning of a work (see the beginning of this chapter).
- For some non-English words and phrases (see also 12.2, Non-English Words, Phrases, and Accent Marks, Accent Marks [Diacritics]) that are not shown among English terms in the current edition of *Merriam-Webster's Collegiate Dictionary* or in accepted medical dictionaries. Italics are not used if words or phrases are considered to have become part of the English language, eg, café au lait, in vivo, in vitro, en bloc.
- For lowercase letters used in alphabetic enumerations of items or topics (the parentheses are set roman): (*a*), (*b*), (*c*), etc.
- For genus and species names of some microorganisms, plants, and animals when used in the singular and the names of a variety or subspecies. Plurals, adjectival forms, taxa above genus (eg, class, order, family) are not italicized (see also 15.14, Nomenclature, Organisms and Pathogens):

  > Bacillaceae
  > *Staphylococcus aureus*
  > *Staphylococcus*
  > staphylococci

staphylococcal
Streptococcus (*But:* organisms, streptococcal, streptococci)

- For portions of restriction enzyme terms (see also 15.6.1, Nomenclature, Genetics, Nucleic Acids and Amino Acids)
- For gene symbols but not gene names (see also 15.6.2, Nomenclature, Genetics, Human Gene Nomenclature; 15.6.3, Nomenclature, Genetics, Oncogenes and Tumor Suppressor Genes; and 15.6.5, Nomenclature, Genetics, Nonhuman Genetic Terms)
- For chemical prefixes (*N*-, *cis*-, *trans*-, *p*-, etc) (see also 15.4.4, Nomenclature, Drugs, Chemical Names, and 15.10, Nomenclature, Molecular Medicine)
- For mathematical expressions such as lines, variables, unknown quantities, and constants (see also 21.0, Mathematical Composition). Numerals or abbreviations for trigonometric functions and differentials are not italicized:

  $\sin x = a/b$

- For some statistical terms (see also 20.10, Study Design and Statistics, Statistical Symbols and Abbreviations):

P	*df*	*z*
r	*U*	R^2

- For the abbreviation for acceleration due to gravity, *g*, to distinguish it from g for gram (see also 14.11, Abbreviations, Clinical, Technical, and Other Common Terms)
- For legal cases (see also 3.16, References, US Legal References), eg, *Roe v Wade*
- For the term *sic* (see also Insertions in Quotations in 8.5.2, Punctuation, Parentheses and Brackets, Brackets)
- In formal resolutions, for *Resolved*
- Sparingly, for emphasis

22.5.5 **Small Caps.** In this typeface style, all the letters take the shape of a capital letter. However, in the place of lowercase letters, smaller capital letters are used. The small caps generally, but not always, align with the same x-height as the regular roman face, in the same typeface. Use small capital letters as follows:

- AM and PM in time (see also 18.5.3, Units of Measure, Conventional Units and SI Units in *JAMA* and the *Archives* Journals, Time)
- BC, BCE, CE, and AD (see also 14.3, Abbreviations, Days of the Week, Months, Eras)
- Some prefixes in chemical formulas (L for levo-, D for dextro-) (see also 15.4.4, Nomenclature, Drugs, Chemical Names, and 15.10, Nomenclature, Molecular Medicine)

ACKNOWLEDGMENTS

Principal author: Annette Flanagin, RN, MA

I thank Karen Adams-Taylor and Mary Ellen Johnston, *JAMA* and *Archives* Journals, for reviewing the manuscript and providing important suggestions for improvement; and Chris Meyer, *JAMA* and *Archives* Journals, for creating the figures.

REFERENCES

1. Wheildon C. *Type & Layout: How Typography and Design Can Get Your Message Across—Or Get in the Way*. Berkeley, CA: Strathmore Press; 1995.
2. Binghurst R. *The Elements of Typographic Style*. Version 3.1. Vancouver, BC: Hartley & Marks; 2005.
3. Keane KA. Ten things editors need to know about magazine design. *Editorial Eye*. 2006;29(5):10-11.
4. Goldberg R. *Digital Typography: Practical Advice for Getting the Type You Want When You Want It*. San Diego, CA: Windsor Professional Information LLC; 2000.

ADDITIONAL RESOURCES AND GENERAL REFERENCES

Ambrose G, Harris P. *The Fundamentals of Typography*. Lausanne, Switzerland: AVA Publishing; 2006.

Appendix A: design and production—basic procedures and key terms. In: *The Chicago Manual of Style*. 15th ed. Chicago, IL: University of Chicago Press; 2003:803-856.

Craig J. *Designing With Type*. 5th ed. New York, NY: Watson-Guptill Publishers; 1999.

Felici J. *The Complete Manual of Typography*. Berkley, CA: Peachpit Press; 2005.

Heller S, Meggs PB. *Texts on Type: Critical Writings on Typography*. New York, NY: Allworth Press; 2001.

Lynch PJ, Horton S. *Web Style Guide: Basic Design Principles for Creating Web Sites*. 2nd ed. New Haven, CT: Yale University; 2001. http://www.webstyleguide.com. Accessed June 14, 2006.

Nielsen J, Loranger H. *Prioritizing Web Usability*. Berkeley, CA: New Riders Press; 2006.

Pocket Pal: A Handy Little Book for Graphic Arts Production. 19th ed. Memphis, TN: International Paper Co; 2003.

Typography. In: Kasdorf WE. *The Columbia Guide to Digital Publication*. New York, NY: Columbia University Press; 2003:227-246.

Web Page Design for Designers. http://www.wpdfd.com. Accessed May 27, 2006.

23 Manuscript Editing and Proofreading

23.1

Editing and Proofreading Marks. Corrections often need to be marked on printed manuscripts and typeset copy. The following marks are common in publishing and used by manuscript editors, proofreaders, and others involved in marking copy to be corrected. Instructions, queries, and clarifications not to be typeset should be circled.

Insertion and Deletion

Caret (insert)	^
Close up space	⁀ ‿
Correct typographical error	corre/kt c
Delete	
Delete and close up	
Delete underline	Word
Spell out	(sp)
Stet text (let stand as set)	(stet)

Positioning

Align	|| or =
Break line	└
Center	] [
Flush left	[or (fl)
Hanging indent	[1]]

Justify	→|
Move left	[
Move right	]
Lower	⊔
Raise	⊓
Transpose	∼ (tr)

Punctuation

Period	⊙	
Comma	^,	
Colon	^:	
Semicolon	^;	
Apostrophe	∨'	
Single quotation marks	∨‘	∨’
Double quotation marks	∨“	∨”
Prime sign	∨′	(prime)
Hyphen	=	
Equals sign	=	(equals)
Minus sign	–	(minus)
Plus sign	+	
Plus/minus sign	±	
Em dash	$\frac{1}{M}$	
En dash	$\frac{1}{N}$	
Parentheses	≠(/)≠	
Brackets	≠[/]≠	

Braces	{ / }
Slash	/
Backslash	\
Bullet	• (bullet)

Queries

Query to author	(Au?)
Set when known	(swk)

Spacing

Insert space	(#)
Insert thin space	(thin #)
Equalize space	(eq #)
Indent 1 em space	[1]
Begin a new paragraph	¶
Run in text (no paragraph)	

Style of Type

Wrong font	(wf)
Lowercase	(lc) or Word
Lowercase with initial capitals	(c + lc) an example
Capitalize	(CAP) word
Set roman or regular type (lightface; not bold or italic)	(rom) or (lf)
Set in *italic* type	(ital) word
Set in **boldface** type	(bf) word

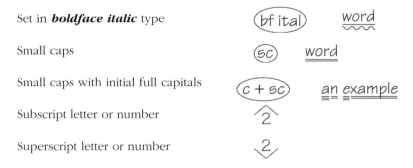

Set in ***boldface italic*** type	(bf ital)	word
Small caps	(sc)	word
Small caps with initial full capitals	(c + sc)	an example
Subscript letter or number	2	
Superscript letter or number	2	

23.2 Proofreading Sample. The following example shows how a proof was marked for corrections and how the corrected text appears in the revised proof.

> Unfortunately, the goal of inducing actual regression of atherosclerosis has remained ellusive. Most atherosclerosis trials have demonstrated that active lipid modulating therapy, primarily using statin drugs, can reduce the rate of disease progression.12-14,19 Two small, single-centre trials have suggested (tr) that statins might induce regression, but methodological issues including small sample size have limited the interpretation and generalization of results.16,17

> Unfortunately, the goal of inducing actual regression of atherosclerosis has remained elusive. Most atherosclerosis trials have demonstrated that active lipid-modulating therapy, primarily using statin drugs, can reduce the rate of disease progression.[12-14,19] Two small, single-center trials have suggested that statins might induce regression, but methodological issues including small sample size have limited the interpretation and generalization of results.[16,17]

23.3 Electronic Text Editing. Many word processing programs have text editing functionality that allows users to view edits and track changes. It is common for insertions to be underlined and deletions to be struck through. Each program offers tools to show or hide the editing marks, notes about formatting, and embedded comments. How reviewers respond to the editing depends not only on the word processing program but also on the technologies and workflow involved. For example, manuscript editors at *JAMA* send authors edited manuscripts as PDF files showing text insertions and deletions as well as embedded comments and questions. Authors can respond by using advanced editing tools directly on the PDF, by printing out and marking up the copy and returning via fax, or by outlining corrections and query answers in an e-mail message.

When manuscript editing is performed electronically, often the editor inserts codes into the electronic file that allow the file to be automatically typeset for initial placement of elements (eg, title, abstract, text, tables, figures, reference list). The coding also allows the content to undergo conversion to another language (eg, HTML or SGML) for publication online. These codes may or may not appear on the edited typescript. The examples below illustrate the same passage of text with the codes hidden and then revealed after the file is run through a process to convert the text to XML code:

In a large cohort of consecutive patients undergoing drug-eluting stent implantation, we noted a 9-month cumulative stent thrombosis incidence of 1.3%, substantially higher than rates reported in major clinical trials (0.4% at 1 year for sirolimus and 0.6% at 9 months for paclitaxel).[3,5] With widespread availability of drug-eluting stents, the scope of percutaneous coronary intervention has been expanded to more complex lesions and patients. In our study, 26% of the population had diabetes and 78% of the lesions were complex. The clinical consequences of stent thrombosis were severe, with a case-fatality rate of 45%.

```
<para>In a large cohort of consecutive patients undergoing
drug-eluting stent implantation, we noted a 9-month
cumulative stent thrombosis incidence of 1.3%, substan-
tially higher than rates reported in major clinical trials
(0.4% at 1 year for sirolimus and 0.6% at 9 months for
paclitaxel).<reflink idref="ref-jbr50003-3 ref-jbr50003-
5"/> With widespread availability of drug-eluting stents,
the scope of percutaneous coronary intervention has been
expanded to more complex lesions and patients. In our
study, 26% of the population had diabetes and 78% of the
lesions were complex. The clinical consequences of stent
thrombosis were severe, with a case-fatality rate of
45%.</para>
```

The examples below illustrate the coding/tagging behind an edited, linked *JAMA* reference. The first paragraph is what the author would see; the second illustrates all the codes behind the tagging.

<jrn>1. Iakovou I, Schmidt T, Bonizzoni E, et al. Incidence, predictors, and outcome of thrombosis after successful implantation of drug-eluting stents. *JAMA*. 2005;293(17):2126-2130. Medline:15870416</jrn>

<refitem id="ref-jle50384-1"><author><first>I</first><last>Iakovou </last></author><author><first>T</first><last>Schmidt</last> </author><author><first>E</first><last>Bonizzoni</last> </author><etal></etal><title>Incidence, predictors, and outcome of thrombosis after successful implantation of drug-eluting stents. </title><jrnlname>JAMA</jrnlname><refcitation><year>2005 </year><volume>293</volume><issueno>17</issueno><fpage>2126 </fpage><lpage>2130</lpage></refcitation><pmid>15870416 </pmid></refitem>

ACKNOWLEDGMENT

Principal author: Stacy Christiansen, MA

24 Glossary of Publishing Terms

This glossary is intended to define terms commonly encountered during editing and publishing as well as those industry terms that also have a more common vernacular meaning. The glossary is not all-inclusive. New terms and new usage of existing terms will emerge with time and advances in technology. Definitions for the terms herein were compiled from the ninth edition of this manual and the sources listed at the end of the chapter. Terms used in definitions that are defined elsewhere in this glossary are shown in a *different font.*

AA: Author's alteration; a change or correction made by an author; used in correcting proofs (compare *EA* and *PE*).

access: The ability to locate specific information in a body of stored data. Data stored on magnetic tape are accessed sequentially; data stored on *disc* may be randomly accessed.

acid-free paper: Paper made by alkaline *sizing*, a treatment that improves the paper's resistance to liquid and vapor and improves the paper's permanence.

advertorial: Promotional or advertising content that has the appearance of editorial content (see 5.12.3, Ethical and Legal Considerations, Advertisements, Advertorials, Supplements, Reprints, and E-prints).

against the grain: See *grain direction*.

AI: Native file format of Illustrator (Adobe).

align: To place *text* and/or graphics to line up horizontally or vertically with related elements.

alphanumeric: Letters, numbers, and symbols used as a code, eg, for a computer command.

ANSI: Acronym for American National Standards Institute, Inc.

API: Abbreviation for application program (or programming) interface, a set of routines, protocols, and tools for building *software applications*. A good API makes it easier to develop a program by providing all the building blocks. A programmer puts the blocks together.

application: A computer *program* that enables the user to perform a specific task, eg, *word processor, Web browsers*, graphic tools.

archive: To copy files from a long-term storage unit for backup purposes.

art repair, art rebuilding: Replacing text, symbols, arrows, and lines on *line art* to produce illustrations that are consistent in format, type, and size.

artwork: Illustrative material, such as photographs, drawings, and graphs, intended for reproduction (see 4.0, Visual Presentation of Data).

ascender: The part of lowercase letters, such as d, f, h, and k, that extends above the midportion or ***x-height*** of the letter (compare ***descender***).

ASCII: Acronym for American Standard Code for Information Interchange (pronounced [ask-ee]); a code representing an alphanumeric group of characters that is recognized by most computers and computer ***programs.***

ASCII file: A computer file containing only ***ASCII***-coded text.

ASTM: Abbreviation for American Society for Testing and Materials.

author's editor: An ***editor*** who substantially edits an author's ***manuscript*** and prepares it to meet the requirements for publication in a particular journal.

backstrip: A strip of paper affixed to the bound edges of paper that form a journal's spine.

back up (v), backup (n): Saving copies of digital files on ***disk***, tape, or other medium; a duplicate file or disk.

bad break: A poor or potentially confusing arrangement of type at the end of a line or the bottom or top of a page or column. Examples include a paragraph ending with 1 or 2 words at the top of a page or column (see ***widow***) or the first line of a paragraph starting at the bottom of a page or column (see ***orphan***), a heading falling on the last line of a page or column, an improperly hyphenated word or acronym, or the second part of a properly hyphenated word starting a page.

bandwidth: The capacity of a communication system in transferring data.

banner: The rectangular graphic at the top of a Web page. Also, in advertising, a banner ad is typically a rectangular advertisement placed on a Web site either above or below (or on the sides of) the site's main content and may be linked to the advertiser's own Web site. Vertical ads are also called towers or skyscrapers.

baseline: The imaginary line on which the letters in a line of ***type*** appear to rest.

basis weight: The weight of paper determined by the weight in pounds of a ream (500 sheets) of paper cut to a standard size for a specific grade. For example, 500 sheets, 25×38 in, of 80-lb coated paper will weigh 80 lb.

baud rate: In telecommunications and electronics, the signaling rate; a baud is the number of changes to the transmission media per second in a modulated signal.

BBS: Abbreviation for bulletin board system.

binary system: A system of numbers using only the digits 1 and 0 for all values; it is the basis for digital computers.

binding: (1) The process by which printed units or pages are attached to form a book, journal, or pamphlet, including operations such as folding, collating, stitching, or gluing (see also ***loose-leaf binding***, ***perfect binding***, ***saddle-stitch binding***, and ***selective binding***). (2) The cover and spine of a book or journal.

BinHex: Coding format that converts binary data into ***ASCII*** characters.

bit: A binary digit, either 0 or 1; the smallest unit of digital information.

bitmap (bmp): Also called *raster* graphic image or digital image, a data file or structure representing a generally rectangular grid of pixels, or points of color, on a computer monitor, paper, or other display device (see also ***tag, tagged***, and *TIFF*); also, the file format built into Windows and native to Microsoft Paint; supports 1- to 24-bit depth and index color.

bitmap fonts: Low-resolution fonts designed for computer screens, whose characters are represented by *bitmaps* or by a pattern of dots.

black: One of the 4 *process printing colors* (see *CMYK*).

blanket: A fabric coated with rubber or other material that is clamped around a printing cylinder to transfer ink from the *press plate* to the paper (see also *offset printing*).

bleed: A printed image that runs off the edge of a printed page. A partial bleed extends above, below, or to the side of the established print area but does not continue off the page (see also *live area*).

blind folio: A page number counted but not printed on the page (see *folio*).

blind image: An image that fails to print because of ink receptivity error.

blog: Abbreviation for weblog. A weblog is a journal-style Web site that is frequently updated and intended for general public consumption. Blogs generally represent the personality of the author.

blueline(s): The *proof* sheet(s) of a book or magazine printed in blue ink that shows exactly how the pages will look when they are printed.

blueprint, blackprint: A photoprint made from film that is used to check position and relative arrangement of text and image elements.

body type: The type characteristics used for the main body text of a work.

boilerplate: A section of text that can be reused without changes.

boldface (bf): A *typeface* that is heavier and darker than the text face used (see 22.0, Typography).

bot: A computer *program* that automates tasks. See also *spider[ing]*.

bouncing reject: A rejected manuscript that is returned to the editorial office with request for reconsideration (see 5.11.5, Ethical and Legal Considerations, Editorial Responsibilities, Roles, Procedures, and Policies, Editorial Responsibility for Rejection).

bps: Abbreviation for bits per second. A measurement of the speed with which data travel from one place to another (compare *baud rate*).

broadside: Printed text or illustrations positioned on the length rather than the width of the page, requiring the reader to turn the publication on its side to read it; usually used for tables and figures that are wider than the normal width of a publication.

browser: See *Web browser*.

bug: Something that causes an error in computer software or hardware (see also *virus*).

bullet: An aligned dot of a heavy weight (•) used to highlight individual elements in a list (see ***centered dot***).

byline: A line of text at the beginning of an article listing the authors' names (compare ***signature*** [2]) (see 2.2, Manuscript Preparation, Bylines and End-of-Text Signatures, and 5.1.1, Ethical and Legal Considerations, Authorship Responsibility, Authorship: Definition, Criteria, Contributions, and Requirements).

byte: A unit of digital information that can code for a single alphanumeric symbol; 1 byte equals 8 to 64 ***bits***.

CAD: Abbreviation for computer-aided design or computer-assisted design.

calibrate: To adjust a device such as a ***scanner*** or a ***monitor, image setter***, or printing press to more precisely reproduce color.

caliper: Thickness of paper or film measured in terms of thousandths of an inch (mils or points); also the tool used to measure the thickness of paper.

call-outs: Quotes of reprinted text, usually bolder and larger than that of the original text, used to place emphasis, improve design, or fill ***white space***. Also called pullout quotes.

camera-ready: Copy, including artwork and text, that is ready to be photographed for reproduction without further composition or alteration.

CAP: (1) Abbreviation for computer-aided publishing or computer-assisted publishing. (2) As a proofreading or editing mark, short for capital letter.

caption: The text accompanying an illustration or photograph. See also ***legend*** and 4.0, Visual Presentation of Data.

CAR: Abbreviation for computer-assisted reading.

case: The ***cover*** of a hardbound book (see also ***lowercase*** and ***uppercase***).

CD: Abbreviation for compact (or computer) ***disc*** containing data or used for storing data.

CDI: Abbreviation for interactive ***compact disc*** containing data.

CD-ROM: Acronym for compact (or computer) ***disc***, read-only memory; a ***compact disc*** containing data that can be read by a computer. Many CD-ROMs are interactive and have sound, graphics, and video.

cell: In tables or spreadsheets, a unit in an array formed by the intersection of a column and a row; in computer terminology, a basic subdivision of a memory that can hold 1 unit of a computer's basic operating data (see also 4.0, Visual Presentation of Data).

centered dot: A heavy dot (•) used to highlight individual elements in a list (see ***bullet***). Also, a lighter centered dot (·) is used in mathematical composition to signify multiplication and in chemical formulas to indicate hydration.

central processing unit (CPU): The component in a digital computer that interprets instructions and processes data contained in ***software***.

CEPS: Acronym for color electronic prepress systems; electronic color equipment used to perform electronic retouching, cloning, and pagination.

character: A letter, numeral, symbol, or punctuation mark.

character count: The process of estimating the amount of space that typed or computer-printed copy will occupy on a published page. A manual character count is made by counting the number of ***characters*** and spaces in an average line of the manuscript, multiplying that number by the number of lines on the ***manuscript*** page, and multiplying that number by the total number of manuscript pages. Most word-processing programs will provide an exact character count and word count.

circulation: The total number of print copies of a publication sold and distributed (see also ***controlled circulation***).

citation analysis: An analysis of the number of times a published article is cited in the reference list of subsequently published articles (see also ***impact factor***).

CMYK: Abbreviation for the 4 ***process printing colors***: cyan, magenta, yellow, and black. See also ***four-color process***.

codes: Combinations of letters, numbers, and symbols entered through a ***keyboard*** that instruct a computer how to format and compose a document or file (see also ***tag*** and ***tagged***).

colophon: A summary of information about the publication or the publication's production methods or specifications; also the publisher's emblem or trademark (see also ***masthead***).

color breaks: Separating elements of a piece of ***artwork*** that will print in more than 1 color. A second or third color ***proof*** may be attached to a black proof to show the color screen on artwork.

color correct: To change the color values in a set of film separations or, using a ***software application***, to correct or compensate for errors in photography, scanning, ***separation***, and output.

color proofs: Photomechanical or digital representations of color.

color separation: The process of separating artwork into component films of cyan, magenta, yellow, and black in preparation for printing (see also ***CMYK***).

compatible: A term describing an environment in which one computer will accept and process data from another computer without conversion of code modifications; also a term describing the ability to use ***hardware*** and ***software*** together on one computer platform.

compilation: A section of a publication that is made up of a group of items, eg, letters or book reviews that are run together with more than 1 per page.

composite figure: A figure that is composed of more than 1 type of element (eg, ***halftone***, ***line art***, 4-color).

composition: The arrangement of ***type*** and typographic characteristics for printing.

compression: A computer technique of eliminating redundant information, such as blank lines from a document or ***white space*** from an image, to reduce the file size for faster transmission or more compact storage of data. See also ***lossy***, ***nonlossy***, and ***LZW compression***.

computer-assisted composition: A process in which text in digital form is recorded on a magnetic medium (magnetic tape, hard disk, ***diskette***, optical drive) and processed through a set of typesetting parameters stored in a computer that dictate the ***type*** size and ***font***, hyphenation and justification, character and word spacing, and all typographical requirements needed to typeset the text. The data stream created from this process is used to drive an image setter for typesetting and printing a page of text.

condensed type: A narrow version of a ***typeface***, designed to fit more text on each line (see 22.0, Typography).

content management system (CMS): ***Software*** that enables management and editing of content on a Web site.

context-sensitive editor: A ***software program*** that uses document structure to determine which elements are appropriate to insert in a particular context within a document (eg, ***XML*** and ***SGML*** editor).

continuous tone: An image that has gradations of tone from dark to light, in contrast to an image formed of pure blacks and whites, such as a pen-and-ink drawing or a page of type (see also ***halftone*** and ***duotone***).

controlled circulation: Copies of a publication distributed to a select list of recipients without charge (see also ***circulation***).

cookie: Message given to a ***Web browser*** by a ***Web server*** to identify users.

copy: Any matter, including a manuscript in handwritten, ***typescript***, or digital format, ***artwork***, photographs, tables, and figures, to be set or reproduced for printing (see also ***hard copy***).

copy editor: An ***editor*** who prepares a document or other copy for publication, making alterations and corrections to ensure accuracy, consistency, and uniformity. Also called ***manuscript editor***.

copy fitting: Estimating the space required to print a given amount of ***copy*** in a specific ***type*** size, ***typeface***, and format. The number of ***characters*** in the manuscript is estimated and divided by the number of characters per ***pica*** for the typeface and type size to be used in the published version; this number is divided by the number of picas of the typeset line, and then by the number of lines of type per page. The result is an estimate of the number of published pages the manuscript will occupy (see also ***character count***).

copyright: The law protecting an author's or publisher's rights to published and unpublished works (see 5.6.3, Ethical and Legal Considerations, Intellectual Property: Ownership, Access, Rights, and Management, Copyright: Definition, History, and Current Law).

corrupted: Refers to data that have been damaged in some way.

cover: The front and back pages of a publication. The 4 pages making up the covers in a publication are often designated covers 1, 2, 3, and 4. Covers 1 and 4 are outside pages, and covers 2 and 3 are inside pages.

cover stock: Paper used for the ***cover***, usually heavier than the paper used for the body of the publication.

CPI: Abbreviation for characters per inch.

CPU: Abbreviation for ***central processing unit***.

crawl, Web crawler : See ***spider[ing]***.

crop: To trim a photograph or illustration to fit a design or to cut off unwanted portions.

crop marks: Lines placed on the sides, top, and bottom of a photograph or illustration indicating the size or area of the image to be reproduced.

CTP: Abbreviation for computer-to-plate; a printing process that transmits a digital image directly from a computer file to a plate used on a press, eliminating the need for film or negatives.

cursor: An on-screen indicator, such as a blinking line, arrow, hollow square, or other image (usually ***mouse*** or keystroke driven), that marks a designated place on the screen and indicates current point of data entry or modification, menu selection, or program function.

cyan: One of the 4 ***process printing colors*** (cyan, magenta, yellow, and black); a shade of blue (see ***CMYK***).

data: Factual information (eg, measurements) used in calculation, analysis, and discussion; information in digital form that can be organized, manipulated, stored, and transmitted.

data bank: A compilation of information stored in a computer for retrieval and use.

database: A collection of stored data from which information can be extracted and organized in various forms and formats, usually for rapid search and retrieval.

debug: To trace and correct errors in a computer ***program***.

demand printing: A part of the publishing industry that creates short-run, customized print publications quickly and on individual request.

demographic versions: Different versions of an issue of a publication containing specific inserts targeted for specific readers; the inserts are usually advertisements.

descender: The part of such letters as p, q, and y that extends below the main body of the letter or ***baseline*** (compare ***ascender*** and see ***x-height***).

desktop color separation: A computer file format that separates an ***EPS*** (***encapsulated PostScript***) color file into the 4 color elements: cyan, magenta, yellow, and black.

desktop publishing (DTP): A microcomputer-based publishing system consisting of a computer, pagination software, ***scanner***, and output device.

digital asset management (DAM): A centralized system for archiving, searching, and retrieving digital files and associated ***metadata***. Also known as enterprise digital asset management, media asset management, or digital asset warehousing.

digitize: To transform a printed character or image into bits or binary digits, so that it can be entered into and manipulated in a computer.

disc, disk: A circular plate coated with a magnetic substance and used for the storage and retrieval of data (see 11.0, Correct and Preferred Usage).

diskette: Another term for a ***disc*** used for storage of information, usually in personal computers.

display type: Type that differs from the ***body type*** of the text of a printed work. Display faces are used in titles, headings, and subheadings and are usually larger than the body type.

doc: Microsoft Word file format and extension (.doc).

document: Organized coherent information in written, printed, or digital format.

document delivery: A service that allows users to search online databases of indexes and tables of contents to identify articles and request copies of those articles to be delivered by mail, by fax, or online.

DOI: Abbreviation for digital object identifier, a means of identifying a ***WWW*** file or ***Internet*** document. A DOI provides a means of persistently identifying a piece of intellectual property on a digital network and associating it with related current data in a structured extensible way.

domain: An ***Internet*** location, and the last part of an ***e-mail*** address indicating the type of business, eg, .com, .net, .edu, .org, .mil, .gov, or letters that indicate a country, eg, .ca, .uk, .fr.

domain name: The name that identifies an ***Internet*** site. Domain names have 2 or more parts (following www.), separated by dots. The part on the left is more specific, and the part on the right is more general, eg, Oxford University Press' domain name is www.oup.co.uk.

DOS: Abbreviation for disk operating system (pronounced [doss]); operating system used by most PC-compatible computers and workstations.

dot: In a ***halftone***, an individual printing element or spot (see also ***dot gain*** and ***dots per inch***).

dot gain: A printing defect that causes dots to print larger than they should, resulting in darker tone and color than intended.

dot matrix printer: A printer that produces ***hard copy*** from a series of wires (pins) that strike against an ink source. The dots created form ***characters***. Quality varies; manuscripts printed on dot matrix printers may not be easily read by some optical scanners for typesetting because the spaces between the dots create an uneven structure (see also ***ink-jet printer, laser printer***, and ***line printer***).

dots per inch (DPI): A measure of the resolution of a printed image (also called spots per inch).

double spread: Printed material (text, tables, illustrations) that extends across 2 pages (left- and right-hand pages); also called a spread or a 2-page spread.

download: The process of transferring digital files from a remote computer to a local computer.

DPI: Abbreviation for ***dots per inch***.

drive: The computer ***hardware***, consisting of the motor, read/write heads, and electronics, that is used with a ***disc***.

DRM: Abbreviation for digital rights management, a system used to protect the copyrights of data distributed or accessed via the ***Internet*** or other digital media. A DRM system protects intellectual property by encrypting the data or marking the content with a digital ***watermark*** so that the content cannot be distributed.

drop cap, dropped cap: The initial letter of a word (usually beginning a ***paragraph***) set in ***boldface***, larger than the body text (see also ***initial***).

drop folio: A page number printed at the bottom of the page (see ***folio***).

DSL: Digital subscriber line that provides an extremely high-speed ***Internet*** connection with the same wires as a regular telephone line.

DSSSL: Abbreviation for document style semantics and specification language; an output ***specification*** standard used with ***SGML***-coded documents and a ***DTD*** to drive a ***typesetter*** or printer.

DTD: Abbreviation for document type definition, which defines the structure of content (ie, journals or books) with a list of elements (ie, title, author, abstract, paragraphs). The DTD is the blueprint for ***SGML*** and ***XML*** documents.

dummy: A layout of a page or an entire journal, to represent the size and appearance after printing.

duotone: A 2-color ***halftone*** reproduction from a black-and-white photograph; usually reproduced in black and 1 other color.

DVD: Abbreviation for digital versatile disc or digital video disc. An optical disc storage media format that can be used for data storage, including movies with high video and sound quality. DVDs resemble compact discs, as their physical dimensions are the same, but they are encoded in a different format and at a much higher density.

EA: Abbreviation for editor's alteration or correction (compare ***AA*** and ***PE***).

e-commerce: Electronic commerce; business that is conducted over the ***Internet*** using any of the applications that rely on the Internet. e-Commerce can be a transaction between 2 businesses, or between a business and a customer.

editor: (1) Someone who directs a publication or heads an editorial staff and/or decides on the acceptability of a document for publication (eg, editor, editor in chief); manages a publication (eg, managing editor); prepares a document for publication by altering, adapting, and refining it (eg, manuscript editor, ***copy editor, author's editor***). (2) In computer terminology, a program used to create text files or make changes to an existing file. Text or full-screen editors allow users to move through a document with direction keys, keystrokes, and a ***mouse***- or command-driven ***cursor***. Line editors allow the user to view the document as a series of numbered lines (see also ***context-sensitive editor*** and ***SGML editor***).

editorial: (1) Of or relating to an ***editor*** or editing. (2) A written expression of opinion that may or may not reflect the official position of the publication. (3) Published material that is not promotional (eg, not an advertisement).

editorial assistant: One who assists in the editorial procedures and processes of editing and publishing.

e-journal: Electronic journal; a journal published in digital format (eg, on the *World Wide Web* or *CD-ROM*) that is accessed via a computer.

elite type: Typewriter type that equals 12 characters to the inch (see also *pica type*).

ellipsis: A series of 3 periods (. . .) used to indicate an omission or that data are not available.

em: A measurement used to specify to the typesetter the amount of space desired for indention, usually equal to the square body of the type size (eg, a 6-point em is 6 points wide).

e-mail: Electronic mail; an online system that allows people to send messages to each other through their computers.

em dash: A punctuation mark (—) used to indicate an interruption or break in thought in a sentence; also used after introductory clauses and before closing clauses or designations (compare *en dash* and see 8.3, Punctuation, Hyphens and Dashes).

EMF: Abbreviation for Enhanced MetaFile, the 32-*bit* file format created by Microsoft Windows.

emulsification: A condition in offset printing that results from a mixing of the water-based fountain solution and oil-based ink on the press (see also *fountain*).

emulsion side: The side of a photographic film to which a chemical coating is applied and on which the image is developed.

en: Half an em (see also *em*).

enamel: The surface of shiny, coated paper.

en dash: A punctuation mark (–) (longer than a hyphen and half the length of an em dash) used in hyphenated or compound modifiers (compare *em dash* and see 8.3, Punctuation, Hyphens and Dashes).

end mark: A symbol, such as a dash (—) or an open square (□), to indicate the end of an article; often used in news stories.

EPS (encapsulated PostScript): A graphics file format. An EPS file is a PostScript file that satisfies additional restrictions for high-resolution graphics. These restrictions are intended to make it easier for software to embed an EPS file within another PostScript document.

e-publication: Electronic publication; a work published in digital format (eg, online, CD-ROM) that is accessed via a computer.

ethernet: A method of networking computers in a local area network (*LAN*).

expanded type: Type in which the characters are wider than normal (see 22.0, Typography).

export: To convert and transfer data from one *application* into another application (compare *import*).

extensible markup language: See *XML*.

face: *Typeface*; style of type (see also *font*).

F&G: Abbreviation for folded and gathered ***signatures*** of a publication for final review before publication.

FAQs: Acronym for frequently asked questions; often used by Web site and home page designers to help users access and search for information and resolve common problems.

fax: Short for facsimile; transmission of printed or digitized material through telephone lines.

figure: An illustration, eg, photograph, drawing, graph (see 4.0, Visual Presentation of Data).

file: A collection of related, digitally stored information that is recognized as a unit by a computer.

filler: (1) Editorial content used to fill ***white space*** created by articles or advertisements not filling an entire page. (2) Chemicals used to fill the spaces between fibers in paper to improve the paper's opacity.

finish: The surface of paper.

firewall: In computer terminology, a security ***software program*** or device that blocks or restricts entry into a local area network from the ***Internet***.

floppy disk: A flexible ***disc*** coated with magnetically sensitive material used for temporary storage of information, usually used with personal computers (see also ***diskette***).

flush: Lines of type aligned vertically along the left ***margin*** (flush left) or the right margin (flush right).

flush and hang: To set the first line ***flush*** left on the ***margin*** and indent the remaining lines.

flyleaf: Any blank page at the front or back of a book.

folio: A page number placed at the bottom or top of a printed page (see also ***drop folio*** and ***blind folio***).

font: The complete assortment of qualities (eg, size, pitch, and spacing) and styles (eg, ***boldface, italic***, etc) of a particular ***typeface*** (see 22.0, Typography).

foot: The bottom of a page (compare ***head***).

footer: See *running foot.*

form, press form: A group of assembled pages (usually 8, 12, 16, or 32 pages), printed at the same time, then folded into consecutively numbered pages (see also ***signature***).

format: The shape, size, style, ***margins***, type, and design of a publication.

FOSI: Acronym for formatted output specification instance (pronounced [foss-ee]). FOSI is a style sheet language for ***SGML*** and ***XML*** (see also ***specifications*** and ***DTD***).

fountain: In offset (lithographic) printing, the part of the press that contains the dampening device and solution (usually water, buffered acid, gum, and alcohol); in nonoffset printing, the part of the press that contains the ink.

four-color process: See *CMYK*.

FPO: Abbreviation meaning for position only; refers to low-resolution graphics used in place of high-resolution graphics to show placement of *artwork* and photographs before printing.

FPS: Abbreviation for frames per second.

FTP: Abbreviation for file transfer protocol. A method for exchanging files between computers on the *Internet*.

function key: A key on a computer *keyboard* that gives an instruction to the machine or computer, as opposed to the keys for letters, numbers, and punctuation marks; often labeled F (eg, F1, F2).

galley proof: A proof of typeset text copy run 1 column wide before being made into a page.

gatefold: A foldout page.

GB: Abbreviation for gigabyte; a unit of computer storage, equal to approximately 1 billion *bytes*.

Gbps: Abbreviation for billions of bits per second; when spelled GBps, it means *gigabytes* per second.

ghost author: An author who meets all criteria for authorship but is not named in the byline of a publication (see 5.1.2, Ethical and Legal Considerations, Authorship Responsibility, Guest and Ghost Authors).

ghosting: Shadows produced by uneven ink coverage (variations are caused by wide contrasts in the colors or tones being printed).

GIF (.gif): Acronym for graphics interchange format. A compressed graphic file normally used for images (eg, logos, cartoons) that do not require many colors (maximum, 256).

gigabyte: See *GB*.

glossy: A photograph or *line art* printed on smooth, shiny paper that traditionally has been required by some publishers for print reproduction.

gopher: An online *Web browser* that allows a user to locate online addresses and topics in text-only format (no graphics).

gradation: A transition of shades between black and white, between one color and another, or between one color and white.

grain direction: The direction of the fibers in a sheet of paper created when the paper is made.

granularity: The level of specificity with which parts of a digital document are identified by a *context-sensitive editor*.

graphical user interface (GUI): Pronounced [goo-ee]; a computer display format that allows the user to select commands, run programs, and view lists of files and other options by pointing a cursor to icons or menus (text lists) of items on the screen.

gray scale: A range of grays with gradations from white to black. A gray-scale image contains various shades of gray.

greeking: (1) A simulation of a reduced-size page used by word-processing *applications* during the print preview function because it is usually not possible to shrink text size in proportion to the page size. The graphic symbols used to represent text resemble Greek letters; hence the term *greeking*. Also called Lorem ipsum, or lipsum. (2) Refers to nonsense text or gray bars inserted in a page to check the layout.

gutter: The 2 inner margins of facing pages of a publication, from printed area to binding.

hairline: The thinnest stroke of a *character*.

hairline rule: A thin rule, usually measuring one-half *point*.

halftone: A black-and-white continuous-tone *artwork*, such as a photograph, that has shades of gray (see also *duotone* and 4.0, Visual Presentation of Data).

halftone screen: A grid used in the halftone process to break the image into dots. The fineness of the screen is denoted in terms of lines per inch (eg, 120, 133, 150).

H&J: Abbreviation for hyphenation and justification; the determination of line breaks and the division of words into lines of prescribed measurement (see *justify*).

handwork: Extra work the printer does by hand, such as stripping in type or making part of a page opaque.

hard copy: Printed copy, in contrast to copy stored in digital format.

hardware: Machinery, circuitry, and other physical entities (compare *software*).

head: The top of a page (compare *foot*).

header: See *running head*.

head margin: Top *margin* of a page.

home page: The first screen a user views when connecting to a specific site on the Web.

HTML: Abbreviation for hypertext markup language; *codes* (*tags*) used to prepare a file containing both text and graphics for placement on the *Internet* via the Web.

http: Abbreviation for hypertext transfer protocol; a computer connection used at the beginning of a Web address to connect with a Web site and transfer information and graphics across the Web.

https: Abbreviation for hypertext transfer protocol, secure. This protocol is used for performing financial and other types of transactions that require secure transmission of information.

hyperlink: (v) The nonlinear relating of information, images, and sounds that allows a computer user to jump quickly from one topic, item, or representation to another by clicking a mouse-driven *cursor* on a highlighted word or *icon*; (n) the highlighted word or icon.

icon: A small graphic image, usually a visual mnemonic, displayed on a computer screen, easily manipulated by the user, that represents common computer commands (eg, a trash can may represent a command for deleting unwanted text or files).

image setter: A device that plots an array of *dots* or *pixels* onto photosensitive material (film) line by line, until an entire page is created (including text, graphics, and color). The film can be output as a negative or positive with resolutions from 300 to 3000 *dots per inch*.

impact factor: A measure of the frequency with which the average article in a journal has been cited in a particular year. It helps to evaluate a journal's relative importance when compared with others in the same field. The impact factor is calculated by dividing the number of current citations to all articles published in the 2 previous years by the total number of "countable" articles published in those 2 years (see also *citation analysis*).

import: Using data produced by one *application* in another, eg, importing data from a spreadsheet and using it to produce a report in a word-processing document (compare *export*).

imposition: The process of arranging pages or press *forms* of a publication so that the pages will be in sequential order when printed, folded, and bound into a publication; a guide or list showing the sequential order of pages.

impression: The transfer of an ink image by pressure from *type*, *plate*, or *blanket* to paper. The speed of a sheet-fed printing press is measured by the number of impressions printed per hour.

imprint: The name of the publishing house or entity that issues a book; the imprint is typically found at the bottom of the title page. It may or may not be the same as the name of the publishing company, and a publishing company may have various imprints.

indent: To set a line of type or paragraph in from the *margin* or margins (see 22.0, Typography).

inferior: See *subscript*.

initial: A large letter, the first letter of a word used to begin a paragraph, chapter, or section. A "sunken" or "dropped" initial cuts 2 or 3 lines down into the text; a "stickup" initial aligns at the bottom with the first line of text and sticks up into the *white space* above (see also *dropped cap*).

ink fountain: Device on the press that supplies the ink to the inking rollers.

ink-jet printer: A device by which ink is forced through a series of nozzles onto paper, commonly used with personal computers. This method of printing is usually used to produce the mailing address or a short message to the subscriber (see also *laser printer*, *line printer*, and *dot matrix printer*).

input: To enter information, instructions, and text into a computer system; or the information that is entered.

in register: See *register*.

insert: Printed material (a piece of paper or multiple pages) that is positioned between the normal pages of a publication during the binding process. The insert is usually printed on different paper than that used in the publication; it is often an advertisement.

instant messaging: Text-based messaging similar to *e-mail* except it allows the user to communicate with others in real time through the *Internet*.

interface: The ability of individual computers to interact; also, the actual *hardware* that performs the function.

international paper sizes: The range of standard metric paper sizes as determined by the International Standards Organization (*ISO*).

Internet: A global network connecting millions of computers for communications purposes, developed in 1969 for the US military, that grew to include educational and research institutions. The Internet facilitates data transfer and communication services, such as remote login, file transfer (*FTP*), electronic mail (*e-mail*), *newsgroups*, and the *World Wide Web.*

Internet service provider (ISP): A commercial entity that provides access to the *Internet*.

intranet: A private network with restricted access to specific users (eg, employees of a company or members of an organization).

ISBN: The International Standard Book Number, a 13-digit number that uniquely identifies books and booklike products published internationally (eg, the ISBN for this manual is 978-0-19-517633-9).

ISO: Abbreviation for International Standards Organization.

ISSN: The International Standard Serial Number, an 8-digit number that identifies periodical publications as such, including electronic serials (eg, the ISSN for *JAMA* is 0098-7484).

IT: Abbreviation for information technology.

italic: A typestyle with characters slanting upward and to the right (*italic*) as opposed to *roman* type (see 22.0, Typography).

JPG or JPEG: Abbreviation for Joint Photographic Experts Group. JPEG is a compressed graphic file (usually with the extension .jpg or .jpeg) normally used for images that require many colors (eg, photographs).

justify: To add or delete space between words or letters to make copy align at the left and right *margins* (see also *unjustified* and 22.0, Typography).

kerning: Modification of spacing between characters, usually to bring letters closer together, to improve overall appearance.

keyboard: Input device of a computer or typesetter, with keys representing letters, numbers, punctuation marks, and functions that give instructions to the computer. See also *function key*.

keyline: Tissue or acetate overlay separating or defining elements and color for *line art* or *halftone artwork*.

ladder: Four or more hyphens appearing at the end of consecutive lines; a typographic pattern to be avoided.

LAN: Acronym for local area network, a computer ***network*** restricted to an local area (eg, a home, office, or small group of buildings such as a college) (compare *WAN*).

laser printer: A high-quality printer that uses a laser beam to produce an image on a drum (see also ***dot matrix printer***, ***ink-jet printer***, and *line printer*).

layout: A drawing showing a conception of the finished product; includes sizing and positioning of the elements.

leaders: A row of dots or dashes designed to guide the reader's eye across space or a page.

leading: Pronounced [led-ding]; the spacing between lines of type (also called line spacing); a carryover term from hot metal composition. For example, 9-point type on 11 points of line space allows 2 points of leading below the type (see 22.0, Typography).

legend: Descriptive text accompanying a ***figure***, photograph, or illustration; also a list (key) that explains symbols on a map or chart (see also ***caption*** and 4.0, Visual Presentation of Data).

ligature: Two or more connected letters, such as æ, set as connected (see 22.0, Typography).

line art: Illustration composed of lines and/or lettering, eg, charts, graphs (see 4.0, Visual Presentation of Data).

line printer: A machine, driven by a computer, that prints out stored data one line at a time (see also ***dot matrix printer***, ***ink-jet printer***, and *laser printer*).

line spacing: See *leading*.

lines per inch (LPI): A unit of measurement for *halftone screens*.

listserve: A digital mailing list program that manages e-mail addresses of an online discussion group. The listserve program duplicates the messages sent by individual users and automatically sends them to every user in the group. Listserv is a registered trademark.

lithographic printing: Formal term for *offset printing*.

live area: The area of a page within the *margins*.

login: The name used to gain access to a computer system or network.

logo: One or more words or other combinations of letters or designs often used for easy recognition and promotion of company names, trademarks, etc.

long page: In *makeup*, a page that runs longer than the *live area* or *margins* of the page (compare *short page*).

loose-leaf binding: Binding that permits pages to be readily removed and inserted (compare ***perfect binding***, ***saddle-stitch binding***, and ***spiral binding***).

lossy: Image compression method that removes minor tonal and/or color variations, causing loss of inforrmation (detail) at high compression ratios.

lowercase: Letters that are not capitalized.

LZW compression: Lempel-Ziv-Welch (not a file format): ***nonlossy*** compression algorithm that allows for compression of image data without loss of quality.

macro: A series of automatically executed computer commands activated by a few programmed keystrokes; useful for repetitive tasks.

magenta: One of the 4 process printing colors (cyan, magenta, yellow, and black); a shade of red (see *CMYK*).

mainframe: A large, powerful central processing computer.

makeready: The part of the printing process that immediately precedes the actual *press run*, in which colors, ink coverage, and ***register*** are adjusted to produce the desired quality; may also apply to the binding process.

makeup: The arrangement of type lines and illustrations into pages or press ***forms*** for review or printing (see also ***imposition***; compare ***live area***).

manuscript: A typed (or occasionally handwritten) composition before it is published.

manuscript editor: See *copy editor*.

margin: The section of white space surrounding typed, composed, or printed copy (see also ***white space***).

mark up: The process of marking manuscript copy with directions for style and composition (see also ***imposition***).

master proof: The set of ***galley proofs*** or ***page proofs*** that carries all corrections and alterations.

masthead: A listing of editorial, production, and publishing staff; editorial boards; contact information; subscription and advertising information; important disclaimers (see also ***boilerplate*** and ***colophon***).

matte finish: The surface of dull-coated paper.

MB: Abbreviation for megabyte; a unit of computer storage, equal to approximately 1 million *bytes*.

measure: The length of the line (width of the column) in which type is composed or set, usually measured in ***picas*** and ***points***.

megabyte: See *MB*.

memory: The part of a computer in which digital information is permanently stored (see also *RAM*).

menu: A series of options in a software program, usually presented on the computer screen as a list of text options.

metadata: Data about data. For example, a library catalog contains information (metadata) about publications (data). Metadata is used in markup languages, such as *HTML*, *SGML*, and *XML*.

MHz: Abbreviation for megahertz, a unit that measures a computer system's cycle speed; 1 MHz equals 1 million cycles per second.

MIME: Abbreviation for multipurpose internal mail extensions, the standard for attaching nontext files to standard Internet mail messages.

modem: Modulator-demodulator; an electronic telecommunication device that converts computer-generated data (digital signals) into analog signals that can be carried over telephone lines.

moiré pattern: An undesirable wavy pattern caused by incorrect screen angles, overprinting halftones, or superimposing 2 geometric patterns.

monitor: A video output device for the display of computer-generated text and graphics.

mouse: A hand-operated device that controls the movement of a *cursor* on a computer screen.

MOV: QuickTime video file format.

MPEG: Abbreviation for Motion Picture Experts Group. MPEG-1 files are used for short animated files on the Web. MPEG-2 files are a much higher resolution format being developed for digital television and movies.

MSL: Abbreviation for must start left, indicating an article must start on a left-hand page. Compare *MSR*.

MSR: Abbreviation for must start right, indicating an article must start on a right-hand page. Compare *MSL*.

multimedia: Interactive electronic products created from digitized data reformatted to include text, images, and sound that allow the user to interact with the information on a computer screen.

multitasking: Performing simultaneous functions or manipulations on one computer or workstation, or performing simultaneous data manipulations in one computer program.

network: Two or more computers connected to share resources (see also *Internet*, *intranet*, *LAN*, and *WAN*).

newsgroup: The common nomenclature for Usenet News, a tool for group discussion on the *Internet*. Newsgroups function as group *e-mail* by providing a posting site for discussion on a particular topic. One can participate by posting a query or by reading answers to queries that have already been posted.

nonlossy: Image compression without loss of quality.

nonproportional spacing: Spacing that does not allow for the adjustment of space between *characters* to eliminate extra *white space*; all letters have the same space, which creates more space around narrow letters and decreases readability.

object: An item or computer representation of something (*icon* or *text*) that a user can select and/or manipulate to perform a task.

oblique: Type that is slightly slanted but not *italic*.

OCR: Abbreviation for optical character reader (or recognition); in digital composition and typesetting, an OCR input device is capable of scanning a *typescript* and replicating the typed characters. An OCR device creates a digital document that can be edited and searched, as opposed to a *scanner*, which simply transfers images from paper to a digital file.

offset, offset printing: Commonly used term for offset *lithographic printing*; a printing method in which an image is transferred from an inked *plate* cylinder to a *blanket* made of rubber or other synthetic material and then onto a sheet of paper.

on-demand printing: See *demand printing*.

opacity: (1) A quality of paper that prevents type or images printed on one side from showing through on the other side. (2) The covering power of ink in printing.

opaque: To block out (on the film negative) those areas that are not to be printed.

operating system (OS): A program that controls the overall operations of a computer system, intermediating between the *application software* programs and the *hardware*, such as MS-DOS, UNIX, Windows, or OS/2.

optical character reader/recognition: See *OCR*.

orphan: One or 2 short words at the end of a paragraph that fall on a separate line at the bottom of a page or column, or a single line of type that starts at the bottom of a page or column (compare *widow*; see also *bad break*).

outline halftone: A portion taken from a *halftone* that is the shape or modified shape of a subject.

out of register: See *register*.

overlay: A hinged flap of paper or transparent plastic covering for a piece of artwork. It may protect the work and/or allow for instructions or corrections to be marked for the printer or camera operator.

overprinting: Printing over an area or page that has already been printed.

overrun: Production of more copies than the number ordered (see also *press run* and *print order*; compare *underrun*).

page proof: A proof that is set or printed in the form of the finished page (see also *proof*).

paginate: To number, mark, or arrange the pages of a document, manuscript, article, or book.

Pantone Matching System colors: See *PMS*.

paragraph: A unit of *text* set off by indention, horizontal space, *bullets*, or other typographical device.

parse: To analyze files by checking *tags* (codes) to ensure that they are used correctly.

password: A private code used to gain access to a locked system.

pasteup: A mock assembly of the elements of ***type*** and ***artwork*** as a guide to the printer for ***makeup***.

PC: Abbreviation for personal computer, usually self-contained (***keyboard***, ***monitor***, printer, ***central processing unit***, and ***memory*** devices), as opposed to a terminal or ***networked*** computer; often used to refer to IBM-compatible computers.

PCT (or PICT): Macintosh graphics file format most commonly used for ***bitmap*** images.

PDA: Abbreviation for personal digital assistant, a handheld device that combines computing, telephone/fax, ***Internet***, and networking features.

PDF: Abbreviation for portable document format, a proprietary file format that captures the elements of a printed document as an electronic image that can be viewed, navigated, or printed.

PDL: Abbreviation for page description language. The code generated by a typesetting or page-layout system that tells the output device, such as a *laser printer* or ***image setter***, where to place elements on a page.

PE: Abbreviation for printer's error or publisher's error; used in correcting ***proofs*** to indicate an error attributable to the printer or publisher (compare *AA* and *EA*).

peer review: The process by which ***editors*** ask experts to read, criticize, and comment on the suitability of a manuscript for publication (see 6.0, Editorial Assessment and Processing, and 5.11.4, Ethical and Legal Considerations, Editorial Responsibilities, Roles, Procedures, and Policies, Editorial Responsibility for Peer Review).

peer-reviewed journal: A journal containing editorial content that is ***peer reviewed***.

penalty copy: Copy that is difficult to typeset (heavily corrected, difficult to read, heavy with tabular material, etc), for which the ***typesetter*** charges more than the regular rate.

perfect binding: Process in which ***signatures*** are collated, the ***gutter*** edge is cut and ground, adhesive is applied to the ***signatures***, and the ***cover*** is applied (compare *loose-leaf binding*, ***saddle-stitch binding***, and ***spiral binding***).

perforate: To punch lines of small holes or slits in a sheet so that it can be torn off with ease.

photostat: A camera process that duplicates graphic matter; also the graphic matter thus produced.

pica: A unit of measure; 1 pica equals approximately $\frac{1}{6}$ inch or 12 points (see also *point*).

pica type: Typewriter type that equals 10 characters to the inch (see also ***elite type***).

pitch: In fixed-pitch ***fonts***, pitch refers to the number of ***characters*** per inch. Common pitch values are 10 and 12. Proportional-pitch fonts have no pitch value because different characters have different widths, eg, the letter M is wider than the letter I.

pixel: A unit in a digital image; the smallest point of a bit-mapped screen that can be assigned independent color and intensity.

plate: (1) A sheet of metal, plastic, rubber, paperboard, or other material used as a printing surface; the means by which an image area is separated from a nonimage area. (2) A full-page, color book illustration, often printed on paper different from that used for the ***text***.

PMID: Abbreviation for PubMed identification number, the unique identifying number assigned to a record when it is entered into ***PubMed***.

PMS (Pantone Matching System) colors: A color identification system matching specific shades of approximately 500 colors with numbers and formulas for the corresponding inks, developed by Pantone Inc.

PNG: Portable (public) network graphic file format.

pockets: Sections on a binder in which individual ***signatures*** are placed and then selected as required for each copy to be bound.

point: The printer's basic unit of measurement, often used to determine type size; 1 point equals approximately $\frac{1}{72}$ inch; 12 points equal 1 ***pica***.

PostScript: A page description language and programming language used primarily in the electronic and desktop publishing areas (see also ***PDL*** and ***EPS***).

PowerPoint: Microsoft software, used to make slide show presentations. File format extensions are the default .ppt (presentation), .pot (template), and .pps (PowerPoint Show).

ppi: Abbreviation for ***pixels*** per inch, unit of measurement for digital images.

preprint: An article or part of a book printed and distributed or transmitted digitally before publication and/or review.

press form: See ***form***.

press plates: The plates used to print multiple copies on the press (see also ***plate***).

press run: The total number of copies of journals, books, or other materials printed.

primary colors: Cyan (C), magenta (M), and yellow (Y). These 3 colors, when mixed with black (K), will closely reproduce all other colors. See ***CMYK***.

print order: The number of copies of printed material ordered.

printout: Paper output of a printer or other device that produces normal-reading copy from computer-stored data.

print run: See ***press run***.

process printing colors: Cyan, magenta, yellow, and black (***CMYK***); used to produce color illustrations in print publications.

program: A set of instructions for a computer. To program is to create such a set of instructions.

programmable key: A key on a computer's ***keyboard*** that, when pressed alone or in combination with other keys, produces a computer command (see also ***macro*** and ***function key***).

proof: A hard copy of the text and graphic material of a document used to check accuracy of text, composition, positioning, and/or typesetting (see also ***hard copy***).

proofreader: One who reads or reviews ***proofs*** for errors.

proportional spacing: Spacing that allows for the adjustment of ***character*** spacing based on character width and increases readability.

protocol: A system for transmitting data between 2 devices that establishes the type of error checking to be used; data compression structures; how the sending device will indicate that it has finished sending a message; and how the receiving device will indicate that it has received a message; also a detailed plan for a scientific study.

PSD: Photoshop (Adobe) file format.

publisher: An entity or person who directs the production, dissemination, and sale of selected information.

PubMed: A searchable database of scientific and biomedical literature compiled by the US National Library of Medicine.

pullout quotes, pull quote: See ***call-outs***.

ragged right: Type set with the right-hand ***margin unjustified*** (or ragged).

RAM: Acronym for random access ***memory***; temporary computer memory used by a computer to hold data currently being processed or created that are lost when the computer is shut down.

raster: A digitized image that is mapped into a grid of ***pixels***; therefore, the image is resolution-dependent. The color of each pixel is defined by a specific number of ***bits***.

raster image processor (RIP): A device that produces a digital ***bitmap*** to show an image's position on a page before printing.

RC (resin-coated) paper: Paper used in composition to produce a type proof of the quality needed for photographic reproduction.

RDF: Abbreviation for resources description framework, a general framework for describing a Web site's ***metadata***.

ream: Five hundred sheets of paper (see also ***basis weight***).

recto: A right-hand page (compare ***verso***).

redlining: A ***software*** program that shows changes made in a document to be seen on screen and on a printed ***typescript*** for review by the ***editor*** and author. Also called revision marking or strikethrough.

register: To print an impression on a sheet in correct relationship to other impressions already printed on the same sheet, eg, to superimpose exactly the various color impressions. When all parts or inks match exactly, they are in register; when they are not exactly aligned, they are out of register.

remake: To alter the makeup of a page or series of pages.

reprint: A reproduction of an original printing in paper or digital format.

reproduction proof: A high-quality proof for use in photoengraving or offset lithography.

resolution: A measurement of the visual quality of an image according to discrimination between distinct elements; the fineness of detail that can be distinguished in an image (see also *dots per inch*).

reverse-out, reverse text, or **reverse image:** Text or image that appears in white surrounded by a solid block of color or black.

RGB: Abbreviation for red, green, blue, the primary additive colors used in color computer *monitors*.

right-reading: Produced to read as original copy from right to left, as in right-reading film (compare *wrong-reading*).

RIP: Abbreviation for *raster image processor*.

river: A streak of white space running down through lines of type, breaking up the even appearance of the page; to be avoided.

ROB: Abbreviation for run-of-book; advertising term meaning a regular page, as opposed to an ad insert (ie, appears in all versions of the publication). Can also refer to placement anywhere space is available in the publication.

roman: A *typestyle* with upright characters, as opposed to *italic* (see 22.0, Typography).

RSS: Abbreviation for Really Simple Syndication, Rich Site Summary, or RDF Site Summary, an XML format for syndicating Web content.

RTF: Abbreviation for rich text format; a generic word-processing format that uses *ASCII* codes to preserve the formatting of a file.

runaround: Type composed or set to fit around an illustration, box, or other design element.

run in: To merge a *paragraph* with the preceding paragraph.

running foot: A line of copy, usually giving publication name, subject, title, date, volume number, and/or authors' names, appearing at the bottom of consecutive pages. Also called footer.

running head: A line of copy, usually giving publication name, subject, title, date, volume number, and/or authors' names, appearing at the top of consecutive pages. Also called header.

runover: Material not fitting in the space allowed (see also *live area* and *long page*).

saddle-stitch binding: Process by which *signatures*, or pages, and *covers* are assembled by inserting staples into the centerfold (see also *loose-leaf binding*, *perfect binding*, and *spiral binding*).

sans serif: An unadorned *typeface*; a letter without a short line projecting from the top or bottom of the main stroke of the letter (compare *serif* and see 22.0, Typography).

scaling: Determining the appropriate size of an image and the amount of reduction or enlargement needed for the image to fit in a specific area.

scanner: A device that uses an electronic reader (eye) to transform *type*, *characters*, and images from a printed page into a digital form; or a device that produces color-separated film or images (see also *OCR*).

score: To indent or mark paper or cards slightly so they can be folded exactly at certain points.

SCORM: Acronym for sharable content object reference model. A standard for Web-based education, it defines how the instruction elements are combined and used.

scribe: Thin strips of nonprinting areas, such as those between figure parts.

scripting language: Programming language used to add additional features to a Web page, such as graphic displays.

search engine: A program that enables users to search for documents on the Web.

selective binding: A method of *binding* in which specific contents of each copy produced are determined by instructions transmitted electronically from a computer. *Signatures*, or specific groups of pages, are selected to produce a copy for a specific recipient or recipient group.

self-cover: A *cover* for a publication that is made of the same paper used for the *text* and printed as part of a larger press *form*.

separation: Converting images to *CMYK* for printing; also used to refer to the actual negatives created for each of the 4 colors (see also *color separation*).

serif: An adorned *typeface*; a short, light line projecting from the top or bottom of a main stroke of a letter (compare *sans serif* and see 22.0, Typography).

server: A computer *software* package or *hardware* that provides specific services to other computers.

SGML: Abbreviation for standard generalized markup language; markup languages are used to capture, or encode, the logical structure of an electronic document, as distinct from its visual presentation. SGML formed the basis for *HTML* and *XML* (see also *ASCII* and *DTD*).

SGML editor: A *context-sensitive editor* based on *SGML*.

short page: In makeup, a page that runs shorter than the established live area (compare *long page*).

show-through: Inking that can be seen on the opposite side of the paper, because of the heaviness of the ink or the thinness of the paper.

sidebar: Text or graphics placed in a box and printed on the right or left side of a page.

signature: (1) A printed sheet comprising several pages that have been folded, so that the pages are in consecutive order according to pagination. (2) A line of text appearing at the bottom of an article that lists the author(s).

signature block: A block of text that automatically appears at the bottom of an *e-mail* message, discussion group, and/or forum post that contains the writer's name and may also include the writer's title, company name, location, e-mail address, and personal message; also sometimes used after letters, book reviews, and other small items of copy.

sink: Starting type below the top line of the *live area*, which leaves an area of *white space*.

site license: (1) A licensing agreement that permits access and use of digital information at a specific site. (2) A fee paid to a software company to allow multiple users at a site to access or copy a piece of *software*.

sizing: Adding material to a paper to make it more resistant to moisture.

slug: A line or lines of copy inserted to draw the attention of the reader, often set between rules in enlarged, bold type.

small caps: Capital letters that are smaller than the typical capital letters of a specific *typeface*, usually the size of the *x-height* of the font (see also 22.0, Typography).

software: Programs and procedures required to enable a computer to perform a specific task, as opposed to the physical components of the system (compare *hardware*).

solid: Style of *type* set with no space between lines.

solidus: A forward slanted line (/) used to separate numbers, letters, or other characters (also called forward slash; see also *virgule* and 8.4, Punctuation, Forward Slash [Virgule, Solidus]).

spacing: Lateral spaces between words, sentences, or columns; also *paragraph* indentions (see *leading*).

spam: Electronic junk mail or *newsgroup* postings.

specifications (specs): Instructions given to the printer that include numbers of copies (*press run* or *print order*); paper stock, coating, and size; and color, typography, and design.

spider[ing]: Software that regularly checks the *Internet* for Web pages to feed a *search engine*. Also called a *bot*, crawler, or Web crawler.

spine: The backbone of a perfect-bound journal or book. The width of the spine depends on the number and thickness of pages in the publication (see also *perfect binding*).

spiral binding: A process of binding a publication with wires or plastic in a spiral form inserted through holes along the binding side (see also *loose-leaf binding*, *perfect binding*, *saddle-stitch binding*, and *selective binding*).

spot color: One or more extra colors on a page.

spread: Two pages, facing each other; see also *double spread*.

sRGB: A color profile with a very limited amount of color values, primarily designed for vivid images displayed over the *Internet*. Not suitable for print reproduction.

standard generalized markup language: See *SGML*.

stet: Instruction that marked or crossed-out copy or type is to be retained as it originally appeared.

STM: Abbreviation for scientific, technical, and medical field of publishing.

stock: Type of paper for printing.

storage: The capability of a device to hold and keep data.

storing data: Placing data in computer storage by recording the data in digital form on magnetic, optical, or other medium, such as ***discs*** and tapes, either inside or outside the computer.

straight copy: Material that can be set in type with no handwork or special programming (copy that contains no mathematical equations, tables, etc).

strapline: The "subtitle" portion of a logo or slogan.

strikethrough: To mark a character or some text for deletion by superimposing a line through the main body of the character(s).

strip: To join film in a unit according to a press ***imposition*** before platemaking.

style: A set of uniform rules to guide the application of grammar, spelling, typography, composition, and design.

subhead: A subordinate heading (see 22.0, Typography).

subscript: A number or symbol that prints partly below the ***baseline***, eg, A_2 (also called inferior).

subscription: The price for a publication; usually set in annual terms.

superior: See ***superscript***.

superscript: A number or symbol that prints partly above the ***baseline***, eg, A^2 (also called superior).

SWK: Abbreviation for "set when known." Used to indicate information (such as page numbers) that will be inserted later in the production process.

SWOP: Abbreviation for specifications for Web ***offset*** publications; a color proofing system used to check color consistency.

syntax: The spelling and grammar of a programming language that communicates to the computer exactly what the user wants. The computer comprehends what is typed only if it is typed in the computer's language.

tag: (v) To insert a style or composition ***code*** in a computer file or document; (n) the ***code*** inserted in a computer file or document.

tagged: Coded, ie, a document or file with the ***codes*** inserted in the text.

TCP/IP: Abbreviation for transmission control protocol/Internet protocol; the language governing communication between computers on the ***Internet***.

tear sheet: A page cut or torn from a book or periodical.

text: The main body of type in a page, manuscript, article, or book. Also used for electronic files that contain only characters, no formatting or illustrations.

text editor: An application used to create, view, and edit ***text*** files.

text wrap: A feature of ***word processors*** that makes it possible to wrap ***text*** around an illustration. Also called text flow.

thumbnail: A miniature display of a page or graphic.

TIFF (or TIF): Acronym for tagged image file format; a file format that allows bitmapped images to be exchanged between different computer ***applications***; the preferred format for images, including photographs and line art.

tints: Various even tone areas of a solid color, usually expressed in percentages.

tip, tip-in, tip-on: A sheet of paper or a ***signature*** glued to another signature before binding.

TOC: Abbreviation for table of contents.

toner: Imaging material or ink used in photocopiers, computer printers, and some off-press proofing systems.

trademark: A legally registered word, name, symbol, slogan, or any combination of these, used to identify and distinguish products and services and to indicate the source and marketer of those products and services (see 5.6.16, Ethical and Legal Considerations, Intellectual Property: Ownership, Access, Rights, and Management, Trademark).

transparency: (1) A transparent object such as a photographic slide that is viewed by shining light through it; color positive film (traditional/conventional). (2) Effect created by pixels turned "off" or by a mask ([alpha channel] digital/electronic).

transpose (tr): A proofreading and editing term meaning to switch the positions of 2 elements (eg, characters, words, sentences, or paragraphs).

trap, trapping: The process of printing one ink on top of another to produce a third color, or to avoid thin white spaces between colors.

trim: The edges that are cut off 3 sides—the top (head), bottom (foot), and right (face)—of a publication after binding.

trim line, trim marks: The line or marks indicated on copy to show where the page ends or needs to be cut.

trim size: The final size of the publication.

TTP: Abbreviation for text transfer protocol; a method for moving ***text*** from one place to another on the ***Internet*** (see also ***FTP***).

turnaround time: The period of time between any 2 events in publishing (eg, between manuscript submission and acceptance, between manuscript scanning and telecommunication to the printer).

type: (n) Printed characters; a small metal block with a raised character on one side, used to produce characters on paper; (v) the act of typing text or entering commands into a computer on a keyboard.

typeface: A named type design, such as Baskerville, Helvetica, or Times Roman, produced as a complete font (see 22.0, Typography).

type gauge: A type-measurement tool calibrated in ***picas*** and ***points***.

typescript: A manuscript output by a computer printer or in typewritten form (see also ***hard copy***).

typesetter: A person, firm, or machine that sets type.

typestyle: The general characteristics of a ***typeface*** (eg, ***roman***, ***boldface***, ***italic***, and ***condensed*** type) (see also 22.0, Typography).

typo: A typographical error in a published work, such as a misspelling or missing letter.

uc/lc: Abbreviation for uppercase/lowercase (letters); as an editing mark, it would indicate using capital and small letters, eg, New York, New York, rather than NEW YORK, NEW YORK.

underrun: Production of fewer printed copies than was ordered (see also ***press run*** and ***print order***; compare ***overrun***).

UNIX (or Unix): A computer operating system designed to be portable, ***multitasking***, and multiuser in a time-sharing configuration. UNIX is characterized by various concepts: plain text files, command line interpreter, hierarchical file system, treating devices and certain types of interprocess communication as files, etc. UNIX is a trademark for a powerful ***operating system***, a suite of ***programs*** that make the computer work.

unjustified: A ragged or uneven margin (compare ***justify*** and see 22.0, Typography).

upload: To transfer a digital file or data from a local computer to a remote computer.

uppercase: A capital letter.

URL: Abbreviation for uniform resource locator; an address for a document or information available via the ***Internet*** or Web (eg, http://www.jama-archives.org).

vector graphics: The use of geometric primitives such as points, lines, curves, and polygons to represent images in computer graphics; resolution-independent graphic images that can be defined by mathematical equations and scaled with no loss of quality.

verso: A left-hand page (compare ***recto***).

virgule: A forward slanted line (/) used to separate numbers, letters, or other characters (also called forward slash; see also ***solidus*** and 8.4, Punctuation, Forward Slash [Virgule, Solidus]).

virus: A computer program, usually hidden in another ***program***, that replicates and inserts itself into other programs without the user's knowledge and that frequently causes harm to the programs or destroys data.

VR: Abbreviation for virtual reality.

WAIS: Abbreviation for wide-area information server (see ***server***).

WAN: Acronym for wide-area ***network***. A WAN is typically made up of 2 or more local area networks (***LANs***); the best-known WAN is the Internet.

watermark: (1) An image or set of characters produced by thinning a specific area of paper that is visible when the paper is held up to light; often used to show a company logo. (2) Faint characters imposed over type or images on a page to prevent unauthorized copying or distribution.

web: (1) An *offset* lithographic printing press. (2) A continuous roll of paper used in printing.

Web: See *World Wide Web*.

Web browser: A *program* for quickly searching and accessing information on the Web.

Web crawler: See *spider[ing]*.

web press: A lithographic press that prints on a continuous roll (web) of paper.

webRGB: A color profile with a very limited number of color values, primarily designed for vivid images displayed over the *Internet*. Not suitable for print reproduction.

Web server: A computer that has Web server software installed and is able to connect to the Internet.

weight: The weight of 500 sheets (a ream) of paper. See *basis weight*.

well: A part of a journal, usually the middle pages, in which advertising is not allowed; usually reserved for important scientific and clinical articles in biomedical journals. Regular features, such as news articles, essays, letters, and book reviews, are typically run outside the editorial well, where ad interspersion may be allowed.

wf: Abbreviation for wrong *font*; incorrect or inconsistent *type size* or *typeface*.

white space: The area of a page that is free of any text or graphics (compare *live area*).

widow: A short line ending a *paragraph* and positioned at the top of a page or column, to be avoided (compare *orphan*; see also *bad break*).

Wi-Fi: The underlying technology of wireless local area networks (*LANs*), first developed for mobile computing devices and now used for increasingly diverse applications.

WMF: Windows MetaFile, a file format created by Microsoft.

word processor: A general term for a computer *program* with which text consisting of words and figures can be input, edited, recorded, stored, and printed.

workstation: Computer used for engineering *applications*, desktop publishing, *software* development, and other types of applications that require a reasonable amount of computing power and high-quality graphics capabilities.

World Wide Web (WWW): The world's biggest *network*, used to access information via the *Internet* with a *Web browser* (also called the Web).

WORM: Acronym for write once, read many, a technology used to write data permanently onto a disk one time and allow it to be read many times.

worm: See *virus*.

WPD: Microsoft WordPerfect file format.

wrong-reading: Produced to read as a mirror image (from left to right) of the original copy; usually refers to film (compare ***right-reading***).

WWW: See *World Wide Web*.

WYSIWYG: Acronym for "what you see is what you get" (pronounced [wizzy-wig]), meaning that which is displayed on the computer screen is essentially how the final product will appear after printing.

x-height: A vertical measurement of a letter, usually equal to the height of a lowercase letter without ***ascenders*** or ***descenders*** (eg, x).

XLS: Microsoft Excel file format.

XML: Abbreviation for extensible markup language. Like ***HTML*** and ***SGML***, XML is a markup language designed to describe content by means of user-defined tags and a *DTD* to describe the content.

yellow: One of the 4 process printing colors (cyan, magenta, yellow, and black) (see *CMYK*).

zip: (n) A compressed file archive that appears as a single file. (v) To compress files by means of a data compression format that allows files to take up less space on a disc or hard drive.

ACKNOWLEDGMENT

Principal author: Jennifer Reiling, *JAMA*

The following reviewed this section and offered suggestions for revision: Monica Mungle and J. D. Neff, *JAMA* and *Archives* Journals; and Nina Sandlin, *American Medical News*.

SOURCES

Ad Up, ad terms and definitions. http://www.ad-up.com/new/adup_ad_defs.html. Accessed February 2005.

African American Literature Book Club. http://aalbc.com/writers/publishing_glossary.htm. Accessed February 2005.

Angelfire glossary. http://www.angelfire.com/ny3/diGi8tech/PGlossary.html. Accessed February 2005.

BMI Global Consultants, Ltd, Web site. http://www.bmiglobal.com. Accessed February 2005.

Brown University computer science glossary. http://www.cascv.brown.edu/compute/cxxmanual/glossary/o.htm. Accessed February 2005.

Carbon Colour. Glossary of printers' terms. http://www.carbon.co.uk/glossary.html. Accessed February 2005.

The Digital Object Identifier System. http://www.doi.org. Accessed February 2005.

ELearning at Bath. Glossary. http://www.bath.ac.uk/e-learning/glossary.htm. Accessed February 2005.

ELearning guru. http://e-learningguru.com/gloss.htm#S. Accessed February 2005.

Frequently asked questions about the ISBN. http://www.isbn.org/standards/home/isbn/us/isbnqa.asp#Q1. Accessed June 2006.

A Glossary of Printing and Paper Terms. Dayton, OH: Mead Corp; 1995.

Hale C, ed. *Wired Style: Principles of English Usage in the Digital Age*. San Francisco, CA: HardWired; 1996.

Hewlett-Packard Upstream CIO. Glossary. http://www.upstreamcio.com/glossary.asp. Accessed February 2005.

Information & Education Technology, University of California. http://iet.ucdavis.edu/glossary.cfm/. Accessed February 2005.

Internetnews.com. http://inews.webopedia.com. Accessed September 2006.

ISSN International Centre. http://www.issn.org/en/node. Accessed June 2006.

John Wiley & Sons Inc. Glossary. http://www.wiley.com/college/busin/icmis/oakman/outline/glossary/glossary.htm. Accessed July 2005.

Kasdorf WE. *The Columbia Guide to Digital Publishing*. New York, NY: Columbia University Press; 2003.

Merriam-Webster's Collegiate Dictionary. 11th ed. Springfield, MA: Merriam-Webster; 2003.

NetLingo: the Internet dictionary. http://www.netlingo.com. Accessed February 2005.

New England Journal of Medicine. Author center: how to prepare your figures. http://authors.nejm.org/Misc/tech.asp. Accessed March 2005.

Noe C. A book collector's glossary. http://www.the-bookman.com/main/Glossary.htm. Accessed February 2005.

Pocketpal. 19th ed. Memphis, TN: International Paper Co; 2003.

Prepressure Page Web site. http://www.prepressure.com. Accessed April 2006.

PubMed tutorial. http://www.nlm.nih.gov/bsd/pubmed_tutorial/glossary.html#p. Accessed February 2005.

Rainwater Press Web site. http://www.rainwater.com. Accessed May 2006.

Red Hat glossary. http://www.redhat.com/docs/glossary/. Accessed February 2005.

Scholarly journals at the crossroads: a subversive proposal for electronic publishing. http://www.arl.org/scomm/subversive/glossary.html. Accessed February 2005.

smallBIZonline. Glossary of Internet terms. http://www.smallbizonline.co.uk/glossary_of_internet_terms.php. Accessed June 2006.

Steven Black Consulting. Glossary of terms. http://www.stevenblack.com/intl%20glossary.html#b. Accessed May 2006.

University of Chicago. http://ccs.uchicago.edu/technotes/misc/Glossary/gloss4.html. Accessed February 2005.

University of Waterloo. http://www.graphics.uwaterloo.ca/content/sidebar/glossary.html. Accessed February 2005.

UNIX tutorial for beginners. http://www.ee.surrey.ac.uk/Teaching/Unix/. Accessed February 2005.

ViMas Technologies. http://www.vimas.com/image_sdk/glossary.htm. Accessed February 2005.

Washington State Department of General Administration. Guidelines for producing materials in large print. http://www.ga.wa.gov/ada/lgprint.htm. Accessed February 2005.

Wĕbopēdia. http://www.webopedia.com. Accessed February 2005.

Wikipedia: The Free Encyclopedia. http://en.wikipedia.org/wiki/Main_Page. Accessed February 2005.

Wiktionary: a multilingual free encyclopedia. http://en.wiktionary.org/wiki/Main_Page. Accessed July 2005.

WordNet: a lexical database for the English language. http://wordnet.princeton.edu. Accessed February 2005.

World Meteorological Organization. Internet glossary of terms. http://www.wmo.ch/web/www/WDM/Guides/Internet-glossary.html. Accessed February 2005.

Yale University Library Information. Licensing digital information: definitions of words and phrases commonly found in licensing agreements. http://www.library.yale.edu/~llicense/definiti.shtml. Accessed July 2005.

25 Resources

The resources listed in this chapter are provided for information only and do not imply an endorsement by the *AMA Manual of Style.*

25.1 General Dictionaries

Acronym Finder. http://www.acronymfinder.com

The American Heritage Dictionary of the English Language. 4th ed. Boston, MA: Houghton Mifflin Co; 2000.

Dictionary.com. http://www.dictionary.com

Merriam-Webster's Collegiate Dictionary. 11th ed. Springfield, MA: Merriam-Webster Inc; 2003. http://www.m-w.com/dictionary.htm

OneLook. http://www.onelook.com

Oxford Dictionaries Online. http://www.askoxford.com

yourDictionary.com. http://www.yourdictionary.com

25.2 Medical and Scientific Dictionaries

BioTech Life Science Dictionary. http://biotech.icmb.utexas.edu/search/dict-search.html

Dorland's Illustrated Medical Dictionary. 30th ed. Philadelphia, PA: Saunders; 2003.

Jablonski S. *Dictionary of Medical Acronyms & Abbreviations.* 5th ed. Philadelphia, PA: Hanley & Belfus Inc; 2004.

Stedman's Medical Dictionary. 28th ed. Baltimore, MD: Lippincott Williams & Wilkins; 2005.

25.3 General Style and Usage

Acronym Finder. http://www.acronymfinder.com

Bernstein T. *The Careful Writer: A Modern Guide to English Usage*. New York, NY: Free Press; 1998.

Brooks BS, Pinson JL. *Working With Words: A Concise Handbook for Media Writers and Editors*. 4th ed. New York, NY: Bedford/St Martins Press; 1999.

The Chicago Manual of Style: The Essential Guide for Writers, Editors, and Publishers. 15th ed. Chicago, IL: University of Chicago Press; 2003.

Follett W, Wensberg E, ed. *Modern American Usage: A Guide*. New York, NY: Hill & Wang; 1998.

Fowler HW, Burchfield RW, ed. *The New Fowler's Modern English Usage*. 3rd rev ed. New York, NY: Oxford University Press; 2000.

Garner BA, ed. *A Dictionary of Modern English Usage*. 2nd ed. New York, NY: Oxford University Press; 1998.

Garner BA. *Garner's Modern American Usage*. 2nd ed. New York, NY: Oxford University Press; 2003.

Kasdorf WE. *The Columbia Guide to Digital Publishing*. New York, NY: Columbia University Press; 2003.

Lederer R, Dowis R. *Sleeping Dogs Don't Lay: Practical Advice for the Grammatically Challenged, and That's No Lie*. New York, NY: St Martins Press; 2001.

McGovern G, Norton R, O'Dowd C. *The Web Content Style Guide: An Essential Reference for Online Writers, Editors and Managers*. London, England: Prentice Hall; 2001.

Pavlicin K, Lyon C. *Online Style Guide: Terms, Usage, and Tips*. St Paul, MN: Elva Resa Publishing; 1998.

Walker JR, Taylor T. *The Columbia Guide to Online Style*. New York, NY: Columbia University Press; 1998.

Webster's Dictionary of English Usage. Reprint ed. Springfield, MA: Merriam-Webster Inc; 2002.

Wissner-Gross E. *Unbiased: Editing in a Diverse Society*. Ames: Iowa State University Press; 1999.

25.4 Medical/Scientific Style and Usage

American Psychological Association. *Publication Manual of the American Psychological Association*. 5th ed. Washington, DC: American Psychological Association; 2001.

ASM Style Manual for Journals and Books. Washington, DC: American Society of Microbiology; 1992.

Cohn V, Cope L. *News & Numbers: A Guide to Reporting Statistical Claims and Controversies in Health and Other Fields*. 2nd ed. Ames: Iowa State University Press; 2001.

Coghill AM, Garson LR, eds. *The ACS Style Guide: Effective Communication of Scientific Information*. 3rd ed. New York, NY: Oxford University Press; 2006.

Davis NM. *Medical Abbreviations: 28,000 Conveniences at the Expense of Communications and Safety*. 13th ed. Huntingdon Valley, PA: Neil M Davis Associates; 2006.

Rubens P, ed. *Science and Technical Writing: A Manual of Style*. 2nd ed. New York, NY: Routledge; 2001.

Style Manual Committee, Council of Science Editors. *Scientific Style and Format: The CSE Manual for Authors, Editors, and Publishers*. 7th ed. New York, NY: Rockefeller University Press, in cooperation with the Council of Science Editors, Reston, VA; 2006.

Sutcliffe AJ, ed. *The New York Public Library Writer's Guide to Style and Usage*. New York, NY: HarperCollins Publishers; 1994.

25.5 Writing

Albert T. *A-Z of Medical Writing*. London, England: BMJ Books; 2000.

Day RA. *How to Write and Publish a Scientific Paper*. 6th ed. Phoenix, AZ: Oryx Press; 1998.

Day RA. *Scientific English: A Guide for Scientists and Other Professionals*. 2nd ed. Phoenix, AZ: Oryx Press; 1995.

Gordon KE. *The Deluxe Transitive Vampire: The Ultimate Handbook of Grammar for the Innocent, the Eager, and the Doomed*. New York, NY: Pantheon Books; 1993.

Gordon KE. *The New Well-Tempered Sentence: A Punctuation Handbook for the Innocent, the Eager, and the Doomed*. Rev ed. New Haven, CT: Ticknor & Fields; 1993.

Huth EJ. *Writing and Publishing in Medicine*. 3rd ed. Baltimore, MD: Lippincott Williams & Wilkins; 1999.

Iles RL. *Guidebook to Better Medical Writing*. Olathe, KS: Island Press; 1997.

Longman Language Activator: Helps You Write and Speak Natural English. 2nd ed. White Plains, NY: Addison Wesley; 2000.

Lunsford AA. *EasyWriter: A Pocket Guide*. 2nd ed. Boston, MA: Bedford/St Martins Press; 2002.

Miller C, Swift K. *The Handbook of Nonsexist Writing*. 2nd ed. Lincoln, NE: Universe; 2001.

Moxley JM. *Publish, Don't Perish: The Scholar's Guide to Academic Writing and Publishing*. Westport, CT: Praeger Publishers; 1992.

O'Conner P. *Woe Is I: The Grammarphobe's Guide to Better English in Plain English*. Expanded ed. New York, NY: Riverhead Books; 2003.

Penrose AM, Katz SB. *Writing in the Sciences: Exploring Conventions of Scientific Discourse*. New York, NY: Longman; 2004.

Strunk W Jr, White EB. *The Elements of Style*. 4th ed. New York, NY: Allyn & Bacon; 2000.

Truss L. *Eats, Shoots and Leaves: The Zero Tolerance Approach to Punctuation*. New York, NY: Gotham Books; 2004.

Wallraff B. *Word Court: Wherein Verbal Virtue Is Rewarded, Crimes Against the Language Are Punished, and Poetic Justice Is Done*. New York, NY: Harcourt Inc; 2000.

Wallraff B. *Your Own Words*. Boulder, CO: Counterpoint Press; 2004.

Walsh B. *Lapsing Into a Comma: A Curmudgeon's Guide to the Many Things That Can Go Wrong in Print—and How to Avoid Them*. Lincolnwood, IL: Contemporary Books; 2000.

Warriner JE. *English Grammar and Composition: Complete Course*. Franklin ed. New York, NY: Harcourt Brace Jovanovich Publishers; 1988.

Williams J. *Style: Ten Lessons in Clarity and Grace*. 6th ed. New York, NY: Longman; 2000.

25.6 Ethical and Legal Concerns

Fischer MA, Perle EG, Williams JT. *Perle and Williams on Publishing Law*. 3rd ed. Englewood Cliffs, NJ: Aspen Law & Business; 2006.

Garner BA. *Elements of Legal Style*. 2nd ed. New York, NY: Oxford University Press; 2002.

Goldstein N, ed. *Associated Press Stylebook and Briefing on Media Law*. Rev and updated ed. Cambridge, MA: Perseus Publishing; 2007.

Goldstein P. *Copyright's Highway: From Gutenberg to the Celestial Jukebox*. Rev ed. Stanford, CA: Stanford University Press; 2003.

Hart JD. *Law of the Web: A Field Guide to Internet Publishing*. Denver, CO: Bradford Publishing Co; 2003.

Hudson Jones A, McLellan F, eds. *Ethical Issues in Biomedical Publication*. Baltimore, MD: Johns Hopkins University Press; 2000.

International Trademark Association. http://www.inta.org/

Maggio R. *Talking About People: A Guide to Fair and Accurate Language*. Phoenix, AZ: Oryx Press; 1997.

Schwartz M; Task Force on Bias-Free Language of the Association of American University Presses. *Guidelines for Bias-Free Writing*. Bloomington: Indiana University Press; 1995.

25.7 Peer Review

Fifth International Congress on Peer Review and Biomedical Publication. http://www.jama-peer.org

Godlee F, Jefferson T, eds. *Peer Review in Health Sciences*. 2nd ed. London, England: BMJ Books; 2003.

Weller A. *Editorial Peer Review: Its Strengths and Weaknesses*. Medford, NJ: Information Today Inc; 2001.

25.8 Illustrations/Displaying Data

Briscoe MH. *Preparing Scientific Illustrations: A Guide to Better Posters, Presentations, and Publications*. 2nd ed. New York, NY: Springer-Verlag; 1996.

Cleveland WS. *The Elements of Graphing Data*. Summit, NJ: Hobart Press; 1994.

Cleveland WS. *Visualizing Data*. Summit, NJ: Hobart Press; 1993.

Frankel F. *Envisioning Science: The Design and Craft of the Science Image*. Cambridge, MA: MIT Press; 2002.

Harris RL. *Information Graphics: A Comprehensive Illustrated Reference*. New York, NY: Oxford University Press; 2000.

Tufte ER. *The Cognitive Style of PowerPoint*. Cheshire, CT: Graphics Press; 2003.

Tufte ER. *Envisioning Information*. Cheshire, CT: Graphics Press; 1990.

Tufte ER. *The Visual Display of Quantitative Information*. Cheshire, CT: Graphics Press; 1983.

Tufte ER. *Visual Explanations: Images and Quantities, Evidence and Narrative*. Cheshire, CT: Graphics Press; 1997.

25.9 Databases

Biosis
http://www.biosis.org
Biological/biochemical information

CABI Publishing
http://www.cabi-publishing.org/
Abstracts/databases

CAS
http://www.cas.org
Chemistry, toxicology, chemical engineering information

Centers for Disease Control and Prevention
http://www.cdc.gov

CINAHL
http://www.cinahl.com
Nursing and allied health information

Cochrane Library
http://www.update-software.com/cochrane

EMBASE.com
http://www.embase.com
Biomedical and pharmacological information

Gale Directory of Online, Portable, and Internet Databases
http://library.dialog.com/bluesheets/html/bl0230.html

GDB Human Genome Database
http://www.gdb.org

Human Genome Organization (HUGO)
http://www.gene.ucl.ac.uk/hugo

Human Genome Variation Society
http://www.hgvs.org

Institute of Medicine
http://www.nas.edu/iom

MEDNDX
http://www.medicalndx.com/
Medical search engine

Medstract.org
http://www.medstract.org
Acronyms and initialisms specific to biology and medicine

The Merck Manual
http://www.merck.com/mrkshared/mmanual/home.jsp

National Academy of Sciences
http://www.nas.edu

OncoLink
http://cancer.med.upenn.edu

Physician's Guide to the Internet
http://physiciansguide.com

ProMED-mail
http://www.promedmail.org
Global electronic reporting system for outbreaks of emerging infectious diseases and toxins, a program of the International Society for Infectious Diseases

PsycINFO
http://www.apa.org/psycinfo
Psychiatry/psychology information (abstracts only)

Thomson Scientific
http://www.isinet.com

US National Library of Medicine Databases
http://www.nlm.nih.gov
Includes MEDLINE, National Center for Biotechnology Information (NCBI), NLM Gateway, and PubMed

World Health Organization
http://www.who.int/en

25.10 Guidelines

CONSORT
http://www.consort-statement.org
A research tool that takes an evidence-based approach to improve the quality of reports of randomized trials

The COPE Report
http://www.publicationethics.org.uk
Committee on Publication Ethics

Declaration of Helsinki
http://www.wma.net/e/policy/b3.htm
Ethical principles for medical research involving human subjects

EMWA Guidelines
http://www.emwa.org/Mum/EMWAguidelines.pdf
European Medical Writers Association

GPP Guidelines
http://www.gpp-guidelines.org
The Good Publication Practice (GPP) guidelines encourage responsible and ethical publication of the results of clinical trials sponsored by pharmaceutical companies.

ICMJE Uniform Requirements
http://www.ICMJE.org
International Committee of Medical Journal Editors

PhRMA Principles
http://www.phrma.org/clinical_trials/
Principles on conduct of clinical trials and communication of clinical trial results

WAME Policy Statements
http://www.wame.org/resources/policies
World Association of Medical Editors

25.11 Professional Scientific Writing, Editing, and Communications Organizations and Groups

American Copy Editors Society (ACES)
38309 Genesee Lake Rd
Oconomowoc, WI 53066
Newsletter: *Newsletter of American Copy Editors Society*
Web site: http://www.copydesk.org

American Medical Writers Association (AMWA)
40 W Gude Dr, Suite 101
Rockville, MD 20850-1192
Telephone: (301) 294-5303
Fax: (301) 294-9006
E-mail: amwa@amwa.org

Journal: *AMWA Journal*
Web site: http://www.amwa.org

Association of Earth Science Editors (AESE)
Newsletter: *Blueline*
Web site: http://www.aese.org

Association of Learned and Professional Society Publishers (ALPSP)
South House, The Street
Clapham, Worthing BN13 3UU
West Sussex, UK
Telephone: +44 (0)1903 871 686
Fax: +44 (0)1903 871 457
E-mail: chief-exec@alpsp.org
Journal: *Learned Publishing*
Newsletter: *ALPSP Alert*
Web site: http://www.alpsp.org/journal.htm

Board of Editors in the Life Sciences (BELS)
Web site: http://www.bels.org

Committee on Publication Ethics (COPE)
BMJ Publishing Group Ltd
BMA House
Tavistock Square
London WC1H 9JR, England
Telephone: +44 (0)20 7383 6602
Fax: +44 (0)20 7383 6668
E-mail: cope@bmjgroup.com
Web site: http://www.publicationethics.org.uk

Copy Editor (Newsletter)
McMurry Inc
McMurry Campus Center
1010 E Missouri Ave
Phoenix, AZ 85014
Telephone: (888) 626-8779
Web site: http://www.copyeditor.com

Council of Science Editors (CSE)
c/o Drohan Management Group
12100 Sunset Hills Rd, Suite 130
Reston, VA 20190-5202
Telephone: (703) 437-4377
Fax: (703) 435-4390
E-mail: CSE@CouncilScienceEditors.org
Journal: *Science Editor*
Web site: http://www.councilscienceeditors.org

The Editorial Eye (Newsletter)
EEI Communications
66 Canal Center Plaza, Suite 200

Alexandria, VA 22314-5507
Telephone: (703) 683-0683
Fax: (703) 683-4915
E-mail: eye@eeicommunications.com
Web site: http://www.eeicommunications.com/eye/index.html

European Association of Science Editors (EASE)
E-mail: secretary@ease.org.uk
Journal: *European Science Editing*
Web site: http://www.ease.org.uk

European Medical Writers Association (EMWA)
Industriestrasse 31
CH-6300 Zug, Switzerland
Telephone: +41 41 720 3306
Fax: +41 41 720 3308
E-mail: info@emwa.org
Web site: http://www.emwa.org

Grammar Hotline Directory
Writing Center
Tidewater Community College
1700 College Cres
Virginia Beach, VA 23456
Telephone: (757) 822-7170
Fax: (757) 427-0327
E-mail: writcent@vblrc2.tc.cc.va.us/
Web site: http://www.tcc.edu/students/resources/writcent/GH/hotlinol.htm

International Committee of Medical Journal Editors (ICMJE)
Christine Laine, MD, MPH
ICMJE Secretariat Office
American College of Physicians
190 N Independence Mall W
Philadelphia, PA 19106-1572
Telephone: 215-351-2660
Fax: (215) 351-2644
E-mail: claine@acponline.org
Web site: http://www.icmje.org

MedLinguistics
Medical Linguistics Consulting
28221 Center Ridge Rd, Suite D-20
Westlake, OH 44145
Telephone: (440) 808-5840
E-mail: medlinguistics@sbcglobal.net
Newsletter: *MedicaLinguistics Update*
Web site: http://www.medlinguistics.com

Society for Scholarly Publishing (SSP)
10200 W 44th Ave, Suite 304
Wheat Ridge, CO 80033-2840

Telephone: (303) 422-3914
Fax: (303) 422-8894
E-mail: ssp@resourcenter.com
Journal: *Journal of Scholarly Publishing*
Web site: http://www.sspnet.org

Society for Technical Communication (STC)
901 N Stuart St, Suite 904
Arlington, VA 22203-1822
Telephone: (703) 522-4114
Fax: (703) 522-2075
E-mail: stc@stc.org
Journals: *Intercom, Technical Communication*
Web site: http://www.stc.org

World Association of Medical Editors (WAME)
Web site: http://www.wame.org

ACKNOWLEDGMENT

Principal author: Jennifer Reiling, *JAMA*.

Index